SIDE EFFECTS OF DRUGS
ANNUAL 25

Side Effects of Drugs Annual 25

SIDE EFFECTS OF DRUGS ANNUAL 25

A worldwide yearly survey of new data and trends in adverse drug reactions

EDITOR

J. K. ARONSON M.A., D.Phil., M.B.Ch.B., F.R.C.P.

Clinical Reader in Clinical Pharmacology
University Department of Clinical Pharmacology
Radcliffe Infirmary, Oxford OX2 6HE, United Kingdom

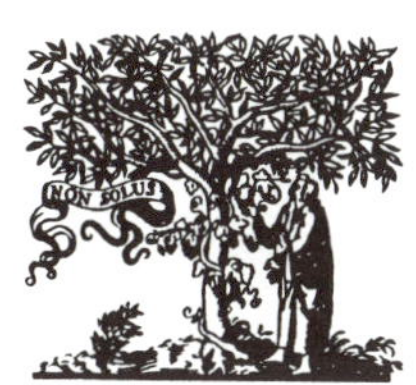

2002
ELSEVIER
Amsterdam – Boston – London – New York – Oxford – Paris
San Diego – San Francisco – Singapore – Sydney – Tokyo

ELSEVIER SCIENCE B.V.
Sara Burgerhartstraat 25
P.O. Box 211, 1000 AE Amsterdam, The Netherlands

First edition 2002

Library of Congress Cataloging in Publication Data
A catalog record from the Library of Congress has been applied for.

ISBN: 0-444-50674-8
ISSN: 0378-6080

♾ The paper used in this publication meets the requirements of ANSI/NISO Z39.48-1992 (Permanence of Paper).

Printed in The Netherlands.

Contributors

M.C. ALLWOOD, B.PHARM., PH.D.
University of Derby, School of Health and Community Studies, Pharmacy Academic Practice Unit, Kingsway House, Derby, DE22 3HL, U.K. E-mail: m.c.allwood@derby.ac.uk

J.K. ARONSON, MA., D.PHIL., M.B.CH.B., F.R.C.P.
University Department of Clinical Pharmacology, Radcliffe Infirmary, Woodstock Road, Oxford, OX2 6HE, U.K. E-mail: jeffrey.aronson@clinpharm.ox.ac.uk

I. AURSNES, M.D.
University of Oslo, Department of Pharmacotherapeutics, P.O. Box 1065 Blindern, N-0316 Oslo, Norway. E-mail: i.a.aursnes@ioks.uio.no

A.M. BALDACCHINO, M.D., M.R.C.PSYCH., M.PHIL., DIP.ADD.BEH.
St. George's Hospital Medical School, Centre for Addiction Studies, 6th Floor, Hunter Wing, Cranmer Terrace, London, SW17 0RE, U.K.

J. BOUSQUET
Hopital Arnaud de Villeneuve, 34295 Montpellier cedex 5, France.
E-mail: bousquet@montp.inserm.fr

A. CARVAJAL, M.D., PH.D.
Instituto de Farmacoepidemiologia, Facultad de Medicine, 47005 Valladolid, Spain.
E-mail: carvajal@ife.uva.es

N.H. CHOULIS, M.D., PH.D.
LAVIPHARM Research Laboratories, Agias Marinas Street, 19002 Peania (Attika), Greece.
E-mail: rizarios-www@ath.forthnet.gr

P. COATES, M.B.B.S., F.R.A.C.P.
University of Pittsburgh, Department of Endocrinology and Metabolism, 1110 Kaufmann Building, 3471 Fifth Avenue, Pittsburgh, PA 15213, U.S.A. E-mail: CoatesP@msx.dept-med.pitt.edu

J. COSTA, M.D.
Universitat Autònoma de Barcelona, Hospital Universitari Germans Trias I Pujol, Clinical Pharmacology Department, Ctra de Canyet, 08916 Badalona, Spain. E-mail: jcosta@cablecat.com

P.J. COWEN, M.D.
University Department of Psychiatry, Warenford Hospital, Oxford, OX3 7JX, U.K.
E-mail: phil.cowen@psychiatry.oxford.ac.uk

S. CURRAN, B.SC., M.B.CH.B., M.MED.SC., M.R.C.PSYCH., PH.D.
Wakefield and Pontefract Community Health NHS Trust, Aberford Centre, Wakefield, WF2 3SP, U.K. E-mail: steve.curran@swyt.nhs.uk

H.J. DE SILVA, M.B.B.S., M.D., D.PHIL, F.R.C.P., F.R.C.P.E., F.C.C.P.
University of Kelaniya, Department of Medicine, Faculty of Medicine, P.O. Box 6, Ragama, Sri Lanka. E-mail: hjdes@sri.lanka.net

F.A. DE WOLFF, M.A., PH.D., M.D.
Leiden University Medical Centre, Toxicology Laboratory, Department of Clinical Chemistry, Pharmacy and Toxicology, P.O. Box 9600, 2300 RC Leiden, The Netherlands.
E-mail: F.A.de_Wolff@lumc.nl

A. DEL FAVERO, M.D.
Istituto di Medicina Interna e Science Oncologiche, Policlinico Monteluce, 06122 Perugia, Italy.
E-mail: delfa@unipg.it

P. DEMOLY
Hopital Arnaud de Villeneuve, 34295 Montpellier cedex 5, France.

J. DESCOTES, M.D., PH.D., PHARM.D.
Hôpital Edouard Herriot, Centre Antipoison—Centre de Pharmacovigilance, 5 Place d'Arsonval, 69347 Lyon cedex 03, France. E-mail: jacques.descotes@chu-lyon.fr

S. DITTMANN, M.D., D.SC.MED.
Vice-Chairman, German Advisory Committee on Immunization, 19 Hatzenporter Weg, 12681 Berlin, Germany. E-mail: sd.internat.immun.consult@t-online.de

M.N.G. DUKES, M.D., M.A., LL.M.
Trosterudveien 19, 0778 Oslo, Norway. E-mail: mngdukes@online.no

I.R. EDWARDS, M.B., F.R.C.P., F.R.A.C.P.
Uppsala Monitoring Centre, The WHO Collaborating Centre for International Drug Monitoring, Stora Torget 3, S-753 20 Uppsala, Sweden. E-mail: ralph.edwards@who-umc.org

H.W. EIJKHOUT, M.D.
Central Laboratory of the Netherlands Red Cross Blood Transfusion Service, Plesmanlaan 125, 1066 CX Amsterdam, The Netherlands. E-mail: H_Eijkhout@CLB.nl

E. ERNST, M.D., PH.D., F.R.C.P. (EDIN)
University of Exeter, School of Postgraduate Medicine and Health Sciences, Division of Community Health Science, Department of Complementary Medicine, 25 Victoria Park Road, Exeter, EX2 4NT, U.K. E-mail: E.Ernst@ex.ac.uk

M. FARRÉ, M.D.
Universitat Autònoma de Barcelona, Institut Municipal d'Investigació Mèdica, Unitat de Farmacologia, Doctor Aiguader 80, 08003 Barcelona, Spain. E-mail: mfarre@imim.es

J.A. FRANKLYN, M.D., PH.D., F.R.C.P., F.MED.SCI.
University of Birmingham, Queen Elizabeth Hospital, Department of Medicine, Edgbaston, Birmingham, B15 2TH, U.K. E-mail: j.a.franklyn@bham.ac.uk

M.G. FRANZOSI, PH.D.
Istituto di Ricerche Farmacologiche "Mario Negri", Department of Cardiovascular Research, Via Eritrea 62, 20157 Milan, Italy. E-mail: franzosi@irfmn.mnegri.it

J. FRASER, M.SC., M.R.C.P., M.B.CH.B.
Beats on Oncology Centre, Western Infirmary, Dumbarton Road, Glasgow, G11 6NT, Scotland.
E-mail: jesuis1@hotmail.com

A.H. GHODSE, M.D., PH.D., F.R.C.P., F.R.C.PSYCH.
St. George's Hospital Medical School, Centre for Addiction Studies, 6th Floor, Hunter Wing, Cranmer Terrace, London, SW17 0RE, U.K. E-mail: h.ghodse@sghms.ac.uk

A.I. GREEN, M.D.
Harvard Medical School, Commonwealth Research Center and Massachusetts Mental Health Center, Department of Psychiatry, 74 Fenwood Road, Boston, MA 02115, U.S.A.
E-mail: alan_green@HMS.harvard.edu

A.H. GROLL, M.D.
Immunocompromised Host Section, Pediatric Oncology Branch, National Cancer Institute, National Institutes of Health, Bldg 10, Rm 13N240, 10, Center Drive MSC, Bethesda, MA 20891, U.S.A.

A.P. HAVRYK, M.B., B.S.
Royal Prince Alfred Hospital, Department of Respiratory Medicine, Camperdown, NSW 2050, Sydney, Australia. E-mail: ahavryk@ozemail.com.au

A. IMHOF, M.D.
University Hospital of Zürich, Department of Medicine, Medical Clinic B, Rämistrasse 100, CH-8091 Zürich, Switzerland. E-mail: alexander.imhof@dim.usz.ch

J.W. JEFFERSON, M.D.
University of Wisconsin Medical School, Madison Institute of Medicine, 7617 Mineral Point Road, Madison, WI 53717, U.S.A. E-mail: jeffj@healthtechsys.com

D.J. JEFFRIES, B.SC., M.B.B.S., F.R.C.P., F.R.C.P.PATH.
St. Bartholomew's and The Royal London School of Medicine and Dentistry, Department of Virology, 51–53 Bartholomew Close, West Smithfield, London, EC1A 7BE, U.K.
E-mail: d.j.jeffries@qmul.ac.uk

H.M.J. KRANS, M.D.
Leiden University Medical Center, Department of Endocrinology and Metabolic Diseases, Building 1 C4-R, Postbus 9600, 2300 RC Leiden, The Netherlands.
E-mail: hmjkrans@wanadoo.nl

S. KRISHNA, B.A., D.PHIL., F.R.C.P.
St. George's Hospital Medical School, Department of Infectious Diseases, Department of Cell and Molecular Sciences, Cranmer Terrace, London, SW17 0RE, U.K.
E-mail: s.krishna@sghms.ac.uk

R. LATINI, M.D.
Istituto di Ricerche Farmacologiche "Mario Negri", Department of Cardiovascular Research, Via Eritrea 62, 20157 Milan, Italy. E-mail: latini@irfmn.mnegri.it

M. LEUWER, M.D.
The University of Liverpool, University Department of Anaesthesia, The Duncan Building, Daulby Street, Liverpool, L69 3GA, U.K. E-mail: mleuwer@liv.ac.uk

P. MAGEE, B.SC., M.SC., M.R.PHARM.S.
Director of Pharmaceutical Sciences, University Hospitals Coventry and Warwickshire NHS Trust, Clifford Bridge Road, Coventry, CV2 2DX, U.K.

A.P. MAGGIONI, M.D.
Istituto di Ricerche Farmacologiche "Mario Negri", Department of Cardiovascular Research, Via Eritrea 62, 20157 Milan, Italy. E-mail: maggioni@anmco.it

L. MARKS, B.A. HONS, D.PHIL.
Health Promotion Unit, London School of Hygiene and Tropical Medicine, Keppel Street, London, WC1, U.K. E-mail: l.marks@ic.ac.uk

L.H. MARTÍN ARIAS, M.D., PH.D.
Instituto de Farmacoepidemiologia, Facultad de Medicina, 47005 Valladolid, Spain. E-mail: lmartin@ife.uva.es

M.M.H.M. MEINARDI, M.D., PH.D.
Academic Medical Centre, Department of Dermatology, Meibergdreef 9, 1105 AZ Amsterdam, The Netherlands. E-mail: m.m.meinardi@amc.uva.nl

R.H.B. MEYBOOM, M.D., PH.D.
Department of Pharmacoepidemiology and Pharmacotherapy, Faculty of Pharmacy, Utrecht University, P.O. Box 80082, 3508 TB Utrecht, The Netherlands.

T. MIDTVEDT, M.D., PH.D.
Karolinska Institutet, Laboratory of Medical Microbial Ecology, Box 60 400, S-171 77 Stockholm, Sweden. E-mail: Tore.Midtvedt@cmb.ki.se

S.K. MORCOS, F.R.C.S., F.F.R.R.C.S.I., F.R.C.R.
Northern General Hospital, Sheffield Teaching Hospitals NHS Trust, Department of Diagnostic Imaging, Sheffield, S5 7AU, U.K. E-mail: Sameh.Morcos@northngh-tr.trent.nhs.uk

W.M.C. MULDER, M.D., PH.D
Academic Medical Center, Department of Dermatology, Meibergdreef 9, 1105 AZ Amsterdam, The Netherlands.

S. MUSA, M.B.CH.B., M.R.C.PSYCH.
Wakefield and Pontefract Community Health NHS Trust, Aberford Centre, Wakefield, WF1 3SP, U.K. E-mail: shabirm@wpch-tr.northy.nhs.uk

L. NICHOLSON, M.B., CH.B.
The University of Auckland, Faculty of Medicine and Health Science, Department of Pharmacology and Clinical Pharmacology, Private Bag 92019, Auckland, New Zealand.

S. OLSSON, M.SCI.PHARM.
Uppsala Monitoring Centre, The WHO Collaborating Centre for International Drug Monitoring, Stora Torget 3, S-753 20 Uppsala, Sweden. E-mail: sten.olsson@who-unc.org

J.N. PANDE, M.D., F.A.M.S.
Professor of Medicine, All India Institute of Medical Sciences, Ansari Nagar, New Delhi 110029, India. E-mail: jnpande@hotmail.com

J.K. PATEL, M.D.
University of Massachusetts Medical School, Department of Psychiatry, 361 Plantation Street, Worcester, MA 01605, U.S.A. E-mail: Patelj@ummhc.org

K. PEERLINCK, M.D.
University of Leuven, Center for Molecular and Vascular Biology and Division of Bleeding and Vascular Disorders, Herestraat 49, B-3000 Leuven, Belgium.
E-mail: Kathelijne.peerlinck@med.kuleuven.ac.be

T. PLANCHE, M.R.C.P.
St. George's Hospital Medical School, Department of Infectious Diseases, Cranmer Terrace, London, SW17 0RE, U.K.

B.C.P. POLAK, M.D.
Vrije Universiteit Medical Center, Department of Ophthalmology, P.O. Box 7057, 1007 MB Amsterdam, The Netherlands. E-mail: bcp.polak@azvu.nl

H.D. REUTER, PH.D.
Siebengebirgsallee 24, D-50939 Köln, Germany. E-mail: ges-phyto@t-online.de

T.D. ROBINSON, M.B., B.S.
Westmead Hospital, Department of Thoracic Medicine, Westmead, NSW 2154, Sydney, Australia. E-mail: traceyr@med.usyd.edu.au

M. SCHACHTER, M.D.
Department of Clinical Pharmacology, Imperial College School of Medicine, National Heart and Lung Institute, St. Mary's Hospital, London, W2 1NY, U.K. E-mail: m.schachter@ic.ac.uk

S.A. SCHUG, M.D., F.A.N.Z.C.A., F.F.P.M.A.N.Z.C.A.
University of Auckland, Division of Anaesthesiology, Faculty of Medicine and Health Sciences, Private Bag 92019, Auckland, New Zealand. E-mail: schug@cyllene.uwa.edu.au

J.P. SEALE, M.B., B.S., PH.D., F.R.A.C.P.
Royal Prince Alfred Hospital, Department of Respiratory Medicine, Camperdown, NSW 2050, Sydney, Australia. E-mail: jpseale@pharmacol.usyd.edu.au

R.P. SEQUEIRA, PH.D.
Arabian Gulf University, College of Medicine and Medical Sciences, Department of Pharmacology and Therapeutics, P.O. Box 22979, Manama, Bahrain. E-mail: sequeira@ns1.agu.edu.bh

T.G. SHORT, MB.CH.B., M.D.
The University of Auckland, Faculty of Medicine and Health Science, Department of Pharmacology and Clinical Pharmacology, Private Bag 92019, Auckland, New Zealand.
E-mail: TimS@ahsl.co.nz

D.A. SICA, M.D.
Medical College of Virginia of Virginia Commonwealth University, Section of Clinical Pharmacology and Hypertension, Division of Nephrology, Box 980160 MCV Station, Richmond, VA 23298-0160, U.S.A. E-mail: dsica@hsc.vcu.edu

A. STANLEY, PH.D., M.R.PHARM.S.
Birmingham Oncology Centre, St. Chad's Unit, City Hospital, Dudley Road, Birmingham, B18 7QH, U.K. E-mail: andrew.stanley@cityhospbham.wmids.nhs.uk

B. SUNDARAM, M.R.C.P.
Northern General Hospital, Sheffield Teaching Hospitals NHS Trust, Department of Diagnostic Imaging, Sheffield, S5 7AU, U.K.

M.C. THORNTON
University of Auckland, Discipline of Anaesthesiology, Faculty of Medicine and Health Sciences, Private Bag 92019, Auckland, New Zealand.

C. TWELVES, B.MED.SCI., F.R.C.P., M.D.
Beats on Oncology Centre, Western Infirmary, Dumbarton Road, Glasgow, G11 6NT, Scotland.

W.G. VAN AKEN, M.D.
Central Laboratory of the Netherlands Red Cross Blood Transfusion Service, Plesmanlaan 125, 1066 CX Amsterdam, The Netherlands. E-mail: WG_van_Aken@clb.nl

G.B. VAN DER VOET, M.D.
Leiden University Medical Centre, Toxicology Laboratory, Department of Clinical Chemistry, Pharmacy and Toxicology, P.O. Box 9600, 2300 RC Leiden, The Netherlands.
E-mail: G.B.van_der_Voet@lumc.nl

P.J.J. VAN GENDEREN, M.D., PH.D.
Habour Hospital and Institute of Tropical Diseases, Department of Internal Medicine, Haringvliet 2, 3011 TD Rotterdam, The Netherlands. E-mail: p.van.genderen@12move.nl

R. VERHAEGHE, M.D.
University of Leuven, Center for Vascular and Molecular Biology, Herestraat 49, 3000 Leuven, Belgium. E-mail: Raymond.Verhaeghe@uz.kuleuven.ac.be

J. VERMYLEN, M.D.
University of Leuven, Center for Molecular and Vascular Biology and Division of Bleeding and Vascular Disorders, Herestraat 49, B-3000 Leuven, Belgium.
E-mail: jozef.vermylen@med.kuleuven.ac.be

T. VIAL, M.D.
Hôpital Edouard Herriot, Centre Antipoison—Centre de Pharmacovigilance, 5 Place d'Arsonval, 69347 Lyon cedex 03, France. E-mail: thierry.vial@chu-lyon.fr

T.J. WALSH, M.D.
Immunocompromised Host Section, Pediatric Oncology Branch, National Cancer Institute, National Institutes of Health, Bldg 10, Rm 13N240, 10, Center Drive MSC, Bethesda, MD 20891, U.S.A. E-mail: walshtj@mail.nih.gov

R. WALTER, M.D.
University Hospital of Zurich, Department of Medicine, Medical Clinic B, Rämistrasse 100, CH-8091 Zurich, Switzerland. E-mail: roland.walter@dim.usz.ch

E.J. WONG, M.D.
Harvard Medical School, Massachusetts Mental Health Center, Department of Psychiatry, Boston, MA 02115, U.S.A. E-mail: Ewong88@juno.com

F. ZANNAD, M.D., PH.D., F.E.S.C.
Centre d'Investigation Clinique INSERM-CHU, Hôpital Jeanne d'Arc, Dommartin les Toul, Nancy, France. E-mail: f.zannad@chu-nancy.fr

O. ZUZAN, M.D.
Royal Liverpool University Hospital, Department of Anaesthesia, Prescot Street, Liverpool, L7 8XP, U.K. E-mail: oliver.zuzan@btinternet.com

Contents

Special reviews

Cumulative index of special reviews, Annuals 16–24

Index of drugs

Note: the format 24.115 refers to SEDA-24, p. 115.

Index of adverse effects

How to use this book

THE SCOPE OF THE ANNUAL

The *Side Effects of Drugs Annual* has been published every year since 1977. It is designed to provide a critical and up-to-date account of new information relating to adverse drug reactions and interactions from the clinician's point of view. It complements the standard encyclopedic work in this field, *Meyler's Side Effects of Drugs*, the 14th edition of which was published in November 2000.

PERIOD COVERED

The present *Annual* reviews all reports that presented significant new information on adverse reactions to drugs during 2000. During the production of this *Annual*, some more recent papers have also been included.

SELECTION OF MATERIAL

In compiling the *Side Effects of Drugs Annual* particular attention is devoted to publications that provide essentially new information or throw a new light on problems already recognized. In addition, some authoritative new reviews are listed. Publications that do not meet these criteria are omitted. Readers anxious to trace all references on a particular topic, including those that duplicate earlier work, or to cross-check an electronic search, are advised to consult *Adverse Reactions Titles*, a monthly bibliography of titles from about 3400 biomedical journals published throughout the world, compiled by the Excerpta Medica International Abstracting Service.

℞ ***SPECIAL REVIEWS***

The special reviews deal in more detail with selected topics, interpreting conflicting evidence and providing the reader with clear guidance. They are identified by the traditional prescription symbol and are printed in italics. This volume includes a Cumulative Index of Special Reviews (SEDA-16 to SEDA-24) and a list of the titles of the Special Reviews published in the current Annual.

CLASSIFICATION OF DRUGS

Drugs are classified according to their main field of use or the properties for which they are most generally recognized. In some cases a drug is included in more than one chapter (for example, lidocaine may be mentioned in Chapter 11 as a local anesthetic and in Chapter 17 as an antidysrhythmic drug). Fixed combinations of drugs are dealt with according to their most characteristic component.

DRUG NAMES

Drugs are usually dealt with under their recommended or proposed International Non-proprietary Names (rINN or pINN); when these are not available, chemical names have been used. If a fixed combination has a generic combination name (e.g. co-trimoxazole for trimethoprim + sulfamethoxazole) that has been used; in some cases brand names have been used instead.

SYSTEM OF REFERENCES

References in the text are tagged in an extended version of the tagging system that has been used in previous editions; the new tagging system is as follows:

M: A meta-analysis or other form of systematic review;
E: An experimental study (animal or in vitro);
A: An anecdote or set of anecdotes (i.e. case histories);
R: A major review, including non-systematic statistical analyses of published studies;
r: A brief commentary (e.g. an editorial or a letter);
C: A major randomized controlled trial or observational study;
c: A minor randomized controlled trial or observational study or a non-randomized study;
S: Official (e.g. Governmental, WHO) statements.

The various editions of *Meyler's Side Effects of Drugs* are cited in the text as SED-13, SED-14, etc; the *Side Effects of Drugs Annuals 1–24* are cited as SEDA-1, SEDA-2, etc.

INDEXES

Index of drugs: this index provides a complete listing of all references to a drug for which adverse effects and/or drug interactions are described.
Index of adverse effects: this index is necessarily selective, since a particular adverse effect may be caused by very large numbers of compounds; the index is therefore mainly directed to adverse effects that are particularly serious or frequent, or are discussed in special detail; before assuming that a given drug does not have a particular adverse effect, consult the relevant chapters.

American spelling has been used throughout, e.g. anemia, estrogen rather than anaemia, oestrogen.

A silver anniversary and a tribute to our contributors

Jeffrey K. Aronson

Traditionally, anniversaries are named according to the substances of which the anniversary presents are supposed to be made (Table 1), a tradition that began in around the middle of the 19th century. Silver is associated with 25th anniversaries, and were it not for the fact that the volumes of the *Side Effects of Drugs Annual* (SEDA) have been bound in silver-coloured cloth since the first volume appeared in 1977, the publishers would have issued a special silver binding for this, the 25th volume in the series.

I have previously reviewed the history of the SEDA volumes (SEDA-23, xxii), but a brief recapitulation of a few details is in order, to explain why the volumes are bound in silver. When Leopold Meyler, the initiator and first editor of *Meyler's Side Effects of Drugs* ("*Meyler*"), died unexpectedly in September 1973, the publishers, Elsevier, invited Graham Dukes to take over the editing of Volume VIII (1976), the latest in what had become a four-yearly series. Dukes persuaded Elsevier that the published literature was too large to be comfortably encompassed in a four-yearly cycle, and he suggested that the volumes should be produced annually instead. The four-yearly volume could then concentrate on providing a complementary critical encyclopaedic survey of the entire field. The first *Side Effects of Drugs Annual* was published in 1977 and was bound in silver to match the binding of Volume VIII of *Meyler*. The first encyclopaedic edition of *Meyler*,

Table 1. *Substances associated with anniversaries*

Anniversary	Associated substance	Anniversary	Associated substance
1	Cotton	14	Ivory
2	Paper	15	Crystal
3	Leather	20	China
4	Flowers	25	Silver
5	Wood	30	Pearl
6	Iron	35	Coral
7	Wool	40	Ruby
8	Bronze	45	Sapphire
9	Copper	50	Gold
10	Tin	55	Emerald
11	Steel	60	Diamond
12	Silk and linen	70	Platinum
13	Lace	75	Diamond

Table 2. *Authors who have contributed to 10 volumes or more*

No. of volumes	Name	SEDA volumes	No. of volumes	Name	SEDA volumes
25	HMJ Krans	1–25	14	TC Jerram	5–18
	RHB Meyboom	1–25		JP Nater	1–14
	BCP Polak	1–25		FJ Richardson	5–18
	H Reuter	1–25		R Verhaeghe	12–25
24	JK Aronson	2–25		J Vermylen	12–25
22	AH Ghodse	4–25		M Verstraete	3–5, 7–17
21	A Del Favero	5–25	13	AGC Bauer	12–24
	J Descotes	4–17, 19–25		B Blackwell	1–13
	T Midtvedt	5–25		G Reybrouck	4–16
20	MNG Dukes	1–18, 24–25	12	GAB Davies-Jones	1–12
	M Schou	2–21		CJ Ellis	13–24
19	AC De Groot	4–22		JC Evreux	4–8, 10–16
	AI Green	7–25		MJS Langman	1–12
18	G Ansell	1–18		GT McInnes	13–24
	FA Nelemans	1–18		RP Sequeira	14–25
17	S Agoston	1–4, 6–18		J Tuomisto	2–13
	P Folb	6–10, 12–23		FA Van Assche	4–14, 16
16	R Bouillon	1–16	11	I Aursnes	15–25
	S Dittmann	10–25		J Elis	2–12
	L Salzman	2–17		A Stanley	15–25
15	AV Astakhova	4–18		JA Steiner	4, 6–15
	NH Choulis	11–25	10	MG Franzosi	16–25
	JA Indänpään-Heikkilä	11–25		IA Jaffe	9–18
	VK Lepakhin	3, 5–18		R Latini	16–25
	I Nir	2–16		AP Maggioni	16–25
				OR Ødegaard	5–14
				K Wierzba	3–12

Table 3. *The editors of SEDA*

Editor	SEDA volumes
MNG Dukes	1–16
L Beeley	12–14
JK Aronson	15–25
CJ van Boxtel	17–19

Table 4. *Regions of publication of articles cited in SEDA-23*

Region of publication	No. of citations in SEDA-23	No. of articles published in 1998	Ratio of citations to articles published ($\times 10^3$)
Australasia	35	5190	6.744
South Africa	2	351	5.698
Asia/Middle East	37	17483	2.116
Europe (non-EU)	90	43539	2.067
European Union*	284	157809	1.800
The Americas	338	192247	1.758
Totals	786	416619	1.887

*Austria, Belgium, Denmark, Finland, France, Greece, Ireland, Italy, Luxembourg, Netherlands, Portugal, Spain, Sweden, UK.

which appeared in 1980, was labelled the ninth edition. Because the ninth edition was bound in red, the four accompanying annuals, bound in silver, were given a red trim. And the trim for each successive four volumes of SEDA has matched the colour of the relevant encyclopaedic edition. Which is why this volume is bound in silver with a red trim, matching the 14th edition of *Meyler* (2000).

It has been the stated aim of the SEDA volumes since their inception to provide a critical and up-to-date account of new information relating to adverse drug reactions and interactions from the clinician's point of view. And in these days of comprehensive computerized databases of references to published bioscience literature, accessible to clinicians at the touch of a button, the SEDA volumes and *Meyler* give added value, since contributors are encouraged not merely to report the existence of the literature but to review it critically and to comment on the extent to which authors have understated or overstated their case, or have even got it plain wrong. In addition, *Meyler* gives clinicians the chance to assess the relevance of individual adverse effects in the light of the overall adverse effects profile.

Meyler and SEDA are thorough and comprehensive: they cover nearly 2000 drugs in all. And such extensive coverage requires a large body of contributors. There have been 284 contributors in all to the 25 volumes of SEDA, a total of 1637 author-years. They have come from countries all round the world, including Australia, Bahrain, Belgium, the Czech Republic, Denmark, Egypt, Finland, France, Germany (West and East), Greece, Hungary, India, Ireland, Israel, Italy, Japan, the Netherlands, New Zealand, Norway, Poland, Russia and the erstwhile Soviet Union, South Africa, Spain, Sri Lanka, Sweden, Switzerland, the UK, and the USA. A list of those (52 in all) who have contributed to 10 volumes or more is given in Table 2; the complete list of all contributors will be found in the *Meyler* website (http://www.elsevier.com/locate/Meyler), as will the list of the 248 authors and editors who have contributed to the various editions of *Meyler*. We owe them an enormous debt of gratitude. The four editors who have overseen their work are listed in Table 3.

The literature covered in the SEDA volumes is also truly international, the language of publication being no barrier. Some of the less familiar journals from which reports have been culled have included *Acta Biomedica de l'Ateneo Parmense, Aktuelle Ernährungsmedizin, Boletin de la Asociacion Medica de Puerto Rico, the Central African Journal of Medicine, Missouri Medicine, and No To Hattatsu*. The countries of publication of the 786 journals that were cited in SEDA-23 (3193 citations in all) are listed in Table 4.

We also owe a debt of gratitude to the distinguished contributors who have enriched the SEDA volumes with an introductory, sometimes controversial, essay on some topic related to adverse drug reactions. They and their topics are also listed in the *Meyler* website.

What then of the future of *Meyler* and the SEDA volumes? Currently each SEDA volume reviews about 3200 citations on adverse drug reactions, and the volume of traffic shows no signs of abating. This means that volumes of SEDA will continue to appear each year, in order to keep clinicians up to date with what is going on [1]. However, it is now customary for printed volumes to be supplemented by electronic versions, and it is therefore planned that the 15th edition of *Meyler* will be issued not only in hard copy but also as a web version. In this way the *Side Effects of Drugs* series will continue to produce critical reviews of the important literature on adverse drug reactions, reporting new reactions and interactions when they occur and reassessing old reactions and interactions when necessary.

REFERENCES

1. Aronson JK, Loke Y, Derry S. Adverse drug reactions: keeping up to date. Fundam Clin Pharmacol 2002; 16: 49–56.

The pill: untangling the adverse effects of a drug

Lara Marks *

Nearly 200 million women have swallowed the contraceptive pill from the time of its first clinical trials to the present, making it one of the most widely consumed drugs in the world. By the end of the 20th century the contraceptive had become a feature of everyday life, with over 70 million women reaching for their pill packet on a daily basis around the globe (1). Within 6 years of its first marketing in the USA, the oral contraceptive had become one of the leading pharmaceutical products sold around the world. By the late 1960s the number of contraceptive pills sold exceeded any other single pharmaceutical product of an ethical nature, and in some cases outsold many proprietary items, such as aspirin. Many contemporaries felt that the pharmaceutical industry had never before seen a product sold so widely or with such a wide impact (2).

Although the pill is commonly cited as one of the factors that triggered the sexual revolution in the developed world in the 1960s, surprisingly few scholars have examined in detail its impact on the overall debate about the safety and efficacy of drugs. Like Librium and thalidomide, the pill was one of several revolutionary new drugs introduced in the 1960s, which reshaped pharmacology, social perceptions of medication, and the regulatory process for new drugs during the second half of the twentieth century. Although not identified as such at the time it was created, the pill can truly be called the first "designer" or "lifestyle" drug. As with many drug firsts there are numerous lessons to be learned from its development and use.

Pharmacologically, the pill is unique. Most drugs are intended for the treatment of organic diseases. By contrast, the pill is aimed at preventing pregnancy, a condition not commonly considered an illness. The fact that it is designed to be consumed by healthy women of reproductive age for long periods of time has magnified concerns about its potential dangers. The pill was also novel in that, unlike all previous forms of contraception, its use was divorced from the moment of intercourse and it had systemic effects.

From the time that it was first marketed as a contraceptive, the pill aroused great debate about its safety. Some physicians were deeply concerned about its long-term impact on women's health. For some, the drug seemed to go against nature and the way that the body worked. As one British doctor asked, in 1961, on the eve of its introduction in Britain (3):

> Are none of my colleagues as apprehensive as I am about the threatened advent of oral contraceptive therapy? The prime function of the human race was to reproduce itself, and we are threatening to strike a blow at the very heart of the process that is responsible for the miracle of life itself. Will Nature let this indignity go unchallenged? Will she allow the creatures to whom she has given the privilege of existence to interfere with the process that gave them the existence?
>
> To prevent contraception by mechanical barriers is a different thing altogether – this is merely controlling the end product of a natural process, not interfering with the process itself. If Nature decides that science has invaded the very heart of her domain, what terrible penalties may she inflict upon

* This year's guest author is Lara Marks, BA Hons, DPhil, who is Visiting Senior Research Associate, Cambridge Group for the History of Population, Cambridge University, and Honorary Senior Lecturer, London School of Hygiene and Tropical Medicine.

the female of the species. Sterility? Ovarian atrophy? Malignant disease?

These fears were heightened when, in November 1961, within months of its initial introduction, a British family doctor from Suffolk wrote to The Lancet of a woman who had developed thrombotic complications after taking the drug (4). By August 1962, the American Food and Drug Administration (FDA) had received reports of 26 women who had had thrombophlebitis, six of whom had died (5–9). Two years later further alarms began to be raised, when a team of researchers at the University of Oregon showed that certain hormones, such as the progestogen and estrogen contained in the first marketed pill, Enovid, promoted the growth of cancers in animals such as rats (10, 11).

The anxieties of the early 1960s were not put to rest in later years. Lingering suspicions about the pill's safety have made it one of the most heavily scrutinized drugs in the world. Moreover, serious concerns about the implications of long-term use by healthy women has led to the implementation of innovative medical approaches to tracking patients for long periods of time, and for detecting and reporting serious adverse reactions to drugs. Focusing on Britain and America and the investigations into thrombosis and cancer, I shall highlight how the contraceptive pill challenged the limits of drug monitoring and surveillance, bringing in its wake new techniques for detecting adverse drug reactions.

Tracking the adverse effects of the pill

The pill posed special dilemmas for those gathering evidence of its possible risks. Although given on prescription, it differed from other medicines because of its pattern of distribution. Monitoring adverse reactions was going to be difficult, because women could obtain prescriptions through a variety of medical practitioners.

Tracking the dissemination of the pill was particularly complex in the USA, where individual doctors were not responsible for the overall care of particular individuals, and coordination between hospitals and practitioners was poor. Women could therefore go from one doctor to another without automatically being monitored, and information was not always passed on between specialists (12, 13). Thus, while some specialists, such as ophthalmologists and neurologists, were seeing women with complaints that seemed to stem from taking the pill, such information was not always channelled back to other specialists, such as the gynecologists or general practitioners who had been responsible for the original prescription (14). In addition, many American doctors were hesitant to report adverse reactions for fear of litigation (15, 16). The transmission of data was also hindered by the diversity of healthcare agencies across different states and the absence of a centralized recording system for patient records and prescriptions, although some states, such as Pittsburgh, had better prescription monitoring than others (17).

The collection of evidence from pharmaceutical companies was also inadequate in the USA. Pharmaceutical companies did not have a uniform policy for gathering reports on deaths that individual doctors notified to them, and the FDA did not provide clear guidelines to manufacturers about the type of investigational evidence they required. The FDA tried to tighten the reporting system for deaths on the part of the pharmaceutical industry in 1966, but such improvements took time to be implemented (18). The situation was not helped by the absence of a consistent method for recording and following patients. Important information was therefore often duplicated or difficult to retrieve (19).

By contrast, Britain had a better infrastructure for monitoring the effects of the pill generally. General practitioners were the first point of call for patients in the National Health Service, were the main coordinators of treatment, and were responsible for keeping a file on a patient's prescription history and other case notes. They could therefore keep track of whether a woman had received a prescription for an oral contraceptive, even when they had not issued it (20). From the mid-1980s a number of computer-based general practice clinical and administrative record systems were established in Britain that made monitoring the effects of the pill even simpler (21). Patient care was also well coordinated between general practitioners and family planning clinics, which was advantageous for tracing patients taking the pill and their adverse effects. British doctors were also less frightened of litigation than their American counterparts, and were therefore more likely to report adverse effects.

Tracking the effects of the pill was complicated by the fact that women did not necessarily stick to one method of contraception, often swapping between oral contraception and mechanical methods. They also took the pill for different lengths of time and often changed their medication or even abandoned the contraceptive. In later years the problem was compounded by the ever-increasing variation in marketed formulations, which contained differing types and doses of hormones and involved different regimens. Under these circumstances it was difficult to isolate which pill, and which of its components, was linked to particular complications (22).

Among the difficulties investigators confronted was the fact that the effects of the pill were difficult to separate from the many factors known to cause thrombotic disease or cancer. While epidemiologists were dissatisfied with methods that did not seem to progress "beyond the clinical impression phase" (23) and stressed the need for good statistically designed studies, other medical experts felt that the epidemiological studies provided an unsatisfactory and inconsistent picture and were "too blunt a tool for the detection of small risks" (23). For these doctors only basic clinical research could yield the answer.

Even when investigators agreed that epidemiological studies were the way forward, it was unclear which technique would produce the best results. One of the major difficulties confronting epidemiologists was finding a large enough sample of women to work with over a long period of time. This was particularly important in the context of thrombosis, given the infrequency of the problem, and in the case of cancer, which can take a long time to manifest. One of the major problems in the early 1960s was that the number of women taking the pill was still relatively small and it was hard to find institutions with adequate concentrations of women for conducting studies on thrombosis and cancer.

The thrombosis puzzle (see also p. 484)

Reports in the 1960s that the pill might cause thrombotic complications took the medical and scientific community by complete surprise. News of the possible links between the contraceptive pill and thrombotic disease were especially worrying in the wake of the thalidomide tragedy that hit the headlines in the early 1960s. While medical practitioners and scientists were keen to unravel the connection between oral contraceptives and thrombotic disease, however, there was great disagreement as to what constituted the most appropriate procedure for investigating the problem and what would be considered affirmative evidence (24).

One of the major problems was that it was unclear that the pill was itself to blame, for many people suffer thrombosis without ever taking oral contraceptives. Pregnancy, operations, obesity, diabetes, and smoking are all risk factors (25).

The quandary was compounded by the absence of reliable statistics concerning the natural occurrence of thrombotic complications in women of various ages. In the early 1960s patients who were hospitalized for thrombotic complications were not always officially reported. In addition, diagnosis was difficult and often inaccurate, and autopsies were not always carried out. Similarly, before August 1962 very few doctors were aware of the possible connection between thrombotic disease and oral contraceptives, and so failed to ask patients presenting with thrombosis whether they were using the pill. This made it difficult to relate the numbers of deaths associated with oral contraceptives to the natural incidence of the disease in women of reproductive age (24, 26–28).

Investigating thrombosis and the pill

During the 1960s various methods were used to investigate the possible thrombotic hazards of the pill, with varying conclusions (29, 30). One of the first studies to suggest a connection between the pill and vascular complications was that of the British Committee on the Safety of Drugs (CSD) in 1965. Based on evidence collected from the receipt of notifications of complications from the pill, the results of this study suggested that thromboembolic death was much higher among oral contraceptive users than among women in general, and that pulmonary embolism was particularly frequent among those taking the pill. Pills containing the synthetic estrogen mestranol were thought to be the most hazardous.

By 1967 two further British studies confirmed the initial findings of the CSD. The first, conducted by the Royal College of General Practitioners (RCGP), compared 147 reported cases of thrombosis among women taking the pill with 294 controls. The second, launched by the Statistical Research Unit of the Medical Research Council (MRC), involved a comparison of 334 deaths from thrombosis and 998 controls. Together these studies showed a very strong correlation between oral contraceptives and thromboembolic disorders. Venous thrombosis (superficial and deep), pulmonary embolism, and myocardial infarction were the most common types of thromboembolic disease in women using the pill, and were three times greater than among non-users (31, 32).

Throughout the 1970s other investigators reinforced such conclusions, adding smoking as a factor that increased the risk. By 1978 enough evidence had been collected in the USA, Britain, and elsewhere to show that the oral contraceptive increased the risk of thrombosis 5- to 10-fold. During the 1970s and 1980s further studies showed that the problem was most commonly associated with oral contraceptives that contained higher doses of estrogen. Moreover, evidence from Sweden suggested that thromboembolic morbidity and mortality reduced significantly after the withdrawal of high-dose oral contraceptives. Table 1 shows the breakdown of different studies.

The pill and cancer

While thrombotic complications of the pill caught the medical and scientific community unawares, from the start many suspected the drug could have carcinogenic effects. Part of the suspicion was fuelled by the fact that as early as the 1930s estrogen had been implicated in the growth of uterine and breast tumors in certain animals, such as mice (57–62). One of the anxieties surrounding the pill was that nobody could be sure of its long-term effects. As one cancer expert advising those running British clinical trials stated in 1960, "The induction period of all cancers in man is long (15–25 years) and therefore the effects of these compounds in cancer induction will not be seen for many years to come" (63). For this reason women who took the pill both in trials and later when it was marketed were recommended to have regular examinations to check for cancer (64).

In 1964 concerns about the potential carcinogenic effects of the pill were reinforced when progestogens and estrogens were found to promote the growth of cancers in experiments on rats (10, 65). Fears continued into the late 1960s and 1970s, when news broke that female dogs had developed breast cancer when given certain oral contraceptives. Anxieties were further heightened when reports began to show links between oral contraceptives and extremely rare non-malignant tumors of the liver (66–72). The issue was not made any easier when in 1975 the FDA withdrew a new form of oral contraceptive, known as sequential pills, from the American market, suspecting that they increased the risk of endometrial cancer (73, 74).

Misgivings about the pill increased further in the 1970s and 1980s with the revelation that stilbestrol had caused vaginal adenocarcinoma in the daughters of women who, from the 1940s, had taken it to prevent miscarriage. Stilbestrol was then being explored for its properties as a morning-after contraceptive; between 1943 and 1959 nearly 6 million American women had been given stilbestrol, and nearly 3 million children had therefore been exposed to it (75–77). Since the possible links between stilbestrol and cancer had taken years to emerge many people wondered how long it would take to prove the oral contraceptive pill unsafe (78).

Such fears were not helped in 1983, when a number of epidemiological investigations showed that the contraceptive might increase the risks of breast and cervical cancer among women in later life. Those most at danger were young women who had taken the pill for many years before the age of 25. Such news was particularly discomfiting, given the rising incidence of breast cancer in many countries in the developed world and the increasing mortality from cervical cancer in the developing world since the 1950s.

The most disturbing aspect of the studies in the 1980s was the fact that progestogens seemed to be the cause of the problem. This was particularly worrying, because many women had switched to pills containing high doses of a progestogen in the wake of the thrombotic scare and the phasing out of high-estrogen pills. Now it seemed that not only was estrogen a problem, but progestogens could also be. This did not leave many pills to choose from.

Table 1. *Selection of different studies undertaken to study effects of oral contraceptives on thrombotic disease**

Type of study and source of data	Sample analysed	Conclusions	Reference
Case-control study using FDA and Searle death reports and clinical records from private gynecologists/obstetricians and planned parenthood centers	350 death reports	Death rate among OC users = 12.1 per million (not significantly different from that expected in non-users, 8.4 million)	(33)
Case-control study in the Metabolic Unit, St Mary's Hospital, London, UK	About 105 OC users, about 78 controls	OC users developed abnormalities of carbohydrate and lipid metabolism similar to steroid-induced diabetes	(34, 35)
US and UK national mortality rates for TE diseases, up to 1964		No direct link between OCs and TE	(36, 37)
US mortality rates		No direct link between OCs and TE	(38)
Case-control study in general practice consultations in Britain, 1961–6	147 cases of TE, 294 controls	OC users had three times greater risk of VT than non-users	(39)
Case-control study of deaths in Britain, 1966	334 deaths and 998 controls	OC users had greater risk of PE and cerebral thrombosis than non-users (8.3 times greater); OC users aged 20–34 = 1.3 per 100 000 users, and aged 35–44 have 3.4 risk of developing PE or cerebral thrombosis; overall thrombotic death rate among OC users, age 20–34 (15 per million) 7.5 times greater than among non-users (2 per million)	(40)
Cohort study by members of Kaiser Foundation Health Plan, Northern California, 1969–71	16 500 cases and controls	Link between OC use and cigarette smoking; no direct link between OC use and cardiovascular disease	(41)
Case-control study of British hospital admissions, 1964–7	58 cases and 116 controls	OC users had a 6–7 times greater risk of idiopathic VT and PE (OC users = 47 per 100 000; non-users = 5 per 100 000); OC users who smoked were at greater risk	(42, 43)
Case-control study of US hospital admissions, 1963–7	175 cases and 175 controls	OC users had 4.4 times greater risk of TE than non-users; High-estrogen pills and sequential pills caused a greater risk of TE	(44, 45)
Case-control study of reports of TE to safety committees in UK, Sweden, and Denmark	1610 reports	Conclusive link between estrogen content and fatal PE and MI; risk of death with mestranol 150 μg increased 2.8 times, with 100 μg increased 1.3 times, and with 50 μg only 0.56 as high as expected; no difference between the two estrogens, ethinylestradiol and mestranol	(46)

Table 1. *Continued*

Type of study and source of data	Sample analysed	Conclusions	Reference
Case-control study of British hospital admissions, 1964–7		OC users had higher risk of postoperative VT or PE than non-users (relative risk 3.8:1)	(47)
Case-control study of Swedish hospital admissions, 1964–8		OC users had 4.5 times higher risk of TE	(48)
Case-control study of US hospital admissions, 1963–7		OC users had 4.4 times higher risk of TE	(49)
Case-control study of US hospital admissions, 1972	43 TE cases, 842 controls	OC users had 11 times higher risk of TE (11 in 100 000); TE attack rate in OC users 60 per 100 000 users per year; risk of thrombotic stroke greater than hemorrhagic stroke in OC users	(50)
Cohort study of general practice consultations (1968–77) and deaths (1968–76) in Britain	46 000 cases and controls	112 of 100 000 users of OCs containing over 50 μg of estrogen would develop DVTs; 80 of 100 000 OC users containing under 50 μg of estrogen would develop DVTs	(51)
Case-control study of deaths in Britain, 1973	153 death reports	OC users had three times higher risk of MI	(52)
Cohort study of hospital referrals (1968–75) and deaths (1968–77) in Britain	17 032 cases and controls	OC users had 6.3 times higher risk than non-users of idiopathic VT; OC users had two times higher risk than non-users of postoperative VT	(53, 54)
Case-control study of US hospital admissions, 1970–73	461	Relative risk of idiopathic thrombosis 7.2 times greater in OC users; relative risk of thrombosis was 1.9 times greater in OC users; women taking OCs containing over 100 μg of estrogen had 10.1 times the risk of thrombotic disease; women taking OCs containing under 100 μg of estrogen had 4.7 times the risk of thrombotic disease	(55)
Case-control/cohort study of US hospital admissions, 1969–76	16 759 cases and controls**	OC users smoking had increased risk of TE and subarachnoid hemorrhage	(56)

* Market research data was used for control purposes in this study.
** Controls based on Walnut Creek cohort study.
OC = oral contraceptive.
DVT = deep venous thrombosis.
PE = pulmonary embolism.
MI = myocardial infarction.
TE = thromboembolism.
VT = venous thrombosis.

Nevertheless, not everyone was pessimistic about the carcinogenic potential of the pill. Indeed, some medical and scientific experts viewed the contraceptive as a potential weapon in the fight *against* cancer. Part of their belief stemmed from the fact that during the 1950s some research had shown that certain hormones, rather than being detrimental, could actually ameliorate certain cancers (60, 61, 79, 80). As early as 1961, just months before news broke associating thrombotic deaths with the pill, Gregory Pincus, one of the developers of the oral contraceptive, argued that it could potentially prevent breast and cervical cancer (81–83). During the late 1970s, a number of epidemiological studies confirmed some of Pincus's theories that the pill might in fact have anticarcinogenic effects. Evidence increasingly suggested that the contraceptive could offer some protection against ovarian and endometrial cancer.

Solving the riddle of the pill and cancer

Nevertheless, many within the medical and scientific communities were unsure about the best method of tackling the contradictory evidence. Several dilemmas confronted them. One of the major difficulties was the fact that cancer was not a reportable disease in the early years of the marketing of the pill. Given the uncertainty of how long it would take for any carcinogenic effects to become apparent, investigators were also uncertain how long it would take for significant results to be obtained and whether the manifestation of such a disease could be definitively ascribed to the pill.

To add to the complexity, the effects of the contraceptive are not universal in their effect on female reproductive organs and other parts of the body, such as the liver. There were also life-cycle questions. Was there, for instance, a difference if the drug was taken earlier rather than later in a woman's reproductive life? It was also extremely difficult to isolate the pill from the genetic, cultural, geographic, and environmental factors known to cause cancer.

Much of the fear about the carcinogenic effects of the pill focused on its potential to cause breast cancer. Breast cancer was the one risk, apart from cardiovascular complications, that many feared might tip the odds against the overall safety of the pill (84). As one epidemiologist pointed out in 1991, breast cancer was so common that "any increase in risk associated with a widely used method of contraception would be a serious concern". He went on to point out that "breast cancer also happens to be a disease that women and their families particularly fear, so any increase in risk might carry a disproportionate weight when choices of contraception are being made" (85).

As early as 1969 breast cancer was calculated to be the leading cause of all early deaths from cancer among women in Britain and America: 10 000 and 29 000 respectively in 1969. By 1987 the lifetime risk of breast cancer had increased in both countries, reaching 1 in 13 in Britain and 1 in 10 in the USA. Between 1955 and 1985 the crude death rate had shot up in Britain from 36 to 52 per 100 000 of the female population. Most of this rise had been among older women. In the USA breast cancer was the most common of all causes of death among women aged 40–44 during the 1980s; at least 37 000 women were dying from the disease each year. Breast cancer had also risen in other parts of Europe and Scandinavia (86–92).

From 1983 onwards one of the major concerns about the pill and breast cancer was the long-term impact on younger women. For instance, one epidemiological study conducted in Los Angeles in 1983 showed that women who took the pill before the age of 25 had a 4-fold increased risk of breast cancer under the age of 37; the risk increased with duration of exposure (93).

Such news was particularly worrying, given the recent increase of younger women taking the pill. In Britain, for instance, the number of sexually active female teenagers (under the age of 20) taking the pill rose from 15% in 1970 to 50% in 1975 and 80% in 1980. The number of women taking the pill under the age of 30 had also increased substantially since its first marketing. In the USA teenage consumption of the pill, although starting later than in Britain, was also high (94–96). By 1987 over 80% of all British general practitioners' prescriptions of the pill were for women under the age of 30 (97, 98).

What really troubled the medical community from 1983 onwards was the thought that the putative higher risk in younger women taking the pill might persist into their middle age. Should this happen, medical experts feared that they would witness an unprecedented rise in the incidence of breast cancer in years to come. In Britain, which already had one of the highest rates of breast cancer in the world, it was estimated in 1981 that such a risk could "eventually produce groups of women with perhaps a one-in-five chance of developing breast cancer in their life-times" (99, 100). Similar concerns surfaced among American experts (91, 101).

By 1988 over 30 epidemiological studies had been undertaken to investigate the links between oral contraceptive use and breast cancer. Yet not a single study had provided a statistically significantly answer (102). In 1992, however, Professor Valerie Beral, director of the Imperial Cancer Research Fund Epidemiology Unit in Oxford, began a collaborative study that was to provide the first conclusive evidence on whether the pill could be linked to breast cancer. Taking data from 54 studies from 25 countries around the world that together had investigated 53 297 women with breast cancer and 100 239 controls, this study represented about 90% of the epidemiological information that had been collected on breast cancer risk and the use of hormonal contraceptives in the previous two decades (103, 104). The data came not only from studies conducted in Britain, the USA, Australia, and New Zealand, but also from Chile, China, Colombia, Kenya, Mexico, Nigeria, the Philippines, and Thailand (105).

The analysis made apparent what no one had seen before: that the carcinogenic effect of the pill on the breast was related to its recent use. Published in 1996, the study showed that the excess mortality from breast cancer occurred among recent users of the pill and for 10 years thereafter, but that past users showed no excess mortality. In the case of women taking the pill the risk was only slight. Tumors in women taking oral contraceptives tended to be localized to the breast and were less clinically advanced. This contrasted with women who had never used oral contraceptives, in whom the cancer was more likely to metastasize. The tumors in women taking the pill were therefore potentially easier to treat.

Most importantly, the carcinogenic effect of the pill on the breast diminished after 10 years of withdrawal. It was therefore unlikely that there would be an epidemic of breast cancer in future years among older women who had taken the pill. The data also indicated that risk was unrelated to any particular estrogen or progestogen. Interestingly, the higher doses of hormones were associated with less risk (104). Physicians were once again reassured in January 1999 when a 25-year follow-up of 46 000 women by the British Royal College of General Practitioners confirmed the earlier findings of the collaborative study (106).

Conclusion

Much of the history of the pill written since the late 1960s has promoted the idea that its early review by the FDA was so inadequate that it allowed a dangerous drug to be marketed. Some critics have gone further, claiming that women were used as guinea-pigs in a massive international experiment (107–110). Written after the cardiovascular risks of the pill were announced, such histories fail to take into account the fact that the drug was reviewed and marketed before 1962, when the worldwide epidemic of birth deformities associated with thalidomide prompted stronger laws governing the regulation and marketing of new drugs in Britain, the USA, and most of Europe. The total number of cases screened by the FDA for premarketing amounted to 897; however, an additional 500 000 women had taken the pill for gynecological treatment (111). My own research and that of Suzanne White Junod has shown that while some of the procedures used during the pill trials might not stand up to the ethical requirements of today, they more than adequately matched those of many drugs tested at the same time.

Moreover, many of the complications later associated with the pill would have been difficult to determine before it was consumed on a large scale. Premarketing testing in the late 1950s was far too limited for the detection of the major but rare adverse reactions, and even today FDA requirements of preclinical testing (about 600 women-years of exposure) of oral contraceptives would provide too little information about the potential long-term lethal risk of cardiovascular or carcinogenic disease. As late as 1990 an IOM publication made the point that women's health would be better served if less money was spent on preclinical trials and some way was found of using money from the sale of the pill to fund postmarketing surveillance. Nevertheless, despite the fact that many of the studies that unravelled the risks of thrombotic problems associated with the pill were government-funded case-control and cohort studies, such research continues to be underfunded to this day. This is paradoxical, given that such studies cost less than the "less useful" preclinical trials.

It was only once thousands of women had been exposed that any conclusions could be drawn. Between 1961 and 1965 the number of women using the pill in the USA rose from under half a million to 5 million, and by 1966 more than 8 million American women were taking it. In Britain the number of women taking the pill rose from 50 000 in 1962 to about half a million in 1966 and 1.1 million in 1969 (112–115). This swift uptake of the pill in the 1960s was crucial in determining the link between the pill and thrombosis.

In later years, however, determining the adverse effects of the pill no longer depended on studying a large enough population, but rather on discovering enough women who had not taken the pill for any length of time, who could act as controls. For example, a survey of sexually active British women aged 16–29 undertaken by the Royal College of General Practitioners in 1985 showed that only 5% had never used it (116).

The introduction of the oral contraceptive led to some of the biggest medical investigations in history, and required international collaboration on a large scale. Conclusive evidence of the relation between the pill and breast cancer, for instance, rested on the examination of over 150 000 women and collaboration with epidemiologists from 25 countries. Much of this work could not have been done without the development of new methods and statistical techniques, including the emergence of meta-analysis since the 1970s (117). Researchers investigating the issue were also aided by the rise of the computer, which was invaluable in analyzing the sheer numbers involved in the studies. The development of new statistical methods combined with the computer made what had seemed an impossible task possible by the 1990s.

REFERENCES

1. Guillebaud G. Introduction. In: Guillebaud J. The pill. Oxford: Oxford University Press, 1980: 3.
2. Lewin H to Guttmacher A, 22 July 1966, Population Council Papers, Box 124, Rockefeller Archive.
3. Glover D. Oral contraception Br Med J 1961; 1: 432.
4. Jordan WM. Pulmonary embolism. Lancet 1961; 2: 1146–7.
5. Memo from GD Searle to Shareowners, Aug 9, 1962, Smithsonian Papers, National Museum of American History, Washington DC.
6. New York Times 1962; 9 August.
7. Memo to PPFA Affiliates from MS Calderone, 6 August 1962, Schlesinger Library, Calderone's Papers, Box 12, fo. 216.
8. Anonymous. Oral contraceptives and thrombophlebitis. Br Med J 1962; 2: 426.
9. Davey J. How safe are the birth control pills? Redbook, Feb 1963, Gregory Pincus' Papers, Library of Congress (GP-LC), Box 60.
10. Anonymous. Do the pills cause cancer? Time 1964; 3 July: 56.
11. Watkins E. On the pill: a social history of oral contraceptives, 1950–1970. Baltimore: Johns Hopkins University Press, 1998: 43–4, 83.
12. Guttmacher AF to Fox T, March 16 1965. Alan Guttmacher's Papers, Francis Countway Library, Boston, Massachusetts (AG-FCL), Box 2.
13. Tietze C. In: Proceedings of a conference: thromboembolic phenomena in women. Chicago: GD Searle, 1962: 12.
14. Seaman B, Seaman G. Women and the crisis in sex hormones: an investigation of the dangerous uses of hormones from birth control to menopause and the safe alternatives. New York: Rawson Associates, 1977: 101.
15. Interview with W Inman by L Marks, 13 Oct 1994, Southampton, transcript 74–5.
16. Inman WHW, Vessey MP. Investigation of deaths from pulmonary, coronary, and cerebral thrombosis and embolism in women of childbearing age. Br Med J 1968; 2: 193–9.
17. FDA Advisory Committee on Obstetrics and Gynecology. Minutes, Second Meeting, 1966; 20 and 21 January: 6.
18. FDA Advisory Committee on Obstetrics and Gynecology. Report on oral contraceptives 1966; 1 Aug: 61, 63–4.
19. FDA Advisory Committee on Obstetrics and Gynecology. Second report on the oral contraceptives 1969; 1 Aug: 2–3.
20. Interview with W Inman by L Marks, 13 October 1994, Southampton, transcript 74–6.
21. Farmer RDT, Preston TD. The risk of venous thromboembolism associated with low oestrogen oral contraceptives. J Obstet Gynaecol 1995; 15: 195–200.
22. Seigel D, Corfman P. Epidemiological prob-

lems associated with studies of the safety of oral contraceptives. J Am Med Assoc 1968; 203: 950–4.
23. GD Searle. Proceedings of a Conference, 1962: 27–8.
24. Tyler ET. Oral contraception and venous thromboembolism. J Am Med Assoc 1963; 185: 131–2.
25. Inman WHW. Don't tell the patient. Hampshire: Highland Park Productions, 1999: Chapter 2.
26. GD Searle. Proceedings of a Conference, 1962: 9, 74, 87.
27. Memo from MS Calderone to all Planned Parenthood–World Population Affiliates, August 1963, Planned Parenthood Federation of America (PPFA) Papers, Sophia Smith Library, Smith College, Northampton, Massachusetts.
28. FDA Advisory Committee on Obstetrics and Gynecology. Minutes, First Meeting 1965; 22 and 25 Nov: 26.
29. Vessey MP, Mann JI. Female sex hormones and thrombosis: epidemiological aspects. Br Med Bull 1978; 34: 157–62.
30. Vessey MP. Female hormones and vascular disease – an epidemiological overview. Br J Fam Plann Suppl 1980; 6: 1–12.
31. Anonymous. Risk of thromboembolic disease in women taking oral contraceptives. A preliminary communication to the Medical Research Council by a Subcommittee. Br Med J 1967; 2: 355–9.
32. Inman WHW. Role of drug–reaction monitoring in the investigation of thrombosis and the "pill". Br Med Bull 1970; 26: 248–56.
33. Department of Health Education and Welfare, USA. FDA report on Enovid. J Am Med Assoc 1963; 185: 776.
34. Wynn V, Doar JWH. Some effects of oral contraceptives on carbohydrate metabolism. Lancet 1966; 2: 715–19.
35. Wynn V, Doar JWH, Mills GL. Some effects of oral contraceptives on serum-lipid and lipoprotein levels. Lancet 1966; 2: 720–3.
36. Swyer GIM. Oral contraceptives, thrombosis, and cyclical factors affecting veins. Br Med J 1966; 1: 355.
37. World Health Organization. Clinical aspects of oral gestogens: report of a WHO scientific group. World Health Organization Technical Report Series No. 326, Geneva, 1966.
38. FDA Advisory Committee on Obstetrics and Gynecology. Report on the oral contraceptives 1966; 1 August.
39. Royal College of General Practitioners. Oral contraception and thrombo-embolic disease. J Coll Gen Pract 1967; 13: 267–79.
40. Inman WHW, Vessey MP. Investigation of deaths from pulmonary coronary and cerebral thrombosis and embolism in women of child-bearing age. Br Med J 1968; 2: 193–9.
41. Ramcharan S. The Walnut Creek Contraceptive Drug Study. A prospective study of the side-effects of oral contraceptives. Volume 1, DHEW Publication No. Washington DC: NIHV, 1974.
42. Vessey MP, Doll R. Investigation of relation between use of oral contraceptives and thromboembolic disease. Br Med J 1968; 2: 199–205.
43. Vessey MP, Doll R. Investigation of relation between use of oral contraceptives and thromboembolic disease. A further report. Br Med J 1969; 1: 651–7.
44. Sartwell P, Masi AT, Arthes FG, Greene GR, Smith HE. Thromboembolism and oral contraceptives: an epidemiological case-control study. Advisory Committee on Obstetrics and Gynecology, FDA Second Report on the Oral Contraceptives, US Government. 1969; 1 Aug: 21–36.
45. Sartwell PE, Masi AT, Arthes FG, Greene GR, Smith HE. Thromboembolism and oral contraceptives: an epidemiologic case-control study. Am J Epidemiol 1969; 90: 365–80.
46. Inman WHW, Vessey MP, Westerholm B, Englelund A. Thromboembolic disease and the steroidal content of oral contraceptives: a report to the Committee on Safety of Drugs. Br Med J 1970; 2: 203–9.
47. Vessey MP, Doll R, Fairbairn AS, Glober G. Postoperative thromboembolism and the use of oral contraceptives. Br Med J 1970; 3: 123–6.
48. Bottinger LE, Westerholm B. Oral contraceptives and thromboembolic disease. Swedish experience. Acta Med Scand 1971; 190: 455–63.
49. Greene GR, Sartwell PE. Oral contraceptive use in patients with thromboembolism following surgery, trauma, or infection. Am J Public Health 1972; 62: 680–5.
50. Anonymous. Oral contraceptives and venous thromboembolic disease, surgically confirmed gall-bladder disease, and breast tumours. Report from the Boston Collaborative Drug Surveillance Programme. Lancet 1973; 1: 1399–404.
51. Royal College of General Practitioners. Oral contraceptives and health: an interim report from the Oral Contraceptive Study of the Royal College of General Practitioners, London, 1974.
52. Mann JI, Inman WHW. Oral contraceptives and death from myocardial infarction. Br Med J 1975; 2: 245–8.
53. Vessey MP, Doll R, Peto R, Johnson B, Wiggins P. A long-term follow-up study of women using different methods of contraception – an interim report. J Biosociol Sci 1976; 8: 373–427.
54. Vessey MP. Steroid contraception, venous thromboembolism, and stroke: data from countries other than the United States. In: Sciarra JJ, Zatuchni GI, JJ Speidel, editors. Risks, benefits, and controversies in fertility control: proceedings of a workshop on risks, benefits, and controversies in fertility control, held in Arlington, Virginia, United States of America. Hagerstown, MD: Harper & Row, 1978: 113–21.
55. Stolley PD, Tonascia JA, Tockman MS, Sartwell PE, Rutledge AH, Jacobs MP. Thrombosis with low-estrogen oral contraceptives. Am J Epidemiol 1975; 102: 197–208.
56. Petitti DB, Wingerd J, Pellegrin F, S Ramcharan. Risk of vascular disease in women. J Am Med Assoc 1979; 242: 1150–4.

57. Gardner WU. Tumors in experimental animals receiving steroid hormones. Surgery 1944; 16: 8–32.
58. Gardner WU. Studies on steroid hormones in experimental carcinogenesis. Recent Prog Horm Res 1946; 1: 217–60.
59. Bielschowsky F, Horning ES. Aspects of endocrine carcinogenesis. Br Med Bull 1958; 14: 106–15.
60. Goodman LS, Gilman A. The Pharmacological Basis of Therapeutics, 2nd edition. New York: The Macmillan Company, 1960: 1594.
61. Sneader W. Drug prototypes and their exploitation. Chichester: John Wiley, 1996: 315.
62. Oudshoorn N. Beyond the natural body: archaeology of sex hormones. London: Routledge, 1994: 107.
63. GM Bonser to E Mears, April 1960, SA/FPA/A5/161/1, Box 251; Council for the Investigation of Fertility Control (CIFC) Minutes, 1960; 21 April: 110. SA/FPA/A5/154, Archives and Manuscripts, Wellcome Library for the History and Understanding of Medicine, London (AM).
64. How safe are the birth control pills? Redbook 1963; February.
65. Watkins ES. On the pill: a social history of oral contraceptives, 1950–1970. Baltimore, London: Johns Hopkins University Press, 1998: 43–4, 83.
66. Anonymous. Further doubts about oral contraception. Br Med J 1970: 1: 252.
67. Anonymous. Volidan 21 and Serial 28 discontinued: new toxicological evidence. Pharm J 1975; 215: 597.
68. Horvath E, Kovacs K, Ross RC. Ultrastructural findings in a well differentiated hepatoma. Digestion 1972; 7: 74.
69. Baum JK, Bookstein JJ, Holtz F, Klein EW. Possible association between benign hepatomas and oral contraceptives. Lancet 1973; 2: 926–9.
70. Mays ET, Christopherson WM, Mahr MM, Williams HC. Hepatic changes in young women ingesting contraceptive steroids. Hepatic hemorrhage and primary hepatic tumors. J Am Med Assoc 1976; 235: 730–2.
71. Edmonsen HA, Henderson B, Benton B. Liver-cell adenomas associated with the use of oral contraceptives. New Engl J Med 1976; 294: 470–2.
72. Vaughan P. The pill turns twenty. The New York Times Magazine 1976; 13 June.
73. Anonymous. Sequential oral contraceptives removed from US market. Pharm J 1976; 217: 257.
74. Prentice RL, Thomas DB. On the epidemiology of oral contraceptives and disease. Adv Cancer Res 1987; 19: 342–59.
75. Seaman B, Seaman G. Women and the crisis in sex hormones: an investigation of the dangerous uses of hormones from birth control to menopause and the safe alternatives. New York: Rawson Associates, 1977: 13–24, 40–2.
76. Direcks A, 't Hoen E. DES: the crime continues. In: Donnell K, editor. Adverse effects: women and the pharmaceutical industry. Toronto: Women's Press, 1986: 41–50.
77. Dutton DB, Preston TA, Pfund NE. Worse than the disease: pitfalls of medical progress. Cambridge: Cambridge University Press, 1988: Chapter 3.
78. Seaman B, Seaman G. Women and the crisis in sex hormones: an investigation of the dangerous uses of hormones from birth control to menopause and the safe alternatives. New York: Rawson Associates, 1977: 116.
79. Gardner WU. Tumors in experimental animals receiving steroid hormones. Surgery 1944; 16: 8–32.
80. Bielschowsky F, Horning ES. Aspects of endocrine carcinogenesis. Br Med Bull 1958; 14: 106–15.
81. G Pincus to D Norman, 1960; 7 June: GP-LC, Box 45.
82. Pincus G, Garcia CR. Studies in vaginal, cervical and uterine histology. Metabolism 1965; 3: 344–7.
83. How safe are the birth control pills? Vogue 1961; 8 January: 90–1, 128.
84. World Health Organization. Fifty facts from The World Health Report 1998: global health situation and trends 1955–2025. Geneva: WHO, 1998.
85. Skegg DCG. Risks and benefits of oral contraceptives: will breast cancer tip the balance? In: Oral contraceptives and breast cancer. Washington: Institute of Medicine, 1991: 166.
86. General Register Office. Registrar General's statistical review of England and Wales, Part 1. London: HMSO, 1969.
87. Anonymous. Doubts about the pill. Newsweek 1969; 19 May: 41.
88. Kalache A, McPherson K, Barltrop K, Vessey M. Oral contraceptives and breast cancer. Br J Hosp Med 1983; 23 October: 278–83.
89. Lincoln R. The pill, breast and cervical cancer, and the role of progestogens in arterial disease. Fam Plann Perspect 1984; 16: 55–63.
90. Hennekens CH, Speizer FE, Lipnick RJ, Rosner B, Bain C, Belanger C, Stampfer MJ, Willett W, Peto R. A case-control study of oral contraceptive use and breast cancer. J Natl Cancer Inst 1984; 72: 39–42.
91. Schlesselman JJ. Oral contraceptives and breast cancer. Am J Obstet Gynecol 1990; 163: 1379–87.
92. World Health Organization. The dimensions of reproductive ill-health. 1990–1995. Geneva: WHO, 1998.
93. Pike MC, Henderson BE, Krailo MD, Duke A, Roy S. Breast cancer in young women and use of oral contraceptives; possible modifying effect of formulation and age at use. Lancet 1983; 2: 926–30.
94. McPherson K. Modeling latent effects in any association between oral contraceptives and breast cancer. In: Morgenstern H, et al., editors. Models of non-communicable diseases: health status and health service requirements. Heidelberg: Springer Verlag, 1992: 74–5.
95. McPherson K, Drife JO. The pill and breast

cancer: why the uncertainty? Br Med J 1986; 293: 709–10.
96. Thorogood M, Vessey M. Trends in use of oral contraceptives in Britain. Br J Fam Plann 1990; 16: 41–53.
97. Thorogood M, Villard-Mackintosh L. Combined oral contraceptives: risks and benefits. Br Med Bull 1993; 49: 124–39.
98. Russell-Briefel R, Ezzati T, Perlman J. Prevalence and trends in oral contraceptive use in premenopausal females ages 12–54 years, United States, 1971–80. Am J Public Health 1985; 75: 1173–6.
99. Anonymous. Breast cancer and the pill – a muted reassurance. Br Med J (Clin Res Ed) 1981; 282: 2075–6.
100. Anonymous. Another look at the pill and breast cancer. Lancet 1985; 2: 985–7.
101. Anonymous. Oral contraceptives: the good news. J Am Med Assoc 1983; 249: 1624–5.
102. Buehring GC. Oral contraceptives and breast cancer: what has 20 years of research shown? Biomed Pharmacother 1988; 42: 525–30.
103. Anonymous. Breast cancer and hormonal contraceptives: collaborative reanalysis of individual data on 53 297 women with breast cancer and 100 239 women without breast cancer from 54 epidemiological studies. Collaborative Group on Hormonal Factors in Breast Cancer. Lancet 1996; 347: 1713–27.
104. Anonymous. Breast cancer and hormonal contraceptives: further results. Collaborative Group on Hormonal Factors in Breast Cancer. Contraception. 1996; 54 Suppl 3: 1S–106S.
105. Interview with Valerie Beral by Lara Marks, 17 and 26 December 1998, London, notes and tape.
106. Beral V, Hermon C, Kay C, Hannaford P, Darby S, Reeves G. Mortality associated with oral contraceptive use: 25 year follow up of cohort of 46 000 women from Royal College of General Practitioners' oral contraception study. Br Med J 1999; 318: 96–100.
107. Moore FD. Ethical boundaries in initial clinical trials. In: Freund PA, editor. Experimentation with human subjects. New York: G Braziller, 1970: 363.
108. Phillips A, Rakusen J. Our bodies, ourselves. Boston: Boston Women's Book Collective, 1984.
109. Grant L. Sexing the millennium: a political history of the sexual revolution. London: HarperCollins, 1993: 54.
110. Hartmann B. Reproductive rights and wrongs: the global politics of population control. New York: Sputh End Press, 1985: 190.
111. White Junod S, Marks L. Women's trials: the approval of the first oral contraceptive in the United States and Great Britain. Bull Hist Med 2002: in press.
112. Anonymous. Syntex symposium. Pharm J 1966; 196: 619–20.
113. Guttmacher AF. The pill around the world. Unpublished paper for IPPF Medical Bulletin, AG-FCL, Box 18, Countway Library 1966; 2 September.
114. Pharm J 1969; 203: 181.
115. Kent A. Thirty years on the pill. The Times 1990; 22 March.
116. Guillebaud J. The pill. Oxford: Oxford University Press, 1980: 20.
117. Cookson C. The nature of things: new conclusions from old studies. Financial Times 1994; 26–27 November: iii.

Reginald P. Sequeira

1 Central nervous system stimulants, drugs that suppress appetite, and drugs used in Alzheimer's disease

METHYLXANTHINES *(SED-14, 1; SEDA-22, 1; SEDA-23, 1; SEDA-24, 1)*

Caffeine

Drug interactions In an open-label, randomized, crossover study in 12 non-smoking healthy volunteers, caffeine 400–1000 mg/day reduced *clozapine* clearance, probably by inhibiting CYP1A2 (1[c]). Differences in habitual caffeine intake can therefore explain some of the large variability in the kinetics of clozapine (2[C]) and should be taken into consideration when clozapine is used. An earlier case report (3[A]) also suggested that caffeine increases plasma concentrations of clozapine, causing toxic symptoms.

Theophylline

Risk factors Based on a retrospective investigation of theophylline-induced convulsions in epileptic children, it was concluded that *infants* under 1 year of age with epilepsy have a higher risk of theophylline-induced convulsions; theophylline should be avoided in this group (4[C]).

Drug interactions *Citalopram* Both theophylline and citalopram are metabolized by CYP1A2. In an open-label, multiple-dose study in 13 healthy non-smoking volunteers, steady-state citalopram therapy had no significant effect on theophylline metabolism. The authors suggested that dosage adjustment of theophylline may not be necessary in patients taking concurrent citalopram (5[c]). The most frequent treatment-related adverse effects were fatigue and nausea.

Corticosteroids and gold salts The kinetic behavior of theophylline given concomitantly with methylprednisolone and auranofin to six women suggested a possible interaction of theophylline with auranofin, although a role of the corticosteroid could not be ruled out. The observed concentrations of theophylline were lower than expected, suggesting the need to measure serum theophylline concentrations in patients who also take steroids and gold salts (6[c]).

Proton pump inhibitors Co-administration of either lansoprazole or pantoprazole in healthy subjects did not affect the steady-state pharmacokinetics of theophylline in therapeutic doses (7[c]).

Tacrolimus An interaction of theophylline with tacrolimus has been described (8[A]).

A 33-year-old man with end-stage renal disease due to diabetic nephropathy received a cadaveric kidney graft. Immunosuppressive therapy after transplantation included tacrolimus (7 mg/day), azathioprine (75 mg/day), and prednisone (7.5 mg/day). He developed erythrocytosis 3 months later and was given drugs that reduce erythropoietin production, first enalapril, without success, and then theophylline (600 mg/day). After a month, his serum creatinine and tacrolimus concentrations were raised. The

Side Effects of Drugs, Annual 25
J.K. Aronson, ed.

dosage of theophylline was therefore reduced to 300 mg/day four times a week. One month later, his serum creatinine and tacrolimus trough blood concentrations increased further. On withdrawal of theophylline, both renal function and tacrolimus trough blood concentration rapidly normalized. Theophylline was then reintroduced in a lower dose and increased the AUC of tacrolimus.

CYP3A4 is primarily responsible for tacrolimus biotransformation in the liver, but it has only a minor role in theophylline metabolism. It is therefore surprising that this tacrolimus–theophylline interaction occurred. The authors suggested that as long as renal function remains stable, low-dose theophylline can be used in transplant patients with erythrocytosis, provided that tacrolimus concentrations are closely monitored.

STIMULANT DRUGS *(SED-14, 12; SEDA-22, 2; SEDA-23, 2; SEDA-24, 2)*

Amphetamines *(SED-14, 16)*

Nervous system A previously healthy 16-year-old schoolboy had *mesencephalic ischemia*, most probably caused by vasospasm, after combined abuse of amphetamine and cocaine (9[A]). There was a close temporal relation between intake of the drug and the onset of symptoms. Thus, combining these drugs, even in small amounts, may be harmful.

Further evidence for *long-term neurotoxicity* associated with methamphetamine abuse has been reported. Magnetic resonance spectroscopy in 26 abstinent methamphetamine abusers with a history of methamphetamine dependence (estimated median lifetime exposure 3640 g; median time since last methamphetamine use, 4.25 months) and 24 healthy subjects without a history of drug abuse, showed that the concentration of *N*-acetylaspartate, a neuronal marker, was significantly reduced in the basal ganglia and frontal white matter, both of which correlated with the duration of methamphetamine use (10[c]). There were also other changes, such as reductions in the concentrations of creatinine, choline-containing compounds, and myoinositol. These findings have given further support to an earlier observation of long-term neurotoxicity associated with methylenedioxymethamphetamine (MDMA, ecstasy) in animals (SEDA-14, 3). However, it is uncertain whether the reported abnormalities suggestive of neuronal damage are reversible despite continued treatment or beyond 21 months of abstinence.

Psychiatric Increased sensitivity to stress may be related to spontaneous recurrence of methamphetamine *psychosis*, triggering flashbacks. Stressful experiences, together with methamphetamine use, induces sensitization to stress associated with noradrenergic hyperactivity, involving increased dopamine release (11[C], 12[C]). This hypothesis has been investigated by determining plasma noradrenaline metabolite concentrations in 26 flashbackers (patients with spontaneous recurrence of methamphetamine psychosis) (11 taking neuroleptic drugs before and during the study and 15 during the course of the study), 18 non-flashbackers with a history of methamphetamine psychosis, eight with persistent methamphetamine psychosis, and 34 controls (23 methamphetamine users and 11 non-users). The 26 flashbackers had had stressful events and/or methamphetamine-induced, fear-related, psychotic symptoms during previous methamphetamine use. Mild psychosocial stressors then triggered flashbacks. During flashbacks plasma noradrenaline concentrations increased markedly. Flashbackers with a history of stressful events, whether or not they had had fear-related symptoms, had a further increase in 3-methoxytyramine concentrations. Thus, robust noradrenergic hyperactivity, involving increased dopamine release in response to mild stress, may predispose to further episodes of flashbacks. The authors pointed out the limitations of their study: (a) plasma noradrenaline concentrations do not accurately reflect central monoamine neurotransmitter function; (b) raised noradrenaline concentrations may reflect heightened autonomic arousal secondary to stress or anxiety; (c) the neuroleptic drugs used may have altered the concentrations of noradrenaline and 3-methoxytyramine; and (d) the study was retrospective and carried out in women in prison.

Reports have suggested that atypical antipsychotic drugs, such as risperidone (13[A]) and olanzapine (14[A]), can be effective in the treatment of acute and residual methamphetamine-induced psychosis. Moreover, adherence to olanzapine for about 8 weeks also effectively controlled cravings for methamphetamine. Rigorous controlled studies are needed to establish the therapeutic efficacy of atypical antipsychotic drugs in the treatment of the psychosis and cravings of methamphetamine addiction.

Teeth In 43 patients who used methamphetamine there were distinct patterns of *tooth wear.* Patients who preferentially snorted methamphetamine had significantly greater tooth wear in the anterior maxillary teeth than patients who injected, smoked, or ingested methamphetamine (15[c]). This difference may be explained anatomically, based on the patterns of regional blood supply. It may be possible to identify methamphetamine abusers from examination of the mouth.

Infection risk A 34-year-old woman who had taken intranasal methamphetamine weekly for 15 years developed *osteomyelitis of the frontal bone and a subperiosteal abscess.* The authors proposed that this was due to chronic abuse of methamphetamine (16[A]).

Death There has been a retrospective investigation of methamphetamine-related fatalities during a 5-year period (1994–1998) in Southern Osaka city in Japan. Among 646 autopsy cases, methamphetamine was detected in 15, most of whom were men in their late thirties. The cause and manner of death were: methamphetamine poisoning ($n = 4$), homicide ($n = 4$), accidental falls and aspiration from drug abuse ($n = 4$), death in an accidental fire, myocardial infarction, and cerebral hemorrhage (one each). Blood methamphetamine concentrations were 23–170 μmol/l in fatal poisoning, 4.4–38 μmol/l in deaths from other extrinsic causes, and 14–22 μmol/l in cardiovascular and cerebrovascular accidents. The common complications were cardiomyopathy, cerebral perivasculitis, and liver cirrhosis/interstitial hepatitis (17[C]). The general profile of patient reported in this series compares with a previous study from Taiwan (SEDA 24, 2).

Drug interactions *Estrogens* There is limited evidence to suggest that the stimulating effects of amphetamine are increased by acute pretreatment with estradiol (18[c]). Two groups of healthy women with regular menstrual cycles participated in two sessions scheduled during the early follicular phases of two menstrual cycles. One group received estradiol patches 0.8 mg, which increased their plasma estradiol concentrations from normal to about 750 pg/ml. Both groups were given amphetamine 10 mg or a placebo in a randomized and counterbalanced order in two sessions. Dependent measures included a self-reported questionnaire, physiological measures, and plasma hormone concentrations. Most of the subjective and physiological effects of amphetamine were not affected by acute estradiol treatment. Nevertheless, estradiol pretreatment increased the magnitude of the effects of amphetamine on subjective ratings of "pleasant stimulation" and reduced ratings of "want more". Estradiol also produced some subjective effects when given alone: it increased the subjective ratings of "feel drug", "energy and intellectual efficiency", and "pleasant stimulation". Some limitations of the study were: (a) plasma amphetamine concentrations were not measured, so an effect of estradiol on the pharmacokinetics of amphetamine cannot be ruled out; (b) only single doses of amphetamine and estradiol were tested; (c) the dose of amphetamine was relatively low, and that of estradiol relatively high, maximizing the chances of detecting estradiol-dependent increases in two subjective effects of amphetamine.

Ritonavir A fatal interaction between ritonavir and methamphetamine has been described (19[A]).

A 49-year-old HIV-positive Caucasian man had taken ritonavir (400 mg bd), saquinavir (400 mg bd), and stavudine (40 mg bd) for 4 months. His CD4 cell count was 617×10^6 cells/l and HIV-1 RNA less than 400 copies/ml. He had previously taken zidovudine for 7 months. He self-injected twice with methamphetamine and sniffed amyl nitrate, and was found dead a few hours later. At autopsy there was no obvious cause of death. Methamphetamine was detected in the bile (0.5 mg/l) and cannabinoids and traces of benzodiazepines were detected in the blood.

Nitric oxide formed from amyl nitrate inhibits cytochrome P450 (20[E]) and ritonavir inhibits CYP2D6 (21[c]), which has a major role in methamphetamine detoxification (22[c]). This interaction could have led to fatal plasma concentrations of methamphetamine. It is therefore suggested that patients who take protease inhibitors are made aware of the potential risk of using any form of recreational drugs metabolized by CYP2D6, particularly methamphetamine.

Ephedrine

Drug interactions An interaction of ephedrine with *entacapone*, a specific, reversible, peripherally-acting inhibitor of catechol-*O*-methyl transferase has been reported (23[A]).

A 76-year-old woman with Parkinson's disease and closed-angle glaucoma was scheduled for eye surgery. She had severe choreoathetoid movements, and 3 weeks before surgery began to take entacapone 200 mg/day, in addition to her five daily doses of co-careldopa. General anesthesia was induced with intravenous propofol 80 mg and fentanyl 25 mg, and maintained with nitrous oxide–oxygen (2:1) and sevoflurane 1–1.5%. After 30 minutes her blood pressure fell from 145/85 to 85/35 mmHg. This was treated with an intravenous bolus of ephedrine 3 mg. The blood pressure immediately rose to 225/125 mmHg; it remained high despite an increase in the dose of sevoflurane, but was controlled by repeated doses of hydralazine 2 mg.

The effect of ephedrine, which is both a direct and indirect sympathomimetic, may have been enhanced by its not being metabolized by catechol-*O*-methyl transferase, because of the action of entacapone.

Methylphenidate

The short-term and long-term efficacy and safety of pharmacological and non-pharmacological interventions in patients with attention deficit hyperactivity disorder (ADHD) have been reviewed in a systematic review of 92 reports of 78 randomized clinical trials (24[M]). There was substantial heterogeneity in the data, and so meta-analysis was not performed. In 22 comparisons of stimulants, the drugs generally did not differ in efficacy. The evidence was too limited to assess the effectiveness of stimulant drugs reliably compared with tricyclic antidepressants. Of six comparisons of drugs and non-drug interventions, five showed that stimulants were more effective. In 20 trials of combined interventions there was no compelling evidence to support combination treatment. Of nine comparisons of tricyclic antidepressants with placebo, six showed benefit of desipramine, whereas the effect of imipramine (three trials) was inconsistent. The study with the highest methodological score showed greater benefit with methylphenidate than placebo. Adverse effects, such as sleep disorders, headache, tics, reduced appetite, abdominal pain, irritability, nausea, and fatigue, were assessed in 29 trials. No evidence was available for more severe, long-term adverse effects, such as the risk of addiction with stimulants, liver toxicity with pemoline, or cardiac dysrhythmias with antidepressants. The authors concluded that in patients with ADHD published studies of treatment regimens provide limited information of effectiveness because of small sample sizes, flawed methods, and heterogeneity across outcomes. Thus, pharmacological interventions in ADHD are consistently more effective than non-pharmacological interventions. Combined interventions are not more beneficial than single interventions.

Nervous system The risk of using methylphenidate for long periods has been highlighted by a case of *stroke* in a child (25[A]).

An 8-year-old boy, who had taken methylphenidate 20 mg/day for 18 months, suddenly developed paresthesia in his left arm, with spontaneous resolution after a few days. Two months later he had more intense paresthesia in the left arm, spreading to the left side of the face; 48 hours later he developed weakness of the arm that extended to the whole of the left side of the body. He remained lucid. The episode resolved spontaneously within 24 hours. After a symptom-free period of 2 months, he had a third episode, similar to the previous ones, but more severe and leaving a residual deficit. Methylphenidate was withdrawn and he did not subsequently relapse. A CT scan showed a hypodense area in the left thalamus, and an MRI scan showed multiple lesions in both thalami. A cerebral angiogram showed enlargement of the basilar artery and the proximal segment of both posterior cerebral arteries.

The authors suggested that in this case the stroke was due to a vasculitis, which has previously been reported with methylphenidate (26[A]).

Metabolism The association between childhood treatment with methylphenidate and adult height and weight has been investigated in 97 boys, aged 4–12 years, who were referred to a child psychiatry outpatient clinic and took methylphenidate for an average of 36 months (27[C]). They were re-evaluated between ages 21 and 23 years. Hierarchical analysis predicted adult height and weight from sets of non-medication and medication-related variables. Medicated individuals who had attained their final stature did not differ in average height or weight from family, community, or non-medicated controls. In some individuals, nausea and vomiting and the use of higher doses of methylphenidate were associated with growth impairment. It has to be emphasized that the correlations in this study do not demonstrate cause and effect relations between medication and ultimate stature.

Drug overdose Of 289 patients exposed to excessive doses of methylphenidate, 31% had symptoms, including most commonly tachycardia, agitation, and lethargy (28[C]). No patient developed severe symptoms, although there was a less favorable outcome with intentional versus unintentional exposure. Peak exposure occurred in 6- to 9-year-old children, in whom therapeutic error was the most common reason for exposure.

Drug interactions Two cases of dyskinesia and bruxism in children have been attributed to an interaction of methylphenidate with *valproic acid*. These adverse effects were severe, occurred a few hours after the ingestion of methylphenidate 5 mg, and lasted for 4 and 7 hours (29[A]).

As an increasing number of adults with ADHD are being treated with methylphenidate, the possibility of drug interactions with methylphenidate increases (30[R]). However, based on a study in extensive and poor CYP2D6 metabolizers, it has been suggested that CYP2D6 is not involved in the metabolism of methylphenidate, and that drugs that are inhibitors of CYP2D6 should not affect methylphenidate plasma concentrations (31[c]).

Modafinil

Modafinil has been shown to be effective in narcolepsy in a 9-week, randomized, placebo-controlled, double-blind, 21-center trial in 271 patients (32[C]). During treatment withdrawal, the patients did not have symptoms associated with amphetamine withdrawal. *Nausea* and *rhinitis* were significantly more common in the treatment group; in contrast, in a previous multicenter study in the USA there was a higher incidence of *headache* (33[C]). Modafinil was also effective in the treatment of somnolence due to pramipexole in a patient with Parkinson's disease (34[A]).

Drug dependence The abuse potential of modafinil is very low and differs from that of methylphenidate (35[c]). The data suggest that the subjective effects of modafinil may be similar to those of drugs such as phenylpropanolamine or caffeine, although a direct comparison with these drugs would be required to draw adequate conclusions. Furthermore, modafinil cannot be injected intravenously or smoked, and its once-daily dosing in the management of excessive daytime sleepiness in patients with narcolepsy suggests that it does not carry the same public health or safety concerns for abuse as amphetamines, since drugs that have a long half-life have less of a tendency to produce a "rush" and hence are less likely to be abused. However, the effects of social responses to the availability of modafinil can only be determined by postmarketing surveillance.

Strychnine

A case of fatal poisoning due to strychnine has been described, and the concentrations of strychnine in various body fluids and organs detailed (36[A]).

DRUGS THAT SUPPRESS APPETITE

Cardiac valvulopathy and primary pulmonary hypertension associated with anorectic drugs

(SEDA-21, 2; SEDA-22, 3; SEDA-23, 2; SEDA-24, 4)

Cardiac valvulopathy *Continued efforts are being made to determine the prevalence of valvulopathy in patients with a history of exposure to fenfluramine and phentermine. Using the FDA case definition of appetite-suppressant related valvulopathy, the prevalence was found to be 31% (60/191) in a selected group of Mayo Clinic patients at Rochester (37[C]). The most common finding was mild aortic regurgitation. Of asymptomatic patients 28% had abnormal echocardiographic findings. This study emphasized the spectrum of diet/drug-related cardiac disease and the potential for valvulopathy in asymptomatic patients.*

Echocardiography is recommended for the detection of valvular regurgitation in asymptomatic users of anorexigens with a heart murmur. The prevalence and diagnostic value of heart murmurs for valvular regurgitation has been determined in 223 patients taking dexfenfluramine for 6.9 months and 189 matched controls. Experienced physicians, non-cardiologists, unaware of the echocardiographic findings took a history and performed cardiac auscultation. Based on their findings the authors have recommended that cardiac auscultation should be the screening method of choice for detecting valvular regurgitation in users of anorexigens (38[C]). In this study, the absence of heart murmurs predicted the absence of clinically important valvular regurgitation in 93% of dexfenfluramine users. These results support the recommendation by the American Heart Association and American College of Cardiology (39[C]) that asymptomatic users of anorexigens without a heart murmur do not warrant echocardiography. The data also suggest that in users of anorexigens with a 10% prevalence of valvular regurgitation and a 10–15% prevalence of heart murmurs, cardiac auscultation will prevent 85–90% of patients from undergoing unnecessary echocardiography. These implications may apply to all users of anorexigens, because the prevalence of valvular regurgitation in recent large series is similar to that in this study (SEDA-24, 4). There are therefore large potential cost savings of cardiac auscultation, by preventing a large proportion of the more than 6 million Americans who are exposed to anorexigens from undergoing initial and follow-up echocardiography or from receiving empiric antibiotic prophylaxis for emergency procedures that preclude further cardiac evaluation.

The lack of detection of predominantly mild regurgitation and morphologically normal valves in a minority of patients is of uncertain relevance. Moreover, the value of antibiotic prophylaxis for infective endocarditis and of regular clinical or echocardiographic follow-up in these patients lacks supportive data. In addition, recent data suggest that valvular regurgitation may regress over time after withdrawal of anorexigens (SEDA-24, 4).

There is further evidence, from an uncontrolled observational study in 85 patients, that the dose and duration of administration of fenfluramine–phentermine affects the risk of significant valvular disease (40[C]). The authors suggested that it would be prudent to consider diagnostic echocardiography in patients who have used fenfluramine–phentermine either in a dosage of 60 mg/day or more or for 9 months or more. They also raised concerns that for patients with mild obesity, the prolonged use of larger cumulative amounts may lead to a higher risk of valve regurgitation.

In patients who had been treated with dexfenfluramine (n = 479) or the combination of phentermine + fenfluramine (n = 455) continuously for 30 days or more in the previous 14 months, there was an increase in the prevalence of aortic regurgitation compared with 539 control subjects (41[C]). There was no increase in the prevalence of moderate or severe aortic regurgitation in treated patients, and no difference in the prevalence of mitral regurgitation between the untreated and treated groups, irrespective of duration of therapy. All evaluations were carried out using the FDA criteria. The authors were careful to point out that their study was not specifically designed or adequately powered to evaluate specific categories of anorexigen therapy duration.

There is further evidence of the relation between the duration of treatment with fenfluramine–phentermine and the prevalence of valvular abnormalities (42[C]). In 1163 patients who had taken anorexigens within the previous 5 years and 672 control patients who had not, valvular abnormalities primarily involved those who had taken anorexigens for more than 6 months, and predominantly resulted in mild aortic regurgitation. The study had some noteworthy limitations: since fenfluramine has been withdrawn from use, a randomized trial was impossible; also the lack of baseline echocardiograms before treatment implies that one cannot be certain that the valvular regurgitation developed subsequent to drug treatment.

Primary pulmonary hypertension Of 579 patients in a prospective surveillance study in patients with pulmonary hypertension at 12 large referral centers in North America, 205 had primary pulmonary hypertension and 374 had secondary pulmonary hypertension (43[C]). Among the drugs surveyed, only fenfluramine had a significant association with primary pulmonary hypertension compared with secondary pulmonary hypertension (adjusted odds ratio for use for more than 6 months = 7.5; 95%

CI = 1.7, 32). The association was stronger with longer duration of use compared with shorter duration of use and was more pronounced in recent users than in remote users. An unexpectedly high (11.4%) number of patients with secondary pulmonary hypertension had used anorexigens. The magnitude of the association with primary pulmonary hypertension, the increased association with increasing duration of use, and the specificity for fenfluramines are consistent with previous studies that suggest that fenfluramines are causally related to primary pulmonary hypertension. In addition, the high prevalence of anorexigen use in patients with secondary pulmonary hypertension also raised the possibility that these drugs precipitate pulmonary hypertension in patients with underlying conditions associated with secondary pulmonary hypertension.

The age-adjusted mortality rates from primary pulmonary hypertension in the years immediately preceding the use of phen/fen were not different from those reported during the years of widespread phen/fen use among patients aged 20–54 years. This analysis failed to support the hypothesis that the widespread use of phen/fen in the years 1992–7 increased the incidence of primary pulmonary hypertension. "If the use of phen/fen during these years created an epidemic of primary pulmonary hypertension, as some have declared, such an epidemic is not reflected in the mortality database maintained by CDC" (44[r]).

A report of pulmonary hypertension associated with the manufacture and ingestion of "recreational" aminorex (4-methylaminorex) by three members of a family has been described (45[A]). The drug is generally synthesized from phenylpropanolamine hydrochloride obtained over the counter, and is smoked as the free base or the hydrochloride salt.

Phentermine/fluoxetine

Following the withdrawal of the fenfluramines, alternative combinations have been explored as appetite suppressants. In an open-label study of the use of a combination of phentermine + fluoxetine in 16 obese patients with binge-eating disorder, in the setting of cognitive behavioral therapy there were significant reductions in weight, binge frequency, and psychological distress by the end of treatment; however, the patients regained most of the weight within 1 year (46[c]). At follow-up at 18 months there was still a reduction in binge eating in patients who continued maintenance treatment. The results did not support the long-term value of adding phentermine/fluoxetine to cognitive behavioral therapy for binge-eating disorder. It is worth emphasizing that it is not known whether phentermine/fluoxetine is also associated with cardiac valvulopathy. Moreover, the recognition that phentermine is a monoamine oxidase inhibitor (47[E]) raises further concern about its safety.

Sibutramine

The safety and efficacy of sibutramine 10 mg/day in 109 obese patients (BMI > 30 kg/m^2, ages 16–65 years) has been evaluated in a double-blind, placebo-controlled, parallel-group, prospective study over a period of 6 months (48[C]). There was a significant loss of body weight, BMI, and waist measurement. There were 45 adverse events in 32 patients taking sibutramine; the most frequent were *dry mouth* (n = 19), *increased blood pressure* (n = 5), *constipation* (n = 5), and *tachycardia* (n = 5); two patients withdrew owing to adverse events. There were 29 adverse events in 23 patients taking placebo, mainly increased blood pressure (n = 11) and dry mouth (n = 10). In contrast, in an earlier study (49[Rc]) there were no significant increases in systolic or diastolic blood pressures or heart rate.

In another study of the efficacy and safety of sibutramine in obese white and African Americans with hypertension the most common adverse event resulting in withdrawal among those taking sibutramine was *hypertension* (5.3% vs 1.4% of patients taking placebo) (50[C]).

DRUGS USED IN ALZHEIMER'S DISEASE *(SED-14, 435; SEDA-22, 7; SEDA-23, 8; SEDA-24, 6)*

Donepezil

The current status of donepezil in the management of Alzheimer's disease has been comprehensively reviewed (51[R]). Several recent studies have confirmed the efficacy and tolerability of donepezil using different doses, study designs, and durations of treatment (52[C]–54[C], 55[cr], 56[C]). Some relevant conclusions were: (a) that younger patients should be targeted for assessment and treatment (57[C]); (b) 6% of patients discontinued medication owing to adverse events (56[C]); (c) sleep disturbances were more common in trials with bed-time dosing of donepezil (55[cr]); (d) long-term safety and realistic improvement was observed over a period of up to 4.9 years (58[C]); (e) the presence of the apolipoprotein E4 allele did not predict donepezil treatment failure (53[C]).

Seven elderly patients with psychotic or non-psychotic behavioral symptoms in Lewy body dementia had some clinical benefit from donepezil (59[A]). Donepezil was withdrawn prematurely in three patients owing to poor response and/or adverse events. The adverse events were *sedation*, *somnolence*, *exacerbated COPD*, *syncope*, *sweating*, and *bradycardia*. These results have to be confirmed in controlled trials.

In two patients with Alzheimer's disease, donepezil provided some benefit for cognitive symptoms, but there were *increased behavioral problems*, such as anxiety, agitation, irritability, and lack of impulse control; these were then successfully controlled by adding gabapentin (60[A]).

The adverse effects of donepezil in general practice have been evaluated in a postmarketing pharmacovigilance study in 1762 patients in the UK (61[C]). This observational cohort study used the technique of "Prescription-Event Monitoring" for a minimum period of 6 months. The commonest adverse events were *nausea*, *diarrhea*, *malaise*, *dizziness*, and *insomnia*. *Aggression*, *agitation*, and *abnormal dreams* were uncommonly associated with the drug. There were no causally-associated cardiac rhythm disturbances or liver disorders. The authors suggested that the abnormal dreams and psychiatric disturbances were possible adverse drug reactions that require further confirmation.

Nervous system *Restless legs*, *mumbling*, and *stuttering* have been reported in a patient taking donepezil (62[A]). According to the Naranjo probability scale, the causality was probable, since rechallenge was positive.

Extrapyramidal effects have been reported in three patients taking donepezil; in two cases the effects disappeared when donepezil was withdrawn (63[A]).

Urinary tract *Urinary incontinence* may often be disregarded as a manifestation of dementia, but it has also been attributed to donepezil.

Of 94 patients with mild to moderate disease treated with recommended dosages of donepezil (3 mg/day during the first week and then 5 mg/day) seven developed urinary incontinence (64[C]). In five of these the incontinence was transient, and there was no need to change the prescription. Incontinence occurred in both sexes, in relatively young and old patients, and in those with very mild to moderate dementia. In six patients the incontinence occurred at the higher dosage of 5 mg/day, in one patient it disappeared when donepezil was withdrawn, and in another an increase in dosage caused the reappearance of incontinence, suggesting a likely causal, dose-dependent relation between donepezil and urinary incontinence.

Urinary incontinence in patients with Down's syndrome treated with donepezil has been described before (SEDA-24, 7). Urinary incontinence can be a major concern and a source of distress, not only for patients but also for caregivers. Clinicians should be alert to the possibility of urinary incontinence when prescribing donepezil for individuals with Alzheimer's disease. The authors emphasized that the incontinence may often be transient and not serious, but it could limit a patient's activities and quality of life, and could also affect therapeutic concordance.

Drug interactions Parkinsonism has been reported in a patient concurrently taking donepezil and *tiapride*, probably through a pharmacodynamic interaction (65[A]).

Metrifonate

In patients with mild to moderate Alzheimer's disease metrifonate significantly improved behavior as well as cognition, function in activities of daily living, and global functional status, as shown by a pooled analysis of four prospective, multicenter, randomized, double-blind, parallel-group, placebo-controlled trials, meeting FDA guidelines (66[M]).

The safety and tolerability of once-daily oral metrifonate has been evaluated in patients with probable mild to moderate Alzheimer's disease in a randomized, double-blind, placebo-controlled, parallel-group study (67[C]). Metrifonate was given to 29 patients as a loading dose (2.5 mg/kg) for 2 weeks, followed by a maintenance dose (1 mg/kg) for 4 weeks; 10 patients received placebo. The proportion of patients who had at least one adverse event was comparable in the two groups: metrifonate 76%, placebo 80%. Selected adverse events, defined as those for which the incidence in the metrifonate and placebo group differed by at least 10%, were *diarrhea*, *nausea*, *leg cramps*, and *accidental injury*. The adverse events were predominantly mild and transient. Those who took metrifonate had a significantly lower heart rate. Metrifonate had no clinically important effect on laboratory tests, such as liver function tests, and did not affect exercise tolerance or pulmonary function.

Rivastigmine

Gastrointestinal Potentially fatal *rupture of the esophagus* has been associated with untitrated use of rivastigmine tablets in a patient with Alzheimer's disease (68[A]).

A 67-year-old Caucasian woman had a 2-year history of progressive memory loss. She had arterial hypertension successfully controlled with lisinopril and no history of ethanol abuse. A diagnosis of probable Alzheimer's disease was made and she was given rivastigmine 1.5 mg/day, increasing to 9 mg/day by weekly increments of 1.5 mg. During the titration period there were no significant adverse effects. After 13 weeks weight loss was observed and rivastigmine was withdrawn. After 8 weeks she developed marked cognitive deterioration and she and her carer were advised to restart rivastigmine 1.5 mg/day. However, she mistakenly took one tablet of 4.5 mg. About 30 minutes later she started to vomit several times. Nearly 2 hours later she complained of severe chest pain, followed by high-grade fever. A chest X-ray showed mediastinal and soft tissue emphysema, and a contrast X-ray showed rupture of the distal part of the esophagus. Emergency surgery was performed and she recovered.

Rivastigmine, and other acetylcholinesterase inhibitors can produce chest pain because of increased esophageal contractions, although consequent rupture of the esophagus has not previously been reported. In this case, the failure to titrate the dosage of rivastigmine could have resulted in rupture secondary to severe vomiting. This confirms the need for careful titration of the dose of rivastigmine, even when re-starting treatment.

Drug interactions Rivastigmine did not interact significantly with a wide range of concomitant medications prescribed for elderly patients with Alzheimer's disease, based on an analysis of 2459 patients (rivastigmine 1696, placebo 763) from four randomized placebo-controlled studies (69[R]). However, the Breslow–Day analysis used in this study detected only differences in the odds ratios of rivastigmine versus placebo among patients taking concomitant medications. Thus, these results have to be cautiously interpreted.

Tacrine

Liver The presence of the combined alleles M1 and T1, which mark deficiencies in glutathione-S-transferase genes, increases susceptibility to tacrine *hepatotoxicity* (70[E]). It would be interesting to use this molecular epidemiological approach to identify the role of combinations of glutathione-S-transferase genotypes in other adverse drug reactions.

REFERENCES

1. Hagg S, Spigset O, Mjorndal T, Dahlqvist R. Effects of caffeine on clozapine pharmacokinetics in healthy volunteers. Br J Clin Pharmacol 2000; 49: 59–63.
2. Jerling M, Merle Y, Mentre F, Mallet A. Population pharmacokinetics of clozapine evaluated with the nonparametric maximum likelihood method. Br J Clin Pharmacol 1997; 44: 447–53.
3. Odom-White J, Leon J. Clozapine levels and caffeine. J Clin Psychiatry 1996; 57: 175–6.
4. Miura T, Kimura K. Theophylline-induced convulsions in children with epilepsy. Pediatrics 2000; 105: 920.
5. Moller SE, Larsen F, Pitsiu M, Rolan PE. Effect of citalopram on plasma levels of oral theophylline. Clin Ther 2000; 22: 1494–1501.
6. Falcao AC, Rocha MJ, Almedia AM, Caramona MM. Theophylline pharmacokinetics with concomitant steroid and gold therapy. J Clin Pharm Ther 2000; 25: 191–5.

7. Pan WJ, Goldwater DR, Zhang Y, Pilmer BL, Hunt RH. Lack of a pharmacokinetic interaction between lansprazole or pantoprazole and theophylline. Aliment Pharmacol Ther 2000; 14: 345–52.
8. Boubenider S, Vincent I, Lambotte O, Roy S, Hiesse C. Interaction between theophylline and tacrolimus in a renal transplant patient. Nephrol Dial Transplant 2000; 15: 1066–8.
9. Strupp M, Hamann GF, Brandt T. Combined amphetamine and cocaine abuse caused mesencephalic ischemia in a 16-year-old boy due to vasospasm? Eur Neurol 2000; 43: 181–2.
10. Ernst T, Chang L, Leonido-Yee M, Speck O. Evidence for long-term neurotoxicity associated with methamphetamine abuse: a 1H MRS study. Neurology 2000; 54: 1344–9.
11. Yui K, Goto K, Ikemoto S, Ishiguro T. Stress induced spontaneous recurrence of methamphetamine psychosis: the relation between stressful experiences and sensitivity to stress. Drug Alcohol Depend 2000; 58: 67–75.
12. Yui K, Ishiguro T, Goto K, Ikemoto S. Susceptibility to subsequent episodes in spontaneous recurrence of methamphetamine psychosis. Ann NY Acad Sci 2000; 914: 292–302.
13. Misra LK, Kofoed L, Oesterheld JR, Richards GA. Risperidone treatment of methamphetamine psychosis. Am J Psychiatry 1997; 154: 1170.
14. Misra LK, Kofoed L, Oesterheld JR, Richards GA. Olanzapine treatment of methamphetamine psychosis. J Clin Psychopharmacol 2000; 20: 393–4.
15. Richards JR, Brofeldt BT. Patterns of tooth wear associated with methamphetamine use. J Periodontol 2000; 71: 1371–4.
16. Banooni P, Rickman LS, Ward DM. Pot puffy tumor associated with intranasal methamphetamine. J Am Med Assoc 2000; 283: 1293.
17. Zhu BL, Oritani S, Shimotouge K, Ishida K, Quan L, Fujita MQ, Ogawa M, Maeda H. Methamphetamine related fatalities in forensic autopsy during 5 years in the southern half of Osaka city and surrounding areas. Forensic Sci Int 2000; 113: 443–7.
18. Justice AJH, De Wit H. Acute effects of estradiol pretreatment on the response to d-amphetamine in women. Neuroendocrinology 2000; 71: 51–9.
19. Hales G, Roth N, Smith D. Possible fatal interaction between protease inhibitors and methamphetamine. Antiviral Ther 2000; 5: 19.
20. Khatsenko O. Interactions between nitric oxide and cytochrome P450 in the liver. Biochemistry 1998; 63: 833–9.
21. Barry M, Mulcahy F, Merry C, Gibbons S, Black D. Pharmacokinetics and potential interactions amongst antiretroviral agents used to treat patients with HIV infection. Clin Pharmacol 1999; 36: 289–304.
22. Lin L, Stefano E, Schmidt D, Hsu L, Ellis S, Lennard M, Tucker G, Cho A. Oxidation of methamphetamine and methylenedioxymethamphetamine by CYP2D6. Drug Metab Dispos 1997; 25: 1059–64.
23. Renfrew C, Dickson R, Schwab C. Severe hypertension following ephedrine administration in a patient receiving entacapone. Anesthesiology 2000; 93: 1562.
24. Jadad AR, Boyle M, Cunningham C. Treatment of attention deficit/hyperactivity disorder. Evid Based Med 2000; 5: 179.
25. Schteinschnaider A, Plaghos LL, Garbugino S, Riveros D. Cerebral arteritis following methylphenidate use. J Child Neurol 2000; 15: 265–7.
26. Trugman JM. Cerebral arteritis and oral methylphenidate. Lancet 1988; 12: 584–5.
27. Kramer JR, Loney J, Ponto LB, Roberts MA, Grossman S. Predictors of adult height and weight in boys treated with methylphenidate for childhood behavior problems. J Am Acad Child Adolesc Psychiatry 2000; 39: 517–24.
28. White SR, Yado CM. Characterization of methylphenidate exposures reported to a regional poison control center. Arch Pediatr Adolesc Med 2000; 154: 1199–203.
29. Gara L, Roberts W. Adverse response to methylphenidate in combination with valproic acid. J Child Adolesc Psychopharmacol 2000; 10: 39–43.
30. Markowitz JS, Morrison SD, De Wane CL. Drug interactions with psychostimulants: a review. Int J Clin Psychopharmacol 1999; 14: 1–18.
31. De Wane CL, Markowitz JS, Carson SW, Boulton DW, Gill HS. Single-dose pharmacokinetics of methylphenidate in CYP2D6 extensive and poor metabolizers. J Clin Psychopharmacol 2000; 20: 347–9.
32. Becker PM, Jamieson AO, Jewel CE, Bogan RK, James DS. Randomized trial of modafinil as a treatment for the excessive daytime somnolence of nacrolepsy. Neurology 2000; 54: 1166–75.
33. US Modafinil in Narcolepsy Multicentre Study Group. Modafinil for the treatment of pathological somnolence in narcolepsy. Ann Neurol 1998; 43: 88–97.
34. Hauser RA, Wahba MN, Zesiewicz TA, Anderson WM. Modafinil treatment of pramipexole-associated somnolence. Mov Disord 2000; 15: 1269–71.
35. Jasinski DR. An evaluation of the abuse potential of modafinil using methylphenidate as a reference. J Psychopharmacol 2000; 14: 53–60.
36. Rosano TG, Hubbard JD, Meola, Swift TA. Fatal strychnine poisoning: application of gas chromatography and tandem mass spectrometry. J Anal Toxicol 2000; 24: 642–7.
37. Teramae CY, Connolly HM, Grogan M, Miller FA Jr. Diet drug related cardiac valve disease: the Mayo Clinic echocardiographic laboratory experience. Mayo Clin Proc 2000; 75: 456–61.
38. Roldan CA, Gill EA, Shively BK. Prevalence and diagnostic value of precordial murmurs for valvular regurgitation in obese patients treated with dexfenfluramine. Am J Cardiol 2000; 86: 535–9.

39. American College of Cardiology/American Heart Association Task Force on Practice Guidelines (Committee on Management of Patients with Valvular Heart Disease). Guidelines for the management of patients with valvular heart disease. Circulation 1998; 98: 1949–84.
40. Lepor NE, Gross SB, Daley WL, Samuels BA, Rizzo MJ, Luko SP, Hickey A, Buchbinder NA, Naqvi TZ. Dose and duration of fenfluramine–phentermine therapy impacts the risk of significant valvular heart disease. Am J Cardiol 2000; 86: 107–10.
41. Gardin JM, Schumacher D, Constantine G, Davis KD, Leung C. Valvular abnormalities and cardiovascular status following exposure to dexfenfluramine or phentermine/fenfluramine. J Am Med Assoc 2000; 283: 1703–9.
42. Jollis JG, Landolfo CK, Kisslo J, Constantine GD, Davis K. Fenfluramine and phentermine and cardiovascular findings: effect of treatment duration on prevalence of valve abnormalities. Circulation 2000; 101: 2071–7.
43. Rich S, Rubin L, Walker AM, Schneeweiss S, Abenheim L. Anorexigens and pulmonary hypertension in the United States. Results from the surveillance of North American Pulmonary Hypertension. Chest 2000; 117: 870–4.
44. Rothman RB. The age-adjusted mortality rate from primary pulmonary hypertension, in age range 20 to 54 years, did not increase during the years of peak "Phen/Fen" use. Chest 2000; 118: 1516–17.
45. Gaine SP, Rubin LJ, Kmetzo JJ, Palevsky HI, Traill TA. Recreational use of aminorex and pulmonary hypertension. Chest 2000; 118: 1496–7.
46. Devlin MJ, Goldfein JA, Carino JS, Wolk SL. Open treatment of overweight binge eaters with phentermine and fluoxetine as an adjunct to cognitive behavioural therapy. Int J Eating Disord 2000; 28: 325–32.
47. Maher TJ, Ulus IH, Wurtman RJ. Phentermine and other monoamine-oxidase inhibitors may increase plasma serotonin when given with fenfluramines. Lancet 1999; 353: 38.
48. Fanghanel G, Cortinas L, Sanchez-Reyes L, Berber A. A clinical trial of the use of sibutramine for the treatment of patients suffering essential obesity. Int J Obes 2000; 24: 144–50.
49. Lean MEJ. Sibutramine – a review of clinical efficacy. Int J Obes 1997; 20 Suppl 1: S30–5.
50. McMahon FG, Fujioka K, Singh BN, Mendel CM, Rowe E, Rolston K, Johnson F, Mooradian AD. Efficacy and safety of sibutramine in obese white and African-American patients with hypertension: a 1-year, double-blind placebo-controlled multicenter trial. Arch Intern Med 2000; 160: 2185–91.
51. Dooley M, Lamb HM. Donepezil. A review of its use in Alzheimer's disease. Drugs Aging 2000; 16: 199–226.
52. Cameron I, Curran S, Newton P, Petty D, Wattis J. Use of donepezil for the treatment of mild–moderate Alzheimer's disease: an audit of the assessment and treatment of patients in routine clinical practice. Int J Geriatr Psychiatry 2000; 15: 887–91.
53. Greenberg SM, Tennis MK, Brown LB, Gomei-Isla T, Hayden D. Donepezil therapy in clinical practice: a randomized crossover study. Arch Neurol 2000; 57: 94–9.
54. Homma A, Takeda M, Imai Y, Udaka F, Hasegawa K, Kameyama M. Clinical efficacy and safety of donepezil on cognitive and global function in patients with Alzheimer's disease: a 24-week, multicentre, double-blind, placebo-controlled study in Japan. Dementia Geriatr Cogn Disord 2000; 11: 299–313.
55. Knopman DS. Management of cognition and function: New results form the clinical trials programme of Aricept (donepezil HCl). Int J Neuropsychopharmacol 2000; 3 Suppl 2: S13–20.
56. Matthews HP, Korbey J, Wilkinson DG, Rowden J. Donepezil in Alzheimer's disease: eighteen month results from Southampton Memory Clinic. Int J Geriatr Psychiatry 2000; 15: 713–20.
57. Evans M, Ellis A, Watson D, Chowdhury T. Sustained cognitive improvement following treatment of Alzheimer's disease with donepezil. Int J Geriatr Psychiatry 2000; 15: 50–3.
58. Rogers SL, Doody RS, Pratt RD, Ieni JR. Long-term efficacy and safety of donepezil in the treatment of Alzheimer's disease: final analysis of a US multicentre open-label study. Eur Neuropsychopharmacol 2000; 10: 195–203.
59. Lancott KL, Herrmann N. Donepezil for behavioural disorders associated with Lewy bodies: a case series. Int J Geriatr Psychiatry 2000; 15: 338–45.
60. Dallochio C, Buffa C, Mazarello P. Combination of donepezil and gabapentin for behavioural disorders in Alzheimer's disease. J Clin Psychiatry 2000; 61: 64.
61. Dunn NR, Pearce GL, Shakir SAW. Adverse effects associated with the use of donepezil in general practice in England. J Psychopharmacol 2000; 14: 406–8.
62. Amouyal-Barkate K, Bagheri-Charabiani H, Montastruc JL, Moulias S, Vellas B. Abnormal movements with donepezil in Alzheimer's disease. Ann Pharmacother 2000; 34: 1347.
63. Carcenac D, Martin-Hunyadi C, Kiesmann M, Demuynck-Roegel C, Alt M, Kuntzmann F. Syndrome extrapyramidal sous donepezil. Presse Med 2000; 29: 992–3.
64. Hashimoto M, Imamura T, Tanimukai S, Kazui H, Mori E. Urinary incontinence: an unrecognized adverse effect with donepezil. Lancet 2000; 356: 568.
65. Arai M. Parkinsonism onset in a patient concurrently using tiapride and donepezil. Intern Med 2000; 39: 863.
66. Farlow MR, Cyrus PA. Metrifonate therapy in Alzheimer's disease: a pooled analysis of four ran-

domized, double-blind, placebo-controlled trials. Dementia Geriatr Cogn Disord 2000; 11: 202–11.
67. Blass JP, Cyrus PA, Bieber F, Gulanski B. Randomized, double-blind, placebo-controlled, multicenter study to evaluate the safety and tolerability of metrifonate in patients with probable Alzheimer disease. The Metrifonate Study Group. Alzheimer Dis Assoc Disord 2000; 14: 39–45.
68. Waziers, Beune P, Funck-Brentano C, Jaillon P. Combined glutathione-S-transferase M1 and T1 genetic polymorphism and tacrine hepatotoxicity. Clin Pharmacol Ther 2000; 67: 432–7.
69. Grossberg GT, Stahelin HB, Messina JC, Anand R, Veach J. Lack of adverse pharmacodynamic drug interactions with rivastigmine and twenty-two classes of medications. Int J Geriatr Psychiatry 2000; 15: 242–7.
70. Simon T, Becquernoni L, Mary-Krause M, De Waziers I, Beune P, Funck-Brentano C, Jaillon P. Combined glutathione-S-transferase M1 and T1 genetic polymorphism and tacrine hepatotoxicity. Clin Pharmacol Ther 2000; 67: 432–7.

P.J. Cowen

2 Antidepressant drugs

TRICYCLIC ANTIDEPRESSANTS
(SED-14, 44; SEDA-22, 11; SEDA-23, 16; SEDA-24, 12)

Drug interactions *Fluconazole* can increase blood concentrations of amitriptyline, presumably by inhibiting cytochrome P450 enzymes (CYP3A4 and CYP2C19) and thus preventing its demethylation. Two case reports (1[A], 2[A]) have described syncope in patients taking combined treatment with amitriptyline and fluconazole, and in one of these subjects (1[A]) concomitant electrocardiographic monitoring showed a prolonged QT interval and torsade de pointes. In neither case were serum amitriptyline concentrations measured, but the symptoms the patients suffered were consistent with tricyclic antidepressant toxicity. Currently the combination of fluconazole and amitriptyline might be particularly likely to be prescribed for patients with immune deficiency syndromes, which can be associated with both fungal infections and neuropathic pain. These case reports suggest that this combination should be used with caution and probably with monitoring of amitriptyline concentrations.

Sodium valproate is increasingly used as a mood stabilizing agent in patients with recurrent mood disorders. It has previously been noted that valproate treatment can increase serum tricyclic concentrations (SEDA-21, 22) and a further patient, a 46-year-old woman, has been reported in whom the addition of valproate (1 g/day) to clomipramine (150 mg/day) led to a substantial increase in serum clomipramine concentrations (185–447 ng/ml); she had feelings of numbness and sleep disturbance, which disappeared when the dose of clomipramine was reduced (3[A]). The increase in tricyclic concentrations following valproate is probably partly due to inhibition of CYP2C enzymes, preventing demethylation of tertiary tricyclic antidepressants to the corresponding secondary amines (desmethylimipramine, in the case of clomipramine). However, valproate can also increase the plasma concentrations of secondary amine tricyclics, such as nortriptyline (3[A]). The current data suggest that the combined use of tricyclic antidepressants and valproate need to be undertaken with caution.

Tricyclic antidepressants lower the seizure threshold and should therefore be used with caution with other agents that can also lower seizure threshold, such as *antipsychotic drugs* (4[A]).

A 34-year-old man with schizophrenia responded well to olanzapine (20 mg/day). However, he then had obsessional hand washing and was given clomipramine, which was increased to a dosage of 250 mg/day. He then reported myoclonic jerks with some dizziness, and 10 days later had a generalized tonic–clonic seizure. The combined clomipramine/desmethylclomipramine concentration was 2212 nmol/l, higher than the upper end of the usual target range (1300 nmol/l). An EEG showed paroxysmal slowing and spike and wave activity. Both olanzapine and clomipramine were withdrawn. Later the clomipramine was restarted as monotherapy and a dose of 300 mg/day was reached, which led to an even higher clomipramine/desmethylclomipramine concentration (3234 nmol/l), but there was no clinical or EEG evidence of seizure activity. However, when olanzapine was added in a dosage of 15 mg/day, myoclonic jerking and abnormal EEG activity recurred within 7 days.

Although the seizures occurred in the presence of high concentrations of clomipramine this case suggests a pharmacodynamic drug interaction, since neither agent given alone provoked seizure activity whereas the combination did. It is, however, possible that clomipramine might have caused a rise in olanzapine blood concentrations, which were not measured.

Side Effects of Drugs, Annual 25
J.K. Aronson, ed.

SELECTIVE SEROTONIN RE-UPTAKE INHIBITORS (SSRIs)

(SED-14, 67; SEDA-22, 11; SEDA-23, 17; SEDA-24, 14)

Nervous system SSRIs can infrequently cause *extrapyramidal movement disorders* and can also worsen established Parkinson's disease (SEDA-22, 23) and another case has been reported (5[A]).

A 68-year-old woman developed major depression. A neurological assessment excluded neurological diseases, including Parkinson's disease. After treatment with citalopram, 20 mg/day for 7 days, she developed severe Parkinsonism, with rigidity, tremor, and bradykinesia, and became unable to walk. The citalopram was withdrawn after a further week and nortriptyline was substituted; however, 10 days later Parkinsonism was still present. Her symptoms eventually responded to co-beneldopa.

The authors concluded that the citalopram had probably precipitated latent Parkinson's disease. Citalopram is the most highly selective SSRI and in anecdotal accounts has been implicated somewhat less often than other SSRIs in extrapyramidal movement disorders. The present case, together with another report of citalopram-induced worsening of pre-existing Parkinson's disease (6[A]), suggests that it should be used with caution in patients with this disorder.

The *serotonin syndrome* is a well-established complication of SSRI treatment. It is usually associated with high doses of SSRIs or the use of SSRIs in combination with other serotonin potentiating agents, such as monoamine oxidase inhibitors (SEDA-22, 24). A case has now been reported in a 45-year-old man who had definite symptoms of serotonin toxicity (hypomania, myoclonus, sweating, and shivering), first when taking a low therapeutic dose of citalopram (20 mg/day) and then with low-dose sertraline (25 mg/day); he was also taking zolpidem (7[A]). The authors speculated that the combination of zolpidem with an SSRI might have predisposed to the serotonin syndrome. It is also possible that some people (e.g. poor metabolizers) are idiosyncratically vulnerable to serotonin toxicity at low doses of SSRIs.

Sensory systems Three patients taking paroxetine for interferon-α-induced depression developed *retinal hemorrhages*, including one with irreversible loss of vision (8[C]).

Electrolyte balance SSRIs can cause *hyponatremia* in elderly patients (SEDA-18, 20, 21). A case of hyponatremia complicated by rhabdomyolysis has been described in a 45-year-old woman taking citalopram and the antipsychotic drug chlorprothixene for depressive psychosis (9[A]). The hyponatremia became apparent 2 weeks after the dose of citalopram was increased to 40 mg/day, when she complained of weakness and lethargy. SSRI-induced hyponatremia is unusual in non-geriatric populations, but the chlorprothixene may have played a role in this case.

Hematologic There have been previous reports of an association between SSRIs and *bleeding disorders* (SEDA-24, 15). Five children, aged 8–15 years, developed bruising or epistaxis 1–12 weeks after starting SSRI treatment (10[A]). In all cases the bleeding problem resolved when the SSRI was withdrawn or the dose lowered. In a review of 30 cases of SSRI-induced bleeding disorders the most common events were bruising, petechiae, purpura, and epistaxis, though gastrointestinal hemorrhage was also reported (11[R]). The mean age of the affected patients was 42 years and the female:male ratio was 3:4. Symptoms were sometimes associated with prolonged bleeding time or platelet aggregation disorders, but often these indices were normal. Possible mechanisms of SSRI-induced bleeding include a defect in platelet aggregation (through platelet serotonin depletion) or an increase in capillary fragility. Some patients appear to have a pre-existing susceptibility, for example, by virtue of treatment with other medications that might predispose to bleeding.

Drug withdrawal Sudden withdrawal of SSRIs causes a characteristic discontinuation syndrome, with *dizziness*, *nausea*, *vivid dreaming*, *fatigue*, *irritability*, *mood instability*, *muscle aches*, *chills*, and *diarrhea* (SEDA-22, 23). In a randomized, placebo-controlled trial sudden withdrawal of paroxetine produced significant abstinence symptoms by as early as the second day, while patients taking fluoxetine remained asymptomatic for the 5-day withdrawal period (12[C]). Patients taking sertraline had an intermediate level of abstinence symptoms.

Both paroxetine-treated and sertraline-treated patients reported impaired functioning during the withdrawal period, while those taking fluoxetine did not. These findings are consistent with earlier reports that suggested that acute withdrawal symptoms after fluoxetine withdrawal are unusual, presumably because of the long half-life of its active metabolite, norfluoxetine.

Abstinence symptoms in the 2 weeks after sudden withdrawal of citalopram have been examined in a double-blind, placebo-controlled study (13[C]). Abstinence symptoms were overall mild, but neurological and psychiatric disturbances were two to three times as common in patients randomized to placebo than in those randomized to continue with citalopram. The authors pointed out that abstinence symptoms were particularly common in patients who were randomized to placebo who also experienced depressive relapse. This shows the difficulty of disentangling the effects of depressive relapse from those of pure treatment withdrawal. However, it is also possible that acute withdrawal of medication induces an abnormal neurobiological state, in which both depression and abstinence symptoms are more likely to occur. Case reports suggest that citalopram withdrawal can cause a typical SSRI withdrawal syndrome. Evidence of the acute effects of withdrawal comes from another recent report (14[A]).

A 45-year-old woman achieved remission from an episode of major depression within 2 weeks of taking citalopram (40 mg/day). After about 3 months of treatment she missed her daily dose of citalopram, and 3 hours later had a sudden episode of dizziness while driving. A similar episode occurred 2 weeks later again after a missed dose of citalopram. The dizziness remitted about an hour after the citalopram was taken.

It would be wise to warn patients about the possible effects of missing doses of the shorter-acting SSRIs.

Fetotoxicity An increasing number of women are exposed to SSRIs during pregnancy. It is therefore important to establish as carefully as possible whether SSRIs have teratogenic effects (SEDA-24, 15). In a retrospective study of the impact on birth outcome of the timing of fluoxetine exposure in 64 pregnant women there were no major differences in birth outcome between infants exposed to fluoxetine early in pregnancy (the first or second trimesters only) and those exposed to fluoxetine throughout the third trimester and delivery (15[c]). However, the infants in the late-exposed group were about twice as likely to be admitted to a special care nursery. No specific pattern of neonatal difficulties could be found to account for this difference, and it is possible that the excess of neonatal problems in the late-onset treatment group was due to worse depression in the women who took antidepressants at around the time of delivery. Poor neonatal adjustment after fluoxetine treatment in pregnancy has been described in a previous study, although the rate of major congenital abnormalities does not seem to be increased.

Lactation Information on breastfeeding difficulties with SSRIs is still incomplete. In a recent case citalopram was reported to cause sleep disturbance in a breastfed infant (16[A]).

A 29-year-old woman took citalopram (40 mg/day) while breastfeeding her 5-week-old daughter. The maternal citalopram concentrations were 99 ng/ml in the serum and 205 ng/ml in the breast milk. The serum concentration in the infant was 13 ng/ml, and the child's sleep was fitful and disturbed. The dosage of citalopram was reduced to 20 mg/day and the two feeds after each daily dose were replaced by artificial nutrition. One week later the infant was sleeping normally, and the serum citalopram concentrations in mother and infant had fallen to 35 ng/ml and 2 ng/ml respectively.

These data suggest that although breastfeeding during citalopram treatment is possible, careful dosing and close observation of mother and infant are necessary.

Drug overdose In general, SSRIs are relatively safe in overdose compared with tricyclic antidepressants. However, there has been concern about possible cardiotoxicity after citalopram overdose (SEDA-21, 12). Various *cardiac effects* have been noted after citalopram overdose, including widened QRS complexes, prolonged QT interval, and ventricular extra beats, and a new report suggests that prolonged sinus bradycardia can also occur (17[A]).

A 32-year-old woman took 800 mg of citalopram, 20 times her usual daily dose, in a suicide attempt. On admission to hospital she had a sinus bradycardia (41 beats/min) but the electrocardiogram was otherwise normal, with a QT interval of 430 ms. Treatment with atropine failed to increase her heart rate and she had hypotension and syncope. A temporary pacemaker was inserted and was required for the next 6 days before it could be safely removed.

One of the largest overdoses of sertraline has been reported (18[A]).

A 51-year-old woman took about 8 g of sertraline, about 80 times the usual daily dose. On admission to hospital she was somnolent but rousable. Her electrocardiogram showed a transiently prolonged QT_c interval (510 ms falling to 470 ms). On the third day she developed agitation, disorientation, myoclonus, and pyrexia (38.5° C), was treated with supportive measures, and recovered over the next 3 days.

While cardiac toxicity was not prominent in this case, the patient developed clear evidence of the serotonin syndrome, which proved self-limiting.

Drug interactions The serotonin syndrome can occur with therapeutic doses of SSRIs (see above), but it occurs most commonly when SSRIs are coadministered with other drugs that also potentiate serotonin function. Recent case reports have suggested that there is a risk of the serotonin syndrome when SSRIs are combined with *buspirone* (19[A]) or *nefazodone* (20[A]).

Rather more unexpected was a report of the serotonin syndrome in a patient taking paroxetine plus an atypical antipsychotic drug, risperidone (21[A]).

A 53-year-old man took paroxetine (40 mg/day) and risperidone (6 mg/day), having previously taken lower doses of both. Within 2 hours he developed ataxia, shivering, and tremor. He had profound sweating but was apyrexial, and was confused, with involuntary jerking movements of his limbs. He recovered without specific treatment over the next 2 days.

While the combination of an SSRI with an antipsychotic drug has been reported to cause delirium, this is the first report of the serotonin syndrome in a patient taking an SSRI and an atypical antipsychotic drug. The reaction is unexpected because risperidone, in addition to being a potent dopamine receptor antagonist, is also a 5-HT_2 receptor antagonist. Recent animal studies have suggested that 5-HT_2 receptor antagonists may increase the firing of serotonergic neurons, perhaps through a postsynaptic feedback loop. This could account for potentiation of the effects of SSRIs by 5-HT_2 receptor antagonists, such as risperidone. The combination of an SSRI and an atypical antipsychotic drug with 5-HT_2 receptor blocking properties, such as risperidone and olanzapine, is being increasingly used. It will be important to determine whether patients taking this combination are at increased risk of serotonin toxicity.

Some SSRIs are potent inhibitors of CYP450 enzymes, including CYP2D6 (SEDA-22, 13). Recent studies have confirmed that paroxetine, presumably through this mechanism, causes clinically important increases in plasma concentrations of *tricyclic antidepressants* (22[c]) and metoprolol (23[c]). In contrast, citalopram is said to be a poor inhibitor of CYP450 and has been used successfully in combination with the tricyclic antidepressant desipramine in a 45-year-old woman who had previously suffered tricyclic toxicity when desipramine had been combined with paroxetine (24[A]).

Fluvoxamine increases plasma concentrations of *clozapine* and its metabolites, probably via inhibition of CYP1A2 (25[c], 26[c]; SEDA-21, 12). It has been suggested that citalopram might be free from this effect. However, in a 39-year-old man, citalopram 40 mg/day produced a 25% increase in combined clozapine and norclozapine concentrations, in association with subjective complaints of sedation, fatigue, hypersalivation, and mild confusion (27[A]). These symptoms settled when the dosage of citalopram was reduced to 20 mg/day. The report suggests that at higher doses, citalopram may produce some inhibition of CYP450 enzymes and should be used with caution in combination with clozapine.

The atypical antipsychotic drug *olanzapine* is also metabolized by CYP1A2. A 21-year-old woman developed Parkinsonism in conjunction with raised olanzapine plasma concentrations when taking fluvoxamine 150 mg/day and olanzapine 15 mg/day (28[A]). Her symptoms settled with a reduction of olanzapine dosage to 5 mg/day. Parkinsonism is rare in patients taking modest doses of olanzapine but it is possible here that coadministration of fluvoxamine raised plasma olanzapine concentrations, thereby producing a high degree of dopamine receptor blockade.

Fluvoxamine increases *methadone* concentrations in patients taking methadone maintenance treatment for the management of opioid dependence (SEDA-19, 11). The addition of sertraline (200 mg/day) produced a modest (16%) increase in methadone concentrations in 31 depressed opioid-dependent subjects after 6 but not 12 weeks of combined treatment (29[C]). The increase in methadone concentrations was more modest than that reported with fluvoxamine, presumably because sertraline is a less potent inhibitor of CYP1A2 and CYP3A4, both of which are involved in methadone metabolism.

Sertraline is itself a substrate for a number of CYP450 enzymes, including CYP2C9, CYP2C19, and CYP3A4. Several case reports have shown loss of antidepressant activity of sertraline at usual therapeutic doses when depressed patients have also taken drugs that induce CYP3A4, including *rifampicin* (30[A]) and *carbamazepine* (31[A]).

OTHER ANTIDEPRESSANTS

Amfebutamone (bupropion)

(SED-14, 60; SEDA-23, 20; SEDA-24, 16)

Nervous system Amfebutamone lowers the *seizure threshold* and can cause paresthesia (32[A]).

A 38-year-old woman who was taking olanzapine (10 mg/day) and lamotrigine (200 mg/day) for the management of a schizoaffective disorder started to take amfebutamone for a depressive mood swing. After 4 weeks the dose of amfebutamone was increased to 300 mg/day, at which point she complained of a twitching pain on the left side of her face. There was hypesthesia of two branches of the left trigeminal nerve, the ophthalmic and maxillary branches, and a reduced left corneal reflex. The amfebutamone was withdrawn and the neurological signs and symptoms disappeared within 8 days. Four weeks later, because of persisting depression, the amfebutamone was reintroduced; again at a dosage of 300 mg/day identical neurological symptoms recurred.

The reason for this unusual reaction is not clear. Amfebutamone may potentiate dopamine neurotransmission, and dopamine D_2 receptors modulate trigeminal nerve function (33[E]).

Immunologic Adverse skin reactions, such as *rash*, *urticaria*, and *pruritus*, have been reported in 1–4% of patients taking amfebutamone. In three patients (two women, one man) a *serum sickness-like reaction* developed 6–21 days after the start of amfebutamone treatment (34[A]). The symptoms, arthralgia, pruritus, and tongue swelling, abated within 2 weeks of treatment with oral corticosteroids.

Nefazodone *(SED-14, 64; SEDA-22, 16; SEDA-23, 20; SEDA-24, 17)*

Nervous system Three men (aged 28–63 years) had troublesome *burning sensations* 3 days to 3 weeks after starting to take nefazodone (35[A]). The burning sensations were not clearly localized to any one area of the body. The episodes lasted for about 30 minutes and recurred several times each day. The symptoms responded to nefazodone withdrawal or dosage reduction. These unpleasant sensations appeared to be linked to nefazodone, but the mechanism was obscure.

Liver Some cases of serious *hepatotoxicity* associated with nefazodone treatment were reviewed in SEDA-24 (p. 17). Two further cases have now been reported (36[A], 37[A]).

A 52-year-old man with a 10-day history of fatigue and jaundice had been taking nefazodone (300 mg/day) for about 6 weeks for depression. Biochemical investigations showed acute liver failure. Infective hepatitis and immune disorders were excluded. He failed to respond to medical treatment, and hepatic transplantation was performed. Histological examination of the liver showed parenchymal necrosis, particularly in centrilobular areas, together with lymphocytic infiltration.

A 46-year-old woman developed fatigue and jaundice about 20 weeks after starting to take nefazodone (300 mg/day). She had raised liver enzymes and bilirubin concentrations. There was no evidence of infectious hepatitis or immune disorders. Liver biopsy showed ballooning degeneration and necrosis of hepatocytes with mixed inflammatory infiltrates. The nefazodone was withdrawn and corticosteroid treatment started. Within 4 months she recovered clinically and her liver function tests returned to normal.

These cases support the notion that nefazodone can rarely cause acute hepatitis with occasional catastrophic liver failure.

Lactation Nefazodone passes into breast milk and has been reported to cause *drowsiness and feeding problems* in a breastfed infant (38[A]).

The mother of a 7-week-old premature girl became depressed and was treated with nefazodone (300 mg/day). Two weeks later the infant became drowsy and lethargic and was not feeding well. No medical condition was found to account for these symptoms and breastfeeding was stopped. The symptoms improved over the following 3 days. The concentrations of nefazodone in breast milk were about 10-fold less than those in maternal plasma, and the total infant dose of nefazodone was calculated to be only 0.45% of the maternal dose. In this case, nefazodone in the breast milk may have caused the infant's drowsiness and feeding problems, despite the fact that the transferred dose of nefazodone would have been very low, since the low gestational age of the infant might have been associated with impaired hepatic and renal clearance, making her susceptible to even very small quantities of nefazodone.

Drug overdose The outcomes of over 1300 poisonings with nefazodone as a sole agent have been reported (39[C]). Generally, the toxic effects were mild, consisting mainly of *drowsiness*, *nausea*, and *dizziness*. Clinical signs developed within 1–4 hours of ingestion and dissipated within the following 24 hours. The most serious toxic effect was *hypotension*, which occurred in 1.6% of cases. Bradycardia occurred in 1.4% of cases. Only one patient had a *seizure* and none required intubation. These data suggest that the toxicity of nefazodone in overdose is low. However, in suicide attempts, antidepressants are often ingested with other agents, particularly alcohol and other sedating drugs. This might increase the toxic effects of nefazodone, particularly with regard to respiratory depression.

Drug interactions Nefazodone inhibits CYP3A4 and so increases plasma concentrations of *carbamazepine* (SEDA-22, 16). In a controlled trial in 12 healthy men the combination of carbamazepine and nefazodone led to increased plasma carbamazepine concentrations and substantially lowered plasma nefazodone concentrations (40[C]). This interaction could lead to difficulties during treatment, since the risk of carbamazepine toxicity would have to be balanced against the loss of therapeutic effect of nefazodone. Except in special circumstances it is probably better to avoid the combination.

Reboxetine *(SED-14, 64; SEDA-24, 18)*

Electrolyte balance A case of *hyponatremia* has been reported with reboxetine (41[A], 42[r]).

A 72-year-old man with diabetes mellitus and cardiovascular disease developed major depression. He was taking aspirin (100 mg/day), enalapril (20 mg/day), and glibenclamide (5 mg/day). His serum sodium was 133 (reference range 134–146) mmol/l. He started to take reboxetine (4 mg/day) and after 8 days experienced malaise and nausea, at which time his serum sodium had fallen to 118 mmol/l. The reboxetine was withdrawn, and both his symptoms and the low serum sodium remitted over the next 6 days. Rechallenge with reboxetine produced a recurrence of both the low sodium and the accompanying symptoms.

It appears that, like SSRIs, reboxetine can also cause hyponatremia in elderly people. In this case the contribution of concomitant general medical illness and its treatment was uncertain.

Venlafaxine *(SED-14, 66; SEDA-22, 17; SEDA-23, 20; SEDA-24, 18)*

Nervous system The *neuroleptic malignant syndrome* has been attributed to venlafaxine (43[A]).

A 44-year-old man with major depression had been taking the antipsychotic drug trifluoperazine (3 mg/day) for anxiety for several years. He was given venlafaxine 75 mg/day, and 12 hours after the first dose developed anxiety and malaise. He was sweating and had tremor and rigidity. His blood pressure fluctuated and his creatine phosphokinase activity was raised at 11 320 IU/l. A diagnosis of neuroleptic malignant syndrome was made and he was treated with dantrolene and bromocriptine. His symptoms settled within 24 hours and trifluoperazine was reintroduced uneventfully.

The neuroleptic malignant syndrome is usually associated with dopamine receptor antagonists, such as trifluoperazine, but the circumstances in this case suggest that the syndrome may have been precipitated by the addition of venlafaxine. Apparently the manufacturer has received a few other reports of neuroleptic malignant syndrome after the addition of venlafaxine to antipsychotic treatment.

Antidepressant drugs, such as tricyclic antidepressants and SSRIs, suppress rapid eye movement (REM) sleep, the period of sleep during which dreaming occurs. Despite this, antidepressant treatment is sometimes associated with *recurrent nightmares*. Venlafaxine also suppresses REM sleep and was associated with nightmares in a 35-year-old woman with body image disturbance; the nightmares remitted when the venlafaxine was withdrawn (44[A]). The authors speculated that indirect activation of 5-HT_2 receptors might have played a causal role, because 5-HT_2 receptor antagonists, such as nefazodone, can be helpful in the treatment of nightmares, for example in patients with post-traumatic stress disorder.

Sexual function Antidepressant drugs can rarely cause *priapism*. The agent most often implicated has been trazodone, perhaps because of its α_1-adrenoceptor antagonist properties. Priapism has now been attributed to venlafaxine (45[A]).

A 16-year-old youth taking venlafaxine (150 mg/day) had several episodes of prolonged erections, which persisted for several hours after intercourse. The episodes remitted after the venlafaxine was withdrawn.

In general venlafaxine has an inhibitory effect on sexual function, but perhaps, like SSRIs, it can rarely cause priapism.

Pain on ejaculation is also a rare adverse effect of tricyclic antidepressants and SSRIs. Painful ejaculation occurred in a 59-year-old man during treatment with venlafaxine (150 mg/day) (46[A]). It remitted when the venlafaxine was withdrawn and did not recur when citalopram (40 mg/day) was used instead.

Drug interactions In six healthy men, venlafaxine (150 mg/day for 10 days) produced an increase of 28% in the systemic availability of a single dose of *imipramine* (100 mg); the availability of the active metabolite of imipramine, desipramine, was also increased (47[c]). These data suggest that venlafaxine inhibits CYP2D6; the effects appear modest relative to those of fluoxetine and are similar to those produced by sertraline.

REFERENCES

1. Dorsey ST, Biblo LA. Prolonged QT interval and torsades de pointes caused by the combination of fluconazole and amitriptyline. Am J Emerg Med 2000; 18: 227–9.
2. Robinson RF, Nahata MC, Olshefski RS. Syncope associated with concurrent amitriptyline and fluconazole therapy. Ann Pharmacother 2000; 34: 1406–9.
3. Fehr C, Gründer G, Hiemke C, Dahmen N. Increase in serum clomipramine concentrations caused by valproate. J Clin Psychopharmacol 2000; 20: 493–4.
4. Deshauer D, Albuquerque J, Alda M, Grof P. Seizures caused by possible interaction between olanzapine and clomipramine. J Clin Psychopharmacol 2000; 20: 283–4.
5. Stadtland C, Erfurth A, Arolt V. De novo onset of Parkinson's disease after antidepressant treatment with citalopram. Pharmacopsychiatry 2000; 33: 194–5.
6. Linazasoro G. Worsening of Parkinson's disease by citalopram. Parkinsonism Relat Disord 2000; 6: 111–13.
7. Voirol P, Hodel P-F, Zullino D, Baumann P. Serotonin syndrome after small doses of citalopram or sertraline. J Clin Psychopharmacol 2000; 20: 713–14.
8. Musselman DL, Lawson DH, Gumnick JF, Manatunga AK, Penna S, Goodkin RS, Greiner K, Nemeroff CB, Miller AH. Paroxetine for the prevention of depression induced by high-dose interferon alfa. New Engl J Med 2001; 344: 961–6.
9. Zullino D, Brauchli S, Horvath A, Baumann P. Inappropriate antidiuretic hormone secretion and rhabdomyolysis associated with citalopram. Therapie 2000; 55: 651–2.
10. Lake MB, Birmaher B, Wassick S, Mathos K, Yelovich AK. Bleeding and selective serotonin reuptake inhibitors in childhood and adolescence. J Child Adolesc Psychopharmacol 2000; 10: 35–8.
11. Nelva A, Guy C, Tardy-Poncet B, Beyens MN, Ratrema M, Benedetti C, Ollagnier M. Bleeding syndromes related to selective serotonin reuptake inhibitors (SSRIs). Seven case reports and literature review. Rev Med Interne 2000; 21: 152–60.
12. Michelson D, Fava M, Amsterdam J, Apter J, Londborg P, Tamura R, Tepner RG. Interruption of selective serotonin reuptake inhibitor treatment. Double-blind, placebo-controlled trial. Br J Psychiatry 2000; 176: 363–8.
13. Markowitz JS, DeVane CL, Liston HL, Montgomery SA. An assessment of selective serotonin reuptake inhibitor discontinuation symptoms with citalopram. Int Clin Psychopharmacol 2000; 15: 329–33.
14. Fernando III AT, Schwader P. A case of citalopram withdrawal. J Clin Psychopharmacol 2000; 20: 581–2.
15. Cohen LS, Heller VL, Bailey JW, Grush L, Ablon JS, Bouffard SM. Birth outcomes following prenatal exposure to fluoxetine. Biol Psychiatry 2000; 48: 996–1000.
16. Schmidt K, Olesen OV, Jensen PN. Citalopram and breast-feeding: serum concentration and side

effects in the infant. Biol Psychiatry 2000; 47: 164–5.
17. Rothenhausler H-B, Haberl C, Ehrentraut S, Kapfhammer H-P, Weber MM. Suicide attempt by pure citalopram overdose causing long-lasting severe sinus bradycardia, hypotension and syncopes: successful therapy with temporary pacemaker. Pharmacopsychiatry 2000; 33: 150–2.
18. Brendel DH, Bodkin JA, Yang JM. Massive sertraline overdose. Ann Emerg Med 2000; 36: 524–6.
19. Manos GH. Possible serotonin syndrome associated with buspirone added to fluoxetine. Ann Pharmacother 2000; 34: 871–4.
20. Smith DL, Wenegrat BG. A case report of serotonin syndrome associated with combined nefazodone and fluoxetine. J Clin Psychiatry 2000; 61: 146.
21. Hamilton S, Malone K. Serotonin syndrome during treatment with paroxetine and risperidone. J Clin Psychopharmacol 2000; 20: 103–5.
22. Leucht S, Hackl H-J, Steimer W, Angersbach D, Zimmer R. Effect of adjunctive paroxetine on serum levels and side-effects of tricyclic antidepressants in depressive inpatients. Psychopharmacology 2000; 147: 378–83.
23. Hemeryck A, Lefebvre RA, De Vriendt C, Belpaire FM. Paroxetine affects metoprolol pharmacokinetics and pharmacodynamics in healthy volunteers. Clin Pharmacol Ther 2000; 67: 283–91.
24. Ashton AK. Lack of desipramine toxicity with citalopram. J Clin Psychiatry 2000; 61: 144.
25. Fabrazzo M, La Pia S, Monteleone P, Mennella R, Esposito G, Pinto A, Maj M. Fluvoxamine increases plasma and urinary levels of clozapine and its major metabolities in a time- and dose-dependent manner. J Clin Psychopharmacol 2000; 20: 708–10.
26. Lu M-L, Lane H-Y, Chen K-P, Jann MW, Su M-H, Chang W-H. Fluvoxamine reduces the clozapine dosage needed in refractory schizophrenic patients. J Clin Psychiatry 2000; 61: 594–9.
27. Borba CP, Henderson DC. Citalopram and clozapine: potential drug interaction. J Clin Psychiatry 2000; 61: 301–2.
28. De Jong J, Hoogenboom B, Doude van Troostwijk L, De Haan L. Interaction of olanzapine with fluvoxamine. Psychopharmacology 2001; 155: 219–20.
29. Hamilton SP, Nunes EV, Janal M, Weber L. The effect of sertraline on methadone plasma levels in methadone-maintenance patients. Am J Addict 2000; 9: 63–9.
30. Markowitz JS, Devane CL. Rifampin-induced selective serotonin reuptake inhibitor withdrawal syndrome in a patient treated with sertraline. J Clin Psychopharmacol 2000; 20: 109–10.
31. Khan A, Shad MU, Preskorn SH. Lack of sertraline efficacy probably due to an interaction with carbamazepine. J Clin Psychiatry 2000; 61: 526–7.
32. Amann B, Hummel B, Rall-Autenrieth H, Walden J, Grunze H. Bupropion-induced isolated impairment of sensory trigeminal nerve function. Int Clin Pyschopharmacol 2000; 15: 115–16.
33. Peterfreund RA, Kosofsky, BE, Fink JS. Cellular localization of dopamine D_2 receptor messenger RNA in the rat trigeminal ganglion. Anesth Analg 1995; 81: 1181–5.
34. McCollom RA, Elbe DHT, Ritchie AH. Bupropion-induced serum sickness-like reaction. Ann Pharmacother 2000; 34: 471–3.
35. Lerner V, Matar MA, Polyakova I. Nefazodone-associated subjective complaints of burning sensations. J Clin Psychiatry 2000; 61: 216–17.
36. Schirren CA, Baretton G. Nefazodone-induced acute liver failure. Am J Gastroenterol 2000; 95: 1596–7.
37. Eloubeidi MA, Gaede JT, Swaim MW. Reversible nefazodone-induced liver failure. Dig Dis Sci 2000; 45: 1036–8.
38. Yapp P, Llett KF, Kristensen JH, Hackett LP, Paech MJ, Rampono J. Drowsiness and poor feeding in a breast-fed infant: association with nefazodone and its metabolites. Ann Pharmacother 2000; 34: 1269–72.
39. Benson BE, Mathiason M, Dahl B, Smith K, Foley MM, Easom LAJ, Butler AY. Toxicities and outcomes associated with nefazodone poisoning: an analysis of 1,338 exposures. Am J Emerg Med 2000; 18: 587–92.
40. Laroudie C, Salazar DE, Cosson J-P, Cheuvart B, Istin B, Girault J, Ingrand I, Decourt J-P. Carbamazepine–nefazodone interaction in healthy subjects. J Clin Psychopharmacol 2000; 20: 46–53.
41. Ranieri P, Franzoni S, Trabucchi M. Reboxetine and hyponatremia. New Engl J Med 2000; 342: 215–16.
42. Schwartz GE, Veith J. Reboxetine and hyponatremia. New Engl J Med 2000; 342: 216.
43. Nimmagadda SR, Ryan DH, Atkin SL. Neuroleptic malignant syndrome after venlafaxine. Lancet 2000; 355: 289–90.
44. Zullino DF, Riquier F. Venlafaxine and vivid dreaming. J Clin Psychiatry 2000; 61: 600.
45. Samuel RZ, Horrigan JP, Barnhill LJ. Priapism associated with venlafaxine use. J Am Acad Child Adolesc Psychiatry 2000; 39: 16–17.
46. Michael A. Venlafaxine-induced painful ejaculation. Br J Psychiatry 2000; 177: 282–3.
47. Albers LJ, Reist C, Vu RL, Fujimoto K, Ozdemir V, Helmeste D,. Poland R, Tang SW. Effect of venlafaxine on imipramine metabolism. Psychiatry Res 2000; 96: 235–43.

J.W. Jefferson

3 Lithium

In a 4-week, placebo-controlled study of lithium in 40 hospitalized children and adolescents (mean age 12.5 years) with aggression related to conduct disorder, lithium was "statistically and clinically superior to placebo" (1[C]). Although there were no dropouts related to adverse events, *nausea*, *vomiting*, and *increased urinary frequency* occurred significantly more often in the lithium group. The 55% incidence of vomiting with lithium (versus 20% with placebo) may have been related to the relatively high mean serum lithium concentration of 1.07 mmol/l (range 0.78–1.55 mmol/l).

In a randomized, placebo-controlled, 12-month maintenance comparison of lithium and divalproex in 372 bipolar I out-patients neither active drug was more effective than placebo on the primary outcome measure – the time to recurrence of any mood episode (2[C]). While a history of intolerance to either lithium or divalproex was an exclusion criterion, it was not stated whether or not prior non-responders were entered and, if so, how many. The following adverse effects were significantly more frequent:

- with lithium than placebo: *nausea*, *diarrhea*, and *tremor*;
- with divalproex than placebo: *tremor*, *weight gain*, and *alopecia*;
- with lithium than divalproex: *polyuria*, *thirst*, *tachycardia*, *akathisia*, and *dry eyes*;
- with divalproex than lithium: *sedation*, *infection*, and *tinnitus*.

Unfortunately, all dropouts were pooled, whether due to adverse events or non-compliance, making overall tolerability comparisons impossible.

Side Effects of Drugs, Annual 25
J.K. Aronson, ed.

ORGANS AND SYSTEMS

Cardiovascular In two studies of 277 and 133 patients taking long-term lithium there was no evidence of increased cardiovascular mortality compared with the general population (3[C], 4[C]). While the latter study reported on 16-year mortality, it did not provide information about which patients continued to take lithium after the first 2 years.

Sinus node dysfunction continues to be associated with lithium. During an episode of lithium toxicity (serum concentration 3.86 mmol/l) a 42-year-old woman developed sinus bradycardia that required a temporary pacemaker (5[A]). There was marked prolongation of sinus node recovery time. Lithium was withdrawn and the patient underwent hemodialysis once daily for 3 days; sinus node recovery time normalized. The presence of non-toxic concentrations of carbamazepine may have contributed.

A 65-year-old man taking lithium for 2 years, with therapeutic concentrations, developed sinus bradycardia (30 beats/min), which remitted when the drug was stopped and recurred when it was restarted (6[A]). Implantation of a permanent pacemaker allowed lithium to be continued. Asymptomatic bradycardia occurred in three of 15 patients treated for mania with a 20 mg/kg oral loading dose of slow-release lithium carbonate (see also Drug dosage regimens) (7[c]).

Abnormalities of the QT_c interval have been explored in 495 psychiatric patients (87 taking lithium but many of them also taking other drugs) and 101 healthy controls (8[C]). There was no association of lithium with QT_c prolongation but it was associated with *non-specific T wave abnormalities* (odds ratio 1.9) and *increased QT dispersion* (odds ratio 2.9). Caution was suggested if lithium is used with drugs associated with QT_c prolongation, such as tricyclic antidepressants, droperidol, and thioridazine.

In a study of 1230 patients with initially unexplained *cardiomyopathy* lithium was implicated in one case (4[C]). Using a data-based mining Bayesian statistical approach to the WHO database of adverse reactions to examine antipsychotic drugs and heart muscle disorders, a significant association was found between lithium and cardiomyopathy, but not myocarditis (9[C]). The authors acknowledged that further study is needed to determine if the association is causal.

Nervous system Since bipolar disorder is a condition for which long-term treatment is usually necessary, both acute and long-term adverse effects are important, especially since patients in remission are often less likely to tolerate them (10[R]). With this in mind, one might consider some speculatively positive findings involving the neurotrophic and neuroprotective effects of lithium (11[R]). The concentration of bcl-2, a cytoprotective protein, was upregulated by lithium in both rodent brains and human neuronal cells, as was the concentration of *N*-acetylaspartate, a marker of neuronal viability and function, in human gray matter (12[Ec]). In addition, a 3-dimensional magnetic resonance imaging study with quantitative brain-tissue segmentation showed that treatment with lithium for 4 weeks increased the total volume of gray matter by about 3% in eight of 10 patients in the depressed phase of bipolar I disorder.

Serotonin syndrome has been reviewed twice, but mention of lithium as a possible contributing factor was scanty (13[R], 14[Ar]).

Neuroleptic malignant syndrome has been reported in a 63-year-old man taking lithium and amoxapine (15[A]), in a 23-year-old woman taking lithium, olanzapine, and fluoxetine (16[A]), and in a 39-year-old woman who had overdosed with lithium and who took a single dose of haloperidol (17[A]).

A brief review of non-Parkinsonian tremor mentioned lithium as a cause of *enhanced physiological tremor* (18[r]). A double-blind study in which 31 patients with breakthrough depression taking lithium received augmentation with either paroxetine or amitriptyline showed a quantitative increase in tremor activity with combined therapy but no significant change in tremor frequency (19[C]).

An 86-year-old man taking lithium monotherapy (serum concentration 0.7 mmol/l) had *asterixis* for several months; it resolved fully within 2 weeks of stopping lithium (20[A]). A 65-year-old woman, after a brief exposure to lithium, developed severe *akathisia* and disabling *Parkinsonism*; within 4 days of stopping lithium the symptoms improved, but orofacial dyskinesia appeared; 10 months later both the Parkinsonism and the dyskinesia had improved but were still present (21[A]).

Twelve patients with affective disorder had EEG recordings before and after 4.4 ± 3.5 months of lithium therapy. Lithium-related changes included:

- increased relative power in the delta and theta band frequencies;
- decreased relative α power;
- decreased dominant α frequency (22[A]).

The clinical implications of these observations, if any, are unclear.

A 66-year-old man presented comatose with an EEG suggestive of Creutzfeldt–Jakob encephalopathy after an 11-month history of progressive dementia and Parkinsonism (23[A]). Lithium (serum concentration 1.3 mmol/l), which he had been taking for 13 years, was withdrawn, and by day 78 clinical examination showed only mild neurological impairment.

A review of *pseudotumor cerebri* devoted one paragraph to induction of this condition by lithium and provided six references but no new information (24[r]).

Neuromuscular function A 51-year-old man developed a *myasthenic syndrome*, which resolved when lithium was withdrawn (25[A]). The authors referred to three other previously reported cases of lithium-induced myasthenia.

A single episode of *acute hypokalemic paralysis* was associated with long-term lithium therapy, but a causal relation was not established (see also Electrolyte balance) (26[A]).

Psychological In a 3-week, double-blind study of the cognitive effects of lithium (serum concentration about 0.8 mmol/l; $n = 15$) versus placebo ($n = 15$) in healthy subjects lithium did not impair implicit recall, ability to process two tasks concurrently and simultaneously, short-term memory, or selective attention, but caused *impaired learning during repeated administration of memory tests* (27[C]). Since neuropsychological testing could not distinguish lithium treatment from pre- and post-treatment in the lithium group, any lithium effects must be considered subtle at best.

A review of minimizing the cognitive effects of lithium and ECT with thyroid hormone suggested benefit in those patients taking lithium who had subclinical hypothyroidism (28[R]).

Psychiatric In a case-control study, lithium was found to be one of several risk factors for *delirium* in 91 psychiatric in-patients (odds ratio 2.23), although the authors concluded that this observation may have been confounded by an association with manic episodes (29[C]). A 38-year-old woman who had tolerated lithium for 20 years developed delirium following a manic episode, despite therapeutic concentrations of lithium (0.7–1.0 mmol/l); the episode remitted fully after lithium was withdrawn (30[A]).

Endocrine *Thyroid* Lithium-induced *hypothyroidism* has been briefly reviewed (31[r]). An abstract reported that 23% of 61 children and adolescents taking lithium and divalproex sodium for up to 20 weeks had a TSH concentration over 10 mU/L (reference range 0.2–6.0); however, no clinical information was provided (32[c]). Another abstract reported that the prevalence of thyroperoxidase antibodies was higher in bipolar out-patients (28% of 226) than in psychiatric in-patients with any diagnosis (10% of 2782) or healthy controls (14% of 225), but this was not related to lithium exposure; on the other hand, hypothyroidism was associated with lithium exposure, especially in the presence of antithyroid antibodies (33[c]).

A 36-year-old woman with lithium-induced hypothyroidism noted that her scalp hair had become thinner and stopping growing (see also Hair) (34[A]).

The observation that Canada, with ample nutritional iodine, has a relatively high rate of lithium-related hypothyroidism compared with relatively low rates in iodine-deficient countries such as Italy, Spain, and Germany led to the suggestion that ambient iodine may play a role in the genesis of this condition (35[r]). This is reminiscent of the association of amiodarone with hypothyroidism or hyperthyroidism in iodine-replete and iodine-deficient areas respectively (SEDA-10, 148).

Reports of *hyperthyroidism* associated with lithium continue to appear; one in a woman who was also hypercalcemic with a normal parathyroid hormone concentration (36[A]) and two discovered while treating lithium toxicity (37[A]).

The action of lithium on the hypothalamic–pituitary–thyroid axis has been discussed in relation to its cognitive effects, as has the use of thyroid hormone to minimize such effects (see also Nervous system) (28[R]).

Lithium has been used, with several other drugs, to treat four patients with amiodarone-associated thyrotoxicosis, but the drugs were ineffective in two patients, who required thyroidectomy (38[A]). One hopes that the authors actually used milligram amounts of lithium carbonate rather than the microgram amounts listed in the article.

Parathyroid Cases of *hyperparathyroidism* in patients taking lithium are occasionally reported.

A 78-year-old woman who had taken lithium for 25 years had hyperparathyroidism (39[A]).

Hyperparathyroidism was considered a possible cause of treatment-resistant manic psychosis in a patient taking lithium (40[A]).

Hypercalcemia and raised parathyroid hormone concentrations improved when a woman who had taken lithium for over 20 years was switched to divalproex (41[A]).

A 64-year-old woman who had taken lithium for over 10 years was admitted with altered consciousness, agitation, and disorientation. The serum calcium was 3.35 (reference range 2.1–2.6) mmol/l and the parathyroid hormone concentration was raised. With hydration and conversion from lithium to valproate, the serum calcium concentration normalized, but 2 years later disorientation and hypercalcemia recurred and a 150 mg parathyroid adenoma was removed surgically (42[A]).

Ovaries When 22 women with bipolar disorder (10 taking lithium alone, 10 taking divalproex alone, and two taking both) were evaluated for polycystic ovary syndrome, none had typical hormonal screening abnormalities (43[C]). Some type of menstrual dysfunction was present in all 10 women taking lithium alone, but it predated use of the drug in all but one.

Prolactin Compared with 17 normal controls, 20 euthymic bipolar patients who had taken lithium for more than 6 months had significantly *lower serum prolactin concentrations* (9.72 vs 15.56 ng/ml), but prolactin concentrations in short-term lithium users ($n = 15$) did not differ from controls (44[C]). Antipsychotic drugs were not involved.

Metabolism *Weight gain* The prevalence of overweight (BMI 25 or more) and obesity (BMI 30 or more) has been evaluated in 89 euthymic bipolar patients and 445 age- and sex-matched controls (45[C]). The bipolar women were more overweight and more obese than the controls and the bipolar men were more obese but not more overweight. Obesity was clearly related to antipsychotic drug use and less so to lithium and anticonvulsants (but patients taking lithium alone had an obesity rate 1.5 times that of the general population).

A review of the effects of mood stabilizers on weight included a section on lithium in which the authors concluded that lithium-related weight gain occurs in one-third to two-thirds of patients, with a mean increase of 4–7 kg; possible mechanisms were discussed (46[R]).

In a 12-month maintenance study, weight gain was an adverse event in 21% of patients taking divalproex, 13% of those taking lithium, and 7% of those taking placebo (2[C]). The divalproex/placebo difference was statistically significant, but the lithium/placebo difference was not.

A review of the effects of obesity on drug pharmacokinetics briefly mentioned that the steady-state volume of distribution of lithium correlated with ideal bodyweight and fat-free mass but not with total bodyweight (47[R]). Lithium clearance was greater in those with obesity than in lean controls, suggesting that obese patients may require larger maintenance doses to maintain target serum concentrations.

The Expert Consensus Guideline Series, *Medication Treatment of Bipolar Disorder 2000*, has recommended "continue present medication, focus on diet and exercise" as the preferred first-line treatment for managing weight gain in patient taking lithium or divalproex. The next approach was to continue medication and add topiramate. Second-line treatments included switching from divalproex to lithium or vice versa, reducing the dosage, and switching to another drug. The addition of an appetite suppressant was a lower second-line recommendation (48[S]).

Electrolyte balance A 25-year-old man who had taken lithium for 5 years awakened from sleep unable to move his limbs and had a generalized flaccid paralysis with a serum potassium concentration of 2.1 mmol/l (26[A]). Lithium was withdrawn and he responded to treatment with intravenous KCl. The diagnosis of acute *hypokalemic paralysis* was attributed to lithium but whether this was causal or coincidental was unclear.

Hematologic Of 39 patients taking lithium, 18% had *neutrophilia* and 15% had *raised activity of polymorphonuclear elastase* (a marker of granulocyte activation) (49[C]). In keeping with these observations, a chart review of 38 patients taking clozapine showed an increase in leukocyte count when lithium was added (50[C]). A man with olanzapine-induced neutropenia (with a prior history of risperidone-induced neutropenia), which normalized with drug withdrawal, had no difficulty when the drug was reintroduced after the patient had been treated with lithium (51[A]).

Mouth A review of drug-induced *oral ulceration* mentioned lithium as a possible cause, based on two older references (52[A], 53[A]), but provided no new information (54[R]).

Gastrointestinal In a 12-month maintenance study, lithium (n = 94) was not unexpectedly associated with more *nausea* (45% vs 31%) and *diarrhea* (46% vs 30%) than placebo (n = 94) (2[C]). A 72-year-old man who had recently started to take lithium developed severe nausea, vomiting, and oliguric renal insufficiency, which was initially attributed to lithium toxicity, until a serum lithium concentration of only 0.35 mmol/l directed evaluation to the correct diagnosis of acute gastric volvulus (55[A]).

Pancreas A 78-year-old woman taking lithium had *hyperamylasemia and hyperlipasemia* in the absence of gastrointestinal symptoms. Ultrasound of the pancreas and liver was normal. She also had hyperparathyroidism and renal dysfunction (see Parathyroid and Urinary) (39[A]).

Urinary tract In a review of the renal and metabolic complications of lithium the example of a 78-year-old woman on long-term lithium who had urinary incontinence, moderate renal insufficiency, a 5–7 liter 24-hour urine volume, and thyroid and parathyroid abnormalities was used to set the scene (39[Ar]).

In a historical cohort study changes in renal function in 86 patients on lithium were evaluated first after a median treatment duration of

5.8 years and again after 16 years (56[C]). *Maximum plasma osmolality was reduced* in nine of 63 patients in the initial study and in 24 of 63 at follow-up. Other findings included *increased serum creatinine* (in one of 76 patients initially and eight of 76 at follow-up) and *reduced GFR* (in three of 29 patients initially and six of 29 at follow-up); only the last of these changes was not significant. The authors noted that this progressive impairment in renal dysfunction was greater than expected for age and advised strict surveillance of renal function in patients taking long-term lithium.

In a retrospective review of 6514 renal biopsies there were 24 patients with renal insufficiency who had taken lithium for a mean duration of 13.6 years (range 2–25); the histological changes included *chronic tubulointerstitial nephropathy* (100%), *cortical and medullary tubular cysts* (63%) or *tubular dilatation* (33%), *global glomerulosclerosis* (100%), and *focal segmental glomerulosclerosis* (50%) (57[C]). Only two had a history of acute lithium toxicity. Clinical findings included *proteinuria* (42%), *nephrotic syndrome* (25%), *nephrogenic diabetes insipidus* (87%), and *hypertension* (33%). Despite lithium withdrawal, either seven (abstract) or eight (text) of nine patients with an initial serum creatinine of over 221 μmol/l (2.5 mg/dl) progressed to *end stage renal insufficiency*, while this occurred in only one of 10 with lower creatinine concentrations. The study design was such that the risk of renal insufficiency with long-term lithium therapy could not be established and the possibility of alternative causes could not be excluded.

A 59-year-old woman with lithium-associated *nephrotic syndrome* (focal segmental glomerulosclerosis on biopsy) had resolution of edema and pleural effusions and marked improvement in albuminemia and proteinuria after withdrawal of lithium (58[A]).

Nephrogenic diabetes insipidus secondary to lithium led to severe dehydration in two patients who required intravenous rehydration followed by a thiazide diuretic to reduce urine volume (59[Ar]). One patient had persistent polyuria (6.7 l/day) 57 months after stopping lithium (41[Ar]).

In a retrospective review of lithium concentrations in 2210 psychiatric hospital patients, 151 (6.8%) had serum concentrations of 1.5 mmol/l or more. Of those with high serum concentrations, 10 (6.6%) had a raised BUN or serum creatinine concentration (60[C]).

In another retrospective study of 114 patients who had taken lithium for 4–30 years and 94 matched unmedicated subjects, 21% of those taking lithium had blood creatinine concentrations greater than 1.5 mg/ml [*sic*]; comparative figures were not given for the controls (61[c]). Raised creatinine concentrations tended to be associated with episodes of lithium toxicity and drugs or diseases that could alter glomerular function.

Carbamazepine-induced renal insufficiency was associated with lithium toxicity in one patient (62[A]), and thyrotoxicosis was considered a possible contributor to lithium toxicity in two patients, possibly by increasing tubular lithium reabsorption through induction of the sodium–hydrogen antiporter (37[A]).

Skin *Secondary skin reactions* were more common in 51 patients taking lithium than in 57 taking other psychotropic drugs (45% vs 25%) and while acne (33% vs 9%) and *psoriasis* (6% vs 0%) were numerically more common in the lithium group, the only statistically significant difference was with acne in men (63[CR]).

Case reports have included lithium-related worsening (and improvement with discontinuation) of *follicular keratosis* (Darier's disease) in a 50-year-old woman (64[A]) and *psoriasis* in a 54-year-old woman (65[A]). A man and a woman developed vegetating plaques with peripheral pustules (*halogenoderma*) after taking lithium for 6 and 8 years respectively (66[A]). No follow-up information was provided and it could not be established whether the lesions were caused by, worsened by, or unrelated to lithium.

Hair A 55-year-old woman who had taken lithium and haloperidol for 11 years presented with a 1-year history of *loss of scalp, axillary, and pubic hair* (67[A]). There were clusters of hyperkeratotic papules over her scalp, extremities, and trunk, and biopsy was suggestive of follicular mycosis fungoides. Thyroid function was normal. She continued to take haloperidol and valproate instead of lithium. Hair regrowth and almost complete resolution of the papules occurred over 3 months.

Hair loss in psychopharmacology has been reviewed (34[Ar]). A 36-year-old woman had taken lithium for 4 months when her scalp hair became thinner and stopped growing. She continued to take lithium, and 2 months later was diagnosed and treated for hypothyroidism, after which her hair became curlier but did not grow longer or fuller.

Reproductive function Compared with 13 women taking placebo, 10 women taking lithium carbonate 900 mg/day for one menstrual cycle had no significant alterations in reproductive hormone concentrations (68[c]).

Lithium at a serum concentration of about 0.6 mmol/l *reduced sperm motility, number, and viability*, and markedly altered testicular histopathology in *Viscacha*, a nocturnal rodent from the pampas of Argentina (69[E]).

Immunologic The very complex antiviral and immunomodulatory effects of lithium have been reviewed (70[R]). In 15 in-patients, lithium produced *changes in a number of histocompatibility antigens*, but whether this has any clinical implications is unknown (71[c]). In vitro studies of monocytes from women with breast cancer showed that lithium chloride *suppressed production of interleukin-8 and induced production of interleukin-15* (72[c], 73[c]). Whether these observations are of clinical importance is unclear.

Multiorgan failure Multisystem organ failure occurred shortly after clozapine was added to a therapeutic dose of lithium in a 23-year-old woman (74[A]). Improvement occurred when clozapine was stopped and the toxicity was attributed to this drug.

Death Diverse literature suggests that lithium saves lives by reducing suicide risk (75[C], 76[R]) and takes lives as a consequence of poisoning (intoxication) (77[C]), with the overall outcome favoring life.

LONG-TERM EFFECTS

Drug abuse Lithium is not a drug of abuse or dependence, although when one bipolar alcohol abuser was prevented from drinking he tried to get a "buzz" by increasing his lithium dose to the point of toxicity (serum concentration 3.0 mmol/l) (78[A]). The only other suggestion of abuse appeared in 1977 when passing mention was made to the "fairly recent (over the past 2 years or so) abuse of lithium" by poly-drug abusers (79[r]).

Drug tolerance In a review of whether the prophylactic efficacy of lithium was transient or persistent the authors concluded that "the balance of evidence does not indicate a general loss of lithium efficacy" (80[R]). A similar conclusion was reached in a study of 22 patients who had taken lithium for at least 20 years (81[C]). There was no change in affective morbidity over the second 10 years compared with the first 10 years. However, individual exceptions could not be excluded.

Drug withdrawal The subject of *manic relapse* after lithium withdrawal has been addressed, with the conclusion that withdrawal mania is "a major and sinister complication of the everyday use of lithium" (82[R]). Withdrawal of effective lithium therapy was associated with an increased risk of suicide and suicidal acts, especially during the first 12 months. Gradual withdrawal (over 15–30 days) was associated with half the rate of suicidal acts compared with more rapid withdrawal (strong trend towards statistical significance) (83[CR]).

Three patients who had taken lithium for 20–25 years relapsed after withdrawal and failed to respond to restarting the drug, once again raising the issue of lithium withdrawal-induced refractoriness (84[A]).

SECOND-GENERATION EFFECTS

Pregnancy Overviews of the effects of lithium during pregnancy and breastfeeding continue to appear (85[R]–89[R]). In 20 infants exposed to lithium during labor and delivery there were higher rates of *perinatal complications* (65%) and *special care nursery admissions* (45%) than in non-exposed infants, although most complications were transient (90[c]). An infant who died shortly after birth had *oromandibular–limb hypogenesis spectrum*, which was speculatively attributed to lithium that the mother had taken during most of her pregnancy (91[A]).

Lactation With regard to breastfeeding, lithium was stated to be "an excellent example of a drug that requires monitoring and case-by-case assessment so that nursing mothers can be successfully treated" (92[r]). A review of mood stabilizers during breastfeeding reaffirmed that there are only two reported cases of infant lithium toxicity associated with breastfeeding (one of which involved both fetal and breast milk exposure). The following recommendations were made in the case of a mother taking lithium who chooses to breastfeed:

- educate her about the manifestations of toxicity;
- explain the risks of dehydration;
- consider partial or total formula supplements during episodes of illness or dehydration;
- suspend breastfeeding if toxicity is suspected;
- check infant and maternal serum lithium concentrations (93[R]).

DRUG ADMINISTRATION

Drug formulations Lithium gamolenate, a compound with in vitro antitumor activity, given intravenously or orally, was ineffective in treating advanced pancreatic adenocarcinoma (n = 278) (94[C]). Adverse effects (type unspecified) attributed to lithium were reported in two of 93 in the oral group (mean serum lithium 0.15 mmol/l), five of 90 with low-dose intravenous administration (mean serum lithium 0.4 mmol/l), and seven of 95 with the high-dose intravenous administration (mean serum lithium 0.8 mmol/l).

In a study of 12 healthy men, there was no food-induced change in the systemic availability of a sustained-release lithium formulation that used an acrylic matrix of Eudragit RSPM as a sustaining agent (95[c]). In 12 bipolar patients, there were higher brain lithium concentrations (measured by magnetic resonance spectroscopy) for any given serum concentration with a sustained-release formulation than a standard formulation (96[c]). Whether this has any clinical importance is unknown.

Following an overdose with a sustained-release formulation (8000 mg of Teralithe 400 LP), the appearance of clinical symptoms (vomiting and dizziness) was delayed for 35 hours, despite a serum lithium concentration of 2.38 mmol/l at 15 hours and 3.12 mmol/l at 25 hours (97[A]).

A woman taking conventional lithium developed lithium toxicity after two doses of a homeopathic formulation "Lithium carb. 30"; a paucity of detail allows no conclusions to be drawn from this observation (98[A]).

Drug dosage regimens Treating acute mania with a 20 mg/kg/day oral loading dose of slow-release lithium carbonate produced at least 50% improvement in nine of 15 patients within 10 days, but three developed new onset *bradycardia* that was severe enough in one to warrant withdrawal of the drug; another patient dropped out because of *tremor*, *fatigue*, and *diarrhea* (7[c]).

Drug overdose A chart review of psychiatric hospital admissions between 1990 and 1996 showed that 6.8% of 2210 patients who were given lithium had at least one serum concentration of 1.5 mmol/l or over (43% of these were increased at admission) and of those only 28% had signs and symptoms of toxicity (60[C]). Of 205 cases of lithium poisoning reported to the Ontario Canada Regional Poison Information Centre in 1996, 12 were acute overdoses (someone else's tablets), 174 were acute-on-chronic poisonings, and 19 were chronic poisonings. Over 80% had no or minimal symptoms, two patients died, and one had persistent renal sequelae (99[C]). In a small number of patients for whom hemodialysis was recommended, the outcomes were similar in those who were actually dialysed and those who were not, leading the authors to conclude that dialysis should be reserved for the more severe cases (100[C]).

Case reports of lithium poisoning include the following:

- a 71-year-old woman who became toxic after urinary diversion with ileal conduits because of absorption of urinary lithium from the bowel (101[A]);
- two women with stormy clinical courses who were found to be hyperthyroid (see also Endorcine) (37[A]);
- a 32-month-old boy who had ingested a relative's tablets (102[A]);
- a 24-year-old woman who survived a lithium carbonate overdose (5600 mg; serum concentration 4.0 mmol/l) with conservative treatment (103[A]);

- a 73-year-old patient with toxic symptoms and moderately severe generalized slowing on the EEG at a therapeutic serum concentration (104[A]);
- a 46-year-old man who became toxic after an initially unrecognized pontine hemorrhage (105[A]);
- a 39-year-old woman who took an overdose of lithium tablets, was given a single dose of haloperidol, and developed neuroleptic malignant syndrome (17[A]);
- a 62-year-old woman with persistent cerebellar and extrapyramidal sequelae (serum concentration 3.61 mmol/l) (106[A]).

In another case, following an overdose with a sustained-release formulation the appearance of clinical symptoms (vomiting and dizziness) was delayed for 35 hours, despite a serum lithium concentration of 2.38 mmol/l at 15 hours and 3.12 mmol/l at 25 hours (97[A]).

Two teenagers with neurological toxicity (serum concentrations 5.4 mmol/l and 4.81 mmol/l) were treated successfully with hemodialysis followed by continuous venovenous hemofiltration, which prevented a postdialysis rebound in serum lithium concentrations (107[A]). An agitated, confused, disoriented 52-year-old woman who took an overdose of lithium recovered fully after high-volume continuous venovenous hemofiltration (108[A]).

The distribution of clinical practice guidelines in Northeast Scotland had no impact on whether appropriate action was taken for high serum lithium concentrations (80% before the guidelines, 82% after). There was no significant difference in proper attention to high concentrations between those in primary care alone (77%) and those in shared care (85%) (109[C]).

DRUG INTERACTIONS

The 2000 *Guide to Psychiatric Drug Interactions* contained a short section on lithium (110[r]). In a review of the differential pharmacokinetics of lithium in the elderly, interactions with diuretics, ACE inhibitors, and NSAIDs were briefly discussed (111[R]).

Antibiotics A 56-year-old man with normal renal function and therapeutic lithium concentrations became toxic (serum concentration 2.53 mmol/l 24 hours after the last dose) with renal impairment (serum creatinine 141 μmol/l; 1.6 mg/dl) within days of starting levofloxacin. Both symptoms and laboratory abnormalities resolved with withdrawal of both lithium and levofloxacin (112[A]).

A 42-year-old woman developed symptoms of lithium toxicity and a raised serum concentration (2.1 mmol/l) while taking trimethoprim (113[A]).

Anticonvulsants A case report suggested an association between lithium and carbamazepine in causing sinus node dysfunction (see also Cardiovascular) (5[A]). Lithium toxicity in a 33-year-old man was attributed to carbamazepine-induced renal insufficiency (see also Overdose and urinary tract) (62[A]). In an open cross-over study in 20 healthy men, the serum lithium concentration was slightly lower (0.65 vs 0.71 mmol/l) when lamotrigine 100 mg/day was added for 6 days, but the difference was not statistically significant (114[c]).

Antidepressants Neuroleptic malignant syndrome occurred in a 63-year-old man taking lithium and amoxapine and resolved with treatment and medication withdrawal (see also Nervous system) (15[A]).

In a placebo-controlled, cross-over study in 12 healthy men lithium and mirtazapine had no effect on the pharmacokinetics of each other and there was no difference in psychometric testing between the addition of lithium and placebo (115[c]).

The authors of a thorough literature review of 503 patients treated with lithium and SSRIs (116[R]) acknowledged that conclusions would be hedged with qualifications and equivocations but suggested the following:

- "when lithium is added to SSRIs new, non-serious, events occur frequently";
- "serotonin syndrome is associated with combined lithium/SSRI therapy but is rare";
- "the evidence for the efficacy of lithium add-on to SSRIs is at best provisional".

There was no systematic evidence that SSRIs alter serum lithium concentrations.

Angiotensin converting enzyme (ACE) inhibitors A 57-year-old man developed confusion, lethargy, ataxia, and myoclonus in conjunction with a serum lithium concentration of 2.6 mmol/l 4 days after starting to take captopril 50 mg tds (117[A]).

In rats ramipril reduced renal lithium clearance and increased fractional lithium reabsorption in association with decreased systolic blood pressure and decreased sodium excretion. These effects were attenuated by icatibant, a specific bradykinin B_2 receptor antagonist (118[E]).

Angiotensin II receptor type-1 (AT_1) antagonists A 58-year-old bipolar woman with previously stable therapeutic lithium concentrations was hospitalized with a 10-day history of confusion, disorientation, and agitation 8 weeks after starting to take candesartan 16 mg/day. Both drugs were withdrawn, the serum lithium concentration fell from a high of 3.25 mmol/l, and she was again maintained on her usual therapeutic concentration of lithium (119[A]). A similar episode occurred in a 51-year-old woman, who developed delirium, confusion, and ataxia shortly after starting valsartan 80 mg/day in association with a serum lithium concentration of 1.4 mmol/l (120[A]).

Anti-inflammatory drugs A review of the psychiatric effects of NSAIDs included a section on renal function and lithium clearance (121[r]).

When celecoxib was co-administered with lithium, celecoxib concentrations were higher for the first 6 hours after the dose but the AUC was not altered significantly (122[r]). In another review it was mentioned that clinically significant interactions with lithium (increased lithium concentrations) had been identified, but no detail was presented (123[r]). The US package insert states that in healthy subjects celecoxib increases mean steady-state plasma lithium concentrations by about 17% (124[S]).

In 16 subjects, meloxicam 15 mg increased plasma lithium concentrations by 21% (range –9 to 59%) and reduced total plasma lithium clearance by 18% (125[c]).

Sulindac, generally believed not to alter lithium pharmacokinetics, was reported to cause a toxic increase in serum lithium concentration in a 23-year-old man and a 27-year-old woman (2.0 and 1.7 mmol/l respectively) (126[A]).

Antipsychotic drugs In a placebo-controlled open-label study in 25 healthy subjects there were no changes in serum lithium concentration or renal lithium clearance when ziprasidone (40–80 mg/day) was added for 7 days (127[C]).

Ciclosporin In rats, lithium chloride alone had no significant renal toxicity, but when it was combined with ciclosporin, the renal toxicity of the latter was worsened (128[E]). There was also a strong ciclosporin dose-dependent increase in serum lithium concentrations (10-fold at the highest dose).

REFERENCES

1. Malone RP, Delaney MA, Luebbert JF, Cater J, Campbell M. A double-blind placebo-controlled study of lithium in hospitalized aggressive children and adolescents with conduct disorder. Arch Gen Psychiatry 2000; 57: 649–54.
2. Bowden CL, Calabrese JR, McElroy SL, Gyulai L, Wassef A, Petty F, Pope HG, Chou JC-Y, Keck PE Jr, Rhodes LJ, Swann AC, Hirschfeld RMA, Wozniak PJ. A randomized, placebo-controlled 12-month trial of divalproex and lithium in treatment of outpatients with bipolar I disorder. Arch Gen Psychiatry 2000; 57; 481–9.
3. Kallner G, Lindelius R, Petterson U, Stockman O, Tham A. Mortality in 497 patients with affective disorders attending a lithium clinic or after having left it. Pharmacopsychiatry 2000; 33: 8–13.
4. Brodersen A, Licht RW, Vestergaard P, Olesen AV, Mortensen PB. Sixteen-year mortality in patients with affective disorder commenced on lithium. Br J Psychiatry 2000; 176: 429–33.
5. Lai C-L, Chen W-J, Huang C-H, Lin F-Y, Lee Y-T. Sinus node dysfunction in a patient with lithium intoxication. J Formos Med Assoc 2000; 99: 66–8.
6. Kähkönen S, Kaartinen M, Juhela P. Permanent pacing-aid to carry out long-term lithium therapy in manic patient with symptomatic bradycardia. Pharmacopsychiatry 2000; 33: 157.
7. Keck PE, Strakowski SM, Hawkins JM, Dunayevich E, Tugrul KC, Bennett JA, McElroy SL. A pilot study of rapid lithium administration in the treatment of acute mania. Bipolar Disorders 2001; 3: 68–72.
8. Reilly JG, Ayis SA, Ferrier IN, Jones SJ, Thomas SHL. QT_c-interval abnormalities and psychotropic drug therapy in psychiatric patients. Lancet 2000; 355: 1048–52.
9. Coulter DM, Bate A, Meyboom RHB, Lindquist M, Edwards IR. Antipsychotic drugs and heart muscle disorder in international pharma-

covigilance: data mining study. Br Med J 2001; 322: 1207–9.
10. Dunner DL. Optimizing lithium treatment. J Clin Psychiatry 2000; 61 Suppl 9: 76–81.
11. Manji HK, Moore GJ, Chen G. Clinical and preclinical evidence for the neurotrophic effects of mood stabilizers: implications for the pathophysiology and treatment of manic-depressive illness. Biol Psychiatry 2000; 48: 740–54.
12. Moore GJ, Bebchuk MJ, Wilds IB, Chen G, Manji HK. Lithium-induced increase in human brain grey matter. Lancet 2000; 356: 1241–2.
13. Keck PE, Arnold LM. The serotonin syndrome. Psychiatr Ann 2000; 30: 333–43.
14. Mason PJ, Morris VA, Balcezak TJ. Serotonin syndrome. Presentation of 2 cases and review of the literature. Medicine 2000; 79: 201–9.
15. Gupta S, Racaniello AA. Neuroleptic malignant syndrome associated with amoxapine and lithium in an older adult. Ann Clin Psychiatry 2000; 12: 107–9.
16. Sierra-Biddle D, Herran A, Diez-Aja S, Gonzalez-Mata JM, Vidal E, Diez-Manrique F, Vazquez-Barquero JL. Neuroleptic malignant syndrome and olanzapine. J Clin Psychopharmacol 2000; 20: 704–5.
17. Lin PY, Wu CK, Sun TF. Concomitant neuroleptic malignant syndrome and lithium intoxication in a patient with bipolar I disorder: case report. Changgeng Yi Xue Za Zhi 2000; 23: 624–9.
18. O'Sullivan JD, Lees AJ. Nonparkinsonian tremors. Clin Neuropharmacol 2000; 23: 233–8.
19. Zaninelli R, Bauer M, Jobert M, Müller-Oerlinghausen B. Changes in quantitatively assessed tremor during treatment of major depression with lithium augmented by paroxetine or amitriptyline. J Clin Psychopharmacol 2001; 21: 190–8.
20. Stewart JT, Williams LS. A case of lithium-induced asterixis. J Am Geriatr Soc 2000; 48: 457.
21. Muthane UB, Prasad BNK, Vasanth A, Satishchandra P. Tardive parkinsonism, orofacial dyskinesia and akathisia following brief exposure to lithium carbonate. J Neurol Sci 2000; 176: 78–9.
22. Schulz C, Mavrogiorgou P, Schröter A, Hegerl U, Juckel G. Lithium-induced EEG changes in patients with affective disorders. Neuropsychobiology 2000; 42 Suppl 1: 33–7.
23. Slama M, Masmoudi K, Blanchard N, Andréjak M. A possible case of lithium intoxication mimicking Creutzfeld–Jakob syndrome. Pharmacopsychiatry 2000; 33: 145–6.
24. Go, KG. Pseudotumour cerebri. Incidence, management and prevention. CNS Drugs 2000; 14: 33–49.
25. Ronzière T, Auzou P, Özsancak C, Magnier P, Sénant J, Hannequiin D. Syndrome myasthénique induit par le lithium. Presse Med 2000; 29: 1043–4.
26. Chémali KR, Suarez JI, Katirji B. Acute hypokalemic paralysis associated with long-term lithium therapy. Muscle Nerve 2001; 24: 297–8.
27. Stip E, Dufresne J, Lussier I, Yatham L. A double-blind, placebo-controlled study of the effects of lithium on cognition in healthy subjects: mild and selective effects on learning. J Affect Disord 2000; 60: 147–57.
28. Tremont G, Stern RA. Minimizing the cognitive effects of lithium therapy and electroconvulsive therapy using thyroid hormone. Int J Neuropsychopharmacol 2000; 3: 175–86.
29. Patten SB, Williams JVA, Petcu R, Oldfield R. Delirium in psychiatric inpatients: a case-control study. Can J Psychiatry 2001; 42: 162–6.
30. Niethammer R, Keller A, Weisbrod M. Delirantes Syndrom als Lithium-nebenwirkung bei normalen Lithiumspiegeln. Psychiatr Prax 2000; 27: 296–7.
31. Jefferson JW. Lithium-associated clinical hypothyroidism. Int Drug Ther Newslett 2000; 35: 84–6.
32. Gracious BL, Findling RL, McNamara NK, Youngstrom EA, Calabrese JR. Elevated TSH in bipolar youth prescribed both lithium and divalproex sodium. Bipolar Disorders 2001; 3 Suppl 1: 38–9.
33. Kupka RW, Nolen WA, Drexhage HA, McElroy SL, Altshuler LL, Denicoff KD, Frye MA, Keck PE, Leverich GS, Rush AJ, Suppes T, Pollio C, Post RM. High rate of autoimmune thyroiditis in bipolar disorder is not associated with lithium. Bipolar Disorders 2001; 3 Suppl 1: 44–5.
34. Mercke Y, Sheng H, Khan T, Lippmann S. Hair loss in psychopharmacology. Ann Clin Psychiatry 2000; 12: 35–42.
35. Leutgeb U. Ambient iodine and lithium-associated clinical hypothyroidism. Br J Psychiatry 2000; 176: 495–6.
36. Ripoll Mairal M, Len Abad Ó, Falcó Ferrer V, Fernández de Sevilla Ribosa T. Hipertiroidismo e hypercalcemia asociados al tratamiento con litio. Rev Clin Esp 2000; 200: 48–9.
37. Oakley PW, Dawson AH, Whyte IM. Lithium: thyroid effects and altered renal handling. Clin Toxicol 2000; 38: 333–7.
38. Claxton S, Sinha SN, Donovan S, Greenaway TM, Hoffman L, Loughhead M, Burgess JR. Refractory amiodarone-associated thyrotoxicosis: an indication for thyroidectomy. Aust NZ J Med 2000; 70: 174–8.
39. Kanfer A, Blondiaux I. Complications rénales et métaboliques du lithium. Nephrologie 2000; 21: 65–70.
40. Collumbien ECA. Een geval van therapieresistente manie. Lithium en hyperparathyreoïdie. Tijdschr Psychiatrie 2000; 42: 851–5.
41. Guirguis AF, Taylor HC. Nephrogenic diabetes insipidus persisting 57 months after cessation of lithium carbonate therapy: report of a case and review of the literature. Endocr Pract 2000; 6: 324–8.
42. Lam P, Tsai S-J, Chou Y-C. Lithium associated hyperparathyroidism with adenoma: a case report. Int Med J 2000; 7: 283–5.

43. Rasgon NL, Altshuler LL, Gudeman D, Burt VK, Tanavoli S, Hendrick V, Korenman S. Medication status and polycystic ovary syndrome in women with bipolar disorder: a preliminary report. J Clin Psychiatry 2000; 61: 173–8.
44. Bastürk M, Karaaslan F, Esel E, Sofuoglu S, Tutus A, Yabanoglu I. Effects of short and long-term lithium treatment on serum prolactin levels in patients with bipolar affective disorder. Prog Neuropsychopharmacol Biol Psychiatry 2001; 25: 315–22.
45. Elmslie JL, Silverstone JT, Mann JI, Williams SM, Romans SE. Prevalence of overweight and obesity in bipolar patients. J Clin Psychiatry 2000; 61; 179–84.
46. Ginsberg DL, Sussman N. Effects of mood stabilizers on weight. Primary Psychiatry 2000; 7: 49–58.
47. Cheymol G. Effects of obesity on pharmacokinetics. Implications for drug therapy. Clin Pharmacokinet 2000; 39: 215–31.
48. Sachs GS, Printz DJ, Kahn DA, Carpenter D, Docherty JP. The Expert Consensus Guideline Series. Medication treatment of bipolar disorder 2000. Postgrad Med 2000; Apr: 1–104.
49. Capodicasa E, Russano AM, Ciurnella E. De Bellis F, Rossi R. Scuteri A, Biondi R. Neutrophil peripheral count and human leukocyte elastase during chronic lithium carbonate therapy. Immunopharmacol Immunotoxicol 2000; 22: 671–83.
50. Wolstein J, Bender S, Hesse A, Jura S, Dittmann-Balíar A. Leukocyte count increases with the addition of lithium to concurrent clozapine treatment. Schizophr Res 2000; 41(NSI): B25.
51. Gajwani P, Tesar GE. Olanzapine-induced neutropenia. Psychosomatics 2000; 41: 150–1.
52. Muniz CE, Berghman DH. Contact stomatitis and lithium carbonate tablets. J Am Med Assoc 1978; 239: 2759.
53. Nathan KI. Development of mucosal ulcerations with lithium carbonate therapy. Am J Psychiatry 1995;152: 956–7.
54. Madinier I, Berry N, Chichmanian R-M. Les ulcerations orales d'origine médicamenteuse. Ann Med Interne (Paris) 2000; 151: 248–54.
55. Ala A, Arnold N, Khin CC, van Someren N. Nausea and vomiting, a cause for concern? Postgrad Med J 2000; 76: 375, 379–80.
56. Bendz H, Aurell M, Lanke J. A historical cohort study of kidney damage in long-term lithium patients: continued surveillance needed. Eur Psychiatry 2001; 16: 199–206.
57. Markowitz GS, Radhakrishnan J, Kambham N, Valeri AM, Hines WH, D'Agati V. Lithium nephrotoxicity: a progressive combined glomerular and tubulointerstitial nephropathy. J Am Soc Nephrol 2000; 11: 1439–48.
58. Schreiner A, Waldherr R, Rohmeiss P, Hewer W. Focal segmental glomerulosclerosis and lithium treatment. Am J Psychiatry 2000; 157: 834.
59. Eustatia-Rutten CFA, Tamsma JT, Meinders AE. Lithium-induced nephrogenic diabetes insipidus. Neth J Med 2001; 58: 137–42.
60. Webb AL, Solomon DA, Ryan CE. Lithium levels and toxicity among hospitalized patients. Psychiatr Serv 2001; 52: 229–31.
61. Lepkifker E, Sverdlik A, Iancu I, Ziv R. Renal failure in long-term lithium treatment. Bipolar Disord 2001; 3 Suppl 1: 45.
62. Mayan H, Golubev N, Dinour D, Farfel Z. Lithium intoxication due to carbamazepine-induced renal failure. Ann Pharmacother 2001; 35: 560–2.
63. Chan HHL, Wing Y-K, Su R, Van Krevel C, Lee S. A control study of the cutaneous side effects of chronic lithium therapy. J Affect Disord 2000; 57: 107–13.
64. Ehrt U, Brieger P. Comorbidity of keratosis follicularis (Darier's disease) and bipolar affective disorder: an indication for valproate instead of lithium. Gen Hosp Psychiatry 2000; 22: 128–9.
65. Miyagawa M, Shimoda K, Danno K, Kato N. Exacerbation of psoriasis during lithium treatment in a patient with bipolar I disorder. Int Clin Psychopharmacol 2000; 15: 368.
66. Alagheband M, Engineer L. Lithium and halogenoderma. Arch Dermatol 2000; 136: 126–7.
67. Francis GJ, Silverman AR, Saleh O, Lee GJ. Follicular mycosis fungoides associated with lithium. J Am Acad Dermatol 2001; 44: 308–9.
68. Baptista T, Lacruz A, De Mendoza S, Guillén MM, Burguera JL, De Burguera M, Hernández L. Endocrine effects of lithium carbonate in healthy premenopausal women: relationship with body-weight reduction. Prog Neuropsychopharmacol Biol Psychiatry 2000; 24: 1–6.
69. Perez Romera E, Muñoz E, Mohamed F, Dominguez S, Scardapane L, Villegas O, Garcïa Aseff S, Guzmán JA. Lithium effect on testicular tissue and spermatozoa of *Viscacha* (*Lagostomus maximus maximus*). A comparative study with rats. J Trace Elem Med Biol 2000; 14: 81–3.
70. Rybakowski JK. Antiviral and immunomodulatory effect of lithium. Pharmacopsychiatry 2000; 33: 159–64.
71. Kang B-J, Park S-W, Chung T-H. Can the expression of histocompatibility antigen be changed by lithium? Bipolar Disord 2000; 2: 140–4.
72. Merendino RA, Arena A, Gangemi S, Ruello A, Losi E, Bene A, Valenti A, Purello D'Ambrosio F. In vitro effect of lithium chloride on interleukin-15 production by monocytes from breast cancer patients. J Chemother 2000; 12: 252–7.
73. Merendino RA, Arena A, Gangemi S, Ruello A, Losi E, Bene A, Purello D'Ambrosio F. In vitro interleukin–8 production by monocytes treated with lithium chloride from breast cancer patients. Tumori 2000; 86: 149–52.
74. Patton S, Remick RA, Isomura T. Clozapine – an atypical reaction. Can J Psychiatry 2000; 45: 393–4.

75. Coppen A. Lithium in unipolar depression and the prevention of suicide. J Clin Psychiatry 2000; 61 Suppl 9: 52–6.
76. Goodwin FK, Ghaemi SN. The impact of mood stabilizers on suicide in bipolar disorder: a comparative analysis. CNS Spectrums 2000; 5 Suppl 1: 12–18.
77. Litovitz TL, Klein-Schwartz W, White S, Cobaugh DJ, Youniss J, Drab A, Benson BE. 1999 Annual report of the American Association of Poison Control Centers Toxic Exposure Surveillance System. Am J Emerg Med 2000; 18: 517–24.
78. O'Boyle M, Emory E. A case of lithium carbonate abuse. Am J Psychiatry 1988; 145: 1036.
79. Lipkin B. Lithium as a drug of abuse. Br Med J 1977; 1: 1411.
80. Kleindienst N, Greil W, Rüger B, Möller H-J. The prophylactic efficacy of lithium – transient or persistent? Eur Arch Psychiatry Clin Neurosci 1999; 249: 144–9.
81. Berghöfer A, Müller-Oerlinghausen B. Is there a loss of efficacy of lithium in patients treated for over 20 years? Neuropsychobiology 2000; 42 Suppl 1: 46–9.
82. Goodwin GM, Phil D. Clinical and biological investigation of mania following lithium withdrawal. In: Manji HK, Bowden CL, Belmaker RH, editors. Bipolar Medications: Mechanisms of Action. Washington, DC: American Psychiatric Press, 2000: 347–56.
83. Tondo L, Baldessarini RJ. Reduced suicide risk during lithium maintenance treatment. J Clin Psychiatry 2000; 61 Suppl 9: 97–104.
84. Oostervink F, Nolen WA, Hoenderboom ACG, Kupka RW. Het risico van lithiumresistentie na stoppen en herstart na langdurig gebruik. Ned Tijsdchr Geneeskd 2000; 144: 401–4.
85. Iqbal MM. The effects of lithium on fetuses, neonates, and nursing infants. Psychiatr Ann 2000; 30: 159–64.
86. Warner JP. Evidence-based psychopharmacology 3. Assessing evidence of harm: what are the teratogenic effects of lithium carbonate? J Psychopharmacol 2000; 14: 77–80.
87. Stowe ZN, Calhoun K, Ramsey C, Sadek N, Newport J. Mood disorders during pregnancy and lactation: defining issues of exposure and treatment. CNS Spectrums 2001; 6: 150–66.
88. Iqbal MM, Gundlapalli SP, Ryan WG, Ryals T, Passman TE. Effects of antimanic mood-stabilizing drugs on fetuses, neonates, and nursing infants. South Med J 2001; 94: 304–22.
89. Williams K, Oke S. Lithium and pregnancy. Psychiatr Bull 2000; 24; 229–31.
90. Viguera AC, Howlett SA, Cohen LS, Nonacs RM, Stoller J. Neonatal outcome associated with lithium use during pregnancy. Presented at the NCDEU 40th Annual Meeting, Boca Raton, Florida, May 30–June 2, 2000. New Clinical Drug Evaluation Unit Program: Poster No. 49.
91. Tekin M, Ellison J. Oromandibular-limb hypogenesis spectrum and maternal lithium use. Clin Dysmorphol 2000; 9: 139–41.
92. Moretti ME, Lee A, Ito S. Which drugs are contraindicated during breastfeeding? Practice guidelines. Can Fam Phys 2000; 46: 1753–57.
93. Chaudron LH, Jefferson JW. Mood stabilizers during breastfeeding: a review. J Clin Psychiatry 2000; 61: 79–90.
94. Johnson CD, Puntis M, Davidson N, Todd S, Bryce R. Randomized, dose-finding phase III study of lithium gamolenate in patients with advanced pancreatic adenocarcinoma. Br J Surg 2001; 88: 662–8.
95. Gai MN, Thielemann AM, Arancibia A. Effect of three different diets on the bioavailability of a sustained release lithium carbonate matrix tablet. Int J Clin Pharmacol Ther 2000; 38: 320–6.
96. Henry ME, Moore CM, Demopolas C, Cote J, Renshaw PF. A comparison of brain lithium levels attained with immediate and sustained release lithium. Biol Psychiatry 2001; 49 Suppl 8: 119S.
97. Astruc B, Petit P, Abbar M. Overdose with sustained-release lithium preparations. Eur Psychiatry 1999; 14: 172–4.
98. Owen D. Interactions between homeopathy and drug treatment. Br Homeopath J 2000; 89: 60.
99. Bailey B, McGuigan M. Lithium poisoning from a poison control center perspective. Ther Drug Monit 2000; 22: 650–5.
100. Bailey B, McGuigan M. Comparison of patients hemodialyzed for lithium poisoning and those for whom dialysis was recommended by PCC but not done: what lesson can we learn? Clin Nephrol 2000; 54: 388–92.
101. Alhasso A, Bryden AA, Neilson D. Lithium toxicity after urinary diversion and ileal conduit. Br Med J 2000; 320: 1037.
102. Ochoa ER, Farrar HC, Shirm SW. Lithium poisoning in a toddler with fever and altered consciousness: case presentation and discussion. J Invest Med 2000; 48: 612.
103. Yoshimura R, Yamada Y, Ueda N, Nakamura J. Changes in plasma monoamine metabolites during acute lithium intoxication. Hum Psychopharmacol 2000; 15: 357–60.
104. Gallinat J, Boetsch T, Padberg F, Hampel H, Herrmann WM, Hegerl U. Is the EEG helpful in diagnosing and monitoring lithium intoxication? A case report and review of the literature. Pharmacopsychiatry 2000; 33: 169–73.
105. Novak-Grubic V, Tavcar R. Lithium intoxication secondary to unrecognized pontine haemorrhage. Acta Psychiatr Scand 2001; 103: 400–1.
106. Roy M, Fond L, Ratrema M, Convers Ph, Lutz MF, Cathébras P. Intoxication au lithium: complications neurologiques sévères. Presse Med 2001; 30: 900–1.
107. Meyer RJ, Flynn JT, Brophy PD, Smoyer WE, Kershaw DB, Custer JR, Bunchman TE. Hemodialysis followed by continuous hemofiltration for

treatment of lithium intoxication in children. Am J Kidney Dis 2001; 37: 1044–7.
108. Van Bommel EFH, Kalmeijer MD, Ponssen HH. Treatment of life-threatening lithium toxicity with high-volume continuous venovenous hemofiltration. Am J Nephrol 2000; 20: 408–11.
109. Eagles JM, McCann I, MacLeod TNN, Paterson N. Lithium monitoring before and after the distribution of clinical practice guidelines. Acta Psychiatr Scand 2000; 101: 349–53.
110. DeVane CL, Nemeroff CB. 2000 Guide to psychotropic drug interactions. Primary Psychiatry 2000; 7: 40–68.
111. Sproule BA, Hardy BG, Shulman KI. Differential pharmacokinetics of lithium in elderly patients. Drugs Aging 2000; 16: 165–77.
112. Takahashi H, Higuchi H, Shimizu T. Severe lithium toxicity induced by combined levofloxacin administration. J Clin Psychiatry 2000; 61: 949–50.
113. De Vries PL. Lithiumintoxicatie bij gelijktijdig gebruik van trimethoprim. Ned Tijdschr Geneeskd 2001; 145: 539–40.
114. Chen C, Veronese L, Yin Y. The effects of lamotrigine on the pharmacokinetics of lithium. Br J Clin Pharmacol 2000; 50: 193–5.
115. Sitsen JMA, Voortman G, Timmer CJ. Pharmacokinetics of mirtazapine and lithium in healthy male subjects. J Psychopharmacol 2000; 14: 172–6.
116. Hawley CJ, Loughlin PJ, Quick SJ, Gale TM, Sivakumaran T, Hayes J, McPhee S. Efficacy, safety and tolerability of combined administration of lithium and selective serotonin reuptake inhibitors: a review of the current evidence. Int Clin Psychopharmacol 2000; 15: 197–206.
117. Ventura JM, Igual MJ, Borrell C, Lozano MD, Maiques FJ, Alós M. Toxicidad de litio inducida por captoprilo. A propósito de un caso. Farm Hosp 2000; 24: 166–9.
118. Bagaté K, Grima M, De Jong W, Imbs J-L, Barthelmebs M. Effects of icatibant on the ramipril-induced decrease in renal lithium clearance in the rat. NS Arch Pharmacol 2001; 363: 281–7.
119. Zwanzger P, Marcuse A, Boerner RJ, Walther A, Rupprecht R. Lithium intoxication after administration of AT1 blockers. J Clin Psychiatry 2001; 62: 208–9.
120. Leung M, Remick RA. Potential drug interaction between lithium and valsartan. J Clin Psychopharmacol 2000; 20: 392–3.
121. Sussman N, Magid S. Psychiatric manifestations of nonsteroidal anti-inflammatory drugs. Prim Psychiatry 2000; 7: 26–30.
122. Davies NM, McLachlan AJ, Day RO, Williams KM. Clinical pharmacokinetics and pharmacodynamics of celecoxib. A selective cyclooxygenase-2 inhibitor. Clin Pharmacokinet 2000; 38: 225–42.
123. Davies NM, Gudde TW, De Leuw MAWC. Celecoxib: a new option in the treatment of arthropathies and familial adenomatous polyposis. Expert Opin Pharmacother 2001; 2: 139–52.
124. Physicians' Desk Reference. Montvale, NJ: Medical Economics Company, Inc, 2001: 2484.
125. Türck D, Heinzel G, Luik G. Steady-state pharmacokinetics of lithium in healthy volunteers receiving concomitant meloxicam. Br J Clin Pharmacol 2000; 50: 197–204.
126. Jones MT, Stoner SC. Increased lithium concentrations reported in patients treated with sulindac. J Clin Psychiatry 2000; 61: 527–8.
127. Apseloff G, Mullet D, Wilner KD, Anziano RJ, Tensfeldt TG, Pelletier SM, Gerber N. The effects of ziprasidone on steady-state lithium levels and renal clearance of lithium. Br J Clin Pharmacol 2000; 49 Suppl 1: 61S–64S.
128. Tariq M, Morais C, Sobki S, Al Sulaiman M, Al Khader A. Effect of lithium on cyclosporin induced nephrotoxicity in rats. Renal Fail 2000; 22: 545–60.

Jayendra K. Patel, Eileen Wong, and Alan I. Green

4 Drugs of abuse

AMPHETAMINES *(SED-14, 100; SEDA-22, 29; SEDA-23, 34; SEDA-24, 32)*

Amphetamine

Nervous system *Intracerebral hemorrhage* associated with amphetamine has been reported for more than five decades. Eight new cases have been associated with amphetamine over a period of 3.5 years (1^{AR}). All had undergone head CT scans and cerebral digital subtraction angiography. Seven had a parenchymal hematoma, three in the frontal lobe and one each in the parietal lobe, frontoparietal region, temporal lobe, and brain stem. One patient had subarachnoid hemorrhage. The time from exposure to onset of symptoms ranged from less than 10 minutes to about 2 months (median 1 day). The authors reviewed the literature and found 37 other cases. They observed that young people, mean age 28 years, were at high risk. While most were repeat abusers, one-third claimed to be first time or infrequent users. Intracerebral hemorrhage was seen with all routes of drug use, 57% from oral use, 34% from intravenous use, and 5% after inhalation. Of those who had a CT scan, 84% had a proven intracerebral hemorrhage, three had subarachnoid hemorrhage, and one had a brainstem hemorrhage. In one patient, with a negative CT scan, the diagnosis of subarachnoid hemorrhage was confirmed by lumbar puncture. In 35 patients who had angiography 20 were normal or showed only mass effect from a hematoma, 16 had vasculitic beading, and one had an arteriovenous malformation. Seven patients died and only 14 had a good recovery.

Psychiatric *Social phobia* has been attributed to amphetamine use (2^{A}).

Side Effects of Drugs, Annual 25
J.K. Aronson, ed.

A 26-year-old woman reported flushing, sweating, palpitation, and shortness of breath, in a range of social situations. She was described as a confident and extraverted woman, with no history of psychiatric problems. She reported daily oral consumption of street amphetamine 1.6 g. At the time of assessment, she had given up her work. Initially, she felt good while taking the drug, but more recently she had been using it to "get going"; there were no symptoms of psychosis or affective disorder.

The authors speculated that dopaminergic dysfunction, reported by some to underlie social phobia, could have resulted in this case from chronic amphetamine-related striatal dopamine depletion.

Methamphetamine

Methamphetamine, a popular drug of abuse, is also known as "speed", "meth", "chalk", "crank", "ice", "crystal", or "glass". In recent years, Japan has experienced an increase in methamphetamine abuse, especially among the young and women. Of 646 forensic autopsy cases between 1994 and 1998 retrospectively studied in the southern half of Osaka City and surrounding areas 15 (2.3%) were positive for methamphetamine (3^{C}). The nine men were older than the six women. Methamphetamine poisoning was the cause of death in four cases, homicide in four, accidental falls in three, and one each was caused by aspiration, house fire, myocardial infarction, and spontaneous intracerebral hemorrhage. Pathological investigations commonly uncovered cardiomyopathy, cerebral perivasculitis, and liver cirrhosis/interstitial hepatitis, irrespective of age.

Nervous system A new report suggests that methamphetamine use may be associated with *neurotoxicity*. The use of proton magnetic resonance scanning (^{1}H MRS) in detecting long-term cerebral metabolite abnormalities in abstinent methamphetamine users has been studied in 26 subjects (13 men) with a history of methamphetamine dependence (mean age 33 years) and 24 healthy subjects with no history of drug dependence (4[C]). The neuronal marker *N*-acetylaspartate was reduced by 6% in the frontal white matter and by 5% in the basal ganglia of the abstinent methamphetamine users. *N*-acetylaspartate is a marker for mature neurons, and reduced *N*-acetylaspartate is thought to indicate reduced neuronal density or neuronal content. According to the authors, these findings suggest neuronal loss or persistent neuronal damage in the absence of significant brain atrophy in methamphetamine users. They speculated that these abnormalities may underlie the persistent abnormal forms of behavior, such as violence, psychosis, and personality changes, seen in some individuals months or even years after their last drug use.

Methamphetamine users in the study also had increased concentrations of choline-containing compounds and myoinositol in the frontal gray matter. Myoinositol is a glial cell marker, while the increase in choline-containing compounds reflects *increased cell membrane turnover*. Thus, these increases in the frontal cortex in drug users may have reflected glial proliferation (astrocytosis). The authors suggested that the finding of reduced *N*-acetylaspartate accompanied by increased myoinositol, which has been observed in many active brain disorders, indicated glial proliferation in response to neuronal injury. However, they noted that neurotoxicity may not be present in subjects who use amounts of the drugs that are much lower than the amounts used by the chronic abusers they studied. They suggested that future studies should observe whether treatments or long periods of abstinence could reverse these abnormalities.

Psychiatry Injection as a method of delivery of illicit drugs carries its own special risks. Methamphetamine-dependent subjects (n = 427) participated in a study to detect differences between injecting methamphetamine users (13%) and non-injecting users (87%) (5[C]). The patients entered treatment at a center in California between 1988 and 1995. Injectors reported significantly more years of heavy use. Psychological problems were more common in the injectors, more of whom reported *depression*, *suicidal ideation*, *hallucinations*, and episodes of *feeling that their body parts "disconnect and leave"*. Moreover, injectors reported more problems concerning sexual functioning and more episodes of loss of consciousness. The injectors were more commonly HIV-positive and they had more felony convictions and were on parole more often than other users. Although individuals who inject methamphetamine use it more often than non-injectors, the number of grams used per week did not differ between the groups. Thus, injectors use a smaller amount of drug per dose than non-injectors. Eighty percent of the injectors were unemployed, possibly reflecting the extent of impairment related to addiction in this group. The injectors, who had more psychiatric and medical morbidity, warrant special attention and carefully designed treatment plans.

Teeth *Dental wear* has been evaluated prospectively in methamphetamine users at an urban university hospital (6[c]). Information was collected from 43 patients (26 men, 40 tobacco smokers), mean age 39 years, who admitted to having used methamphetamine for more than 1 year. Patients who regularly snorted methamphetamine had higher "tooth-wear" scores for anterior maxillary teeth than patients who injected, smoked, or ingested methamphetamine. The authors suggested that the anatomy of the blood supply to this area possibly explained the association of the regional differences in tooth wear with snorted methamphetamine. The anterior maxillary teeth and the nasal mucosa have a common blood supply. Thus, snorting may cause vasoconstriction impairing the blood supply both to the nasal mucosa as well as the teeth.

Infection risk A rare case of *Pott's puffy tumor*, anterior extension of a frontal sinus infection that results in frontal bone osteomyelitis and subperiosteal abscess, has been associated with methamphetamine use (7[A]).

A 34-year-old woman presented with a 9-day history of fever, chills, photophobia, and neck pain. Nine months earlier, she had developed a swelling on her forehead, which enlarged and spontaneously drained pus. Over the next weeks, a fistula developed at the site of the swelling, accompanied by an intermittent bloody purulent drainage that lasted for about 9 months. She had either inhaled methamphetamine or had used it intranasally weekly for 15 years, and reported continued use immediately before the development of the forehead lesion. She had a sinocutaneous fistula in the midline of the forehead, with seropurulent discharge but no local erythema or tenderness. A CT scan of the head showed complete opacification of all sinuses, with a 1 cm connection between the anterior frontal sinus and the skin. Cultures grew *Streptococcus milleri* and *Candida albicans*. She responded to extensive medical and surgical treatment.

The authors proposed that intranasal methamphetamine had contributed to chronic sinus inflammation and subsequent complications. Furthermore, the vasoconstriction induced by methamphetamine in the mucosal vessels may have resulted in ischemic injury to the sinus mucosa, providing an environment conducive to bacterial growth.

Drug overdose There has been a new report of two deaths from methamphetamine overdose in Thailand, which has experienced a recent increase in methamphetamine abuse (8[A]).

A 43-year-old male drug dealer swallowed a number of methamphetamine tablets at the time of his arrest. When seen in the emergency room, he was comatose with reactive pupils. He died 6 hours after consuming the tablets. The autopsy findings were non-specific.

Another 33-year-old female drug dealer, while at the police station, swallowed a number of methamphetamine pills that had been hidden in her undergarments. At the hospital, a gastric lavage was done but she died 10 hours after ingestion.

Methamphetamine related deaths are rare; however, as described in these cases, there may be an increased risk of death in drug dealers who, in attempting to avoid arrest, may consume toxic amounts without anticipating the consequences.

Drug interactions The interaction between the protease inhibitor *ritonavir* and methamphetamine has been discussed (9[A]).

A 49-year-old HIV-positive Caucasian had been taking an antiretroviral regimen, including ritonavir, for 4 months. His friends witnessed him injecting methamphetamine twice before they left him asleep lying naked prone on the floor. He was found dead in the same position the next day. Autopsy did not show the cause of death. Toxicology analyses showed amphetamines, methamphetamine, cannabinoids, and diazepam.

The authors reported that ritonavir inhibits the cytochrome enzyme CYP2D6, which is primarily involved in methamphetamine metabolism. This interaction could have led to a fatal plasma concentration of methamphetamine. They suggested that patients taking antiretroviral drugs should be cautioned about potential drug interactions and the risks of combining them with recreational drugs that are metabolized by CYP2D6.

Methylenedioxymethamphetamine (MDMA, ecstasy)

The pharmacological and pharmacokinetic effects of ecstasy have been studied in healthy volunteers (10[c]). In the pilot phase, two subjects each took ecstasy 50, 100, and 150 mg. In the second phase, eight subjects took ecstasy 75 and 125 mg. All were CYP2D6 extensive metabolizers. The ecstasy plasma concentrations were not proportional to dose, probably indicating non-linear kinetics in the dosage range usually taken recreationally. While the results were not conclusive (owing to problems in the study design) and require further exploration, the finding that relatively small increases in the dose of ecstasy ingested can translate to disproportionate rises in ecstasy plasma concentrations, if confirmed, would be important.

Cardiovascular Extensive *aortic dissection* with cardiac tamponade and mesenteric ischemia has been attributed to ecstasy (11[A]).

A 29-year-old man who ingested ecstasy and alcohol at a rave had no immediate adverse effects, slept well later on, and was in good health until he suddenly collapsed to the floor about 2 hours after waking. When seen 36 hours after the last dose of ecstasy he was short of breath, and had abdominal pain, diarrhea, and vomiting. He had a loose bloody bowel movement but refused further investigation. He was discharged with a diagnosis of gastroenteritis, only to be readmitted 8 hours later after sudden deterioration and hypertension. Despite extensive efforts, his condition deteriorated and he died 5 hours later. At autopsy, there was a type I aortic dissection, starting at the root and spreading to the bifurcation, which had resulted in cardiac tamponade. The dissection had involved the mesenteric arteries, resulting in bowel ischemia.

Since this condition is rare in young adults, diagnosis can be difficult. The authors believed that this was the first case report of aortic dissection secondary to ecstasy.

Ecstasy has been associated with *sudden death* and *cardiovascular complications*. Eight healthy self-reported ecstasy users participated in a four-session, ascending-dose, double-blind, placebo-controlled comparison of the echocardiographic effects of ecstasy and those of dobutamine (12[C]). Ecstasy 1.5 mg/kg increased the mean heart rate by 28 beats/min, systolic blood pressure by 25 mmHg, diastolic blood pressure by 7 mmHg, and cardiac output by 2 l/min. The effects of ecstasy were similar to those produced by dobutamine (40 μg/kg/min), except that ecstasy had no measurable inotropic effects. Thus, ecstasy increases systolic and diastolic blood pressures in the absence of a significant change in cardiac contractility and end-systolic wall thickness. The resulting increase in the tension of the ventricular wall leads to disproportionately higher myocardial oxygen consumption than would be expected from the observed changes in the heart rate and blood pressure. The authors commented that the behavioral and environmental factors accompanying the use of ecstasy – sustained exercise from dancing, often in crowded nightclubs with high ambient temperature and humidity – could further potentiate toxicity. They recommended a combination of β-blockers and vasodilators for the emergency treatment of ecstasy-associated vascular instability.

Nervous system An unusual case of *bilateral sixth nerve palsy* associated with ecstasy has been reported (13[A]).

A 17-year-old man developed horizontal diplopia in all directions of gaze while using ecstasy tablets every 5–7 days for 2 months. A diagnosis of bilateral sixth nerve palsy was confirmed. Ocular movements returned to normal within 5 days without treatment. There was no evidence of inflammation or degenerative disease of the central nervous system.

The authors speculated that the most likely cause of the lesion was either an interaction of ecstasy with serotonergic neurons or cerebral edema (albeit not detected by MRI) secondary to ecstasy.

Mineral and fluid balance Yet another case of the *syndrome of inappropriate antidiuretic hormone secretion* (SIADH) (SEDA-23, 36) has been reported (14[A]).

An 18-year-old woman developed impaired consciousness, psychomotor shaking, hallucinations, tics, and delirium. Her serum sodium concentration was low at 120 mmol/l with a plasma osmolality of 242 mosm/kg and urine osmolality of 562 mosm/kg, suggesting SIADH. Most other blood tests were within the reference ranges, except for a raised creatine kinase. Urine screen was positive for amphetamines. Treatment with hypertonic saline brought about resolution of symptoms. The patient recalled taking three ecstasy tablets over 6 hours.

Drug formulations In New Zealand, "Herbal Ecstasy" is a term used for many different herbal formulations, none of which contains ecstasy. Some of the names for these herbs (which may be sold in stores) include "The Bomb", "Reds", and "Sublime". Analysis of "The Bomb" showed substantial amounts of ephedrine; the Ministry of Health in New Zealand removed it from the market. Some symptoms associated with herbal ecstasy include headache, dizziness, palpitation, tachycardia, and raised blood pressure. Thus, in countries where the term "Herbal Ecstasy" is commonly used, it is important that those who see patients who have taken Herbal Ecstasy should not confuse it with ecstasy, as toxicity and medical management may be quite different (15[c]).

OPIATES *(SED-14, 198; SEDA-22, 35; SEDA-24, 36)*

Deaths from opiate abuse

R

Opiates are widely used all over the world, but recently concerns about opiate use (and deaths from such use) have increased in Australia and the UK (16[C]). The rate of opiate overdose deaths in these countries increased dramatically between 1985 and 1995. Throughout that period, it was four to 10 times higher in Australia than the UK, but the rate of increase may have been greater in the UK in the latter half of the period, since the difference in rate narrowed substantially during that time. Methadone maintenance treatment, established in Australia in 1969 and in the UK in 1970, has become the main treatment for opiate dependence in both countries. About half of the opiate deaths in the UK were attributed at least in part to methadone. By contrast, considerably fewer (18%) opiate overdose deaths in Australia were attributed to methadone. The authors suggested that the discrepancy in the rates between the two countries could be artefacts of the differ-

ences in (a) the documentation of these deaths, (b) the rate of opiate dependence, (c) the route of opiate administration, (d) opiate purity, and most importantly (e) the method of delivery of methadone maintenance treatment.

Methadone-related fatalities have been reported from all countries in which methadone has been used for either detoxification or maintenance treatment of opiate users. These fatalities are often defined as cases of poisoning due to methadone or as polydrug intoxication with methadone as the leading cause of death. Methadone maintenance treatment was introduced in Germany in 1989, and 1396 drug-related deaths were reported from 1990 to 1999 in Hamburg (17[C]). While the absolute numbers of drug-related deaths by poisoning did not change over this period, the rise in methadone-associated deaths paralleled a fall in the number of heroin-associated deaths. From 1990 to 1998, the rate of monovalent heroin intoxication in cases of poisoning fell from 60% to 11%, while the rate of polydrug intoxication increased. Poisoning caused by methadone combined with other substances first gained significance 4 years after methadone maintenance treatment was introduced in Hamburg. Since 1994, methadone-related deaths have increased steadily, and by 1997–8 the numbers had increased exponentially. In the first 6 months of 1999, 60% of all cases of poisoning among drug addicts showed the presence of methadone. When strict guidelines for describing such poisonings were used, 39 poisonings in 1998 (40%) were predominantly caused by methadone, six of them being monovalent methadone intoxication. About two-thirds of all methadone-related poisonings concerned drug addicts who never stayed in methadone maintenance treatment, implying that they obtained methadone from outside of regular treatment. Almost 10 years after the introduction of methadone maintenance treatment in Hamburg, methadone replaced heroin as the leading cause of death due to poisoning. At the same time, however, the absolute number of drug-related deaths and poisonings fell slightly.

While methadone maintenance treatment has clearly reduced overall morbidity and mortality in addicts globally, some issues remain unresolved. There are significant differences in the delivery of methadone maintenance treatment from one country to another. The authors reported that in some patients the starting doses of methadone are quite high and potentially lethal. This is especially so when the patients are also using other drugs and attempting to wean off them. Thus, continued polydrug use in treatment is an important risk factor for mortality. Many patients receive take-home doses for a week at a time. While this is useful in a select group of patients, it is not useful in those who sell methadone to buy heroin and combine the two drugs without knowledge of their half-lives and potential complications. The authors suggested changes in methadone maintenance treatment policy, in order to reduce the chances of accidental overdose/poisoning. Specifically, they recommended: a substantial improvement in quality assurance; a more restrictive methadone take-home policy (at least for patients with evidence for concomitant opiate use); and evaluating heroin or long-acting acetylmethadol as alternatives.

Another report from Australia reviewed all the accidental illicit drug deaths that occurred in the Sydney area in 1995–7 (18[C]). There were 3559 autopsies, of which 4% were considered accidental illicit drug deaths; of these deaths, 121 were men and 22 were women. While the highest number of male deaths occurred in the 25–35 year age group, female deaths were evenly spread from ages 20 to 35. Almost half (49%) of the deaths occurred from morphine poisoning, 27% from multiple drug toxicity, and 21% from heroin toxicity combined with alcohol. Methadone was detected in 19 cases (13%); 12 of these people were enrolled in a methadone maintenance program. Methadone intoxication alone was responsible for two deaths (1%) only. Methadone was present in the blood in a potentially fatal concentration in 13 cases, while 113 people (80%) had a heroin concentration in the fatal range and 91% had detectable concentrations of heroin. There were no significant neurological findings in the 143 cases studied. More than 50% of those with methadone detected also had heroin in their blood. Unfortunately, this appears to show that some people who participate in a methadone program may still die from accidental heroin overdose. Thus, the authors emphasized the importance of education of heroin users about the risk of accidental overdose.

There is excess mortality in heroin users compared with the general population. The prevalence and experience of heroin overdose in drug users in a general practice in Ireland were examined during 5 months (19[c]). Of the 33 patients identified, 24 agreed to participate. They had had their first overdose on average 5 years after starting to use heroin. Ten had taken an overdose themselves, 23 had witnessed an overdose, 22 knew a victim of fatal overdose, and four had been present at a fatal overdose. However, they reported poor understanding of how to deal with an overdose. Despite maintenance treatment with methadone, a significant proportion continued to inject heroin; 17% admitted to the use of illicit methadone, but methadone was not implicated in overdose in any case. The authors suggested that overdose prevention and management should become a priority for general practitioners who care for opiate-dependent patients. Factors implicated in overdose include too high a dose, use after a period of abstinence, and mixing with other drugs.

Clostridium novyi type A, a bacterium that was associated with serious infection during the two world wars, killed 35 injecting heroin users in Britain and Ireland (20[r]). C novyi type A is present in soil and dust and is a well-recognized cause of infection in sheep, cattle, and other animals. Contaminated batches of heroin from a common source were believed to be responsible for the recent outbreak. The bacteria were able to survive the process of preparation for injection. All recent cases occurred after intramuscular injection, which provides the requisite anerobic conditions for infection. This was the first time that this organism caused an outbreak of infection in drug injectors. A total of 74 cases with the same clinical features were reported.

Diamorphine (heroin)

Respiratory Heroin-induced *pulmonary edema* ("heroin lung"), though first described in 1880, is still not very well understood pathophysiologically. In a retrospective case-control study there were 23 heroin fatalities and 12 controls with sudden cardiac deaths (21[c]). The authors tried to verify that defects of the alveolar capillary membranes and/or an acute anaphylactic reaction can lead to pulmonary congestion, edema, and hemorrhages. There were defects of the epithelial and endothelial basal laminae of the alveoli in both groups. There was an insignificant increase in IgE-positive cells in the heroin group. The findings suggested that heroin-associated lung edema is generally not caused by an anaphylactic reaction.

Nervous system *Myelopathy* has been reported after intranasal insufflation of diamorphine (22[A]).

> A 52-year-old man with a history of diamorphine abuse presented with sudden paraplegia a few hours after intranasal insufflation. He had flaccid paralysis of both legs, acute urinary retention, and reduced rectal tone. Deep tendon reflexes were absent and plantar responses were extensor. MRI scanning of the spine and immunoglobulin profile supported the conclusion that this was a case of acute myelopathy with an immunopathological cause, involving a protein specific to spinal cord parenchyma, triggering acute local inflammation, ischemia, and tissue damage. Seven weeks later he recovered normal neurological function.

This case of heroin myelopathy is similar to other reported cases, except that this case occurred with intranasal rather than intravenous use. The MRI findings were consistent with transverse myelitis. The authors suggested that hypersensitivity and an immune-mediated attack on the spinal cord was the likely mechanism of injury.

Urinary tract In Australia heroin use is increasing, as are cases of overdose and deaths. Following an observation that many patients develop *acute renal insufficiency* after using heroin, the authors identified 27 patients (mostly men, average age 29 years) who developed renal insufficiency after intravenous heroin use (23[c]). *Rhabdomyolysis* was the likely cause of renal insufficiency in all cases. Twelve had a history of polydrug abuse and all had a history of intravenous diamorphine use in the 24 hours before presentation. Eight patients required renal dialysis for an average of 14 days. Patients who required dialysis had a higher admission creatine kinase, a higher peak creatine kinase, and a lower urine output in the initial 24 hours. They also had a longer hospital stay. Some had positive tests for hepatitis B (10%), hepatitis C (74%), and HIV (5%); viral infections can compound rhabdomyolysis and subsequent renal impairment through glomerulonephritis. No patient died and all patients recovered normal renal function. Rhabdomyolysis is a recognized cause of renal insufficiency, but its pathogenesis after heroin use is not fully understood.

In most of 19 renal specimens from autopsies of intravenous diamorphine users there was severe *lymphomonocytic glomerulonephritis* as a result of activation of the classical pathway of the complement binding system (24[C]). This could have been a result of diamorphine itself, adulterants, or active hepatitis B and/or C infection.

Musculoskeletal *Myopathy* has been attributed to heroin (25[A]).

A 36-year-old man developed progressive, painless stiffness of both knee joints over 3 months. It had started 4 weeks after he began to give himself heroin injections two to three times a day in alternate thigh muscles. He had a broad-based stiff gait, and he walked without bending his knees. Because of contractures of the quadriceps muscles, which were indurated, active and passive knee flexion was limited to an angle of 5–10 degrees. Electromyography of the right quadriceps muscle showed firm fibrous resistance to needling without insertional activity. Ultrasound showed a preserved but enlarged muscle structure and thickening of the connective tissue. A muscle biopsy showed variation in fiber size with scattered collection of atrophic fibers and perivascular and endomysial infiltrates comprised chiefly of lymphocytes and macrophages. The serum creatine kinase activity was normal. After 7 weeks of physiotherapy, MRI of the thighs showed severe fibrosis of the muscle, suggesting a possible inflammatory component. Following treatment with prednisone and D-penicillamine, he was entirely normal, except for slightly limited knee flexion on both sides.

This patient's main symptoms were progressive stiffness, due to contractures of the quadriceps muscles induced by chronic heroin injections. The findings made it very likely that heroin caused a primarily vascular lesion leading to non-specific inflammatory changes and subsequent fibrosis. Clinically, weakness was minimal and there was painless contracture. This presumably reflects the predominantly fibrotic process within muscle tissue. Combination therapy with prednisone and D-penicillamine led to significant improvement. The regenerating process was confirmed by the second muscle biopsy, and electromyography showed reinnervation. The second biopsy did not show inflammatory cells, indicating absence of the inflammatory component. Thus, this case suggests that heroin-induced fibrotic myopathy is reversible.

COCAINE *(SED-14, 106; SEDA-22, 31; SEDA-23, 37; SEDA-24, 37)*

Cardiovascular Cocaine users often present with complaints suggestive of *acute cardiac ischemia* (chest pain, dyspnea, syncope, dizziness, and palpitation). Two recent studies have shown that the risk of actual acute cardiac ischemia among cocaine users with such symptoms was low (26[CR], 27[C]). The first study reviewed the clinical database from the Acute Cardiac Ischemia–Time Insensitive Predictive Instrument Clinical Trial, a multicenter prospective clinical trial conducted in the USA in 1993 (26[CR]). Among 10 689 enrolled patients, 293 (2.7%) had cocaine-associated complaints. This rate varied from 0.3 to 8.4% in the 10 participating hospitals. Only six of these patients had a diagnosis of acute cardiac ischemia (2.0%), four with unstable angina and two with acute myocardial infarction. The cocaine users were admitted to the coronary care unit as often as other study participants (14% vs 18%), but were much less likely to have confirmed unstable angina (1.4% vs 9.3%).

A second study also suggested that cocaine users who present with chest pain have a very low risk of adverse cardiac events (27[C]). Emergency departments have instituted centers for the evaluation and treatment of patients with chest pain who are at low to moderate risk of acute coronary syndromes. In this particular study, patients with a history of coronary artery disease or presentations that included hemodynamic instability, electrocardiographic changes consistent with ischemia, or clinically unstable angina were directly admitted to hospital. In a retrospective study of 179 patients with reliable 30-day follow-up in chest pain centers, there was one cardiac complication due to cocaine.

Possible predictors of cardiovascular responses to smoked cocaine have been studied in 62 crack cocaine users (24 women and 38 men, aged 20–45 years) who used a single dose of smoked cocaine 0.4 mg/kg (28[C]). Physiological responses to smoked cocaine, such as changes in heart rate and blood pressure, were monitored. The findings suggested that higher baseline blood pressure and heart rate, a greater amount and frequency of current cocaine use, and current cocaine snorting predicted a reduced cardiovascular response to cocaine. By contrast, factors such as male sex, African–American race, higher bodyweight, and current marijuana use were associated with a greater cardiovascular response.

Vasculitis causing peripheral vascular disease in the arm has been attributed to cocaine (29[A]).

A 48-year-old man who smoked cigarettes and used cocaine developed ischemia of the right index finger due to occlusion of the distal ulnar artery. He had a history of recurrent deep vein thrombosis. A venous bypass graft was performed. Two years later he had non-healing gangrene of the left index finger. His blood pressure was normal in both arms. Urine toxicology was positive for cocaine. Angiography of the left arm showed small-vessel vasculitis.

A young man had an *ischemic stroke* after the combined use of cocaine and amphetamine (30[A]).

A previously healthy 16-year-old man developed an unsteady gait and double vision. His symptoms began 5 minutes after intranasal "amphetamine" (actually amphetamine cut with cocaine). He had a left-sided internuclear ophthalmoplegia, an incomplete fascicular paresis of the left oculomotor nerve, and saccadic vertical smooth pursuit. Cranial MRI showed a left-sided hyperintense lesion near the midline of the mesencephalon. A repeat MRI 9 days later showed that the lesion was much smaller. He made a full recovery within 3 weeks.

Respiratory Some of the pulmonary complications of crack cocaine, including *coughing*, *chest pain*, and *palpitation*, as well as *end-stage lung disease*, *eosinophilic infiltrates in the lungs*, *pulmonary infarction*, and *pneumothorax*, have been outlined in previous Annuals (SEDA-20, 21; SEDA-21, 25; SEDA-22, 31; SEDA-23, 37). Cocaine can also cause *exacerbation of the course of asthma*. All adult visits to an urban emergency room for an asthma attack during a 7-month period have been reviewed (31[C]). Of 163 patients (aged 18–55 years), 116 agreed to participate in a facilitated questionnaire and 103 provided urine samples for drug screening. African–Americans made up 89% of the group and 35% were cigarette smokers. Urine toxicology was positive for cocaine in 13% and for opiates in 5.8%. The severity of the exacerbation of asthma was greatest in the cocaine-positive group, 38% of whom were admitted to hospital (compared with 20% of the non-cocaine users). The length of stay was significantly longer in the cocaine-positive patients. Most of the patients did not use inhaled corticosteroids according to the treatment guidelines.

Nervous system The association of cocaine with cerebrovascular events, such as *transient ischemic attacks* (SEDA-24, 24) and *cerebral infarction* (SEDA-22, 23; SEDA-20, 26; SEDA-20, 21), has been documented. "Spontaneous" acute *subdural hematoma* related to cocaine abuse has been described for the first time (32[A]).

A 38-year-old man with a 10-year history of cocaine use became comatose. He had had an acute severe headache and progressive deterioration after abusing cocaine. His Glasgow Coma Scale was 3 and his pupils were dilated but reactive to light. He had hypertension and bradycardia. Routine toxicology was positive for cocaine. Blood tests, including coagulation profile, were normal. A CT scan of the brain showed a left acute subdural hematoma with midline shift and obliteration of the basal cisterns. During emergency craniotomy the source of the bleed was identified as a pinhole rupture of a parietal cortical artery. The patient had no history of head injury and there were no intraoperative findings of head injury. He died 24 hours later without evidence of clot reaccumulation. An autopsy was not performed.

Psychological The possible effect of cocaine on neuropsychological performance is an area of current research (SEDA-24, 25; SEDA-23, 21). Neurolinguistic functioning has been assessed in six African–American male cocaine abusers undergoing drug rehabilitation (33[c]). A test battery to assess language, cognition, and memory skills was administered at 1 week and 1 month of cocaine abstinence. Participants' performances were compared with the normative data for each test. There was *reduced ability for general language knowledge*, *memory*, and *verbal learning ability* during the period of early abstinence. The sample size was small and the duration of study short, and the authors suggested that more studies are needed in this area.

Psychiatric The possible genetic basis of cocaine-induced *paranoia* has been studied in 45 European Americans with cocaine dependency (34[c]). Low activity of the enzyme dopamine β-hydroxylase (DBH, the enzyme that catalyses the conversion of dopamine to noradrenaline) in the serum or cerebrospinal fluid was positively associated with the occurrence of positive psychotic symptoms in several psychiatric disorders. The activity of dopamine β-hydroxylase is a stable, genetically determined trait that is regulated by genes located at the DBH locus. The haplotype associated with low dopamine β-hydroxylase activity, Del-a, occurred more often in 29 subjects with cocaine-induced paranoia than in 16 without. These findings may have implications for the pharmacological treatment of cocaine dependence.

The rate of co-morbid conditions has been studied in 208 female African–American crack cocaine users, of whom 148 were in drug treatment and 54 were active crack users, and of whom 61% reported a history of sexual abuse (35[C]). Many had co-morbid depression (48%) and eating disorders (11%).

Endocrine Cocaine addiction is associated with *altered endocrine responses to hyperthermic stress* during abstinence (36[C]). In a prospective study, 10 male cocaine users (assessed after 4 weeks of abstinence and again after 1 year of abstinence) sat in a sauna for 30 minutes at a temperature of 90° F and a relative humidity of 10%. At the end of the sauna, they rested for another 30 minutes at room temperature. Sublingual temperature, pulse rate, and blood pressure were recorded just before and immediately after the sauna and 30 minutes after the period at room temperature. Venous β-erythropoietin, ACTH, metenkephalin, prolactin, and cortisol were also measured. There were no significant differences between the two groups in heart rate and blood pressure. At baseline and after 1 year of abstinence, plasma prolactin concentrations were higher in the cocaine users than in the controls. Moreover, the hormonal responses in cocaine users were different from those in controls. Concentrations of all the hormones, except for metenkephalin, were significantly lower in the cocaine users than in the controls at the end of the sauna; the cocaine users did not have significant hormonal changes to hyperthermia, after either 4 weeks or 1 year of abstinence. The authors concluded that cocaine abuse produces alterations in the hypothalamic–pituitary axis, which persist during abstinence.

Liver *Acute hepatitis* induced by intranasal cocaine, with transient increases in liver enzymes, has been reported in three HIV-positive patients (37[A]). All had non-active chronic viral hepatitis with normal immunologic status; one was seropositive for hepatitis B virus and two were positive for hepatitis C virus. A few days after intranasal cocaine use, serum aminotransferases rose to high values, and two of the patients had fever, stiffness, sweats, and hepatomegaly. Alcohol and hepatotoxic agents were ruled out. Within a few days, the clinical and laboratory signs of hepatitis improved in all three cases.

Fetotoxicity In a recent study, 158 cocaine-exposed (82 heavily and 76 lightly exposed) and 161 non-cocaine exposed infants were administered the Neurobehavioral Assessment at 43 weeks after conception (38[C]). Mediating factors (the timing and amount of drug exposure) and maternal psychological distress as a confounding factor were considered in the design and statistical analysis. The infants with heavy cocaine exposure had significantly more *jitteriness* and *attentional difficulties.* They were also more likely to be identified with an abnormality and less likely to cooperate with testing procedures than infants in the other groups. Higher concentrations of cocaine metabolites, cocaethylene and benzoylecgonine, were associated with a higher incidence of movement and tone abnormalities, jitteriness, and the presence of any abnormality. Higher cocaethylene concentrations were associated with attentional abnormalities; higher concentrations of meta-hydroxybenzoylecgonine were associated with jitteriness.

In another study cognitive, motor, and behavior development, as measured by the Mullen Scales of Early Learning and the Bayley Scales of Infant Development-II, were compared in 56 prenatally cocaine-exposed infants and toddlers (aged 1–3 years) and 56 non-exposed matched controls (39[C]). There were *developmental problems in expressive and receptive language areas* in those who had been exposed prenatally.

An infant born at 37 weeks gestation to a mother who had engaged in discontinuous cocaine abuse during the first and second trimesters of pregnancy had *microcrania* (below the 10th percentile), *a closed anterior fontanelle*, and *overlapping of all sutures* (40[A]). The infant was of *low birth weight* (2290 g; 25th percentile). There were *deep scalp rugae, a prominent occipital bone*, and normal hair pattern. MRI of the brain showed *enlargement of the lateral ventricles and pericerebral spaces, with severe reduction of the cerebral and cere-*

bellar parenchyma, and *white matter abnormalities*. These findings are part of the recognizable pattern of defects in the rare condition termed *fetal brain disruption sequence*. The presence of a normal hair pattern suggests normal brain development during the first 18 weeks of gestation. At a later stage partial destruction of the brain results in reduced intracranial pressure and subsequent collapse of the fetal skull.

Another unusual congenital malformation, the *cloverleaf skull*, has been associated with cocaine exposure in utero (41[A]). In this condition, the cranium is trilobed, with severe brain deformity and hydrocephalus, because of premature fusion of the coronal and lambdoid sutures.

A girl born by cesarean section at 38 weeks gestation weighed 3515 g and measured 54 cm in length. Cardiopulmonary resuscitation was performed. She had feeding and respiratory problems. Cranial sonography on day 11 showed a trilobed cranial mass with ventricular enlargement. She was discharged on day 35. The mother, a 24-year-old cocaine user, had engaged in active drug use in the 2 years before and during the first 2 months of pregnancy; she had also used alcohol (three units per day) and smoked marijuana (1–2 cigarettes per day) during the first 5 months, and she had smoked 10 cigarettes per day throughout the entire pregnancy. The father was a marijuana smoker. The infant failed to thrive (bodyweight at 6 months 3120 g, height 57 cm), developed sepsis, and died. Autopsy showed adrenal infarction secondary to systemic infection.

Drug overdose A case of fatal "crack" cocaine ingestion in an infant has been reported (42[A]).

A 10-month-old girl developed apnea, ventricular fibrillation, and a metabolic acidosis, and died shortly afterwards. Her 2-year-old brother had fed her "crack" cocaine. At autopsy the brain had a thinned corpus callosum, ranging in thickness from 0.2 to 0.5 cm. There were two pieces of "crack" cocaine in the duodenum and high concentrations of cocaine in the blood and other tissues.

The authors noted that the thinned corpus callosum suggested that the infant had been exposed to cocaine in utero or during the early postnatal period.

Body packing, the act of swallowing packets holding illegal drugs in order to hide the evidence from legal authorities, can cause symptoms of drug intoxication or overdose (SEDA-22, 44) (43[c]). In a recent analysis of all cases of cocaine body packers reported to a metropolitan poisons control center from January 1993 to May 1994, 34 of 46 patients were symptom-free. Eight patients had mild symptoms (hypertension and tachycardia) that resolved with decontamination (activated charcoal or whole body irrigation) or tranquilizers (one received benzodiazepines). Two had severe symptoms, including seizures and cardiac dysrhythmias, and both died.

CANNABINOIDS *(SED-14, 95; SEDA-23, 41; SEDA-24, 36)*

Although marijuana may be considered by drug-users to be relatively safe, reports of adverse outcomes associated with its use continue to appear.

Cardiovascular A sustained *cardiac dysrhythmia* has been attributed to marijuana (44[A]).

A 14-year-old African–American man with no cardiac history had palpitation and dizziness, resulting in a fall, within 1 hour of smoking marijuana. After vomiting several times he had a new sensation of skipped heartbeats. The only remarkable finding was a flow murmur. The electrocardiogram showed atrial fibrillation. Echocardiography was normal. Serum and urine toxicology showed cannabis. He was given digoxin, and about 12 hours later his cardiac rhythm converted to sinus rhythm. Digoxin was withdrawn. He abstained from marijuana over the next year and was symptom free.

The authors noted that marijuana's catecholaminergic properties can affect autonomic control, vasomotor reflexes, and conduction-enhancement of perinodal fibers in cardiac muscle, and thus lead to an event such as this.

Respiratory A possible role of marijuana use in the formation of large *lung bullae* has been discussed (45[A]). Four men who smoked both tobacco and marijuana developed large, multiple, bilateral, peripheral bullae at their lung apices, with normal parenchymal tissue elsewhere. While the pulmonary effects of long-term tobacco smoking are well documented, including the possible development of large emphysematous bullae and an uncommon type of bullous disease, similar effects from chronic marijuana use have not been described. While δ-9-tetrahydrocannabinol (the active component of marijuana) may not contribute directly to this finding, it is possible that the respiratory dynamics of smoking the drug may explain it. Typically, a draw on a marijuana "joint" has, on average, a depth of inspiration that is one-third greater, a volume two-thirds greater, and a breath-holding time four times longer than a draw on a cigarette. The marijuana "joint" lacks a filter tip, and the practice of smoking "leads to a 4-fold greater delivery of tar and a five times greater increase in carboxyhemoglobin per cigarette smoked" (46[C]). Smoking three to four "joints" of marijuana per day is reported to produce a symptom profile and damage to the respiratory airways similar to that caused by smoking 20 tobacco cigarettes daily.

Nervous system The effects of chronic marijuana smoking on human brain function and cognition have been further investigated (47[C]). Normalized regional brain blood flow and regional brain metabolism, measured using PET scanning with ^{15}O, were compared in 17 frequent marijuana users and 12 non-users. Testing was performed after at least 26 hours of monitored abstention in all subjects. Marijuana users had *hypoactivity or reduced brain blood flow* in a large region of the posterior cerebellum compared with controls. This is consistent with what was reported in the only previous PET study of chronic marijuana use (48[C]). The cerebellum is hypothesized to have input to aspects of cognition, specifically timing, the processing of sensory information, and attention and prediction of real-time events. Users often report that marijuana smoking is followed by alterations in the sense of time and less efficient cognitive processing.

Immunologic Marijuana, the pollen of the cannabis plant, and δ-9-tetrahydrocannabinol, the active ingredient of marijuana, can cause hypersensitivity reactions and skin test reactivity. A severe *allergic reaction* after intravenous marijuana has been reported (49[A]).

A 25-year-old man with intermittent methamphetamine use developed facial edema, pruritus and dyspnea 45 minutes after injecting a mixture of crushed marijuana leaves and heated water. He was anxious, and had tachypnea, respiratory stridor, wheezing, edema of the face and oral mucosa, and truncal urticaria. There was mild prerenal uremia and urine toxicology was positive for methamphetamine and marijuana. Skin testing was not done. With appropriate medical intervention there was resolution of symptoms within a day.

The authors noted that marijuana may have contaminants, including *Aspergillus*, *Salmonella*, herbicides, and mercury, which can trigger allergic reactions.

Fetotoxicity The effect of maternal and prenatal marijuana exposure on offspring from birth to adolescence is being investigated (50[C]). The Ottawa Prenatal Prospective Study (OPPS), a longitudinal project begun in 1978, recently reported its findings in 146 low-risk, middle-class children aged 9–12 years. Their performances on neurobehavioral tasks that focus on visuoperceptual abilities (ranging from basic skills to those requiring integration and cognitive manipulation of such skills) were analysed. Performance outcomes were different in children with prenatal exposure to cigarette smoking and those with prenatal exposure to marijuana. Maternal cigarette smoking affected fundamental visuoperceptual functioning. Prenatal marijuana use had a *negative effect on performance in visual problem solving*, which requires integration, analysis, and synthesis. In a second prospective study, the effects of prenatal marijuana exposure and child behavior problems were studied in 763 subjects aged 10 years (51[C]). Prenatal maternal marijuana exposure was associated with *increased hyperactivity*, *impulsivity*, and *inattention* in the children. There was also *increased delinquency* and *externalizing problems*. The authors suggested a possible pathway between prenatal marijuana exposure and delinquency, which may be mediated by the effects of marijuana exposure on symptoms of inattention.

REFERENCES

1. Buxton N, McConachie NS. Amphetamine abuse and intracranial hemorrhage. J R Soc Med 2000; 93: 472–7.
2. Williams K, Argyropoulos S, Nutt DJ. Amphetamine misuse and social phobia. Am J Psychiatry 2000; 157: 834–5.

3. Zhu B, Oritini S, Shimotouge K, Ishida K, Quan L, Fujita MQ, Ogawa M, Maeda H. Methamphetamine-related fatalities in forensic autopsy during 5 years in the southern half of Osaka city and surrounding areas. Forensic Sci Int 2000; 113: 443–7.
4. Ernst T, Chang L, Leonido-Yee M, Speck O. Evidence for long-term neurotoxicity associated with methamphetamine abuse: a ^{1}H MRS study. Neurology 2000; 54: 1344–9.
5. Domier CP, Simon SL, Rawson RA, Huber A, Ling W. A comparison of injecting and noninjecting methamphetamine users. J Psychoact Drugs 2000; 32: 229–32.
6. Richards JR, Brofeldt BT. Patterns of tooth wear associated with methamphetamine use. J Periodontol 2000; 71: 1371–4.
7. Banooni P, Rickman LS, Ward DM. Pott puffy tumor associated with intranasal methamphetamine. J Am Med Assoc 2000; 283: 1293.
8. Sribanditmongkol P, Chokjamsai M, Thampitak S. Methamphetamine overdose and fatality: 2 case reports. J Med Assoc Thailand 2000; 83: 1120–3.
9. Hales G, Roth N, Smith D. Possible fatal interaction between protease inhibitors and methamphetamine. Antiviral Ther 2000; 5: 19.
10. De la Torre R, Farre M, Ortuno J, Mas M, Brenneisen R, Roset PN, Segura J, Cami J. Non-linear pharmacokinetics of MDMA ('ecstasy') in humans. Br J Clin Pharmacol 2000; 49: 104–9.
11. Duflou J, Mark A. Aortic dissection after ingestion of 'ecstasy' (MDMA). Am J Forensic Med Pathol 2000; 21: 261–3.
12. Lester SJ, Baggott M, Welm S, Schiller NB, Jones RT, Foster E, Mendelson J. Cardiovascular effects of 3,4-methylenedioxymethamphetamine: a double-blind, placebo-controlled trial. Ann Intern Med 2000; 133: 969–73.
13. Schroeder B, Brieden S. Bilateral sixth nerve palsy associated with MDMA ('ecstasy') abuse. Am J Opthalmol 2000; 129: 408–9.
14. Gomez-Balaguer M, Pena H, Morillas C, Henandez A. Syndrome of inappropriate antidiuretic hormone secretion and "designer drugs" (ecstasy). J Pediatr Endocrinol Metab 2000; 13: 437–8.
15. Yates KM, O'Connor A, Horsley CAE. 'Herbal ecstasy': a case series of adverse reactions. NZ Med J 2000; 113: 315–17.
16. Hall W, Lynskey M, Degenhardt L. Trends in opiate-related deaths in the UK and Australia, 1985–1995. Drug Alcohol Depend 2000; 57: 247–54.
17. Heineman A. Iwersen-Bergmann S, Stein S, Schmoldt A, Puschel K. Methadone-related fatalities in Hamburg 1990–1999: implications for quality standards in maintenance treatment? Forensic Sci Int 2000; 113: 449–55.
18. Garrick TM, Sheedy D, Abernethy J, Hodda AE, Harper CG. Heroin-related deaths in Sydney, Australia. How common are they? Am J Addict 2000; 9: 172–8.
19. Cullen W, Bury G, Langton D. Experience of heroin overdose among drug users attending general practice. Br J Gen Pract 2000; 50: 546–9.
20. Christie B. Gangrene bug killed 35 heroin users. West J Med 2000; 173: 82–3.
21. Dettmeyer R, Schmidt P, Musshoff F, Dreisvogt C, Madea B. Pulmonary edema in fatal heroin overdoses: immunohistological investigations with IgE, collagen IV and laminin – no increase of defects of alveolar-capillary membranes. Forensic Sci Int 2000; 110: 87–96.
22. McCreary M, Emerman C, Hanna J, Simon J. Acute myelopathy following intranasal insufflation of heroin: a case report. Neurology 2000; 55: 316–17.
23. Rice EK, Isbel NM, Becker GJ, Atkins RC, McMahon LP. Heroin overdose and myoglobinuric acute renal failure. Clin Nephrol 2000; 54: 449–54.
24. Dettmeyer R, Stojenovski G, Modea B. Pathogenesis of heroin-associated glomerulonephritis. Correlation between the inflammatory activity and renal deposits of immunoglobulin and complement? Forensic Sci Int 2000; 113: 227–31.
25. Weber M, Diener HC, Voit T, Neuen-Jacob E. Focal myopathy induced by chronic heroin injection is reversible. Muscle Nerve 2000; 23: 274–7.
26. Feldman JA, Fish SS, Beshansky JR, Griffith JL. Acute cardiac ischemia in patients with cocaine-associated complaints: results of a multicenter trial. Ann Emerg Med 2000; 36: 469–76.
27. Kushman SO, Storrow AB, Liu T, Gibler WB. Cocaine-associated chest pain in a chest pain center. Am J Cardiol 2000; 85: 394–6.
28. Sofluoglu M, Nelson D, Dudish-Poulsen S, Lexau B, Pentel PR. Predictors of cardiovascular response to smoked cocaine in humans. Drug Alcohol Depend 2000; 57: 239–45.
29. Kumar PD, Smith HR. Cocaine-related vasculitis causing upper-limb peripheral vascular disease. Ann Intern Med 2000; 133: 923–4.
30. Strupp M, Hamann GF, Brandt T. Combined amphetamine and cocaine abuse caused mesencephalic ischemia in a 16-year-old boy – due to vasospasm? Eur Neurol 2000; 43: 181–2.
31. Rome LA, Lippmann ML, Dalsey WC, Taggart P. Prevalence of cocaine use and its impact on asthma exacerbation in an urban population. Chest 2000; 117: 1324–9.
32. Alves OL. Gomes O. Cocaine-related acute subdural hematoma: an emergent cause of cerebrovascular accident. Acta Neurochir 2000; 142: 819–21.
33. Butler LF, Frank EM. Neurolinguistic function and cocaine abuse. J Med Speech-Lang Path 2000; 8: 199–212.
34. Cubells JF, Kranzler HR, McCance-Katz, Anderson GM. A haplotype at the DBH locus, associated with low plasma dopamine beta-hydroxylase activity, also associates with cocaine-induced paranoia. Mol Psychiatry 2000; 5: 56–63.
35. Ross-Durow PL, Boyd CJ. Sexual abuse, depression, and eating disorders in African American

women who smoke cocaine. J Subst Abuse Treat 2000; 18: 79–81.
36. Vescovi PP. Cardiovascular and hormonal responses to hyperthermic stress in cocaine addicts after a long period of abstinence. Addict Biol 2000; 5: 91–5.
37. Peyriere H, Mauboussin J-M. Cocaine-induced acute cytologic hepatitis in HIV-infected patients with nonactive viral hepatitis. Ann Intern Med 2000; 132: 1010–11.
38. Singer LT, Arendt R, Minnes S, Farkas K. Neurobehavioral outcomes of cocaine-exposed infants. Neurotoxicol Teratol 2000; 22: 653–66.
39. Chapman JK. Developmental outcomes in two groups of infants and toddlers: prenatal cocaine exposed and noncocaine exposed part 1. Infant–Toddler Intervention 2000; 10: 19–36.
40. Bellini C, Massocco D, Serra G. Prenatal cocaine exposure and the expanding spectrum of brain malformations. Arch Intern Med 2000; 160: 2393.
41. Esmer MC, Rodriguez-Soto G, Carrasco-Daza D, Iracheta ML. Cloverleaf skull and multiple congenital anomalies in a girl exposed to cocaine in utero: case report and review of the literature. Child's Nerv Syst 2000; 16: 176–80.
42. Havlik DM, Nolte KB. Fatal "crack" cocaine ingestion in an infant. Am J Forensic Med Pathol 2000; 21: 245–8.
43. June R, Ask SE, Keys N, Wahl M. Medical outcome of cocaine bodystuffers. J Emerg Med 2000; 18: 221–4.
44. Singh GK. Atrial fibrillation associated with marijuana use. Pediatr Cardiol 2000; 21: 284.
45. Johnson MK, Smith RP, Morrison D, Laszlo G. Large lung bullae in marijuana smokers. Thorax 2000; 55: 340–2.
46. Wu TC, Tashkin DP, Djahed B, Rose JE. Pulmonary hazards of smoking marijuana as compared with tobacco. New Engl J Med 1988; 318: 347–51.
47. Block RI, O'Leary DS, Hichwa RD, Augustinack JC. Cerebellar hypoactivity in frequent marijuana users. Neuroreport 2000; 11: 749–53.
48. Volkow ND, Gillespie H, Mullani N, Tancredi L, Grant C, Valentine A, Hollister L. Brain glucose metabolism in chronic marijuana users at baseline and during marijuana intoxication. Psychiatry Res 1996; 67: 29–38.
49. Perez JA. Allergic reaction associated with intravenous marijuana use. J Emerg Med 2000; 18: 260–1.
50. Fried PA, Watkinson B. Visuoperceptual functioning differs in 9- to 12-year olds prenatally exposed to cigarettes and marihuana. Neurotoxicol Teratol 2000; 22: 11–20.
51. Goldschmidt L, Day NL, Richardson GA. Effects of prenatal marijuana exposure on child behavior problems at age 10. Neurotoxicol Teratol 2000; 22: 325–36.

Stephen Curran and Shabir Musa

5 Hypnosedatives and anxiolytics

Insomnia is a common and distressing condition caused by a range of physical, psychological and physiological factors. Painful disorders in particular are associated with insomnia, but other less obvious physical causes, e.g. Parkinson's disease (1[A]), vasospastic syndrome (2[A]), and hypothalamic–pituitary–adrenal axis abnormalities (3[A]), are important. Psychological disorders, including depression and anxiety, frequently cause sleep disturbance. It is essential that a thorough physical and psychological assessment is undertaken to identify specific causes, and treatments aimed at these will lead to improved sleep and often avoid the need for hypnotic medication. Other non-pharmacological treatments are also becoming increasingly important, including cognitive behavior (4[c]). Drugs such as tricyclic antidepressants have also been suggested, because of their sedative effects and low risk of dependence (5[c]), but they should be avoided because of their adverse effects profile, including cardiotoxicity. However, benzodiazepines continue to be widely used for the treatment of insomnia (6[M]).

BENZODIAZEPINES *(SED-14, 122; SEDA-22, 40; SEDA-23, 44; SEDA-24, 46)*

In a case-control study using the Systematic Assessment of Geriatric Drug Use via Epidemiology (SAGE) database, the records of 9752 patients hospitalized for fracture of the femur during the period 1992–6 were extracted and matched by age, sex, state, and index date to the records of 38 564 control patients (7[C]). Among older individuals, the use of benzodiazepines slightly increased the risk of *fracture of the femur*. Overall, non-oxidative benzodiazepines do not seem to confer a lower risk than oxidative agents. However, the latter may be more dangerous among very old individuals (85 years of age or older), especially if used in high dosages.

The role of different types of benzodiazepines in the risk of *falls* in a hospitalized geriatric population has been examined in a prospective study of 7908 patients, consecutively admitted to 58 clinical centers during 8 months (8[C]). Over 70% of the patients were older than 65 years, 50% were women, and 24% had a benzodiazepine prescription during the hospital stay. The findings suggested that benzodiazepines with short and very short half-lives form an important and independent risk factor for falls. Their prescription for older hospitalized patients should be carefully evaluated.

Alprazolam

Psychological Several case reports have suggested that treatment with alprazolam can result in *behavioral disinhibition* (9[C]). In one study covering the period January 1989 to June 1990, the medical records of 323 psychiatric in-patients treated with alprazolam, clonazepam, or no benzodiazepine were reviewed (10[C]). The frequency of behavioral disturbances were not significantly different in the different groups, suggesting that alprazolam does not have unique disinhibitory activity. In addition, the data suggested that disinhibition may not be an important clinical problem associated with benzodiazepine use. The study design did not allow the establishment of a relation between the prescription of the benzodiazepine and worsening behaviors, and the findings need to be interpreted conservatively, because it was a retrospective review of a heterogeneous population.

Drug interactions There have been two studies of the effects of repeated ingestion of *grapefruit juice* on the pharmacokinetics and

Side Effects of Drugs, Annual 25
J.K. Aronson, ed.

pharmacodynamics of both single and multiple oral doses of alprazolam in a total of 19 subjects (11[c]). Grapefruit juice altered neither the steady-state plasma concentration of alprazolam nor its clinical effects.

The inhibitory effect of *ritonavir* (a viral protease inhibitor) on the metabolism of alprazolam, a CYP3A-mediated reaction in humans, has been investigated in a double-blind study (12[c]). Ten subjects took alprazolam 1.0 mg concurrent with low-dose ritonavir (four doses of 200 mg) or placebo. Ritonavir reduced alprazolam clearance by 60%, prolonged its half-life and magnified benzodiazepine agonist effects, such as sedation and performance impairment.

The effect of *sertraline* on alprazolam metabolism has been studied in a randomized, double-blind, placebo-controlled study in 10 healthy volunteers (13[C]). Sertraline (50–150 mg/day) did not alter the single-dose kinetics or dynamics of alprazolam.

Bentazepam

Liver There have been three cases in which *chronic hepatocellular injury* developed with oral bentazepam (14[A]). These findings provide further evidence for the hepatotoxicity of bentazepam.

Clonazepam

Endocrine A 43-year-old man underwent an incomplete transcranial removal of a pituitary growth hormone-secreting macroadenoma (15[A]). His daily insulin dose was reduced from more than 300 to 104 units/day and he was given hydrocortisone and levothyroxine replacement therapy, together with lanreotide injections. A month after discharge, he was given high-dose clonazepam. Three months later, the clonazepam was withdrawn abruptly and he developed hypoglycemic coma. The author concluded that interruption of benzodiazepine treatment had caused *reduced growth hormone secretion and insulin requirements*.

Drug interactions In a randomized, double-blind, placebo-controlled, cross-over study in 13 subjects *sertraline* did not affect the pharmacokinetics or pharmacodynamics of clonazepam (16[C]).

Diazepam

Nervous system In an open study in 104 patients with acute stroke diazepam 10 mg bd for 3 days was well tolerated (17[C]).

In a multicenter double-blind study 310 patients with generalized anxiety disorder were treated for 6 weeks with abecarnil, diazepam, or placebo at mean daily doses of 12 mg of abecarnil or 22 mg of diazepam administered three times daily (18[C]). Major adverse events for both abecarnil and diazepam were *drowsiness*, *dizziness*, *fatigue*, and *coordination difficulties*.

Skin *Sweet's syndrome* has been attributed to diazepam (19[A]).

A 70-year-old white man, with no significant preceding medical history, developed an acute painful rash, a fever (38.4° C), and severe arthralgia. Five days before he had taken diazepam 10 mg bd for lumbar muscular contracture due to hard physical exercise. He had taken no other medications. There were well-defined purple-red skin plaques, surmounted by vesicular and hemorrhagic blisters. He had a leukocytosis. Sweet's syndrome was confirmed by punch biopsy of a lesion. Diazepam was withdrawn, and prednisolone 30 mg/day was given for 2 weeks and then tapered. The patient improved quickly and the eruption cleared in 10 days.

Fetotoxicity Diazepam has been reported to cause *inappropriate ADH secretion* in a neonate (20[A]).

A female infant was delivered vaginally at 41 weeks. Her 30-year-old mother had taken diazepam for epilepsy and hysterical attacks throughout the pregnancy. The pregnancy and delivery were uneventful. The baby was admitted to the neonatal ward in anticipation of neonatal drug withdrawal syndrome. On the first day of life, milk feeding was stopped because of poor sucking, vomiting, and increased gastric aspirate volume. On the same day oliguria was reported and the urine osmolality was increased. Secretion of antidiuretic hormone was suspected as the cause of the oliguria, and so fluid intake was restricted and a diuretic was given. Subsequently the urine output increased and the urine osmolality gradually fell. The patient's condition became stable and she was discharged on day 16.

Flunitrazepam

Psychiatric A 69-year-old man developed acute benzodiazepine withdrawal delirium after a short course of flunitrazepam following an acute exacerbation of chronic obstructive pulmonary disease (21[A]). He was not an alcohol- or drug-abuser and he had not previously been taken benzodiazepines. Six days after withdrawal of flunitrazepam he became *agitated and confused*, and had *visual hallucinations*, *disorganized thinking*, *insomnia*, *increased psychomotor activity*, *disorientation in time and place*, and *memory impairment*. *Tachycardia* and significant *anxiety* were also noted. He fulfilled the criteria for DSM IV withdrawal syndrome and delirium, and had spontaneous relief of symptoms within 48 hours.

Triazolam

Drug interactions The inhibitory effect of *ritonavir* on the biotransformation of triazolam and zolpidem has been investigated (22[C]). Short-term low-dose ritonavir produced a large and significant impairment of triazolam clearance and enhancement of its clinical effects. In contrast, ritonavir produced small and clinically unimportant reductions in zolpidem clearance. The findings are consistent with the complete dependence of triazolam clearance on CYP3A activity, compared with the partial dependence of zolpidem clearance on CYP3A.

In a randomized, four-phase, cross-over study, the effect of *grapefruit juice* on the metabolism of triazolam interaction was investigated. Even one glass of grapefruit juice increased plasma triazolam concentrations and chronic consumption produced a significantly greater increase. The half-life of triazolam is prolonged by repeated consumption of grapefruit juice, probably due to inhibition of hepatic CYP3A4 activity (23[c]).

OTHER HYPNOSEDATIVES AND ANXIOLYTICS *(SEDA-14, 133; SEDA-22, 42; SEDA-23, 46; SEDA-24, 49)*

Clomethiazole

Nervous system A placebo-controlled trial of clomethiazole (75 mg/kg by 24-hour intravenous infusion) has been undertaken in 95 patients with hemorrhagic stroke (24[C]). Mortality at 90 days was 19% in the clomethiazole group and 23% in the placebo group. *Sedation* was the most common adverse event (clomethiazole 53%, placebo 17%), followed by *rhinitis* and *coughing*. The incidence and pattern of serious adverse events was similar between the groups. The authors concluded that clomethiazole is safe to use in patients with hemorrhagic stroke.

A recent case report has illustrated the dangers of driving a motor vehicle whilst taking clomethiazole (25[A]).

A 53-year-old male car driver was followed by the police for about 2 km, while he drove in an unsafe manner, until the car crashed into the owner's garage. Analysis of his blood showed a clomethiazole concentration of 3.3 μg/ml. Neither alcohol nor any other drug could be detected. One day later he committed suicide by swallowing at least 60 capsules of clomethiazole.

Chloral hydrate

Gastrointestinal *Pneumatosis cystoides coli* has been attributed to long-term chloral hydrate (26[A]).

A 69-year-old man had daily loose stools with mucous discharge. Repeated stool cultures were negative. Histology confirmed the appearances of pneumatosis cystoides coli. Various treatments had little effect on his symptoms. He had taken chloral hydrate for insomnia for 10 years. Subjectively, his symptoms were worse while taking the drug and resolved after withdrawal. With his consent, an unblinded controlled challenge with chloral hydrate was performed. The results, recorded meticulously in a symptoms diary, were dramatic. Before chloral hydrate, his bowels opened 18 times per week and only two motions contained mucus. After one tablet of chloral hydrate on days 1, 2, 5, and 7 he passed 49 stools in 1 week, 35 containing mucus. Two weeks later his bowel habit had returned to normal, with 15 movements per week, and only one stool contained mucus. Subsequently his bowel frequency fell to 8–10 times per week with considerable colonoscopic improvement.

Lesopitron

Lesopitron is a non-benzodiazepine anxiolytic drug. Its structure is similar to that of buspirone, and it is an agonist at central serotonin ($5\text{-}HT_{1A}$) receptors. A 6-week, double-blind, randomized, parallel, phase II, single-center, outpatient study has been performed to study the efficacy and safety of lesopitron 40–80 mg/day compared with lorazepam 2–4 mg/day and placebo in 161 patients with generalized anxiety disorder (27[C]). The most common adverse events with lesopitron were *somnolence*, *head-*

ache, and *dyspepsia*, compared with headache, somnolence, and insomnia with lorazepam. Patients treated with placebo mainly experienced headache, somnolence, and pharyngitis.

Zolpidem

Psychiatric *Delirium* has been attributed to zolpidem (28[A])

A 26-year-old woman was treated at a psychiatric in-patient unit for psychotic depression. She had no formal thought disorder and no perceptual disturbances and was cognitively intact. Ten days later she was stabilized on fluoxetine, risperidone, and benzatropine. She then developed flu-like symptoms, and 3 days later took zolpidem 10 mg to help her to sleep. After 30 minutes she was found agitated, confused, and rambling, and wanted to go to the beach. Her speech was disorganized and she had visual hallucinations. Her gait was ataxic. There were no signs of meningeal irritation. Her temperature was 37.3° C, her pulse 114 beats/min, and her blood pressure 116/78 mmHg. When she was evaluated the next morning, her delirium had cleared and she made a full recovery.

Drug abuse A literature review has been undertaken to evaluate the abuse potential of zolpidem (29[R]). To date, 15 cases of abuse or dependence have been published. In six patients, the abuse was secondary to other forms of abuse or dependence. The authors concluded that the abuse potential of zolpidem is much less than with other hypnotics and that it is also a relatively safe drug compared with conventional hypnotics. Patients with a history of other substance abuse may be considered as being at risk of later abuse of zolpidem.

Four cases of former drug or alcohol abusers with personality disorders have been described; all developed dependence while taking high doses of zolpidem (30[A]).

Withdrawal-induced *seizures* have been described in a woman taking various benzodiazepines and zolpidem (31[A]).

A 43-year-old woman had had insomnia since she was a child. At the age of 15 benzodiazepine therapy improved her sleeping, but when she gradually stopped taking benzodiazepines the insomnia returned after a few days. At the age of 26 she was abusing several benzodiazepines, including diazepam and flunitrazepam. At the age of 30 she was taking high doses of bromazepam every evening before going to sleep. After 1 month, she abruptly stopped taking bromazepam and during withdrawal had an epileptic seizure. During the next few years, she had periods of relative well-being, but also two further periods of benzodiazepine abuse, both resulting in seizures after withdrawal. Finally, a physician prescribed zolpidem. Two months later she increased the dose to 450–600 mg/day. After another month of abuse, she was forced by an unexpected event to discontinue the zolpidem and 4 hours later had an epileptic seizure, similar to the previous ones. She started taking zolpidem again, the drug abuse continued, and her fits settled. Six months later she underwent a planned program of zolpidem withdrawal.

Zaleplon

Nervous system Zaleplon is a pyrazolopyrimidine, non-benzodiazepine hypnotic, which is indicated for short-term management of insomnia. The pharmacokinetics and pharmacodynamics of zaleplon (10 or 20 mg) and zolpidem (10 or 20 mg) have been investigated in a randomized, double-blind, cross-over, placebo-controlled study in 10 healthy volunteers with no history of sleep disorder (32[C]). The half-life of zaleplon was significantly shorter than that of zolpidem. Zaleplon produced less sedation than zolpidem at the two doses studied, and the sedation scores in the zaleplon groups returned to baseline sooner than in the zolpidem groups. Zaleplon had no effect on recent or remote recall, whereas zolpidem had a significant effect on both measures.

Zaleplon and triazolam have been compared in two concurrent multicenter, randomized, double-blind, placebo-controlled crossover studies in chronic insomniacs (33[C]). Study 1 compared zaleplon (10 and 40 mg) with triazolam (0.25 mg) and placebo; study 2 compared zaleplon (20 and 60 mg) with triazolam (0.25 mg) and placebo. All doses of zaleplon produced significant reductions in sleep latency, and triazolam 0.25 mg reduced sleep latency comparable with zaleplon 10 mg. Only triazolam and zaleplon 60 mg produced significant increases in total sleep time compared with placebo. Zaleplon 40 and 60 mg and triazolam also reduced the percentage of REM sleep compared with placebo. There was no evidence of residual daytime impairment with zaleplon, but triazolam produced significant impairment in performance on a digit copying test. There were more adverse events with zaleplon 60 mg compared with triazolam 0.25 and placebo. The most frequently reported adverse events with all treatments included *headache*, *dizziness*, and *somnolence*.

Three doses of zaleplon have been compared with placebo in out-patients with insomnia in a 4-week study (34[C]). During week 1, sleep latency was significantly shorter with zaleplon 5, 10, and 20 mg compared with placebo. The significant reduction in sleep latency persisted to week 3 with zaleplon 10 mg and to week 4 with zaleplon 20 mg. Compared with placebo, zaleplon 10 mg and 20 mg also had significant positive effects on sleep duration, number of awakenings, and sleep quality. Pharmacological tolerance did not develop with zaleplon and there were no indications of rebound insomnia or withdrawal symptoms after discontinuation. There was no significant difference in the frequency of adverse events with zaleplon compared with placebo. The authors concluded that zaleplon provides effective treatment of insomnia with a favorable safety profile.

Drug interactions The interaction of zaleplon with *ibuprofen* has been investigated in 17 subjects (35[C]). Healthy adult volunteers were given zaleplon 10 mg alone, ibuprofen 600 mg alone, or zaleplon 10 mg plus ibuprofen 600 mg in an open-label, randomized, crossover study. The adverse effects were mild and resolved without intervention. The authors concluded that there was no evidence of a significant interaction between zaleplon and ibuprofen.

The interaction of zaleplon with *digoxin* has been investigated in 20 subjects (36[C]). There were one or more adverse effects in 18% of those who took digoxin alone and 35% of those who took digoxin plus zaleplon, but these were all mild and resolved quickly. Zaleplon had no significant effects on selected pharmacokinetic and pharmacodynamic properties of digoxin.

REFERENCES

1. Larsen JP, Tandberg E. Sleep disorders in patients with Parkinson's disease; epidemiology and management. CNS Drugs 2001; 15: 267–75.
2. Pache M, Krauch, K, Cajochen C, Wirz-Justice A, Dubler B, Kaiser HJ. Cold feet and prolonged sleep-onset latency in vasospastic syndrome. Lancet 2001; 358: 125–6.
3. Vgontzas AN, Bixler EO, Lin HM, Prolo P, Mastorakos G, Vela-Bukales A, Chrousos GP. Chronic insomnia is associated with nyctohemeral activation of the hypothalamic–pituitary–adrenal axis; clinical implications. J Clin Endocrinol Metab 2001; 86: 3787–94.
4. Edinger JD, Wohlgemuth WK, Radtke RA, Marsh GR, Quillian RI. Does cognitive–behavioural insomnia therapy alter dysfunctional beliefs about sleep? Sleep 2001; 24: 591–9.
5. Hajak G, Rodenbeck A, Voderholzer U, Riemann D, Cohrs S, Hoha-Berger M, Ruther E. Doxepin in the treatment of primary insomnia; a placebo-controlled, double-blind, polysomnographic study. J Clin Psychiatry 2001; 62: 453–63.
6. Holbrook A, Crowther R, Lotter A, Endeshaw Y. The role of benzodiazepines in the treatment of insomnia: meta-analysis of benzodiazepine use in the treatment of insomnia. J Am Geriatr Soc 2001; 49: 824–6.
7. Sgadari A, Lapane KL, Mor V, Landi F, Bernabei R, Gambassi G. Oxidative and nonoxidative benzodiazepines and the risk of femur fracture. J Clin Psychopharmacol 2000; 20: 234–9.
8. Passaro A, Volpato S, Romagnoni F, Manzoli N, Zuliani G, Fellin R. Benzodiazepines with different half-life and falling in a hospitalized population: the GIFA study. J Clin Epidemiol 2000; 53: 1222–9.
9. Cowdrey RW, Gardener DL. Pharmacotherapy of borderline personality disorders. Arch Gen Psychiatry 1988; 45: 111–20.
10. Rothschild AJ, Shindul-Rothschild JA, Viguera A, Murray M, Brewster S. Comparison of the frequency of behavioral disinhibition on alprazolam, clonazepam, or no benzodiazepine in hospitalized psychiatric patients. J Clin Psychopharmacol 2000; 20: 7–11.
11. Yasui N, Kondo T, Furukori H, Kaneko S, Ohkubo T, Uno T, Osanai T, Sugawara K, Otani K. Effects of repeated ingestion of grapefruit juice on the single and multiple oral-dose pharmacokinetics and pharmacodynamics of alprazolam. Psychopharmacology 2000; 150: 185–90.
12. Greenblatt DJ, Von Moltke LL, Harmatz JS, Durol ALB, Daily JP, Graf JA, Mertzanis P, Hoffman, JL, Shader RI. Alprazolam–ritonavir interaction: implications for product labeling. Clin Pharmacol Ther 2000; 67: 335–41.
13. Hassan PC, Sproule BA, Naranjo CA, Herrmann N. Dose-response evaluation of the interaction between sertraline and alprazolam in vivo. J Clin Psychopharmacol 2000; 20: 150–8.
14. Andrade RJ, Lucena MI, Aguilar J, Lazo MD, Camargo R, Moreno P, Garcia-Escano MDP, Marquez A, Alcantara R, Alcain G. Chronic liver injury related to use of bentazepam: an unusual instance of benzodiazepine hepatotoxicity. Dig Dis Sci 2000; 45: 1400–4.
15. Shuster J. Benzodiazepines and glucose control; mycophenolate mofetil-induced dyshidrotic eczema; concomitant use of bupropion and amantadine causes neurotoxicity; intra-articular steroids and acute adrenal crisis. Hosp Pharm 2000; 35: 489–91.
16. Bonate PL, Kroboth PD, Smith RB, Suarez

E, Oo C. Clonazepam and sertraline: absence of drug interaction in a multiple-dose study. J Clin Psychopharmacol 2000; 20: 19–27.
17. Lodder J, Luijckx GJ, Van Raak L, Kessels F. Diazepam treatment to increase the cerebral GABAergic activity in acute stroke: a feasibility study in 104 patients. Cerebrovasc Dis 2000; 10: 437–40.
18. Rickels K, DeMartinis N, Aufdembrinke B. A double-blind, placebo-controlled trial of abecarnil and diazepam in the treatment of patients with generalized anxiety disorder. J Clin Psychopharmacol 2000; 20: 12–18.
19. Guimera FJ, Garcia-Bustinduy M, Noda A, Saez M, Dorta S, Sanchez R, Martin-Herrera A, Garcia-Montelongo R. Diazepam-associated Sweet's syndrome. Int J Dermatol 2000; 39: 795–8.
20. Nako Y, Tachibana A, Harigaya A, Tomomasa T, Morikawa A. Syndrome of inappropriate secretion of antidiuretic hormone complicating neonatal diazepam withdrawal. Acta Paediatr 2000; 89: 488–9.
21. Diehl, J-L, Guillibert E, Guerot E, Kimounn E, Labrousse J. Acute benzodiazepine withdrawal delirium after a short course of flunitrazepam in an intensive care patient. Ann Med Interne 2000; 151 Suppl A: A44–6.
22. Greenblatt DJ, Von Moltke LL, Harmatz JS, Durol ALB, Daily JP, Graf JA, Mertzanis P, Hoffman JL, Shader RI. Differential impairment of triazolam and zolpidem clearance by ritonavir. J Acquired Immune Defic Syndr 2000; 24: 129–36.
23. Lilja JJ, Kivisto KT, Backman JT, Neuvonen PJ. Effect of grapefruit juice dose on grapefruit juice-triazolam interaction: repeated consumption prolongs triazolam half-life. Eur J Clin Pharmacol 2000; 56: 411–15.
24. Wahlgren NG, Diez-Tejedor E, Teitelbaum J, Arboix A, Leys D, Ashwood T, Grossman E. Results in 95 haemorrhagic stroke patients included in CLASS, a controlled trial of clomethiazole versus placebo in acute stroke patients. Stroke 2000; 31: 82–5.
25. Logemann E. Risks for driving under the influence of clomethiazole. Probl Forens Sci 2000; XLIII: 144–7.
26. Shand AG, Penman ID, Ghosh S. Effects of a controlled challenge of chloral hydrate in pneumatosis cystoides coli – further evidence of a causal link? Am J Gastroenterol 2000; 95: 3654–5.
27. Fresquet A, Sust M, Lloret A, Murphy MF, Carter FJ, Campbell GM, Marion-Landais G. Efficacy and safety of lesopitron in outpatients with generalized anxiety disorder. Ann Pharmacother 2000; 34: 147–53.
28. Freudenreich O, Menza M. Zolpidem-related delirium: a case report. J Clin Psychiatry 2000; 61: 449–50.
29. Soyka M, Bottlender R, Möller H-J. Epidemiological evidence for a low abuse potential of zolpidem. Pharmacopsychiatry 2000; 33: 138–41.
30. Vartzopoulos D, Bozikas V, Phocas C, Karavatos A, Kaprinis G. Dependence on zolpidem in high dose. Int Clin Psychopharmacol 2000; 15: 181–2.
31. Aragona M. Abuse, dependence, and epileptic seizures after zolpidem withdrawal: review and case report. Clin Neuropharmacol 2000; 23: 281–3.
32. Drover D, Lemmens H, Naidu S, Cevallos W, Darwish M, Stanski D. Pharmacokinetics, pharmacodynamics, and relative pharmacokinetic/pharmacodynamic profiles of zaleplon and zolpidem. Clin Ther 2000; 22: 1443–61.
33. Drake CL, Roehrs TA, Mangano RM, Roth T. Dose-response effects of zaleplon as compared with triazolam 0.25 mg and placebo in chronic primary insomnia. Hum Psychopharmacol 2000; 15: 595–604.
34. Fry J, Scharf M, Mangano R, Fujimori M. Zaleplon improves sleep without producing rebound effects in outpatients with insomnia. Int Clin Psychopharmacol 2000; 15: 141–52.
35. Garcia PS, Carcas A, Zapater P, Rosendo J, Paty I, Leister CA, Troy SM. Absence of an interaction between ibuprofen and zaleplon. Am J Health-Syst Pharmacol 2000; 57: 1137–41.
36. Garcia PS, Paty I, Leister CA, Guerra P, Frias, J, Perez LEG, Darwish M. Effect of zaleplon on digoxin pharmacokinetics and pharmacodynamics. Am J Health-Syst Pharmacol 2000; 57: 2267–70.

Alfonso Carvajal and Luis H. Martín Arias

6 Antipsychotic drugs

Comparing antipsychotic drugs

Typical versus atypical drugs *There is no clear evidence that atypical antipsychotic drugs are more effective or better tolerated than conventional antipsychotic drugs; conventional antipsychotic drugs should therefore usually be used in the initial treatment of schizophrenia, unless the patient has previously not responded to these drugs or has unacceptable extrapyramidal adverse effects. This has been concluded from a meta-analysis of 52 randomized comparisons of atypical antipsychotic drugs with conventional antipsychotic drugs (12 649 patients) or alternative atypical antipsychotic drugs (1[M]). After correction for the higher than recommended doses of conventional antipsychotic drugs that are used in some trials, there was a modest advantage of atypical antipsychotic drugs in terms of extrapyramidal adverse effects, but the differences in efficacy and overall tolerability disappeared, suggesting that many of the perceived benefits of atypical antipsychotic drugs are really due to excessive doses of the comparator drugs used in trials.*

When compared with typical antipsychotic drugs, risperidone may be more acceptable to those with schizophrenia and have marginal benefits in terms of limited clinical improvement and adverse effects profile. The superiority of risperidone in these respects may have been overestimated, owing to possible publication bias in favor of risperidone. Any marginal benefit has to be balanced against the greater cost of risperidone and its increased tendency to cause other adverse effects, such as weight gain. Similar conclusions arose from an independent cross-sectional survey, not sponsored by the pharmaceutical industry, in schizophrenic out-patients clinically stabilized on an antipsychotic drug for a period of 6 months: quality-of-life measures and Global Assessment of Functioning did not show any significant differences between the conventional antipsychotic drugs (n = 44) and the novel ones (risperidone, n = 50; olanzapine, n = 48; quetiapine, n = 42; clozapine, n = 46) (2[C]).

Several reviews of atypical antipsychotic drugs have appeared, but have not added anything new (3[R], 4[R]). Both types of antipsychotic drugs have serious shortcomings, particularly their adverse effects on the extrapyramidal and endocrine systems. A prospective 6-month open study, promoted by Lilly, the market authorization holder of olanzapine, has been conducted, in which olanzapine (n = 2128), risperidone (n = 417), and haloperidol (n = 112) were compared (5[C]). Age, sex, and duration of disease did not differ among the groups. The initial and overall mean daily doses were respectively: olanzapine 12.2 and 13.0 mg; risperidone 5.2 and 5.4 mg; haloperidol 13.9 and 13.6 mg. The improvements were similar in the three groups. A lower proportion of patients taking olanzapine had extrapyramidal symptoms (37%) compared with risperidone (50%) and haloperidol (76%). Weight gain was significantly more common with olanzapine (6.9%) than risperidone (1.9%) or haloperidol (0.9%).

Since atypical antipsychotic drugs have been said to have fewer adverse effects than typical drugs in schizophrenic patients, adverse effects have been studied in people with mental retardation treated with atypical antipsychotic drugs (n = 17), typical antipsychotic drugs (n = 17), or no drugs (n = 17) (6[c]). The patients taking atypical antipsychotic drugs did not have different overall adverse events from those taking no medications, and both had significantly fewer overall adverse effects than those taking typical antipsychotic drugs. However, the study had some important flaws: patients taking typical antipsychotic drugs were on average 7 years older than those taking atypical drugs;

Side Effects of Drugs, Annual 25
J.K. Aronson, ed.

they had also taken medication for longer and had more stereotypic movement disorders at baseline. This jeopardizes the conclusions.

The global efficacy of olanzapine was not substantially different from that of haloperidol in two of three comparative trials involving 2500 patients, according to a comprehensive review of the safety and efficacy of olanzapine; in addition, the only relevant comparative trial failed to demonstrate superiority of olanzapine over risperidone (7[R]). Olanzapine has fewer adverse neurological effects than haloperidol, but there is no evidence that it differs from other recent neuroleptic drugs in this respect.

A 6-week, multicenter, double-blind, randomized comparison of quetiapine (mean dose 455 mg/day) and haloperidol (8 mg/day) has been carried out in 448 schizophrenic patients (8[C]). At day 42, the total score on the Positive and Negative Symptom Scale (PNSS) was equally reduced in the two groups. There were 69 withdrawals among the 221 patients who took quetiapine and 80 among the 227 who took haloperidol. Of the patients who took quetiapine, 154 (70%) had one or more spontaneously reported adverse events, whereas 171 (75%) of the haloperidol-treated patients reported adverse events. Motor and extrapyramidal effects were much more frequent among haloperidol users. In the quetiapine group the most common adverse events were somnolence (20%), insomnia (13%), and dry mouth (10%); in the haloperidol group the most frequent adverse events were akathisia (20%), insomnia (15%), and hypertonia (13%). The overall mean weight gain was 1.9 kg in those who took quetiapine and 0.3 kg in those who took haloperidol. With quetiapine, there was a fall in prolactin concentration from baseline by more than 16 μg/l and with haloperidol a rise of just under 6 μg/l during the same period. There was one death from acute heart failure in the haloperidol group.

Another similarly designed comparison of quetiapine and haloperidol in schizophrenic patients with a partial response to other antipsychotic drugs gave similar results (9[C]). Patients with a history of partial response to conventional antipsychotic drugs and who displayed a partial or no response to fluphenazine (20 mg/day) for 1 month were randomly allocated to haloperidol 20 mg/day (n = 145) or quetiapine 600 mg/day (n = 143). At 8 weeks the total score on the Positive and Negative Symptom Scale was reduced to the same extent in the two groups. Similar numbers of patients withdrew during the randomized phase of the trial in the quetiapine (n = 32) and haloperidol (n = 28) treatment arms. The proportions of patients who were taking anticholinergic drugs at the end of the study were 44% and 60% for quetiapine and haloperidol respectively. The most frequently reported adverse events with quetiapine were somnolence (9.8%), postural hypotension/dizziness (7.7%), dry mouth (5.6%), increased muscle tone (5.6%), and akathisia (5.6%). In contrast, the most common adverse events with haloperidol were related to extrapyramidal signs: tremor (12%), akathisia (9.0%), hypertonia (6.9%), extrapyramidal syndrome (6.3%), and insomnia (6.2%). The mean increase in bodyweight was 1.4 kg with quetiapine and 0.7 kg with haloperidol.

Tiapride has been assessed for the treatment of agitation and aggressiveness in elderly patients with cognitive impairment in a multicenter, double-blind study, in which patients were randomly allocated to tiapride 100 mg/day (n = 102), haloperidol 2 mg/day (n = 101), or placebo (n = 103) (10[C]). The percentage of responders after 21 days, according to the Multidimensional Observation Scale for Elderly Subjects (MOSES) irritability/aggressiveness subscale, was significantly greater in both of the active treatment groups (haloperidol 63%, tiapride 69%) than in the placebo group (49%). The numbers of dropouts were 10 in the tiapride group, 21 in the haloperidol group, and 16 in the placebo group. The number of patients with at least one extrapyramidal symptom was significantly smaller with tiapride (16%) than haloperidol (34%) and identical to that with placebo group (17%); there was no significant difference across the groups in the numbers of patients with endocrinological adverse events. Four deaths were reported: one with placebo (stroke), one with tiapride (pneumonia), and two with haloperidol (stroke and heart failure).

Intramuscular ziprasidone has recently been compared with intramuscular haloperidol in the treatment of acute psychosis for a very short period (11[C]). Patients were randomly allocated to intramuscular ziprasidone for up to 3 days of flexible dosing (n = 90; last oral daily dose 91 mg) or haloperidol (n = 42; last oral daily dose 14 mg) followed by oral treatment to day 7. Mean reductions from baseline in all efficacy variables were significantly greater with ziprasidone than with haloperidol at the end of the study. The percentage of patients who had any adverse event was lower with ziprasidone (46%) than haloperidol (60%); most of the adverse effects were mild or moderate. Four patients discontinued ziprasidone owing to adverse events compared with one in the haloperidol group.

In a trial funded by Knoll Pharmaceuticals, the market authorization holder, zotepine was compared with chlorpromazine and placebo (12[C]). Patients with exacerbation of schizophrenia were randomly allocated to zotepine 150–300 mg/day (n = 53), chlorpromazine 300–600 mg/day (n = 53), or placebo (n = 53) for 8 weeks. Mean Brief Psychiatric Rating Scale (BPRS) scores improved statistically significantly more with zotepine than chlorpromazine or placebo. During the study, 14 patients reported extrapyramidal symptoms, five taking zotepine, four taking chlorpromazine, and five taking placebo. In all, 99 patients (zotepine 43; chlorpromazine 33; placebo 23) reported a total of 257 adverse events (zotepine 120; chlorpromazine 85; placebo 52) during the study. The mean weight reduction with placebo (1.4 kg) was significantly different from the mean weight gain with zotepine (2.4 kg) and chlorpromazine (1.4 kg). Two patients (one taking zotepine, one taking chlorpromazine) with suspected myocardial infarction required hospitalization, but both subsequently recovered.

Case series and reviews have suggested superior effectiveness of zuclopenthixol acetate in the acute management of disturbed behavior caused by serious mental illness. However, this seems not to have been supported by the evidence from an analysis of randomized controlled trials (13[M]). A meta-analysis of five randomized comparisons of zuclopenthixol acetate with other neuroleptic drugs in patients with considerable behavioral disturbance showed that in all studies there was some improvement in mental state scores (BPRS; CGI), but none showed statistically significant differences between zuclopenthixol acetate and "standard treatment". In three studies there was more sedation in those who took zuclopenthixol acetate than in those allocated to haloperidol. With regard to adverse effects, the studies were not homogeneous: one study showed that people who took zuclopenthixol acetate were more likely to need antiparkinsonian drugs (OR = 6.4; CI = 1.5–17); other studies did not show any differences in this particular outcome.

Comparing different atypical drugs There have been some interesting systematic reviews from the Cochrane Collaboration (www.cochrane.org.uk). Head-to-head comparisons of atypical antipsychotic drugs in non-treatment-resistant schizophrenia have been carried out. For instance, olanzapine and risperidone seem to be broadly similar, according to the numbers of patients who respond to treatment (40% reduction in Positive and Negative Syndrome Scale (PANSS) scores: n = 339, RR = 1.14, 95% CI = 0.99, 1.32). Olanzapine caused fewer people to withdraw early (n = 404, RR = 1.31, 95% CI = 1.06, 1.60; NNT = 8, 95% CI = 4, 32) and caused fewer extrapyramidal adverse effects (n = 339, RR = 1.67, 95% CI = 1.14, 2.46; NNH = 8, 95% CI = 5, 33), although comparative doses of risperidone were higher than those recommended in practice.

The benefits of the atypical antipsychotic drugs in patients with bipolar disorder and the possibility that risperidone, quetiapine, olanzapine, and clozapine caused tardive dyskinesia have been studied (14[c]), and there has been a retrospective comparison of clozapine (5 trials), risperidone (25 trials), and olanzapine (20 trials) using data from consecutive treatment trials in the Massachusetts General Hospital (15[c]). The overall results suggested equivalent efficacy of the novel antipsychotic drugs according to changes in Clinical Global Impressions Scale scores. Extrapyramidal symptoms occurred in about 29% of cases in all groups. There were no prolactin-related adverse effects. Substantial weight gain of more than 4.5 kg was significantly more frequent in patients taking olanzapine.

Clozapine and risperidone have also been compared in 10 patients with psychosis in Parkinson's disease, who were randomized to risperidone or clozapine for 12 weeks (16[C]). The mean improvement in the total BPRS score was 3.0 with clozapine (mean dose 62.5 mg/day) and 6.0 with risperidone (mean dose 1.2 mg/day). The white blood cell count fell below 3.0×10^9/l after 10 weeks in one subject taking clozapine and rose to 5.0×10^9/l after withdrawal. One subject taking clozapine had a marked increase in rigidity and incontinence of urine after 4 weeks, and there were similar *effects in a patient who took risperidone for 10 weeks. All three adverse events resolved on withdrawal.*

Risperidone has been compared with clozapine in a random, open-label study in schizophrenic patients for 10 weeks; treatment outcomes were assessed blindly and 19 patients entered the randomized phase (17[C]). There were no significant differences between the groups in baseline or endpoint positive or negative symptoms, disease severity, or global or social functioning scores, and patients' opinion on the two drugs did not differ. These results have corroborated previous evidence that risperidone may be as effective as clozapine, but it is probable that this study did not have enough power to detect a difference.

Comparing different typical drugs *The long-term safety and efficacy of amisulpride in subchronic and chronic schizophrenia have been assessed in an open, multicenter study in 489 patients randomly allocated to amisulpride (mean dose, 605 mg/day; n = 370) or haloperidol (mean dose, 14.6 mg/day; n = 119) for 12 months (18[C]). Improvement in mean total score on the Brief Psychiatric Rating Scale was significantly greater with amisulpride than haloperidol. The proportion of patients with at least one treatment-emergent adverse event was similar in the two groups, 69% with amisulpride and 70% with haloperidol, but extrapyramidal symptoms occurred more often with haloperidol (41%) than with amisulpride (26%); endocrine disorders occurred in of 4% those taking amisulpride and 3% of those taking haloperidol. Amenorrhea (6% vs 0%) and weight increase (11% vs 4%) were more frequent with amisulpride. There were serious adverse events in 10% of the patients taking amisulpride and 7% of those taking haloperidol.*

Antipsychotic drugs versus other types of drugs *There has been a randomized, placebo-controlled comparison of haloperidol (mean dose 1.8 mg/day), trazodone (200 mg/day), and behavior management techniques in 149 patients with Alzheimer's disease (19[C]). Although 34% of the subjects improved relative to baseline, there were no significant differences on outcome among the four arms; there were significantly fewer cases of bradykinesia and parkinsonian gait in those given behavioral therapy. These results suggest that other treatments for agitation in dementia need to be considered and evaluated; likewise, they are consistent with the results of an important meta-analysis (20[M]) and a clinical trial (21[C]).*

Cardiovascular *Dysrhythmias* QT interval prolongation, *torsade de pointes*, and sudden death are associated with antipsychotic drugs (SEDA-24, 54). Several regulatory measures (see www.mca.gov.uk; www.medsafe.govt.nz; www.imb.ie; www.hc-sc.gc.ca; www.bpfk.org; www.fda.gov; www.who.int/medicines) have been adopted in different countries with regard to thioridazine, which has a high risk. A further four cases, in which thioridazine in standard doses was implicated as the cause of death or as a contributing factor, have been reported (22[Ar]). Several factors increase the risk of thioridazine toxicity: female sex, pre-existing cardiac disease, age, hypokalemia, glucose load, alcohol intake, exercise, increased serum concentrations in poor CYP2D6 metabolizers, and concomitant therapy with tricyclic antidepressants, erythromycin, co-trimoxazole, cisapride, risperidone, hydroxyzine, and drugs that inhibit CYP2D6 (some SSRIs, fluphenazine, and perphenazine).

Further case reports have appeared.

A 75-year-old man developed ventricular fibrillation and cardiac arrest after intravenous haloperidol (23[A]). His past history included coronary bypass surgery and coronary angioplasty. As he continued to have severe chest pain, emergency angioplasty was performed. On day 3 he received haloperidol by infusion 2 mg/hour, with 2 mg increments every 10 minutes (up to 20 mg in 6 hours) as needed for relief of agitation. Before haloperidol his QT_c interval was normal; after haloperidol it increased to 570 ms. The next day he developed ventricular fibrillation. Subsequent electrocardiograms showed prolonged QT_c intervals of 579 and 615 ms, and haloperidol was withdrawn; the QT_c returned to normal.

A 76-year-old man developed torsade de pointes while taking tiapride 300 mg/day; the QT_c interval 1 day after starting treatment was 600 ms; the dysrhythmia resolved when tiapride was withdrawn (24[A]).

However, malignant dysrhythmias can occur without changes in the QT interval (SEDA-24, 54), and further cases have been reported.

A 64-year-old woman underwent coronary artery bypass surgery and was given intravenous haloperidol for agitation and to avoid postoperative delirium; she developed torsade de pointes (25[A]).

Asystolic cardiac arrest occurred in a 49-year-old woman after she had received haloperidol 10 mg intramuscularly for 2 days; no previous QT_c prolongation had been observed (26[A]).

Hypotension Attention must be paid to hypotension with antipsychotic drugs, particularly in elderly patients (SED-14, 141; SEDA-24, 54). Hypotension has been newly reported in two patients who were taking thioridazine (27[A]). The patients, men aged 68 and 70 years, had traumatic brain injury and were taking oral thioridazine 25 mg/day for agitation. A few days later they developed mild hypotension (100/50 and 100/60 mmHg respectively).

Nervous system *Sleep* Patients with Alzheimer's disease, as well as having impaired cognitive function and a change in personality, have a tendency to develop sleep–wake cycle disturbances that may be aggravated by classical neuroleptic drugs. This has been observed when haloperidol was given to a 54-year-old patient with dementia; 10 days later, the circadian rest–activity cycle began to disintegrate and there was total dysrhythmicity for over 2 months; deterioration was progressive (28[A]). Because of extrapyramidal symptoms, haloperidol 40 mg/day was changed to clozapine 50 mg/day and treatment with donepezil was begun. Two weeks later there was sudden and rapid normalization of the rest–activity cycle, started by an apparent shift of wake-up time to earlier each day, until it attained a new stable timing; orientation and memory also improved.

Extrapyramidal movements A comprehensive review of antipsychotic drug-induced abnormal movements has focused on older patients (29[R]). Since there is no effective treatment for patients with tardive dyskinesia once it develops, attention should be paid to its prevention and close monitoring. It has been confirmed that striatal D_2 receptor occupancy is an important mediator of response and adverse effects in antipsychotic treatment (30[C]). In a double-blind study, 22 patients with first-episode schizophrenia were randomly assigned to a starting dose of haloperidol 1 or 2.5 mg/day. After 2 weeks D_2 receptor occupancy was determined with raclopride and positron emission tomography; the clinical response, extrapyramidal adverse effects, and prolactin concentrations were also measured. The patients had a wide range of D_2 receptor occupancy (38–87%). The likelihoods of clinical response, hyperprolactinemia, and extrapyramidal adverse effects and akathisia increased significantly as D_2 receptor occupancy exceeded 65, 72, and 78% respectively. Since 65–70% D_2 receptor occupancy was obtained with haloperidol 2.5 mg/day in most of the patients, the authors suggested that a dose of 2–3 mg/day should be the optimal starting dose for first-episode patients, which contrasts with the 10–20 mg/day reported in other studies.

Akathisia In 192 consecutive patients attending an emergency department for nausea/vomiting or headache, akathisia occurred in 16% of those treated with prochlorperazine (5–10 mg intravenously or intramuscularly); 4% (all of them women) developed dystonia (31[c]).

Akathisia has been associated with iron deficiency (SEDA-17, 49). However, the rationale for iron supplementation in the treatment of akathisia is poor, and there are potential long-term adverse consequences (SEDA-20, 38). A new study has addressed this issue in patients with acute psychotic disorders who received antipsychotic drugs; 33 patients who developed akathisia were compared with 23 who did not (32[c]). Serum iron was similar in the two groups but ferritin concentrations were significantly lower in akathisia; nevertheless, iron and ferritin concentrations were within the reference ranges.

Following the development of akathisia, biperiden 5 mg was given intravenously to 17 patients and intramuscularly to six (33[c]). The mean times to onset of effect were 1.6 and 31 minutes respectively and the maximum effects occurred at 9.2 and 50 minutes. Adverse effects occurred in six patients after intravenous biperiden (slight or mild confusion, drowsiness, dizziness, palpitation, and dry mouth) and in two after intramuscular biperiden (drowsiness and dry mouth).

Dystonia A man in his late twenties, with a several-year history of intravenous heroin use, developed diplopia after he had received single doses of chlorpromazine 100 mg and ibuprofen 400 mg for anxiety (34[A]). There was no extraocular muscle paresis and neurological examination was unremarkable. The diplopia resolved after 6–8 hours.

Tardive dystonia Tardive dystonia, a variant of tardive dyskinesia, consists of persistent dystonic movements, usually after months or years of neuroleptic drug exposure (SEDA-23, 53). There were no differences in responses to injections of botulinum toxin in patients with tardive oromandibular dystonia (n = 24) or idiopathic oromandibular dystonia (n = 92) (35[c]). Patients seen in a movement disorder clinic, who satisfied the inclusion criteria for tardive oromandibular dystonia (chronicity and onset after neuroleptic treatment) or idiopathic dystonia, were retrospectively studied; those with tardive dystonia had more orofaciolingual stereotypis.

Neuroleptic malignant syndrome Neuroleptic malignant syndrome is characterized by muscle rigidity, hyperthermia, altered consciousness, autonomic dysfunction, and rhabdomyolysis (SED-14, 147; SEDA-20, 41). New cases with particular features have emerged. Five patients had residual catatonia after withdrawal; two recovered gradually with supportive treatment (36[Ar]). Three patients were treated with electroconvulsive therapy; two had an initial positive response, but one died later of intercurrent pneumonia; the third did not respond.

It has been suggested that neurotransmitter abnormalities other than reduced dopaminergic function may be responsible for neuroleptic malignant syndrome, in the light of three cases in which the syndrome occurred after antipsychotic drug administration during benzodiazepine withdrawal (37[A]). Benzodiazepines potentiate GABA transmission and their long-term use is associated with a compensatory reduction in GABA activity; since nigral dopaminergic neurons are modulated through the action of GABAergic projection neurons, reduced GABA could facilitate the occurrence of the syndrome.

Risk factors that have been proposed for the development of neuroleptic malignant syndrome include, among others, a history of prior episodes (SEDA-22, 52). A case report has further illustrated that possibility (38[A]).

A 19-year-old man with bipolar disorder received intramuscular haloperidol 30 mg/day and chlorpromazine 300 mg/day and developed neuroleptic malignant syndrome; the neuroleptic drugs were withdrawn. One month later he had a recurrence. It transpired that he had discontinued his medication 2 weeks after discharge, but because his manic symptoms recurred his relatives had started to give him haloperidol 10 mg/day again, which led to the recurrence.

It is said that the risk of recurrence on re-exposure to neuroleptic drugs (about 15–30%) can be minimized by delaying rechallenge by 2 weeks or by using a neuroleptic drug of an alternative class.

Lithium intoxication has been associated with neuroleptic malignant syndrome in a patient with bipolar disorder (39[A]).

A 39-year-old woman taking lithium 900 mg/day became agitated and was given sulpiride 400 mg/day. The next day she was still agitated and received intramuscular haloperidol 5 mg. She then attempted suicide by taking 20–30 tablets of lithium carbonate (300 mg/tablet). She had severe muscle rigidity, difficulty in swallowing, disorientation in time and place, ataxia, and fluctuating consciousness; her blood pressure fell to 70/58 mmHg, her body temperature was 38–39° C, and her pulse rate was 110 beats/min; her serum creatine kinase activity was 4000 U/l (normal 7–87 U/l). All medications were stopped and she improved within 4–7 days.

Psychological In schizophrenia there is *reduced cognitive function*, and antipsychotic drugs can cause additional impairment (SEDA-21, 43). Visuomotor testing has been performed in 76 patients with schizophrenia or a schizophreniform disorder receiving haloperidol (n = 23; mean dose, 10 mg/day), olanzapine (n = 26; 10.6 mg/day), or risperidone (n = 27; 4.4 mg/day) (40[C]). Cognitive function was better in patients receiving risperidone or olanzapine compared with those receiving haloperidol; patients receiving haloperidol or risperidone had more severe extrapyramidal signs than those receiving olanzapine. The authors concluded that the benefits on cognitive functioning had resulted from a direct effect and were not related to reduced extrapyramidal effects. However, the patients receiving haloperidol were older and had a longer duration of illness than those receiving olanzapine or risperidone; this precludes any firm conclusions.

Musculoskeletal *Rhabdomyolysis* has been described in a handicapped child without other symptoms of neuroleptic malignant syndrome (41[A]).

A 6-year-old boy who was taking clonazepam 2.6 mg/day, diazepam 10 mg/day, and phenobarbital 50 mg/day was given oral haloperidol (0.3 mg/day) plus biperiden (0.3 mg/day) for choreoathetosis. After haloperidol had been introduced, his mother noticed that his urine sometimes became dark brown. He had myoglobinuria (660 ng/ml; normal under 10 ng/ml) but no renal insufficiency. Haloperidol and biperiden were withdrawn and 2 days later his urine was normal.

A marked increase in creatine kinase without neuroleptic malignant syndrome has been previously described (SEDA-21, 48), and a recent report has further emphasized this possibility (42[A]).

A 19-year-old schizophrenic patient taking risperidone 6 mg/day and olanzapine 20 mg/day had a creatine kinase activity of 6940 U/l without clinical manifestations of neuroleptic malignant syndrome; when switched to clozapine (dose not stated) the creatine kinase fell to about 300 U/l. He developed granulocytopenia, quetiapine was started, and the creatine kinase again rose to 3942 U/l but fell after 4 days to 389 U/l without withdrawal of quetiapine.

The authors concluded that the mechanism by which creatine kinase increases is not comparable for olanzapine, quetiapine, and clozapine, and that the increase could be self-limiting.

Hematologic There is greater variability in the reference ranges for all white blood cell indices in patients with schizophrenia than in the healthy population (43[c]). This suggests that abnormal hematological findings in patients with schizophrenia should be assessed in the context of a reference range specifically determined in schizophrenic patients.

Skin Abnormal *skin pigmentation* has been reported with some neuroleptic drugs (SEDA-19, 49). A 45-year-old schizophrenic woman with blue eyes and blond hair who had received a lifetime exposure of at least 1748 g of chlorpromazine had blue discoloration of the skin by age 36 (44[A]). Chlorpromazine was withdrawn and clozapine substituted (up to a maximum of 600 mg/day). The skin pigmentation resolved over 4 years.

Sexual function *Sexual dysfunction* had been reported in association with antipsychotic drugs (SED-14, 149; SEDA-22, 54; SEDA-23, 56; SEDA-24, 59), and another case has been published (45[A]).

A 49-year-old man with bipolar disorder had erectile dysfunction shortly after starting to take haloperidol 50 mg/day and lithium 1500 mg/day. Before this he had had normal sexual function. After 2 months the dosage of haloperidol was reduced to 20 mg/day, but the sexual dysfunction persisted and did not improve with sildenafil. He was then switched to olanzapine 10 mg/day and lithium 1200 mg/day and 1 week later his sexual dysfunction had disappeared.

Body temperature In spite of the fact that antipsychotic drugs can cause neuroleptic malignant syndrome, whose main feature is fever, they commonly cause a *reduction in body temperature*. This has been observed in a study of 14 drug-free and seven schizophrenic patients taking different antipsychotic drugs (46[c]). The temperature fell by about 0.36° C at 24 hours after the drug-free subjects started to take antipsychotic drugs.

Drug withdrawal There has been a randomized controlled study of the factors that affect antipsychotic drug withdrawal or dosage reduction among people with learning disabilities, who were being treated for behavioral problems with typical antipsychotic drugs (47[C]). Of 36 patients, 12 completed full withdrawal and a further seven achieved and maintained at least a 50% reduction. Drug withdrawal or dosage reduction was not associated with increased maladaptive behavior. This result reinforces concerns that antipsychotic drug treatment for maladaptive behavior reduction is often ineffective and inappropriate.

Fetotoxicity A neonate had severe *hypothermia* after antenatal exposure to haloperidol (48[A]). He weighed 3710 g at birth and did not need resuscitation; his axillary temperature was 35° C and he had severe generalized hypotonia. His temperature rose to 36.5° C after 6 hours of rewarming with an overhead radiant heater.

Drug administration route Injectable depot neuroleptic drugs are important for compliance in schizophrenic out-patients. Emphasis has been placed on the benefits of long-acting depot formulations along with the risks (SEDA-23,

73). In a retrospective study in a tertiary center in Riyadh, 69 patients (38 men) had been given depot neuroleptic drugs during 1991–2000 (49[c]). The mean age was 35 years and the mean duration of illness 11 years. Of the 69, only 24 were still receiving their depot injections regularly in that clinic; the authors suggested that negative family and society attitude towards mental illness and interference with psychiatric treatment by traditional and faith healers could have accounted for this lack of compliance. Although the use of depot neuroleptic drugs is advocated as maintenance treatment for patients with bipolar disorders, no such patients were identified. The authors pointed out that in spite of the fact that patients had been clinically stable 7% had been receiving their depot neuroleptic drugs for more than 8 years, with no attempts to reduce the dosage or to increase the interval of administration.

Drug overdose Of the 524 inquiries received by the National Poisons Information Service concerning new antipsychotic drugs over 9 months, only 45 cases involved overdose with a single agent (olanzapine, $n = 10$; clozapine, $n = 8$; risperidone, $n = 10$; sulpiride, $n = 16$) (50[C]). There were no deaths or cases of convulsions. Cardiac dysrhythmias occurred only with sulpiride. Symptoms were most marked with clozapine: most patients had agitation, dystonia, central nervous system depression, and tachycardia. Most of the patients who had taken risperidone were asymptomatic.

Neuroleptic drug poisoning in 86 children has been retrospectively studied in two pediatric hospitals in the USA (1987–97), with about 9000 and 11 000 annual admissions (51[C]). Most (70%) occurred in children under 6 years of age; over two-thirds of the cases (78%) were unintentional. The owner of the antipsychotic medication, when identified (85% of cases), was the grandmother (22%), another family member (21%), the patient (13%), or a non-family caregiver (8%); the most common sites where ingestion occurred were the patient's home (64%) and the relative's home (22%). There was a depressed level of consciousness in 91% and a dystonic reaction in 51%; there were no deaths.

Fatal intoxication has been reported with melperone (52[A]).

A 36-year-old woman was found dead in her flat about 2 days after her last contact with one of her relatives. Besides melperone, she was known to take diazepam and carbamazepine. The police found four empty containers of 100 melperone tablets (100 mg per tablet). Post-mortem blood concentration analysis showed melperone, diazepam, nordiazepam, and carbamazepine; the melperone concentration in venous blood was very high (17.1 mg/l).

A 46-year-old woman took amisulpride (12 g), alprazolam (40 mg), and sertraline (1 g) with suicidal intent and 3 hours later was still unconscious and was intubated (53[A]). Her body temperature rose from 37.1° C on admission to 38° C soon after. She was discharged on the third day.

In contrast, a 50-year-old man who took an overdose of ziprasidone 3120 mg (52 tablets) had no serious effects; he was a little drowsy and his speech was slightly slurred (54[A]). Ziprasidone blood concentrations were not measured.

Drug interactions A 40-year-old man with schizophrenia developed a raised plasma concentration of haloperidol in combination with chlorpromazine and during overlap treatment with clozapine (55[A]). Like haloperidol, chlorpromazine is a competitive inhibitor of CYP2D6; however, clozapine appears to be largely metabolized by CYP1A2.

INDIVIDUAL ATYPICAL DRUGS

Clozapine *(SED-14, 140; SEDA-22, 56; SEDA-23, 59; SEDA-24, 61)*

Of 656 Danish patients who were taking clozapine, 35% were taking concomitant neuroleptic drugs, 28% benzodiazepines, 19% anticholinergic drugs, 11% antidepressants, 8% antiepileptic drugs, and 2% lithium (56[C]). The rationale for supplementing clozapine treatment in refractory schizophrenia in this way has been thoroughly reviewed following a bibliographic search covering 1978–98 (57[M]). In all 70 articles were retrieved but only a few were controlled studies, most being case reports/series. Among the many possible drug combinations, the evidence suggests that clozapine plus sulpiride is the most efficacious combination. The combined use of benzodiazepines and clozapine can cause cardiorespiratory collapse; valproate can cause hepatic dysfunction, and more so with clozapine; lithium can cause neurotoxicity and seizures, and more so with clozapine; and at least some SSRIs appear to raise plasma clozapine concentrations to above the usual target range.

A 37-item survey covering a variety of somatopsychic domains has been administered to 130 schizophrenic patients taking a stable clozapine regimen (mean dose 464 mg/day; mean duration 34 months) (58[c]). Most of them reported an improvement in their level of satisfaction, quality of life, compliance with treatment, thinking, mood, and alertness. Most reported worse *nocturnal salivation* (88%); *weight gain* (35%) came second; fewer patients reported a worsening of various *gastrointestinal and urinary symptoms*.

Benefit has previously been obtained in mentally retarded patients treated with clozapinc (SEDA-23, 59). In a retrospective review, 33 such patients were evaluated; adverse effects were mild and transient, *constipation* being the most common ($n = 10$) (59[c]). There were no significant cardiovascular adverse effects and no seizures; no patient discontinued treatment because of agranulocytosis. However, the small sample size and the lack of a control group precluded definitive conclusions.

Cardiovascular Cardiovascular adverse effects of clozapine are not uncommon. Clozapine has been particularly associated with *cardiomyopathy* (SED-14, 142; SEDA-21, 52; SEDA-24, 62), *changes in blood pressure* (SEDA-21, 52; SEDA-22, 57; SEDA-23, 59), *electrocardiographic changes* (SEDA-22, 57; SEDA-23, 60; SEDA-24, 62), and *venous thromboembolism* (SEDA-20, 47).

Data from the Swedish Reactions Advisory Committee have newly suggested that the use of clozapine is associated with venous thromboembolic complications (60[c]). Between 1 April 1989, and 1 March 2000, 12 cases of venous thromboembolism were collected; in five the outcome was fatal. Symptoms occurred in the first 3 months of treatment in eight patients; the mean clozapine dose was 277 mg/day (75–500). Although during the study total antipsychotic drug sales, excluding clozapine, accounted for 96% of all antipsychotic drug sales, only three cases of thromboembolism associated with those antipsychotic drugs were reported. The reported risk of thromboembolism associated with clozapine is estimated to be 1 per 2000–6000 treated patients, the true risk being higher owing to under-reporting. These conclusions are consistent with those from an important observational study (61[C]).

A substantial portion of patients taking clozapine develop electrocardiographic abnormalities, but most of them are benign and do not need treatment. This was the conclusion reached in a study in 61 schizophrenic patients taking clozapine, in which a retrospective chart review was conducted to identify electrocardiographic abnormalities (62[C]). The prevalence of electrocardiographic abnormalities in those who used antipsychotic drugs other than clozapine was 14% (6/44), while that in the antipsychotic drug-free patients was 12% (2/17); when treatment was switched to clozapine, the prevalence of electrocardiographic abnormalities rose to 31% (19/61).

Nervous system In patients taking clozapine, *seizures* are said to be dose-related (SEDA-24, 62), and several anticonvulsants have been shown to be helpful in prevention and treatment. A 15-year-old boy with refractory schizophrenia had seizures with clozapine; he was given gabapentin, and several years later was free of seizures (63[A]).

Clozapine is said to cause less *tardive dyskinesia* and fewer extrapyramidal adverse effects than haloperidol (SEDA-22, 56). Moreover, it is believed that clozapine can improve pre-existing tardive dyskinesia (SEDA-23, 60). Nevertheless, 46 patients taking clozapine had higher tardive dyskinesia scores compared with 127 taking typical neuroleptic drugs (64[C]). In a multiple regression analysis, there was a significant relation between the total score on the Abnormal Involuntary Movement Scale (AIMS) as a dependent variable and current neuroleptic drug dose, duration of treatment, age, sex, diagnosis, current antiparkinsonian therapy, and illness duration. There was no beneficial effect of clozapine on the prevalence of tardive dyskinesia, and the authors' conclusion was that certain patients develop tardive dyskinesia in spite of long-term intensive clozapine treatment; however, since most clozapine users were past users of typical neuroleptic drugs, this conclusion must be regarded with caution. Tardive dyskinesia has been attributed to clozapine in a 44-year-old man, who had discontinued haloperidol 24 days before the event (65[A]).

Clozapine has little or no potential to cause *tardive dystonia*, and it has even been speculated that it may be effective for this adverse effect (SEDA-24, 63); however, there was no evidence of a beneficial effect of clozapine in *primary dystonia*, the most common form of dystonia and a difficult disorder to treat, until the recent report of a 56-year-old woman with severe and persistent primary cranial dystonia (Meige's syndrome), who responded to clozapine (50–100 mg) (66[A]).

Neuroleptic malignant syndrome has occasionally been associated with clozapine (SED-14, 147; SEDA-22, 58; SEDA-23, 60), although the presentation can be different from that associated with traditional antipsychotic drugs (SEDA-24, 63). Now, neuroleptic malignant syndrome and subsequent acute interstitial nephritis has been reported in a 44-year-old woman (67[A]). This patient met the main criteria for neuroleptic malignant syndrome, although she did not develop rigidity or a rise in creatine kinase activity. On the other hand, abnormal creatine kinase activity and signs of myotoxicity were respectively found in 14% and 2.1% of patients who took clozapine for an average of 18 months ($n = 94$) (68[C]).

Psychiatric *Panic disorder* has been attributed to clozapine (69[A]).

A 34-year-old woman taking clozapine 400 mg/day for psychiatric symptoms had recurrent attacks of sudden chest pressure, dizziness, fear of dying, and intense anxiety; reducing the dose of clozapine to 250 mg/day led to modest improvement. Olanzapine 10 mg/day was then substituted, without recurrence, and her panic symptoms progressively improved.

Endocrine *Hyperglycemia, diabetic ketoacidosis*, and *insulin-dependent hyperglycemia* have been associated with clozapine therapy (SEDA-22, 58; SEDA-23, 60; SEDA-24, 64). Now three cases of new-onset diabetes mellitus have been reported in patients who were taking clozapine (70[A], 71[A]).

Metabolic *Weight gain*, commonly associated with clozapine (SEDA-23, 61), has again been reported (72[A]).

A 29-year-old man taking clozapine 800 mg/day gained 46 kg in weight after 25 months, and had myoclonic jerks in both hands, arms, and shoulders; he was treated with the antiepileptic drug topiramate (which also causes weight loss). The myoclonic jerks disappeared completely. He lost 21 kg over 5 months, with no significant change in eating habits or food consumption, and felt more energetic, more active, and more motivated to exercise.

Hematologic Clozapine-induced *thrombocytosis* (774×10^9/l) has been reported in a middle-aged man (73[A]).

In contrast, a 43-year-old man developed *thrombocytopenia* (platelet count 60×10^9/l), which persisted for 40 months after clozapine treatment (74[A]). There was increased in vitro platelet [^{14}C] serotonin release in the presence of clozapine. The authors suggested an immune mechanism and pointed out that the manufacturers recommend withdrawing clozapine when the platelet count falls below 100×10^9/l.

The incidence of *agranulocytosis* with clozapine has been extensively studied, and data from different countries have been published (SEDA-23, 62). Agranulocytosis in a 45-year-old man was successfully treated with granulocyte colony-stimulating factor (75[A]). On the other hand, both negative and positive rechallenge in patients with previous agranulocytosis can occur (SEDA-22, 59; SEDA-23, 61). A 29-year-old woman developed agranulocytosis after taking clozapine 300 mg/day for 5 years; 4 months after withdrawal, the clozapine was reintroduced (500 mg/day), and after 8 months the leukocyte count was still within the reference range (76[A]).

The underlying mechanisms of agranulocytosis are unknown, but hemopoietic cytokines, such as granulocyte colony-stimulating factor (G-CSF), are likely to be involved (77[A]).

In a 26-year-old woman who developed granulocytopenia twice, first when taking clozapine and again when taking olanzapine, G-CSF concentrations, but not those of other cytokines, closely paralleled the granulocyte count.

In a 73-year-old patient who developed granulocytopenia while taking clozapine, G-CSF and leukocyte counts were reliable indicators of the evolution of the condition, showing an abortive form of toxic bone-marrow damage with subsequent recovery (78[A]).

So, monitoring G-CSF concentrations may be useful in following patients in whom clozapine-induced marrow damage is suspected.

Some of the genetic aspects of clozapine-induced agranulocytosis have been further evaluated (79[C]). Polymorphisms of specific clozapine metabolizing enzyme systems were determined in 31 patients with agranulocytosis and in 77 without. Genotyping of a recently discovered G^{-463} A polymorphism of the myeloperoxidase gene and CYP2D6 showed no evidence of an association.

Gastrointestinal *Hypersalivation* is a common and well-known adverse effect of clozapine (SEDA-22, 60). Ten patients with sialorrhea associated with clozapine, who did not respond to anticholinergic or adrenergic drugs, received intranasal ipratropium bromide (80[c]). At 6 months, six patients maintained improvement.

Constipation is an adverse effect that has often been associated with clozapine; it may be serious and even fatal (SEDA-22, 60). A 49-year-old man taking clozapine developed a *perforated colon* and *peritonitis* (81[A]). He survived, albeit with a markedly reduced quality of life. The authors suggested that diet modification and regular exercise should be encouraged in patients taking clozapine, in order to prevent constipation.

Urinary tract *Enuresis* has been associated with clozapine (SEDA-22, 60) and is not related to age, sex, clozapine dosage, duration of clozapine use, duration of hospitalization, duration of illness, age at onset of schizophrenia, or concurrent treatment with other psychiatric drugs (SEDA-24, 64). A recent report has suggested that polymorphism of the α_{1a}-adrenoceptor gene plays no major role in the pathogenesis of schizophrenia or in clozapine-induced urinary incontinence (82[A]).

Drug withdrawal In susceptible patients, abrupt or rapid withdrawal of clozapine can be accompanied by severe symptoms (SEDA-23, 63). The withdrawal syndrome associated with clozapine may be of considerable clinical significance (83[r]).

Drug overdose A 40-year-old man who took 3–4 g of clozapine became unconscious, with constricted pupils, sinus tachycardia, and twitching; peak clozapine and norclozapine concentrations were 3.5 mg/l and 0.7 mg/l respectively, with secondary peaks at about 36 hours (84[A]). Recovery was uneventful, and he was well 2 days after admission.

Drug interactions *Erythromycin*, an inhibitor of CYP3A4, can increase plasma clozapine concentrations, and adverse effects have been reported; however, it has been suggested that the metabolism of clozapine is not altered by erythromycin, because CYP3A4 is a relatively minor pathway for clozapine metabolism, in contrast to CYP1A2 (SEDA-24, 66). In a case of neutropenia the authors suggested that an interaction of clozapine with erythromycin had been the precipitating factor (85[A]).

Inhibitors of CYP1A2, such as caffeine, have been previously associated with changes in the metabolism of clozapine (SEDA-23, 63). A possible pharmacokinetic interaction between a CYP1A2 inhibitor, *ciprofloxacin*, and clozapine, with moderately increased serum concentrations of clozapine has been reported (86[A]).

Selective serotonin re-uptake inhibitors increase plasma clozapine concentrations (SEDA-22, 62; SEDA-23, 63; SEDA-24, 65). The effects of paroxetine and sertraline on steady-state plasma concentrations of clozapine and its metabolites have been studied in 17 patients taking clozapine (200–400 mg/day), nine of whom took additional paroxetine (20–40 mg/day) and eight sertraline (50–100 mg/day) (87[c]). The metabolism of clozapine was not affected by sertraline, but paroxetine, a potent inhibitor of CYP2D6, appeared to inhibit its metabolism, possibly by affecting a pathway other than *N*-desmethylation and *N*-oxidation. After 3 weeks of paroxetine, mean plasma concentrations of clozapine and norclozapine increased significantly by 31% and 20% respectively, while concentrations of clozapine *N*-oxide were unchanged.

A possible interaction of clozapine with citalopram has also been reported, with increased serum clozapine concentrations, perhaps dose-related (88[c]). On the other hand, combined therapy with clozapine and fluvoxamine (n = 11), and clozapine monotherapy (n = 12) have been monitored before and during the first 6 weeks of medication (89[c]). The coadministration of fluvoxamine attenuated and delayed the clozapine-induced increase in plasma concentrations of tumor necrosis factor-α, enhanced and accelerated the clozapine-induced increase in leptin plasma concentrations without a significant effect on clozapine-induced weight gain, and reduced granulocyte counts.

Valproic acid can increase the sedative effect of clozapine, but it also has been reported that this interaction has only a small effect on plasma clozapine concentrations (SEDA-24, 66). In a 33-year-old woman taking clozapine and valproic acid the serum concentrations of clozapine fell significantly (90[A]). The authors suggested that valproic acid had induced the metabolism of clozapine.

Olanzapine *(SEDA-22, 64; SEDA-23, 64; SEDA-24, 66)*

Olanzapine has *anticholinergic adverse effects* and often causes *weight gain*, subclinical cases of *raised transaminase activities*, *increased blood pressure*, and *QT interval prolongation*. This is in part consistent with the results of an observational prospective study sponsored by Lilly, in which 2128 patients were treated with olanzapine as monotherapy (mean dose 13 mg/day) or combined with other drugs, and 821 were treated with other antipsychotic drugs as monotherapy or combined with other drugs (control group) (91[C]). Olanzapine was well tolerated and effective, and the overall incidence of adverse events was significantly lower than in controls, although weight gain (6.9%) was significantly more frequent. Dropouts were statistically similar in the two groups. To evaluate anticholinergic effects, differences among patients taking olanzapine (n = 12; average dose, 15 mg/day) or clozapine (n = 12; average dose, 444 mg/day) for at least 8 weeks were measured in an unblinded study (92[c]). *Altered salivation* was significantly more common with clozapine (increased salivation) and olanzapine (decreased salivation), whereas *constipation*, *urinary disturbances*, and *tachycardia/palpitation* were significantly more common with clozapine. There were no global cognitive problems in either group.

The efficacy and safety of olanzapine in particular disorders have been studied (SEDA-24, 67). Its use in patients with Gilles de la Tourette syndrome has been explored in a 52-week, double-blind, cross-over comparison of olanzapine (5 and 10 mg/day) and low-dose pimozide (2 and 4 mg/day) in four patients (aged 19–40 years) with a high frequency of tics (2–10/min), vocalizations, and lack of co-morbidity (93[c]). There was a highly significant reduction in rating scale scores for the syndrome with olanzapine 10 mg versus baseline and versus pimozide 2 mg, and a significant reduction with olanzapine 5 mg versus pimozide 4 mg; only moderate *sedation* was reported by one patient during olanzapine treatment while three complained of *minor motor adverse effects and sedation* during pimozide treatment.

Nervous system *Seizures* associated with olanzapine in premarketing studies have been estimated to occur in 0.9% of patients, which is probably comparable to the incidence with many conventional agents; status epilepticus and seizures have previously been reported (SEDA-24, 67). Now, seizures caused by a possible interaction of olanzapine with *clomipramine* have been reported in a 34-year-old man with schizophrenia complicated by obsessive–compulsive disorder (94[A]).

Anecdotal reports of olanzapine-induced *tardive dyskinesia* have been previously described as occurring in 1% of treated patients (SEDA-22, 65; SEDA-24, 68), although olanzapine may also improve pre-existing tardive dyskinesia (SEDA-22, 65; SEDA-23, 66; SEDA-24, 68). A further case of remission of tardive dyskinesia after changing from flupenthixol to olanzapine has been reported (95[A]).

Several cases of *neuroleptic malignant syndrome* associated with olanzapine have previously been reported (SEDA-23, 66; SEDA-24, 68), and new cases have appeared (96[A]–99[A]).

A 23-year-old woman had some of the features of the serotonin syndrome (mental status changes, sweating, tremor, and fever); however, the large rise in creatine kinase activity, extreme lead-pipe rigidity, and the abrupt onset suggested neuroleptic malignant syndrome rather than the serotonin syndrome (96[A]).

An 85-year-old man developed fever, muscle rigidity, and changes in mental state, but his serum creatine kinase activity was not increased (97[A]).

A 42-year-old man took olanzapine for 3 weeks and developed hyperpyrexia, tremor, labile blood pressure, and mental changes; he had a metabolic acidosis and an escalating creatine kinase activity (98[A]).

A 78-year-old woman developed fulminant neuroleptic malignant syndrome complicated by pneumonia while taking olanzapine and levomepromazine. When the neuroleptic drugs were withdrawn she recovered; however, when the combination was restarted later, because of severe agitation and hallucinations, the symptoms of neuroleptic malignant syndrome recurred (99[A]).

In contrast to these cases, a 34-year-old man, who had had clozapine-induced neuroleptic malignant syndrome, was successfully treated with olanzapine (100[A]).

Sensory systems *Esotropia* (an inward squint) has been reported, purportedly for the first time, in a patient taking olanzapine and fluoxetine for psychosis; it resolved promptly on withdrawal of olanzapine (101[A]).

A 14-year-old girl with psychotic depression took fluoxetine 40 mg/day and olanzapine 5 mg/day and 6 months later developed a severe headache, menorrhagia, diplopia, and eye irritation; her mother had also noted a "lazy eye". She had corrected visual acuity of 20/20 in both eyes, and intermittent esotropia of 14–16 diopters when fixing at 6 meters, and 8 diopters when fixing at 1/3 meters. A month later, her deviation had increased to 20 and 14 diopters respectively. Olanzapine was withdrawn and within 1 week the diplopia and headaches cleared, and the esotropia resolved.

Psychiatric *Mania* has been previously associated with olanzapine (SEDA-23, 66; SEDA-24, 68). A new case of manic symptoms induced by olanzapine has been reported in an 85-year-old woman with a 3-year history of delusional disorder; her florid manic symptoms resolved 2 weeks after withdrawal (102[A]).

Olanzapine can cause both de novo and worsening *obsessive–compulsive symptoms* (SEDA-23, 67; SEDA-24, 68). Three cases have recently been reported in which olanzapine caused significant exacerbation of obsessive–compulsive symptoms in schizophrenia (two cases) and obsessive–compulsive disorder (one case) (103[A]). In contrast, in another study 23 patients with obsessive–compulsive disorder who had not responded to a 6-month, open-label trial of fluvoxamine (300 mg/day) entered a 3-month open-label trial of augmentation with olanzapine (5 mg/day) (104[c]). There was a significant reduction in the mean score on the Yale–Brown Obsessive–Compulsive Scale; concomitant schizotypal personality disorder was the only factor significantly associated with a response. The most common adverse effects were mild to moderate *weight gain* and *sedation*.

Endocrine and metabolic Significant *weight gain* occurs more often with olanzapine than either haloperidol or risperidone (SEDA-22, 64; SEDA-23, 67). Average weight gain was 8 kg in patients with refractory schizophrenia (n = 8) who were taking olanzapine in high doses (20–40 mg over an average of 40 weeks) (105[A]). *Hyperglycemia and diabetes* have also been associated with olanzapine (SEDA-23, 67; SEDA-24, 69). The effects of olanzapine on glucose–insulin homeostasis have been studied in 14 patients in an attempt to elucidate the possible mechanisms of olanzapine-associated weight gain (106[c]). Olanzapine caused weight gain of 1–10 kg in 12 patients and raised concentrations of insulin, leptin, and blood lipids, as well as insulin resistance; three patients developed diabetes mellitus. The authors concluded that both increased insulin secretion and hyperleptinemia may be mechanisms behind olanzapine-induced weight gain. They also suggested that the metabolite *N*-desmethylolanzapine has a normalizing effect on the metabolic abnormalities.

A 54-year-old woman developed severe glucose dysregulation with exacerbation of type 2 diabetes 12 days after starting to take olanzapine 10 mg/day; she also gained 13 kg (107[A]).

Histamine H_2 receptor antagonists, like nizatidine, can control appetite in overweight patients (108[A]). This has been observed in a 23-year-old man who had had repeated episodes of weight gain during olanzapine treatment and had good control and subsequent weight reduction after 4–5 weeks of therapy with nizatidine.

Hematologic Olanzapine is relatively free of hematological adverse effects (SEDA-24, 69), although it has occasionally been associated with reduced hematological values (unspecified) (SEDA-23, 67). A case of olanzapine-induced *neutropenia* has been reported (109[A]).

A 20-year-old man with schizophrenia took olanzapine 5 mg/day increasing to 10 mg/day after 3 days. His total leukocyte count fell to 3.9×10^9/l on the 5th day, with an absolute neutrophil count of 1.52×10^9/l. Olanzapine was withdrawn and the leukocyte count normalized within 72 hours. A few days later rechallenge was positive. He was given lithium 900 mg/day and continued to take olanzapine 20 mg/day.

Olanzapine has also been associated with prolonged granulocyte depression in patients with previously reduced clozapine-induced granulocyte counts. It has been suggested that it would be prudent to avoid starting olanzapine in patients with clozapine-induced granulocyte depression until the leukocyte count has normalized (SEDA-22, 65; SEDA-23, 67).

Prolonged granulocytopenia due to olanzapine occurred in a 39-year-old woman after clozapine withdrawal (110[A]). In contrast, two patients with severe clozapine-induced granulocytopenia and agranulocytosis were successfully treated with olanzapine in a dose greater than 25 mg/day (111[A]). Furthermore, a 65-year-old man who had previously developed leukopenia and neutropenia, first with clozapine and then also with risperidone, took olanzapine (20 mg/day) for 2 years with only a transient reduction in leukocyte and neutrophil (but not erythrocyte or platelet) counts during a flu-like illness (112[A]).

Genetic determinants may be associated with olanzapine-induced agranulocytosis (SEDA-24, 70). Olanzapine-induced blood disorders have been reviewed and compared with clozapine-induced agranulocytosis (113[r]). There is some evidence for an association of human leukocyte antigen (HLA) type with clozapine-induced agranulocytosis, but this may vary in different ethnic groups. It has been stated that if there is also an HLA association for olanzapine-induced agranulocytosis, it seems to be different from the HLA antigens incriminated for clozapine. However, the number of cases with olanzapine-induced agranulocytosis is far too small to allow meaningful conclusions.

Thrombocytopenia, with a platelet count of 20×10^9/l, possibly associated with olanzapine and subsequently with benzatropine mesylate, has been reported, purportedly for the first time, in a 38-year-old woman (114[A]).

Pancreas Acute *pancreatitis* has been reported, purportedly for the first time, in a patient who did not take alcohol and who had undergone a cholecystectomy in the past; other medical causes of pancreatitis were ruled out (115[A]).

Urinary tract A 61-year-old man with bipolar disorder treated with olanzapine and lithium developed *urinary incontinence* 4 days later (116[A]). He was successfully treated with ephedrine 25 mg/day. The authors suggested that the α-blocking effect of olanzapine was involved and that an α-adrenoceptor agonist (such as ephedrine) would reduce urinary incontinence in such cases.

Sexual function *Priapism* has been reported in association with olanzapine (SEDA-23, 68; SEDA-24, 70), and a new case of recurrent priapism during clozapine and then olanzapine therapy has been reported in a 43-year-old man (117[A]).

Drug overdose Deaths and non-fatal cases of overdose of olanzapine have been previously reported (SEDA-22, 68; SEDA-24, 70), and two further fatal cases have been published (118[A]). Blood olanzapine concentrations were 237 ng/ml in one and 675 ng/ml in the other. In a third case a 22-year-old man took about 800 mg of olanzapine; his olanzapine serum concentration reached a maximum of 200 ng/ml (usual target serum concentrations are about 10 ng/ml) (119[A]). His vital signs were stable at all times, but he started to become progressively somnolent, with short periods of aggressive agitation. Gastric lavage was performed and after 10 hours he was alert and oriented.

Drug interactions Seizures in a 34-year-old man were attributed to an interaction of olanzapine with *clomipramine* (94[A]). Clomipramine and olanzapine are both metabolized by CYP1A2 and CYP2D6, and it is therefore possible that raised concentrations of both compounds resulted from coadministration.

Quetiapine *(SEDA-22, 65; SEDA-23, 68; SEDA-24, 71)*

Nervous system Although quetiapine seems to cause a lower incidence of extrapyramidal symptoms, a case of neuroleptic malignant syndrome has recently been described (120[A]).

A 40-year-old man with chronic schizophrenia and borderline intelligence presented with an acute psychotic decompensation. He had previously taken several different antipsychotic drugs and had had significant extrapyramidal symptoms but never neuroleptic malignant syndrome. He was given quetiapine 25 mg bd increasing to 250 mg bd by day 13. He then had increasing symptoms of restlessness, agitation, and episodic sweating. Loxapine 25 mg and lorazepam 2 mg were added. On day 14 he developed confusion, lead-pipe muscle rigidity, a temperature of 38.2° C, a labile blood pressure, tachypnea, and tachycardia; creatine kinase activity was 18 354 IU/l and he had myoglobinuria. Quetiapine was withdrawn and supportive treatment was instituted. He recovered 5 days after withdrawal.

Risperidone *(SEDA-22, 66; SEDA-23, 68; SEDA-24, 71)*

Objections have been raised on the ways in which some clinical trials are interpreted (121[r]). Furthermore, it has been stated that a major problem with the risperidone literature is that the original data can be very difficult to decipher or even obtain. Huston and Moher have described their frustration in trying to perform a meta-analysis of the effects of risperidone; they found "obvious redundancy in the results of a single-center trial being published twice", as well as problems with "changing authorship, lack of transparency in reporting, and frequent citation of abstracts and unpublished reports" (122[r]). These concerns have been reiterated in a recent editorial (123[r]).

The safety and tolerability of a rapid oral loading regimen for risperidone, developed to achieve therapeutic doses within 24 hours, have been evaluated (124[c]). Risperidone was initiated in a dose of 1 mg, increasing by 1 mg every 6–8 hours up to 3 mg. Dose increases were contingent on the tolerance of the last administered dose. Of 11 consecutive in-patients who were treated with this protocol, seven tolerated the most rapid titration, achieving a dose of 3 mg bd in 16 hours; three required slightly slower titration and achieved the target dose in 24 hours; one could not tolerate the 3 mg dose but tolerated 2 mg tds; no patient had serious extrapyramidal adverse effects, sedation, or any other adverse event during the rapid titration, and in no case did risperidone have to be withdrawn. The authors concluded that aggressive dosing with risperidone is well tolerated in most psychiatric in-patients.

The optimal dose of risperidone in first-episode schizophrenia has been studied in 17 drug-naive patients (12 women, 5 men; mean age 29 years) (125[c]). The mean optimal dosage of risperidone was 2.70 mg/day. All the patients reached the optimal dose before developing extrapyramidal adverse effects; four developed *parkinsonism* and one developed *akathisia* at a mean dosage of 5.20 mg/day. In contrast, acute exacerbations of schizophrenia may require a higher dose.

In a prospective, 6-week open trial in 31 Chinese patients with acute exacerbation of schizophrenia risperidone doses were titrated to 6 mg/day (if tolerated) over 3 days, but were reduced thereafter if adverse effects occurred (126[c]). Efficacy and adverse effects were assessed on days 0, 4, 14, 28, and 42. Endpoint steady-state plasma concentrations of risperidone and 9-hydroxyrisperidone were analysed. Of the 30 patients who completed the trial, 17 tolerated the 6 mg dose well, while the other 13 received lower final doses (mean 3.6 mg) for curtailing adverse effects. At endpoint, 92% of the 13 low-dose patients had responded to treatment (a 20% or more reduction in the total score on the Positive and Negative Syndrome Scale), compared with 53% of the 17 high-dose subjects. There were no significant between-group differences in other minor efficacy measures. Endpoint plasma concentrations of the active moieties (risperidone plus 9-hydroxyrisperidone) were 40 ng/ml in the low-dose group and 50 ng/ml in the high-dose group; this difference was not significant, suggesting that the different responses were pharmacokinetic in origin. The results of this preliminary trial suggest that up to 6 mg/day of risperidone is efficacious in treating patients with an acute exacerbation of schizophrenia. Nearly 60% of the patients tolerated 6 mg; in the other 40%, reducing the dosage to relieve adverse effects still yielded efficacy.

The efficacy and safety of risperidone have been previously studied in special groups of patients, such as adults with autism and in children and adolescents (SEDA-23, 69). Now, the efficacy and safety of long-term risperidone have been assessed in children and adolescents ($n = 11$) in a prospective study (127[c]). Subjects with autism or pervasive developmental disorder not otherwise specified took risperidone for 6 months, after which their parents were given the option of continuing for a further 6 months. *Weight gain* was common, although the rate of increase abated with time. After 6 months two patients developed *facial dystonias*, which disappeared after reducing the dosage in one case and after withdrawal in the other. *Amenorrhea* was also observed, but there were no changes in liver function, bloods tests, or electroencephalography. The authors concluded that risperidone may be effective and relatively safe in the long-term treatment of behavioral disruption in autistic children and adolescents.

Table 1. *The results of two 12-week, randomized, double-blind studies of risperidone in elderly patients with behavioral symptoms associated with dementia*

Mean age (y)	*n*	Dose (mg/day)	Response (%)	EPS* (%)	Reference
81	344	Risperidone 1.1	54	15	(132[C])
		Haloperidol 1.2	63	22	
		Placebo	47	11	
83	625	Risperidone 1	45	12.8	(133[C])
		Risperidone 2	50	21.2	
		Placebo	33	7.4	

* Extrapyramidal symptoms.

Youths with behavioral disorders (128[c], 129[c]) and patients with disturbing neuroleptic drug-induced extrapyramidal symptoms (130[C]) have also been studied. Ten youths (aged 6–14 years) were randomly assigned to receive placebo and 10 to receive risperidone (0.75–1.50 mg/day) for conduct disorder in a preliminary study lasting 10 weeks (128[c]). Of those assigned to risperidone, six completed the course; three completed placebo. Those who took risperidone were significantly less aggressive during the last weeks of the study than those who did not. Eight youths who took risperidone and four who took placebo had at least one adverse effect, including *increased appetite* (*n* = 3 for risperidone), *sedation* (*n* = 3 for risperidone; *n* = 2 for placebo), *headache* (*n* = 1 for risperidone; *n* = 1 for placebo), *insomnia* (*n* = 1 for risperidone), *restlessness* (*n* = 1 for risperidone), *irritability* (*n* = 1 for risperidone), *enuresis* (*n* = 1 for placebo), and *nausea/vomiting* (*n* = 1 for risperidone; *n* = 1 for placebo). These adverse effects were mild and transient.

There was marked reduction in aggression in 14 of 26 subjects (10–18 years old) in an open study of risperidone (0.5–4 mg/day) for 2–12 months (129[c]). Two subjects had marked *weight gain* (8 and 10 kg) in the first 8 weeks; another participant who took lithium (1400 mg/day, serum concentration 0.9 mmol/l) presented with moderate *akathisia* and *hand tremor*; in seven, *tiredness* and *sedation* occurred after week 8.

In patients aged 18–73 years with disturbing extrapyramidal symptoms during previous neuroleptic drug treatment (*n* = 77), there was a greater reduction of parkinsonism over 8 weeks with risperidone (*n* = 40; average dose 7.4 mg/day) than with haloperidol (*n* = 37; average dose 9.9 mg/day) (130[C]). With risperidone the most frequently mentioned adverse effects were *headache* (*n* = 4), *oculogyric crisis* (*n* = 3), and *hypersalivation* (*n* = 3); with haloperidol the adverse effects were *sleep disorders* (*n* = 4), *tremor* (*n* = 4), and *vomiting* (*n* = 3).

Agitated and demented elderly patients should not be treated with neuroleptic drugs, unless they have pronounced psychotic symptoms (see General section above). According to a recent thorough review, risperidone is more effective than placebo in patients with dementia (131[R]). Notwithstanding, the results of the two major controlled clinical trials have not been conclusive (see Table 1). There was no statistical difference between the treatments in the first study, although there was in the second; extrapyramidal symptoms were notably more common with risperidone. In both studies, there was a high rate of placebo response, which implies that these patients responded favorably to the increased care that is given during a clinical trial. Long-term data in patients with dementia are lacking, but they are crucial in identifying tardive dyskinesia.

Nervous system *Tardive dyskinesia* has previously been reported with risperidone (SEDA-22, 68; SEDA-23, 70), and new cases have emerged.

A 16-year-old girl developed buccolingual masticatory tardive dyskinesia after taking risperidone 6 mg/day (134[A]); when she restarted risperidone 2 mg/day, increasing to 6 mg/day later on, the dyskinesia improved.

A 74-year-old woman developed persistent tardive dyskinesia following a short trial (3 weeks) of a low dose (0.5 mg bd) of risperidone (135[A]).

Advanced age and dementia may have been contributing factors in several previously reported cases of risperidone-induced tardive dyskinesia (see above and SEDA-23, 70). This adverse effect has now been studied in 330 elderly patients with dementia (mean age 83 years) (136[C]). They were enrolled in a 1-year, open-label study, in which the modal risperidone dose was 0.96 mg/day and the median length of use was 273 day. The 1-year cumulative incidence of persistent tardive dyskinesia among the 225 patients without dyskinesia at baseline was 2.6%, and patients with dyskinesia at baseline had significant reductions in severity.

Dyskinesia occurred for 5 days in an 82-year-old woman after withdrawal of risperidone and citalopram, which she had taken for about 3 months (137[A])

Attention deficit hyperactivity disorder (ADHD) may be a risk factor for risperidone-induced tardive dyskinesia as much as withdrawal dyskinesia. Both conditions have occurred in patients with a past or recent history of attention deficit hyperactivity disorder: a 34-year-old woman who developed dyskinesia after starting risperidone, with a marked increase in prolactin concentrations (138[A]), and a 13-year-old boy who developed mild mouth movements, neck twisting, and intermittent upward gaze approximately 2 weeks after withdrawal of risperidone (1.5 mg and then 0.5 mg) (139[A]).

Dystonia and tardive dystonia have been reported.

A 23-year-old man taking risperidone 8 mg/day developed blepharospasm (140[A]).

A 25-year-old man who had never taken any other psychotropic medication, developed tardive dyskinesia with severe blepharospasm and tardive dystonia 2 months after withdrawal of risperidone (141[A]).

Possible risperidone-induced tardive dystonia has been reported in a 47-year-old man (142[A]).

Conversely, it has been reported, purportedly for the first time, that a 28-year-old woman simultaneously developed four types of tardive extrapyramidal symptoms (dystonia, dyskinesia, choreoathetotic movements, and myoclonus) while taking haloperidol; the symptoms were subsequently relieved by the use of low-dose risperidone (3 mg/day) (143[A]).

Neuroleptic malignant syndrome has previously been reported in patients taking risperidone; most cases occurred within the first months, even within 12 hours (SEDA-22, 68; SEDA-23, 70). Delayed risperidone-induced neuroleptic malignant syndrome has been reported in a 27-year-old man after 21 months (144[A]), and in a 17-year-old girl who took risperidone 0.5 mg bd (145[A]). Risperidone-induced neuroleptic malignant syndrome has been reported in a 63-year-old woman with probable Lewy body dementia, who had previously had an episode of neuroleptic malignant syndrome with trifluoperazine (146[A]).

Whether risperidone should be used in patients with Parkinson's disease is a subject of debate (SEDA-23, 70). The efficacy and safety of risperidone have recently been evaluated in 39 patients (25 women and 19 men) with Parkinson's disease (147[c]). There was either complete or near-complete resolution of hallucinations in 23, but an unsatisfactory response ($n = 6$) or worsening of Parkinsonism ($n = 6$) in 12. Excluding patients with diffuse Lewy body disease, there was no significant worsening of scores on the Unified Parkinson's Disease Rating Scale after either 3 or 6 months of treatment, and the presence of dementia did not predict the response to treatment.

Psychiatric An association of *obsessive–compulsive symptoms* with risperidone has previously been reported (SEDA-22, 69; SEDA-23, 71; SEDA-24, 72). In a recent case reintroduction of risperidone did not cause obsessive–compulsive symptoms to re-emerge in a 29-year-old man who had previously developed obsessive–compulsive features when first treated with risperidone (148[A]).

Visual distortion with generalized anxiety and panic attacks has been attributed to risperidone (SEDA-22, 69). Visual disturbance resembling hallucinogen persistent perception disorder occurred after each of three consecutive risperidone dosage increases in a 55-year-old woman; there was absence of substance abuse (149[A]).

Endocrine *Hyperprolactinemia* and *galactorrhea* associated with risperidone have previously been reported (SED-14, 148; SEDA-22, 69; SEDA-23, 71; SEDA-24, 72). Galactorrhea with gynecomastia has recently been reported in a 38-year-old hypothyroid man who took risperidone for 14 days (150[A]). The authors suggested that men with primary hypothyroidism may be particularly sensitive to neuroleptic drug-induced increases in prolactin concentrations. On the other hand, five patients (four women and one man, aged 30–45 years), who were evaluated for risperidone-induced hyperprolactinemia, had significant hyperprolactinemia, with prolactin concentrations of 66–209 μg/l (151[c]). All but one had manifestations of hypogonadism, and in these four patients risperidone was continued and a dopamine receptor agonist (bromocriptine or cabergoline) was added; in three patients this reduced the prolactin concentration and alleviated the hypogonadism. In a meta-analysis of two independent studies (n = 404), prolactin was greatly increased by risperidone (mean change 45–80 ng/ml), a larger effect than with olanzapine and haloperidol (152[M]).

Metabolic Pathological *weight gain* has been increasingly identified as a problem, particularly when risperidone is given to children (SEDA-22, 69, SEDA-23, 71). In a recent review, 37 children and adolescent in-patients treated with risperidone for 6 months were compared with 33 psychiatric in-patients who had not taken atypical neuroleptic drugs (153[c]). Risperidone was associated with significant weight gain in 78% of the treated children and adolescents (as opposed to 24% of those in the comparison group); risperidone dosage, concomitant medicaments, and other demographic characteristics (such as age, sex, pubertal status, and baseline weight and body mass index) were not associated with an increased risk of morbid weight gain.

Endocrine There has been a recent report of *diabetic ketoacidosis* in a 42-year-old man, without a prior history of diabetes mellitus, who took risperidone (2 mg bd) (154[A]). The authors pointed out that in premarketing studies of risperidone diabetes mellitus occurred in 0.01–1% of patients.

Urinary tract Several cases of *urinary incontinence* have been associated with risperidone, and the package insert lists this adverse effect in up to 1% of patients (SEDA-22, 70). The authors of a recent report stated that at least 28% of patients developed transient urinary incontinence after starting risperidone, and they reported two cases, in both of which the adverse effect was clearly temporally related to the drug (155[A]).

Sexual function *Erectile dysfunction* has previously been described (SEDA-24, 71). Now, *priapism* associated with risperidone has been reported in a 19-year-old man who had taken 2 mg/day for 4 days (156[A]).

Lactation The distribution and excretion of risperidone and 9-hydroxyrisperidone into the breast milk of a young woman with puerperal psychosis, who was treated with risperidone, has been reported (157[A]).

A 21-year-old woman with a 2-year history of bipolar disorder stopped all of her medication when she discovered that she was pregnant; she was given risperidone 2.5 months after childbirth, gradually increasing to a steady-state dosage of 6 mg/day. Risperidone and 9-hydroxyrisperidone concentrations in plasma and breast milk were quantified, and calculations indicated that a suckling infant would receive only 0.84% of the maternal dose as risperidone and 3.46% as 9-hydroxyrisperidone.

Drug interactions A potential pharmacokinetic interaction of risperidone with *carbamazepine* (SEDA-22, 71; SEDA-23, 72) and a pharmacokinetic or an additive pharmacodynamic interaction of risperidone with *serotonin re-uptake inhibitors* (SEDA-23, 72; SEDA-24, 74) have previously been described. A 23-year-old man had high risperidone plasma concentrations secondary to concurrent thioridazine use, and raised 9-hydroxyrisperidone concentrations in association with carbamazepine dosage reduction and concomitant fluvoxamine therapy (158[A]).

To further evaluate the pharmacokinetic interaction between risperidone and carbamazepine or valproic acid, plasma concentrations of risperidone and 9-hydroxyrisperidone were measured in 44 patients (aged 26–63 years) treated with risperidone alone (n = 23) or co-medicated with carbamazepine (n = 11) or sodium valproate (n = 10) (159[c]). Carbamazepine markedly reduced the plasma concentrations of risperidone and 9-hydroxyrisperidone, probably by inducing CYP3A4; this interaction is likely to be clinically significant. Conversely, valproic acid did not have any major effect on plasma risperidone concentrations.

The serotonin syndrome, an acute condition characterized by mental changes, restlessness, myoclonus, hyper-reflexia, and autonomic instability, caused by a hyperserotonergic state of the central and peripheral nervous system, has been reported during treatment with *paroxetine* and risperidone (160[A]). In addition, a case of edema in a patient taking risperidone and paroxetine has also been reported (161[A]).

Sertindole

Sertindole is an antipsychotic drug that was approved in several countries in 1997. However, it was suspended in January 2000, following concerns about reports of cardiac dysrhythmias and sudden cardiac death (SEDA-22, 71). The Committee for Proprietary Medicinal Products (CPMP) of The European Agency for the Evaluation of Medicinal Products has recently recommended lifting the ban on sertindole-containing medicinal products on the basis of additional data provided by the marketing authorization holders (see monthly report from October, 2001: www.emea.eu.int).

Tiapride *(SEDA-19, 56)*

Tiapride is a substituted benzamide derivative with dopamine antagonistic effects, specifically on dopamine D_2 and D_3 receptors. From a clinical point of view, it can be considered as an atypical neuroleptic drug. A recent comparison of tiapride and haloperidol is described above.

Ziprasidone *(SEDA-23, 73; SEDA-24, 74)*

Ziprasidone is a dibenzotheolylpiperazine compound with a receptor binding profile similar to that of other atypical antipsychotic drugs, and high affinity for serotonin ($5\text{-}HT_{2A}$) and dopamine (D_2) receptors; it also has potent affinity for $5\text{-}HT_{1A}$, $5\text{-}HT_{1D}$, and $5\text{-}HT_{2C}$ receptors and inhibits serotonin and noradrenaline re-uptake. On 5 February 2000, the FDA approved ziprasidone for the treatment of schizophrenia (www.fda.gov).

Cardiovascular Over the past several years, the FDA has been concerned with the possibility that ziprasidone and a number of other drugs might increase the risk of the specific potentially fatal cardiac dysrhythmia, torsade de pointes. The FDA did not approve ziprasidone in 1998, because of evidence that it can cause *prolongation of the QT interval*, which predisposes to torsade de pointes, and they asked that specific safety data be gathered. The safety data were submitted in 1999. Although QT prolongation predisposing to torsade is still a theoretical concern, over 4000 patients have been treated in clinical trials without evidence of this dysrhythmia. In addition, overall mortality in the trials was similar to that seen with placebo and other antipsychotic drugs. The FDA labeling does not include a so-called "black-box warning" and does not require an electrocardiogram before or during treatment. However, the labeling does warn physicians and patients about QT interval prolongation and the possible risk of sudden death. The labeling suggests that doctors use their best judgment, based on the health status of the individual, as to whether to use ziprasidone as first-line treatment or only after other available drugs have failed. There is no requirement that patients have regular heart check-ups while taking this drug.

Metabolic Two extensive reviews of the clinical pharmacology of ziprasidone have recently appeared (162[R], 163[R]). Emphasis has been put on weight gain; ziprasidone is said to be associated with less weight gain than the other atypical drugs and than most conventional antipsychotic drugs.

Ziprasidone has been used in 28 children and adolescents (aged 7–17 years) with Tourette's syndrome in an 8-week pilot study (164[C]). They were randomly assigned to ziprasidone (5–40 mg/day; $n = 16$) or placebo ($n = 12$). Ziprasidone significantly reduced tic frequency. There was one case each of *somnolence* and *akathisia*, both with the highest dose of ziprasidone; these were considered to be severe but did not necessitate withdrawal.

Drug interactions Pfizer, the marketing authorization holder of ziprasidone, has promoted several pharmacokinetic studies. Neither *oral contraceptives* (ethinylestradiol 30 μg/day and levonorgestrel 150 μg/day) (165[c]), *lithium* 900 mg/day (166[c]), *ketoconazole* 400 mg/day

(167[c]), nor *carbamazepine* (100–400 mg/day) (168[c]) induced clinically significant changes in the pharmacokinetics of ziprasidone (40 mg/day).

Zotepine *(SEDA-22, 72; SEDA-23, 73)*

The efficacy and safety of zotepine have been explored in a 1-year open study in 253 schizophrenic patients (mean age 38 years, range 18–65) who took zotepine 75–450 mg/day (169[C]). The mean total BPRS score was reduced from 52 at baseline to 41. Since concomitant treatment was allowed, 173 patients reported 205 ongoing and 448 new antipsychotic medicaments during the study. A total of 826 adverse events were reported by 220 patients; 50 had serious adverse events and five died during the study, two taking zotepine; one death was a suicide and the other was due to a ventricular dysrhythmia. In all, 138 patients (55%) withdrew from the study (60 because of adverse events). The most frequently reported adverse events were *weight gain* (28%; mean weight gain 4.3 kg), *somnolence* (15%), and *weakness* (13%). There were adverse events that could be related to extrapyramidal effects in 5%. In 14 patients with normal baseline electrocardiography there were abnormalities at the end of the study, most commonly *sinus tachycardia*; there were no reports of torsade de pointes.

Zuclopenthixol

Hematologic *Neutropenia* and *agranulocytosis* are complications of antipsychotic drug therapy (SED-14, 149), and a case of neutropenia associated with zuclopenthixol has been reported (170[A]).

A 66-year-old schizophrenic man, took zuclopenthixol 10 mg tds for 18 days and developed mild leukopenia (2.9×10^9/l) and thrombocytopenia (109×10^9/l). He was asymptomatic, with no evidence of infection or bleeding tendency. Zuclopenthixol was withdrawn, without any change in the rest of his drug therapy (glibenclamide 5 mg tds, biperiden 2 mg bd, oxazepam 10 mg tds, dipyridamole 75 mg tds, and ranitidine 150 mg od). The leukocyte and platelet counts rose over the next 5 days.

REFERENCES

1. Geddes J, Freemantle N, Harrison P, Bebbington P. Atypical antipsychotics in the treatment of schizophrenia: systematic overview and meta-regression analysis. Br J Med 2000; 321: 1371–6.
2. Voruganti L, Cortese L, Oyewumi L, Cernovsky Z, Zirul S, Awad A. Comparative evaluation of conventional and novel antipsychotic drugs with reference to their subjective tolerability, side-effect profile and impact on quality of life. Schizophr Res 2000; 43: 135–45.
3. Worrel JA, Marken PA, Beckman SE, Ruehter VL. Atypical antipsychotic agents: a critical review. Am J Health-Syst Pharm 2000; 57: 238–58.
4. Beaumont G. Antipsychotics – the future of schizophrenia treatment. Curr Med Res Opin 2000; 16: 37–42.
5. Sacristán JA, Gómez JC, Montejo AL, Vieta E, Gregor KJ. Doses of olanzapine, risperidone, and haloperidol used in clinical practice: results of a prospective pharmacoepidemiologic study. Clin Ther 2000; 22: 583–99.
6. Advokat CD, Mayville EA, Matson JL. Side effect profiles of atypical antipsychotics, typical antipsychotics, or no psychotropic medications in persons with mental retardation. Res Dev Disabil 2000; 21: 75–84.
7. Anonymous. Keep an eye on this neuroleptic. Can Fam Phys 2000; 46: 322–6.
8. Copolov DL, Link CGG, Kowalcyk B. A multicentre, double-blind, randomized comparison of quetiapine (ICI 204,636, "Seroquel") and haloperidol in schizophrenia. Psychol Med 2000; 30: 95–105.
9. Emsley RA, Raniwalla J, Bailey PJ, Jones AM. A comparison of the effects of quetiapine ("Seroquel") and haloperidol in schizophrenic patients with a history of and a demonstrated, partial response to conventional antipsychotic treatment. Int Clin Phychopharmacol 2000; 15: 121–31.
10. Allain H, Dautzenberg PHJ, Maurer K, Schuck S, Bonhomme D, Gérard D. Double blind study of tiapride versus haloperidol and placebo in agitation and aggressiveness in elderly patients with cognitive impairment. Psychopharmacology 2000; 148: 361–6.
11. Brook S, Lucey JV, Gunn KP. Intramuscular ziprasidone compared with intramuscular haloperidol in the treatment of acute psychosis. J Clin Psychiatry 2000; 61: 933–41.
12. Cooper SJ, Tweed J, Raniwalla J, Butler A, Welch C. A placebo-controlled comparison of zotepine versus chlorpromazine in patients with acute exacerbation of schizophrenia. Acta Psychiatr Scand 2000; 101: 218–25.
13. Al-Sughayir MA. Depot antipsychotics: patient characteristics and prescribing pattern. Saudi

Med J 2000; 21: 1178–81.
14. Dunayevich E, McElroy SL. Atypical antipsychotics in the treatment of bipolar disorder: pharmacological and clinical effects. CNS Drugs 2000; 13: 433–41.
15. Guille C, Sachs GS, Ghaemi SN. A naturalistic comparison of clozapine, risperidone, and olanzapine in the treatment of bipolar disorder. J Clin Psychiatry 2000; 61: 638–42.
16. Ellis T, Cudkowicz ME, Sexton PM, Growdon JH. Clozapine and risperidone treatment of psychosis in Parkinson's disease. J Neuropsychiatry Clin Neurosci 2000; 12: 364–9.
17. Wahlbeck K, Cheine M, Tuisku K, Ahokas A, Joffe G, Rimón R. Risperidone versus clozapine in treatment-resistant schizophrenia: a randomized pilot study. Prog Neuro-Psychopharmacol Biol Psychiatry 2000; 24: 911–22.
18. Colonna L, Saleem P, Dondey-Nouvel L, Rein W. Long-term safety and efficacy of amisulpride in subchronic or chronic schizophrenia. Int Clin Psychopharmacol 2000; 15: 13–22.
19. Teri L, Logsdon RG, Peskind E, Raskind M, Weiner MF, Tractenberg RE, Foster NL, Schneider LS, Sano M, Whitehouse P, Tariot P, Mellow AM, Auchus AP, Grundman M, Thomas RG, Schafer K, Thal LJ. Treatment of agitation in AD: a randomized, placebo-controlled clinical trial. Neurology 2000; 55: 1271–8.
20. Schneider LS, Ollock VE, Lyness SA. A meta-analysis of controlled clinical trials of neuroleptic treatment in dementia. J Am Geriatr Soc 1990; 38: 553–63.
21. Sultzer DL, Gray KF, Gunay I, Berisford MA, Mahler ME. A double-blind comparison of trazodone and haloperidol for treatment of agitation in patients with dementia. Am J Geriatr Psychiatry 1997; 5: 60–9.
22. Timell AM. Thioridazine: re-evaluating the risk/benefit equation. Ann Clin Psychiatry 2000; 12: 147–51.
23. Douglas PH, Block PC. Corrected QT interval prolongation associated with intravenous haloperidol in acute coronary syndromes. Catheter Cardiovasc Interventions 2000; 50: 352–5.
24. Iglesias E, Esteban E, Zabala S, Gascon A. Tiapride-induced torsade de pointes. Am J Med 2000; 109: 509.
25. Perrault LP, Denault AY, Carrier M, Cartier R, Belisle S. Torsades de pointes secondary to intravenous haloperidol after coronary bypass grafting surgery. Can J Anaesth 2000; 47: 251–4.
26. Johri S, Rashid H, Daniel PJ, Soni A. Cardiopulmonary arrest secondary to haloperidol. Am J Emerg Med 2000; 18: 839.
27. Rampello L, Raffaele R, Vecchio I, Pistone G, Brunetto MB, Malaguarnera M. Behavioural changes and hypotensive effects of thioridazine in two elderly patients with traumatic brain injury: post-traumatic syndrome and thioridazine. Gaz Med Ital Arch Sci Med 2000; 159: 121–3.
28. Wirz-Justice A, Werth E, Savaskan E, Knoblauch V, Gasio PF, Müller-Spahn F. Haloperidol disrupts, clozapine reinstates the circadian rest–activity cycle in a patient with early-onset Alzheimer disease. Alzheimer Dis Assoc Disord 2000; 14: 212–15.
29. Caligiuri MP, Jeste DV, Lacro JP. Antipsychotic-induced movement disorders in the elderly: epidemiology and treatment recommendations. Drugs Aging 2000; 17: 363–84.
30. Kapur S, Zipursky R, Jones C, Remington G, Houle S. Relationship between dopamine D_2 occupancy, clinical response, and side effects: a double-blind PET study of first-episode schizophrenia. Am J Psychiatry 2000; 157: 514–20.
31. Olsen JC, Keng JA, Clark JA. Frequency of adverse reactions to prochlorperazine in the ED. Am J Emerg Med 2000; 18: 609–11.
32. Hofmann M, Seifritz E, Botschev C, Kräuchi K, Müller-Spahn F. Serum iron and ferritin in acute neuroleptic akathisia. Psychiatry Res 2000; 93: 201–7.
33. Hirose S, Ashby CR. Intravenous biperiden in akathisia: an open pilot study. Int J Psychiatry Med 2000; 30: 185–94.
34. Iqbal N. Heroin use, diplopia, Largactil. Saudi Med J 2000; 21: 1194.
35. Tan E-K, Jankovic J. Tardive and idiopathic oromandibular dystonia: a clinical comparison. J Neurol Neurosurg Psychiatry 2000; 68: 186–90.
36. Caroff S, Mann SC, Keck PE, Francis A. Residual catatonic state following neuroleptic malignant syndrome. J Clin Psychopharmacol 2000; 20: 257–9.
37. Bobolakis I. Neuroleptic malignant syndrome after antipsychotic drug administration during benzodiazepine withdrawal. J Clin Psychopharmacol 2000; 20: 281–3.
38. Askin R, Herken H, Derman H. Recurrent neuroleptic malignant syndrome: a case report. Int Med J 2000; 7: 287–8.
39. Lin P-Y, Wu K, Sun T-F. Concomitant neuroleptic malignant syndrome and lithium intoxication in a patient with bipolar I disorder: case report. Chang Gung Med J 2000; 23: 624–9.
40. Weiser M, Shneider-Beeri M, Nakash N, Brill N, Bawnik O, Reiss S, Hocherman S, Davidson M. Improvement in cognition associated with novel antipsychotic drugs: a direct drug effect or reduction of EPS. Schizophr Res 2000; 46: 81–9.
41. Yoshikawa H, Watanabe T, Abe T, Oda Y, Ozawa K. Haloperidol-induced rhabdomyolysis without neuroleptic malignant syndrome in a handicapped child. Brain Dev 2000; 22: 256–8.
42. Boot E, De Haan L. Massive increase in serum creatine kinase during olanzapine and quetiapine treatment, not during treatment with clozapine. Psychopharmacology 2000; 150: 347–8.
43. Voss SN, Sanger T, Beasley C. Hematologic reference ranges in a population of patients with schizophrenia. J Clin Psychopharmacol 2000; 20: 653–7.
44. Lal S, Lal S. Chlorpromazine-induced cutaneous pigmentation – effect of replacement with clozapine. J Psychiatry Neurosci 2000; 25: 281.

45. Tsai S-J, Hong C-J. Haloperidol-induced impotence improved by switching to olanzapine. Gen Hosp Psychiatry 2000; 22: 391–2.
46. Shiloh R, Hermesh H, Weizer N, Dorfman-Etrog P, Weizman A, Munitz H. Acute antipsychotic drug administration lowers body temperature in drug-free male schizophrenic patients. Eur Neuropsychopharmacol 2000; 10: 443–5.
47. Ahmed Z, Fraser W, Kerr MP, Kiernan C, Emerson E, Robertson J, Felce D, Allen D, Baxter H, Thomas J. Reducing antipsychotic medication in people with a learning disability. Br J Psychiatry 2000; 176: 42–6.
48. Mohan MS, Patole SK, Whitehall JS. Severe hypothermia in a neonate following antenatal exposure to haloperidol. J Paediatr Child Health 2000; 36: 412.
49. Hirshberg B, Gural A, Caraco Y. Zuclopenthixol-associated neutropenia and thrombocytopenia. Ann Pharmacother 2000; 34: 740–2.
50. Capel MM, Colbridge MG, Henry JA. Overdose profiles of new antipsychotic agents. Int J Neuropsychopharmacol 2000; 3: 51–4.
51. James LP, Abel K, Wilkinson J, Simpson PM, Nichols MH. Phenothiazine, butyrophenone, and other psychotropic medication poisonings in children and adolescents. Clin Toxicol 2000; 38: 615–23.
52. Stein S, Schmoldt A, Schulz M. Fatal intoxication with melperone. Forensic Sci Int 2000; 113: 409–13.
53. Dorne R, Pommier C, Manchon M, Berny C. Intoxication par l'amisulpride (Solian®): à propos d'une observation avec documentation toxicologique. Thérapie 2000; 55: 319–28.
54. Burton S, Heslop K, Harrison K, Barnes M. Ziprasidone overdose. Am J Psychiatry 2000; 157: 835.
55. Allen SA. Effect of chlorpromazine and clozapine on plasma concentrations of haloperidol in a patient with schizophrenia. J Clin Pharmacol 2000; 40: 1296–7.
56. Peacok L, Gerlach J. Clozapine treatment in Denmark: concomitant psychotropic medication and haematologic monitoring system with liberal usage practices. J Clin Psychiatry 1994; 55: 44–9.
57. Chong SA, Remington G. Clozapine augmentation: safety and efficacy. Schizophr Bull 2000; 26: 421–40.
58. Waserman J, Criollo M. Subjective experiences of clozapine treatment by patients with chronic schizophrenia. Psychiatr Serv 2000; 51: 666–8.
59. Antonacci DJ, De Groot CM. Clozapine treatment in a population of adults with mental retardation. J Clin Psychiatry 2000; 61: 22–5.
60. Hägg S, Spigset O, Söderström TG. Association of venous thromboembolism and clozapine. Lancet 2000; 355: 1155–6.
61. Walker AM, Lanza LL, Arellano F, Rothman KJ. Mortality in current and former users of clozapine. Epidemiology 1997; 8: 671–7.
62. Ung GK, Jun SK, Yong MA, Sun JC, Jee HH, Young JK, Yong SK. Electrocardiographic abnormalities in patients treated with clozapine. J Clin Psychiatry 2000; 61: 441–6.
63. Usiskin SI, Nicolson R, Lenane M, Rapoport JL. Gabapentin prophylaxis of clozapine-induced seizures. Am J Psychiatry 2000; 157: 482–3.
64. Modestin J, Stephan PL, Erni T, Umari T. Prevalence of extrapyramidal syndromes in psychiatric inpatients and the relationship of clozapine treatment to tardive dyskinesia. Schizophr Res 2000; 42: 223–30.
65. Elliott ESR, Marken PA, Ruehter VL. Clozapine-associated extrapyramidal reaction. Ann Pharmacother 2000; 34: 615–18.
66. Sieche A, Giedke H. Treatment of primary cranial dystonia (Meige's syndrome) with clozapine. J Clin Psychiatry 2000; 61: 949.
67. Doan RJ, Callaghan WD. Clozapine treatment and neuroleptic malignant syndrome. Can J Psychiatry 2000; 45: 394–5.
68. Reznik I, Volcheck L, Mester R, Kotler M, Sarova-Pinhas I, Spivak B, Weizman A. Myotoxicity and neurotoxicity during clozapine treatment. Clin Neuropharmacol 2000; 23: 276–80.
69. Bressan RA, Monteiro VBM, Dias CC. Panic disorder associated with clozapine. Am J Psychiatry 2000; 157: 2056.
70. Rigalleau V, Gatta B, Bonnaud S, Masson M, Bourgeois ML, Vergnot V, Gin H. Diabetes as a result of atypical anti-psychotic drugs – a report of three cases. Diabet Med 2000; 17: 484–6.
71. Wehring H, Alexander B, Perry PJ. Diabetes mellitus associated with clozapine therapy. Pharmacotherapy 2000; 20: 844–7.
72. Dursun SM, Devarajan S. Clozapine weight gain, plus topiramate weight loss. Can J Psychiatry 2000; 45: 198.
73. Hampson ME. Clozapine-induced thrombocytosis. Br J Psychiatry 2000; 176: 400.
74. Gonzales MF, Elmore J, Luebbert C. Evidence for immune etiology in clozapine-induced thrombocytopenia of 40 months' duration: a case report. CNS Spectr 2000; 5: 17–18.
75. Marcos F, Solano F, Arbol F, Caballero L, Maldonado G, López P, Durán A. Clozapine-induced agranulocytosis. SN 2000; 5: 27–9.
76. Silvestrini C, Arcangeli T, Biondi M, Pancheri P. A second trial of clozapine in a case of granulocytopenia. Hum Psychopharmacol Clin Exp 2000; 15: 275–9.
77. Schuld A, Kraus T, Hinze-Selch D, Haack M, Pollmächer T. Granulocyte colony-stimulating factor plasma levels during clozapine- and olanzapine-induced granulocytopenia. Acta Psychiatr Scand 2000; 102: 153–5.
78. Jauss M, Pantel J, Werle Eschröder J. G-CSF plasma levels in clozapine-induced neutropenia. Biol Psychiatry 2000; 48: 1113–15.
79. Dettling M, Sachse C, Müller-Oerlinghausen B, Roots I, Brockmöller J, Rolfs A, Cascorbi I. Clozapine-induced agranulocytosis and hereditary polymorphisms of clozapine metabolizing enzymes: no association with myeloperoxidase and

cytochrome P4502D6. Pharmacopsychiatry 2000; 33: 218–20.
80. Calderon J, Rubin E, Sobota WL. Potential use of ipratropium bromide for the treatment of clozapine-induced hypersalivation: a preliminary report. Int Clin Psychopharmacol 2000; 15: 49–52.
81. Freudenreich O, Goff DC. Colon perforation and peritonitis associated with clozapine. J Clin Psychiatry 2000; 61: 950–1.
82. Hsu JW, Wang YC, Lin CC, Bai YM, Chen JY, Chiu HJ, Tsai SJ, Hong CJ. No evidence for association of alpha 1a adrenoceptor gene polymorphism and clozapine-induced urinary incontinence. Neuropsychobiology 2000; 42: 62–5.
83. Goudie AJ. What is the clinical significance of the discontinuation syndrome seen with clozapine? J Psychopharmacol 2000; 14: 188–92.
84. Renwick AC, Renwick AG, Flanagan RJ, Ferner RE. Monitoring of clozapine and norclozapine plasma concentration-time curves in acute overdose. Clin Toxicol 2000; 38: 325–8.
85. Usiskin SI, Nicolson R, Lenane M, Rapoport JL. Retreatment with clozapine after erythromycin-induced neutropenia. Am J Psychiatry 2000; 157: 1021.
86. Raaska K, Neuvonen PJ. Ciprofloxacin increases serum clozapine and N-desmethylclozapine: a study in patients with schizophrenia. Eur J Clin Pharmacol 2000; 56: 585–9.
87. Spina E, Avenoso A, Salemi M, Facciolá G, Scordo MG, Ancione M, Madia A. Plasma concentrations of clozapine and its major metabolites during combined treatment with paroxetine or sertraline. Pharmacopsychiatry 2000; 33: 213–17.
88. Borba CP, Henderson DC. Citalopram and clozapine: potential drug interaction. J Clin Psychiatry 2000; 61: 301–2.
89. Hinze-Selch D, Deuschle M, Weber B, Heuser I, Pollmächer T. Effect of coadministration of clozapine and fluvoxamine versus clozapine monotherapy on blood cell counts, plasma levels of cytokines and body weight. Psychopharmacology 2000; 149: 163–9.
90. Conca A, Beraus W, König P, Waschgler R. A case of pharmacokinetic interference in comedication of clozapine and valproic acid. Pharmacopsychiatry 2000; 33: 234–5.
91. Gómez JC, Sacristán JA, Hernández J, Breier A, Carrasco PR, Saiz CA, Carbonell EF. The safety of olanzapine compared with other antipsychotic drugs: results of an observational prospective study in patients with schizophrenia (EFESO study). J Clin Psychiatry 2000; 61: 335–43.
92. Chengappa KNR, Pollock BG, Parepally H, Levine J, Kirshner MA, Brar JS, Zoretich RA. Anticholinergic differences among patients receiving standard clinical doses of olanzapine or clozapine. J Clin Psychopharmacol 2000; 20: 311–16.
93. Onofrj M, Paci C, D'Andreamatteo G, Toma L. Olanzapine in severe Gilles de la Tourette syndrome: a 52-week double-blind cross-over study vs. low-dose pimozide. J Neurol 2000; 247: 443–6.
94. Deshauer D, Albuquerque J, Alda M, Grof P. Seizures caused by possible interaction between olanzapine and clomipramine. J Clin Psychopharmacol 2000; 20: 283–4.
95. Haberfellner EM. Remission of tardive dyskinesia after changing from flupenthixol to olanzapine. Eur Psychiatry 2000; 15: 338–9.
96. Sierra-Biddle D, Herran A, Díez-Aja S, González-Mata JM, Vidal E, Díez-Manrique F, Vázquez-Barquero JL. Neuroleptic malignant syndrome and olanzapine. J Clin Psychopharmacol 2000; 20: 704–5.
97. Nyfort-Hansen K, Alderman CP. Possible neuroleptic malignant syndrome associated with olanzapine. Ann Pharmacother 2000; 34: 667.
98. Stanfield SC, Privette T. Neuroleptic malignant syndrome associated with olanzapine therapy: a case report. J Emerg Med 2000; 19: 355–7.
99. Järventausta K, Leinonen E. Neuroleptic malignant syndrome during olanzapine and levomepromazine treatment. Acta Psychiatr Scand 2000; 102: 231–3.
100. Nemets B, Geller V, Grisaru N, Belmaker RH. Olanzapine treatment of clozapine-induced NMS. Hum Psychopharmacol Clin Exp 2000; 15: 77–8.
101. Singh HK, Markowitz GD, Myers G. Esotropia associated with olanzapine. J Clin Psychopharmacol 2000; 20: 488.
102. Narayan G, Puranik A. Olanzapine-induced mania. Int J Psychiatry Clin Pract 2000; 4: 333–4.
103. Lykouras L, Zervas IM, Gounellis R, Malliori M, Rabavilas A. Olanzapine and obsessive–compulsive symptoms. Eur Neuropsychopharmacol 2000; 10: 385–7.
104. Bogetto F, Bellino S, Vaschetto P, Ziero S. Olanzapine augmentation of fluvoxamine-refractory obsessive-compulsive disorder (OCD): a 12-week open trial. Psychiatry Res 2000; 96: 91–8.
105. Bronson BD, Lindenmayer JP. Adverse effects of high-dose olanzapine in treatment-refractory schizophrenia. J Clin Psychopharmacol 2000; 20: 382–4.
106. Melkersson KI, Hulting Al, Brismar KE. Elevated levels of insulin, leptin, and blood lipids in olanzapine-treated patients with schizophrenia or related psychoses. J Clin Psychiatry 2000; 61: 742–9.
107. Bettinger TL, Mendelson SC, Dorson PG, Crismon ML. Olanzapine-induced glucose dysregulation. Ann Pharmacother 2000; 34: 865–7.
108. Sacchetti E, Guarneri L, Bravi D. H_2 antagonist nizatidine may control olanzapine-associated weight gain in schizoprenic patients. Biol Psychiatry 2000; 48: 167–8.
109. Gajwani P, Tesar GE. Olanzapine-induced neutropenia. Psychosomatics 2000; 41: 150–1.
110. Konakanchi R, Grace JJ, Szarowicz R, Pato MT. Olanzapine prolongation of granulocytopenia after clozapine discontinuation. J Clin Psychopharmacol 2000; 20: 703–4.
111. Oyewumi LK, Al-Semaan Y. Olanzapine: safe during clozapine-induced agranulocytosis. J Clin Psychopharmacol 2000; 20: 279–81.

112. Dernovsek MZ, Tavcar R. Olanzapine appears haematologically safe in patients who developed blood dyscrasia on clozapine and risperidone. Int Clin Psychopharmacol 2000; 15: 237–8.
113. Felber W, Naumann R, Schuler U, Fülle M, Reuster T, Garcia K, Heilemann H. Are there genetic determinants of olanzapine-induced agranulocytosis? Pharmacopsychiatry 2000; 33: 197–9.
114. Bogunovic O, Viswanathan R. Trombocytopenia possibly associated with olanzapine and subsequently with benztropine mesylate. Psychosomatics 2000; 41: 277–8.
115. Doucette DE, Grenier JPMS, Robertson PS. Olanzapine-induced acute pancreatitis. Ann Pharmacother 2000; 34: 1128–31.
116. Vernon LT, Fuller MA, Hattab H, Varnes KM. Olanzapine-induced urinary incontinence: treatment with ephedrine. J Clin Psychiatry 2000; 61: 601–2.
117. Compton MT, Saldivia A, Berry SA. Recurrent priapism during treatment with clozapine and olanzapine. Am J Psychiatry 2000; 157: 659.
118. Gerber JE, Cawthon B. Overdose and death with olanzapine. Am J Forensic Med Pathol 2000; 21: 249–51.
119. Bosch RF, Baumbach A, Bitzer M, Erley CM. Intoxication with olanzapine. Am J Psychiatry 2000; 157: 304–5.
120. Al-Waneen R. Neuroleptic malignant syndrome associated with quetiapine. Can J Psychiatry 2000; 45: 764–5.
121. Meibach RC, Mazurek MF, Rosebush P. Neurologic side effects in neuroleptic-naive patients treated with haloperidol or risperidone. Neurology 2000; 55: 1069.
122. Huston P, Moher D. Redundancy, disaggregation, and the integrity of medical research. Lancet 1996; 347:1024–6.
123. Rennie D. Fair conduct and fair reporting of clinical trials. J Am Med Assoc 1999; 282: 1766–8.
124. Feifel D, Moutier CY, Perry W. Safety and tolerability of a rapidly escalating dose-loading regimen for risperidone. J Clin Psychiatry 2000; 61: 909–11.
125. Kontaxakis VP, Havaki-kontaxaki BJ, Stamouli SS. Optimal risperidone dose in drug-naive, first-episode schizophrenia. Am J Psychiatry 2000; 157: 1178–9.
126. Lane HY, Chiu WC, Chou JC, Wu ST, Su MH, Chang WH Risperidone in acutely exacerbated schizophrenia: dosing strategies and plasma levels. J Clin Psychiatry 2000; 61: 209–14.
127. Zuddas A, Di Martino A, Muglia P, Cianchetti C. Long-term risperidone for pervasive developmental disorder: efficacy, tolerability, and discontinuation. J Child Adolesc Psychopharmacol 2000; 10: 79–90.
128. Findling RL, McNamara NK, Branicky LA, Schluchter MD, Lemon E, Blumer JL. A double-blind pilot study of risperidone in the treatment of conduct disorder. J Am Acad Child Adolesc Psychiatry 2000; 39: 509–16.
129. Buitelaar JK. Open-label treatment with risperidone of 26 psychiatrically-hospitalized children and adolescents with mixed diagnoses and aggressive behavior. J Child Adolesc Psychopharmacol 2000; 10: 19–26.
130. Heck AH, Haffmans PMJ, De Groot IW, Hoencamp E. Risperidone versus haloperidol in psychotic patients with disturbing neuroleptic-induced extrapyramidal symptoms: a double-blind, multi-center trial. Schizophr Res 2000; 46: 97–105.
131. Bhana N, Spencer CM. Risperidone. A review of its use in the management of the behavioural and psychological symptoms of dementia. Drugs Aging 2000; 16: 451–71.
132. De Deyn PP, Rabheru K, Rasmussen A, Bocksberger JP, Dautzenberg PL, Eriksson S, Lawlor BA. A randomized trial of risperidone, placebo, and haloperidol for behavioural symptoms of dementia. Neurology 1999; 53: 946–55.
133. Katz IR, Jeste DV, Mintzer JE, Clyde C, Napolitano J, Brecher M. Comparison of risperidone and placebo for psychosis and behavioral disturbances associated with dementia: a randomized, double-blind trial. Risperidone Study Group. J Clin Psychiatry 1999; 60: 107–15.
134. Kumar S, Malone DM. Risperidone implicated in the onset of tardive dyskinesia in a young woman. Postgrad Med J 2000; 76: 316–17.
135. Spivak M, Smart M. Tardive dyskinesia from low-dose risperidone. Can J Psychiatry 2000; 45: 202.
136. Jeste DV, Okamoto A, Napolitano J, Kane JM, Martinez RA. Low incidence of persistent tardive dyskinesia in elderly patients with dementia treated with risperidone. Am J Psychiatry 2000; 157: 1150–5.
137. Miller LJ. Withdrawal-emergent dyskinesia in a patient taking risperidone/citalopram. Ann Pharmacother 2000; 34: 269.
138. Silver H, Aharon N, Schwartz M. Attention deficit–hyperactivity disorder may be a risk factor for treatment-emergent tardive dyskinesia induced by risperidone. J Clin Psychopharmacol 2000; 20: 112–14.
139. Lore C. Risperidone and withdrawal dyskinesia. J Am Acad Child Adolesc Psychiatry 2000; 39: 941.
140. Mullen A, Cullen M. Risperidone and tardive dyskinesia: a case of blepharospasm. Aust NZ J Psychiatry 2000; 34: 879–89.
141. Bassitt DP, De Souza Lobo García L. Risperidone-induced tardive dyskinesia. Pharmacopsychiatry 2000; 33: 155–6.
142. Narendran R, Young CM, Pato MT. Possible risperidone-induced tardive dystonia. Ann Pharmacother 2000; 34: 1487–8.
143. Suenaga T, Tawara Y, Goto S, Kouhata SI, Kagaya A, Horiguchi J, Yamanaka Y, Yamawaki S. Risperidone treatment of neuroleptic-induced tardive extrapyramidal symptoms. Int J Psychiatry Clin Pract 2000; 4: 241–3.
144. Lee MS, Lee HJ, Kim L. A case of delayed

NMS induced by risperidone. Psychiatr Serv 2000; 51: 254–5.
145. Robb AS, Chang W, Lee HK, Cook MS. Risperidone-induced neuroleptic malignant syndrome in an adolescent. J Child Adolesc Psychopharmacol 2000; 10: 327–30.
146. Sechi G, Agnetti VA, Masuri R, Deiana GA, Pugliatti M, Paulus KSM, Rosati G. Risperidone, neuroleptic malignant syndrome and probable dementia with Lewy bodies. Prog Neuro-Psychopharmacol Biol Psychiatry 2000; 24: 1043–51.
147. Leopold NA. Risperidone treatment of drug-related psychosis in patients with parkinsonism. Mov Disord 2000; 15: 301–4.
148. Sinha BNP, Duggal HS, Nizamie SH. Risperidone-induced obsessive-compulsive symptoms: a reappraisal. Can J Psychiatry 2000; 45: 397–8.
149. Lauterbach EC, Abdelhamid A, Annandale JB. Posthallucinogen-like visual illusions (palinopsia) with risperidone in a patient without previous hallucinogen exposure: possible relation to serotonin $5HT_{2A}$ receptor blockade. Pharmacopsychiatry 2000; 33: 38–41.
150. Mabini R, Wergowske G, Baker FM. Galactorrhea and gynecomastia in a hypothyroid male being treated with risperidone. Psychiatr Serv 2000; 51: 983–5.
151. Tollin SR. Use of the dopamine agonists bromocriptine and cabergoline in the management of risperidone-induced hyperprolactinemia in patients with psychotic disorders. J Endocrinol Invest 2000; 23: 765–70.
152. David SR, Taylor CC, Kinon BJ, Breier A. The effects of olanzapine, risperidone, and haloperidol on plasma prolactin levels in patients with schizophrenia. Clin Ther 2000; 22: 1085–96.
153. Martin A, Landau J, Leebens P, Ulizio K, Cicchetti D, Scahill L, Leckman JF. Risperidone-associated weight gain in children and adolescents: a retrospective chart review. J Child Adolesc Psychopharmacol 2000; 10: 259–68.
154. Croarkin PE, Jacobs KM, Bain BK. Diabetic ketoacidosis associated with risperidone treatment? Psychosomatics 2000; 41: 369–70.
155. Agarwal V. Urinary incontinence with risperidone. J Clin Psychiatry 2000; 61: 219.
156. Sirota P, Bogdanov I. Priapism associated with risperidone treatment. Int J Psychiatry Clin Pract 2000; 4: 237–9.
157. Hill RC, McIvor RJ, Wojnar-Horton RE, Hackett LP, Ilett KF. Risperidone distribution and excretion into human milk: case report and estimated infant exposure during breast-feeding. J Clin Psychopharmacol 2000; 20: 285–6.
158. Alfaro CL, Nicolson R, Lenane M, Rapoport JL. Carbamazepine and/or fluvoxamine drug interaction with risperidone in a patient on multiple psychotropic medications. Ann Pharmacother 2000; 34: 122–3.
159. Spina E, Avenoso A, Facciolà G, Salemi M, Scordo MG, Giacobello T, Madia AG, Perucca E. Plasma concentrations of risperidone and 9-hydroxyrisperidone: effect of comedication with carbamazepine or valproate. Ther Drug Monit 2000; 22: 481–5.
160. Hamilton S, Malone K. Serotonin syndrome during treatment with paroxetine and risperidone. J Clin Psychopharmacol 2000; 20: 103–5.
161. Masson M, Elayli R, Verdoux H. Rispéridone et øedème: à propos d'un cas. Encéphale 2000; 26: 91–2.
162. Buckley PF. Ziprasidone: pharmacology, clinical progress and therapeutic promise. Drugs Today 2000; 36: 583–9.
163. Daniel DG, Copeland LF. Ziprasidone: comprehensive overview and clinical use of a novel antipsychotic. Expert Opin Investig Drugs 2000; 9: 819–28.
164. Sallee FR, Kurlan R, Goetz CG, Singer H, Scahill L, Law G, Dittman VM, Chappell PB. Ziprasidone treatment of children and adolescents with Tourette's syndrome: a pilot study. J Am Acad Child Psychiatry 2000; 39: 292–9.
165. Muirhead GJ, Harness J, Holt PR, Oliver S, Anziano RJ. Ziprasidone and the pharmacokinetics of a combined oral contraceptive. Br J Clin Pharmacol 2000; 49 Suppl 1: 49S–56S.
166. Apseloff G, Mullet D, Wilner KD, Anziano RJ, Tensfeldt TG, Pelletier SM, Gerber N. The effects of ziprasidone on steady-state lithium levels and renal clearance of lithium. Br J Clin Pharmacol 2000; 49 Suppl 1: 61S–64S.
167. Miceli JJ, Smith M, Robarge L, Morse T, Lauent A. The effects of ketoconazole on ziprasidone pharmacokinetics – a placebo-controlled crossover study in healthy volunteers. Br J Clin Pharmacol 2000; 49 Suppl 1: 71S–76S.
168. Miceli JJ, Anziano RJ, Robarge L, Hansen RA, Lauent A. The effect of carbamazepine on the steady-state pharmacokinetics of ziprasidone in healthy volunteers. Br J Clin Pharmacol 2000; 49 Suppl 1: 65S–70S.
169. Palmgren K, Wighton A, Reynolds CW, Butler A, Tweed JA, Raniwalla J, Welch CP, Bratty JR. The safety and efficacy of zotepine in the treatment of schizophrenia: results of a one-year naturalistic clinical trial. Int J Psychiatry Clin Pract 2000; 4: 299–306.
170. Coutinho E, Fenton M, Adams C, Campbell C. Zuclopenthixol acetate in psychiatric emergencies: looking for evidence from clinical trials. Schizophr Res 2000; 46: 111–18.

Jeffrey K. Aronson

7 Antiepileptic drugs

GENERAL TOPICS *(SED-14, 164; SEDA-22, 81; SEDA-23, 83; SEDA-24, 82)*

R

Comparisons of different antiepileptic drugs

The clinical pharmacology and adverse effects of some new antiepileptic drugs (ganaxolone, levetiracetam, losigamone, pregabalin, remacemide, rufinamide, stiripentol, and zonisamide) have been reviewed (1[R]).

The uses and adverse effects of antiepileptic drugs in the treatment of painful peripheral neuropathy have been reviewed (2[r]).

Quality of life *The effects of carbamazepine and lamotrigine on health-related quality of life have been compared for 1 year in 260 patients with newly diagnosed epilepsy randomized to 48 weeks of treatment (3[C]). Patients taking carbamazepine had significantly worse quality of life at week 4 but not later. They also had more cognitive adverse effects in general and more changes in energy and affect during the first 4 weeks of treatment.*

Cost-effectiveness *The cost-effectiveness of four antiepileptic drugs used to treat newly diagnosed adult epilepsy has been studied by cost minimization analysis in 12 European countries (4[C]). The analysis took account of each drug's adverse effects and tolerability profiles. Lamotrigine incurred higher costs than carbamazepine, phenytoin, and valproate, whose costs were similar.*

Withdrawal of therapy *Gabapentin, lamotrigine, topiramate, and vigabatrin have been compared using Kaplan-Meier survival analysis in 61 patients to see how long they chose to keep taking each drug, and if they stopped, why they stopped (5[c]). The results are shown in Table 1. Lamotrigine seemed to be the best tolerated of the four drugs and topiramate the least. These results have been mirrored by those of two larger retrospective studies (6[c], 7[c]) (Table 1).*

The efficacy and safety of gabapentin and vigabatrin as first-line add-on treatment have been compared in 102 patients with partial epilepsy (8[C]). The improvement rate was 48% with gabapentin and 56% with vigabatrin. There were seven withdrawals in each group because of adverse events. Of the serious adverse events only one was thought to be drug-related – depression and weight gain in a patient taking vigabatrin.

General adverse effects *Carbamazepine and valproic acid have been compared in a randomized study in 30 patients (9[C]). Significantly more patients taking carbamazepine reported adverse events, including nausea and vomiting, dizziness, lethargy, and ataxia and tremors.*

In a comparison of carbamazepine and lamotrigine for trigeminal neuralgia in 18 patients with multiple sclerosis, lamotrigine was more effective (10[C]). After withdrawal of carbamazepine, drowsiness resolved in 16 patients; cerebellar signs improved partially in five patients and completely in two; brainstem signs improved partially in four patients and completely in three; ambulation improved in 11. In one patient taking lamotrigine a skin rash forced withdrawal.

The use of antiepileptic drugs (gabapentin, lamotrigine, and topiramate) as mood-stabilizers has been reviewed (11[R]). The authors concluded that the benefit:harm ratios of these drugs have not been well enough established for their routine use in bipolar disorder.

Nervous system *The risk of aggravating ju-*

Side Effects of Drugs, Annual 25
J.K. Aronson, ed.

Table 1. *Persistence with therapy with different antiepileptic drugs in different studies*

	Gabapentin	Lamotrigine	Tiagabine	Topiramate	Vigabatrin
Number (6[c])	36	37	–	28	26
Median time to 50% drop out (months)	13	>43	–	9.5	29
Withdrawn owing to lack of efficacy (%)	58	24	–	25	62
Number (7[c])	146	122	88	70	37
Withdrawn owing to lack of efficacy (%)	25	16	30	30	46
Withdrawn owing to adverse effects (%)	16	15	26	42	16
Number (8[c])	158	424	–	393	–
Withdrawn owing to lack of efficacy (%)	39	34	–	19	–
Withdrawn owing to adverse effects (%)	37	22	–	40	–

venile myoclonic epilepsy with carbamazepine and phenytoin has been assessed in a retrospective study of 170 patients, of whom 40 had taken carbamazepine or phenytoin (12[c]). There was aggravation of seizures in 23 patients, six benefited, and there was no effect in the other 11. Of the 28 patients who used carbamazepine, 19 had aggravated symptoms, including myoclonic status in two. Of the 16 patients who used phenytoin, six had aggravated symptoms, including one in association with phenobarbital. Vigabatrin was given in only one case, in association with carbamazepine, and provoked mixed absence and myoclonic status.

Psychiatric *In a retrospective study of 89 patients who developed psychiatric symptoms during treatment with tiagabine, topiramate, or vigabatrin, the psychiatric problem was either an affective or a psychotic disorder (not including affective psychoses) (13[c]). All but one of the patients had complex partial seizures with or without secondary generalization. More than half were taking polytherapy. Nearly two-thirds had a previous psychiatric history, and there was a strong association between the type of previous psychiatric illness and the type of emerging psychiatric problem. Patients taking vigabatrin had an earlier onset of epilepsy and more neurological abnormalities than those taking topiramate.*

The routine drug management of epilepsy by community health nurses without prior training in epilepsy management has been evaluated by neurologists in Zimbabwe (14[C]). Of 114 patients (aged 8–56 years, 84% with generalized seizures), 40% had been seizure-free for at least 6 months, 72% took phenobarbital, 36% took carbamazepine, and 20% took phenytoin; 68% took monotherapy. Specialist interventions were required in 60% of consultations. Serum drug concentrations were measured in 38 patients; 58% were below the target range and 16% were above. Increased dosage was required in 29% of patients and dosage reduction or withdrawal in 18%. In several cases drug withdrawal was undertaken to convert polytherapy to monotherapy.

Special senses *Visual field defects* associated with various antiepileptic drugs (carbamazepine, diazepam, gabapentin, phenytoin, tiagabine, and vigabatrin) have been reviewed (15[Rc]). The true frequency is unknown, but in a retrospective study in 158 patients with partial epilepsy visual field defects were detected in 21 (13%); 13 patients had concentric visual field constriction without subjective spontaneous manifestations. Of these 13 patients, nine were taking vigabatrin.

Visual-evoked potentials and brainstem auditory-evoked potentials have been measured in 58 children and adolescents taking carbamazepine, phenobarbital, or sodium valproate monotherapy and 50 sex- and age-matched controls (16[C]). After 1 year the patients taking carbamazepine had significantly prolonged visual-evoked P100 latencies compared with both baseline and control values; they also had significantly prolonged peak latencies of auditory waves I–III–V and interpeak interval I–V. Those taking sodium valproate had significantly prolonged visual-evoked P100 latencies. In contrast, children taking phenobarbital had no changes.

Metabolism Lipoprotein(a) concentrations have been measured in 51 patients taking long-term carbamazepine, phenobarbital, phenytoin, or valproate and 51 age- and sex-matched controls (17[C]). Lipoprotein(a) concentrations were above 450 mg/l in 11 patients compared with only four controls, and the mean serum lipoprotein(a) concentrations were 330 and 169 mg/l respectively. The epileptic patients also had a thicker intima media of the common carotid artery. These results suggest that patients taking antiepileptic drugs may be at a higher risk of atherosclerosis.

Skin A *psoriasiform eruption* has been reported in a 28-year-old woman taking carbamazepine and valproate (18[A]). Rechallenge was not attempted, and the association with either of these drugs was not clear.

In three patients who had *toxic epidermal necrolysis* after taking phenytoin or carbamazepine there was an increase in $CD3^+CLA^+$ cells, paralleling the severity of the disease in both peripheral blood and skin, tending to normalize as the condition improved (19[A]). E selectin was detected in endothelial vessels in parallel with CLA expression on lymphocytes. There was overexpression of TNF-α, interferon-γ, and interleukin-2 in peripheral monocytes. These results suggest an important role for T cells in the production of drug-induced toxic epidermal necrolysis.

Musculoskeletal system Anticonvulsant therapy causes changes in calcium and bone metabolism and can lead to *reduced bone mass* with the risk of osteoporotic fractures. Both phenytoin and carbamazepine have direct effects on bone cells. Bone mineral density has been measured in 59 patients and 55 age- and sex-matched controls (20[C]). Bone mineral density in the lumbar spine (L2–4) and femora was lower in the patients, significantly so in the former case. This reduction depended on the duration of therapy. Excretion of pyridinoline cross-links was markedly increased and 25-hydroxycholecalciferol and 1,25-dihydroxycholecalciferol were significantly reduced. The proliferation rate of human osteoblast-like cells was increased by phenytoin in low doses.

Reproductive system The incidence of *polycystic ovary syndrome* in women taking antiepileptic drugs has been studied in a prospective cohort analysis of premenopausal women (aged 20–53 years) with focal epilepsy (21[C]). Of 93 women, 38 were taking one antiepileptic drug (18 valproate, 20 carbamazepine), 36 were taking more than one drug, and 19 were taking no medications. Polycystic ovary syndrome was identified in two of the 19 patients taking no medication, four of the 38 patients taking monotherapy, and one of the patients taking more than one antiepileptic drug. The incidence of polycystic ovary syndrome in patients taking valproate monotherapy (11%) was similar to that in those taking carbamazepine (10%) and those not taking antiepileptic drugs (11%). These results suggest that polycystic ovary syndrome in women with focal epilepsy is not related to valproate or carbamazepine.

Teratogenicity The teratogenic effects of antiepileptic drugs have been assessed through the use of a surveillance system (MADRE) of infants with malformations (22[C]). Exposure was defined by the use of antiepileptic drugs during the first trimester of pregnancy. Of 8005 cases of malformations, 299 infants had been exposed in utero to antiepileptic drugs. Of those exposed to monotherapy, 65 were exposed to phenobarbital, 10 to methylphenobarbital, 80 to valproic acid, 46 to carbamazepine, 24 to phenytoin, and 16 to other antiepileptic drugs. The following associations were found:

- carbamazepine: cardiac malformations;
- methylphenobarbital: oral clefts and cardiac malformations;
- phenobarbital: oral clefts and cardiac malformations;
- valproate: spina bifida, cardiac malformations, hypospadias, porencephaly, and other specified anomalies of the brain, anomalies

of the face, coarctation of the aorta, and limb reduction defects.

Risk factors *Children* Febrile seizures are the most common seizure disorder in childhood, occurring in 2–5% of children, but there is no unanimity regarding the need for long-term antiepileptic drug therapy. A subcommittee of the American Academy of Pediatrics has recently concluded that there are no long-term adverse effects of simple febrile seizures, and that although there is evidence that continuous antiepileptic therapy with phenobarbital or valproate and intermittent therapy with diazepam are effective in reducing the risk of recurrence, the potential adverse effects associated with antiepileptic drugs outweigh the relatively minor risks associated with simple febrile seizures (23[R]). They recommended that long-term treatment is not indicated.

Drug formulations The rationale and use of modified-release formulations of antiepileptic drugs (carbamazepine, valproic acid, and tiagabine) have been reviewed (24[R]). The authors concluded that modified-release formulations afford the advantages of better patient compliance, fewer adverse effects, and less fluctuation in plasma concentrations, making monitoring of drug concentrations easier. They concluded that these advantages should lead to better seizure control and improved quality of life.

Drug interactions Patients taking carbamazepine or phenytoin are resistant to steroid neuromuscular blocking drugs. The effect of cisatracurium on the onset, duration, and speed of recovery from neuromuscular blockade has been studied in 24 patients taking antiepileptic drugs and 14 controls (25[c]). The onset and duration of neuromuscular blockade were not different among the groups, but the speed of recovery was significantly faster in those taking antiepileptic drugs.

Monitoring therapy The use of serum antiepileptic drug concentrations has been reviewed (26[R]). The authors suggested that there is still no evidence that specific target drug concentrations are valid in determining appropriate therapy.

INDIVIDUAL DRUGS

Benzodiazepines *(SED-14, 186; SEDA-23, 84; SEDA-24, 84) (see also Chapter 5)*

Respiratory A previous report that rectal and intravenous diazepam can cause *respiratory depression* in children with seizures (SEDA-24, 84) has been challenged (27[r], 28[r]). The authors of the second comment stated that this complication does not occur when rectal diazepam gel is used without other benzodiazepines; they also recommended that during long-term therapy families should be instructed not to give rectal diazepam more than once every 5 days or five times in 1 month.

Nervous system Benzodiazepines can provoke *seizures* and occasionally precipitate status epilepticus. A 28-year-old man with complex partial status, which lasted for 2 months, had a paradoxical worsening of seizure activity in response to diazepam and midazolam (29[A]).

Skin *Bullae with sweat gland necrosis* rarely complicate coma, but have recently been reported in association with clobazam, used as adjunctive therapy for resistant epilepsy in a 4-year-old girl (30[A]).

Carbamazepine *(SED-14, 172; SEDA-22, 85; SEDA-23, 85; SEDA-24, 84)*

Usual target range for plasma concentrations: 17–42 μmol/l (4–10 mg/l)

In 10 children with chorea (eight girls and two boys; aged 7–16 years), nine with rheumatic fever, carbamazepine (4–10 mg/kg/day; plasma concentrations 12–34 μmol/l) produced improvement within 2–14 days (31[c]). The chorea disappeared within 2–12 weeks. There were no adverse effects.

Nervous system Retrospective studies have suggested that antiepileptic drugs can be associated with *peripheral nerve dysfunction*. This has now been prospectively studied in 81 patients (aged 13–67 years) without polyneuropathy who took sodium valproate (n = 44) or carbamazepine (n = 37) as monotherapy in standard daily doses (32[C]). After 2 years one patient had clinical signs of polyneuropathy and six patients had symptoms of polyneuropathy, but electrophysiology did not show significant changes or trends. Only one patient had abnormal electrophysiological findings, which were only subclinical, and eight patients had abnormal values at two subsequent visits. There were no consistent patterns, and the data were unaffected when the drugs were examined separately or when patients were grouped according to whether or not they had symptoms of polyneuropathy. The authors concluded that previously untreated young to middle-aged patients who take valproic acid or carbamazepine for 2 years are not at risk of polyneuropathy.

Combined *phonic and motor tics* occurred in a 7-year-old boy with Down's syndrome when he took carbamazepine 19 mg/kg for suspected focal epilepsy (33[A]). Carbamazepine concentrations were within the usual target range. The symptoms resolved completely after withdrawal.

Carbamazepine can cause *altered visual evoked potentials and brainstem evoked potentials* (34[C]). In 100 epileptic patients aged 8–18 years taking carbamazepine in a modified-release formulation interpeak latencies of I–III and III–V of brainstem evoked potentials were significantly delayed and N75/P100 and P100/N145 amplitudes in the visual evoked potentials were reduced.

Relatively low doses of carbamazepine (300–600 mg/day) have been reported to have caused serious *worsening of disability* in five patients with multiple sclerosis (35[A]). The authors suggested that this effect was due to blockade of sodium channels by carbamazepine.

Sensory systems There was *abnormal color perception* in 28% of 18 patients taking carbamazepine monotherapy; in one case there was an abnormality in the blue–yellow axis (36[c]). In the same patients carbamazepine has no effect on contrast sensitivity or glare sensitivity (37[C]).

Auditory disturbance is rarely associated with carbamazepine. A 25-year-old woman had falsely higher pitch perception after starting carbamazepine for schizoaffective disorder (38[A]). Her serum carbamazepine concentration was in the usual target range. The symptom resolved on withdrawal.

Psychiatric A 9-year-old boy with seizures developed intermittent complex *visual hallucinations* during therapy with fosphenytoin and, on a separate occasion, carbamazepine (39[A]).

Metabolism Changes in bodyweight have been evaluated in 349 patients taking carbamazepine, phenytoin, or tiagabine. Carbamazepine add-on therapy caused significant mean weight gain of 1.5% (40[C]). Tiagabine add-on therapy caused no significant weight change when added to either phenytoin or carbamazepine.

Nutrition Concentrations of plasma homocysteine, plasma pyridoxal 5′-phosphate (active vitamin B_6), serum folate, erythrocyte folate, and serum vitamin B_{12} have been measured both fasting and after methionine in 60 epileptic patients (aged 14–18 years) and 63 sex- and age-matched controls before therapy and after 1 year of therapy with valproate or carbamazepine (41[C]). After 1 year the patients who took valproate and carbamazepine had significantly *increased plasma homocysteine concentrations* compared with both baseline and control values and there was a significant fall in serum folate and plasma pyridoxal 5′-phosphate. Serum vitamin B_{12} and erythrocyte folate were unchanged.

The genetic determinants of this effect on homocysteine have been determined in 136 epileptic children taking carbamazepine or valproate as monotherapy (42[C]). Nutritional determinants (folate and vitamins B_6 and B_{12}) and genetic determinants (MTHFR 677CT) of plasma homocysteine were studied in a random sample of 59 of those children. Total homocysteine concentrations were significantly increased and folate and vitamin B_6 concentrations were significantly reduced. Carbamazepine lowered folate concentrations in association with hyperhomocysteinemia, which seemed to be related to the homozygous MTHFR 677CT mutation. Valproate, although also associated with hyperhomocysteinemia, only reduced vitamin B_6 concentrations, independent of the MTHFR genotype.

Gastrointestinal *Lymphocytic colitis* has been attributed to carbamazepine in a 77-year-old man, who had taken it for 6 months (43[A]).

Skin A 17-year-old girl developed *Stevens–Johnson syndrome* after using carbamazepine 400 mg/day for 2 weeks (44[A]). She was treated with intravenous immunoglobulin and intravenous methylprednisolone and recovered completely.

Immunologic The *carbamazepine hypersensitivity syndrome* has been reviewed (45[R]). Some of the following cases are examples of the different manifestations of this syndrome.

A 12-year-old boy developed a maculopapular rash on two occasions after taking carbamazepine (46[A]). A patch test was positive, but an in vitro lymphocyte transformation test was negative. However, T cells incubated with carbamazepine produced an excess of interferon-γ.

The author proposed that this had been a delayed hypersensitivity response, perhaps mediated by a reactive metabolite.

A 45-year-old man developed acute cardiac tamponade due to systemic lupus erythematosus associated with carbamazepine, which he had taken for 8 months (47[A]).

An 11-year-old girl developed a skin rash, fever, lymphadenopathy, and arthralgia after taking carbamazepine (plasma concentration 21 μmol/l) for 3 weeks (48[A]). She had a lymphocytosis, mild thrombocytopenia, marked eosinophilia, and high transaminases. She was given betametasone, and carbamazepine was gradually withdrawn. The fever and rash gradually abated and all the laboratory tests normalized by 2 weeks after the disappearance of the skin rash.

Lactation In seven lactating women the mean concentrations of carbamazepine in milk and plasma samples were 15 and 26 μmol/l respectively; the concentrations of carbamazepine 10,11-epoxide were 5 and 8 μmol/l respectively (49[c]). The mean milk/plasma ratios were 0.64 and 0.79 respectively. The amounts of carbamazepine and carbamazepine 10,11-epoxide that a breastfeeding child is likely to consume are thus very small.

Drug overdose Acute massive carbamazepine intoxication has been reported in a 27-year-old man (50[A]). The plasma concentration was 147 μmol/l. He had a sinus tachycardia and a leukocytosis.

In 14 children under the age of 5 years with peak serum carbamazepine concentrations of 76–134 μmol/l after acute accidental overdose there was nystagmus in 12, drowsiness in 10, ataxia in four, and mild tachycardia in two (51[c]). None died.

Three drug dispensing errors causing carbamazepine overdose have been reported (52[A]). In each case carbamazepine was given instead of another drug with a similar name – Tegretol instead of Trental (pentoxifylline, two cases) and carbamazepine–neuroxpharm instead of piracetam–neuraxpharm. All three developed mild cerebellar symptoms and two had increased wakefulness. All three had high carbamazepine concentrations (50–55 μmol/l).

The post-mortem blood concentration of carbamazepine has been reported in a case of suicide attributed to "mixed drug toxicity" with carbamazepine, lamotrigine, paroxetine, and thioridazine (53[A]). It was 76 μmol/l.

Drug interactions *Antiretroviral protease inhibitors* Some drugs of this group inhibit CYP3A4, which is mostly responsible for the metabolism of carbamazepine. Failure of antiretroviral drug therapy has been attributed to an interaction of carbamazepine with *indinavir* in a 48-year-old man taking indinavir, zidovudine, and lamivudine; his HIV–RNA viral load became undetectable after less than 2 months and he developed a *Herpes zoster* infection (54[A]). Lower doses of carbamazepine are also required during coadministration of *ritonavir*, as has been shown in two recent cases.

Within 4 days of the introduction of ritonavir in a 49-year-old woman taking carbamazepine 600 mg/day the serum carbamazepine concentration rose from 29 to 84 μmol/l and ataxia occurred (55[A]). The dosage of carbamazepine was reduced to 300 mg/day and the serum concentration fell but then rose again. Finally, a serum carbamazepine concentration in the target range was achieved with a dosage of 100 mg/day.

The serum carbamazepine concentration rose from 27 to 76 μmol/l after ritonavir was introduced in a 36-year-old man (56[A]). Dizziness and a gait disorder resolved when carbamazepine was withdrawn. The serum phenytoin concentration was unaffected by ritonavir.

Lithium A 42-year-old woman developed sinus node dysfunction during lithium toxicity (serum concentration 3.4 mmol/l) (57[A]). The authors suggested that concomitant carbamazepine therapy (serum concentration 22 μmol/l) had exacerbated the effect of lithium on the sinus node.

Nefazodone The pharmacokinetic interaction of nefazodone 200 mg bd with steady-state carbamazepine has been investigated in 12 healthy men (58[C]). Nefazodone increased the steady-state plasma AUC of carbamazepine by 23% and reduced the AUC of active carbamazepine-10,11-epoxide by 20%. The steady-state AUC of nefazodone fell 14-fold and the AUCs of its metabolites (hydroxynefazodone, meta-chlorophenylpiperazine, and triazoledione) also fell significantly. Thus nefazodone had a small inhibitory effect on carbamazepine metabolism, while carbamazepine greatly increased the metabolism of nefazodone.

Phenprocoumon Carbamazepine reduces the effects of coumarin anticoagulants (SED-14, 1185), including phenprocoumon (SEDA-22, 86), by inducing cytochrome P450 enzymes, and another case has been reported (59[A]).

A 53-year-old woman taking phenprocoumon had a large reduction in prothrombin time when carbamazepine was added. After withdrawal of carbamazepine, the prothrombin time returned to target values. Valproate had no effect on phenprocoumon.

Risperidone Steady-state plasma concentrations of risperidone and 9-hydroxyrisperidone have been measured in 23 patients taking risperidone alone and in 11 patients co-medicated with carbamazepine (60[C]). Carbamazepine markedly reduced the concentrations of both compounds, although the difference was significant only for the metabolite.

St. John's wort St. John's wort contains an enzyme inducer that can reduce the plasma concentrations of drugs that are substrates of CYP3A4, such as indinavir and ciclosporin. However, in eight healthy volunteers aged 24–43 years, St. John's wort 300 mg/day (0.3% hypericin standardized tablet) for 14 days had no effect on the pharmacokinetics of carbamazepine (61[c]).

Sertraline Loss of antidepressant activity of sertraline can occur at usual therapeutic doses when depressed patients have also taken drugs that induce CYP3A4, including carbamazepine, as has been reported in two cases, a 33-year-old woman and a 25-year-old man (62[A]).

Ziprasidone The effect of steady-state carbamazepine administration on the steady-state pharmacokinetics of ziprasidone has been studied in 25 healthy young adults, in a randomized, placebo-controlled study (63[C]). Carbamazepine caused small reductions in ziprasidone $AUC_{0\to 12}$ and C_{max} (36% and 27% respectively). The authors concluded that carbamazepine had increased ziprasidone clearance by induction of CYP3A4.

Monitoring therapy The relations between plasma concentrations of carbamazepine and its two major metabolites, carbamazepine-10, 11-epoxide and carbamazepine-10,11-diol, and antimanic efficacy and adverse effects in patients with schizoaffective disorder have been studied in 10 patients (64[C]). There were positive relations between plasma concentrations of the epoxide and the degree of clinical improvement and adverse effects, but not with plasma concentrations of carbamazepine or its diol.

Gabapentin *(SED-14, 188; SEDA-22, 87; SEDA-23, 87; SEDA-24, 86)*

The use of gabapentin has been reviewed (65[r]). Its adverse effects are limited to neuropsychological disorders, namely *dizzy spells*, *drowsiness*, *fatigue*, and *headache*. The risk of interactions is also limited.

The efficacy of gabapentin in dosages up to 3600 mg/day as adjunctive therapy has been studied in 2016 patients with partial seizures (66[C]). The four most commonly reported adverse events were *somnolence* (15%), *dizziness* (10%), *weakness* (5.8%), and *headache* (4.5%).

The effectiveness of gabapentin has been studied in 22 patients with bipolar disorder who had an incomplete response to other mood stabilizers (67[c]). *Somnolence* was common (six patients); adverse events that occurred in two patients each included *irritability*, *memory impairment*, *headache*, and *tremor*. One patient dropped out because of a mild *rash*.

Nervous system In a comparison of twice- and thrice-daily gabapentin, 29 stable responders were selected and followed for 3 months (68[C]). The mean number of seizures per month was 4.2 at baseline, 1.0 during the thrice-daily and 0.9 during the twice-daily period. Adverse effects were reported by 11 patients during the thrice-daily period and by five patients during the twice-daily period; *sedation* and *vertigo* were the most frequent.

The efficacy and safety of gabapentin in relieving the symptoms of panic disorder have been studied in 103 patients in a randomized, placebo-controlled, double-blind study for 8 weeks (69[C]). Adverse events included *somnolence*, *headache*, and *dizziness*. One patient had a serious adverse event, a car accident, while taking gabapentin.

Myoclonus has been studied in 104 patients taking gabapentin for epilepsy (70[c]). There were 13 cases of mild myoclonus, which did not significantly interfere with daily activities. All the patients had refractory epilepsy and were taking other antiepileptic drugs. Six had a severe chronic static encephalopathy; five had no medical diagnosis other than seizures. Ten developed multifocal myoclonus and three developed focal myoclonus, contralateral to their epileptic focus. Two had an exacerbation of pre-existing myoclonus. Withdrawal led to rapid resolution.

Of 12 patients with moderate to severe dementia and severe behavioral disorders given gabapentin (200–1200 mg/day) for 8 weeks five had adverse events such as *gait instability*, *emotional instability*, and *sedation*; two patients discontinued treatment prematurely because of severe adverse effects (71[c]).

The role of gabapentin in neuropathic pain has been evaluated in a systematic review (72[M]). The most common adverse events were *dizziness* and *somnolence*, which occurred in about 25% of patients; ataxia occurred in about 8%. Adverse effects were dose related.

A 68-year-old man with essential tremor who was taking propranolol 80 mg/day had several daily episodes of *paroxysmal dystonic movements* in both hands 2 days after the addition of gabapentin 900 mg/day (73[A]). The dose of propranolol was reduced to 40 mg/day and the dystonic movements resolved. The authors suggested that there had been a synergistic effect between propranolol and gabapentin.

A 60-year-old woman with postherpetic neuralgia developed *asterixis* after having taken gabapentin for 4 days (74[A]). The authors proposed that the mechanism was GABAergic.

Psychiatric Two women, aged 37 and 38 years, took gabapentin and after a few days developed behavioral changes associated with *euphoria* (75[A]). In one case the symptoms were transient and in the other they resolved after withdrawal. The behavioral changes were not related to seizure activity.

Urinary tract A renal transplant recipient with a long-term stable functioning allograft developed reversible *acute renal dysfunction* after beginning gabapentin therapy for chronic pain in diabetic neuropathy (76[A]). The authors suggested that this was due to renal afferent vasoconstriction.

Sexual function A 25-year-old man taking gabapentin 900 mg/day reported *anorgasmia* during sexual intercourse (77[A]). He was given valproate instead and his symptom resolved within 12 days.

Body temperature Gabapentin may be effective in the treatment of hot flushes (hot flashes), and by the same token has been reported to have increased the frequency of *hypothermic episodes* in a 38-year-old man with hypothalamic dysfunction (78[A]).

Lamotrigine *(SED-14, 188; SEDA-22, 88; SEDA-23, 87; SEDA-24, 87)*

Usual target range for plasma concentrations: 4–16 μmol/l (1–4 mg/l)

The pharmacology, clinical pharmacology, adverse effects, and interactions of lamotrigine have been reviewed (79[R]). Its adverse events are primarily neurological, gastrointestinal, and dermatological and are typically mild or moderate and transient, with the exception of a potentially serious rash. Maculopapular or erythematous *skin rashes* occur in about 12% of children and are the most common reason for withdrawal. More severe forms of rash, including Stevens–Johnson syndrome, occur occasionally, with a 3-fold higher incidence in children (about 1%) than adults (about 0.3%).

In 126 patients with carbamazepine- or valproate-resistant epilepsy given lamotrigine 50% during add-on therapy and 53% during lamotrigine monotherapy had at least 50% reduction in total seizures (80[C]). There were adverse events in 49 patients, including *respiratory tract infections* (n = 11), *dizziness* (n = 8), *headache* (n = 7), *diplopia* (n = 5), *tremor*

(n = 5), *somnolence* (n = 4), *insomnia* (n = 4), *nausea* (n = 4), and *weakness* (n = 3). Treatment was discontinued in nine patients because of adverse events, in five cases because of *rash*.

The effectiveness of lamotrigine as monotherapy has been studied retrospectively in 83 children (mean age 8.7 years) with focal epilepsy (n = 43), generalized epilepsy (n = 32), or not classified (n = 8) (81[c]). The median follow-up period was 8 months (mean = 8.5). *Rash* was the most common adverse effect, in five patients; two patients discontinued treatment. There were no cases of Stevens–Johnson syndrome.

Lamotrigine has been used as maintenance monotherapy for rapid-cycling bipolar disorder in 324 patients (open label) and 182 patients (double-blind) (82[C]). In all, 265 patients reported adverse events during the open-label phase. The most common adverse events (over 10%) were *headache*, *infection*, *influenza*, *nausea*, *abnormal dreams*, *dizziness*, and *rash*. During the double-blind phase 122 patients reported adverse events, equally with lamotrigine and placebo. The most common of those that were related to drug therapy were *nausea* (n = 4) and *headache* (n = 6).

In 44 patients with profound mental retardation a retrospective assessment of adjunctive lamotrigine (272 mg/day) showed a significant reduction in seizure frequency from 10.1 to 5.8 seizures per month (83[c]). There were no treatment-related changes in laboratory parameters, vital signs, or bodyweight and no serious rashes. In three of five patients there was *worsened self-injurious behavior*, requiring drug withdrawal.

Lamotrigine has been studied in 32 children with epilepsy refractory for at least 1 year to other antiepileptic drugs (84[c]). Adverse effects were uncommon, and there were no skin rashes.

The efficacy and safety of lamotrigine have been prospectively evaluated in 41 children and young adults (aged 3–25 years) with drug-resistant partial epilepsies (85[C]). Lamotrigine withdrawal was mainly due to lack of efficacy (46%); only two patients developed a transient *skin rash*, which did not require withdrawal.

Nervous system A retrospective survey yielded five cases of *tics* in three boys and two girls aged 2.5–12 years) within the first 10 months of therapy (4–17 mg/kg/day) (86[A]). Four had simple motor tics and one had mostly vocal tics (gasping sounds) with normal laryngoscopic evaluation. In three cases the tics resolved completely within 1 month of drug withdrawal and recurred in two after reintroduction. A fourth had gradual improvement over 4 months after withdrawal; in the fifth, simple motor tics improved spontaneously with a reduction in dose.

Two young men (aged 18 and 22 years) with epilepsy had disabling *myoclonic jerks* after taking lamotrigine after 2–3 years of therapy when their plasma lamotrigine concentrations rose to about 70 μmol/l (87[A]).

Endocrine In two children with cranial diabetes insipidus desmopressin requirements fell while they were taking lamotrigine (88[A]). Lamotrigine may act at voltage-sensitive sodium channels and reduce calcium conductance. Both of these mechanisms of action are shared by carbamazepine, which can cause hyponatremia secondary to *inappropriate secretion of antidiuretic hormone*.

Hematologic Lamotrigine rarely causes hematological adverse effects. A 29-year-old woman with Blackfan–Diamond anemia developed an *erythroblastopenic crisis* after taking phenytoin on two separate occasions and then again after taking lamotrigine (89[A]). The proposed mechanism was inhibition of dihydrofolate reductase, and the crisis responded to treatment with folinic acid. Lamotrigine was then continued without ill effect.

Reversible *agranulocytosis* developed in a 30-year-old woman who had taken lamotrigine 100 mg/day for 6 weeks and valproate 250 mg/day for 2 weeks (90[A]). Her white cell count fell from 6.7×10^9/l at 4 weeks to 2.6×10^9/l at 6 weeks and the absolute neutrophil count was 580×10^6/l. The white cell count recovered after withdrawal of lamotrigine; the valproate was continued.

Liver Reversible *hepatotoxicity* occurred in three children taking lamotrigine (91[Ar]). In one there was severe hepatic failure. The liver abnormalities resolved after withdrawal.

Skin In 12 patients with probable Alzheimer's disease and seizures and 16 with other neurological disorders, lamotrigine caused three cases of mild *rashes* (92[c]).

Safe reintroduction of lamotrigine proved possible in seven young people (aged 5–19 years) who had previously had a mild rash associated with a first course (93[c]). The lamotrigine was withdrawn immediately when the rash was identified and was subsequently reintroduced after 47–236 days using a slow escalation regimen, starting with 0.1 mg/day. Lamotrigine was successfully reintroduced without recurrence of persistent rash and without any adverse effects in all seven cases.

The analgesic efficacy of lamotrigine in painful HIV-associated distal sensory polyneuropathy has been studied, given anecdotal reports of its efficacy, in a randomized, double-blind, placebo-controlled study (94[C]). Of 42 subjects, 13 did not complete the 14-week study. Of those who took lamotrigine five dropped out because of *rashes* and one because of a gastrointestinal infection. The rashes were mild or moderate morbilliform rashes and resolved after withdrawal.

Although lamotrigine-induced rashes are usually mild, more severe rashes can occur.

A 33-year-old woman, who had taken valproate for 3 years, developed Stevens–Johnson syndrome soon after starting to take lamotrigine 150 mg/day (95[A]). Lamotrigine was withdrawn and prednisolone given; the signs and symptoms progressively resolved over 10 days.

Immunologic A 17-year-old girl with a history of bipolar disorder developed fever, lymphadenopathy, skin rash, diarrhea, and acute renal failure requiring dialysis after taking lamotrigine for 4 weeks (96[A]). Renal biopsy showed acute *interstitial nephritis* with focal granulomas and colonic biopsy showed *colitis and ileitis* with non-necrotizing epithelioid granulomas.

Drug-induced *lupus-like syndrome* has been associated with lamotrigine (97[A]).

A 57-year-old woman, who had taken lamotrigine 2 mg/kg/day for about 2 years developed arthralgia affecting the small joints of the hands, wrists, and knees, an erythematous skin rash, myalgia, and Raynaud's phenomenon. Serum antinuclear antibodies were positive (1:320, speckled pattern), as was anti-Ro/SSA. Rheumatoid factor and anticardiolipin antibodies were negative and serum complement was normal. Lamotrigine was withdrawn and the symptoms and abnormal tests gradually normalized.

Severe hypersensitivity affecting the skin, lymph nodes, and liver has been reported with lamotrigine in a 36-year-old man, who had taken high doses of sodium valproate and lamotrigine for about a month (98[A]). Skin tests were negative with both drugs, but lymphocyte stimulation tests were twice positive with lamotrigine. Later re-exposure to sodium valproate was tolerated.

Risk factors *Children* The effects of lamotrigine in children have been reviewed (99[M]). Its efficacy has been demonstrated in 13 studies in 1096 children with a variety of seizure types. Generally, lamotrigine treatment in these trials was at higher initial doses and faster dose escalations than are currently recommended. Most adverse events associated with lamotrigine were mild to moderate and did not result in withdrawal. In placebo-controlled, add-on trials 85% of those who took lamotrigine had an adverse event compared with 83% of those who took placebo. Lamotrigine was associated with an increased risk of adverse events in the nervous system (*dizziness*, *tremor*, *ataxia*, and *diplopia*), gastrointestinal tract (*nausea*), and urinary tract (*infection*). *Skin rash* was reported more often with lamotrigine than placebo and more often by children than by adults. The simultaneous use of valproate was associated with an increased incidence of rash.

Drug overdose Post-mortem blood and tissue concentrations of lamotrigine have been reported in a case of suicide attributed to "mixed drug toxicity" with carbamazepine, lamotrigine, paroxetine, and thioridazine (53[A]). The blood lamotrigine concentration was 155 μmol/l. Two other individuals with high post-mortem blood lamotrigine concentrations, who did not die of overdoses, were also taking valproate.

Drug interactions The effects of other antiepileptic drugs on the pharmacokinetics of lamotrigine have been studied in 62 patients with epilepsy (100[C]). *Carbamazepine*, *phenytoin*, and *phenobarbital*, all enzyme inducers, increased the oral clearance of lamotrigine, individually by 58% and in combination by nearly 200%. *Valproate* reduced the oral clearance of lamotrigine by about 70%, but the effect was not related to the concentration of valproate (hence the rather misleading title of the paper). There was no effect on lamotrigine clearance when a single enzyme inducer was combined with valproate, but combinations of enzyme inducers had almost the same effect in the presence or absence of valproate. Consistent with this result, it has also been shown that the effect of valproate on the clearance of lamotrigine is independent of valproate dose and steady-state concentration in 28 patients with intractable epilepsy (101[C]). However, in contrast to these findings, there were good relations between the dose of valproate 200–1000 mg/day and the increase in lamotrigine AUC and the prolongation of half-life in eight patients with epilepsy (102[c]). It would be surprising if this interaction were not dose-related.

The interaction of *methsuximide* with lamotrigine has been studied in 16 patients (aged 9–19 years) with a variety of seizure types and syndromes (103[c]). The mean lamotrigine serum concentration before starting or after stopping methsuximide was 54 μmol/l and the mean concentration while taking methsuximide was 25 μmol/l. Methsuximide lowered the serum lamotrigine concentration in every case, with a mean fall of 53% (range 36–72%). In some patients this led to a deterioration in seizure control when methsuximide was added or an improvement in seizure control after methsuximide was withdrawn. The mechanism is thought to be induction of metabolism.

Cimetidine The effect of cimetidine on the pharmacokinetics of lamotrigine has been studied in 10 healthy men (104[C]). Cimetidine had no effect on the pharmacokinetics of lamotrigine.

Ketamine Because some of the cognitive effects of ketamine may be mediated through increased glutamate release, lamotrigine, which inhibits glutamate release, has been used to reduce the neuropsychiatric effects of ketamine in 16 healthy subjects (105[c]). Lamotrigine significantly reduced ketamine-induced perceptual abnormalities and increased its immediate mood-elevating effects.

Lithium The effect of lamotrigine on steady-state lithium pharmacokinetics has been studied in 20 healthy adult men (106[C]). Lamotrigine did not significantly change the pharmacokinetics of lithium.

Rifampicin The effect of rifampicin on the pharmacokinetics of lamotrigine have been studied in 10 healthy men (104[C]). Rifampicin induced the glucuronidation of lamotrigine, increasing total clearance about 2-fold.

Levetiracetam *(SED-14, 190; SEDA-24, 90)*

The pharmacology, clinical pharmacology, uses, and adverse reactions and interactions of levetiracetam have been reviewed (1[R], 107[R], 108[R], 109[r], 110[r]).

The efficacy and tolerability of levetiracetam monotherapy in refractory partial seizures has been studied in a double-blind, placebo-controlled study in 286 patients (111[C]). Adverse events that were more common with levetiracetam and that occurred in more than 5% of cases included *weakness*, *infection*, and *somnolence*. Of 181 patients who took levetiracetam, 36 completed the study compared with only 10 of 105 who took placebo.

The tolerability and efficacy of levetiracetam, 2 or 4 g/day, as add-on therapy have been studied in 119 patients with refractory epilepsy (112[C]). *Somnolence* was the most common reason for withdrawal and occurred more often with levetiracetam than placebo, as did *weakness*. Somnolence was more common with the higher dose, which was not more effective than the lower dose. *Nausea*, *dizziness*, and *urinary tract infections* were also more common with the higher dose.

The efficacy and safety of levetiracetam 1 and 3 g/day as adjunctive therapy for refractory partial seizures have been studied in a double-blind, randomized, placebo-controlled trial in 294 patients with uncontrolled partial seizures (113[C]). Treatment-associated adverse events that occurred in at least 10% of patients and had incidences higher than placebo were *weakness*, *dizziness*, *a flu-like syndrome*, *headache*, *infection*, *rhinitis*, and *somnolence*. These effects were mostly mild to moderate.

The efficacy and tolerability of levetiracetam 1–4 g/day as add-on treatment for refractory epilepsy have been studied in 29 patients with refractory epilepsy (114[c]). The most common adverse events were *somnolence* and *weakness*, the frequency and severity of which increased with increasing doses.

The efficacy and tolerability of levetiracetam 1–2 g/day as add-on therapy have been studied in 324 patients with refractory partial seizures (115[C]).

Levetiracetam did not affect the plasma concentrations of other antiepileptic drugs or alter vital signs or laboratory measurements. The most commonly reported adverse effects in patients taking levetiracetam were *weakness*, *headache*, and *somnolence*.

Oxcarbazepine *(SED-14, 190; SEDA-23, 88; SEDA-24, 90)*

The pharmacology, clinical pharmacology, and adverse reactions and interactions of oxcarbazepine have been reviewed (107[R], 110[r], 116[R]–118[R]).

Oxcarbazepine has an adverse effects profile similar to that of carbamazepine. It has not been associated with hepatotoxicity or hematological toxicity. It is less likely than carbamazepine to cause hypersensitivity reactions, but may be more often associated with *hyponatremia*. It is less likely than carbamazepine to induce CYP450 enzymes, but it may significantly increase the clearance of oral contraceptives and significantly induce CYP450 at higher doses.

The safety and efficacy of oxcarbazepine 600–2400 mg/day as adjunctive therapy for uncontrolled partial seizures has been studied in a randomized, double-blind, placebo-controlled study in 694 patients aged 15–65 years (119[C]). During the double-blind phase, 76%, 84%, 90%, and 98% of patients taking placebo or oxcarbazepine 600, 1200, or 2400 mg/day respectively, reported one or more adverse events. The most common adverse events were related to the nervous and gastrointestinal systems.

The safety and efficacy of oxcarbazepine 300 and 2400 mg/day have been studied in patients with refractory partial epilepsy in a double-blind, randomized trial (120[C]). *Dizziness*, *fatigue*, *somnolence*, and *nausea*, mostly transient and mild to moderate, were the most frequent adverse events.

The safety and efficacy of oxcarbazepine have been studied in a randomized, placebo-controlled trial in 267 children with inadequately controlled partial seizures (121[C]). There was at least one adverse event in 91% of those who took oxcarbazepine and 82% of those who took placebo; *vomiting*, *somnolence*, *dizziness*, and *nausea* occurred more often (2-fold or more) with oxcarbazepine.

Phenobarbital and primidone *(SED-14, 186; SEDA-23, 89)*

The use and adverse effects of primidone in the treatment of essential tremor has been reviewed (122[r]). Acute reactions include *vertigo*, *nausea*, and *unsteadiness*; chronic reactions include *worsening of depression*.

Pretreating patients with phenobarbital can reduce the impact of adverse events when primidone is introduced. Of 30 patients with intractable partial epilepsy pretreated with phenobarbital before starting primidone (500 mg/day increasing by 125–250 mg/day every 3 weeks until adverse events or a seizure-free state was reached), 26 tolerated the introduction of primidone with minimal or no adverse events (123[c]). Only one patient had to discontinue primidone during the initial 4 weeks because of severe *dizziness*. Three other patients had dizziness severe enough to interfere with their activities and this disappeared in two patients after the dose was lowered.

Nervous system In a study of 114 patients, of whom 72% took phenobarbital, one had *ataxia* due to phenobarbital toxicity (14[C]).

Skin *Toxic epidermal necrolysis* has been reported in a 62-year-old woman and a 72-year-old man who had taken phenobarbital 100 and 150 mg/day respectively (124[A]).

Immunologic *Giant cell myocarditis* has been reported in a patient taking phenytoin, phenobarbital, and mephobarbital and in one taking primidone (125[A]).

Death The efficacy of a single intramuscular dose of phenobarbital (20 mg/kg) in preventing seizures in childhood cerebral malaria has been the subject of a randomized, placebo-controlled study in 340 children in Kenya (126[C]). Seizure frequency was significantly lower with phenobarbital than placebo: 18 vs 46 children had three or more seizures of any duration (OR = 0.32; 95% CI = 0.18, 0.58). However, *mortality* was doubled (30 vs 14 deaths; OR = 2.39; CI = 1.28, 4.64). The frequency of respiratory arrest was higher with phenobarbital than placebo, and mortality was greatly increased in children who received phenobarbital plus three or more doses of diazepam (OR = 32; CI = 1.2, 814). The authors felt that although phenobarbital was effective, the risks were too high to recommend using it.

Fetotoxicity After prenatal exposure to antiepileptic drugs, *small head size* has been observed in neonates and *cognitive impairment* in infancy. However, it is currently unknown whether these effects are permanent or disappear later in life. Head size and cognition have now been studied in adults who had been exposed in utero to phenobarbital plus phenytoin and who as neonates had a significantly smaller occipitofrontal circumference than neonates who had been exposed to phenobarbital alone or controls (mean difference 0.7 cm) (127[C]). There was no difference in cognitive functioning between the exposed and the control groups, and most of the exposed subjects had normal intellectual capacity. However, 12% of the exposed subjects versus 1% of the controls had persistent learning problems. In addition, more of the exposed subjects were mentally retarded. The authors concluded that the combination of phenobarbital plus phenytoin reduced neonatal head size, which was not associated with reduced cognitive functioning in adulthood, but was associated with learning problems and mental retardation.

Phenytoin *(SED-14, 180; SEDA-22, 90; SEDA-23, 89; SEDA-24, 90)*

Usual target range for plasma concentrations: 40–80 μmol/l (10–20 mg/l)

The effects of phenytoin have been studied in 39 patients with acute mania (128[c]). One patient dropped out because of *tachycardia* and one required a dosage reduction because of *nystagmus*.

Cardiovascular In 775 patients who received intravenous phenytoin, valproate, or placebo, intravenous site reactions occurred in 25% of patients who received phenytoin (129[M]). Most of the events (70%) occurring in the first intravenous site and all occurred in peripheral administration sites. When patients who received the drug by central line were excluded, the estimated incidence was 30%. There were fewer adverse events when phenytoin was given alone than when it was given together with valproate.

Nervous system Retrospective studies have suggested that antiepileptic drugs may be associated with *peripheral nerve dysfunction*. This has now been studied prospectively in 81 patients (aged 13–67 years) without polyneuropathy who took sodium valproate (n = 44) or carbamazepine (n = 37) as monotherapy in standard daily doses (32[C]). After 2 years one patient had clinical signs of polyneuropathy and six patients had symptoms of polyneuropathy, but electrophysiology did not show significant changes or trends. Only one patient had abnormal electrophysiological findings, which were only subclinical, and eight patients had abnormal values at two subsequent visits. There were no consistent patterns, and the data were unaffected when the drugs were examined separately or when patients were grouped according to whether or not they had symptoms of polyneuropathy. The authors concluded that previously untreated young to middle-aged patients who take valproic acid or carbamazepine for 2 years are not at risk of polyneuropathy.

Cerebellar atrophy has been reported in association with phenytoin intoxication (130[A]).

Psychiatric A 9-year-old boy with seizures developed intermittent complex *visual hallucinations* during therapy with fosphenytoin and, on a separate occasion, carbamazepine (36[A]).

Mouth *Gingival hyperplasia* is a well-known adverse effect of phenytoin, and can on occasion be extensive, as in the case of a 17-year-old boy who took 300 mg/day unsupervised for 2 years and developed coarsening of the facial features, extensive gingival hyperplasia, and cerebellar ataxia (131[A]). The gingival hyperplasia resolved within 3 months of withdrawal but the ataxia persisted.

In a study of 114 patients, of whom 20% took phenytoin, five taking phenytoin had gingival hyperplasia (14[C]).

Liver A 51-year-old woman developed hepatitis while taking phenytoin 300 mg/day (132[A]). The authors did not discuss the possible role of paracetamol, which was coadministered in a dosage of 4 g/day (see Drug interactions below).

Skin *Toxic epidermal necrolysis* has been reported in a 28-year-old woman who had taken phenytoin for 20 days (133[A]). Phenytoin was cytotoxic in vitro to the patient's lymphocytes.

A 49-year-old man with post-traumatic epilepsy taking phenytoin developed severe *rhinophyma*; he also had *gingival hyperplasia* (134[A]). Nothing in the history of this case pointed definitively to a cause-and-effect association.

An unusual effect of phenytoin, termed the *purple glove syndrome*, has been reported (135[A]).

A 10-year-old boy took phenytoin 100 mg/day and his seizures were well controlled. However, a pharmacist gave him about 1000 mg of phenytoin instead of the prescribed dose, and several hours later he became drowsy and his hands and feet turned dark purple with marked swelling. Phenytoin was withdrawn after 4 days and the swelling and discoloration of his hands and feet improved gradually and disappeared 11 days later.

Purple glove syndrome has been reported after intravenous phenytoin but not, until this report, after oral administration.

Immunologic *Giant cell myocarditis* has been reported in a patient taking phenytoin, phenobarbital, and mephobarbital (125[A]).

A *lupus-like syndrome* has been attributed to phenytoin (136[A]).

A 67-year-old white man who had taken phenytoin 300 mg/day for about 15 years developed fever, pericarditis, severe abdominal pain, malaise, and weight loss. He had a positive antinuclear antibody in a titer of 1:80 in a homogeneous pattern, a strongly positive antihistone antibody test, a raised erythrocyte sedimentation rate (115 mm/hour), and a neutrophilia (21×10^9/l). All these abnormalities resolved within a few weeks of withdrawal. Rechallenge was not performed.

The long delay between the start of therapy and the clinical presentation makes it highly likely that phenytoin was not implicated in this case and that recovery was spontaneous.

Drug administration route Intravenous phenytoin has been associated with fatal hemodynamic complications and serious reactions at the injection site, including skin necrosis and amputation of extremities. Fosphenytoin, a phenytoin prodrug, has the same pharmacological properties but none of the injection site and cardiac rhythm complications after intravenous administration (137[R]).

Drug overdose Serum phenytoin concentrations in overdose have been studied in nine patients aged 20–66 years (138[c]). The serum phenytoin concentrations were initially 136–230 μmol/l and fell linearly (i.e. with zero-order kinetics); the elimination rate varied from 19 to 41 μmol/l/day. In those with the highest serum concentrations at presentation there was a delay before the fall in concentrations began.

The effectiveness of charcoal hemoperfusion has been reported in a 19-year-old woman who took about 5 g of phenytoin (139[A]). The plasma concentrations of total and unbound phenytoin fell rapidly, from 160 and 14 μmol/l to 65 and 6 μmol/l respectively, after 3 hours of hemoperfusion. The total phenytoin half-life was 3.9 hours. The protein-bound fraction was constant (91%) throughout.

Phenytoin poisoning has been reported in a patient who took Chinese proprietary medicines containing phenytoin, carbamazepine, and valproate (140[A]). The manufacturer's information leaflet did not mention any of these prescription drugs.

Drug interactions It has been proposed that phenytoin can exacerbate the hepatotoxic effects of paracetamol (141[Ar]).

A 55-year-old woman with a community-acquired pneumonia had unexplained, moderate rises in hepatic enzyme activities while taking paracetamol 1300–6200 mg/day and phenytoin 350 mg/day. Paracetamol was withdrawn, and her chemistry normalized within 2 weeks.

The authors suggested that induction of CYP3A4 by phenytoin had encouraged the formation of a hepatotoxic metabolite of paracetamol.

The interaction of oral phenytoin and *enteral feeding formulations* has been reviewed (142[M]). Four prospective, randomized, controlled trials in healthy volunteers showed no interaction. However, numerous anecdotal reports and studies have shown dramatic reductions in serum phenytoin concentrations in patients receiving enteral feeding formulations. The authors therefore concluded that this interaction occurs in patients but not in healthy volunteers.

Remacemide

Remacemide hydrochloride is a low-affinity, non-competitive *N*-methyl-D-aspartate

(NMDA) channel blocker that has been used in epilepsy, Parkinson's disease, Huntington's chorea, and neuroprotection after stroke. Its pharmacology, clinical pharmacology, uses, and adverse effects and interactions have been reviewed (1[R], 143[R]).

The adverse effects of remacemide have been studied in 40 patients with refractory epilepsy randomized to placebo or ascending weekly doses of remacemide in a twice or four times a day regimen for up to 1 month (144[C]). There were adverse events in 38 patients; the most common were *dizziness*, *abdominal pain*, *headache*, *diplopia*, *fatigue*, *dyspepsia*, and *abnormal vision*.

The efficacy, safety, and pharmacokinetics of adjunctive remacemide have been investigated in a randomized, double-blind, placebo-controlled, cross-over study in 28 adult patients with refractory epilepsy (145[C]). The mean plasma carbamazepine concentration increased by about 15%. Three patients withdrew owing to adverse events (two remacemide, one placebo). Adverse events that occurred more often with remacemide than placebo included *dyspepsia*, *dizziness*, *abnormal gait*, *diplopia*, *abnormal vision*, *somnolence*, *chest pain*, and *fatigue*.

In a randomized, double-blind, placebo-controlled study of remacemide in 200 patients with early Parkinson's disease who were not yet taking levodopa or dopamine agonists, remacemide did not produce improvement in signs or symptoms (146[C]). Significantly fewer patients taking remacemide 600 mg/day were able to tolerate 5 weeks of their assigned treatment on a twice-daily schedule compared with patients taking placebo (64% vs 94%). However, most patients who had intolerable adverse effects with the twice-daily schedule could tolerate the same daily dosage given in four parts during the day. The most common adverse events were *dizziness* and *nausea*. There were no serious adverse events or clinically significant treatment-related changes in vital signs, laboratory values, or electrocardiograms.

Drug interactions Remacemide delays the absorption of *levodopa* and increases the concentrations of drugs that are metabolized by CYP3A4 (143[R]).

Stiripentol *(SEDA-24, 91)*

The clinical pharmacology and adverse effects of stiripentol have been reviewed (1[R]).

The effects of stiripentol have been studied in 41 children with severe myoclonic epilepsy in infancy in a randomized, placebo-controlled, add-on trial (147[C]). There were adverse effects in 21 patients taking stiripentol (*drowsiness* and *loss of appetite*) compared with five taking placebo, and the adverse effects disappeared when the doses of other antiepileptic drugs were reduced in 12 of the 21 cases.

Sulthiame *(SED-14, 187; SEDA-24, 91)*

The efficacy and tolerability of sulthiame as monotherapy have been studied in a double-blind, placebo-controlled trial for 6 months in 66 children with benign childhood epilepsy with centrotemporal spikes (148[C]). The number of adverse events per day of exposure was similar with sulthiame and placebo, and no patient withdrew because of adverse effects.

Tiagabine *(SED-14, 190; SEDA-22, 91; SEDA-23, 89; SEDA-24, 91)*

The safety of long-term tiagabine has been studied retrospectively in 42 patients with refractory partial epilepsy who took tiagabine for longer than 6 months (149[c]). The most common adverse events were *tiredness* (56%), *headache* (46%), *dizziness* (44%), *visual symptoms* (blurring, difficulty in focusing, and diplopia; 39%), *altered thinking* (32%), and *tremor* (31%). The adverse events profile was comparable among those who had taken tiagabine for 6–12, 12–24 months, and more than 24 months.

The use of tiagabine 4–16 mg/day in preventing migraine has been studied in 41 patients who had failed treatment with divalproex sodium because of adverse effects or lack of efficacy (150[c]). There was at least a 50% reduction in the frequency of migraine headaches in 33 patients. There were adverse events in 12 patients, most commonly *tiredness*; a few patients had *weight gain* or *confusion*.

The effects of tiagabine have been studied in a 4-month, single-blind study in 52 children over the age of 2 years with different syndromes of refractory epilepsy (151[c]). Adverse events, mostly mild to moderate, were reported by 39% of the children during the single-blind placebo period and by 83% of the children during tiagabine treatment. The events predominantly affected the nervous system; *weakness* (19%), *nervousness* (19%), *dizziness* (17%), and *somnolence* (17%) were the most common. One child had *hallucinations* that responded to dosage reduction. Only three children withdrew because of adverse events.

Nervous system There have recently been some cases of *generalized non-convulsive status epilepticus* in patients with chronic partial epilepsy treated with tiagabine, and another case has been reported, on this occasion specifically associated with frontal lobe discharges, which does not seem to have been previously reported (152[A]).

A 12-year-old boy with familial bilateral perisylvian polymicrogyria, mental retardation, and refractory partial seizures was given tiagabine in addition to sodium valproate, and the dosage was increased to 10 mg tds (1 mg/kg/day). This produced complete seizure control. After 1 week he developed hypoactivity, reduced reactivity, and affective detachment. An electroencephalogram showed subcontinuous sharp-wave discharges, with irregular runs of atypical spike–wave complexes over the anterior regions of both hemispheres, consistent with a diagnosis of frontal non-convulsive status epilepticus. The dosage of tiagabine was reduced to 15 mg/day and there was complete regression of the behavioral and affective changes and normalization of the electroencephalogram.

Tiagabine 0.45–0.57 mg/kg/day was also associated with long-standing non-convulsive status epilepticus in three girls, two aged 12 years and one aged 17 years, with refractory localization-related epilepsy (153[A]). Resolution followed withdrawal of tiagabine or a reduction in dosage.

Sensory systems The effect of tiagabine on visual function has been studied in 15 patients with chronic partial epilepsy treated for 23–55 months with tiagabine monotherapy after failure with standard antiepileptic drug monotherapy (154[c]). Three patients had localized field losses (two quadrantanopic and one hemianopic) from earlier brain lesions. Tiagabine had no effect on visual fields but acquired *color vision defects* were found in seven of 14 patients; contrast sensitivity was unaffected.

Metabolism Changes in bodyweight have been evaluated in 349 patients taking carbamazepine, phenytoin, or tiagabine. Carbamazepine add-on therapy caused significant mean weight gain of 1.5% (40[C]). Tiagabine add-on therapy caused no significant weight change when added to either phenytoin or carbamazepine.

Topiramate *(SED-14; 191; SEDA-22, 91; SEDA-23, 90; SEDA-24, 92)*

In an open-label study of the effects of topiramate 100–1600 mg/day in 292 adults (mean age 33 years) with partial and/or generalized seizures previously resistant to antiepileptic drug therapy over 50% of the patients achieved at least a 50% reduction in seizures (155[c]). The most commonly reported adverse events were related to the central nervous system, including *headache, difficulty in concentrating, somnolence, anorexia, fatigue, dizziness, nervousness, nausea, confusion*, and *paresthesia*; 32% discontinued because of adverse events.

Topiramate had a beneficial effect on benign essential tremor in an open-label study in nine patients (156[c]). Six patients complained of *fatigue* and two discontinued therapy; four complained of *paresthesia*.

The effectiveness and tolerability of topiramate has been studied in an open-label study in 56 patients with bipolar disorder (157[c]). The most common adverse effects were neurological and gastrointestinal, including *reduced appetite* ($n = 11$), *cognitive impairment* ($n = 10$), *fatigue* ($n = 5$), and *sedation* ($n = 5$). Six patients dropped out during acute treatment and four during maintenance therapy because of adverse effects (*cognitive impairment, poor appetite and weight loss, sedation, paresthesia, psychosis, anxiety, tremor, nausea, altered taste*, and *rash*).

In a 3-year retrospective review of the use of topiramate in 51 children aged 3–16 years with partial and generalized epilepsy, 15 children had a greater than 50% reduction in their seizure frequency and four became seizure free (158[c]). Adverse effects were reported in 29 patients; most were related to *behavioral and cognitive difficulties*; less common effects included *anorexia*, *weight loss*, and *headache*. Topiramate was withdrawn in 25 patients, in 20 cases because of adverse effects.

In 18 patients with severe myoclonic epilepsy in infancy topiramate caused reduced seizure frequency in most (159[c]). There were adverse effects in nine patients, eight with a weekly titration schedule and one with a fortnightly schedule. They were usually minor and transient *nervous system effects*, except for *weight loss*, which lasted longer and occurred in four patients.

The results of six double-blind, placebo-controlled trials with topiramate in adults with treatment-resistant partial-onset seizures with or without secondary generalization have been analyzed (160[M]). Seizures were reduced by at least 50% in 43% of topiramate-treated patients and in 12% of placebo-treated patients. The most common treatment-related adverse events were *dizziness*, *somnolence*, *fatigue*, *psychomotor slowing*, *nervousness*, *paresthesia*, *ataxia*, *memory difficulty*, and *speech problems*. These effects were generally mild to moderate, usually occurred early in treatment, often during titration, and resolved with continued treatment. Other adverse effects were *weight loss* and, in a few patients, *renal calculi*.

Among the adverse effects of topiramate are *reduced appetite* and *weight loss*, and this has been put to use in the treatment of binge eating in an open-label study in 13 patients (161[c]). Nine patients had a moderate or better response, two had moderate or marked responses that subsequently diminished, and two had a mild response or none. *Neurological adverse effects* were the most common. Three patients discontinued topiramate because of adverse effects, and two resumed at a later date without significant recurrence.

The efficacy and tolerability of topiramate have been studied in 170 patients with refractory epilepsy (162[c]). The most common adverse effects resulting in withdrawal were *fatigue*, *weight loss*, *irritability*, *paresthesia*, *depression*, and *headache*. Three patients developed renal calculi but continued therapy.

The effect of topiramate for 6–18 months in 34 children with drug-resistant epilepsy has been studied (163[c]). Adverse effects were reported in nine patients, *appetite suppression* in five, *behavioral disturbances* in three, *somnolence* in two, and *poor concentration* in one.

In an open-label, long-term extension to a double-blind, placebo-controlled trial of topiramate in 83 children with partial-onset seizures, with or without secondary generalization, seizure frequency over the last 3 months of therapy was reduced by at least 50% in 47 children (164[c]). *Anorexia* was common during long-term therapy. Five children withdrew because of adverse events.

The efficacy and safety of topiramate has been studied in 46 adult Chinese patients with refractory partial epilepsy in a randomized, double-blind, placebo-controlled study (165[C]). Adverse events were mostly mild and transient, with no significant differences between treatment groups. Two patients taking topiramate had *weight loss*.

Respiratory Topiramate inhibits carbonic anhydrase isoenzymes II and IV, which are present in the central nervous system. *Respiratory alkalosis* in a 15-year-old girl, who presented with hyperpnea, was not therefore surprising (166[A]). The problem resolved within 24 hours of withdrawal.

Nervous system In the comparison of four antiepileptic drugs mentioned above, the commonest adverse effect of topiramate in 28 patients was *irritability*, which occurred in seven of 10 patients who discontinued therapy because of adverse effects (5[c]).

The response to topiramate has been evaluated in 97 patients with Lennox–Gastaut syndrome in a long-term, open-label extension to a double-blind, placebo-controlled trial (167[c]). The most common adverse events, apart from childhood illnesses, were *somnolence* and *anorexia*.

The factors associated with *behavioral and cognitive abnormalities* in children taking topiramate have been studied retrospectively (168[c]). There were behavioral or cognitive abnormalities in 11 of 75 children at 2–4 months after the start of therapy. The mean dosage (4.6 mg/kg/day) at which these abnormalities were observed was similar to the mean final dose (5.8 mg/kg/day) in children without abnormalities. Five of the 11 children with behavioral or cognitive abnormalities had a previous history of behavioral or cognitive abnormalities, but only nine of the 64 children without abnormalities had a previous history of behavioral or cognitive abnormalities.

Angelman's syndrome, a genetic disorder that involves a defect in the DNA coding for subunits of the $GABA_A$ receptor, is often associated with intractable epilepsy. Topiramate was effective in five children with Angelman's syndrome and epilepsy (169[c]). One patient had transient *insomnia* and one had *akathisia and insomnia* that persisted until topiramate was withdrawn.

Psychological Topiramate can cause *altered cognitive function*, and its effects on tests of intellect and other cognitive processes have been studied in 18 patients (170[c]). Repeat assessments in those taking topiramate were associated with a significant deterioration in many domains, which were not seen in controls. The greatest changes were for verbal IQ, verbal fluency, and verbal learning. There were improvements in verbal fluency, verbal learning, and digit span in patients who had topiramate withdrawn or reduced.

The cognitive effects of topiramate and valproate as adjunctive therapy to carbamazepine have been compared in 53 patients (171[C]). Topiramate was given in an initial dose of 25 mg and increased weekly by 25 mg/day increments to a minimum of 200 mg/day. Cognition was significantly worsened by topiramate and improved by valproate. Gradual introduction of topiramate reduced the extent of cognitive impairment.

Acid base balance Mental status changes and *metabolic acidosis* can occur with topiramate, through inhibition of carbonic anhydrase (172[A]).

A 20-year-old man taking topiramate, valproate, and phenytoin had acute mental changes with hyperchloremic metabolic acidosis. He had been receiving a modest dose of topiramate for 9 months. His mental status returned to normal within 48 hours of withdrawal

Gastrointestinal *Weight loss* is common with topiramate and can occasionally be extensive (173[A]).

A 37-year-old obese white woman with affective instability and obesity taking topiramate (up to 275 mg/day) lost 10 kg over 10 weeks, although she remained obese (BMI 52 kg/m^2). She also improved mentally.

In this case the weight loss was a beneficial side effect of topiramate.

Drug interactions The clinical pharmacology of topiramate has been reviewed in relation to its interactions (174[R]). The metabolism of topiramate can be enhanced by enzyme inducing drugs, such as *carbamazepine* and *phenytoin*, and inhibited by *valproate*. Topiramate may cause a small rise in plasma phenytoin concentrations by inhibition of CYP2C19. It increases plasma estrogen concentrations in women taking *oral contraceptives*, by an unknown mechanism. It slightly impairs *digoxin* clearance but the interaction is probably not clinically significant.

Valproate sodium *(SED-14, 182; SEDA-22, 91; SEDA-23, 90; SEDA-24, 93)*

Tentative target range for plasma concentrations: 350–700 μmol/l (50–100 mg/l)

The therapeutic uses of valproate in psychiatric conditions have been reviewed (175[R], 176[R]). The major adverse effects in one study of 150 patients were *tremor* (9.3%), *gastrointestinal effects* (8.9%), *drowsiness* (8.6%), *hair loss* (7.9%), *weight gain* (6.9%), *weakness* (6.9%), *dizziness* (4.1%), *thrombocytopenia* (2.9%), and *headache* (2.7%).

Cardiovascular In 775 patients who received intravenous phenytoin, valproate, or placebo, *intravenous site reactions* occurred in 18% of patients who received valproate (129[M]). Most of the events (70%) occurring in the first intravenous site and all occurred in peripheral administration sites. When patients who received the drug by central line were excluded, the estimated incidence was 21%. There were fewer adverse events when phenytoin was given alone than when it was given together with valproate.

Respiratory Fatal *pulmonary hemorrhage* occurring during high-dose valproate monotherapy in a 30-year-old woman (177[A]). It was accompanied by a low platelet count (15×10^9/l).

Nervous system Valproate can cause *altered visual evoked potentials and brainstem evoked potentials* (34[C]). In 100 epileptic patients aged 8–18 years taking valproate in a modified-release formulation interpeak latencies of I–III and III–V of brainstem evoked potentials were significantly delayed and N75/P100 and P100/N145 amplitudes in the visual evoked potentials were reduced.

Valproate toxicity has been reported to have caused a *neurodegenerative condition* that mimicked multisystem atrophy in a 67-year-old woman (178[A]).

Psychological There has been a randomized, double-blind, single cross-over study of the effects of sodium valproate on cognitive performance and behavior in eight children with learning and behavioral problems associated with electroencephalographic epileptiform discharges but without clinical seizures (179[c]). The children became *more distractible*, had *increased delay in response time*, and had *lower memory scores* while taking valproate. Their parents reported higher internalizing scores on the Child Behavior Checklists.

Metabolism *Hyperammonemic encephalopathy* accompanied by triphasic waves has been attributed to valproate (180[A]).

A 61-year-old man with epilepsy had altered consciousness after his dose of valproate was increased because of poor seizure control. Electroencephalography showed triphasic waves and high-amplitude δ-wave activity with frontal predominance. Although serum AsT and AlT, were normal, the serum ammonium concentration was high at 960 μg/l (reference range 30–470). Serum amino acid analysis showed multiple minor abnormalities. Valproate was withdrawn. He improved within 4 days and the electroencephalogram, serum ammonium concentration, and amino acid profile were normal by day 8.

In two other cases the addition of topiramate was thought to have precipitated valproate-induced hyperammonemic encephalopathy (181[A]). Recovery occurred after withdrawal of valproate or topiramate. The authors suggested that topiramate may have contributed to the hyperammonemia by inhibiting carbonic anhydrase and cerebral glutamine synthetase.

Fluid balance Severe *peripheral edema* occurred in a 42-year-old man taking valproate 1.5 g/day and resolved on withdrawal (182[A]). The authors proposed that increased GABA activity had inhibited natriuresis by altering the action of nitric oxide in the kidneys or by inhibiting the central production of C-type natriuretic peptide.

Hematologic A 5-year-old girl with acquired protein C deficiency suffered a stroke while taking valproate (183[Ac]). The authors then measured protein C concentrations in 20 children taking valproate monotherapy and 20 children taking other antiepileptic drugs. There were significantly *lower protein C concentrations* in those taking valproate. Protein S and antithrombin III were not affected. Despite this, there is no known association between valproate therapy and a risk of thromboembolic disease, and the clinical relevance of this effect on protein C is not clear.

There was a small *reduction in platelet count* (from 150 to 110 × 10^9/l) in association with gastrointestinal symptoms in a 45-year-old man when he took valproate 750 mg tds, but not when he took the same dose of divalproex, an enteric-coated formulation (184[A]). In another case a small reduction in platelet count (from 170 to 110 × 10^9/l) in a 37-year-old woman was associated with disproportionate perioperative bleeding (185[A]). An antiplatelet antibody was also detected and the authors therefore proposed that valproate must also have caused reduced platelet aggregation. Small reductions in red cell, white cell, and platelet counts occurred in a 65-year-old man taking valproate; the changes were dose-related but did not merit the description of pancytopenia that the authors used in the title of their paper (186[A]).

Gastrointestinal The suggestion that divalproex (valproate semisodium) causes fewer gastrointestinal adverse reactions than valproate (SEDA-23, 94; 184[A]) has been challenged (187[r]). In other cited studies divalproex was associated with a higher risk of gastrointestinal effects.

Liver Fatal *hepatitis* has been reported in a child taking valproate (188[A]).

An 8-year-old boy with complex partial seizures had taken valproate for more than 3 years. His sister developed uncomplicated hepatitis A, and 1 month later he became jaundiced, went into fulminant hepatic failure, quickly became encephalopathic, and died, despite discontinuation of valproate, aggressive supportive therapy, and treatment with carnitine. He had positive hepatitis A IgM; other causes for acute hepatitis were ruled out. Liver pathology showed distended hepatocytes with cholestasis and microvesicular changes.

The authors thought that valproate-induced hepatotoxicity may have exacerbated this child's infective hepatitis.

Hepatotoxicity due to valproate has been attributed to reactive hepatotoxic metabolites of valproate, which are normally detoxified by glutathione conjugation followed by mercapturic acid metabolism to their respective *N*-acetylcysteine conjugates (189[E]).

The Alpers–Huttenlocher syndrome, progressive neuronal degeneration of childhood, which is associated with seizures and abnormal liver function tests, can lead a clinician to use valproate, which can then precipitate acute liver damage, as has been reported in five cases (190[A]). In all cases liver transplantation for valproate-induced liver damage was then associated with worsening neurological function. In another case Alpers–Huttenlocher syndrome was misdiagnosed as valproate toxicity (191[A]).

Reproductive system Three women taking valproate developed *hyperandrogenism* and *polycystic ovaries*, associated in two cases with weight gain and menstrual disorders (192[A]). Valproate was replaced by lamotrigine, and the serum testosterone concentrations fell in all three women, the polycystic changes disappeared from the ovaries in two, and the two women who had gained weight and developed amenorrhea lost weight and started menstruating. In the light of this report others have clarified the distinction between polycystic ovary syndrome and polycystic ovary morphology, and have pointed out that it was not clear which of these valproate had actually caused (193[r], 194[r]). The report also contrasts with a report that polycystic ovary syndrome was identified in two of 19 patients taking no medications, four of 38 patients taking valproate or carbamazepine monotherapy, and one of 36 patients taking more than one antiepileptic drug, suggesting that polycystic ovary syndrome in women with focal epilepsy is not related to valproate or carbamazepine (21[C]).

Body temperature Valproate can cause *reduced body temperature* and in four cases this led to hypothermia (195[A]).

Risk factors The importance of *hypoalbuminemia* as a risk factor in valproate toxicity has been emphasized (196[A]).

A 53-year-old woman had a heart transplantation and developed worsening cardiac function, possible rejection, and increased lethargy. Her dose of valproate had been adjusted based on the total serum valproate concentration, but hypoalbuminemia prompted the measurement of the unbound serum valproate concentration, which was high. When the dose of valproate was adjusted based on the unbound rather than the total serum concentration she eventually improved.

Non-linear protein binding of valproate can result in disproportionate increases in unbound drug; adverse effects can then result when dosage adjustments are based solely on measurement of total valproate serum concentrations in patients with hypoalbuminemia.

Teratogenicity There has been a case-control study of the relation between prenatal exposure to valproate and the presence of limb deficiencies in newborn infants, using data from the Spanish Collaborative Study of Congenital Malformations (ECEMC) (197[C]). Of 22 294 consecutive malformed infants (excluding genetic syndromes) and 21 937 control infants with specified data on antiepileptic drugs during gestation, 57 malformed infants and 10 control infants had been exposed to valproate during the first trimester of pregnancy. Of the malformed infants who had been exposed to valproate 21 had *congenital limb defects* of different types (including overlapping digits, talipes, clubfoot, clinodactyly, arachnodactyly, hip dislocation, and pre- and postaxial polydactyly); three had limb deficiencies. After controlling for potential confounding factors there was an odds ratio of limb deficiencies of 6.2 (CI = 1.3, 30). The estimated risk for women taking valproate of having a baby with limb deficiencies was around 0.42%.

Drug administration route The successful use of intravenous valproate in psychiatric practice has been described (198[Ar]). The safety of rapid infusion of valproate has been studied in 20 patients with acute repetitive seizures, who received 20 mg/kg loading doses at rates of 33–555 mg/min (199[c]). Consciousness and respiratory function were not affected. There was no significant local irritation. Two patients with significant contributing factors developed *hypotension* and required vasopressors.

Drug overdose A beneficial effect of high-flux hemodialysis without hemoperfusion has been described in valproate overdose (200[A]).

A 25-year-old white woman took an unknown amount of valproic acid, became comatose, and developed hypotension and lactic acidosis. Her valproic acid concentrations rose to over 8400 μmol/l. High-flux hemodialysis was performed for 4 hours; the calculated half-life during the procedure was 2.7 hours, compared with a posthemodialysis value of 23 hours, suggesting that high-flux hemodialysis had increased the clearance rate of valproic acid. Her hemodynamic status and mental function improved in conjunction with the acute reduction in valproic acid concentrations.

Drug interactions Steady-state plasma concentrations of risperidone and 9-hydroxyrisperidone have been measured in 23 patients taking risperidone alone and in 10 co-medicated with sodium valproate (201[C]). Valproate had no effect on the kinetics of risperidone.

Vigabatrin *(SED-14, 192; SEDA-22, 92; SEDA-23, 92; SEDA-24, 94)*

Vigabatrin has been studied in an open 1-year extension of a randomized, double-blind, placebo-controlled Canadian trial in 97 adults with resistant partial epilepsy (202[c]). There was a mean weight gain of 3.7 kg by the end of the study. Treatment was discontinued in 12% because of adverse effects. Neurological/psychiatric adverse effects were the most common reason for withdrawal, including three *behavioral reactions* attributed to the drug.

Nervous system Acute *encephalopathy* has previously been attributed to vigabatrin in adults. There has now also been a case in a child (203[A]).

A 6-month-old girl with infantile Alexander disease with hydrocephalus developed apathy, somnolence, and sopor, with slowing of background encephalographic activity, 3 days after starting vigabatrin, which was withdrawn. During the next 2 days her symptoms abated and after 10 days her electroencephalogram normalized.

℞ *Adverse effects of vigabatrin on the eyes*

Vigabatrin causes a variety of changes in visual function, including reductions in visual field, visual acuity, color vision, and electroretinographic and electro-oculographic amplitudes.

Frequency and general reports *Visual field defects have been commonly reported in patients taking vigabatrin (10–30%; SEDA-24, 95), but in a recent observational cohort study the prevalence was relatively low, at 0.8% of 7228 patients (204[C]). However, this result has been challenged as a probable underestimate, because of the use of a questionnaire to elicit the diagnosis (205[r]–207[r]).*

Visual field loss due to vigabatrin has been studied in 18 patients taking long-term treatment (0.5–9.5 years) and five controls (208[c]). Of the 18 patients taking vigabatrin, there were mild visual field defects in six right eyes and eight left eyes, and severe defects in nine right eyes and eight left eyes. Most of the defects were peripheral constriction with nasal predominance.

The efficacy and adverse effects of steroids and vigabatrin in children with infantile spasms have been reviewed (209[M]). The authors found a high rate of visual field defects and concluded that although vigabatrin is efficacious it does not seem to be more effective than steroids or corticotrophin, and that the benefits of vigabatrin do not justify the associated risks of possible irreversible visual changes.

In a double-blind, randomized study in patients with partial epilepsy three of 32 patients taking vigabatrin had abnormal visual perimetry after the end of the study (210[C]).

Dose-relatedness *Visual function has been studied in 21 epileptic patients taking vigabatrin and compared with visual function in 11 similar epileptic patients who had never taken it, in order to investigate whether the severity of visual field defect is related to the dose of vigabatrin and to consider other factors that may correlate with severity (211[C]). Nine of 20 patients taking vigabatrin complained of blurring of vision compared with two of 11 controls. Four patients taking vigabatrin described flickering lights compared with one control. None had a posterior vitreous detachment. Three of 30 eyes of patients taking vigabatrin had distant visual acuity of 6/12 or worse compared with three of 22 controls, and five of 30 had near visual acuity worse than N6 compared with one of 22 controls. A mean of 1.73 Ishihara plates were misread by patients taking vigabatrin compared with 0.18 in the controls. There was a significant correlation between the severity of visual field defect and the total dose of vigabatrin.*

Pathophysiological studies *Because of this adverse effect, visual fields have been studied in eight patients with vigabatrin-attributed visual field loss; six were no longer taking vigabatrin (212[c]). Seven patients had marked visual field constriction with some sparing of the temporal visual field; the eighth had concentric constriction. Two patients had subnormal Arden electro-oculography indices; one patient had an abnormally delayed photopic b wave; five patients had delayed 30-Hz flicker b waves; and seven patients had delayed oscillatory potentials. Multifocal electroretinography confirmed that the effects occurred at the retinal level.*

Visual fields, visual evoked potentials, and electroretinography have also been assessed in 24 children treated with vigabatrin; 13 had at least one abnormal study (213[c]). There was visual field constriction in 11 of 17 patients who had perimetry; five of 15 patients who underwent visual evoked potential testing and four of 11 who underwent electroretinography had abnormal examinations. Abnormal visual evoked potentials and electroretinograms were mostly found in children who also had visual field constriction. Of five patients who were taking vigabatrin alone, three had abnormalities; however, all the other patients were taking other antiepileptic drugs and additive effects could not be ruled out.

In another study the retinal electrophysiologic markers associated with vigabatrin-attributed visual field loss have been distinguished from those associated with current vigabatrin therapy in eight previous and 18 current vigabatrin users (214[C]). They underwent electro-oculography, electroretinography, and automated static threshold perimetry and 22 healthy subjects underwent electroretinography. Of 26 patients exposed to vigabatrin, 18 had visual field loss; none taking other antiepileptic drugs had this type of visual field abnormality. The presence and severity of the visual field loss was significantly associated with the latency (implicit time) and amplitude of the electroretinographic cone function. The amplitude of the cone flicker response was the strongest predictor of visual field loss. The electro-oculogram, the photopic and scotopic electroretinogram, and the latency of the electroretinographic second oscillatory potential were not significantly related to the presence of visual field loss. Vigabatrin was significantly associated with the photopic amplitude, the scotopic a-wave latency, and the latency of the second oscillatory potential.

There was abnormal color perception in 32% of 32 patients taking vigabatrin monotherapy; in four cases there was an abnormality in the blue–yellow axis (37[c]). In the same patients there was a positive correlation between visual contrast sensitivity and the size of the visual field; macular photo-stress and glare tests were equal in both groups and did not differ from normal values; there was no effect on glare sensitivity (38[C]).

Causative factors *Concentric visual field loss found in the presurgical evaluation of patients with drug-resistant temporal lobe epilepsy taking vigabatrin has been studied and related to potential causative factors in 157 consecutive patients with drug-resistant temporal lobe epilepsy (215[C]). There was absolute concentric contraction of the visual field of 10–30 degrees presurgically in 20 of 118 patients who had ever used vigabatrin and in none of 39 who had not. Men were significantly more often affected than women (15 of 72 vs 5 of 85). The degree of visual field loss correlated with the duration of vigabatrin medication. There was no correlation of visual field contraction with a history of meningitis as potential cause of the epilepsy, duration of the epilepsy, status epilepticus in the medical history, or histological abnormality of the brain tissue removed. Ophthalmological examination of the patients with concentric contraction showed no abnormalities. None of the patients with concentric contraction complained spontaneously of their visual field loss.*

Reversibility *Long-term changes in the concentric contraction of the visual field have been studied in 27 patients with temporal lobe epilepsy taking vigabatrin (216[c]). Concentric contraction of the visual field did not change in 16 patients who stopped taking vigabatrin before the first examination but there was slight but significant worsening of visual field loss in 11 patients who continued taking vigabatrin. The authors concluded that vigabatrin-associated visual field loss is not reversible and that progression can occur when vigabatrin is continued.*

The reversibility of visual function loss from vigabatrin has been studied in 13 patients who had discontinued the drug up to a year be-

fore because of lack of efficacy or reductions in visual field (217[C]). Although electroretinographic cone implicit time improved, most of the patients did not have improvement in either clinical measures of visual function (i.e. visual acuity, color vision, visual fields) or in electroretinographic amplitudes. However, several patients who had minimal visual field loss while taking vigabatrin had substantial recovery of the electroretinographic amplitudes. There was no association between recovery of function and either duration of treatment or cumulative dosage. Multifocal electroretinography showed a diffuse loss of function that was not isolated to the periphery.

In contrast, in another study there was partial reversibility of visual field constriction and retinal function after withdrawal in two patients (218[A]).

Of 30 children with epilepsy (14 boys and 16 girls, aged 4–20 years) taking vigabatrin for infantile spasms and simple and complex partial epilepsy, who had never complained of ophthalmologic disturbances, four had visual field constriction in the nasal hemifield (219[c]). In one child, visual abnormalities were stable even 10 months after vigabatrin withdrawal, while in another there was improvement 5 months after withdrawal.

Effects of other antiepileptic drugs and interaction with vigabatrin *Other antiepileptic drugs can also alter visual evoked potentials and brainstem evoked potentials.*

Visual field defects associated with various antiepileptic drugs (carbamazepine, diazepam, gabapentin, phenytoin, tiagabine, and vigabatrin) have been reviewed (15[Rc]). The true frequency is unknown, but in a retrospective study in 158 patients with partial epilepsy visual field defects were detected in 21 (13%); 13 patients had concentric visual field constriction without subjective spontaneous manifestations. Of these 13 patients, nine were taking vigabatrin.

Visual-evoked potentials and brainstem auditory-evoked potentials have been measured in 58 children and adolescents taking carbamazepine, phenobarbital, or sodium valproate monotherapy and 50 sex- and age-matched controls (16[C]). After 1 year the patients taking carbamazepine had significantly prolonged visual-evoked P100 latencies compared with both baseline and control values; they also had significantly prolonged peak latencies of auditory waves I–III–V and interpeak interval I–V. Those taking sodium valproate had significantly prolonged visual-evoked P100 latencies. In contrast, children taking phenobarbital had no changes.

In 100 epileptic patients aged 8–18 years taking carbamazepine or valproate in modified-release formulations either alone or with added vigabatrin interpeak latencies of I–III and III–V of brainstem evoked potentials were significantly delayed and N75/P100 and P100/N145 amplitudes in the visual evoked potentials were reduced (34[C]). However, the addition of vigabatrin did not worsen the effects caused by the other two drugs alone.

Mouth *Gingival overgrowth* has been reported in a 29-year-old man who had taken vigabatrin for 5 years for partial epileptic seizures (220[A]).

Drug overdose After an overdose of vigabatrin 45 g, a 17-year-old girl developed a *behavioral disorder* (221[A]). A CT scan of the brain was normal but an electroencephalogram showed abnormal δ waves.

Drug interactions Although vigabatrin is not metabolized by liver enzymes it increased serum carbamazepine concentrations by at least 10% in 66 epileptic patients aged 10–66 years with focal seizure onset with or without secondary generalization (222[c]).

Zonisamide *(SED-14, 193; SEDA-22, 93)*

The pharmacology, clinical pharmacology, and adverse effects of zonisamide have been reviewed (1[R], 107[R]).

Psychiatric Of 74 epileptic patients who had taken zonisamide 14 had *psychotic episodes*, diagnosed retrospectively (223[c]). The authors estimated that the incidence of psychotic episodes during zonisamide treatment was several times higher than the previously reported prevalence of epileptic psychosis, and that the risk was higher in young patients. In 13 patients, psychotic episodes occurred within a few years of starting zonisamide. In children, obsessive–compulsive symptoms were related to psychotic episodes.

A unique form of *paramnesia* has been attributed to zonisamide (224[A]).

After an episode of zonisamide-induced psychosis a 28-year-old man with epilepsy consistently mistook people who were unknown to him, such as hospital staff, for people whom he had met long ago. However, he did not misidentify their names or other attributes, such as their occupations.

The authors could not fit this extraordinary form of misidentification into any known subcategory of misidentification syndromes, but rather thought that it fitted Kraepelin's description of "assoziierende Erinnerungsfälschungen".

Acid base balance *Metabolic acidosis* has been reported in patients taking zonisamide (225[A]). Zonisamide inhibits carbonic anhydrase (226[E]), which might have contributed, as has been suggested by another case of metabolic acidosis in a 7-year-old boy, in which the mechanism was renal tubular acidosis.

Ammonium chloride, bicarbonate, and furosemide loading tests in an epileptic man with metabolic acidosis and episodic hypokalemia taking zonisamide showed evidence of distal renal tubular acidosis (227[A]). On re-examination 7 weeks after zonisamide had been replaced with phenytoin, the renal tubular acidosis had resolved.

Urinary tract Further cases of *nephrolithiasis* have been reported in patients taking zonisamide (228[A]).

A 13-year-old boy who had taken zonisamide and acetazolamide for 2 months developed abdominal pain due to left-sided hydronephrosis, which resolved after the passage of a stone. He had an alkaline urine, and acetazolamide was withdrawn. However, 2 months later he formed another stone. Zonisamide was withdrawn and he formed no more stones.

A 7-year-old boy took zonisamide for 3 months and then formed a thick sludge of calcium phosphate in the bladder when dehydrated because of pneumonia.

A 15-year-old girl, who had a history of recurrent urinary obstruction, formed a thick sludge of calcium oxalate in the bladder.

In all three patients the urine was alkaline and there was hypercalciuria.

Skin Zonisamide can cause lack of sweating (229[A]).

A 10-year-old boy who had taken zonisamide for about 9 months noticed that he had a dry skin and that he seldom sweated. His zonisamide blood concentration was very high. He discontinued zonisamide and became able to sweat.

The authors suggested that this effect was due to ion channel blockade.

In 16 patients taking zonisamide, acetylcholine stimulation testing after about 1 month was normal in four cases and reduced in 12 (230[c]). There was reduced sweating in four of the 12 who had a reduced test response, but not in the four with a normal response.

REFERENCES

1. Willmore J. Clinical pharmacology of new antiepileptic drugs. Neurology 2000; 55 Suppl 3: S17–24.
2. Politsky JM. Painful diabetic neuropathy: treatment with modern anticonvulsants. Mature Med Can 2000; 3: 60–3.
3. Gillham R, Kane K, Bryant-Comstock L, Brodie MJ. A double-blind comparison of lamotrigine and carbamazepine in newly diagnosed epilepsy with health-related quality of life as an outcome measure. Seizure 2000; 9: 375–9.
4. Heaney DC, Shorvon SD, Sander JWAS, Boon P, Komarek V, Marusic P, Dravet C, Perucca E, Majkowski J, Lima JL, Arroyo S, Tomson T, Ried S, Van Donselaar C, Eskazan E, Peeters P, Carita P, Tjong-a-Hung I, Myon E, Taieb C. Cost minimization analysis of antiepileptic drugs in newly diagnosed epilepsy in 12 European countries. Epilepsia 2000; 41 Suppl 5: S37–44.
5. Collins TL, Petroff OAC, Mattson RH. A comparison of four new antiepileptic medications. Seizure 2000; 9: 291–3.
6. Datta PK, Crawford PM. Refractory epilepsy: treatment with new antiepileptic drugs. Seizure 2000; 9: 51–7.
7. Lhatoo SD, Wong ICK, Polizzi G, Sander JWAS. Long-term retention rates of lamotrigine, gabapentin, and topiramate in chronic epilepsy. Epilepsia 2000; 41: 1592–6.
8. Lindberger M, Alenius M, Frisen L, Johannessen SI, Larsson S, Malmgren K, Tomson T. Gabapentin versus vigabatrin as first add-on for patients with partial seizures that failed to respond to monotherapy: a randomized, double-blind, dose titration study. Epilepsia 2000; 41: 1289–95.
9. Vasudev K, Goswami U, Kohli K. Carbamazepine and valproate monotherapy: feasibility, relative safety and efficacy, and therapeutic

drug monitoring in manic disorder. Psychopharmacology 2000; 150: 15–23.
10. Leandri M, Lunardi G, Inglese M, Messmer-Uccelli M, Mancardi GL, Gottlieb A, Solaro C. Lamotrigine in trigeminal neuralgia secondary to multiple sclerosis. J Neurol 2000; 247: 556–8.
11. Ghaemi SN, Gaughan S. Novel anticonvulsants: A new generation of mood stabilizers? Harv Rev Psychiatry 2000; 8: 1–7.
12. Genton P, Gelisse P, Thomas P, Dravet C. Do carbamazepine and phenytoin aggravate juvenile myoclonic epilepsy? Neurology 2000; 55: 1106–9.
13. Trimble MR, Rusch N, Betts T, Crawford PM. Psychiatric symptoms after therapy with new antiepileptic drugs: psychopathological and seizure related variables. Seizure 2000; 9: 249–54.
14. Adamolekun B, Mielke J, Ball D, Mundanda T. An evaluation of the management of epilepsy by primary health care nurses in Chitungwiza, Zimbabwe. Epilepsy Res 2000; 39: 177–81.
15. Stefan H, Bernatik J, Knorr HLJ. Visual field constriction and antiepileptic drug treatment. Neurol Psychiatry Brain Res 2000; 7: 185–90.
16. Verrotti A, Trotta D, Cutarella R, Pascarella R, Morgese G, Chiarelli F. Effects of antiepileptic drugs on evoked potentials in epileptic children. Pediatr Neurol 2000; 23: 397–402.
17. Schwaninger M, Ringleb P, Annecke A, Winter R, Kohl B, Werle E, Fiehn W, Rieser PA, Walter-Sack I. Elevated plasma concentrations of lipoprotein(a) in medicated epileptic patients. J Neurol 2000; 247: 687–90.
18. Brenner S, Golan H, Lerman Y. Psoriasiform eruption and anticonvulsant drugs. Acta Derm-Venereol 2000; 80: 382.
19. Leyva L, Torres MJ, Posadas S, Blanca M, Besso G, O'Valle F, Del Moral RG, Santamaria LF, Juarez C. Anticonvulsant-induced toxic epidermal necrolysis: monitoring the immunologic response. J Allergy Clin Immunol 2000; 105 I: 157–65.
20. Feldkamp J, Becker A, Witte OW, Scharff D, Scherbaum WA. Long-term anticonvulsant therapy leads to low bone mineral density – evidence for direct drug effects of phenytoin and carbamazepine on human osteoblast-like cells. Exp Clin Endocrinol Diabetes 2000; 108: 37–43.
21. Bauer J, Jarre A, Klingmuller D, Elger CE. Polycystic ovary syndrome in patients with focal epilepsy: a study in 93 women. Epilepsy Res 2000; 41: 163–7.
22. Arpino C, Brescianini S, Robert E, Castilla EE, Cocchi G, Cornel MC, De Vigan C, Lancaster PAL, Merlob P, Sumiyoshi Y, Zampino G, Renzi C, Rosano A, Mastroiacovo P. Teratogenic effects of antiepileptic drugs: use of an international database on Malformations and Drug Exposure (MADRE). Epilepsia 2000; 41: 1436–43.
23. Baumann RJ, Duffner PK. Treatment of children with simple febrile seizures: the AAP practice parameter. Pediatr Neurol 2000; 23: 11–17.
24. Collins RJ, Garnett WR. Extended release formulations of anticonvulsant medications clinical pharmacokinetics and therapeutic advantages. CNS Drugs 2000; 14: 203–12.
25. Koenig HM, Edwards TL. Cisatracurium-induced neuromuscular blockade in anticonvulsant treated neurosurgical patients. J Neurosurg Anesthesiol 2000; 12: 314–18.
26. Snodgrass SR, Parks BR. Anticonvulsant blood levels: historical review with a pediatric focus. J Child Neurol 2000; 15: 734–46.
27. Mackereth S. Use of rectal diazepam in the community. Dev Med Child Neurol 2000; 42: 785.
28. Kriel RL, Cloyd JC, Pellock JM. Respiratory depression in children receiving diazepam for acute seizures: a prospective study. Dev Med Child Neurol 2000; 42: 429.
29. Al Tahan A. Paradoxic response to diazepam in complex partial status epilepticus. Arch Med Res 2000; 31: 101–4.
30. Setterfield JF, Robinson R, MacDonald O, Calonjet E. Coma-induced bullae and sweat gland necrosis following clobazam. Clin Exp Dermatol 2000; 25: 215–18.
31. Harel L, Zecharia A, Straussberg R, Volovitz B, Amir J. Successful treatment of rheumatic chorea with carbamazepine. Pediatr Neurol 2000; 23: 147–51.
32. Bogliun G, Di Viesti P, Monticelli LM, Beghi E, Zarrelli M, Simone P, Airoldi L, Frattola L. Anticonvulsants and peripheral nerve function results of prospective monitoring in patients with newly diagnosed epilepsy. Clin Drug Invest 2000; 20: 173–80.
33. Holtmann M, Korn-Merker E, Boenigk HE. Carbamazepine-induced combined phonic and motor tic in a boy with Down's syndrome. Epileptic Disord 2000; 2: 39–40.
34. Zgorzalewicz M, Galas-Zgorzalewicz B. Visual and auditory evoked potentials during long-term vigabatrin treatment in children and adolescents with epilepsy. Clin Neurophysiol 2000; 111: 2150–4.
35. Ramsaransing G, Zwanikken C, De Keyser J. Worsening of symptoms of multiple sclerosis associated with carbamazepine. Br Med J 2000; 320: 1113.
36. Nousiainen I, Kalviainen R, Mantyjarvi M. Color vision in epilepsy patients treated with vigabatrin or carbamazepine monotherapy. Ophthalmology 2000; 107: 884–8.
37. Nousiainen I, Kalviainen R, Mantyjarvi M. Contrast and glare sensitivity in epilepsy patients treated with vigabatrin or carbamazepine monotherapy compared with healthy volunteers. Br J Ophthalmol 2000; 84: 622–5.
38. Miyaoka T, Seno H, Itoga M, Horiguchi J. Reversible pitch perception deficit caused by carbamazepine. Clin Neuropharmacol 2000; 23: 219–21.
39. Benatar MG, Sahin M, Davis RG. Antiepileptic drug-induced visual hallucinations in a child. Pediatr Neurol 2000; 23: 439–41.
40. Hogan RE, Bertrand ME, Deaton RL, Sommerville KW. Total percentage body weight

changes during add-on therapy with tiagabine, carbamazepine and phenytoin. Epilepsy Res 2000; 41: 23–8.
41. Verrotti A, Pascarella R, Trotta D, Giuva T, Morgese G, Chiarelli F. Hyperhomocysteinemia in children treated with sodium valproate and carbamazepine. Epilepsy Res 2000; 41: 253–7.
42. Vilaseca MA, Monrós E, Artuch R, Colomé C, Farré C, Valls C, Cardo E, Pineda M. Antiepileptic drug treatment in children: hyperhomocysteinaemia, B-vitamins and the 677CT mutation of the methylenetetrahydrofolate reductase gene. Eur J Paediatr Neurol 2000; 4: 269–77.
43. Linares Torres P, Fidalgo Lŏpez I, Castaón López A, Martinez Pinto Y. Colitis linfocítica como causa de diarrea crónica: posible relación con carbamazepina. Aten Prim 2000; 25: 366–7.
44. Straussberg R, Harel L, Ben-Amitai D, Cohen D, Amir J. Carbamazepine-induced Stevens–Johnson syndrome treated with IV steroids and IVIG. Pediatr Neurol 2000; 22: 231–3.
45. Elstner S, Sperling W. The carbamazepine-hypersensitivity-syndrome – aspects of differential diagnoses with a representative case history. Fortschr Neurol Psychiatr 2000; 68: 188–92.
46. Koga T, Kubota Y, Nakayama J. Interferon-gamma production in the peripheral lymphocytes of a patient with carbamazepine hypersensitivity syndrome. Acta Derm-Venereol 2000; 80: 73.
47. Verma SP, Yunis N, Lekos A, Crausman RS. Carbamazepine-induced systemic lupus erythematosus presenting as cardiac tamponade. Chest 2000; 117: 597–8.
48. Verrotti A, Feliciani C, Morresi S, Coscione G, Morgese G, Toto P, Chiarelli F. Carbamazepine-induced hypersensitivity syndrome in a child with epilepsy. Int J Immunopathol Pharmacol 2000; 13: 49–53.
49. Shimoyama R, Ohkubo T, Sugawara K. Monitoring of carbamazepine and carbamazepine 10,11-epoxide in breast milk and plasma by high-performance liquid chromatography. Ann Clin Biochem 2000; 37: 210–15.
50. Campany Herrero D, Mateu De Antonio J, Del Villar Ruiz De La Torre JA, Grau Cerrato S, Salas Sánchez E, Ortiz Sagristà P. Intoxicación aguda por carbamazepina. Farm Hosp 2000; 24: 43–6.
51. Lifshitz M, Gavrilov V, Sofer S. Signs and symptoms of carbamazepine overdose in young children. Pediatr Emerg Care 2000; 16: 26–7.
52. Rösel T, Schneider J, Fischer JTh, Druschky K-F. "Carbamazepin Intoxikation" durch Verwechslung von Medikamenten. Dtsch Med Wochenschr 2000; 125: 352–6.
53. Pricone MG, King CV, Drummer OH, Opeskin K, McIntyre IM. Postmortem investigation of lamotrigine concentrations. J Forensic Sci 2000; 45: 11–15.
54. Hugen PWH, Burger DM, Brinkman K, Ter Hofstede HJM, Schuurman R, Koopmans PP, Hekster YA. Carbamazepine–indinavir interaction causes antiretroviral therapy failure. Ann Pharmacother 2000; 34: 465–70.
55. Burman W, Orr L. Carbamazepine toxicity after starting combination antiretroviral therapy including ritonavir and efavirenz. AIDS 2000; 14: 2793–4.
56. Garcia AB, Ibarra AL, Etessam JP, Salio AM, Martinez DAP, Diaz RS, Heras MT. Protease inhibitor-induced carbamazepine toxicity. Clin Neuropharmacol 2000; 23: 216–18.
57. Lai C-L, Chen W-J, Huang C-H, Lin F-Y, Lee Y-T. Sinus node dysfunction in a patient with lithium intoxication. J Formos Med Assoc 2000; 99: 66–8.
58. Laroudie C, Salazar DE, Cosson J-P, Cheuvart B, Istin B, Girault J, Ingrand I, Decourt J-P. Carbamazepine-nefazodone interaction in healthy subjects. J Clin Psychopharmacol 2000; 20: 46–53.
59. Schlienger R, Kurmann M, Drewe J, Muller-Spahn F, Seifritz E. Inhibition of phenprocoumon anticoagulation by carbamazepine. Eur Neuropsychopharmacol 2000; 10: 219–21.
60. Spina E, Avenoso A, Facciola G, Salemi M, Scordo MG, Giacobello T, Madia AG, Perucca E. Plasma concentrations of risperidone and 9-hydroxyrisperidone: effect of comedication with carbamazepine or valproate. Ther Drug Monit 2000; 22: 481–5.
61. Burstein AH, Horton RL, Dunn T, Alfaro RM, Piscitelli SC, Theodore W. Lack of effect of St John's wort on carbamazepine pharmacokinetics in healthy volunteers. Clin Pharmacol Ther 2000; 68: 605–12.
62. Khan A, Shad MU, Preskorn SH. Lack of sertraline efficacy probably due to an interaction with carbamazepine. J Clin Psychiatry 2000; 61: 526–7.
63. Miceli JJ, Anziano RJ, Robarge L, Hansen RA, Laurent A. Effect of carbamazepine on the steady-state pharmacokinetics of ziprasidone in healthy volunteers. Br J Clin Pharmacol 2000; 49 Suppl 1: 65S–70S.
64. Yoshimura R, Nakamura J, Eto S, Ueda N. Possible relationships between plasma carbamazepine-10,11-epoxide levels and antimanic efficacy and side effects in patients with schizoaffective disorder. Hum Psychopharmacol 2000; 15: 237–40.
65. Anonymous. Gabapentin monotherapy – sometimes helpful. Prescrire Int 2000; 9: 40–2.
66. Morrell MJ, Mclean MJ, Willmore LJ, Privitera MD, Faught RE, Holmes GL, Magnus L, Bernstein P, Rose-Legatt A. Efficacy of gabapentin as adjunctive therapy in a large, multicenter study. Seizure 2000; 9: 241–8.
67. Vieta E, Martinez-Aran A, Nieto E, Colom F, Reinares M, Benabarre A, Gasto C. Adjunctive gabapentin treatment of bipolar disorder. Eur Psychiatry 2000; 15: 433–7.
68. Muscas GC, Chiroli S, Luceri F, Del Mastio M, Balestrieri F, Arnetoli G. Conversion from thrice daily to twice daily administration of gabapentin (GBP) in partial epilepsy: analysis of clinical efficacy and plasma levels. Seizure 2000; 9: 47–50.
69. Pande AC, Pollack MH, Crockatt J, Greiner M, Chouinard G, Lydiard RB, Taylor CB, Dager SR, Shiovitz T. Placebo-controlled study of gabapentin

treatment of panic disorder. J Clin Psychopharmacol 2000; 20: 467–71.
70. Asconape J, Diedrich A, DellaBadia J. Myoclonus associated with the use of gabapentin. Epilepsia 2000; 41: 479–81.
71. Herrmann N, Lanctôt K, Myszak M. Effectiveness of gabapentin for the treatment of behavioral disorders in dementia. J Clin Psychopharmacol 2000; 20: 90–3.
72. Laird MA, Gidal BE. Use of gabapentin in the treatment of neuropathic pain. Ann Pharmacother 2000; 34: 802–7.
73. Palomeras E, Sanz P, Cano A, Fossas P. Dystonia in a patient treated with propranolol and gabapentin. Arch Neurol 2000; 57: 570–1.
74. Jacob PC, Chand RP, Omeima E-S. Asterixis induced by gabapentin. Clin Neuropharmacol 2000; 23: 53.
75. Trinka E, Niedermuller U, Thaler C, Doering S, Moroder T, Ladurner G, Bauer G. Gabapentin-induced mood changes with hypomanic features in adults. Seizure 2000; 9: 505–8.
76. Gallay BJ, De Mattos AM, Norman DJ. Reversible acute renal allograft dysfunction due to gabapentin. Transplantation 2000; 70: 208–9.
77. Brannon GE, Rolland PD. Anorgasmia in a patient with bipolar disorder type 1 treated with gabapentin. J Clin Psychopharmacol 2000; 20: 379–81.
78. Guttuso TJ Jr. Gabapentin's effects on hot flashes and hypothermia. Neurology 2000; 54: 2161–3.
79. Culy CR, Goa KL. Lamotrigine: a review of its use in childhood epilepsy. Paediatr Drugs 2000; 2: 299–330.
80. Jozwiak S, Terczynski A. Open study evaluating lamotrigine efficacy and safety in add-on treatment and consecutive monotherapy in patients with carbamazepine- or valproate-resistant epilepsy. Seizure 2000; 9: 486–92.
81. Barron TF, Hunt SL, Hoban TF, Price ML. Lamotrigine monotherapy in children. Pediatr Neurol 2000; 23: 160–3.
82. Calabrese JR, Suppes T, Bowden CL, Sachs GS, Swann AC, McElroy SL, Kusumakar V, Ascher JA, Earl NL, Greene PL, Monaghan ET. A double-blind, placebo-controlled, prophylaxis study of lamotrigine in rapid-cycling bipolar disorder. J Clin Psychiatry 2000; 61: 841–50.
83. Gidal BE, Walker JK, Lott RS, Shaw R, Speth J, Marty KJ, Rutecki P. Efficacy of lamotrigine in institutionalized, developmentally disabled patients with epilepsy: a retrospective evaluation. Seizure 2000; 9: 131–6.
84. Léthel V, Chabrol B, Livet MO, Mancini J. Intérêt de la lamotrigine therapy en pédiatrie. Étude rétrospective chez 32 enfants. Arch Pédiatr 2000; 7: 234–42.
85. Parmeggiani L, Belmonte A, Ferrari AR, Perucca E, Guerrini R. Add-on lamotrigine treatment in children and young adults with severe partial epilepsy: an open, prospective, long-term study. J Child Neurol 2000; 15: 671–4.
86. Sotero De Menezes MA, Rho JM, Murphy P, Cheyette S. Lamotrigine-induced tic disorder: report of five pediatric cases. Epilepsia 2000; 41: 862–7.
87. Janszky J, Rasonyi G, Halasz P, Olajos S, Perenyi J, Szucs A, Debreczeni J. Disabling erratic myoclonus during lamotrigine therapy with high serum level – report of two cases. Clin Neuropharmacol 2000; 23: 86–9.
88. Mewasingh L, Aylett S, Kirkham F, Stanhope R. Hyponatraemia associated with lamotrigine in cranial diabetes insipidus. Lancet 2000; 356: 656.
89. Pulik M, Lionnet F, Genet P. Successful treatment of lamotrigine-induced erythroblastopenic crisis with folinic acid. Neurology 2000; 55: 1235–6.
90. Solvason HB. Agranulocytosis associated with lamotrigine. Am J Psychiatry 2000; 157: 1704.
91. Fayad M, Choueiri R, Mikati M. Potential hepatotoxicity of lamotrigine. Pediatr Neurol 2000; 22: 49–52.
92. Tsolaki M, Kourtis A, Divanoglou D, Bostanzopoulou M, Kazis A. Monotherapy with lamotrigine in patients with Alzheimer's disease and seizures. Am J Alzheimer's Dis 2000; 15: 74–9.
93. Besag FMC, Ng GYT, Pool F. Successful re-introduction of lamotrigine after initial rash. Seizure 2000; 9: 282–6.
94. Simpson DM, Olney R, McArthur JC, Khan A, Godbold J, Ebel-Frommer K. A placebo-controlled trial of lamotrigine for painful HIV-associated neuropathy. Neurology 2000; 54: 2115–19.
95. Yalçin B, Karaduman A. Stevens–Johnson syndrome associated with concomitant use of lamotrigine and valproic acid. J Am Acad Dermatol 2000; 43 Suppl: 898–9.
96. Fervenza FC, Kanakiriya S, Kunau RT, Gibney R, Lager DJ. Acute granulomatous interstitial nephritis and colitis in anticonvulsant hypersensitivity syndrome associated with lamotrigine treatment. Am J Kidney Dis 2000; 36: 1034–40.
97. Sarzi-Puttini P, Panni B, Cazzola M, Muzzupappa S, Turiel M. Lamotrigine-induced lupus. Lupus 2000; 9: 555–7.
98. Schaub N, Bircher AJ. Severe hypersensitivity syndrome to lamotrigine confirmed by lymphocyte stimulation in vitro. Allergy Eur J Allergy Clin Immunol 2000; 55: 191–3.
99. Messenheimer JA, Giorgi L, Risner ME. The tolerability of lamotrigine in children. Drug Saf 2000; 22: 303–12.
100. Gidal BE, Anderson GD, Rutecki PR, Shaw R, Lanning A. Lack of an effect of valproate concentration on lamotrigine pharmacokinetics in developmentally disabled patients with epilepsy. Epilepsy Res 2000; 42: 23–31.
101. Kanner AM, Frey M. Adding valproate to lamotrigine: a study of their pharmacokinetic interaction. Neurology 2000; 55: 588–91.
102. Morris RG, Black AB, Lam E, Westley IS. Clinical study of lamotrigine and valproic acid in patients with epilepsy: Using a drug interaction to advantage? Ther Drug Monit 2000; 22: 656–60.

103. Besag FMC, Berry DJ, Pool F. Methsuximide lowers lamotrigine blood levels: a pharmacokinetic antiepileptic drug interaction. Epilepsia 2000; 41: 624–7.
104. Ebert U, Thong NQ, Oertel R, Kirch W. Effects of rifampicin and cimetidine on pharmacokinetics and pharmacodynamics of lamotrigine in healthy subjects. Eur J Clin Pharmacol 2000; 56: 299–304.
105. Anand A, Charney DS, Oren DA, Berman RM, Hu XS, Cappiello A, Krystal JH. Attenuation of the neuropsychiatric effects of ketamine with lamotrigine: support for hyperglutamatergic effects of N-methyl-D-aspartate receptor antagonists. Arch Gen Psychiatry 2000; 57: 270–6.
106. Chen C, Veronese L, Yin Y. The effects of lamotrigine on the pharmacokinetics of lithium. Br J Clin Pharmacol 2000; 50: 193–5.
107. Schachter SC. The next wave of anticonvulsants: focus on levetiracetam, oxcarbazepine and zonisamide. CNS Drugs 2000; 14: 229–49.
108. Abou-Khalil B. Levetiracetam – a new therapeutic option for epilepsy. Today's Ther Trends 2000; 18: 241–54.
109. Genton P, Van Vleymen B. Piracetam and levetiracetam: close structural similarities but different pharmacological and clinical profiles. Epileptic Disord 2000; 2: 99–105.
110. Anonymous. Two new drugs for epilepsy. Med Lett Drugs Ther 2000; 42: 33–5.
111. Ben-Menachem E, Falter U, for the European Levetiracetam Study Group. Efficacy and tolerability of levetiracetam 3000 mg/d in patients with refractory partial seizures: a multicenter, double-blind, responder-selected study evaluating monotherapy. Epilepsia 2000; 41: 1276–83.
112. Betts T, Waegemans T, Crawford P. A multicentre, double-blind, randomized, parallel group study to evaluate the tolerability and efficacy of two oral doses of levetiracetam, 2000 mg daily and 4000 mg daily, without titration in patients with refractory epilepsy. Seizure 2000; 9: 80–7.
113. Cereghino JJ, Biton V, Abou-Khalil B, Dreifuss F, Gauer LJ, Leppik I, and the United States Levetiracetam Study Group. Levetiracetam for partial seizures. Results of a double-blind, randomized clinical trial. Neurology 2000; 55: 236–42.
114. Grant R, Shorvon SD. Efficacy and tolerability of 1000–4000 mg per day of levetiracetam as add-on therapy in patients with refractory epilepsy. Epilepsy Res 2000; 42: 89–95.
115. Shorvon SD, Löwenthal A, Janz D, Bielen E, Loiseau P, for the European Levetiracetam Study Group. Multicenter double-blind, randomized, placebo-controlled trial of levetiracetam as add-on therapy in patients with refractory partial seizures. Epilepsia 2000; 41: 1179–86.
116. Lott RS, Helmboldt K. A carbamazepine analogue for partial seizures in adults and children with epilepsy. Formulary 2000; 35: 219–33.
117. Shorvon S. Oxcarbazepine: a review. Seizure 2000; 9: 75–9.
118. Kramer G. Oxcarbazepine (Trileptal): a new antiepileptic drug for mono- and add-on-therapy. Aktuel Neurol 2000; 27: 59–71.
119. Barcs G, Walker EB, Elger CE, Scaramelli A, Stefan H, Sturm Y, Moore A, Flesch G, Kramer L, D'Souza J. Oxcarbazepine placebo-controlled, dose-ranging trial in refractory partial epilepsy. Epilepsia 2000; 41: 1597–607.
120. Beydoun A, Sachdeo RC, Rosenfeld WE, Krauss GL, Sessler N, Mesenbrink P, Kramer L, D'Souza J. Oxcarbazepine monotherapy for partial-onset seizures: a multicenter, double-blind, clinical trial. Neurology 2000; 54: 2245–51.
121. Glauser TA, Nigro M, Sachdeo R, Pasteris LA, Weinstein S, Abou-Khalil B, Frank LM, Grinspan A, Guarino T, Bettis D, Kerrigan J, Geoffroy G, Mandelbaum D, Jacobs T, Mesenbrink P, Kramer L, D'Souza J, Andrews RV, Barros MD, Bebin M, Beierwaltes P, Berkovic S, Bonet HB, Bourgeois BFD, Carmant L, Clark P, Cooper A, D'Cruz O, De Arbelaiz R, et al. Adjunctive therapy with oxcarbazepine in children with partial seizures. Neurology 2000; 54: 2237–44.
122. Koller WC, Hristova A, Brin M. Pharmacologic treatment of essential tremor. Neurology 2000; 54 Suppl 4: S30–8.
123. Kanner AM, Parra J, Frey M. The "forgotten" cross-tolerance between phenobarbital and primidone: it can prevent acute primidone-related toxicity. Epilepsia 2000; 41: 1310–14.
124. Devidal R, Guy C, Perrot JL, Cathebras P, Ferron C, Ollagnier M. Syndrome de Lyell et phénobarbital: à propos de deux cas. Thérapie 2000; 55: 225–7.
125. Daniels PR, Berry GJ, Tazelaar HD, Cooper LT Jr. Giant cell myocarditis as a manifestation of drug hypersensitivity. Cardiovasc Pathol 2000; 9: 287–91.
126. Crawley J, Waruiru C, Mithwani S, Mwangi I, Watkins W, Ouma D, Winstanley P, Peto T, Marsh K. Effect of phenobarbital on seizure frequency and mortality in childhood cerebral malaria: a randomised, controlled intervention study. Lancet 2000; 355: 701–6.
127. Dessens AB, Cohen-Kettenis PT, Mellenbergh GJ, Koppe JG, Van de Poll NE, Boer K. Association of prenatal phenobarbital and phenytoin exposure with small head size at birth and with learning problems. Acta Paediatr Int J Paediatr 2000; 89: 533–41.
128. Mishory A, Yaroslavsky Y, Bersudsky Y, Belmaker RH. Phenytoin as an antimanic anticonvulsant: a controlled study. Am J Psychiatry 2000; 157: 463–5.
129. Anderson GD, Lin Y, Temkin NR, Fischer JH, Winn HR. Incidence of intravenous site reactions in neurotrauma patients receiving valproate or phenytoin. Ann Pharmacother 2000; 34: 697–702.
130. Hironishi M. [Cerebellar atrophy associated with phenytoin intoxication.] Brain Nerve 2000; 52: 264–5.
131. Sharma S, Dasroy SK. Gingival hyperplasia

induced by phenytoin. New Engl J Med 2000; 342: 5.

132. Colombo-Arnet E. Phenytoin-induzierte Hypersensitivitätsreaktion mit Leberversagen. Schweiz Rundsch Med Prax 2000; 89: 675–7.

133. Eisen ER, Fish J, Shear NH. Management of drug-induced toxic epidermal necrolysis. J Cutaneous Med Surg 2000; 4: 96–102.

134. Jaramillo MJ, Stewart KJ, Kolhe PS. Phenytoin induced rhinophyma treated by excision and full thickness skin grafting. Br J Plast Surg 2000; 53: 521–3.

135. Yoshikawa H, Abe T, Oda T. Purple glove syndrome caused by oral administration of phenytoin. J Child Neurol 2000; 15: 762.

136. Siragusa RJ, Ramos-Caro FA, Edwards NL, Flowers FP. Drug-induced lupus due to phenytoin. J Pharm Technol 2000; 16: 5–7.

137. DeToledo JC, Ramsay RE. Fosphenytoin and phenytoin in patients with status epilepticus. Improved tolerability versus increased costs. Drug Saf 2000; 22: 459–66.

138. Chua HC, Venketasubramanian N, Tjia H, Chan SP. Elimination of phenytoin in toxic overdose. Clin Neurol Neurosurg 2000; 102: 6–8.

139. Kawasaki C, Nishi R, Uekihara S, Hayano S, Otagiri M. Charcoal hemoperfusion in the treatment of phenytoin overdose. Am J Kidney Dis 2000; 35: 323–6.

140. Lau KK, Lai CK, Chan AYW. Phenytoin poisoning after using Chinese proprietary medicines. Hum Exp Toxicol 2000; 19: 385–6.

141. Brackett CC, Bloch JD. Phenytoin as a possible cause of acetaminophen hepatotoxicity: case report and review of the literature. Pharmacotherapy 2000; 20: 229–33.

142. Yeung SCSA, Ensom MHH. Phenytoin and enteral feedings: does evidence support an interaction? Ann Pharmacother 2000; 34: 896–905.

143. Schachter SC, Tarsy D. Remacemide: current status and clinical applications. Expert Opin Invest Drugs 2000; 9: 871–83.

144. Chadwick D, Smith D, Crawford P, Harrison B. Remacemide hydrochloride: a placebo-controlled, one month, double-blind assessment of its safety, tolerability and pharmakinetics as adjunctive therapy in patients with epilepsy. Seizure 2000; 9: 544–50.

145. Richens A, Mawer G, Crawford P, Harrison B. A placebo-controlled, double-blind cross-over trial of adjunctive one month remacemide hydrochloride treatment in patients with refractory epilepsy. Seizure 2000; 9: 537–43.

146. Shoulson I, Greenamyre T, Kieburtz K, Schwid S, McDermott M, Kayson E, Chase T, Fahn S, Lang A, Penney J. A multicenter randomized controlled trial of remacemide hydrochloride as monotherapy for PD. Neurology 2000; 54: 1583–8.

147. Chiron C, Marchand MC, Tran A, Rey E, D'Athis P, Vincent J, Dulac O, Pons G, and the STICLO Study Group. Stiripentol in severe myoclonic epilepsy in infancy: a randomised placebo-controlled syndrome-dedicated trial. Lancet 2000; 356: 1638–42.

148. Rating D, Wolf C, Bast T. Sulthiame as monotherapy in children with benign childhood epilepsy with centrotemporal spikes: a 6-month randomized, double-blind, placebo-controlled study. Epilepsia 2000; 41: 1284–8.

149. Fakhoury T, Uthman B, Abou-Khalil B. Safety of long-term treatment with tiagabine. Seizure 2000; 9: 431–5.

150. Freitag FG, Diamond S, Diamond ML, Urban GJ, Pepper BJ. An open use trial of tiagabine in migraine. Headache Q 2000; 11: 133–4.

151. Uldall P, Bulteau C, Pedersen SA, Dulac O, Lyby K. Tiagabine adjunctive therapy in children with refractory epilepsy: a single-blind dose escalating study. Epilepsy Res 2000; 42: 159–68.

152. Piccinelli P, Borgatti R, Perucca E, Tofani A, Donati G, Balottin U. Frontal nonconvulsive status epilepticus associated with high-dose tiagabine therapy in a child with familial bilateral perisylvian polymicrogyria. Epilepsia 2000; 41: 1485–8.

153. Balslev T, Uldall P, Buchholt J. Provocation of non-convulsive status epilepticus by tiagabine in three adolescent patients. Eur J Paediatr Neurol 2000; 4: 169–70.

154. Nousiainen I, Mantyjarvi M, Kalviainen R. Visual function in patients treated with the GABAergic anticonvulsant drug tiagabine. Clin Drug Invest 2000; 20: 393–400.

155. Abou-Khalil B and the Topiramate YOL Study Group. Topiramate in the long-term management of refractory epilepsy. Epilepsia 2000; 41 Suppl: S72–6.

156. Galvez-Jimenez N, Hargreave M. Topiramate and essential tremor. Ann Neurol 2000; 47: 837–8.

157. McElroy SL, Suppes T, Keck PE Jr, Frye MA, Denicoff KD, Altshuler LL, Brown ES, Nolen WA, Kupka RW, Rochussen J, Leverich GS, Post RM. Open-label adjunctive topiramate in the treatment of bipolar disorders. Biol Psychiatry 2000; 47: 1025–33.

158. Mohamed K, Appleton R, Rosenbloom L. Efficacy and tolerability of topiramate in childhood and adolescent epilepsy: a clinical experience. Seizure 2000; 9: 137–41.

159. Nieto-Barrera M, Candau R, Nieto-Jimenez M, Correa A, Ruiz del Portal L. Topiramate in the treatment of severe myoclonic epilepsy in infancy. Seizure 2000; 9: 590–4.

160. Reife R, Pledger G, Wu S-C. Topiramate as add-on therapy: pooled analysis of randomized controlled trials in adults. Epilepsia 2000; 41 Suppl: S66–71.

161. Shapira NA, Goldsmith TD, McElroy SL. Treatment of binge-eating disorder with topiramate: a clinical case series. J Clin Psychiatry 2000; 61: 368–72.

162. Stephen LJ, Sills GJ, Brodie MJ. Topiramate in refractory epilepsy: a prospective observational study. Epilepsia 2000; 41: 977–80.

163. Yeung S, Ferrie CD, Murdoch-Eaton DG, Livingston JH. Topiramate for drug-resistant epilep-

sies. Eur J Paediatr Neurol 2000; 4: 31–3.
164. Ritter F, Glauser TA, Elterman RD, Wyllie E, and the Topiramate YP Study Group. Effectiveness, tolerability, and safety of topiramate in children with partial-onset seizures. Epilepsia 2000; 41 Suppl: S82–5.
165. Yen D-J, Yu H-Y, Guo Y-C, Chen C, Yiu C-H, Su M-S. A double-blind, placebo-controlled study of topiramate in adult patients with refractory partial epilepsy. Epilepsia 2000; 41: 1162–6.
166. Laskey AL, Korn DE, Moorjani BI, Patel NC, Tobias JD. Central hyperventilation related to administration of topiramate. Pediatr Neurol 2000; 22: 305–8.
167. Glauser TA, Levisohn PM, Ritter F, Sachdeo RC, and the Topiramate YL Study Group. Topiramate in Lennox–Gastaut syndrome: open-label treatment of patients completing a randomized controlled trial. Epilepsia 2000; 41 Suppl: S86–90.
168. Gerber PE, Hamiwka L, Connolly MB, Farrell K. Factors associated with behavioral and cognitive abnormalities in children receiving topiramate. Pediatr Neurol 2000; 22: 200–23.
169. Franz DN, Glauser TA, Tudor C, Williams S. Topiramate therapy of epilepsy associated with Angelman's syndrome. Neurology 2000; 54: 1185–8.
170. Thompson PJ, Baxendale SA, Duncan JS, Sander JWAS. Effects of topiramate on cognitive function. J Neurol Neurosurg Psychiatry 2000; 69: 636–41.
171. Aldenkamp AP, Baker G, Mulder OG, Chadwick D, Cooper P, Doelman J, Duncan R, Gassmann-Mayer C, De Haan GJ, Hughson C, Hulsman J, Overweg J, Pledger G, Rentmeester TW, Riaz H, Wroe S. A multicenter, randomized clinical study to evaluate the effect on cognitive function of topiramate compared with valproate as add-on therapy to carbamazepine in patients with partial-onset seizures. Epilepsia 2000; 41: 1167–78.
172. Stowe CD, Bolliger T, James LE, Haley TM, Griebel ML, Fartar III HC. Acute mental status changes and hyperchloremic metabolic acidosis with long-term topiramate therapy. Pharmacotherapy 2000; 20 I: 105–9.
173. Teter CJ, Early JJ, Gibbs CM. Treatment of affective disorder and obesity with topiramate. Ann Pharmacother 2000; 34: 1262–5.
174. Garnett WR. Clinical pharmacology of topiramate: a review. Epilepsia 2000; 41 Suppl: S61–5.
175. Lennkh C, Simhandl C. Current aspects of valproate in bipolar disorder. Int Clin Psychopharmacol 2000; 15: 1–11.
176. Davis LL, Ryan W, Adinoff B, Petty F. Comprehensive review of the psychiatric uses of valproate. J Clin Psychopharmacol 2000; 20/1 Suppl: 1S–17S.
177. Sleiman C, Raffy O, Roue C, Mal H. Fatal pulmonary hemorrhage during high-dose valproate monotherapy. Chest 2000; 117: 613.
178. Shill HA, Fife TD. Valproic acid toxicity mimicking multiple system atrophy. Neurology 2000; 55: 1936–7.
179. Ronen GM, Richards JE, Cunningham C, Secord M, Rosenbloom D Can sodium valproate improve learning in children with epileptiform bursts but without clinical seizures? Dev Med Child Neurol 2000; 42: 751–5.
180. Kifune A, Kubota F, Shibata N, Akata T, Kikuchi S. Valproic acid-induced hyperammonemic encephalopathy with triphasic waves. Epilepsia 2000; 41: 909–12.
181. Hamer HM, Knake S, Schomburg U, Rosenow F. Valproate-induced hyperammonemic encephalopathy in the presence of topiramate. Neurology 2000; 54: 230–2.
182. Haviv YS, Kuper A. Severe peripheral oedema associated with valproic acid. Clin Drug Invest 2000; 19: 385–7.
183. Gruppo R, DeGrauw A, Fogelson H, Glauser T, Balasa V, Gartside P. Protein C deficiency related to valproic acid therapy: a possible association with childhood stroke. J Pediatr 2000; 137: 714–18.
184. Levine J, Chengappa KNR, Parepally H. Side effect profile of enteric-coated divalproex sodium versus valproic acid. J Clin Psychiatry 2000; 61: 680–1.
185. Proulle V, Masnou P, Cartron J, Kaplan C, Ajzenberg N, Tchernia G, Dreyfus M. GPIaIIa as a candidate target for anti-platelet autoantibody occurring during valproate therapy and associated with peroperative bleeding. Thromb Haemost 2000; 83: 175–6.
186. Oluboka OJ, Haslam D, Gardner DM. Pancytopenia and valproic acid: a dose-related association. J Am Geriatr Soc 2000; 48: 349–50.
187. Wagner PG, Welton SR, Hammond CM. Gastrointestinal adverse effects with divalproex sodium and valproic acid. J Clin Psychiatry 2000; 61: 302–3.
188. Fayad M, Choueiri R, Mikati M. Fatality from hepatitis a in a child taking valproate. J Child Neurol 2000; 15: 135–6.
189. Gopaul SV, Farrell K, Abbott FS. Identification and characterization of N-acetylcysteine conjugates of valproic acid in humans and animals. Drug Metab Dispos 2000; 28: 823–32.
190. Thomson MA, Lynch S, Strong R, Shepherd RW, Marsh W. Orthotopic liver transplantation with poor neurologic outcome in valproate-associated liver failure: a need for critical risk-benefit appraisal in the use of valproate. Transplant Proc 2000; 32: 200–3.
191. Delarue A, Paut O, Guys J-M, Montfort M-F, Lethel V, Roquelaire B, Pellissier J-F, Sarles J, Camboulives J. Inappropriate liver transplantation in a child with Alpers–Huttenlocher syndrome misdiagnosed as valproate-induced liver failure. Pediatr Transplant 2000; 4: 67–71.
192. Isojärvi JIT, Tapanainen JS. Valproate, hyperandrogenism, and polycystic ovaries. A report of 3 cases. Arch Neurol 2000; 57: 1064–8.
193. Reuber M, Goulding PJ, for the APOS-

Investigators. Valproate, polycystic ovary syndrome and the need for a prospective study. Seizure 2000; 9: 235–6.
194. Betts T. Editorial comment. Seizure 2000; 9: 236.
195. Zachariah SB, Zachariah A, Ananda R, Stewart JT. Hypothermia and thermoregulatory derangements induced by valproic acid. Neurology 2000; 55: 150–1.
196. Haroldson JA, Kramer LE, Wolff DL, Lake KD. Elevated free fractions of valproic acid in a heart transplant patient with hypoalbuminemia. Ann Pharmacother 2000; 34: 183–7.
197. Rodriguez-Pinilla E, Arroyo I, Fondevilla J, Garcia MJ, Martinez-Frias ML. Prenatal exposure to valproic acid during pregnancy and limb deficiencies: a case-control study. Am J Med Genet 2000; 90: 376–81.
198. Norton JW, Quarles E. Intravenous valproate in neuropsychiatry. Pharmacotherapy 2000; 20 I: 88–92.
199. Limdi NA, Faught E. The safety of rapid valproic acid infusion. Epilepsia 2000; 41: 1342–5.
200. Kane SL, Constantiner M, Staubus AE, Meinecke CD, Sedor JR. High-flux hemodialysis without hemoperfusion is effective in acute valproic acid overdose. Ann Pharmacother 2000; 34: 1146–51.
201. Spina E, Avenoso A, Facciola G, Salemi M, Scordo MG, Giacobello T, Madia AG, Perucca E. Plasma concentrations of risperidone and 9-hydroxyrisperidone: effect of comedication with carbamazepine or valproate. Ther Drug Monit 2000; 22: 481–5.
202. Guberman A, Bruni J. Long-term open multicentre, add-on trial of vigabatrin in adult resistant partial epilepsy. Seizure 2000; 9: 112–18.
203. Haas-Lude K, Wolff M, Riethmuller J, Niemann G, Krageloh-Mann I. Acute encephalopathy associated with vigabatrin in a six-month-old girl. Epilepsia 2000; 41: 628–30.
204. Wilton LV, Stephens MOB, Mann RD. Visual field defect associated with vigabatrin: observational cohort study. Br Med J 1999; 319: 1165–6.
205. Comaish IF, Gorman C, Galloway NR. Visual field defect associated with vigabatrin. Br Med J 2000; 320: 1403.
206. Manuchehri K. Visual field defect associated with vigabatrin. Br Med J 2000; 320: 1403–4.
207. Midelfart A. Visual field defect associated with vigabatrin. Br Med J 2000; 320: 1403–4.
208. Midelfart A, Midelfart E, Brodtkorb E. Visual field defects in patients taking vigabatrin. Acta Ophthalmol Scand 2000; 78: 580–4.
209. Riikonen RS. Steroids or vigabatrin in the treatment of infantile spasms? Pediatr Neurol 2000; 23: 403–8.
210. Lindberger M, Alenius M, Frisen L, Johannessen SI, Larsson S, Malmgren K, Tomson T. Gabapentin versus vigabatrin as first add-on for patients with partial seizures that failed to respond to monotherapy: a randomized, double-blind, dose titration study. Epilepsia 2000; 41: 1289–95.
211. Manuchehri I, Goodman S, Siviter L, Nightingale S. A controlled study of vigabatrin and visual abnormalities. Br J Ophthalmol 2000; 84: 499–505.
212. Harding GFA, Wild JM, Robertson KA, Lawden MC, Betts TA, Barber C, Barnes PMF. Electro-oculography, electroretinography, visual evoked potentials, and multifocal electroretinography in patients with vigabatrin-attributed visual field constriction. Epilepsia 2000; 41: 1420–31.
213. Gross-Tsur V, Banin E, Shahar E, Shalev RS, Lahat E. Visual impairment in children with epilepsy treated with vigabatrin. Ann Neurol 2000; 48: 60–4.
214. Harding GFA, Wild JM, Robertson KA, Rietbrock S, Martinez C. Separating the retinal electrophysiologic effects of vigabatrin: treatment versus field loss. Neurology 2000; 55: 347–52.
215. Hardus P, Verduin WM, Postma G, Stilma JS, Berendschot TTJM, Van Veelen CWM. Contraction of the visual field in patients with temporal lobe epilepsy and its association with the use of vigabatrin medication. Epilepsia 2000; 41: 581–7.
216. Hardus P, Verduin WM, Postma G, Stilma JS, Berendschot TTJM, Van Veelen CWM. Long term changes in the visual fields of patients with temporal lobe epilepsy using vigabatrin. Br J Ophthalmol 2000; 84: 788–90.
217. Johnson MA, Krauss GL, Miller NR, Medura M, Paul SR. Visual function loss from vigabatrin: effect of stopping the drug. Neurology 2000; 55: 40–5.
218. Krakow K, Polizzi G, Riordan-Eva P, Holder G, Macleod WN, Fish DR. Recovery of visual field constriction following discontinuation of vigabatrin. Seizure 2000; 9: 287–90.
219. Iannetti P, Spalice A, Perla FM, Conicella E, Raucci U, Bizzarri B. Visual field constriction in children with epilepsy on vigabatrin treatment. Pediatrics 2000; 106 I: 838–42.
220. Mesa Aguado FL, Lopez Leyva C, Gonzalez Moles MA, Del Moral RG, O'Valle Ravassa FJ. Clinical and histopathological description of a new case of vigabatrin-induced gingival overgrowth. Med Oral 2000; 5: 133–7.
221. Mouton P, Defer G-L. Troubles comportmentaux par intoxication aiguë au vigabatrin. Rev Neurol 2000; 156: 184–6.
222. Jedrzejczak J, Dlawichowska E, Owczarek K, Majkowski J. Effect of vigabatrin addition on carbamazepine blood serum levels in patients with epilepsy. Epilepsy Res 2000; 39: 115–20.
223. Miyamoto T, Kohsaka M, Koyama T. Psychotic episodes during zonisamide treatment. Seizure 2000; 9: 65–70.
224. Murai T, Kubota Y, Sengoku A. Unknown people believed to be known: the "assoziierende Erinnerungsfälschungen" by Kraepelin. Psychopathology 2000; 33: 52–4.
225. Imai K, Mario T, Shimono K, Ueda H, Okinaga T, Yanagihara K, Li Z, Okada S. Three cases of hypoactivity and poor appetite with zonisamide-

induced metabolic acidosis. No To Hattatsu 2000; 32: 75–7.
226. Masuda Y, Karasawa T. Inhibitory effect of zonisamide in human carbonic anhydrase in vitro. Arzneimittelforschung 1993; 43: 416–18.
227. Inoue T, Kira R, Kaku Y, Ikeda K, Gondo K, Hara T. Renal tubular acidosis associated with zonisamide therapy. Epilepsia 2000; 41: 1642–4.
228. Kubota M, Nishi-Nagase M, Sakakihara Y, Noma S, Nakamoto M, Kawaguchi H, Yanagisawa M. Zonisamide-induced urinary lithiasis in patients with intractable epilepsy. Brain Dev 2000; 22: 230–3.
229. Matsuoka Y, Nakai N, Tada M, Nishigaki T, Onoe S. A case of hidropoietic disorder caused by zonisamide, antiepileptic drug. Skin Res 2000; 42: 58–62.
230. Okumura A, Ishihara N, Kato T, Hayakawa F, Kuno K, Watanabe K. Predictive value of acetylcholine stimulation testing for oligohidrosis caused by zonisamide. Pediatr Neurol 2000; 23: 59–61.

A.H. Ghodse and A.M. Baldacchino

8 Opioid analgesics and narcotic antagonists

OPIOID AGONISTS

Alfentanil *(SED-14, 211; SEDA-22, 97; SEDA-23, 98; SEDA-24, 104)*

Respiratory The severity of *respiratory depression* with alfentanil has been assessed in 49 patients undergoing abdominal hysterectomy under general anesthetic, who were randomly allocated to three groups (1^c). Group 1 did not receive alfentanil during surgery, group 2 received alfentanil 30 μg/kg, and group 3 received a bolus dose of alfentanil 10–20 μg/kg and an increasing alfentanil infusion by increments of 0.25–0.5 mg/kg/min. In this randomized double-blind study alfentanil had respiratory depressant effects (measured by plethysmography and pulse oximetry). In one patient in group 1 and three each in groups 2 and 3), but there were no cases of clear-cut recurrent respiratory depression.

Fetotoxicity Alfentanil 10 μg/kg in normal parturients does not reduce Apgar scores, but a higher dose (15–30 μg/kg) is recommended for attenuation of the "stress" response in non-pregnant patients. In a randomized, placebo-controlled, double-blind study alfentanil was used in 40 patients in a dose of 10 μg/kg 1 minute before induction of anesthesia in 40 uncomplicated cesarean deliveries to determine whether it would reduce the maternal stress response after tracheal intubation without subsequent neonatal depression (2^c). There was a small but significant improvement in maternal hemodynamic stability in the alfentanil group at the expense of early but transient *neonatal depression*.

Side Effects of Drugs, Annual 25
J.K. Aronson, ed.

Codeine *(SED-14, 212; SEDA 22, 98)*

Pancreas Four cases of acute pancreatitis related to codeine have been reported (3^A).

A 65-year-old man presented with severe abdominal pain 90 minutes after ingesting codeine and low-dose paracetamol. Serum amylase and lipase were significantly raised. Liver function tests were moderately abnormal. Abdominal ultrasound and CT scan showed edematous pancreatitis. Endoscopic retrograde cholangiography showed a papilla with a spastic appearance and an abnormal bile duct. The patient recovered completely. Three months later, he took codeine and paracetamol after a hemorrhoidectomy; abdominal pain recurred 1 hour later and acute pancreatitis was confirmed.

A 26-year-old woman developed abdominal pain 2 days after taking codeine for a respiratory tract infection. Three hours later, she complained of epigastric pain and vomiting. Her serum amylase and lipase were raised. Her symptoms resolved and the diagnosis was mild idiopathic pancreatitis. One week later she took codeine for similar respiratory symptoms. Two hours later she developed similar symptoms, and CT scan showed an enlarged and heterogeneous pancreas, with necrosis of the tail of the pancreas involving the left kidney. She responded to conservative treatment.

A 53-year-old woman developed severe central abdominal and epigastric pain 90 minutes after taking codeine for migraine. Pancreatic amylase, lipase, and liver function tests were mildly raised. Abdominal ultrasound was consistent with acute pancreatitis.

A 57-year-old woman developed severe abdominal pain 2 hours after taking codeine. She had had two similar episodes in the past, once with loperamide and once with codeine. Abdominal CT scan showed an edematous acute pancreatitis.

In three cases, unintentional rechallenge with codeine resulted in recurrence of the symptoms, and the diagnosis was confirmed radiologically and biochemically. All the patients had previously had a cholecystectomy, suggesting that this may increase the likelihood of codeine-induced pancreatitis. The authors speculated that codeine could cause a rise in biliary and/or pancreatic sphincter pressure in cholecystectomized patients, either by exacerbating preexisting disease of the sphincter of Oddi or as a consequence of reduced storage capacity of the biliary tract, initiating acute pancreatitis. They cautioned that codeine-associated acute pancreatitis can be misconstrued – it may seem as if patients are taking codeine for pancreatic pain when in fact the codeine is producing the pain.

Skin Two reports have highlighted the importance of using an oral provocation test and not a patch test to determine if codeine is the causative agent in non-urticarial skin lesions (4[A], 5[A]).

A 58-year-old man developed a pruritic rash on the body and face, with periorbital swelling 3 hours after taking codeine 20 mg, acetylcysteine 600 mg, and acetylsalicylic acid 500 mg. An oral provocation test over 2 hours with codeine phosphate (1 mg, 4 mg, and 8 mg) precipitated a pruritic scarlatiniform rash for 24 hours, with swelling of the arms, starting 7 hours after the 8 mg dose. A rechallenge test confirmed the effect of codeine. Throughout this period histamine release tests (CAST-ELISA with codeine) were negative.

A 57-year-old patient presented with generalized malaise, fever, pruritus, and palpebral and labial angio-edema 6 hours after taking a tablet containing paracetamol 500 mg, saccharin 10 mg, and codeine phosphate 30 mg. There was complete resolution in 8 hours, after treatment with prednisolone, hydroxyzine, and metamizole. Later a patch test with 1% codeine and an oral provocation test with paracetamol were both negative. Following an oral provocation test with codeine 5 mg, the patient developed similar symptoms.

Dextromethorphan *(SED-14, 212; SEDA-22, 98; SEDA-23, 99; SEDA-24, 104)*

Dextromethorphan is the dextrorotatory isomer of the synthetic opioid levorphanol and is thought to act as a central nervous system antitussive (6[C]). It binds to CNS sigma opioid binding sites and increases 5-HT concentrations by inhibiting uptake and by enhancing the release of 5-HT, as well as antagonizing NMDA receptors.

The role of dextromethorphan in acute and chronic pain control has been reviewed (7[R]). There is a clear beneficial role of oral dextromethorphan (in doses of 30–90 mg) in acute pain management; it has no or few adverse effects and even reduces the need for analgesic adjuncts. However, the results of the few double-blind studies of dextromethorphan in chronic and neuropathic pain have shown it to be associated with unsatisfactory analgesia.

In a randomized, placebo-controlled study in 60 patients given dextromethorphan 10, 20, or 40 mg intramuscularly before abdominal surgery there was a dose-dependent effective postoperative analgesic effect, with lower total consumption of rescue morphine during the 3-day observation period (8[c]). There were no opioid-related adverse effects in those who were given dextromethorphan 40 mg.

Psychiatric Another case of dextromethorphan-induced psychosis has been reported (9[A]).

An 18-year-old student had dissociative phenomenon, nihilistic and paranoid delusions, vivid visual hallucinations, thought insertion, and broadcasting after having consumed 1–2 bottles of cough syrup (dextromethorphan 711 mg per bottle) every day for several days. The psychotic symptoms completely remitted without any treatment 4 days after withdrawal of dextromethorphan. He was hospitalized twice more over the next 2 months with similar symptoms; each time he had consumed large doses of dextromethorphan.

Endocrine During a double-blind placebo-controlled study of the effect of high-doses dextromethorphan in children with bacterial meningitis, two of four patients developed type 1 *diabetes mellitus*; they had received dextromethorphan and the other two placebo (10[A]).

A 10-year-old boy received dextromethorphan 36 mg/kg/day by nasogastric tube. He developed hyperglycemia with ketoacidosis after 5 days and required insulin. The dose of dextromethorphan was reduced over the next 4 days and withdrawn. Insulin was withdrawn 4 days later.

A 14-year-old girl received dextromethorphan 26 mg/kg/day by nasogastric tube. She developed hyperglycemia after 2 days and needed insulin for 6 days. A later glucose tolerance test was normal.

Pancreatic β cells in rats express NMDA receptors, stimulation of which leads to insulin secretion (11[c]). The authors postulated that dextromethorphan inhibits insulin secretion by blocking NMDA receptors and thus impairs glucose tolerance. Both patients had reduced insulin concentrations, implying that peripheral insulin resistance was unlikely to have been the cause of diabetes.

Drug interactions Dextromethorphan is metabolized by CYP2D6 to dextrorphan, which binds to phencyclidine receptors and is thought to account for the adverse effects of hallucinations, ataxia, and nystagmus. Individuals who are slow metabolizers or take long-acting dextromethorphan formulations, and those taking *5-HT re-uptake inhibitors* or *monoamine oxidase inhibitors* are at increased risk of serotonergic adverse effects, as well as the narcotic adverse effects of coma and respiratory depression.

In a randomized, double-blind, placebo-controlled, cross-over study, seven healthy volunteers who took *quinidine* (50 mg quinidine sulfate orally) or a placebo followed by either dextromethorphan 50 mg or a placebo were assessed for changes in pharmacodynamics and antinociceptive and neuromodulatory effects (12[c]). Quinidine inhibited CYP2D6, reducing the conversion of dextromethorphan to dextrorphan in rapid metabolizers to the rate seen in poor metabolizers. The accumulation of dextromethorphan caused by quinidine increased subjective and objective pain thresholds by 35 and 45% respectively. This study suggests that debrisoquine/sparteine-type polymorphisms account for important differences in the effect of dextromethorphan and the balance between the analgesic effect of dextromethorphan and the hallucinogenic effect of dextrorphan. Concomitant use of quinidine or other inhibitors of CYP2D6 could further affect this balance, increasing the risk of serotonergic and narcotic-related adverse effects.

Morphi Dex® contains morphine sulfate and dextromethorphan in a 1:1 ratio. Double-blind, single-dose analgesic efficacy studies in over 800 patients with postsurgical pain have shown superior analgesic activity for the combination (60:60 mg) than separate doses of the individual components (13[R], 14[C]). In double-blind, multiple-dose studies in 321 patients with chronic pain the combination provided satisfactory pain control with a significantly lower mean daily dose of morphine sulfate. Other studies have shown similar responses (13[R]) and an adverse events profile similar to that of a similar dose of morphine sulfate (15[C]). The most common adverse events seen in a multiple-dose, non-placebo-controlled study of 1400 subjects were *nausea*, *dizziness*, *vomiting*, *somnolence*, *confusion*, and *pruritus*. There was a significant trend towards lower incidence of constipation with the combination than with morphine sulfate alone (16[C], 17[C]).

Dextropropoxyphene *(SED-14, 212; SEDA-23, 99; SEDA-24, 104)*

Skin *Acute generalized pustulosis* attributed to dextropropoxyphene has been reported for the first time (18[A]).

A 43-year-old woman, who had taken antibiotics and analgesics, including dextropropoxyphene, for parotitis, developed, generalized erythema with numerous pustules on the trunk followed by a pyrexia. Patch testing was positive with dextropropoxyphene only and negative with paracetamol, spiramycin, aspirin, and tenoxicam.

Diamorphine (heroin) *(SED-14, 214; SEDA-21, 87; SEDA-24, 105)*

In a randomized, placebo-controlled, double-blind study of the relative efficacies of patient-controlled analgesia (PCA) regimens (19[C]) 60 patients undergoing elective total hip or knee replacement were randomly allocated to receive epidural diamorphine 2.5 mg followed by a PCA bolus 1 mg with a 20-minute lockout (group 1), subcutaneous diamorphine 2.5 mg followed by a PCA bolus 1 mg with a 10-minute lockout (group 2), or epidural diamorphine 2.5 mg in 4 ml of 0.125% bupivacaine followed by a PCA bolus of 1 mg diamorphine in 4 ml 0.125% bupivacaine with a 20-minute lockout (group 3). Diamorphine demands were significantly higher in group 2 in the first postoperative 24-hour period, but pain scores were only significantly higher in group 2 in the first 3 hours postoperatively compared with group 3 and group 1. There were also fewer opioid-related adverse effects in group 2, and group 3 reported higher incidences of various adverse effects. The conclusion was that PCA diamorphine given with or without bupivacaine provides analgesia of similar efficacy once adequate pain relief has been achieved. Taking the incidences of adverse effect profiles into account, diamorphine subcutaneous PCA was a simple and effective method of providing analgesia.

In another randomized double-blind study, 14 patients, undergoing elective surgery for correction of bilateral arthritic deformities of the feet received 15 ml of 0.9% saline containing diamorphine 2.5 mg into the cannula in one foot and 15 ml of saline into the other foot (20[C]). Intravenous regional diamorphine did not improve postoperative pain relief or secondary hyperalgesia. There were no significant adverse effects.

Nervous system Focal myopathy has been reported after intramuscular diamorphine (21[A]).

A 36-year-old man developed progressive stiffness of both knees and a broad-based stiff gait over 3 months. Electromyography of the right quadriceps muscles showed firm fibrous resistance and a muscle biopsy showed scattered collections of atrophic fibers and prominent endomysial fibrosis. This was confirmed by MRI scanning of the thigh, suggesting focal myopathy with prominent muscle fibrosis and inflammatory changes. There was clinical improvement within 2 weeks of starting prednisolone and D-penicillamine. However, it is also possible that even without treatment the course would have been unchanged.

Fentanyl *(SED-14, 213; SEDA-22, 98; SEDA-23, 100; SEDA-24, 105)*

Effective postoperative pain relief can be obtained with a mixture of fentanyl and bupivacaine, which not only provides better analgesia than either drug alone, but fewer adverse effects. There have been several studies of the efficacy of this mixture, using different doses and routes of administration, the addition of clonidine, and in comparison with morphine.

In a randomized, double-blind study in 56 patients continuous infusion of fentanyl (1 or 0.5 μg/kg/hour) and bupivacaine 0.1 mg/kg/hour, with intravenous morphine patient-controlled analgesia (PCA) as rescue analgesia, produced better pain relief after knee ligament operations than epidural saline combined with intravenous morphine PCA (22[c]). There was a non-significant increase in *nausea* in the fentanyl group.

In another randomized double-blind study 84 parturients requesting epidural analgesia were given either bupivacaine 20 ml only followed by intravenous fentanyl 60 μg or bupivacaine 20 ml with fentanyl 60 μg followed by intravenous saline (23[C]). The minimum local analgesia concentration (MLAC) of bupivacaine + intravenous fentanyl was 0.064% w/v and the MLAC of bupivacaine + epidural fentanyl was 0.034% w/v. The epidural fentanyl solution significantly increased the analgesic potency of bupivacaine by a factor of 1.88 compared with intravenous fentanyl. This was associated with increased *pruritus* with epidural fentanyl.

Women scheduled for cesarean section (n = 32) were given spinal bupivacaine 10 mg (0.5%) or spinal bupivacaine 5 mg (0.5%) plus fentanyl 25 μg (24[c]). Those given fentanyl had adequate spinal anesthesia for cesarean section with fewer adverse effects (nausea and hypotension). This observation was reproduced by spinal anesthesia with bupivacaine 4 mg plus fentanyl 20 μg, which provided adequate spinal anesthesia for surgical repair of hip fracture in elderly patients, with fewer adverse effects than bupivacaine 10 mg (25[c]).

In a randomized, placebo-controlled study a mixture of ropivacaine 0.2% and fentanyl 2 μg/ml plus a background infusion of 5 ml/hour was given to 20 patients for postoperative patient-controlled epidural analgesia after gynecological surgery. Another 21 patients were given the same mixture without the background infusion. Both groups were monitored hourly for arterial blood pressure, heart rate, and respiratory rate, and pain, sedation, motor blockade, and sensory levels were monitored every 6 hours (26[c]). There was no difference in pain scores or patient satisfaction scores between the two groups, but the patients who received the background infusion had a higher incidence of adverse effects (71% vs 30%). The authors suggested that there was no additional benefit in using a background infusion.

The addition of droperidol 2.5 mg to fentanyl 0.4 mg in 40 ml of 0.125% bupivacaine lowered the incidence of postoperative *nausea and vomiting* compared with a solution without droperidol or with butorphanol added instead, in patients undergoing anorectal surgery in a prospective randomized single-blind study (27[c]).

There was no difference in analgesic efficacy or the incidence of adverse effects when fentanyl 100 μg was compared with sufentanil 20 μg in women in labor who requested epidural analgesia (28[c]).

Cardiovascular Fentanyl plus droperidol (neuroleptanalgesia) was more effective than morphine in relieving anginal pain during unstable angina. However the patients who received the neuroleptanalgesia also had longer hospital stays, because of significantly more *cardiac instability* and *anginal episodes*, and a higher total mortality (29[c]).

Nervous system A 55-year-old man was given fentanyl 0.05 mg for treatment of left chest pain and immediately developed an *acute confusional state and fluctuating tetraparesis* (30[A]). The symptoms abated 12 hours after withdrawal. A provocation test confirmed that fentanyl 0.1 mg was enough to cause myoclonic and dystonic reactions with increased agitation. Administration of intravenous naloxone 0.8 mg improved the condition.

A 14-year-old girl developed a *dystonic reaction* to fentanyl 50 μg given as a general anesthesia for dental extraction; her abnormal movements stopped completely after 3 days (31[A]).

Neuromuscular function There have been three reports and a prospective study of *muscle rigidity* after fentanyl administration in neonates (32[A], 33[A]).

Two neonates had transient (0.5–2 minutes) chest wall rigidity after intravenous boluses of fentanyl 2 and 4 μg/kg. They were already compromised, one with a respiratory distress syndrome and one with a diaphragmatic hernia. The third case was a premature male infant of 28 weeks gestation. An intravenous bolus of fentanyl 3 μg/kg was given before intubation and was followed by isolated rigidity of the tongue lasting 20 seconds (32[A]).

In a prospective case series study of 89 preterm and term infants who received fentanyl out of a total of 404 neonatal intensive care patients in 1 year, eight neonates (9%) had chest wall rigidity (33[A]). The spectrum of neuromuscular activity extends from mild muscle rigidity through abnormal muscle movements (chewing) to tonic–clonic movements. In two cases there was laryngospasm with chest wall rigidity. In all cases low-dose fentanyl (3–6 μg/kg) had been given for analgesia or sedation.

Drug administration route Opioids have traditionally been given intramuscularly and intravenously. Other methods of administration are oral, subcutaneous, rectal, intrathecal, and extradural. Novel routes include intranasal, inhalational, intra-articular, and transdermal. A good review of the last of these (34[R]) has considered the possibilities and techniques available for acute and/or chronic pain relief.

Transdermal administration of fentanyl has been extensively reviewed (35[R]). Fentanyl is a good choice for transdermal application, owing to its low molecular weight, adequate solubility in oil and water, high analgesic potency, and fewer adverse effects, especially gastrointestinal symptoms. In systemic availability studies, 92% of the fentanyl dose delivered from the TTS into the skin reached the systemic circulation as unchanged unmetabolized fentanyl (36[c]). Morphine, codeine, and hydromorphone are not good candidates for transdermal administration. Pethidine has a high transdermal permeability but poor analgesic potency. Besides fentanyl, only sufentanil and buprenorphine would be suitable transdermal opioid products (37[c]).

There are three techniques used for the transdermal administration of fentanyl. The transdermal therapeutic system (TTS) is a membrane-controlled system designed to release fentanyl at a constant rate for up to 3 days, and is useful in patients with chronic cancer pain (38[c]). There are still limited and predominantly uncontrolled studies that show that TTS fentanyl is useful in chronic pain of neuropathic or somatic origin. The latest open randomized cross-over trial in 18 patients with painful chronic pancreatitis concluded that TTS fentanyl should not be the first-choice analgesic, because of a high incidence of skin adverse effects and low analgesic effects compared with morphine (39[c]).

TTS fentanyl is not useful in acute or postoperative pain, because of the risk of respiratory depression due to the long delay and decay time, which do not allow adequate dose finding (35[R]). Some patients have acute symptoms of morphine withdrawal, in spite of adequate pain control, when they are converted from morphine to transdermal fentanyl. The mechanism has not yet been determined (40[A], 41[A]).

Transdermal fentanyl was the cause of an opioid overdose when a 77-year-old man with a history of severe arthritis developed respiratory failure after starting epidural diamorphine–bupivacaine mixture for postoperative pain (42[A]). The fentanyl patch was removed, the epidural infusion was stopped, and naloxone was given to counteract the excessive opioid effects.

Fentanyl transdermal delivery systems (FTDS) use an unsealed multilaminate system containing a solid matrix, in which fentanyl is embedded instead of the reservoir designed in the TTS. FTDS is not to be recommended for routine postoperative pain treatment, even though it has a faster onset of action (4–6 hours) after cases of fentanyl toxicity, especially respiratory depression. FTDS has not been investigated adequately in chronic pain and is not expected to be superior to the TTS technique.

Iontophoretic transdermal application of opioids is another technique that is currently being tested. The factors that affect the delivery of opioids like fentanyl and sufentanil by this technique include the physicochemical nature of the drug solution, the voltage used, and the duration and nature of the current used (43[c], 44[c]).

An *electrotransport therapeutic system* (ETS) for fentanyl has been developed. Preliminary studies show that ETS of fentanyl may be useful for the treatment of acute pain (45[c]).

Drug overdose A 24-year-old woman with a history of polysubstance abuse and extensive psychiatric history, presented with acute opioid overdose caused by the intentional oral ingestion of a fentanyl patch (Duragesic) (46[A]).

Hydrocodone

Ear, nose, and throat In a retrospective review in a specialized otological center 12 patients were identified with rapidly progressive *hearing loss* and a concurrent history of hydrocodone overuse with paracetamol (47[c]). These patients were helped by cochlear implantation.

Methadone *(SED-14, 214; SEDA-21, 88; SEDA-23, 103; SEDA-24, 106)*

Methadone is being used increasingly for treating chronic pain and cancer pain (neuropathic and somatic) that is non-responsive or has lost responsiveness because of tolerance to high-dose μ opioid agonists (e.g. morphine, fentanyl, oxycodone) (48[R]). There are several protocols for converting from morphine to methadone and for initiating and stabilizing maintenance dosages.

In a randomized, double-blind, placebo-controlled trial of the efficacy of intravenous methylnaltrexone (0.015–0.095 mg/kg) in treating chronic methadone-induced *constipation* in 22 patients attending a methadone maintenance program (oral methadone linctus 30–100 mg/day), methylnaltrexone induced immediate bowel movements in all subjects (49[C]). There were no opioid withdrawal symptoms or significant adverse effects.

A risk-benefit analysis of methadone maintenance treatment for diamorphine dependence has shown lower mortality and morbidity with improvement in quality of life (50[C]). The risks of methadone treatment include an increased risk of opiate overdosage during induction into treatment and adverse effects of methadone in some patients. However, with careful management the benefits of prescribing methadone outweigh the risks.

The validity of self-reported opiate and cocaine use has been studied in 175 veterans enrolled in a methadone treatment program (51[C]). Urine analysis showed higher rates of substance use than the patients themselves reported. The authors encouraged the development of more objective measures for assessing patient progress and the performance of the methadone program.

There has been a cross-sectional survey of 238 patients in New South Wales who died during a methadone maintenance program in a 5-year period (52[C]). There were 50 *deaths* (21%) in the first week of methadone maintenance treatment, 88% of which were drug related. These findings reinforce the importance of a thorough drug and alcohol assessment of people seeking methadone maintenance treatment, cautious prescribing of methadone, frequent clinical review of patients, and tolerance to methadone during stabilization.

Morphine *(SED-14, 215; SEDA-22, 100; SEDA-23, 103; SEDA-24, 107)*

In a randomized double-blind study in 94 patients with acute renal colic, morphine had equal analgesic efficacy to pethidine and a similar adverse effects profile (53[C]).

Low-dose intrathecal morphine (0.3 mg) plus 0.5% spinal bupivacaine and patient-controlled intravenous morphine (given as a 1 mg bolus with a 5-minute lockout period) has been compared with patient-controlled intravenous morphine alone in 38 patients undergoing knee surgery in a randomized double-blind study (54[C]). The former combination provided effective analgesia with a low and non-significant incidence of *emesis*, *pruritus*, and *respiratory depression*.

In a dose-response study of the effects of epidural morphine after cesarean section the quality of analgesia increased with the dose of morphine to a ceiling dose of 3.75 mg (55[C]). Adverse effects were not dose related.

Perioperative administration of morphine is another way of enhancing its analgesic properties during the transition from total remifentanil-based anesthesia to the postoperative period, when adequate analgesia is sometimes difficult. In a randomized study in 245 patients undergoing abdominal or urological surgery the effect of perioperative morphine was evaluated (56[C]). Patients were given a bolus of 0.15 or 0.25 mg/kg 30 minutes before the end of surgery. The results suggested that intraoperative morphine administration did not preclude the need for more morphine in the immediate postoperative period. The 0.25 mg/kg dose was slightly more effective but caused more respiratory depression.

Nervous system Intravenous patient-controlled administration of morphine (total 56 mg in 9 hours) was associated with *downbeat nystagmus* in a 61-year-old man with a Grade 3 adenocarcinoma of the gastroesophageal junction and a previous small cerebellar infarct (57[A]). Withdrawal of the analgesia led to complete resolution of all signs and symptoms within 12 hours.

Biliary tract Morphine can cause *choledochal sphincter spasm*, especially if there is a previous history of cholecystectomy (58[A]).

A 60-year-old man received intramuscular morphine 10 mg with scopolamine 0.4 mg as premedication and 40 minutes later complained of sharp right upper quadrant pain radiating to the back. The symptoms were identical to the gall-bladder pain he had experienced in the past and for which he had had a cholecystectomy 25 years before. He had complete relief from intravenous naloxone 0.9 mg.

Management of adverse drug reactions The use of adjunctive pharmacological agents to reduce the incidence of morphine-induced *pruritus* has again been documented (59[C], 60[C]).

The effectiveness of intravenous *ondansetron* in preventing intrathecal morphine-induced pruritus has been investigated in a randomized, double-blind, placebo-controlled study in 60 consecutive women undergoing cesarean section (59[C]). All were given spinal anesthesia with bupivacaine and intrathecal morphine 0.15 mg and then randomly divided into three groups. Group 1 received intravenous saline injections as placebo, group 2 received diphenhydramine 30 mg intravenously, and group 3 received ondansetron 0.1 mg/kg intravenously. Group 3 had a significantly lower incidence of pruritus (25%) than both group 1 (85%) and group 2 (80%), with no difference in postoperative pain scores between the groups.

In another randomized double-blind study, 140 patients undergoing cesarean section had anesthesia with epidural bupivacaine 100 mg and adrenaline to which was added morphine 2 mg and *droperidol* 0, 1.25, 2.5, or 5.0 mg (60[C]). Previous evidence had suggested that intravenous droperidol reduces morphine-induced pruritus, but that the effect disappeared when the dose was increased from 2.5 to 5.0 mg (61[C]). However, in this study, epidural droperidol caused a dose-dependent reduction in morphine-induced pruritus even at a dose of 5 mg.

Intravenous droperidol 1.25 mg and intravenous dexamethasone 8 mg, given at the end of cesarean section, have been compared in reducing the incidence of nausea and vomiting caused by epidural morphine 3 mg in 120 women in a randomized, double-blind, placebo-controlled study (62[C]). The incidence of nausea and vomiting was 18% with dexamethasone, 21% with droperidol, and 51% with saline. About 11–13% of the women who were given dexamethasone or droperidol required rescue antiemetic therapy compared with 41% in the saline group. The incidence of pruritus was similar among the three groups (26–42%). Six women (16%) given droperidol reported restlessness compared with none in the other two groups.

Oxycodone *(SED-14, 216; SEDA-23, 104; SEDA-24, 107)*

Oxycodone is 1.5 times as potent as morphine and has a longer duration of action.

The postoperative analgesic effects of intravenous ketamine 10 mg and oxycodone 2 mg have been compared in a randomized double-blind study in 40 tonsillectomized men (63[c]). There were no significant differences between the two analgesics. The patients found ketamine more acceptable than oxycodone. Oxycodone was associated with more skin problems, especially pruritus. Oxycodone also caused a significantly *lower respiratory rate* with lower oxygen saturation throughout the recovery period and increased sedation throughout the study.

The effects of modified-release oxycodone in osteoarthritic pain have been evaluated in a placebo-controlled, double-blind trial in 133 patients (64[c]). Oxycodone was effective, and although opioid-related adverse effects were frequent they were considered acceptable by the authors.

Pethidine (meperidine) *(SED-14, 217; SEDA-21, 89; SEDA-24, 107)*

There has been a systematic review of the postoperative analgesic efficacy and adverse effects of pethidine and ketorolac compared with placebo in published randomized, controlled, double-blind studies (65[M]). The authors of this meta-analysis reviewed studies of moderate to severe postoperative pain relief and the use of single doses by injection (intravenously or intramuscularly) or orally. Studies of epidural, intrathecal, or intravenous administration using patient-controlled analgesia were excluded. Of the 24 placebo-controlled pethidine studies, only eight met the inclusion criteria and these generated 10 pethidine versus placebo comparisons and 254 patients given pethidine 50 or 100 mg intramuscularly. No studies of oral or intravenous pethidine at any dose met the inclusion criteria. Only the eight comparisons of pethidine 100 mg versus placebo ($n = 203$) had sufficient information available for analysis of adverse effects. The overall conclusion was that opioids carry a small but finite risk of serious adverse effects, such as respiratory depression, and a greater risk of minor adverse effects than single-dose injected or oral NSAIDs like ketorolac. Analgesia from the injected opioid or NSAID was equivalent to that achieved with oral NSAIDs. For those who cannot swallow, the choice is injected opioids like pethidine.

Cardiovascular A 70-year-old patient with a metastatic carcinoid tumor of the liver presented with a hypertensive crisis after being given pethidine 10 mg/hour by continuous intravenous infusion (66[A]). The patient remained hypertensive with a systolic blood pressure of 210 mmHg, even after chemoembolization of the tumor. The blood pressure fell when pethidine was withdrawn and nitroprusside was given. The serum 5-HT concentration was 15 (reference range 0.17–0.26) μmol/l and the urine 5-hydroxyindoleacetic acid concentration was 1311 (reference range less than 10) mg/g of creatinine. The authors postulated that the *hypertensive crisis* had occurred from the release of 5-HT from the tumor and blockade by pethidine of 5-HT re-uptake.

Nervous system Further cases of *seizures* due to norpethidine toxicity have been reported (67[A]–69[A]). Two of the patients had renal disease.

A 46-year-old woman with previous extensive urological problems, including ureteric stricture and recurrent urinary tract infections, was given pethidine in a total cumulative dose of 1500 mg postoperatively over 12 hours when she presented with a single tonic-clonic seizure that lasted 30 s. The pethidine concentration was 1200 ng/ml and the norpethidine concentration 2100 ng/ml.

A 72-year-old patient with end-stage renal insufficiency undergoing peritoneal dialysis developed myoclonic contractions and a generalized tonic–clonic seizure 48 hours after having been given pethidine in a total cumulative dose of 250 mg intravenously and 600 mg orally. The neurotoxicity resolved after withdrawal of pethidine and 4 hours of hemodialysis.

A 2-month-old boy presented with muscle rigidity of the arms and legs, catatonia, and an exaggerated startle reflex after being erroneously given a single dose of pethidine 1 mg/kg. The symptoms subsided without any active intervention.

Two case reports have highlighted the potential danger injecting pethidine into the lateral thigh region, which can cause *injury to the femoral nerve branch to the vastus lateralis*, causing muscle atrophy (70[A]).

Gastrointestinal A study in which it was intended to recruit 90 women in labor for a comparison of intrathecal bupivacaine 2.5 mg, fentanyl 25 μg, pethidine 15 mg, and pethidine 25 mg was stopped prematurely after only 34 had been recruited, because of a significant increase in the incidence of *nausea and vomiting* in the patients who received the two doses of pethidine (71[C]).

Immunologic A 42-year-old patient presented with generalized pruritus, erythema, urticaria, facial angio-edema, dysphagia, dysphonia, and dizziness 15 minutes after a single intramuscular dose of pethidine 100 mg for severe renal colic (72[A]). Prick tests and intradermal tests with pethidine and other compounds confirmed an *allergic reaction* to pethidine.

Remifentanil *(SED-14, 217; SEDA-22, 101; SEDA-23, 105; SEDA-24, 108)*

The role of remifentanil-based anesthesia in gynecological and obstetric procedures has been reviewed (73[R]). Because it is very short-acting, remifentanil provides adequate, titratable, predictable analgesia.

Cardiovascular Most of the recent studies on remifentanil have concentrated on its hemodynamic effects in different operative settings.

Three groups of 20 women due to undergo elective surgery were recruited into a randomized, double-blind study (74[C]). Group 1 received a bolus dose of remifentanil 1 μg/kg and an infusion of remifentanil (0.5 μg/kg/min); groups 2 and 3 received remifentanil 0.5 μg/kg and an infusion of 0.25 μg/kg/min. Groups 1 and 2 received pretreatment with glycopyrrolate 200 μg whilst group 3 did not. Cardiovascular responses to laryngoscopy and orotracheal intubation were measured. There were no significant differences in the three groups, except that there was a significantly *lower heart rate* in group 3 after induction of anesthesia and after intubation.

The hemodynamic effects of bolus intravenous remifentanil 0.2, 0.33, and 1 μg/kg/min have been studied in patients scheduled for coronary artery bypass grafting (75[c]). The study was terminated after only eight patients had been recruited, because of severe *hypotension, bradycardia*, and/or evidence of *myocardial ischemia*. The authors concluded that remifentanil should not be given as a bolus dose of 1 μg/kg but as an infusion at a low rate. An editorial response to this article suggested that the hemodynamic instability reported may have resulted from other contributing factors, such as hypovolemia, impairment of venous return, or excessive anesthesia due to remifentanil toxicity (76[r]).

In a prospective study in 12 men undergoing elective coronary artery bypass grafting remifentanil 0.5 and 2.0 μg/kg/min combined with propofol preserved hemodynamic stability and reduced myocardial blood flow and metabolism to a similar extent (77[C]).

Sufentanil *(SED-14, 217; SEDA-22, 101; SEDA-23, 105; SEDA-24, 109)*

In a prospective dose-finding study, 170 women with cervical dilatation of 3–5 cm were randomized to receive intrathecal sufentanil 0, 2.5, 5.0, 7.5, or 10 μg combined with bupivacaine 5 mg (78[C]). Bupivacaine combined with 2.5 μg sufentanil provided analgesia comparable to higher doses with a lower incidence of *nausea and vomiting* and less severe *pruritus*.

In a randomized double-blind study in 243 parturients who received three doses of sufentanil (0.5, 0.75, and 1 μg/ml) in combination with bupivacaine 0.625 mg/ml and adrenaline 1.25 μg/ml by continuous epidural infusion there were no differences in analgesic effects, but there was significantly more *pruritus* in those who received the highest dose of sufentanil (79[C]). The authors suggested using the lowest dose of sufentanil (0.5 μg/ml) with bupivacaine solution to minimize the risk of adverse effects on the mother and neonate, with optimal analgesia.

In another randomized, double-blind study in 40 primiparous women in labor at less than 5 cm cervical dilatation who requested epidural analgesia, the addition of clonidine 75 μg to epidural sufentanil 20 μg did not provide any advantages in analgesic efficacy or adverse effects (80[c]).

In a randomized double-blind study in 120 patients undergoing major abdominal surgery the combination of sufentanil 0.75 μg/ml with ropivacaine 0.2% provided optimal postoperative patient-controlled epidural analgesia with the fewest adverse effects of the regimens used (ropivacaine alone or ropivacaine plus sufentanil 0.5, 0.75, or 1.00 μg/ml) (81[C]).

The addition of 3.5% dextrose to sufentanil 10 μg given intrathecally in a randomized double-blind study of 48 women in early labor produced a significant reduction in the incidence of clinically important *pruritus* (82[c]). Dextrose did not compromise the quality and duration of analgesia.

Nervous system There have been three reports of *neurological changes* after the intrathecal administration of sufentanil plus bupivacaine (83[A], 84[A]).

An 18-year-old nulliparous woman with an uncomplicated pregnancy developed difficulty in swallowing, respiratory abnormalities, and excessive tiredness 13 minutes after receiving sufentanil 5 μg with bupivacaine 1.25 mg as a spinal analgesic and disappearing over 20 minutes. A 36-year-old nulliparous woman complained of dyspnea and sensory block extending to the face 15 minutes after an intrathecal injection of sufentanil 5 μg with bupivacaine 1.25 mg. In neither case was there motor blockade or neonatal sequelae (83[A]).

A 40-year-old pregnant woman developed acute confusion, aphasia, increased salivation, and difficulty in swallowing 15 minutes after intrathecal administration of sufentanil 10 μg with bupivacaine 2.5 mg. There was spontaneous resolution 1 hour later with no need for pharmacological intervention (84[A]).

Such adverse effects can be caused by sufentanil, bupivacaine, or both. Regardless of which drug caused these events, the intrathecal administration of a hypobaric solution to a patient in the sitting position might have contributed, since rostral spread of intrathecal drugs is accelerated in this setting. The use of smaller doses of sufentanil (2.5 or 5 μg) will also prevent such adverse effects.

Tramadol *(SED-14, 218; SEDA-22, 103; SEDA-23, 107; SEDA 24, 109)*

In a randomized double-blind study in 20 patients with severe postoperative pain given either intravenous tramadol 1 mg/kg or morphine 0.1 mg/kg both drugs were effective analgesics but higher dosages than those usually administered were necessary (85[c]). Tramadol did not cause any severe adverse effects, but with morphine there was one case each of severe *sedation* and *respiratory depression*. Further studies are needed to determine whether tramadol has significant advantages over morphine in patients with severe postoperative pain.

The analgesic efficacy of tramadol can be further enhanced by adding injectable lysine acetylsalicylate (aspirin) after orthopedic surgery with no significant increase in adverse effects (86[c]).

In a comparison of tramadol (1 or 2 mg/kg) and fentanyl (2 μg/kg) for postoperative analgesia after pediatric anesthesia the two drugs had equal analgesic potency and produced similar hemodynamic stability and a similar incidence of adverse effects (87[C]).

The role of tramadol in the treatment of rheumatological pain has been reviewed (88[R]). Tramadol causes fewer opioid adverse effects for a given level of analgesia compared with traditional opioids. Common adverse effects, such as *nausea* and *dizziness*, usually occur only at the beginning of therapy, abate with time, and are further minimized by up-titrating the dosage over several days (89[C]).

In two randomized double-blind studies tramadol provided effective and safe long-term relief of pain in diabetic neuropathy (90[C]) and fibromyalgia (91[CR]). The adverse effects (*constipation*, *nausea*, and *headache*) were well tolerated.

Respiratory The effect of oral tramadol on the ventilatory response to acute isocapnic hypoxia has been studied in 20 healthy volunteers. Tramadol had a small but significant *depressive effect on the hypercapnic ventilatory response* but no effect on the hypoxic ventilatory response (92[c]). This is in contrast to morphine, which causes 50–60% suppression of the hypoxic ventilatory response.

Nervous system Tramadol-associated *seizures* have been studied retrospectively in 9218 adult tramadol users and 37 232 non-users (93[c]). Seizures occurred in under 1% of all tramadol users, but the risk of seizure was increased 2- to 6-fold among users adjusted for selected co-morbidities and polydrug prescription. The risk of seizure was higher in those aged 25–54 years, those who had more than four tramadol prescriptions, and those who had a history of alcohol abuse, stroke, or head injury.

In a nested case-control study of 11 383 patients, there were 21 cases of idiopathic seizures, only three of whom had been exposed to tramadol alone, the other having taken other analgesics (opioids or others) (94[c]). The findings did not suggest an increased risk of seizures among patients taking tramadol alone.

Psychiatric *Auditory hallucinations* have been attributed to tramadol (95[A]).

A 74-year-old man with lung cancer took tramadol 200 mg/day for chest pain. Soon afterwards (time not specified) he had vivid auditory hallucinations in the form of "two voices singing accompanied by an accordion and a banjo". They resolved 48 hours after withdrawal.

Gastrointestinal In a randomized double-blind placebo-controlled study of 76 women undergoing abdominal hysterectomies tramadol 100 mg was a more effective analgesic than ketorolac 30 mg given every 6 hours intravenously (96[c]). However, of those given tramadol 38% had *vomiting* compared with only 8% of those who were given ketorolac.

Drug interactions The death of a 36-year-old patient with a history of alcohol dependence who was taking tramadol, venlafaxine, trazodone, and quetiapine has highlighted the increased risk of seizures with concomitant use of tramadol and *selective serotonin re-uptake inhibitors* (97A[R]).

PARTIAL OPIOID AGONISTS

Buprenorphine *(SED-14, 220; SEDA-22, 103; SEDA-23, 108; SEDA-24, 110)*

In a 3-day randomized placebo-controlled study 40 patients with acute pancreatitis or acute-on-chronic pancreatitis were given either buprenorphine 2.4 mg/day or procaine hydrochloride 2 g/day by constant intravenous infusion (98[c]). The patients who received buprenorphine had significantly lower pain scores than those given procaine and were significantly less likely to demand additional analgesia. The adverse effect profiles were similar in the two groups, with the exception of a significantly higher rate of *sedation* in those who were given buprenorphine. The authors suggested that intravenous buprenorphine is more effective and safer than procaine in acute pancreatitis.

There have been three studies of the use of buprenorphine to treat opiate dependence.

The authors of a randomized, multicenter, placebo-controlled, double-blind study of 72 opioid-dependent individuals, who were given either buprenorphine 8 mg/day or methadone 60 mg/day for 6 months, claimed that there were no significant differences in adverse effects during induction or maintenance (99[C]). Buprenorphine provided an alternative to methadone, with equal improvement in quality of life, psychopathology, and compliance. The results of this study should be interpreted with care, because of the unusual experimental design, which did not reflect practices in ordinary methadone maintenance programs. However, similar observations were observed during an open-label, flexible-dose study involving in-patient induction and out-patient maintenance in 15 opioid-dependent pregnant women (100[c]). Sublingual buprenorphine (1–10 mg/day) was well accepted by the women, and there was a low incidence of *neonatal abstinence syndrome*. Further controlled and larger studies need to be done to substantiate these observations.

Liver With increasing use of buprenorphine in the treatment of opioid dependence, it has been confirmed that the use of buprenorphine in opioid-dependent individuals with a history of hepatitis causes significant *increases in AST and ALT activities* (101[c]). Liver enzymes should be monitored before giving buprenorphine to patients with hepatitis.

Drug formulations A sublingual formulation that combines buprenorphine and naloxone is thought to be an ideal agent for reducing parental buprenorphine abuse. In a small pilot study in nine opioid-dependent individuals already stabilized on buprenorphine 8 mg/day naloxone 0, 4, or 8 mg was added (102[c]). The addition of naloxone did not precipitate opiate withdrawal.

Nalbuphine *(SEDA-23, 98; (SED-14, 222; SEDA-22, 104; SEDA-24, 110)*

In a double-blind placebo-controlled study in 24 elderly patients scheduled for elective total hip replacement who were randomized to either intrathecal morphine 160 μg or nalbuphine 400 μg postoperatively when the pain score was greater than 3 cm on a visual analogue scale nalbuphine produced significantly faster onset and shorter duration of analgesia (103[c]). Both opioids produced adequate maximal pain relief in all patients. The adverse effects profile was unremarkable in both groups.

In a randomized, double-blind, multicenter comparison of three different intrathecal doses of nalbuphine (0.2, 0.8, or 1.6 mg) and a single intrathecal dose of morphine (0.2 mg) for post-operative pain relief after cesarean section in 90 parturients, intrathecal nalbuphine 0.8 mg provided rapid and effective analgesia, with minimal adverse effects but a shorter duration of action, reinforcing morphine's position as an analgesic that provides long-lasting analgesia (104[C]).

OPIOID ANTAGONISTS

Nalmefene *(SED-14, 219; SEDA-22, 104; SEDA-23, 109; SEDA-24, 110)*

The Cervene Stroke Study Investigation Group conducted a phase III study to assess the efficacy and safety of nalmefene (Cervene) in patients with acute ischemic strokes and also the safety of combined recombinant tissue plasminogen activator and nalmefene in a subset of patients (105[C]). It was a randomized, placebo-controlled, double-blind study of a 24-hour infusion of nalmefene on 368 patients who received 60 mg nalmefene administered as 10 mg bolus over 15 minutes and then a 50 mg infusion over 24 hours or placebo. Even though nalmefene appeared safe and well tolerated, the study failed to find any benefit in stroke patients treated with nalmefene within 6 hours.

Naltrexone *(SED-14, 220; SEDA-22, 104; SEDA-23, 110; SEDA-24, 111)*

Gastrointestinal The risk factors for naltrexone-induced *nausea* have been studied in 120 alcohol-dependent patients in an open-label trial (106[c]). After 5–30 days of abstinence, they received a bolus dose of naltrexone 25 mg followed by 50 mg/day for 10 weeks. Moderate to severe nausea was reported in 15%. The risk of nausea was significantly predicted by poor medication compliance, intensity of drinking during treatment, short duration of abstinence, young age, and female sex.

Gastrointestinal adverse effects of naltrexone were also observed in 183 alcohol-dependent individuals who received either naltrexone or nefazodone (107[C]). These adverse effects predicated early termination of naltrexone used to treat alcohol dependence (108[C])

Biliary tract A woman with chronic cholestasis and disabling pruritus had severe but transient opioid withdrawal-like reactions after oral naltrexone 12.5 mg and 2 mg (109[A]). This observation suggests the hypothesis that increased central opioidergic tone is a component of the pathophysiology of cholestasis.

REFERENCES

1. Snijdelaar DG, Katz J, Clairoux M, Sandler AN. Respiratory effects of intraoperative alfentanil infusion in post-abdominal hysterectomy patients: a comparison of high versus low dose. Acute Pain 2000; 3: 131–9.
2. Gin T, Ngan-Kee WD, Siu YK, Stuart JC, Tan PE, Lam KK. Alfentanil given immediately before the induction of anaesthesia for elective caesarean delivery. Anesth Analg 2000; 90: 1167–72.
3. Hastier P, Buckley MJM, Peten EP, Demuth N, Dumas R, Demarquay J, Caroli-Bosc F, Delmont J. A new source of drug-induced acute pancreatitis: codeine. Am J Gastroenterol 2000; 95: 3295–8.
4. Mohrenschleger M, Glockner A, Jessberger B, Worret WI, Ollert M, Rakoski J, Ring J. Codeine caused pruritic scarlatiniform exanthemata: patch test negative but positive to oral provocation test. Br J Dermatol 2000; 143: 663–4.
5. Vidal C, Pèrez Leiros, P, Bugarin R, Armisen M. Fever and urticaria to codeine. Allergy Eur J Allergy Clin Immunol 2000; 55: 416–17.
6. Shaul WL, Wandell M, Robertson WO, Dextromethorphan toxicity: reversal by naloxone. Pediatrics, 1977; 59: 117–18.
7. Weinbroum AA, Rudick V, Poret G, Ben-Abraham R. The role of dextromethorphan in pain control. Can J Anaesth 2000; 47: 585–96.
8. Wu CT, Yu J-C, Liu S-T, Yen C-C, Li C-Y, Wong C-S. Preincisional dextromethorphan treatment for post-operative pain management after upper abdominal surgery. World J Surg 2000; 24: 512–17.
9. Price LH, Lebel J. Dextromethorphan-induced psychosis. Am J Psychiatry 2000; 157: 304.
10. Konrad D, Sobetzko D, Schmidt, B, Schaenk EJ. Insulin-dependent diabetes mellitus induced by the antitussive agent dextromethorphan. Diabetologia 2000; 43: 261–2.
11. Molnar E, Varadi A, McIlhinney RAJ, Ashcroft SJH. Identification of functional ionotropic glutamate receptor proteins in pancreatic beta-cells and in islets of Langerhans. FEBS Lett 1995; 371: 253–7.

12. Desmeules JA, Oestreicher MK, Piguet V, Allaz A-F, Dayer P. Contribution of cytochrome P-4502D6 phenotype to the neuromodulatory effects of dextromethorphan. J Pharmacol Exp Ther 1999; 288: 607–12.
13. Caruso FS, Goldblum R, for the MorphiDex Group. Dextromethorphan, an NMDA receptor antagonist, enhances the analgesic properties of morphine. Inflammopharmacology 2000; 8: 161–73.
14. Caruso FS. MorphiDex®. Pharmacokinetic studies and single-dose analgesic efficacy studies in patients with postoperative pain. J Pain Symptom Manage 2000; 19: 531–6.
15. Katz NP. MorphiDex® (MS:DM) double-blind multiple-dose studies in chronic pain patients. J Pain Symptom Manage 2000; 19: 537–41.
16. Goldblum R. Long term safety of MorphiDex®. J Pain Symptom Manage 2000; 19: 550–6.
17. Chevlon E: Morphine with dextromethorphan: conversion from other opioid analgesics. J Pain Symptom Manage 2000; 19: 542–9.
18. Machet L, Martin L, Machet MC, Lovette G, Vaillent L. Acute generalised exanthematous pustulosis induced by dextropropoxyphene and confirmed by patch testing. Acta Dermatol-Venereol 2000; 80: 224–5.
19. Gopinathen C, Sockalingham I, Fung MA, Peat S, Hanna MH. A comparative study of patient-controlled epidural diamorphine, subcutaneous diamorphine and an epidural diamorphine/bupivacaine combination for post-operative pain. Eur J Anaesthesiol 2000; 17: 189–96.
20. Serpell MG, Anderson E, Wilson D, Dawson N. I.v. regional diamorphine for analgesia after foot surgery. Br J Anaesth 2000; 84: 95–6.
21. Weber M, Diener H-C, Voit T, Neuen-Jacob E. Focal myopathy induced by chronic heroin injection is reversible. Muscle Nerve 2000; 23: 274–7.
22. Silvasti M, Pitkanen M. Continuous epidural analgesia with bupivacaine–fentanyl versus patient-controlled analgesia with i.v. morphine for postoperative pain relief after knee ligament surgery. Acta Anaesthesiol Scand 2000; 44: 37–42.
23. Polley LS, Columb MO, Naughton NN, Wagner DS, Dovantes DM, Van de Ven CJM. Effect of intravenous versus epidural fentanyl on the minimum local analgesic concentration of epidural bupivacaine in labor. Anesthesiology 2000; 93: 122–8.
24. Ben-David B, Miller G, Garriel R, Gurevitch A. Low-dose bupivacaine–fentanyl spinal anesthesia for cesarean delivery. Reg Anesth Pain Med 2000; 25: 235–9.
25. Ben-David B, Frankel R, Arzumonov T, Marchevesky Y, Volpin G. Minidose bupivacaine–fentanyl spinal anesthesia for surgical repair of hip fracture in the aged. Anesthesiology 2000; 92: 6–10.
26. Wong K, Chong JL, Lo WK, Sia ATH. A comparison of patient-controlled epidural analgesia following gynaecological surgery with and without a background infusion. Anaesthesia 2000; 55: 212–16.
27. Kotake Y, Matsumoto M, Al K, Morisaki H, Takeda J. Additional droperidol, not butorphenol, augments epidural fentanyl analgesia following anorectal surgery. J Clin Anesth 2000; 12: 9–13.
28. Connelly NR, Parker RK, Vallurupelli V, Bhopatkal S, Dunn S. Comparison of epidural fentanyl versus epidural sufentanil for analgesia in ambulatory patients in early labor. Anesth Analg 2000; 91: 374–8.
29. Burduk P, Guzik P, Piechoska M, Bronisz M, Rozek A, Jozdon M, Jordan MR. Comparison of fentanyl and droperidol mixture (neuroleptanalgesia 11) with morphine on clinical outcomes in unstable angina patients. Cardiovasc Drugs Ther 2000; 14: 259–69.
30. Stuerenberg HJ, Claassen J, Eggers C, Hansen HC. Acute adverse reaction to fentanyl in a 55 year old man. J Neurol Neurosurg Psychiatry 2000; 69: 281–2.
31. Bragonier R, Bartle D, Langton-Hewer S. Acute dystonia in a 14-yr-old following propofol and fentanyl anaesthesia. Br J Anaesth 2000; 84: 828–9.
32. Müller P, Vogtmann C. Three cases with different presentation of fentanyl-induced muscle rigidity – a rare problem in intensive care of neonates. Am J Perinatol 2000; 17: 23–6.
33. Fahnenstich H, Steffan J, Kau N, Bartmann P. Fentanyl-induced chest wall rigidity and laryngospasm in preterm and term infants. Crit Care Med 2000; 28: 836–9.
34. Williams-Alexander JM, Rowbotham DJ. Novel routes of opioid administration. Br J Anaesth 1998; 81: 3–7.
35. Grond S, Radburch L, Lehmann KA. Clinical pharmacokinetics of transdermal opioids. Focus on transdermal fentanyl. Clin Pharmacokinet 2000; 38: 59–89.
36. Varvel JR, Shafer SL, Hwang SS, Coen PA, Stanski DR. Absorption characteristics of transdermally administered fentanyl. Anesthesiology 1989; 70: 928–34.
37. Roy SD, Flynn GL. Transdermal delivery of narcotic analgesics: comparative permeabilities of narcotic analgesics through human cadaver skin. Pharm Res 1989; 6: 825–32.
38. Vilevoye-Kerkmeer APE, Mattern C, Vitendaal MP. Transdermal fentanyl in opioid-naïve cancer pain patients. An open trial using transdermal fentanyl for the treatment of chronic cancer pain in opioid-naïve patients and a group using codeine. J Pain Symptom Manage 2000; 19: 185–92.
39. Niemann T, Madsen LG, Larsen S, Thorsgaard N. Opioid treatment of painful chronic pancreatitis. Transdermal fentanyl versus sustained-release morphine. Int J Pancreatol 2000; 27: 235–40.
40. Davies AN, Bond C. Transdermal fentanyl and the opioid withdrawal syndrome. Palliative Med 1996; 10: 348.

41. Zenz M, Donner B, Strumpf M. Withdrawal symptoms during therapy with transdermal fentanyl (Fentanyl TTS)? J Pain Symptom Manage 1994; 9: 54–5.
42. Alsahaf MH, Stockwell M. Respiratory failure due to the combined effects of transdermal fentanyl and epidural bupivacaine/diamorphine following radical nephrectomy. J Pain Symptom Manage 2000: 20: 210–13.
43. Vanbever R, Le Boulenge E, Preet V. Transdermal delivery of fentanyl by electroporation I. Influence of electrical factors. Pharm Res 1996; 13: 559–65.
44. Vanbever R, De Morre N, Preat V. Transdermal delivery of fentanyl by electroporation II. Mechanisms involved in drug transport. Pharm Res 1996; 13: 1360–6.
45. Dunn C. "Touch of a button" delivers transdermal fentanyl. In Pharm 1997; 1087: 19–20.
46. Purucker M, Swan W. Potential for Duragesic patch abuse. Ann Emerg Med 2000; 35: 314.
47. Friedman RA, House JW, Luxford WM, Gherini S, Mills D. Profound hearing loss associated with hydrocodone/acetaminophen abuse. Am J Otol 2000; 21: 188–91.
48. Ayonrinde OT, Bridge DT. The rediscovery of methadone for cancer pain management. Med J Aust 2000; 173: 536–40.
49. Yvan C-S, Foss JF, O'Connor M, Osinski J, Karrison T, Moss J, Roizen MF. Methylnaltrexone for reversal of constipation due to chronic methadone use. A randomised controlled trial. J Am Med Assoc 2000; 283: 367–72.
50. Bell J, Zador D. A risk-benefit analysis of methadone maintenance treatment. Drug Saf 2000; 22: 179–90.
51. Chermack, ST, Roll J, Reilly M, Davis L, Kilaru U, Grabowski J. Comparison of patient self-reports and urinalysis results obtained under naturalistic methadone treatment conditions. Drug Alcohol Depend 2000; 59: 43–9.
52. Zador D, Sunjic S. Deaths in methadone maintenance treatment in New South Wales, Australia 1990–1995. Addiction 2000; 95: 77–84.
53. O'Connor A, Schug S, Cardwell H. A comparison of the efficacy and safety of morphine and pethidine as analgesia for suspected renal colic in the emergency setting. J Accid Emerg Med 2000; 17: 261–4.
54. Cole PJ, Craske DA, Wheatley RG. Efficacy and respiratory effects of low-dose spinal morphine for postoperative analgesia following knee arthroplasty. Br J Anaesth 2000; 85: 233–7.
55. Palmer CM, Nogani WM, Maren GV, Alves DM. Post cesarean epidural morphine: a dose-response study. Anesth Analg 2000; 90: 887–91.
56. Fletcher D, Pinaud M, Scherpereel P, Clyto N, Chauvin M. The efficacy of intravenous 0.15 versus 0.25 mg/kg intraoperative morphine for immediate postoperative analgesia after remifentanil-based anaesthesia for major surgery. Anesth Analg 2000; 90: 666–71.
57. Henderson RD, Wijdicks EFM. Downbeat nystagmus associated with intravenous patient-controlled administration of morphine. Anesth Analg 2000; 91: 691–2.
58. Ho AMH. Previous cholecystectomy and choledochal sphincter spasm after morphine sedation. Can J Anaesth 2000; 47: 50–2.
59. Yeh H-M, Chen L-K, Lin C-J, Chan W-H, Chen Y-P, Lin C-S, Sun W-Z, Wang M-J, Tsai S-K. Prophylactic intravenous ondansetron reduces the incidence of intrathecal morphine-induced pruritus in patients undergoing cesarean delivery. Anesth Analg 2000; 91: 172–5.
60. Horta ML, Ramos L, Gonçalves ZR. The inhibition of epidural morphine-induced pruritus by epidural droperidol. Anesth Analg 2000; 90: 638–41.
61. Horta ML, Ramos L, Goncalves Z da R, De Oliveira MA, Tonellotto D, Teixeira JP, De Melo PR. Inhibition of epidural morphine-induced pruritus by intravenous droperidol. The effect of increasing the doses of morphine and of droperidol. Reg Anesth 1996; 21: 312–17.
62. Tzeng JI, Wang JJ, Host, Tang CS, Liu YC, Lee SC. Dexamethasone for prophylaxis of nausea and vomiting after epidural morphine for post-caesarean section analgesia: comparison of droperidol and saline. Br J Anaesth 2000; 85: 865–8.
63. Levanen J. Ketamine and oxycodone in the management of postoperative pain. Mil Med 2000; 165: 450–5.
64. Roth SH, Fleischmenn RM, Burch FX, Dietz F, Bockow B, Repopart RJ, Rustein J, Lacouture PG. Around-the-clock, controlled-release oxycodone therapy for osteoarthritis-related pain: placebo-controlled trial and long-term evaluation. Arch Intern Med 2000; 160: 853–60.
65. Smith LA, Carroll D, Edwards JE, Moore RA, McQuay HJ. Single dose ketorolac and pethidine in acute postoperative pain: systematic review with meta-analysis. Br J Anaesth 2000; 84: 48–58.
66. Balestretro LM, Beaver CR, Rigas J. Hypertensive crisis following meperidine administration and chemoembolization of a carcinoid tumour. Arch Intern Med 2000; 160: 2394–5.
67. Knight B, Thomson N, Perry G. Seizures due to norpethidine toxicity. Aust NZ J Med 2000; 30: 513.
68. Hassan H, Bastani B, Gellens M. Successful treatment of normeperidine neurotoxicity by hemodialysis. Am J Kidney Dis 2000; 35: 146–9.
69. Baris S, Karakeya D, Sarchasan B. A dose of 1 mg/kg meperidine causes muscle rigidity in infants? Paediatr Anaesth 2000; 10: 684.
70. Haber M, Kovan E, Andary M, Honet J. Postinjection vastus lateralis atrophy: 2 case reports. Arch Phys Med Rehabil 2000; 81: 1229–33.
71. Booth JV, Lindsay DR, Olufolabi AJ, El-Moalem HE, Penning DH, Reynolds JD, The Duke Women's Anesthesia Research Group. Subarachnoid meperidine (pethidine) causes signific-

ant nausea and vomiting during labor. Anesthesiology 2000; 93: 418–21.
72. Anibarro B, Vila C, Seoane J. Urticaria induced by meperidine allergy. Allergy Eur J Allergy Clin Immunol 2000; 55: 305.
73. Buerkle H, Wilhelm W. Remifentanil for gynaecological and obstetric procedures. Curr Opin Anaesthesiol 2000; 13: 271–5.
74. Hall AP, Thompson JP, Leslie AP, Kumar N, Rowbotham DJ. Comparison of different doses of remifentanil on the cardiovascular response to laryngoscopy and tracheal intubation. Br J Anaesth 2000; 84: 100–2.
75. Elliott P, O'Hare R, Bill KM, Phillips AS, Gibson FM, Mirakhur RK. Cardiovascular depression with remifentanil. Anesth Analg 2000; 91: 58–61.
76. Michelsen LG. Hemodynamic effects of remifentanil in patients undergoing cardiac surgery. Anesth Analg 2000; 91: 1563.
77. Kazmauer S, Hanekop GG, Buhre W, Weyland A, Busch T, Redke OC, Zoelflel R, Sonntag H. Myocardial consequences of remifentanil in patients with coronary artery disease. Br J Anaesth 2000; 84: 578–83.
78. Wong CA, Scavone BM, Loffredi M, Wang WY, Peeceman AM, Ganchiff JN. The dose-response of intrathecal sufentanil added to bupivacaine for labor analgesia. Anesthesiology 2000; 92: 1553–8.
79. Eriksson SL, Frykolm P, Stenlund P-M, Olofsson Ch. A comparison of three doses of sufentanil in combination with bupivacaine–adrenaline in continuous epidural analgesia during labour. Acta Anaesthesiol Scand 2000; 44: 919–23.
80. Connelly NR, Mainkar T, El-Mansouri M, Manikantan P, Genketa RR, Dunn S, Parker RK. Effect of epidural clonidine added to epidural sufentanil for labor pain management. Int J Obstet Anesth 2000; 9: 94–8.
81. Brodner G, Mertes N, Aken HV, Mollhoff T, Zahl M, Wirtz S, Marcus MAE, Buerkle H. What concentration of sufentanil should be combined with ropivacane 0.2% wt/vol for postoperative patient-controlled epidural analgesia? Anesth Analg 2000; 90: 649–57.
82. Abouleish AE, Portnoy D, Abouleish EL. Addition of dextrose 3.5% to intrathecal sufentanil for labour analgesia reduces pruritus. Can J Anaesth 2000; 47: 1171–5.
83. Abu Abdou W, Aveline C, Bonnet F. Two additional cases of excessive extension of sensory blockade after intrathecal sufentanil for labor analgesia. Int J Obstet Anesth 2000; 9: 48–50.
84. Fragneto RY, Fisher A. Mental status change and aphasia after labor analgesia with intrathecal sufentanil/bupivacaine. Anesth Analg 2000; 90: 1175–6.
85. Wiebalck A, Tryba M, Hoell T, Strumpf M, Kulka P, Zenz M. Efficacy and safety of tramadol and morphine in patients with extremely severe postoperative pain. Acute Pain 2000; 3: 112–18.
86. Pang W-W, Huang S, Tung C-C, Huang M-H. Patient-controlled analgesia with tramadol versus tramadol plus lysine acetyl salicylate. Anesth Analg 2000; 91: 1226–9.
87. De Oliveira EDS, Micheletti LG, Sakata RW, Iwata NM, Do Amarel JLG. A comparative study of postoperative analgesia of tramadol or fentanyl in pediatric patients anaesthetic induction. Rev Bras Med 2000; 57: 89–92.
88. Desmeules JA. The tramadol option. Eur J Pain 2000; 4: 15–21.
89. Schnitzer TJ, Gray WL, Paster RZ, Kamin M. Efficacy of tramadol in treatment of chronic low back pain. J Rheumatol 2000; 27: 772–8.
90. Harati Y, Gooch C, Swenson M, Edelman SV, Greene D, Raskin P, Donofrio P, Cornblath D, Olson WH, Kamin M. Maintenance of the long-term effectiveness of tramadol in treatment of the pain of diabetic neuropathy. J Diabetes Complications 2000; 14: 65–70.
91. Russell IJ, Kamin M, Bennett RM, Schnitzer TJ, Green JA, Katz WA. Efficacy of tramadol in treatment of pain in fibromyalgia. J Clin Rheumatol 2000; 6: 250–7.
92. Warren PM, Taylor JH, Nicholson KE, Wraith PK, Drummond GB. Influence of tramadol on the ventilatory response to hypoxia in humans. Br J Anaesth 2000; 85: 211–16.
93. Gardner JS, Blough D, Drinkard CR, Shatin D, Anderson G, Graham D, Alderfer R. Tramadol and seizures: a surveillance study in a managed care population. Pharmacotherapy 2000; 20: 1423–31.
94. Gasse C, Derby L, Scaramozza-Verilekus C, Jick H. Incidence of first-time idiopathic seizures in users of tramadol. Pharmacotherapy 2000; 20: 629–34.
95. Keeley PW, Foster G, Whitelaw L. Hear my song: auditory hallucinations with tramadol hydrochloride. Br Med J 2000; 321: 1608.
96. Fortuny GO, Julia LO, Riera FO, Palleres MS, Montesa RC, Roca IC. Ketorolac versus tramadol: comparison of analgesic efficacy for pain after abdominal hysterectomy. Rev Esp Anestesiol Reanim 2000; 47: 162–7.
97. Ripple MG, Pestaner JP, Levine BS, Smielek JE. Lethal combination of tramadol and multiple drugs affecting serotonin. Am J Forens Med Pathol 2000; 21: 370–4.
98. Jakobs R, Adamek MU, Von Bubnoff AC, Riemann JF. Buprenorphine or procaine for pain relief in acute pancreatitis: a prospective randomised study. Scand J Gastroenterol 2000; 35: 1319–23.
99. Panc PP, Maremmani I, Pirastu R, Tagliamonte A, Gessa GL. Buprenorphine: a controlled clinical trial in the treatment of opioid dependence. Drug Alcohol Depend 2000; 60: 39–50.
100. Fischer G, Johnson RE, Eder H, Jegsch R, Peternell A, Weninger M, Langer M, Aschaver HN. Treatment of opioid-dependent pregnant women with buprenorphine. Addiction 2000; 95: 239–44.
101. Petry NM, Bickel WK, Piasecki D, Morsch LA, Badger GJ. Elevated liver enzyme levels in opioid-dependent patients with hepatitis treated

with buprenorphine. Am J Addict 2000; 9: 265–9.
102. Harns DS, Jones RT, Welm S, Upton RA, Lin E, Mendelson J. Buprenorphine and naloxone co-administration in opiate-dependent patients stabilised on sublingual buprenorphine. Drug Alcohol Depend 2000; 61: 85–94.
103. Fournier R, Van Gessel E, Macksay M, Gamulin Z. Onset and offset of intrathecal morphine versus nalbuphine for postoperative pain relief after total hip replacement. Acta Anaesthesiol Scand 2000; 44: 940–5.
104. Culebras X, Gaggero G, Zatlovkel J, Kern C, Masti, R-A. Advantages of intrathecal nalbuphine, compared with intrathecal morphine, after cesarean delivery: an evaluation of postoperative analgesia and adverse effects. Anesth Analg 2000; 91: 601–5.
105. Clark WM, Raps EC, Tong DC, Kelly RE, Cervene Stroke Study Investigators. Cervene (nalmefene) in acute ischaemic stroke. Final results of a Phase III efficacy study. Stroke 2000; 31: 1234–9.
106. O'Malley S, Krishnan-Sarin S, Farren C, O'Conner PG. Naltrexone-induced nausea in patients treated for alcohol dependence: clinical predictors and evidence of opioid-mediated effects. J Clin Psychopharmacol 2000; 20: 69–76.
107. Kranzler HR, Modesto-Lowe V, Van Kirk J. Naltrexone vs nefazadone for treatment of alcohol dependence. A placebo-controlled trial. Neuropsychopharmacology 2000; 22: 493–503.
108. Robsenow DJ, Colby SM, Monti PM, Swift RM, Martin RA, Mueller TI, Gordon A, Eaton CA. Predictors of compliance with naltrexone among alcoholics. Alcohol Clin Exp Res 2000; 24: 1542–9.
109. Jones EA, Dekker LRC. Florid opioid withdrawal-like reaction precipitated by naltrexone in a patient with chronic cholestasis. Gastroenterology 2000; 118: 431–2.

A. Del Favero

9 Anti-inflammatory and antipyretic analgesics and drugs used in gout

Controversies in assessing the safety profiles of the new COX-2 inhibitors

In the concluding comments in my previous review of this topic (SEDA-24, 115) I stated that a number of questions needed to be addressed before COX-2 selective inhibitors could be considered to be safer than traditional NSAIDs. Among these questions the most important were related to possible gastrointestinal, cardiovascular, and renal problems. Here I shall assess recent data that can help to clarify these problems.

Gastrointestinal *Two large trials have addressed the efficacy of COX-2 selective inhibitors and the associated risk of gastrointestinal complications: the Celecoxib Long-term Arthritis Safety Study (CLASS) and the Vioxx Gastrointestinal Outcomes Research (VIGOR) trial (1[C], 2[C]).*

CLASS consisted of two separate studies, in which celecoxib was compared with ibuprofen and diclofenac; the results obtained from the two traditional NSAIDs were pooled for analysis. Overall, 3987 patients with osteoarthritis and rheumatoid arthritis took celecoxib (400 mg bd), 1985 patients took ibuprofen (800 mg tds), and 1996 took diclofenac (75 mg bd). The study lasted 13 months, but only the data from 6 months of follow-up have been published.

There was no statistically significant difference between the two groups in the incidence of the primary endpoint of complicated ulcers (upper gastrointestinal bleeding, ulcer perforation, gastric outlet obstruction); the annualized incidence of complicated ulcers in patients taking celecoxib was 0.76% (11 events per 1441 patient-years) versus an incidence of 1.45% (20 events per 1384 patient-years) in patients taking the non-selective NSAIDs, a non-significant difference. However, for the composite endpoint of upper gastrointestinal ulcer complications plus symptomatic gastroduodenal ulcers, celecoxib was significantly better tolerated than traditional NSAIDs; the annualized incidence was 2.08% (30 events per 1441 patient-years) with celecoxib versus 3.54% (49 events per 1384 patient-years) for patients taking traditional NSAIDs, significantly different.

The lack of difference in the rate of ulcer complications between the two treatments appeared to be a function of the higher-than-expected rate of complicated ulcers in those taking celecoxib compared with previous studies (3[C]). Further analysis showed that this increase in complications was likely to be attributable to concurrent low-dose aspirin; the annualized incidence of upper gastrointestinal tract ulcer complications and of symptomatic gastroduodenal ulcers in patients not taking low-dose aspirin was significantly lower with celecoxib than with non-selective NSAIDs (0.44% or 5 events per 1143 patient-years versus 1.27% or 14 events per 1101 patient-years respectively). In patients taking aspirin the annualized incidence of upper gastrointestinal complications and symptomatic ulcers were not significantly different (4.7% or 14 events per 298 patient-years in patients taking celecoxib versus 6.0% or 17 events per 283 patient-years in those taking traditional NSAIDs).

Side Effects of Drugs, Annual 25
J.K. Aronson, ed.

Moreover, the overall incidence of gastrointestinal symptoms in patients taking celecoxib was only slightly lower than those suffered by patients taking the traditional NSAIDs, as was the rate of withdrawal due to gastrointestinal intolerance in both users and non-users of low-dose aspirin.

This subgroup analysis shows what might be called "competing co-morbidity"; that is, in the subgoup of patients taking aspirin as prophylaxis against ischemic heart disease, the gastrointestinal safety advantage of celecoxib over traditional NSAIDs was almost totally wiped out by the use of aspirin (4[r]).

Despite that, the authors of CLASS concluded by stating that celecoxib caused fewer symptomatic ulcers and ulcer complications than ibuprofen or diclofenac at 6 months.

These conclusions are not only contradicted by the published data (1[C]), but are also called into question by subsequent information on the trial available to the FDA (5[S], 6[S]). As described on the FDA web site, the published account of CLASS differed from the original protocol in many respects (in primary outcomes, statistical analysis, and trial duration). In particular, the published article represented selective reporting of the combined analysis of only the first 6 months of two separate protocols of longer duration: the first a 12-month comparison of celecoxib with diclofenac and the other a 16-month comparison of celecoxib with ibuprofen. The unpublished data show that by week 65 celecoxib was associated with a similar number of ulcer complications as diclofenac and ibuprofen and that the relative risks of both complicated ulcers and all serious gastrointestinal adverse events were higher at 12–16 months than they were at 6 months, suggesting an increased risk of serious adverse events with celecoxib long-term therapy.

It is unfortunate that important information from CLASS may not be widely known because it is not published, and this bias can mislead physicians and patients.

In the VIGOR study 8076 patients with rheumatoid arthritis were randomly assigned to receive rofecoxib 50 mg/day or naproxen 500 mg bd. The primary endpoint was a confirmed clinical upper gastrointestinal event (gastroduodenal perforation or obstruction, upper gastrointestinal bleeding, and symptomatic gastroduodenal ulcer).

Overall, confirmed upper gastrointestinal events occurred in 177 patients, 56 with rofecoxib (n = 4047) and 121 in those taking naproxen (n = 4029). In 53 of these patients the event was complicated, 16 taking rofecoxib and 37 taking naproxen. That means that during a median follow-up of 9.0 months, there were 2.1 confirmed gastrointestinal events per 100 patient-years with rofecoxib compared with 4.5 per 100 patient-years with naproxen (RR = 0.5; 95% CI = 0.2, 0.8). The respective rates of complicated ulcers (perforation, obstruction, and bleeding) were 0.6 per 100 patient-years and 1.4 per 100 patient-years (RR = 0.4; 95% CI = 0.2, 0.8).

It is also worthy of note that the most common adverse events that led to withdrawal of treatment, excluding the primary gastrointestinal endpoints, were dyspepsia, abdominal pain, epigastric discomfort, nausea, and heartburn and that significantly fewer patients discontinued treatment as a result of any one of these five upper gastrointestinal symptoms in the rofecoxib group (3.5%) than in the naproxen group (4.9%).

What are the clinical implications of these studies? Proof that the gastrointestinal toxicity of selective COX-2 inhibitors is significantly less than that of traditional NSAIDs was achieved, at least in part, in the VIGOR study, but CLASS failed to show a significant safety advantage over comparator NSAIDs. Despite the evidence that COX-2 inhibitors may cause less gastrointestinal toxicity than non-selective NSAIDs, there are some caveats (7[R]).

First, the results of these large clinical trials need confirmation. In fact, despite the large number of patients studied the numbers of observed serious gastrointestinal events were relatively small and the likelihood of a gastrointestinal complication in patients who are taking NSAIDs depends on pre-existing risk factors, which are likely to be relevant to the gastrointestinal effects of COX-2 inhibitors. The role of aspirin, found in CLASS, is a clear example of a possible confounding factor.

Second, the population selected for clinical trials and the type of treatment (i.e. duration of treatment or intermittent vs continuous use) may not be fully representative of daily practice and the results of these trials must therefore be verified in clinical practice.

Third, the roles of the two cyclooxygenase isoenzymes are not fully understood, and we still have much to learn about the potential risks *of the inhibition of COX-2 in the gastrointestinal tract and in other systems or organs (7[R], 8[c]–11[c]). In particular, the risk of inhibiting COX-2 in the large bowel in patients with inflammatory bowel disease should be carefully considered. Whether a COX-2 selective inhibitor can harm the intestine in the presence of gastrointestinal inflammation will depend on whether COX-2 is induced to the extent that it becomes the predominant source of prostaglandins (12[r]). However, we have no data yet on the safety of COX-2 inhibitors in patients with inflammatory bowel disease.*

Fourth, it is imperative to consider the overall safety profile of these new compounds. Both cyclooxygenase enzymes have important roles in physiological conditions and in various pathological syndromes, and therefore the beneficial effects of selective COX-2 inhibition in the stomach may be offset by the risk of COX-2 inhibition in other organs or physiologic processes. Competition between gastroprotection and cardioprotection with traditional NSAIDs and selective COX-2 inhibitors is a good example of this (4[R]).

Cardiovascular *Among the questions raised by the availability of selective COX-2 inhibitors, those regarding their prothrombotic potential are of major concern.*

COX-2 inhibitors act by inhibiting the synthesis of prostacyclin in the vascular wall but not platelet thromboxane production. They could therefore theoretically increase the risk of cardiovascular events by shifting the hemostatic balance toward a prothrombotic state. However, it is not clear that theory has much impact on reality.

Information about this topic comes from the two large studies (CLASS and VIGOR) already mentioned, from a pooled cardiovascular safety analysis using individual patient data derived from all rofecoxib phase IIb to V trials conducted by the manufacturer that lasted at least 2 weeks, and from the adverse events reporting system in the USA (13[M]).

In VIGOR, based on the excess of cardiovascular adverse effects in one group of enrolled patients found in an interim analysis, the data and safety monitoring committee of the study recommended blinding adjudication of cardiovascular events: 45 patients taking rofecoxib and 20 taking naproxen were judged to have serious thrombotic cardiovascular adverse events, including myocardial infarction, unstable angina, cardiac thrombus, resuscitated cardiac arrest, sudden or unexpected death, ischemic stroke, and transient ischemic attacks. The rate of myocardial infarction was 0.1% with naproxen versus 0.4% with rofecoxib, a statistically significant difference, primarily accounted for by the high rate of myocardial infarction among the 4% of study population with the highest risk of a myocardial infarction for whom low-dose aspirin would have been indicated. The difference in the rates of myocardial infarction between the two groups was not significant among the patients without indications for aspirin as secondary prophylaxis. Overall mortality and cardiovascular mortality were similar in the two groups.

In contrast, in CLASS there was no significant difference in the incidence of major cardiovascular events between celecoxib and non-selective NSAIDs. However, patients were allowed to use low-dose aspirin (20% of enrolled patients) and this may have protected them from adverse cardiovascular events.

The results of VIGOR can be explained by either a significant prothrombotic effect of rofecoxib and/or an antithrombotic effect of naproxen, which may have a significant antiplatelet effect. To clarify this, the annualized myocardial infarction rates in both VIGOR and CLASS were compared with those found in placebo-treated patients with similar cardiac risk factors enrolled in three meta-analyses of four aspirin primary prevention trials (13[M], 14[M]). The analysis showed 0.24 and 0.30% increases over placebo in cardiovascular events for rofecoxib and celecoxib respectively, suggesting a prothrombotic potential of both COX-2 inhibitors. However, these results have been heavily criticized (15[r]–21[r]), because of many potential pitfalls in the comparisons of patient populations in different trials. The results from a recently reported pooled analysis of individual patient data combined across rofecoxib phase IIb to phase V trials seem to be more reliable (22[M]). Cardiovascular events were assessed across 23 studies. Comparisons were made between patients taking rofecoxib and those taking placebo, naproxen, or other nonselective NSAIDs (diclofenac, ibuprofen, and nabumetone). The major outcome measure was the combined endpoint used by the Anti-platelet Trialist Collaboration, which includes cardio-

vascular death, hemorrhagic death, death of unknown cause, non-fatal myocardial infarction, and non-fatal stroke. More than 28 000 patients, representing more than 14 000 patient-years at risk, were analysed. The relative risk for any endpoint was 0.84 (95% CI = 0.51, 1.38) when comparing rofecoxib with placebo; 0.79 (95% CI = 0.40, 1.55) when comparing rofecoxib with non-selective NSAIDs; and 1.69 (95% CI = 1.07, 2.69) when comparing rofecoxib with naproxen. These data provide no evidence for an excess of cardiovascular events for rofecoxib relative to either placebo or the non-selective NSAIDs that were studied. Instead, the difference between rofecoxib and naproxen showed that naproxen was associated with a reduced risk of cardiovascular events.

This might be the result of the antiplatelet effects of this non-selective NSAID. However, although the data are suggestive, neither the VIGOR results nor this analysis provide sufficient evidence to establish the potential cardioprotective benefits of naproxen. More information is needed on the cardiovascular effects of selective COX-2 inhibitors and their combination with antiplatelet drugs.

The shift in hemostatic balance toward a prothrombotic state might not be the only mechanism by which COX-2 inhibitors could increase the risk of cardiovascular adverse effects. In fact, non-selective NSAIDs can raise blood pressure and antagonize the hypotensive effect of antihypertensive medications to an extent that may increase hypertension-related morbidity (23[M], 24[R]). The problem is clinically relevant, as arthritis and hypertension are common co-morbid conditions in elderly people, requiring concurrent therapy.

Information on the effect of COX-2 selective inhibitors on arterial blood pressure is scanty. In VIGOR more patients developed hypertension with rofecoxib than naproxen. For rofecoxib, the mean increase in blood pressure was 4.6/1.7 mmHg compared with a 1.0/0.1 mmHg increase with naproxen (13[M]). Noteworthy previous work has shown that a 2 mmHg reduction in diastolic blood pressure can result in about a 40% reduction in the rate of stroke and a 25% reduction in the rate of myocardial infarction (25[R]). The effect of celecoxib on blood pressure was evaluated in a post-hoc analysis using the safety database generated during the celecoxib clinical development program in more than 13 000 subjects (26[M]). The incidence of hypertension after celecoxib was greater than that after placebo but similar to that after non-selective NSAIDs. Hypertension and exacerbation of pre-existing hypertension respectively occurred in 0.8 and 0.6% of patients. Furthermore, there was no evidence of drug–drug interactions between celecoxib and other antihypertensive drugs.

The cardiorenal safety profiles of celecoxib (200 mg/day) and rofecoxib (25 mg/day) have recently been compared in a 6-week, randomized, parallel-group, double-blind trial in 810 patients with osteoarthritis aged 65 years or over taking antihypertensive drugs (27[C]). The primary endpoints were edema and changes in systolic and diastolic blood pressures, measured at baseline and after 1, 2, and 6 weeks.

Systolic blood pressure rose significantly in 17% of rofecoxib-treated patients (n = 399) compared with 11% of celecoxib-treated patients (n = 411), a statistically significant difference, at any time in the study. Diastolic blood pressure rose in 2.3% of rofecoxib-treated patients compared with 1.5% of celecoxib-treated patients, a non-significant difference. At week 6, the change from baseline in mean systolic blood pressure was +2.6 mmHg for rofecoxib compared with –0.5 mmHg for celecoxib, a highly significant difference. Nearly twice as many rofecoxib-treated than celecoxib-treated patients had edema.

Despite some limitations, this study provides some evidence that COX-2 selective inhibitors may differ in their ability to alter arterial blood pressure.

What are the implications of these observations with respect to the increased risk of thrombotic events with COX-2 selective inhibitors? Patients who have had a major cardiovascular event should be treated with low-dose aspirin (if indicated). For such patients the use of a COX-2 selective or of a traditional NSAID probably does not make any difference. In any case, careful control of arterial blood pressure is mandatory.

Urinary tract *Renal dysfunction after therapy with COX-2 inhibitors is not unexpected. COX-2 is expressed in the normal human kidney, especially in endothelial and smooth muscle cells of the vasculature and glomerular epithelial cells. Angiotensin II and endothelin induce and upregulate COX-2 and prostaglandin synthesis. Furthermore, it seems reasonable* *to hypothesize that intrarenal dependence on COX-2-synthesized prostaglandins increases in heart failure, liver failure, volume depletion, and chronic renal disease (28[R]).*

As experience with these drugs accumulates, it appears that the pattern of nephrotoxicity of COX-2 selective inhibitors is similar to that of traditional NSAIDs (29[Ar]). The evidence comes from different sources: clinical trials, case reports, and analysis of spontaneous reports in international safety databases.

The incidence of adverse effects related to renal function in CLASS and VIGOR was low and similar (0.9% with celecoxib and 1.2% with rofecoxib). The incidence of increased creatinine and urea nitrogen concentrations was slightly lower in patients taking celecoxib than in those taking ibuprofen or diclofenac. Similar results have been documented in two other clinical trials. The first compared celecoxib with diclofenac in long-term management of rheumatoid arthritis in 430 patients (30[C]). There were only small increases in serum creatinine concentration (from 93.3 μmol/l at baseline to 95.5 μmol/l at the final visit) and serum urea concentration (from 6.0 to 6.4 mmol/l). There was a similar increase in patients taking diclofenac. The second trial, in 1149 patients, compared celecoxib with naproxen; serum creatinine concentrations were not affected by either celecoxib or naproxen (31[C]).

However, data from these clinical trials must be interpreted with caution, as patients at major risk of renal adverse events were likely to be excluded.

In contrast, published case reports and case series have provided more insight into the potential nephrotoxicity associated with COX-2 selective inhibitors. Taken together, these case reports suggest that COX-2 inhibitors, like non-selective NSAIDs, produce similar and consistent renal adverse effects in patients with one or more risk factors that induce prostaglandin-dependent renal function (i.e. patients with renal and cardiovascular disease and taking a number of culprit medications, such as diuretics and ACE inhibitors). Acute renal insufficiency, disturbances in volume status (edema, heart failure), metabolic acidosis, hyperkalemia, and hyponatremia have been commonly described. The duration of treatment with COX-2 inhibitors before the development of clinically recognized renal impairment ranged from a few days to 3–4 weeks. Withdrawal of COX-2 inhibitors and supportive therapy most often resulted in resolution of renal dysfunction, but in some patients hemodialysis was required (29[Ar], 32[A]–36[A]).

The renal safety of rofecoxib and celecoxib has been studied using the database of spontaneous reports of adverse drug reactions in the WHO Monitoring Center in Uppsala (37[C]). Disproportionality in the association between COX-2 selective inhibitors and renal-related adverse drug reactions was evaluated using a Bayesian confidence propagation neural network method, in which a statistical parameter (the information component: IC) was calculated for each drug–reaction combination. In this method an IC value significantly greater than 0 implies that the association of a drug–reaction pair is stronger than background; the higher the IC value, the more the combination stands out from the background. As with non-selective NSAIDs, both COX-2 selective inhibitors were associated with renal-related adverse drug reactions. IC values were significantly different for the following comparisons: water retention, abnormal renal function, renal insufficiency, cardiac failure, and hypertension. However, the adverse renal impact of rofecoxib was significantly greater than that of celecoxib. Renal-related events for rofecoxib were 2- to 4-fold higher than for celecoxib and the severity of these reported adverse reactions was also more serious. Studies based on spontaneous reports have many limitations and their results must therefore be confirmed by additional epidemiological studies that can provide more accurate information on incidence rates and risk factors.

In conclusion, potential renal toxicity in certain high-risk patients from the COX-2 selective inhibitors seems to be similar to that found with traditional NSAIDs with respect to renal regulation of sodium excretion and glomerular filtration rate.

Whether celecoxib offers any distinct safety advantage with respect to rofecoxib in clinical practice remains to be seen.

In the mean time selective COX-2 inhibitors, like other NSAIDs, must be used cautiously in patients with predisposing diseases (i.e. reduced renal function, cardiac decompensation, hepatic failure) or who are taking some other medications (ACE inhibitors, diuretics).

Possible association of NSAIDs with inflammatory bowel disease

The evidence that NSAIDs can cause exacerbation of inflammatory bowel disease is at best scanty (SEDA-10, 76; SEDA-15, 92; SEDA-17, 102). In the few studies in which drugs as a cause of relapse of chronic inflammatory bowel disease have been investigated NSAIDs have not be shown to be major contributors.

However, well-documented published series of patients with quiescent inflammatory bowel disease whose colitis became active shortly after they were given NSAIDs make the causal relation probable, at least in some patients (38[A]–41[A]). Because the pathogenesis of inflammatory bowel disease is unknown, it is difficult to say whether episodes of colitis are exacerbations of the underlying disease or unrelated events caused by NSAIDs in predisposed patients.

Two studies of the possible association between NSAIDs and the onset or exacerbation of inflammatory bowel disease have given contrasting results.

In the first study (42[C]) the authors interviewed 60 patients (mean age 42 years) with either Crohn's disease or ulcerative colitis who required admission to hospital owing to symptoms of their disease, and 62 matched controls (mean age 46 years) with irritable bowel syndrome who did not require hospitalization. Patients were asked about their use of NSAIDs and the relation in time and duration to the exacerbation or onset of the inflammatory bowel disease. There was an association with the use of NSAIDs in 31% of the patients with inflammatory bowel disease, but in only 2% of those with irritable bowel syndrome.

Compared with patients with irritable bowel syndrome the odds ratio (OR) for an exacerbation or new onset of symptoms of inflammatory bowel disease after recent use of NSAIDs (defined as use within 1 month of symptom exacerbation or onset of disease) was 20 (95% CI = 2.6, 160).

In contrast, the second study (43[C]) showed that the use of NSAIDs was not associated with a higher incidence of active inflammatory bowel disease. The authors retrospectively examined the records of 192 out-patients with inflammatory bowel disease: 112 with Crohn's disease (mean age 53 years) and 80 with ulcerative colitis (mean age 61 years). The use of NSAIDs was more common in patients with inactive inflammatory bowel disease than in those with active disease. Of 40 patients with active Crohn's disease, three were using NSAIDs compared with 14 of 72 with inactive disease. Of 58 patients with active ulcerative colitis eight were using NSAIDs compared with five of 21 patients with ulcerative colitis in remission.

These contrasting results may have been due to different patient populations studied (in-patient vs out-patients) or to other limitations: in the case-control study, the number of patients enrolled was small and the confidence intervals of the odds ratio were very large; in the observational study, the analysis was retrospective and the possibility of use of over-the-counter NSAIDs by some patients could not be excluded.

Despite the clinical importance of the problem we lack a firm answer to the question of whether patients with inflammatory bowel disease should refrain from using NSAIDs.

Drug interactions To explore the frequency of continuous use of over-the-counter (OTC) drugs and the potential for harmful interactions between OTC drugs and prescribed drugs, a population-based interview survey was conducted in 10 477 subjects (44[C]). Daily use of OTC drugs was reported by 7% of the subjects and 4% of those who used OTC drugs had taken combinations with potential for clinically significant interactions. Interactions were most common for NSAIDs such as ketoprofen (15% of ketoprofen users), ibuprofen (10%), and aspirin (6%). Unfortunately, this study did not provide information on whether the potential interactions led to actual clinical problems.

Acetylsalicylic acid (aspirin) and related compounds *(SED-14, 223; SEDA-22, 113; SEDA-23, 16; SEDA-24, 121)*

Fluid balance Severe *fluid retention*, possibly due to impaired renal tubular secretion, has been reported in a 29-year-old woman taking aspirin (1.5 g/day for several days) for persistent headache (45[C]). During rechallenge with aspirin (0.5 g tds for 3 days) a dynamic renal scintigram showed a substantial fall in tubular filtration. Withdrawal was followed by complete uneventful recovery. Pulmonary edema is a feature of salicylate intoxication, but this patient was taking a therapeutic dosage.

Gastrointestinal The question of whether the risk of *gastrointestinal hemorrhage* with long-term aspirin is dose related (SEDA-12, 100) merits further attention, as more data on the toxicity of low-dose aspirin have recently become available (46[C], 47[M]). In a meta-analysis of the incidence of gastrointestinal hemorrhage associated with long-term aspirin and the effect of dose in 24 randomized controlled clinical trials including almost 66 000 patients exposed for an average duration of 28 months to a wide range of different doses of aspirin (50–1500 mg/day), gastrointestinal hemorrhage occurred in 2.47% of patients taking aspirin compared with 1.42% taking placebo (OR = 1.68; 95% CI = 1.51, 1.88). In patients taking low doses of aspirin (50–162.5 mg/day; n = 49 927) gastrointestinal hemorrhage occurred in 2.3% compared with 1.45% taking placebo (OR = 1.56; 95% CI = 1.40, 1.81). The pooled OR for gastrointestinal hemorrhage with low-dose aspirin was 1.59 (95% CI = 1.4, 1.81). A meta-regression to test for a linear relation between the daily dose of aspirin and the risk of gastrointestinal hemorrhage gave a pooled OR of 1.015 (95% CI = 0.998, 1.047) per 100 mg dose reduction. The reduction in the incidence of gastrointestinal hemorrhage was estimated to be 1.5% per 100 mg dose reduction, but this was not significant.

These data are in apparent contrast with others previously reported (48[M]) (SEDA-21, 100) which showed that gastrointestinal hemorrhage was dose related. Many reasons may explain these contrasting results, the most important being differences in the definition of the hemorrhagic events, in study design, in the population studied, and in the presence of accessory risk factors (49[C], 50[C], 51[r]).

The recent trends towards the use of lower doses of aspirin have been driven by the belief that these offer a better safety profile while retaining equivalent therapeutic efficacy. Despite the large number of patients enrolled in randomized clinical trials and included in meta-analyses, there is no firm evidence that dose reduction significantly lowers the risk of gastrointestinal bleeding. Patients and doctors therefore need to consider the trade-off between the benefits and harms of long-term treatment with aspirin. Meanwhile it seems wise to use the lowest dose of proven efficacy.

ANILINE DERIVATIVES

Paracetamol *(SED-14, 240; SEDA-22, 114; SEDA-23, 116; SEDA-24, 122)*

Skin *Fixed drug eruptions* from paracetamol are infrequent (SEDA-23, 116), but an unusual non-pigmented fixed drug eruption has recently been described (52[A]).

Immunologic *Acute hypersensitivity reactions* due to paracetamol are rare (SEDA-22, 114), but can be life threatening (53[A]).

Drug interactions Paracetamol is metabolized in part by CYP2E1, and inducers of CYP2E1 predispose patients to paracetamol hepatotoxicity. However, a possible interaction leading to hepatotoxicity with *phenytoin* has been reported in a 55-year-old woman taking paracetamol 1300–6200 mg/day over 10 days (54[A]). Phenytoin induces CYP2C and CYP3A4 but not CYP2E1. As CYP3A4 may participate in paracetamol metabolism the induction of this isoform may also be responsible for paracetamol-induced hepatotoxicity.

ANTHRANILIC ACID DERIVATIVES

Mefenamic acid *(SED-14, 261; SEDA-23, 118)*

Gastrointestinal *Esophageal injury* is a rare adverse effect of NSAIDs. The published evidence comprises only a few specific studies and a small number of single case reports regarding various NSAIDs (SEDA-15, 92). A report of esophageal ulceration associated with mefenamic acid capsules has now been published (55[A]).

Five days before he presented with esophageal ulceration, a 35-year-old man took two capsules of mefenamic acid (total dose 500 mg) in bed with a small amount of water. The following morning he noted severe retrosternal pain, which persisted until he was seen 4 days later. Endoscopy showed a 3-cm esophageal ulcer near the aortic arch. Within a few days there was complete resolution of ulceration.

All NSAIDs should be taken while standing or sitting, rather than lying, and with about 200 ml of water.

ARYLALKANOIC ACID DERIVATIVES *(SED-14, 268; SEDA-22, 115; SEDA-23, 119; SEDA-24, 122)*

Diclofenac

Immunologic Cutaneous tests with diclofenac were not useful in diagnosing *hypersensitivity* in a series of 12 non-atopic patients who had severe symptoms of hypersensitivity (56[A]). However, oral challenge in patients who had had only cutaneous symptoms was diagnostic.

Risk factors The Japanese Health Authority has sent a "Dear Doctor" letter warning against the use of diclofenac in patients with *encephalitis* or *encephalopathy* related to influenza, which may be associated with higher mortality (57[S]).

Ketoprofen

Urinary tract A 62-year-old woman developed *acute renal insufficiency* after using topical ketoprofen for 5 days (58[A]). She had several predisposing factors to NSAID-induced acute renal insufficiency, such as advanced age, chronic renal impairment due to polycystic kidney disease, and treatment with an ACE inhibitor and furosemide. As topical NSAIDs can be absorbed via the skin, they cannot considered safe in high-risk patients, in whom all NSAIDs are contraindicated.

Skin Several reports have documented the *photosensitizing potential* of topical ketoprofen. In some cases ketoprofen can be responsible for very prolonged photosensitivity after only a single application (59[A]).

Ketorolac

There are contrasting data on the benefit:harm ratio of parenteral ketorolac as an analgesic (SEDA-21, 105). This prompted regulatory review of ketorolac in many countries, leading to revision of labeling, dosage recommendations, and prescribing practices. The use of ketorolac should be limited in dosage and duration; in some patients (i.e. the elderly) it should probably be restricted altogether. It is important for prescribers to understand that increasing the dosage of ketorolac beyond the label recommendations (60–120 mg/day for a maximum of 2–5 days) will not provide better efficacy, but will increase the risk of serious adverse reactions (60[R]).

Loxoprofen

Liver The Japanese Health Authority has tightened the hepatic warnings for loxoprofen after eight reports of serious hepatic adverse events since 1997, including two deaths (61[S]).

Drug interactions Loss of consciousness due to marked bradycardia caused by severe hyperkalemia has been described in an 85-year-old woman who took loxoprofen for several days and long-term *imidapril* (an ACE inhibitor). The combination of an NSAID with an ACE inhibitor can produce serious adverse effects in high-risk patients (62[A]).

Nabumetone

Skin Nabumetone-induced *pseudoporphyria* has been described (SEDA 22, 117), and a further five cases in four adults and a child have been reported (63[A], 64[C], 65[A]).

Drug interactions Concomitant therapy with warfarin and NSAIDs is of concern, owing to the potential for increasing bleeding. In a 72-year-old man the concomitant use of nabumetone and warfarin led to an increased international normalized ratio and hemarthrosis (66[A]). Previous reports suggested a lack of interaction of nabumetone with warfarin, but close monitoring is advisable when these two drugs are coadministered.

Naproxen

Skin Severe skin reactions occur infrequently with naproxen. However, there have been recent reports of a *leukocytoclastic vasculitis* in a

62-year-old woman with skin, peripheral nerve, and renal involvement (67[A]) and a linear IgA bullous dermatosis in a 69-year-old man (68[A]). In both cases long-term corticosteroid treatment caused gradually resolution.

Piketoprofen *(SEDA-21, 107)*

Skin A *photoallergic contact dermatitis* followed topical administration of piketoprofen in a 46-year-old man after 3 days; photopatch testing for piketoprofen was positive (69[A]).

COXIBS

Celecoxib

Psychiatric A 78-year-old woman had *auditory hallucinations* while taking celecoxib for osteoarthritis (70[A]). Her symptoms occurred after she had taken celecoxib (200 mg bd) for 48 hours and progressed over the next 8 days. Celecoxib was withdrawn and her hallucinations gradually disappeared over the next 4 days. Rechallenge with a lower dose (100 mg bd) caused recurrence.

Hematologic A recent report has raised the possibility that patients with a known prothrombotic state and raised platelet thromboxane A2 production may be at high risk of *thrombosis* when selective COX-2 inhibitors are used (71[A]).

Thrombosis occurred during celecoxib therapy (400 mg/day) in four women (aged 37–56 years) with connective tissue diseases and conditions that predisposed them to thrombosis, including Raynaud's phenomenon, raised anticardiolipin antibody titers, lupus anticoagulant, and a previous history of thrombosis. Peripheral artery thrombosis (three patients) and pulmonary embolism (one patient) were documented after starting celecoxib. Symptoms of thrombosis began to appear within 1 week of starting celecoxib in three patients and 2 months after the starting celecoxib in the fourth patient.

A causal relation between celecoxib and these thrombotic events cannot be established with certainty on the basis of the available evidence. However, the temporal relation between the start of treatment and the thrombotic event was impressive, at least in three patients, and the findings were consistent with the hypothesis that thrombosis is an adverse consequence of reduced production of systemic prostaglandin I_2 brought about by COX-2 inhibition. Reduced synthesis of prostaglandin I_2 may act in concert with other thrombotic risk factors (such as those occurring in this series of patients) to precipitate acute vascular occlusion.

The use of COX-2 inhibitors in patients with connective tissue diseases and other prothrombotic states must be carefully considered.

Liver A 67-year-old woman developed acute *hepatocellular and cholestatic liver damage* after taking celecoxib (100 mg/day) for 1 week (72[A]). Celecoxib was withdrawn and the liver function tests normalized within 2 weeks.

Skin Skin reactions, including *rashes*, *urticaria*, and other allergic reactions, are not uncommon, according to data reported to the Australian Adverse Reactions Advisory Committee (73[S]) and other reports (74[A]–76[A]).

Drug interactions Celecoxib can potentiate the anticoagulant effects of *warfarin*. Although concomitant administration of celecoxib and warfarin had no significant effect on prothrombin time or the steady-state pharmacokinetics of S- or R-warfarin in 24 healthy volunteers (77[c]), serious bleeding complications have been reported to adverse drug reactions monitoring systems (78[A]) and in journals (79[A]–81[A]). These data suggest that celecoxib potentiates the anticoagulant effects of warfarin in some patients. Patients taking warfarin must be fully monitored when celecoxib is added, changed, or withdrawn.

INDOMETHACIN AND RELATED COMPOUNDS *(SED-14, 279; SEDA-22, 118)*

Indomethacin

Nervous system Low-dose indomethacin (0.1 mg/kg) begun in the first 24 hours of life and given every 24 hours for 6 doses was not associated with adverse neurodevelopmental outcome at 36 months corrected age (82[C]).

Fetotoxicity The possible association of indomethacin tocolysis with *neonatal necrotizing* *enterocolitis* has been the subject of a case-control study (83[C]). All cases of proven necrotizing enterocolitis were ascertained and four controls for each case were randomly identified. During 18 months there were 24 cases of necrotizing enterocolitis. Indomethacin as a single tocolytic agent was not associated with necrotizing enterocolitis (OR = 1.0, 95% CI = 0.2, 4.8).

Sulindac *(SED-14, 284; SEDA-24, 122)*

Drug interactions Unlike other NSAIDs, sulindac does not seem to interact with *lithium* (SEDA-10, 82). However, a recent report has suggested that it may increase serum lithium concentrations (84[A]).

MISCELLANEOUS COMPOUNDS

Nimesulide *(SED-14, 294; SEDA-24, 123)*

Liver *Severe hepatitis* can occur in patients taking nimesulide (SEDA-23, 121). Two recent case reports have provided further evidence of this. In one case (85[A]) fatal hepatitis occurred after 8 months of treatment and in the other (86[A]) treatment for 5 days precipitated fulminant hepatitis.

Pregnancy A new report has confirmed the potential danger of using nimesulide as a tocolytic agent (SEDA 24, 123). Nimesulide (100 mg bd) was prescribed for postoperative preterm labor prophylaxis and severe *oligohydramnios* was identified 3 weeks later (87[A]). After withdrawal the amniotic fluid volume returned to normal over 2 weeks. There were no adverse neonatal renal effects.

DRUGS USED IN THE TREATMENT OF GOUT

Allopurinol *(SED-14, 310; SEDA-23, 122)*

Hypersensitivity is a well known complication of allopurinol therapy and requires drug withdrawal because of its severity. However, in some patients allopurinol is needed to control tophaceous gout. One way to overcome this problem is desensitization, strategies for which allow patients to resume allopurinol therapy without any further problem (88[A], 89[A]).

REFERENCES

1. Silverstein FE, Faich G, Goldstein JL, Simon LS, Pincus T, Whelton A, Makuch R, Eisen G, Agrawal NM, Stenson WF, Burr AM, Zhao WW, Kent JD, Lefkowith JB, Verburg KM, Geis GS. Gastrointestinal toxicity with celecoxib vs nonsteroidal anti-inflammatory drugs for osteoarthritis and rheumatoid arthritis. The CLASS study: a randomized controlled trial. J Am Med Assoc 2000; 284: 1247–55.
2. Bombardier C, Laine L, Reicin A, Shapiro D, Burgos-Vargas R, Davis B, Day R, Bosi Ferraz M, Hawkey CJ, Hochberg MC, Kvien TK, Schnitzer TJ. Comparison of upper gastrointestinal toxicity of rofecoxib and naproxen in patients with rheumatoid arthritis. New Engl J Med 2000; 343: 1520–8.
3. Goldstein JL, Silverstein FE, Agrawal NM, Hubbard RC, Kaiser J, Maurath CJ, Verburg KM, Geis GS. Reduced risk of upper gastrointestinal ulcer complications with celecoxib, a novel COX-2 inhibitor. Am J Gastroenterol 2000; 95: 1681–90.
4. Boers M. NSAIDs and selective COX-2 inhibitors: competition between gastroprotection and cardioprotection. Lancet 2001; 357: 1222–3.
5. Hrachovec JB, Mora M. Reporting of 6-month vs 12-month data in a clinical trial of celecoxib. J Am Med Assoc 2001; 286: 2398.
6. Wright JM, Perry TL, Bassett KL, Chambers GK. Reporting of 6-month vs 12-month data in a clinical trial of celecoxib. J Am Med Assoc 2001; 286: 2398–400.
7. FitzGerald GA, Patrono C. Drug therapy: the coxibs, selective inhibitors of cyclooxygenase-2. New Engl J Med 2001; 345: 433–42.
8. Mizuno H, Sakamoto C, Matsuda K, Wada K, Uchida T, Noguchi H, Akamatsu T, Kasuga M. Induction of cyclooxygenase 2 in gastric mucosal lesions and its inhibition by the specific antagonist delays healing in mice. Gastroenterology 1997; 112: 645–8.
9. Prescott SM. Is cyclooxygenase-2 the alpha and the omega in cancer? J Clin Invest 2000; 105: 1511–13.
10. Newberry RD, Stenson WF, Lorenz RG. Cyclooxygenase-2-dependent arachidonic meta-

bolities are essential modulators of the intestinal immune response to dietary antigen. Nat Med 1999; 8: 900–6.
11. Morteau O, Morham SG, Sellon R, Dieleman LA, Langenbach R, Smithies O, Sartor RB. Impaired mucosal defense to acute colonic injury in mice lacking cyclooxygenase-1 or cyclooxygenase-2. J Clin Invest 2000; 105: 469–78.
12. Hawkey CJ. COX-2 inhibitors. Lancet 1999; 353: 307–14.
13. Mukherjee D, Nissen SE, Topol EJ. Risk of cardiovascular events associated with selective COX-2 inhibitors. J Am Med Assoc 2001; 286: 954–9.
14. Sanmuganathan PS, Ghahramani P, Jackson PR, Wallis EJ, Ramsay LE. Aspirin for primary prevention of coronary heart disease: safety and absolute benefit related to coronary risk derived from meta-analysis of randomised trials. Heart 2001; 85: 265–71.
15. Fleming M. Cardiovascular events and COX-2 inhibitors. J Am Med Assoc 2001; 286: 2808.
16. Burnakis TG. Cardiovascular events and COX-2 inhibitors. J Am Med Assoc 2001; 286: 2808.
17. Konstam MA, Demopoulos LA. Cardiovascular events and COX-2 inhibitors. J Am Med Assoc 2001; 286: 2809.
18. Grant KD. Cardiovascular events and COX-2 inhibitors. J Am Med Assoc 2001; 286: 2809.
19. Haldey EJ, Pappagallo M. Cardiovascular events and COX-2 inhibitors. J Am Med Assoc 2001; 286: 2808–13.
20. McGeer PL, McGeer EG, Yasojima K. Cardiovascular events and COX-2 inhibitors. J Am Med Assoc 2001: 286; 2810.
21. White WB, Whelton A. Cardiovascular events and COX-2 inhibitors. J Am Med Assoc 2001; 286: 2811–12.
22. Konstam MA, Weir MR, Reicin A, Shapiro D, Sperling RS, Barr E, Gertz BJ. Cardiovascular thrombotic events in controlled clinical trials of rofecoxib. Circulation 2001; 104: 1–9.
23. Johnson AG, Nguyen TV, Day RO. Do nonsteroidal anti-inflammatory drugs affect blood pressure? A meta-analysis. Ann Intern Med 1994; 121: 289–300.
24. Whelton A. Renal and related cardiovascular effects of conventional and COX-2-specific NSAIDs and non-NSAID analgesics. Am J Ther 2000; 7: 63–74.
25. Collins R, Peto R, MacMahon S, Hebert P, Fiebach NH, Eberlein KA, Godwin J, Qizilbash N, Taylor JO, Hannekens CH. Blood pressure, stroke, and coronary heart disease. Part 2. Short-term reductions in blood pressure: overview of randomised drug trials in their epidemiological context. Lancet 1990; 335: 827–38.
26. Whelton A, Maurath CJ, Verburg KM, Geis GS. Renal safety and tolerability of celecoxib, a novel cyclooxygenase-2 inhibitor. Am J Ther 2000; 7: 159–75.
27. Whelton A, Fort JG, Puma JA, Normandin D, Bello AE, Verburg KM. Cyclooxygenase-2-specific inhibitors and cardiorenal function: a randomized, controlled trial of celecoxib and rofecoxib in older hypertensive osteoarthritis patients. Am J Ther 201; 8: 85–95.
28. Dunn MJ. Are COX-2 selective inhibitors nephrotoxic? Am J Kidney Dis 2000; 35: 976–7.
29. Perazella MA, Tray K. Selective cyclooxygenase-2 inhibitors: a pattern of nephrotoxicity similar to traditional nonsteroidal anti-inflamatory drugs. Am J Med 200; 111: 64–7.
30. Emery P, Zeidler H, Kvien TK, Guslandi M, Naudin R, Stead H, Verburg KM, Isakson PC, Hubbard RC, Geis GS. Celecoxib versus diclofenac in long-term management of rheumatoid arthritis: randomised double-blind comparison. Lancet 1999; 354: 2106–11.
31. Simon LS, Weaver AL, Graham DY, Kivitz AJ, Lipsky PE, Hubbard RC, Isakson PC, Verburg KM, Yu SS, Zhao WW, Geis GS. Anti-inflammatory and upper gastrointestinal effects of celecoxib in rheumatoid arthritis: a randomized controlled trial. J Am Med Assoc 1999; 282: 1921–8.
32. Boyd IW, Mathew TH, Thomas MC. COX-2 inhibitors and renal failure: the triple whammy revisited. Med J Aust 2000; 274: 173–5.
33. Perazella MA, Eras J. Are selective COX-2 inhibitors nephrotoxic? Am J Kidney Dis 2000; 35: 937–40.
34. Pfister AK, Crisalli RJ, Carter WH. Cyclooxygenase-2 inhibition and renal function. Ann Intern Med 2001; 134: 1077.
35. Graham MG. Acute renal failure related to high-dose celecoxib. Ann Intern Med 2001; 135: 69–70.
36. Wolf G, Porth J, Stahl RAK. Acute renal failure associated with rofecoxib. Ann Intern Med 2000; 133: 394.
37. Zhao SZ, Reynolds MW, Lejkowith J, Whelton A, Arellano FM. A comparison of renal-related adverse drug reactions between rofecoxib and celecoxib, based on the World Health Organization/Uppsala Monitoring Centre safety database. Clin Ther 2001; 23: 1478–91.
38. Giardiello FM, Hansen FC 3rd, Lazenby AJ, Hellman DB, Milligan FD, Bayless TM, Yardley JH. Collagenous colitis in setting of nonsteroidal antiinflammatory drugs and antibiotics. Dig Dis Sci 1990; 35: 257–60.
39. Rampton DS, McNeil NI, Sarner M. Analgesic ingestion and other factors preceding relapse in ulcerative colitis. Gut 1983; 24: 187–9.
40. Rampton DS, Sladen GE. Relapse of ulcerative proctocolitis during treatment with non-steroidal anti-inflammatory drugs. Postgrad Med J 1981; 57: 297–9.
41. Kaufmann HJ, Taubin HL. Nonsteroidal anti-inflammatory drugs activate quiescent inflammatory bowel disease. Ann Intern Med 1987; 107: 513–16.
42. Felder JB, Korelitz BI, Rajapakse R, Schwarz S, Horatagis AP, Gleim G. Effects of nonsteroidal antiinflammatory drugs on inflammatory bowel dis-

ease: a case-control study. Am J Gastroenterol 2000; 95: 1949–54.
43. Bonner GF, Walczak M, Kitchen L, Bayona M. Tolerance of nonsteroidal antiinflammatory drugs in patients with inflammatory bowel disease. Am J Gastroenterol 2000; 95: 1946–8.
44. Sihvo S, Klaukka T, Martikainen J, Hemminki E. Frequency of daily over-the-counter drug use and potential clinically significant over-the-counter-prescription drug interactions in the Finnish adult population. Eur J Clin Pharmacol 2000; 56: 495–9.
45. Manfredini R, Ricci L, Giganti M, La Cecilia O, Kuwornu Afi H, Chierici F, Gallerani M. An uncommon case of fluid retention simulating a congestive heart failure after aspirin consumption. Am J Med Sci 2000; 320: 72–4.
46. Sorensen HT, Mellemkjaer L, Blot WJ, Nielsen GL, Steffensen FH, McLaughlin JK, Olsen JH. Risk of upper gastrointestinal bleeding associated with use of low-dose aspirin. Am J Gastroenterol 2000; 95: 2218–24.
47. Derry S, Loke YK. Risk of gastrointestinal haemorrhage with long term use of aspirin: meta-analysis. Br Med J 2000; 321: 1183–7.
48. Roderick PJ, Wilkes HC, Meade TW. The gastrointestinal toxicity of aspirin: an overview of randomised controlled trials. Br J Clin Pharmacol 1993; 35: 219–26.
49. Tramer MR, Moore RA, Reynolds DJ, McQuay HJ. Quantitative estimation of rare adverse events which follow a biological progression: a new model applied to chronic NSAID use. Pain 2000; 85: 169–82.
50. Weil J, Langman MJ, Wainwright P, Lawson DH, Rawlins M, Logan RF, Brown TP, Vessey MP, Murphy M, Colin-Jones DG. Peptic ulcer bleeding: accessory risk factor and interactions with non-steroidal anti-inflammatory drugs. Gut 2000; 46: 27–31.
51. Tramer MR. Aspirin, like all other drugs, is a poison. Br Med J 2000; 321: 1170–1.
52. Galindo PA, Borja J, Feo F, Gomez E, Encinas C, Garcia R. Nonpigmented fixed drug eruption caused by paracetamol. J Invest Allergol Clin Immunol 1999; 9: 399–400.
53. Ayonrinde OT, Saker BM. Anaphylactoid reactions to paracetamol. Postgrad Med J 2000; 76: 501–2.
54. Brackett CC, Bloch JD. Phenytoin as a possible cause of acetaminophen hepatotoxicity: case report and review of the literature. Pharmacotherapy 2000; 20: 229–33.
55. Katsinelos P, Dimiropoulos S, Vasiliadis T, Fotiadis G, Xiarchos P, Eugenidis N. Oesophageal ulceration associated with ingestion of mefenamic acid capsules. Eur J Gastroenterol Hepatol 1999; 11: 1431–2.
56. Del Pozo MD, Lobera T, Blasco A. Selective hypersensitivity to diclofenac. Allergy Eur J Allergy Clin Immunol 2000; 55: 412–13.
57. Anonymous. Diclofenac Dear Doctor letter issue in Japan. Scrip 2000; 17: 2597.
58. Krummel T, Dimitrov Y, Moulin B, Hannedouche T. Acute renal failure induced by topical ketoprofen. Br Med J 2000; 320: 93.
59. Offidani AM, Cellini A, Amerio P, Simonetti O, Bossi G. A case of persistent light reaction phenomenon to ketoprofen? Eur J Dermatol 2000; 10: 153–4.
60. Reinhart DJ. Minimising the adverse effects of ketorolac. Drug Saf 2000; 22: 487–97.
61. Anonymous. Loxoprofen hepatic warning tightened in Japan. Scrip 2000; 24: 2544.
62. Kurata C, Uehara A, Sugi T, Yamazaki K. Syncope caused by nonsteroidal anti-inflammatory drugs and angiotensin-converting enzyme inhibitors. Jpn Circ J 1999; 63: 1002–3.
63. Antony F, Layton AM. Nabumetone-associated pseudoporphyria. Br J Dermatol 2000; 142: 1067–9.
64. Checketts SR, Morgan GJ Jr. Two cases of nabumetone induced pseudoporphyria. J Rheumatol 1999; 26: 2703–5.
65. Cron RQ, Finkel TH. Nabumetone induced pseudoporphyria in childhood. J Rheumatol 2000; 27: 1817–18.
66. Dennis VC, Thomas BK, Hanlon JE, Potentiation of oral anticoagulation and hemarthrosis associated with nabumetone. Pharmacotherapy 2000; 20: 234–9.
67. Schapira D, Balbir-Gurman A, Nahir AM. Naproxen-induced leukocytoclastic vasculitis. Clin Rheumatol 2000; 19: 242–4.
68. Bouldin MB, Clowers-Webb HE, Davis JL, McEvory MT, Davis MD. Naproxen-associated linear IgA bullous dermatosis: case report and review. Mayo Clin Proc 2000; 75: 967–70.
69. Bujan JJ, Morante JM, Guemes MG, Del Pozo Losada J, Capdevila EF. Photoallergic contract dermatitis from piketoprofen. Contact Dermatitis 2000; 43: 315.
70. Lantz MS, Giambanco V. Acute onset of auditory hallucinations after initiation of celecoxib therapy. Am J Psychiatry 2000; 157: 1022–3.
71. Crofford LJ, Oates JC, McCune WJ, Gupta S, Kaplan MJ, Catella Lawson F, Morrow JD, McDonagh KT, Schmaier AH. Thrombosis in patients with connective tissue diseases treated with specific cyclooxygenase 2 inhibitors: a report of four cases. Arthritis Rheum 2000; 43: 1891–6.
72. Nachimuthu S, Volfinoz L, Gopal LN. Acute liver injury induced by celecoxib. Gastroenterology 2000; 118: 1471.
73. Anonymous. Celecoxib: early Australian reporting experience. Aust Adv Drug React Bull 2000; 19: 6.
74. Grob M, Scheidegger P, Wuthrich B,. Allergic skin reaction to celecoxib. Dermatology 2000; 201: 383.
75. Crouch TE, Stafford CT. Urticaria associated with COX-2 inhibitors. Ann Allergy Asthma Immunol 2000; 84: 140.
76. Cummins R, Wagner-Weiner L. Paller A. Pseudoporphyria induced by celecoxib in a patient

with juvenile rheumatoid arthritis. J Rheumatol 2000; 27: 2938–40.
77. Karim A, Tolbert D, Piergies A, Hubbard RC, Harper K. Celecoxib does not significantly alter the pharmacokinetics or hypoprothrombinemic effect of warfarin in healthy subjects. J Clin Pharmacol 2000; 40: 655–63.
78. McMorran M, Morawiecka I. Celecoxib (Celebrex^{TM}): 1 year later. Can Med Assoc J 2000; 162: 1044–6.
79. Linder JD, Monkemuller KE, Davis JV, Wilcox CM. Cyclooxygenase-2 inhibitor celecoxib: a possible cause of gastropathy and hypoprothrombinemia. South Med J 2000; 93: 930–2.
80. Mersfelder TL, Stewart LR. Warfarin and celecoxib interaction. Ann Pharmacother 2000; 34: 325–7.
81. Haase KK, Rojas-Fernandez Ch, Lane L, Frank DA. Potential interaction between celecoxib and warfarin. Ann Pharmacother 2000; 34: 666–7.
82. Couser RJ, Hoekstra RE, Ferrara TB, Wrigth GB, Cabalka AK, Connett JE. Neurodevelopmental follow-up at 36 months' corrected age of preterm infants treated with prophylactic indomethacin. Arch Pediatr Adolesc Med 2000; 154: 598–602.
83. Parilla BV, Grobman WA, Holtzman RB, Thomas HA, Dooley SL. Indomethacin tocolysis and risk of necrotizing enterocolitis. Obstet Gynecol 2000; 96: 120–3.
84. Jones MT, Stoner SC. Increased lithium concentrations reported in patients treated with sulindac. J Clin Psychiatry 2000; 61: 527–8.
85. Andrade RJ, Lucena MI, Fernandez MC, Gonzales M. Fatal hepatitis associated with nimesulide. J Hepatol 2000; 32: 174.
86. Schattner A, Sokolovskaya N, Cohen J. Fatal hepatitis and renal failure during treatment with nimesulide. J Intern Med 2000; 247: 153–5.
87. Holmes RP, Stone PR. Severe oligohydramnios induced by cyclooxygenase-2 inhibitor nimesulide. Obstet Gynecol 2000; 96: 810–11.
88. Tanna SB, Barnes JF, Seth SK. Desensitization to allopurinol in a patient with previous failed desensitization. Ann Pharmacother 1999; 33: 1180–3.
89. Vàzquez-Mellado J, Guzmàn Vàzquez S, Cazarín Barrientos J, Gòmez Ríos V, Burgos-Vargas R. Desensitisation to allopurinol after allopurinol hypersensitivity syndrome with renal involvement in gout. J Clin Rheumatol 2000; 6: 266–8.

T.G. Short and L. Nicholson

10 General anesthetics and therapeutic gases

ANESTHETIC VAPORS *(SED-14, 318; SEDA-22, 125; SEDA-23, 126; SEDA-24, 128)*

Sevoflurane is pleasant to breathe and has a rapid onset and offset of action. It is challenging the tradition of intravenous anesthetic induction in adult patients, sevoflurane 7–8% inhalation was compared to bolus doses of propofol for anesthetic induction (1[M]). Anesthesia maintenance included nitrous oxide 50–70% and either propofol infusion or sevoflurane inhalation, and spontaneous ventilation via a laryngeal mask. Patients in the sevoflurane group were significantly more likely to have postoperative *nausea* and *vomiting* (odds ratios 4.2 and 3.2). There were non-significant trends towards greater patient dissatisfaction and a longer induction time in the sevoflurane group, and more frequent apnea in the propofol group. There were no significant complications in either group. Both agents are suitable for anesthetic induction, but propofol retains a small advantage in having better recovery characteristics.

Single-agent induction and maintenance of anesthesia has been compared in a randomized study of 44 patients undergoing elective spinal surgery (2[c]). Patients received either propofol 4–6 μg/ml via a target controlled infusion or sevoflurane 8% for induction, and sevoflurane 3.5 with 67% nitrous oxide for maintenance plus alfentanil as required. Patients in the propofol group required a significantly larger dose of opiate during the procedure (2.2 vs 0.3 mg). Two patients who received propofol complained of *pain on injection*. There was no significant breath holding or laryngospasm in either group. Heart rate was significantly lower in the sevoflurane group compared with propofol both before and after incision. The number of adjustments to the patient's depth of anesthesia were similar in both groups. The authors concluded that either technique was suitable for spinal surgery. The inclusion of nitrous oxide in the sevoflurane group accounted for the differences in opioid requirements.

A combination of midazolam plus propofol has been compared with midazolam only for sedation in colonoscopy (3[c]). Midazolam alone produced less profound amnesia, and patients took longer to recover. There were no differences in cardiovascular or respiratory parameters. Oxygen saturation was poor in both groups, with saturations less than 85% in 22% of patients given midazolam and in 19% of patients given propofol, although the patients did not initially receive supplementary oxygen. In a similar comparison of midazolam and propofol as sedative agents for diagnostic endoscopy in 80 patients, endoscopy was judged successful in 98% of patients given propofol (mean total dose 354 mg) and 80% of patients given midazolam (mean total dose 8 mg) (4[c]). Patients in the propofol group recovered consciousness more quickly and had complete amnesia. One patient in the propofol group suffered an *apneic phase* with *impaired circulation*, requiring manual ventilation and drug therapy.

Anesthetist-administered midazolam and patient-controlled propofol have been compared for sedation during vitreoretinal surgery (5[c]). The patients received propofol 15–18 mg according to age, with a 1-minute lockout, or 0.25–0.5 mg of midazolam as judged necessary by the anesthetist. Few patients were amnesic for the procedure and both techniques produced satisfactory sedation and comfort. Non-anesthetists need to be extremely wary if using propofol for sedation, since propofol has a low therapeutic index and commonly causes *unconsciousness*, *respiratory depression*, and

Side Effects of Drugs, Annual 25
J.K. Aronson, ed.

cardiovascular collapse, particularly when it is used in combination with either midazolam or alfentanil (6[r]). Adequate staff, training, and facilities for resuscitation of patients must be available before considering propofol sedation. Propofol can cause *deep sedation*, and the episode reported in one of these studies is not surprising. Extreme caution must be exercised in recommending these techniques to non-anesthetists.

The effects of hypercapnia on cerebral autoregulation during sevoflurane or propofol anesthesia have been studied in a randomized cross-over study in eight healthy patients (7[c]). Hypercapnia began to inhibit cerebral autoregulation as measured by transcranial Doppler at a mean value of 56 mmHg P_aCO_2 with sevoflurane 1.0–1.1% and at 61 mmHg P_aCO_2 with propofol 140 μg/kg/min. Patients also received remifentanil for analgesia, a drug with no known effects on cerebral autoregulation. The study is important, because one advantage of both propofol anesthesia and sevoflurane anesthesia is the lack of inhibition of cerebral autoregulation at standard doses. Clearly, careful control of ventilation is required for this to be true.

The effects of isoflurane, sevoflurane, and propofol on jugular venous oxygen saturation (SjO_2) in patients undergoing coronary artery bypass surgery have been studied (8[c]). SjO_2 values were significantly lower in the propofol group 1 hour after bypass, suggesting an imbalance of oxygen supply and demand with propofol. Because anesthetic agents also reduce the cerebral metabolic rate, the implications of this finding are uncertain. However low SjO_2 values have previously been associated with postoperative neuropsychiatric dysfunction after cardiopulmonary bypass.

Respiratory The effects of desflurane and sevoflurane on bronchial smooth muscle reactivity have been compared in a randomized study of 40 patients (9[c]). Induction of anesthesia was with thiopental, followed by muscle relaxation and ventilation. Airway pressures were recorded during administration of desflurane or sevoflurane at one minimal alveolar concentration (MAC). Airway resistance increased by 5% in the desflurane group and fell by 15% in the sevoflurane group. The increase in airways resistance was greater in smokers and with desflurane, but did not differ with sevoflurane. The result was a surprise, given that desflurane stimulates the sympathetic nervous system. Thiopental also increased airways resistance by 10%. The result is important, because induction of anesthesia can cause bronchospasm and desflurane could exacerbate this.

Nervous system *Convulsions* during anesthesia are of concern because with the use of muscle relaxants they may go unrecognized. The epileptogenic properties of isoflurane and sevoflurane have been compared under a range of different ventilatory conditions in 24 ASA I or II mentally handicapped patients undergoing dental operations (10[c]). Half had a history of epilepsy and half did not. Each patient was ventilated with 100% oxygen and an end-tidal carbon dioxide (ET_{CO_2}) of 40 mmHg (A), then 50% oxygen 50% nitrous oxide ET_{CO_2} = 40 mmHg (B), then 100% oxygen ET_{CO_2} = 20 mmHg (C), at one MAC of isoflurane then at 1.5 and 2.0 MAC with each different mode of ventilation. The process was repeated 3 months later with sevoflurane. The electroencephalogram was concurrently recorded. The spike and wave index increased significantly from 2.0% during 1.0 MAC sevoflurane to 6.1% during 2.0 MAC in group A in the epilepsy group, while no spike activity was seen in the non-epilepsy group. Only a few spikes were observed in the isoflurane group in A with none in B or C. Supplementation with nitrous oxide or hyperventilation suppressed the occurrence of spikes. The authors concluded that sevoflurane has stronger epileptogenic properties than isoflurane, but that this can be counteracted by nitrous oxide or hyperventilation.

Halothane

Cardiovascular *Pulsus alternans* in association with hypercapnia occurred in a study of 120 patients who breathed spontaneously during halothane anesthesia (11[c]). End-tidal carbon dioxide concentration was allowed to rise freely until pulsus alternans or other cardiac dysrhythmias occurred. Ten of the patients developed pulsus alternans, which was promptly relieved on institution of positive pressure ventilation and the return of end-tidal carbon dioxide concentration to normal. The mechanism and the significance of this phenomenon are not well understood.

Respiratory A child who underwent induction of anesthesia with halothane developed *pulmonary edema* associated with hiccups (12[A]).

An 8-year-old girl with a history of seizures and cerebral ischemic strokes secondary to moya moya disease underwent anesthetic induction with halothane and 70% nitrous oxide. She had had three previous uneventful anesthetics. Hiccups started within seconds of induction of anesthesia and did not cease until 20 minutes later, when she was paralysed, intubated, and ventilated. During the next 20 minutes a period of hemodynamic instability ensued, with increasing oxygen requirements. The procedure was stopped and pulmonary edema was confirmed on chest X-ray. The child was transferred to the intensive care unit and ventilated overnight. Further recovery was uneventful.

Hiccups during anesthesia are often thought to be benign. Negative pressure pulmonary edema is usually associated with an obstructed airway, as occurs with laryngospasm, or other causes of upper airway obstruction, but was presumably the cause in this child.

Isoflurane

Liver A case of fatal *hepatotoxicity* associated with isoflurane has been reported (13[A]).

A 76-year-old woman with previous exposure to isoflurane 3 years earlier underwent an above-knee amputation for a liposarcoma using isoflurane anesthesia. On day 3 postoperatively she became febrile and confused. Bacterial cultures later showed *Staphylococcus aureus* in the sputum and *Escherichia coli* in the urine. Associated hypotension for 2 hours resolved with inotropic support, and renal function remained normal. On day 6 she became jaundiced and developed further hypotension. Despite intensive care treatment she died on day 7. An autopsy showed centrilobular necrosis consistent with drug-induced hepatitis. All other liver serology was negative.

The clinical details in this case were similar to those seen in halothane hepatitis. The authors concluded that although there was no direct evidence that isoflurane was the causative agent, it was the most likely agent to have caused this type of hepatitis. Unfortunately trifluoroacetic acid antibodies titers were not measured, because this test, if positive, would have confirmed the diagnosis. There is now a significant number of case reports of severe hepatitis associated with isoflurane, but the frequency appears to be significantly lower than for halothane.

Sevoflurane

Cardiovascular The effects of sevoflurane on cardiac conduction have been studied in 60 healthy unpremedicated infants (14[c]). Patients received sevoflurane either 8% from a primed circuit or at incremental increasing doses. *Nodal rhythm* occurred in 12 cases. The mean duration of the nodal rhythm was 62 seconds in the incremental group and 90 seconds in the 8% group. All of the dysrhythmias were self-limiting and there were no ventricular or supraventricular dysrhythmias. No adverse events occurred as a result of the dysrhythmias. This study highlights the importance of using electrocardiographic monitoring when inducing anesthesia with volatile agents.

Nervous system A *generalized tonic–clonic seizure* has been reported in association with the use of sevoflurane (15[A]).

A 19-year-old man with a history of metamphetamine abuse 3 weeks earlier, but no personal or family history of seizure activity had anesthesia induced with midazolam 1 mg, nitrous oxide 50%, and sevoflurane 8%. The sevoflurane was subsequently reduced to 2%. After radical orchidectomy the sevoflurane and nitrous oxide were withdrawn and oxygen 100% was given and 2 minutes later rhythmic jerking movements began in the legs and quickly spread to the rest of the body. The movements were accompanied by an arched back and a stiff neck. Arterial oxygen saturation dropped to 50% and ventilation was controlled, again using sevoflurane 8%. The duration of the seizure was about 4 minutes. The sevoflurane was again withdrawn 3 minutes later, and a similar seizure occurred. This time it was controlled with midazolam 1 mg and propofol 30 mg. Recovery was marked only by mild disorientation. Postoperative computerized tomography showed a ganglioneuroma in the posterior cortex. The electroencephalogram was normal.

Epileptiform activity on the electroencephalogram in association with sevoflurane has also been reported in two children aged 3 and 5 years in a center in which EEG monitoring is routine (16[A]). In both cases the activity occurred after several minutes of anesthesia, when the sevoflurane concentrations were increased to 7–8%. The epileptiform activity resolved after a reduction in sevoflurane concentrations. No seizure activity was noted.

Sevoflurane can cause epileptiform activity on the electroencephalogram, especially during emergence from anesthesia. It has also been associated with epileptiform discharges in volunteer studies, but clinical convulsions appear to be very rare. These cases show that clinicians need to be aware of the possibility of generalized seizures, especially in patients who are predisposed to seizures.

Urinary tract Sevoflurane can reportedly contribute to the development of *renal insufficiency*. The two mechanisms proposed are toxicity from compound A or fluoride ions. Compound A is a breakdown product of sevoflurane, which may occur in carbon dioxide absorbers and has been proven to be nephrotoxic in rats but not in humans. Fluoride ions are produced as a result of metabolism of sevoflurane and may reach high concentrations following prolonged anesthesia.

This topic has been reviewed in a meta-analysis of 22 controlled trials in 3436 patients (82% ASA I or II, 16% ASA III, and 2% ASA IV) (17[M]). The trials had compared sevoflurane for anesthesia maintenance with isoflurane, propofol, or enflurane. Serum creatinine and blood urea nitrogen were used to assess preoperative and postoperative renal function. The duration of anesthesia was 0.5–11 hours. Most patients (97%) were exposed to less than 4 MAC-hours of volatile agent. Reductions in the serum creatinine and blood urea nitrogen were significantly smaller with isoflurane than with sevoflurane. In patients who received concurrent aminoglycosides, sevoflurane was associated with a small increase in serum creatinine. The following factors had no effect on renal function: type of anesthetic circuit, choice of carbon dioxide absorber, inorganic fluoride ion concentration, duration of anesthesia, use of nitrous oxide, or how sick patients were. When all patients were considered, the incidences of clinically significant increases in serum creatinine were the same between agents. In patients with baseline creatinine values greater than 132 μmol/l (1.5 mg/daily) the incidence of clinically important increases in serum creatinine was significantly higher in both treatment groups compared with baseline. This meta-analysis has provided strong evidence that sevoflurane does not contribute to clinically significant renal insufficiency. More data are needed on its use for low-flow anesthesia.

Musculoskeletal *Prolongation of rapacuronium-induced neuromuscular blockade* by sevoflurane has been studied in a randomized placebo-controlled comparison with suxamethonium in 40 children (18[c]). Patients received sevoflurane and nitrous oxide anesthesia followed by rapacuronium 2 mg/kg. The study was stopped after only seven patients had been recruited, because the mean time to return of twitch height to 25% of baseline was 26 minutes. This time represents a stage at which neuromuscular blockade can be reversed and was twice as long as predicted from experience in adult patients. The authors suggested that the prolonged neuromuscular relaxation was due to the interaction of sevoflurane with rapacuronium, because this prolongation has not been observed using other inhalation agents.

NITROUS OXIDE *(SED-14, 325; SEDA-22, 128; SEDA-23, 129; SEDA-24, 132)*

Cardiovascular Nitrous oxide inhibits methionine synthase, thereby preventing the conversion of homocysteine to methionine. A high homocysteine concentration has also been identified as an independent risk factor for coronary artery and cerebrovascular disease. The effect of nitrous oxide on homocysteine concentrations and myocardial ischemia has been studied in a randomized controlled study in 90 patients, ASA grade 1–3, who received a standardized anesthetic consisting of propofol induction, an opioid, and either inhalational isoflurane or isoflurane and 50% nitrous oxide (19[C]). They underwent carotid endarterectomy (average operation duration 3.3 hours). Electrocardiographic monitoring consisted of a three-channel Holter monitor (leads II, V2, and V5), which was later examined for periods of ischemia by a physician blinded to treatment group. Myocardial enzyme activities were not measured. Baseline homocysteine concentrations (12.7 μmol/l) were significantly increased in the recovery room and at 48 hours to 15.5 and 18.8 μmol/l respectively. The concentrations did not increase in those not given nitrous oxide. Periods of preoperative and intraoperative ischemia did not differ. Postoperatively the nitrous oxide group had more patients with ischemia (19 vs 11), longer ischemic events in the first 24 hours (54 vs 17 minutes), and more episodes of ischemia lasting more than 30 minutes (23 vs 14). The authors concluded that nitrous oxide is associated with *increased myocardial ischemia*. They conceded that they had not shown causality. Previous studies have not shown this outcome, but were less sensitive, using only two-channel or once daily 12-lead electrocardiography, or not monitoring patients postoperatively. The subject warrants a major study before a firm conclusion can be drawn.

Nervous system A case of *myelopathy* associated with nitrous oxide abuse has been reported (20[A]).

A 23-year-old man presented with a 5-day history of gait disturbance and incoordination. He had severe loss of proprioception in his legs and could not walk. He was hypomanic. Severe posterior column myelopathy was diagnosed using MRI scanning. His nitrous oxide use had consisted of 40–60 whipped cream bulbs per day for 6 months. He also admitted to intermittent diamorphine abuse, but not for the 3 weeks before admission. He was treated with hydroxocobalamin and methionine, but still had minor abnormalities 3 months later.

The authors noted that although the evidence is scant, treatment should consist of both vitamin B_{12} and methionine.

INTRAVENOUS AGENTS

BARBITURATE ANESTHETICS

(SED-14, 327; SEDA-22, 129; SEDA-23, 131)

Thiopental

Endocrine Thiopental given for cerebral protection after cardiac arrest to patients in intensive care caused *altered thyroid function* (21[c]). Five patients received 5 mg/kg as a bolus followed by 3 mg/kg/hour for 48–72 hours. Free T_3 concentrations fell dramatically in three of them and remained near normal in the other two. In those in whom T_3 concentrations fell they returned to near normal on withdrawal of thiopental. Reverse T_3 concentrations increased in these patients. Although the study was not controlled, the authors speculated that thiopental causes conversion of T_3 to reverse T_3, and that this may intensify the euthyroid sick syndrome after cardiac arrest.

MISCELLANEOUS NON-BARBITURATE ANESTHETICS

Ketamine *(SED-14, 329; SEDA-22, 130; SEDA-23, 130; SEDA-24, 134)*

The addition of ketamine to bupivacaine for spinal anesthesia has been studied in 60 patients undergoing spinal anesthesia for insertion of intracavitory brachytherapy implants for cervical carcinoma (22[c]). They were randomly assigned to receive either bupivacaine 10 mg or bupivacaine 7.5 mg plus ketamine 25 mg. Motor recovery was significantly quicker in the ketamine group. *Blood pressure was significantly lower* in the bupivacaine group 5 minutes after administration, and *perioperative intravenous fluid requirements were significantly higher*. Patients given ketamine reported more *sedation* and *dizziness*, both intraoperatively and postoperatively. There were no nightmares or dissociative features. Overall satisfaction was better with bupivacaine. The study was abandoned after 30 patients, because of the high rate of adverse effects with ketamine. Although ketamine had local anesthetic sparing properties, its adverse effects made it unsuitable for intrathecal administration.

Nervous system There have been several attempts to attenuate the unpleasant adverse effects (*unpleasant dreams* and *hallucinations*) that occur after sedation with ketamine. The latest involve the use of clonidine (23[c]), midazolam (24[c]), and lamotrigine (25[c]).

Oral clonidine, 2.5 or 5.0 μg/kg, 90 minutes before ketamine 2 mg/kg has been compared with placebo in 39 patients (23[c]). In those given clonidine 2.5 μg/kg, heart rate responses were reduced compared with placebo (maximum heart rate 97 vs 76 beats/min). In those given clonidine 5 μg/kg, heart rate responses were less (maximum heart rate 97 vs 77 beats/min) and mean arterial pressure was lower (121 vs 141 mmHg), and there were fewer nightmares and less drooling. The psychomotor symptoms with this dose of ketamine were minimal and clonidine mainly limited the hemodynamic adverse effects.

The effect of intravenous midazolam 0.05 mg/kg on *emergence phenomena* after ketamine 1.5 mg/kg intravenously for painful procedures has been assessed in a randomized, double-blind, placebo-controlled study in 104 children (24[c]). Midazolam was given 2 minutes after the ketamine. There was no significant difference between the two groups in levels of agitation. The overall rate of agitation was low, but probably high enough to detect any significant differences between the groups.

The neuropsychiatric effects of ketamine were modulated by lamotrigine, a glutamate release inhibitor, in 16 healthy volunteers (25[c]). Lamotrigine 300 mg was given 2 hours before ketamine 0.26 and 0.65 mg/kg on two separate days. There were fewer ketamine-induced *perceptual abnormalities*, fewer *schizophreniform symptoms*, and less *learning and memory impairment*. Mood elevating effects were increased with lamotrigine. The authors commented that the results were experimental and that further studies are needed to confirm the potential benefits in a larger group of patients.

The pharmacological effects of the R- and S-enantiomers of ketamine have been compared in 11 subjects who received R-ketamine 0.5 mg then S-ketamine 0.15 mg, separated by 1 week (26[c]). Before and after each drug administration they were subjected to a painful stimulus using a nerve stimulator applied to the right central incisor tooth. Pain suppression was equal with the two drugs. The subjects reported more unpleasant *psychotomimetic effects* with S-ketamine and more pleasant effects with R-ketamine. Seven of 11 subjects preferred R-ketamine, while none preferred S-ketamine. These results suggest that the neuropsychiatric effect of ketamine may be predominantly due to the S-enantiomer, and that R-ketamine may be a better alternative. This study is in direct distinction to earlier work suggesting that R-ketamine is responsible for most of the undesirable neuropsychiatric side effects of ketamine.

Propofol *(SED-14, 330; SEDA-22, 130; SEDA-23, 132; SEDA-24, 135)*

Nervous system *Acute dystonia* has been reported in a 14-year-old girl after the administration of propofol 150 mg and fentanyl 50 mg for a dental anesthetic (27[A]). The intraoperative course was uneventful, but she developed non-rhythmic and non-symmetrical shaking in her upper limbs, unresponsive to diazepam and paraldehyde. A CT brain scan was normal. Her symptoms were eventually relieved by procyclidine 2.5 mg. This adverse effect has been reported many times in adults, but this is the first reported case of dystonia associated with propofol in a child.

Metabolic Propofol 2% has been compared with midazolam for sedation in 63 ventilated patients in intensive care (28[c]). They were randomly assigned to either propofol 1.5–6 mg/kg/hour or midazolam 0.1–0.35 mg/kg/hour. Sedation was considered a failure if greater rates were required or if triglyceride concentrations were over 5.7 mmol/l (500 mg/dl) on one occasion or greater than 4.0 mmol/l (350 mg/dl) on two occasions. Hemodynamic, respiratory, and neurological variables were similar. Sedation failure occurred in 15 patients given propofol, three with increased triglyceride concentrations and 12 with poor sedation. In comparison, sedation failed in only one of the patients given midazolam. Average *serum triglyceride concentrations were higher* in the propofol group. In a separate retrospective comparison triglyceride concentrations were lower than in similar patients treated with 1% propofol, and the sedation failure rate was lower using 2% propofol (9% vs 36%). The authors concluded that 2% propofol is safe but may be less efficient than midazolam. It should be noted that the dose ranges that they used may not have been comparable, leading to an artificially high failure to provide adequate sedation in the propofol group.

Musculoskeletal *Rhabdomyolysis* has been reported in two patients receiving propofol for sedation while being ventilated for severe asthma (29[A]).

A 47-year-old woman had an infusion of propofol 200 μg/kg/min for 4 days. On day 2 she developed hematuria, and laboratory investigations showed renal insufficiency with hyperkalemic metabolic acidosis. She died as a result of rhabdomyolysis with cardiac involvement.

A 41-year-old man who received propofol at rates of up to 222 μg/kg/min for 2 days developed oliguria and the propofol was withdrawn. He was also receiving fentanyl and low molecular weight heparin for deep vein thrombosis prophylaxis. He subsequently developed a very high creatine kinase activity (over 170 000 IU/l). Echocardiography showed globally depressed myocardial dysfunction. He subsequently recovered. The rates of propofol infusion were high and this was thought to be a contributing factor.

A similar death, possibly relating to propofol, has been reported in an 18-year-old man who suffered multiple trauma (30[A]). He was sedated for 98 hours with propofol 530–700 mg/hour. On day 5 he developed a metabolic acidosis with hyperkalemia and his serum was lipemic. An echocardiogram showed global hypokinesia. He deteriorated and died shortly afterwards.

Although in none of these cases was a definitive link between propofol and the pathology established, the authors pointed out that several other cases have been reported, especially in children. Clinicians should be more aware that propofol may cause rhabdomyolysis, which appears to occur particularly at high doses.

Infection risk Shortly after the introduction of propofol in 1989, clusters of infection related to its use were reported, and there have been several new reports (31[r], 32[r]). The complications include *hypotension*, *tachycardia*, *septic shock*, *convulsions*, and *death*. Ethylenediaminetetra-acetic acid (EDTA) has been added to the formulation to retard microbial growth. However, there have been concerns over the effects of this additive on trace element homeostasis, particularly when it is used in intensive care units for long-term sedation. Five randomized controlled trials have been reviewed, and minimal or no effects have been found on zinc, magnesium, or calcium homeostasis. However, there is no evidence to suggest that cluster infection has been or will be reduced with this formulation and there is still a need for care with sterility when using this product.

BENZODIAZEPINES *(SED-14, 327; SEDA-22, 129; SEDA-23, 131; SEDA-24, 133; see also Chapter 5)*

Diazepam

Cardiovascular Inadvertent intra-arterial injection of diazepam (2.5 mg in 0.5 ml) has been reported in an 8-year-old girl (33[A]). *Gangrene* resulted and amputation of the 4th and 5th fingers was required. This complication has been previously reported with diazepam and is also well known with other classes of drugs, such as barbiturates and phenothiazines. It appears to be caused by the drug rather than the solvent used in the intravenous formulations.

Nervous system A paradoxical response to diazepam has been reported in a 20-year-old man with complex partial seizures who presented with exacerbation of his disease (34[A]). He was taking phenytoin and sodium valproate, with plasma concentrations in the target ranges. During a video electroencephalogram recording he was given diazepam 10 mg, and the partial seizures developed into frequent *generalized seizures*. The same response was seen on a subsequent occasion. The authors commented that although paradoxical reactions to benzodiazepines are rare, they should be considered in cases of refractory epilepsy.

Endocrine The *syndrome of inappropriate secretion of antidiuretic hormone* (SIADH) has been described in a neonate born to a mother taking diazepam chronically for epilepsy (35[A]). The baby was delivered at 41 weeks by normal vaginal delivery and had Apgar scores of 8 and 10 at 1 and 5 minutes after delivery. The baby was admitted to a neonatal intensive care unit in anticipation of drug withdrawal. SIADH was diagnosed on clinical and laboratory evidence. Recovery was uneventful. This is the first described case of SIADH caused by neonatal drug withdrawal when only a benzodiazepine has been given.

Skin *Sweet's syndrome*, an inflammatory dermatitis associated with a high white blood cell count and fever, has been described in a 70-year-old man who took diazepam 10 mg bd for 5 days (36[A]). He had taken no other medications in the preceding days. The diazepam was withdrawn and prednisone 30 mg/day, tapering over 2 weeks, was prescribed. The lesions cleared within 10 days.

Flunitrazepam

Withdrawal syndrome and delirium has been attributed to flunitrazepam (37[A]).

A 69-year-old man in intensive care received flunitrazepam 13 μg/kg/hour for 36 hours. The diagnosis of drug withdrawal and delirium, 6 days after withdrawal of flunitrazepam, was made on clinical and laboratory evidence. No other sedatives or analgesics were given throughout his stay. Recovery was uneventful.

The authors commented that physicians should be more aware of drug withdrawal syndromes, even after limited periods of administration of sedative drugs.

Midazolam

A cherry-flavored midazolam syrup has been evaluated for premedication in 85 children requiring general anesthesia (38[c]). The patients received a randomly assigned dose of 0.25, 0.5, or 1 mg/kg. All clinicians and observers were blinded to the treatment group. There was satisfactory dose-related sedation in 81%, and 83% had satisfactory non-dose-related anxiolysis at separation from parents and at anesthetic induction. One or more adverse events occurred in 36%, but only 31% of these were judged as possibly related to midazolam (*hiccups* 6%, *hypoxemia* 6%, *vomiting* 5%, *hallucinations* 4%, *drooling* 4%, *agitation* 2%, *coughing* 2%, *diplopia* 2%, *dizziness* 2%, and *hypotension* 2%). The authors suggested that although adverse effects were common they were minor, and that midazolam premedication allowed for successful anesthesia without high levels of anxiety.

Ear, nose, throat Midazolam nasal spray 2 mg/kg has been compared with a citric acid placebo for conscious sedation in children undergoing painful procedures (39[c]). Citric acid was added to the placebo so that the sensation of nasal burning caused by midazolam did not unblind the observers. The procedure consisted of intravenous cannulation, with the use of EMLA cream for topical analgesia. Parents and nurses judged the procedure to be more comfortable with midazolam, but children rated the discomfort of the procedure similar in the two groups. Anxiety was significantly reduced by midazolam. There was *nasal discomfort* in 43% of the midazolam group. The authors concluded that midazolam intranasal spray effectively reduces anxiety, but that its use may be limited by nasal discomfort.

Nervous system Midazolam can cause paradoxical reactions, including increased *agitation* and *poor cooperation* (40[c], 41[r]). Often other drugs are required to continue the procedure successfully. Reversal of the phenomena by flumazenil, a benzodiazepine antagonist, has been reported. In 30 patients flumazenil 0.15–0.5 mg resulted in cessation of the agitation without reversal of sedation. Adverse effects of flumazenil were not reported. Care must be taken when considering the use of flumazenil for reversal of midazolam-induced agitation, as these data are anecdotal and no controlled trials have been published.

REFERENCES

1. Joo HS, Perks WJ. Sevoflurane versus propofol for anesthetic induction: a meta analysis. Anesth Analg 2000; 91: 213–19.
2. Watson KR, Shah MV. Clinical comparison of "single agent" anaesthesia with sevofurane versus target controlled infusion of propofol. Br J Anaesth 2000; 85: 541–6.
3. Reimann FM, Samson U, Derad M, Schiefer B, Stange EF. Synergistic sedation with low-dose midazolam and propofol for colonoscopies. Endoscopy 2000; 32: 239–44.
4. Jung M, Hofmann C, Kiecclich R, Brackertz A. Improved sedation in diagnostic and therapeutic ERCP: propofol is an alternative to midazolam. Endoscopy 2000; 32: 233–8.
5. Morley HR, Karagiannis A, Schultz DJ, Walker JC, Newland HS. Sedation for vitreoretinal surgery: a comparison of anaesthetist administered midazolam and patient controlled sedation with propofol. Anaesth Intensive Care 2000; 28: 37–42.
6. Bell GD, Charlton JE. Colonoscopy – is sedation necessary and is there any role for intravenous propofol? Endoscopy 2000; 32: 264–7.
7. McCulloch TJ, Visco E, Lam AM. Graded hypercapnia and cerebral autoregulation during sevoflurane or propofol anesthesia. Anesthesiology 2000; 93: 1205–9.
8. Nandate K, Vuylsteke A, Ratsep I, Messahel S, Oduro-Dominah A, Menon DK, Matta BF. Effects of isoflurane, sevoflurane and propofol anaesthesia on jugular venous oxygen saturation in patients undergoing coronary artery bypass surgery. Br J Anaesth 2000; 84: 631–3.
9. Goff MJ, Arain SR, Ficke DJ, Uhrich TD, Ebert TJ. Absence of bronchodilation during desflurane anesthesia: a comparison to sevoflurane and thiopentone. Anesthesiology 2000; 93: 404–8.
10. Iijima T, Nakamura Z, Iwao Y, Sankawa H. The epileptogenic properties of the volatile anesthetics

sevoflurane and isoflurane in patients with epilepsy. Anesth Analg 2000; 91: 989–95.
11. Saghaei M, Mortazavian M. Pulsus alternans during general anesthesia with halothane. Anesthesiology 2000; 93: 91–4.
12. Stuth EAE, Stucke AG, Berens RJ. Negative-pressure pulmonary edema in a child with hiccups during induction. Anesthesiology 2000; 93: 282–4.
13. Turner GB, O'Rourke D, Scott GO, Beringer TRO. Fatal hepatotoxicity after re-exposure to isoflurane: a case report and review of the literature. Eur J Gastroenterol Hepatol 2000; 12: 955–9.
14. Green DH, Townsend P, Bagshaw O, Stokes MA. Nodal rhythm and bradycardia during inhalational induction with sevoflurane in infants: a comparison of incremental and high-concentration techniques. Br J Anaesth 2000; 85: 368–70.
15. Hilty CA, Drummond JC. Seizure-like activity from sevoflurane anesthesia. Anesthesiology 2000; 93: 1357–9.
16. Schultz A, Schultz B, Grouven U, Korsch G. Epileptiform activity in the EEGs of two nonepileptic children under sevoflurane anaesthesia. Anaesth Intensive Care 2000; 28: 205–7.
17. Mazze RI, Callan CM, Galvez ST, Delgado-Herrera L, Mayer DB. The effects of sevoflurane on serum creatinine and blood urea nitrogen concentrations: a retrospective twenty-two-center, comparative evaluation of renal function in adult surgical patients. Anesth Analg 2000; 90: 683–8.
18. Cara DM, Armory P, Mahajan RP. Prolonged duration of the neuromuscular block with rapacuronium in the presence of sevoflurane. Anesth Analg 2000; 91: 1392–3.
19. Badner NH, Beattie WS, Freeman D, Spence JD. Nitrous oxide-induced increased homocysteine concentrations are associated with increased postoperative myocardial ischaemia in patients undergoing carotid endarterectomy. Anesth Analg 2000; 91: 1073–9.
20. Butzkueven H, King JO. Nitrous oxide myelopathy in an abuser of whipped cream bulbs. J Clin Neurosci 2000; 7: 73–5.
21. Kotake Y, Matsumoto M, Takeda J. Thiopental intensifies the euthyroid sick syndrome after cardiopulmonary resuscitation. J Anesth 2000; 14: 38–41.
22. Kathirvel S, Sadhasivam S, Saxena A, Kannan TR, Ganjoo P. Effects of intrathecal ketamine added to bupivacaine for spinal anaesthesia. Anaesthesia 2000; 55: 899–910.
23. Handa F, Tanaka M, Nishikawa T, Toyooka H. Effects of oral clonidine premedication on side effects of intravenous ketamine anesthesia: a randomised double-blind, placebo-controlled study. J Clin Anesth 2000; 12: 19–24.
24. Sherwin TS, Green SM, Khan A, Chapman DS, Dannanburg B. Does adjunctive midazolam reduce recovery agitation after ketamine sedation for pediatric procedures? A randomised, double-blind, placebo-controlled trial. Ann Emerg Med 2000; 35: 229–38.
25. Anand A, Charney DS, Oren DA, Berman RM, Hu XS, Cappiello A, Krystal JH. Attenuation of the neuropsychiatric effects of ketamine with lamotrigine. Arch Gen Psychiatry 2000; 57: 270–6.
26. Rabben T. Effects of the NMDA receptor antagonist ketamine in electrically induced Ad-fiber pain. Methods Find Exp Clin Pharmacol 2000; 22: 185–9.
27. Bragonier R, Bartle D, Langton-Hewer S. Acute dystonia in a 14-yr-old following propofol and fentanyl anaesthesia. Br J Anaesth 2000; 84: 828–9.
28. Camps AC, Riera JASI, Vazquez DT, Borges MS, Rodriguez JP, Lopez EA. Midazolam and 2% propofol in long-term sedation of traumatized, critically ill patients: efficacy and sedation. Crit Care Med 2000; 28: 3612–19.
29. Stelow EB, Johari VP, Smith SA, Crosson JT, Apple FS. Propofol-associated rhabdomyolysis with cardiac involvement in adults: chemical and anatomic findings. Clin Chem 2000; 46: 577–81.
30. Perrier ND, Baerga-Varela Y, Murray MJ. Death related to propofol use in an adult patient. Crit Care Med 2000; 28: 3071–4.
31. Zaloga GP, Teres D. The safety and efficacy of propofol containing EDTA: a randomised clinical trial programme focusing on cation and trace metal homeostasis in critically ill patients. Intensive Care Med 2000; 26: S398–9.
32. Mehta U, Gunston GD, O'Connor N. Serious consequences to the misuse of propofol anaesthetic. S Afr Med J 2000; 90: 240.
33. Derakshan MR, Amputation due to inadvertent intra-arterial diazepam injection. Iran J Med Sci 2000; 25: 84–6.
34. Al Tahan A. Paradoxical response to diazepam in complex partial status epilepticus. Arch Med Res 2000; 31: 101–4.
35. Nako Y, Tachibana A, Harigaya A, Tomomasa T, Morikawa A. Syndrome of inappropriate secretion of antidiuretic hormone complicating neonatal diazepam withdrawal. Acta Paediatr 2000; 89: 488–95.
36. Guimera FJ, Garcia-Bustinduy M, Noda A, Saez M, Dorta S, Sanchez R, Martin-Herrera A, Garcia-Montelongo R. Diazepam related Sweet's syndrome. Int J Dermatol 2000; 39: 795–800.
37. Diehl JL, Guillibert E, Guerot E, Kimounn E, Labousse J. Acute benzodiazepine withdrawal delirium after a short course of flunitrazepam in an intensive care patient. Ann Med Interne 2000; 151 Suppl A: 44–6.
38. Marshall J, Rodarte A, Blumer J, Khoo KC, Akbari B, Kearns G. Pediatric pharmacodynamics of midazolam oral syrup. J Clin Pharmacol 2000; 40: 578–89.
39. Ljungman G, Kreuger A, Andréasson S, Gordh T, Sörensen S. Midazolam nasal spray reduces procedural anxiety in children. Paediatrics 2000; 105: 73–8.
40. Fulton SA, Mullen KD. Completion of upper endoscopic procedures despite paradoxical reac-

tion to midazolam: a role for flumazenil? Am J Gastroenterol 2000; 95: 809–11.
41. Saltik IN, Ozen H. Role of flumazenil for paradoxical reaction to midazolam during endoscopic procedures in children. Am J Gastroenterol 2000; 3011–12.

Stephan A. Schug and Malcolm C. Thornton

11 Local anesthetics

GENERAL TOPICS

Immunologic A 23-year-old woman developed an *allergic contact dermatitis* after applying an over-the-counter proprietary antipruritic jelly containing 0.1% dibucaine chloride, and a "caine" mixture (5% benzocaine, 1% dibucaine hydrochloride, 1% procaine hydrochloride) (1[A]). She had positive patch testing to both components.

EFFECTS RELATED TO DIFFERENT MODES OF USE

Brachial plexus anesthesia

Patient-controlled interscalene analgesia (PCIA) with ropivacaine 0.2% has been compared with patient-controlled intravenous analgesia (PCIVA) with opioid in 35 patients after elective major shoulder surgery (2[c]). Although *hemidiaphragmatic excursion* on the non-operated side was increased in the PCIA group 24 and 48 hours after the initial block, pulmonary function was similar in both groups. Pain was significantly better controlled in the PCIA group at 12 and 24 hours and the PCIA group had a lower incidence of *nausea* and *vomiting* (5.5% vs 60%).

Respiratory A 55-year-old man with newly diagnosed non-small-cell lung cancer developed *difficulty in breathing*, *cyanosis*, *agitation*, and *confusion* 10 minutes after interscalene supplementation of an axillary nerve block with only 3 ml of 2% mepivacaine with adrenaline (3[A]). He was anesthetized, intubated, and ventilated. Surgery proceeded and postoperative radiographic examination of the lungs showed ipsilateral elevation of the diaphragm with reduced respiratory excursion. Phrenic nerve block after the interscalene injection was the postulated cause of the deterioration in respiratory function. He was successfully extubated at the end of the procedure.

Caudal, epidural, and spinal anesthesia

Caudal anesthesia

In a 31-day-old neonate inadvertent *venous cannulation* with a caudally placed epidural catheter was detected by a positive test dose with adrenaline containing local anesthetic (4[A]).

Epidural anesthesia

A 1-year-old boy inadvertently received ropivacaine 6 mg intravenously over 2 hours when his epidural infusion was incorrectly connected to his intravenous cannula (5[A]). He had already received ropivacaine 28 mg via his epidural catheter. He suffered no overt adverse effects.

Patient controlled epidural analgesia using either 0.125% ropivacaine with fentanyl 2 μg/ml or 0.125% bupivacaine with fentanyl 2 μg/ml was studied in 50 patients during labor. Significantly more patients receiving bupivacaine developed motor blockade; 68% of patients in the bupivacaine group developed minimal *motor block* (Bromage score = 1), while the majority (68%) of patients in the ropivacaine group had no motor blockade. The incidences of adverse effects were similar in both groups. *Hypotension* occurred in 24% of the ropivacaine group and 16% of the bupivacaine group. *Pruritus* occurred in 56% of the ropivacaine group and 52% of the bupivacaine group (6[c]).

Cardiovascular A 27-year-old woman de-

Side Effects of Drugs, Annual 25
J.K. Aronson, ed.

veloped significant *myocardial depression* and *pulmonary edema* after administration of 5 ml of bupivacaine 0.5% via an epidural catheter (7[A]). The bupivacaine followed a test dose of 3 ml lidocaine 2%. Although initial aspiration on the epidural catheter was negative, the most likely explanation must be inadvertent intravascular administration of lidocaine and bupivacaine.

Nervous system *Total spinal anesthesia* was the reason for potentially life-threatening complications of epidural anesthesia in three cases.

A 68-year-old man developed total spinal anesthesia after the administration of 20 ml of ropivacaine 1% without a prior test dose via an epidural catheter, which was inadvertently placed intrathecally (8[A]). Initial aspiration of both the Touhy needle and the catheter failed to identify the intrathecal position of the catheter. The patient noted weakness in his right leg immediately after the end of the injection. This was followed by weakness in his right arm, asystole, apnea, and loss of consciousness. Ventricular escape beats were noted and sinus rhythm returned after mask ventilation with 100% oxygen and the administration of atropine 1 mg and ephedrine 50 mg. He was able to open his eyes, but remained apneic and was therefore intubated and ventilated. Cardiovascular stability was maintained with incremental boluses of ephedrine to a total of 60 mg. He regained consciousness and was successfully extubated 145 minutes later. All sensory and motor deficits had resolved within 8 hours and no neurological deficit or transient neurological symptoms were detected 5 days later.

This complication emphasizes the fact that aspiration is not sufficient to identify an intrathecal catheter position and that a large dose of a local anesthetic should be never administered without a prior test dose.

Total spinal anesthesia was suspected in a 46-year-old man who was found unconscious and apneic with no palpable cardiac output 20 minutes after a high thoracic (T2/3) epidural injection of 3 ml lidocaine 1% and 3 ml bupivacaine 0.125% (9[A]). Following initial cardiopulmonary resuscitation he was admitted to the intensive care unit, where treatment included mechanical lung ventilation, thiamylal infusion, and cooling to a core temperature of 33–34° C. The thiamylal was withdrawn after 17 days and he was warmed and successfully extubated the next day. He was discharged after a further 4 months of rehabilitation with no relevant neurological consequences.

Delayed onset, prolonged coma, and flaccid quadriplegia occurred in a 22-year-old woman 2 hours after an injection of fentanyl 100 μg and 10 ml bupivacaine 0.25%, given in divided doses (4, 3, and 3 ml) via an epidural catheter (10[A]). At the time of the initial attempt at insertion she had complained of severe cervico-occipital pain with loss of resistance to air injection. Despite negative aspiration of CSF the physician suspected intrathecal injection of air and abandoned the attempt at epidural catheter placement at that level. An epidural catheter was successfully inserted one level higher. Within 1 hour of the original epidural injection she developed hypotension requiring ephedrine, and a surprisingly high sensory block to T6 with profound lower limb motor blockade. This progressed 2 hours later to upper limb weakness, with respiratory failure requiring intubation and ventilation. She remained unconscious for 9 hours after the initial intubating dose of thiopental. She was able to move all of her limbs 26 hours later and was successfully extubated 43 hours later.

In the last case the authors felt that although the initial picture looked like the effects of subdural injection of bupivacaine and fentanyl, the prolonged coma with high motor blockade was more reminiscent of total spinal injection. They postulated that delayed total spinal anesthesia had occurred in this patient as a result of the epidural administration of a large quantity of bupivacaine and fentanyl via a hole made in the dura during the first attempt at epidural insertion.

An 85-year-old woman undergoing elective right total knee replacement had *prolonged motor blockade* of her left leg when her epidural ropivacaine (0.2% at 8–10 ml/hour) infusion was discontinued on the third postoperative day; normal motor function had returned by the sixth postoperative day (11[A]).

Transient neurological symptoms, previously only described after spinal anesthesia, have been reported in two parturients who received lidocaine 45 mg with adrenaline 5 μg/ml as a test dose followed by bupivacaine (12[A]). One patient received a single dose of bupivacaine 12.5 mg and the other received a total of 62 mg bupivacaine administered as two 5 ml and one 3 ml bolus of 0.25% bupivacaine followed by an infusion of 0.125% bupivacaine at 5 ml/hour for 4 hours 40 minutes. Both patients later developed reversible burning lower back, buttock pain, and leg pain; there was nothing to suggest intrathecal administration of local anesthetic in either case. Both patients gave birth in the lithotomy position, which may have been contributory.

Severe burning pain in the buttocks, thighs, and calves has been described in a 5-year-old boy who was given 0.25% bupivacaine and morphine epidurally for perioperative and postoperative analgesia (13[A]). The authors made the diagnosis of transient neurological symptoms, a first in a child.

Horner's syndrome has been reported after lumbar epidural block on two separate occasions in two patients who were having lumbar epidural anesthesia for chronic pain treatment (14[A]). The authors suggested that this complication had probably occurred through anatomical changes in the epidural space, leading to a high degree of sympathetic blockade.

A watershed *cerebral infarct* with subsequent full recovery has been described in a 70-year-old man 8 hours after a hypotensive event following an incremental bolus of 1% lidocaine 10 ml via an established epidural catheter (15[A]). A cause and effect relation cannot be established in such cases.

Endocrine Symptomatic hypoglycemia occurred in a healthy 30-year-old primigravida after a second 5 ml bolus of 0.25% bupivacaine administered epidurally during labor (16[A]). She developed an altered mental state, which responded rapidly to 50 ml of 50% dextrose administered intravenously.

Intrathecal (spinal) anesthesia

Intrathecal isobaric ropivacaine (15 mg) has been compared with intrathecal isobaric bupivacaine (10 mg) in 100 patients having transurethral resection of the bladder or prostate (17[C]). Median cephalad spread of blocks was two segments higher for both pinprick and cold with bupivacaine compared with ropivacaine. Onset time to anesthesia was the same in both groups. Significantly more patients in the ropivacaine group complained of painful sensations at the surgical site (16% vs 0%). There was no difference in anesthetic duration, the incidence, intensity, onset, and duration of motor blockade, or the incidence of hypotension in the two groups. There were no cases of transient neurological symptoms. The authors concluded that ropivacaine 15 mg is less potent than bupivacaine 10 mg for intrathecal analgesia.

In 80 patients undergoing lower extremity or lower abdominal surgery randomized to receive hyperbaric bupivacaine 10 mg alone or in combination with fentanyl 12.5 μg intrathecally, those given fentanyl had significantly longer duration of analgesia with no reported sedation or respiratory depression (18[C]). *Pruritus* occurred in 20% of patients given fentanyl and *shivering* occurred significantly more often in those given bupivacaine only (30% vs 12.5%).

The addition of low doses of clonidine and neostigmine to intrathecal bupivacaine–fentanyl in 30 patients in labor significantly increased the duration of analgesia but was associated with significantly more *emesis* (19[c]).

In a comparison of intrathecal bupivacaine 10 mg and bupivacaine 7.5 mg combined with ketamine 25 mg in 30 healthy women, there was no extension of postoperative analgesia or reduction in postoperative analgesic requirements in those given ketamine (20[c]). Those given ketamine had a shorter duration of motor blockade, but had an increased incidence of adverse effects, and the study was abandoned after 30 patients.

Intrathecal blockade with 0.5% isobaric bupivacaine 10 mg has been compared with 0.5% isobaric bupivacaine 5 mg combined with fentanyl 25 μg (diluted to 2 ml with isotonic saline) in 32 patients undergoing elective cesarean section (21[c]). The bupivacaine–fentanyl combination was associated with significantly less *hypotension* than bupivacaine alone (31% vs 94%) and a near 10-fold reduction in the mean ephedrine requirement (2.8 vs 23.8 mg). There were also significant differences in the incidence of *nausea* (31% vs 69%) and the median time to peak block (8 vs 10 minutes) with bupivacaine plus fentanyl. The authors advised further large-scale studies to quantify the minimum dose of bupivacaine plus fentanyl for single-dose spinal anesthesia.

Cardiovascular Isobaric bupivacaine 4 mg combined with fentanyl 20 μg has been compared with isobaric bupivacaine 10 mg alone in 20 patients over the age of 70 undergoing surgery for fractured neck of femur (21[c]). Hypotension was defined as a systolic blood pressure less than 90 mmHg or a fall in mean arterial pressure of more than 25%. Significantly more patients given bupivacaine only had *hypotension* (90% vs 10%). The mean dosage requirement of ephedrine was higher with bupivacaine only (32 vs 0.5 mg) and two patients in this group required phenylephrine, while no patient given bupivacaine plus fentanyl did. No patient in either group complained of perioperative pain or required supplementary analgesia intraoperatively.

Nervous system A 40-year-old woman developed *acute aphasia* and a *change in mental status* 15 minutes after the intrathecal administration of sufentanil 10 μg and isobaric bupivacaine 2.5 mg as part of a combined spinal epidural anesthetic for analgesia during labor (22[A]). She appeared to be in a *dissociated state*, had apparent *difficulty swallowing* and was *aphasic*, but able to follow simple commands. She had sensory block to T6 on the right and T8 on the left, with no motor block. The neurological picture resolved about 100 minutes after the anesthetic; an exact etiology could not be established.

A similar case has been reported 20 minutes after the intrathecal administration of 0.5% hyperbaric bupivacaine 2 ml for cesarean section (23[A]). She became unresponsive then apneic for a short time. There were no changes in heart rate or blood pressure and no loss of airway protection. She slowly regained consciousness over the next hour without any consequences. The authors were unclear about the cause and suggested subdural injection, as the slow onset, stable hemodynamics, and rapid recovery were suggestive of this complication. However, other causes, including a psychogenic response, are possibilities.

A 36-year-old man had two *generalized tonic–clonic convulsions* after receiving intrathecal tetracaine 8 mg to supplement inadequate block established by intrathecal administration of tetracaine 10 mg (24[A]). His seizures were controlled with intravenous thiamylal sodium. He regained consciousness, but complained of dizziness and blurred vision. He had a sensory block to T4–5. The authors excluded total spinal anesthesia as a cause of the seizures, on the basis of the sensory level and the lack of hypotension.

New onset, severe lightning pain after repeated subarachnoid blockade occurred in a 48-year-old man with pre-existing neuropathic pain after incomplete spinal cord injury, similar to previous reports in patients with phantom limb pain (25[A]).

A 30-year-old patient developed aseptic meningitis 24 hours after spinal anesthesia with bupivacaine plus fentanyl; it resolved without sequelae within 48 hours (26[A]).

Transient neurological symptoms and intrathecal local anesthetics

Neurological sequelae of intrathecal anesthesia are rare and usually minor. However, in recent years there has been a growing number of reports of transient neurological symptoms associated with the use of both isobaric and hyperbaric solutions of local anesthetics. In previous years hyperbaric lidocaine 5% dominated the literature, but there are now reports with most other local anesthetics.

Incidence *Transient neurological symptoms have been studied in patients given intrathecal lidocaine 2% or intrathecal prilocaine 2%. In one study of 70 patients transient neurological symptoms occurred in 20% of patients given lidocaine, with no cases in those given prilocaine (27[C]). In another study in 70 patients given intrathecal procaine or lidocaine in a 2:1 dose ratio there were significantly more transient neurological symptoms with lidocaine than with procaine (31% vs 6%) (28[C]). However, in a similar study of 100 patients there was no significant difference in the incidence of transient neurological symptoms, although the trend suggested a lower incidence with prilocaine (4% vs 14.3%) (29[C]).*

In 110 patients presenting for knee arthroscopy who were randomized to receive either 1% hypobaric lidocaine 50 mg or 1% hypobaric lidocaine 20 mg + fentanyl 25 μg complaints of transient neurological symptoms were nearly 10 times more frequent in those given lidocaine 50 mg (32.7% vs 3.6%) (30[C]). Patients given lidocaine 50 mg also had a greater fall in systolic blood pressure and a greater need for ephedrine.

Effect of position *Transient neurological symptoms occurred in five of 12 volunteers given 5% lidocaine 50 mg intrathecally and then placed in the low lithotomy position (31[c]). No consistent abnormalities were detected by prespinal and postspinal electromyography, nerve conduction studies, or somatosensory evoked potentials. This is in line with the current opinion that transient neurological symptoms constitute neither a neurological syndrome nor an expression of the neurotoxicity of local anesthetics.*

In 70 patients undergoing surgery in the supine position there were transient neurological symptoms in 26% of patients after intrathecal lidocaine, compared with 3% after intrathecal bupivacaine (32[C]). The incidence of transient neurological symptoms after intrathecal lidocaine 5% in patients undergoing surgery in the supine position is therefore similar to the previously reported incidence in the lithotomy position.

Mechanism *A high concentration of tetracaine given intrathecally in rabbits caused neuronal injury and glutamate release in the CSF (33[E]). The authors postulated that this might give some insight into the mechanisms of neurotoxicity of intrathecal local anesthetics.*

Cervical plexus anesthesia

Two cases of *recurrent laryngeal nerve blockade* during deep cervical plexus anesthesia for carotid endarterectomy have been reported. One patient complained of being unable to clear secretions effectively from her throat, had a paroxysm of coughing, and developed a large neck hematoma requiring surgical reexploration (34[A]).

Respiratory A 71-year-old man complained of *difficulty in breathing* and was desaturated on pulse oximetry for 5 minutes after cervical plexus blockade (35[A]). He required tracheal intubation, was ventilated for 110 minutes, and was then successfully extubated. It was thought that the most likely diagnosis was cardiorespiratory failure exacerbated by phrenic nerve blockade.

Nervous system A 67-year-old man developed transient *hemiparesis* and *facial nerve palsy* before becoming *unconscious* and *apneic* 10 minutes after a right cervical plexus block (35[A]). His trachea was intubated without the need for anesthetic drugs and he was ventilated. *Hypotension* was treated with intravenous ephedrine. He woke up, started breathing, and was extubated 75 minutes later. The authors postulated brainstem anesthesia following accidental injection of local anesthetic into a dural cuff as a cause of loss of consciousness.

Dental anesthesia

Sensory systems A 45-year-old man developed temporary *monocular blindness*, *ophthalmoplegia*, *ptosis*, and *mydriasis* immediately after a mandibular block injection (36[A]). Unidentified intra-arterial injection into the maxillary artery, with backflow of the local anesthetic solution to the middle meningeal artery was the postulated cause.

Ophthalmological complications after intraoral anesthesia occurred in 14 cases over 15 years (37[A]). The most common symptom was *diplopia*. Three patients developed *Horner's syndrome*, with ptosis, enophthalmos, and miosis on the same side as the anesthesia. Three patients developed *mydriasis* and *ptosis*. There was complete resolution in all patients. The authors postulated that direct diffusion of anesthetic solution from the pterygomaxillary fossa through the sphenomaxillary cavity to the orbit had caused the ophthalmological effects.

Infiltration anesthesia

Prilocaine 3% plus felypressin 0.03 IU/ml has been compared with lidocaine 2% plus adrenaline 12.5 μg/ml in 300 women having large-loop excision of the cervical transformation zone (38[C]). Those who received lidocaine had significantly less blood loss, but were more likely to have adverse effects, including shaking and feeling faint.

Nervous system A *stroke* occurred after infiltration of the tonsillar bed with bupivacaine subsequent to tonsillectomy (39[A]).

A 16-year-old girl undergoing adenotonsillectomy had cardiac asystole for 10 seconds after injection of her adenoid bed with 0.5% bupivacaine 1 ml with adrenaline 5 μg/ml. She had already been given an unstated quantity of bupivacaine with adrenaline 5 μg/ml injected into her tonsillar fossae. Her cardiac output returned spontaneously, but she had a central medullopontine infarction, confirmed on MRI and CT brain scans. Magnetic resonance angiography showed an abnormal circle of Willis, with absence of both posterior communicating vessels. The authors were unclear as to the exact cause of the cardiac event and stroke, which resulted in a persistent neurological deficit.

Intravenous regional anesthesia (IVRA)

Methods of reducing the dose of lidocaine used in IVRA by adding fentanyl 0.05 mg, pancuronium bromide 0.5 mg, or both, have been evaluated in 60 patients undergoing elective forearm, wrist, and hand surgery; the dose of lidocaine used was 100 mg (40[C]). None of the patients had signs of drug toxicity on release of the tourniquet; those who were given all three agents had better anesthesia and muscle relaxation. A separate group of volunteers, in whom the tourniquet was released immediately after injection of the lidocaine/fentanyl/pancuronium mixture, complained of minor adverse effects, including mild dizziness and transient visual disturbances and one case of vomiting and moderate hypotension.

A study of lidocaine toxicity in IVRA showed that two of 24 patients who were given 0.5% lidocaine 40 ml for carpal tunnel decompression had serum lidocaine concentrations above the target range 2 minutes before and 2, 5, and 10 minutes after distal tourniquet deflation (41[c]). However, no patients had signs of central nervous system or cardiovascular toxicity.

Nervous system A 56-year-old man developed unexplained acute *aphasia* when the tourniquet was released 20 minutes after the infusion of 0.75% lidocaine 20 ml for wrist surgery (42[A]). He also had *light-headedness*, but no circumoral numbness or visual or auditory disturbances. He made a spontaneous recovery 20 hours later with no sequelae.

Laryngeal anesthesia

Nervous system A 22-year-old man had a *generalized tonic–clonic convulsion* and *loss of consciousness* after an attempted superior laryngeal nerve block using 2% lidocaine 2 ml (43[A]). The seizure was not terminated by intravenous diazepam 10 mg and he was intubated after intravenous thiopental and suxamethonium. He required two boluses of ephedrine 10 mg to maintain his blood pressure. Surgery proceeded uneventfully and he recovered without any sequelae. The authors postulated vertebral artery injection of local anesthetic as the cause of the seizure and loss of consciousness.

Ocular anesthesia

Local infiltration with prilocaine 2% was significantly more comfortable than lidocaine 2% in a prospective randomized study in 125 patients undergoing minor eyelid procedures (44[c]).

Peribulbar anesthesia with 1% etidocaine, 0.5% bupivacaine, and hyaluronidase has been evaluated in 300 patients (45[C]). The mean volume administered was 17 ml. There was adequate analgesia in 85% of cases, and the other 15% required supplementation with a subtenon block. Akinesia occurred in 82% of cases. Two patients developed *generalized seizures*, and four developed severe *hypotension*.

Cardiovascular In addition to complications arising from the local anesthetic used during ocular anesthesia, complications can arise as a direct result of the injection. An *arteriovenous fistula* has been reported (46[A]).

An arteriovenous fistula of the supraorbital vessels developed in a 75-year-old man after peribulbar anesthesia with a supplementary supranasal injection. He elected to have conservative management and the lesion remained asymptomatic and static in size over 10 months follow-up.

Sensory systems Two cases of *transient blindness* after subconjunctival injection of 2% mepivacaine 2 ml were reported in patients with advanced refractory glaucoma undergoing diode laser cyclophotocoagulation (47[A]). The authors hypothesized that in patients with advanced optic neuropathy, even subconjunctival anesthesia can result in optic nerve block.

Differences in the manufacture of unpreserved lidocaine formulations have been postulated as a cause of *transient corneal clouding* in patients who were given intraocular unpreserved lidocaine 1% as an adjunct to topical anesthesia (48[r]). Independent analysis of the lidocaine solution associated with corneal clouding found it to be hypotonic and not buffered with bicarbonate compared with the solution that did not cause corneal clouding.

Nine patients developed prolonged symptomatic *diplopia* (predominantly vertical) after peribulbar anesthesia with ropivacaine 1% plus hyalase 750 units (49[c]). The mean time to resolution of the diplopia was 24 hours. The authors stressed the importance of warning patients undergoing peribulbar blockade with ropivacaine of the possibility of prolonged diplopia and queried its future use in routine cataract surgery.

A retrobulbar injection in a 45-year-old woman with high myopia was complicated by *globe perforation* with vitreous and submacular *hemorrhage* (50[A]).

Hematologic A 27-year-old woman with diabetes mellitus, complicated by diabetic retinopathy and chronic renal insufficiency with anemia, developed *methemoglobinemia* (11.2%) after peribulbar blockade with prilocaine 80 mg, bupivacaine 30 mg, hyaluronidase, and naphazoline (51[A]). She recovered uneventfully after methylene blue 1.5 mg/kg. The authors concluded that she may have been at increased risk of methemoglobinemia as a result of the metabolic acidosis associated with renal insufficiency, since impaired protein binding of prilocaine could have increased the concentrations of ionized prilocaine. Furthermore, the patient was also taking isosorbide dinitrate, which may have predisposed her to methemoglobinemia.

Topical anesthesia

Respiratory Unilateral *bronchospasm* has been described in a 19-year-old woman after the administration of lidocaine 4% 5 ml into the larynx via a Laryngojet injector (52[A]).

Nervous system An 84-year-old woman had three *generalized tonic–clonic seizures* after repeated applications of EMLA (17 applications of 10 g over 23 weeks) (53[A], 54[r]).

Errors by pharmacists or parents continue to contribute to severe complications, such as *seizures*, after the use of EMLA cream in overdose in children (55[A]).

A 21-month-old girl had four generalized tonic-clonic seizures after inadvertent overuse of EMLA before curettage of skin lesions of molluscum contagiosum. Because of a pharmacy error, 30 g tubes of EMLA were dispensed instead of 5 g tubes. The toddler's mother applied 75 g under occlusive dressing, covering about 350 cm^2 of the child's surface area. This dose significantly exceeds the recommendations for a 14 kg child – maximum 10 g on a maximum area of 100 cm^2. Two doses of intravenous lorazepam (0.1 mg/kg) did not control the seizures, which stopped only after phenobarbital (20 mg/kg) was given. The child then required intubation and ventilation for respiratory depression. The lidocaine concentration 4 hours after the first of application EMLA was 2.5 μg/ml and the methemoglobin concentration was 8%.

Hematologic A 4-day-old boy had methemoglobinemia (16%) after the application of EMLA cream to his penis before circumcision (56[A]).

Death A 21-year-old developed *seizures*, *respiratory distress* requiring tracheal intubation, severe *hypotension*, and then *bradycardia* culminating in asystole and *death* while gargling with 4% lidocaine 20 ml (800 mg) (57[A]). The authors strongly advised against exceeding the maximum recommended dose of lidocaine (200 mg), even when using it topically.

INDIVIDUAL COMPOUNDS

Benzocaine

Hematologic There have been many further reports of *methemoglobinemia* after the administration of topical benzocaine formulations (58[A], 59[r], 60[A], 61[A], 62[c], 63[A]). All of these patients made a complete recovery without sequelae after the intravenous administration of methylene blue 1–2 mg/kg.

A 69-year-old man developed methemoglobinemia (68%) after pharyngeal anesthesia using 20% benzocaine 15 ml (swish and swallow) for transesophageal echocardiography (64[A]). He responded to intravenous methylene blue, but a diagnosis of non-Q wave myocardial infarction was made on the basis of raised cardiac enzymes and a normal electrocardiogram.

Whether benzocaine-induced methemoglobinemia is idiosyncratic or dose-dependent remains controversial. There has been a retrospective review of 188 benzocaine exposures in children under 18 years of age, reported to four regional poison information centers, in 1993–6 (65[R]). Mean and median ingested dosages were 87 and 50 mg/kg respectively and 55% patients had an exposure over 40 mg/kg. In all, 92% patients were asymptomatic. Reported symptoms included *oral numbness* (eight patients), *vomiting* (three patients), and *oral irritation*, *dizziness*, and *nausea* (one patient each). *Methemoglobin* concentrations were measured in eight patients, seven of whom had concentrations over 1%. One child, who had had 5–10 applications of over-the-counter teething gel applied in 24 hours, had a methemoglobin concentration of 19% and was the only patient to have *cyanosis*. The authors concluded that accidental ingestion of over-the-counter benzocaine-containing products rarely causes cyanosis and that adverse reactions are not dose related.

Immunologic Benzocaine can cause *sensitization*, and being a para-aminobenzoic acid derivative can cross-react with paraphenylenediamine, sulfonamides, aniline dyes, and related local anesthetics. However, in a recent retrospective study of 5464 patients it was concluded that benzocaine allergy is not common in the UK, confirming earlier reports that benzocaine should not be used as a single screening agent for local anesthetic allergy (66[C]).

Bupivacaine

Cardiovascular *Ventricular dysrhythmias* and seizures were reported in a patient who received 0.5% bupivacaine 30 ml with adrenaline 5 μg/ml for lumbar plexus block, after a negative aspiration test (67[A]). The patient developed ventricular fibrillation and required advanced cardiac life support for 1 hour, including 15 defibrillations, and adrenaline 40 mg before sinus rhythm could be restored. There were no neurological sequelae.

Drug interactions There have been two studies of the effects of adding *clonidine* to solutions of bupivacaine.

The analgesic efficacy of the addition of clonidine to an epidural solution of bupivacaine plus fentanyl has been subjected to a randomized double-blind study in 61 parturients who received bupivacaine plus fentanyl with or without clonidine (median dose 28 μg/hour). There was no difference between the groups in pruritus or nausea score, but those given clonidine had less shivering and better analgesia (68[c]).

In another randomized double-blind study a combination of clonidine and neostigmine was added to intrathecal bupivacaine plus fentanyl in 45 parturients (69[c]). The combination increased the duration of labor analgesia by 83%, but was associated with significantly more nausea. However, the results were equivocal, and larger studies are needed.

Mepivacaine

Severe *bradypnea* and *bradycardia* requiring external ventricular pacing occurred in a previously asymptomatic 30-year-old woman with a known cardiac conduction defect 85 minutes after a paracervical block with mepivacaine 400 mg (70[A]).

Ropivacaine

Nervous system Two episodes of *central nervous system* toxicity without significant cardiovascular toxicity have been described in a patient who had brachial plexus blocks with excessively high doses of ropivacaine (and lidocaine in the second case) 6 weeks apart (71[A]). This again confirms the notion that ropivacaine has a safer toxicity profile than bupivacaine; as reported above, the latter can cause significant cardiotoxicity with difficulty in resuscitation.

A 45-year-old woman with rheumatoid arthritis asked for regional anesthesia for arthrodesis of her wrist. An interscalene block was performed with ropivacaine 300 mg (6 mg/kg). After 3 minutes she complained of *circumoral numbness* and *twitching* in her throat. She developed *irrational speech* and *perioral twitching* and 15 minutes after injection developed *involuntary clonic twitching* in her left upper arm. She was anesthetized with thiopental and ventilated with 100% oxygen via a bag and mask. She regained consciousness within 20 minutes and at 135 minutes was fully conscious, with complete sensorimotor block of her left upper limb. Six weeks later she had an axillary nerve block with ropivacaine 225 mg (4.5 mg/kg) and lidocaine 200 mg (4 mg/kg) with adrenaline. After 25 minutes she complained of a strange feeling in her tongue and became *dysarthric* and *unresponsive to voice*. She was anesthetized with propofol and the arthrodesis was performed under general anesthetic. Postoperatively she had a complete brachial plexus block, which resolved after 6 hours. In both instances the only cardiovascular effect noted was *sinus tachycardia* (150–170 beats/min).

REFERENCES

1. Nakada T, Iijima M. Allergic contact dermatitis from dibucaine hydrochloride. Contact Dermatitis 2000; 42: 283.
2. Borgeat A, Perschak H, Bird P, Hodler J, Gerber C. Patient-controlled interscalene analgesia with ropivacaine 0.2% versus patient-controlled intravenous analgesia after major shoulder surgery: effects on diaphragmatic and respiratory function. Anesthesiology 2000; 92: 102–8.
3. Koscielniak-Nielsen Z. Hemidiaphragmatic paresis after interscalene supplementation of insufficient axillary block with 3 ml of 2% mepivacaine. Acta Anaesthesiol Scand 2000; 44: 1160–2.
4. Mancuso TJ, Bacsik J, Overbey E. Positive test dose in a neonate with a caudally placed epidural catheter. Paediatr Anaesth 2000; 10: 565–6.
5. Thong WY, Pajel V, Khalil SN. Inadvertent administration of intravenous ropivacaine in a child. Paediatr Anaesth 2000; 10: 563–4.
6. Meister GC, D'Angelo R, Owen M, Nelson K, Gaver R. A comparison of epidural analgesia with 0.125% ropivacaine with fentanyl versus 0.125% bupivacaine with fentanyl during labor. Anesth Analg 2000; 90: 632–7.
7. Cotileas P, Myrianthefs P, Haralambakis A, Cotsopoulos P, Stamatopoulou C, Ladakis C, Baltopoulos G. Bupivacaine-induced myocardial depression and pulmonary edema: a case report. J Electrocardiol 2000; 33: 291–6.
8. Esteban JL, Gomez A, Gonzalez-Miranda F. Unintended total spinal anaesthesia with ropivacaine. Br J Anaesth 2000; 84: 697–8.
9. Taga K, Tomita M, Watanabe I, Sato K, Awamori K, Fujihara H, Shimoji K. Complete recovery of consciousness in a patient with decorticate rigidity following cardiac arrest after thoracic epidural injection. Br J Anaesth 2000; 85: 632–4.
10. Evron S, Krumholtz S, Wiener Y, Brohorov T, Bahar M. Prolonged coma and quadriplegia after accidental subarachnoid injection of a local anesthetic with an opiate. Anesth Analg 2000; 90: 116–18.
11. Baldwin ES, Turner MA. Profound motor blockade with epidural ropivacaine. Anaesthesia 2000; 55: 91.
12. Markey J, Naseer O, Bird D, Rabito S, Winnie A. Transient neurologic symptoms after epidural analgesia. Anesth Analg 2000; 90: 437–9.
13. Bourlon-Figuet S, Dubousset AM, Benhamou D, Mazoit J. Transient neurologic symptoms after epidural analgesia in a five-year-old child. Anesth Analg 2000; 91: 856–7.
14. Hogagard JT, Djurhuus H. Two cases of reiterated Horner's syndrome after lumbar epidural block. Acta Anaesthesiol Scand 2000; 44: 1021–3.
15. Wu C, Francisco D, Benesch C. Perioperative stroke associated with postoperative epidural analgesia. J Clin Anesth 2000; 12: 61–3.
16. Jacobs J, Vallejo R, DeSouza G, TerRiet M. Severe hypoglycemia after labor epidural analgesia. Anesth Analg 2000; 90: 892–3.
17. Malinovsky JM, Charles F, Kick O, Lepage JY, Malinge M, Cozian A, Bouchot O, Pinaud M. Intrathecal anesthesia: ropivacaine versus bupivacaine. Anesth Analg 2000; 91: 1457–60.
18. Karakan M, Tahtaci N, Goksu S. The effects of intrathecal bupivacaine and fentanyl in combined spinal epidural anesthesia. Int Med J 2000; 7: 145–9.
19. Owen M, Ozsarac O, Sahin S, Uckunkaya N, Kaplan N, Magunaci I. Low-dose clonidine and neostigmine prolong the duration of intrathecal bupivacaine–fentanyl for labor analgesia. Anesthesiology 2000; 92: 361–6.
20. Kathirvel S, Sadhasivam S, Saxena A, Kannan T, Ganjoo P. Effects of intrathecal ketamine added to bupivacaine for spinal anaesthesia. Anaesthesia 2000; 55: 899–904.
21. Ben-David B, Miller G, Gavriel R, Gurevitch A. Low-dose bupivacain–fentanyl spinal anesthesia for cesarean delivery. Reg Anesth Pain Med 2000; 25: 235–9.
22. Fragneto R, Fisher A. Mental status change and aphasia after labor analgesia with intrathecal sufentanil/bupivacaine. Anesth Analg 2000; 90: 1175–6.
23. Chan Y, Gopinathan R, Rajendram R. Loss of consciousness following spinal anaesthesia for Caesarean section. Br J Anaesth 2000; 85: 474–6.
24. Chen IC, Lin CS, Chou HM, Peng TH, Liu C, Wang CF, Lin I. Unexpected recurrent seizures following repeated spinal injections of tetracaine – a case report. Acta Anaesthesiol Sinica 2000; 38: 103–6.
25. Wajima Z, Shitara T, Inoue T, Ogawa R. Severe lightning pain after subarachnoid block in a patient with neuropathic pain of central origin: which drug is best to treat the pain? Clin J Pain 2000; 16: 265–9.
26. Robles Romero M, Gonzalez Mesa JM, De las Heras Rosas MA, Rojas C. Meningitis aseptica tras anestesia intradura. Rev Esp Anestesiol Reanim 2000; 47: 226.
27. De Weert K, Traksel M, Gielen M, Slappendel R, Weber E, Dirksen R. The incidence of transient neurological symptoms after spinal anaesthesia with lidocaine compared to prilocaine. Anaesthesia 2000; 55: 1020–4.
28. Hodgson PS, Liu SS, Batra MS, Gras TW, Pollock JE, Neal JM. Procaine compared with lidocaine for incidence of transient neurologic symptoms. Reg Anesth Pain Med 2000; 25: 218–22.
29. Ostgaard G, Hallaraker O, Ulveseth OK, Flaatten H. A randomised study of lidocaine and prilocaine for spinal anaesthesia. Acta Anaesthesiol Scand 2000; 44: 436–40.
30. Ben-David B, Maryanovsky M, Gurevitch A, Lucyk C, Solosko D, Frankel R. A comparison of minidose lidocaine–fentanyl and conventional-dose lidocaine. Anesth Analg 2000; 91: 865–70.
31. Pollock JE, Burkhead D, Neal JM, Liu SS, Friedman A, Stephenson C. Spinal nerve function

in five volunteers experiencing transient neurologic symptoms after lidocaine subarachnoid anesthesia. Anesth Analg 2000; 90: 658–65.
32. Keld DB, Hein L, Dalgaard M, Krogh L, Rodt SA. The incidence of transient neurologic symptoms (TNS) after spinal anaesthesia in patients undergoing surgery in the supine position. Hyperbaric lidocaine 5% versus hyperbaric bupivacaine 0.5%. Acta Anaesthesiol Scand 2000; 44: 285–90.
33. Ohtake K, Matsumoto M, Wakamatsu H, Kawai K, Nakakimura K, Sakabe T. Glutamate release and neuronal injury after intrathecal injection of local anesthetics. Neuroreport 2000; 11: 1105–9.
34. Harris RJD, Benveniste G. Recurrent laryngeal nerve blockade in patients undergoing carotid endarterectomy under cervical plexus block. Anaesth Intensive Care 2000; 28: 431–3.
35. Carling A, Simmonds M. Complications from regional anaesthesia for carotid endarterectomy. Br J Anaesth 2000; 84: 797–800.
36. Wilkie GJ. Temporary uniocular blindness and ophthalmoplegia associated with a mandibular block injection. A case report. Aust Dent J 2000; 45: 131–3.
37. Penarrocha-Diago M, Sanchis-Bielsa JM. Ophthalmologic complications after intraoral local anesthesia with articaine. Oral Surg Oral Med Oral Pathol Oral Radiol Endod 2000; 90: 21–4.
38. Howells RE, Tucker H, Millinship J, Foden Shroff J, Dhar KK, Jones PW, Redman CW. A comparison of the side effects of prilocaine with felypressin and lignocaine with adrenaline in large loop excision of the transformation zone of the cervix: results of a randomised trial. Br J Obstet Gynaecol 2000; 107: 28–32.
39. Alsarraf R, Sie K. Brain stem stroke associated with bupivacaine injection for adenotonsillectomy. Otolaryngol Head Neck Surg 2000; 122: 572–3.
40. Abdulla W, Kroll S, Eckhardt-Abdulla R. Intravenous regional anaesthesia – a new approach in clinical application. Anästhesiol Intensivmed 2000; 41: 94–103.
41. Kireker HD, Aynacioglu AS, Goksu S. Determination of 0.5% lidocaine serum concentrations and evaluation for toxicity in intravenous regional anaesthesia. Turk Anesteziyol Reanim 2000; 28: 211–16.
42. Cherng CH, Wong CS, Ho ST. Acute aphasia following tourniquet release in intravenous regional anesthesia with 0.75% lidocaine. Reg Anesth Pain Med 2000; 25: 211–12.
43. Hsu CH, Lin TC, Yeh CC, Ho ST, Wong CS. Convulsions during superior laryngeal nerve block – a case report. Acta Anaesthesiol Sinica 2000; 38: 93–6.
44. Burton AM, Backhouse O, Metcalfe T. Prilocaine versus lignocaine for minor lid procedures. Eye 2000; 14: 594–6.
45. Calenda E, Olle P, Muraine M, Brasseur G. Peribulbar anesthesia and subtenon injection for vitreoretinal surgery: 300 cases. Acta Ophthalmol Scand 2000; 78: 196–9.
46. To EW, Chan DT. Arteriovenous fistula induced by a peribulbar nerve block. J Cataract Refractive Surg 2000; 26: 1253–5.
47. Schlote T, Freudenthaler N, Von Eicken J, Rohrbach JM. Transient blindness after subconjunctival anaesthesia for diode laser cyclophotocoagulation of advanced glaucoma. Klin Monatsbl Augenheilkd 2000; 217: 296–8.
48. Spalton DJ. Problems with unpreserved lignocaine for intraocular use. J Cataract Refractive Surg 2000; 26: 633.
49. Wells A, Maslin K. Diplopia from peribulbar ropivicaine. Clin Exp Ophthalmol 2000; 28: 32–3.
50. Lam DS, Tam BS, Chan WM, Bhende P. Combined cataract extraction and submacular blood clot evacuation for globe perforation caused by retrobulbar injection. J Cataract Refractive Surg 2000; 26: 1089–91.
51. Eltzschig H, Rohrbach M, Schroeder TH. Methaemoglobinaemia after peribulbar blockade: an unusual complication in ophthalmic surgery. Br J Ophthalmol 2000; 84: 442.
52. Farmery AD. Severe unilateral bronchospasm mimicking inadvertent endobronchial intubation: a complication of the use of a topical lidocaine Laryngojet injector. Br J Anaesth 2000; 85: 917–19.
53. Boulinguez S, Sparsa A, Bouyssou-Gauthier M, Bedane C, Bonnetblanc J. Adverse effects associated with EMLA cream used as topical anesthetic for the mechanical debridement of leg ulcers. J Am Acad Dermatol 2000; 42: 146–7.
54. Lok C. Adverse effects associated with EMLA cream used as topical anesthetic for the mechanical debridement of leg ulcers. Reply. J Am Acad Dermatol 2000; 42: 147–8.
55. Rincon E, Baker R, Iglesias A, Duarte AM. CNS toxicity after topical application of EMLA cream on a toddler with molluscum contagiosum. Pediatr Emerg Care 2000; 16: 252–4.
56. Couper R. Methaemoglobinaemia secondary to topical lignocaine/prilocaine in a circumcised neonate. J Paediatr Child Health 2000; 36: 406–7.
57. Zuberi B, Shaikh M, Jatoi NUN, Shaikh W. Lidocaine toxicity in a student undergoing upper gastrointestinal endoscopy. Gut 2000; 46: 435.
58. Haynes JM. Acquired methemoglobinemia following benzocaine anesthesia of the pharynx. Am J Crit Care 2000; 9: 199–201.
59. Gregory P, Matsuda K. Cetacaine spray-induced methemoglobinemia after transesophageal echocardiography. Ann Pharmacother 2000; 34: 1077.
60. Nguyen S, Cabrales R, Bashour C, Rosenberger TJ, Michener J, Yared JP, Starr N. Benzocaine-induced methemoglobinemia. Anesth Analg 2000; 90: 369–71.
61. Kern K, Langevin P, Dunn B. Methemoglobinemia after topical anesthesia with lidocaine and benzocaine for a difficult intubation. J Clin Anesth 2000; 12: 167–72.
62. Gupta P, Lala D, Arsura E. Benzocaine-induced methemoglobinemia. South Med J 2000; 93: 83–6.
63. Gunaratnam N, Vazquez-Sequeiros E, Gostout C, Alexander G. Methemoglobinemia related to

topical benzocaine use: is it time to reconsider the empiric use of topical anesthesia before sedated EGD? Gastrointest Endosc 2000; 52: 692–3.
64. Wurdeman R, Mohiuddin S, Holmberg M, Shalaby A. Benzocaine-induced methemoglobinemia during an outpatient procedure. Pharmacotherapy 2000; 20: 735–8.
65. Spiller H, Revolinski D, Winter M, Weber J, Gorman S. Multi-center retrospective evaluation of oral benzocaine exposure in children. Vet Hum Toxicol 2000; 42: 228–31.
66. Sidhu SK, Shaw S, Wilkinson JD. A 10-year retrospective study on benzocaine allergy in the United Kingdom. Am J Contact Dermatitis 1999; 10: 57–61.
67. Pham-Dang C, Beaumont S, Floch H, Bodin J, Winer A, Pinaud M. Acute toxic accident following lumbar plexus block with bupivacaine. Ann Fr Anesth Reanim 2000; 19: 356–9.
68. Peach JM, Pavy TJG, Orlikowski CEP, Evans SF. Patient-controlled epidural analgesia in labor: the addition of clonidine to bupivacain–fentanyl. Reg Anesth Pain Med 2000; 25: 34–40.
69. Owen MD, Özsaraç Ö, Sahin S, Uçkunkeya N, Kaplan N, Magunaci I. Low-dose clonidine and neostigmine prolong the duration of intrathecal bupivacain–fentanyl for labor analgesia. Anesthesiology 2000; 92: 361–6.
70. Ayestaran C, Matorras R, Gomez S, Arce D, Rodriguez-Escudero F. Severe bradycardia and bradypnea following vaginal oocyte retrieval: a possible toxic effect of paracervical mepivacaine. Eur J Obstet Gynecol Reprod Biol 2000; 91: 71–3.
71. Ala-Kokko T, Lopponen A, Alahuhta S. Two instances of central nervous system toxicity in the same patient following repeated ropivacaine-induced brachial plexus block. Acta Anaesthesiol Scand 2000; 44: 623–6.

O. Zuzan and M. Leuwer

12 Neuromuscular blocking agents and skeletal muscle relaxants

NON-DEPOLARIZING NEUROMUSCULAR BLOCKING AGENTS *(SED-14, 371; SEDA-22, 149; SEDA-23, 150; SEDA-24, 159)*

The most striking recent event with regard to the adverse effects of neuromuscular blocking agents was the withdrawal of rapacuronium from the US market in March 2001. The manufacturers informed the FDA in an open letter about postmarketing reports of severe *bronchospasm* and some *deaths* of unknown origin associated with rapacuronium. The severity of the incidents recently reported to the manufacturers was impressive enough to cause fears about patient safety. This event highlights the need for continued surveillance, not only during clinical trials but also during the routine use of approved drugs. Appropriate reporting pathways must be available.

Immunologic A number of reports of *hypersensitivity reactions* after rocuronium administration have been published during recent years (1[A]–7[A]). In one hospital, the incidence of such reactions was 1 in 3000 (5[A]) and in another 1 in 6000 (1[A]), which prompted the authors to suggest that the frequency of reactions to rocuronium should be monitored. On the other hand, it had been previously assumed that rocuronium had a low potential for anaphylaxis (8[C]). In Australia and the UK, the incidence of anaphylaxis to rocuronium was found to follow the increase in its usage over the last few years (9[C], 10[C]). In France, where a nationwide reporting system has been in use for several years, 41 cases among 452 reported cases of anaphylaxis due to neuromuscular blocking agents were attributed to rocuronium (11[C]). This proportion compared well with the frequency of use of rocuronium in France at that time. However, the incidence of anaphylaxis to all muscle relaxants in that survey was 1 in 6500 anesthetics. Therefore, an incidence of 1 in 3000 for one particular agent in one hospital should raise concern. This might be just coincidental, but it might also reflect a higher degree of sensitization in that region, owing to increased exposure to cross-reactive allergens contained, for example, in cosmetics or household products (12[c]).

The Norwegian Medicines Agency has recently recommended that rocuronium bromide should be withdrawn from routine practice, referring to 29 reported cases of anaphylaxis or anaphylactoid reactions among 150 000 administrations over 2.5 years. In response, and with regard to the paucity of reported cases of anaphylaxis to rocuronium in other Nordic countries, the statistical problems of surveying such rare adverse drug reactions have been highlighted (13[cR]).

Drug interactions *Bambuterol* has been reported to alter the metabolism of mivacurium (14[C]). Bambuterol has a dose-dependent inhibitory effect on plasma cholinesterase activity and prolongs the effects of succinylcholine. Bambuterol 10 mg was given to 28 patients 2 hours before an elective operation requiring general anesthesia. The patients given bambuterol had a 67–97% fall in plasma cholinesterase activity, leading to reduced clearance of mivacurium. This resulted in a shorter onset

Side Effects of Drugs, Annual 25
J.K. Aronson, ed.

and a 3- to 4-fold prolongation of action of the neuromuscular blockade produced by standard doses of mivacurium.

DEPOLARIZING NEUROMUSCULAR BLOCKING AGENTS *(SED-14, 361; SEDA-22, 147; SEDA-23, 150; SEDA-24, 158)*

Succinylcholine

Cardiovascular Some controversial correspondence has followed the report of four cases of *fatal cardiac arrest* among 150 patients who were given succinylcholine by paramedics in out-of-hospital emergencies (15[C]). The authors suggested that this might militate against succinylcholine-facilitated endotracheal intubation in this setting. Others, however, have argued that there was no evidence for a causal role of succinylcholine in those cases (16[r]). Patients with critical conditions, such as respiratory failure requiring endotracheal intubation, may have a cardiac arrest without being given succinylcholine. Furthermore, undetected esophageal intubation was considered to be an alternative explanation of cardiac arrest. Indeed, when endotracheal intubation is attempted in these often dramatic and stressful circumstances by healthcare providers who have no routine practice in this there may be a high rate of esophageal intubation. In one study 18 of 108 patients who had been intubated by paramedics were found to have the tube in their esophagus (17[C]). So the role of succinylcholine in the above report is questionable. On the other hand succinylcholine is part of the protocol for emergency intubation in many centers worldwide and succinylcholine-associated cardiac arrest, apart from anecdotal instances, has not been reported to be a relevant problem (18[C]). Succinylcholine may increase the success rate of emergency intubations while reducing the incidence of traumatic intubations (19[C]). Therefore, we believe that rapid-sequence intubation with an induction agent such as etomidate and succinylcholine is still the technique of choice for airway management in emergencies. Whoever uses this technique must be aware of contraindications to succinylcholine and must have frequent practice in endotracheal intubation.

Electrolyte balance Recently a large number of cases of cardiac arrest associated with *hyperkalemia* have been reported in critically ill patients after prolonged immobilization (20[A]–27[A]) and a recent report has extended the list (28[A]). There is evidence to suggest that complete immobilization may result in alterations of the muscle cell surface, which imitate those seen after denervation. Extrajunctional spread of acetylcholine receptors has particularly been demonstrated and is believed to result in massive release of intracellular potassium once succinylcholine is injected. Given the growing number of reports and the potentially fatal effects, it is increasingly recommendable to regard succinylcholine as being contraindicated in critically ill patients who have been immobilized in an intensive care unit for more than 48 hours.

Similarly, extrajunctional spread of acetylcholine receptors might have caused hyperkalemic cardiac arrest in a patient with wound botulism (29[A]).

A 28-year-old previously healthy man was admitted with a 4-week history of progressive symmetrical muscle weakness that had started in his neck and descended to both arms and legs. He also complained of diplopia, dysphonia, and dysphagia. On the day of admission, he noted difficulty in breathing. He had a history of intermittent diamorphine abuse, and had been injecting "black tar" heroin subcutaneously for the past month. Several hours after admission he had to be intubated, and was given etomidate 20 mg plus succinylcholine 80 mg. Within 60 seconds he developed a wide complex tachycardia, which degenerated into ventricular fibrillation refractory to electrical countershock and standard resuscitative measures. His serum potassium concentration 10–12 minutes after the onset of cardiocirculatory arrest was 6.8 mmol/l, having been 4.7 mmol/l several hours before. Calcium chloride, sodium bicarbonate, and glucose/insulin were given, and 25 minutes after the arrest began the heart rhythm converted to sinus tachycardia. The electrocardiogram subsequently showed no structural abnormalities. A serological test taken on the day of admission was positive for botulinum toxin type A. The patient eventually survived without any residual deficits and was discharged from hospital after 63 days.

The authors suggested that succinylcholine should be avoided in patients with suspected botulism and in patients with muscle weakness of unknown origin. Wound botulism had been observed before in drug users who have injected black tar heroin (30[c]). Botulinum toxin inhibits presynaptic acetylcholine release, resulting in muscle weakness. In animals chronic administration of botulinum toxin caused an increase in the number of postsynaptic acetylcholine receptors with distribution across the muscle surface (31[E]) and postsynaptic acetylcholine receptors converted into the immature type with prolonged channel opening times (32[E]). With huge numbers of muscle fibers altered in that way, succinylcholine may cause hyperkalemic cardiac arrest by producing massive potassium efflux.

One major concern for anesthetists is succinylcholine-associated hyperkalemia in apparently fit patients without obvious risk factors. In line with that, there is a report from Japan of life-threatening hyperkalemia in three women who underwent cesarean section (33[A]).

Cardiac arrest occurred in a 34-year-old woman who was given succinylcholine 120 mg. She had been immobilized and treated with high-dose magnesium sulfate and ritodrine for 5 weeks before the event because of preterm uterine contractions. Her preoperative creatine kinase activity was 4050 IU/l. After rapid-sequence induction of anesthesia and injection of succinylcholine she became cyanotic and pulseless and the electrocardiogram showed ventricular fibrillation. The serum potassium concentration after 25 minutes of cardiopulmonary resuscitation, which included the administration of adrenaline, sodium bicarbonate, and calcium chloride, was 5.7 mmol/l. During resuscitation vaginal vacuum delivery was performed. Finally, she was defibrillated successfully and made a full recovery.

Two other patients had been immobilized and treated with magnesium and ritodrine for several weeks. Preoperative creatine kinase activities were 2120 IU/l and 630 IU/l. In both cases, serum potassium increased by 2.3 mmol/l within 2–3 minutes after succinylcholine injection (from 4.0 to 6.3 mmol/l and from 4.9 to 7.2 mmol/l). This was accompanied by tall peaked T waves and a short period of ventricular tachycardia in one case and by tall peaked T waves and widened QRS complexes in the other.

The authors suggested that the combined effects of immobilization and prolonged magnesium administration might have resulted in a denervation-like state of large groups of skeletal muscles. The drawback of that explanation is that an awake and healthy person will always move normally even when confined to bed. As long as muscle cells receive physiological stimulation via the neuromuscular junction in patients without muscle weakness, denervation-like changes should not occur to a significant extent. In addition, denervation alone is not known to be associated with an increase in plasma creatine kinase activity, a strong indicator of muscle cell damage, which was found in all the patients reported here. Unfortunately, the authors did not document creatine kinase activities or myoglobin concentrations after succinylcholine, which might have given some idea about additional succinylcholine-induced rhabdomyolysis.

It can be assumed that these three patients had some form of myopathy, either acquired during their previous course or pre-existing. It would have been interesting to know if they had any clinical symptoms, such as muscle pain or weakness. Pre-existing myopathy would be unlikely if plasma creatine kinase activities had been normal before. However, this information was not given in the paper. On the other hand, myopathy could have been acquired during the course of pregnancy and hospital treatment. Various drugs and toxins have been associated with myopathies (34[R]). Hypermagnesemia can produce muscle weakness but magnesium sulfate has not so far been reported to cause myopathy. Therefore, the role of ritodrine in these cases should be questioned. This selective β_2-adrenoceptor agonist has previously been linked to myopathic changes in a patient treated for preterm labor (35[A]). In addition, glucocorticoid treatment, probably used to promote fetal lung development, might be a contributory factor. Long-term glucocorticoid treatment is associated with myopathic changes (34[R]).

In the end, the exact mechanism of succinylcholine-associated hyperkalemia in these cases can not be determined. To our knowledge, this is the first report linking this phenomenon to this specific scenario. Given the huge numbers of patients who receive succinylcholine during rapid-sequence induction of anesthesia for cesarean section, even after some time of treatment for preterm labor without adverse effects, it would be overzealous to call for a restricted use of succinylcholine in these patients. Rather, this report is in support of preoperative screening of plasma creatine kinase activity. We suggest that succinylcholine should not be used in patients with raised plasma creatine kinase activity. It is a good idea to check creatine kinase activity preoperatively in women due to undergo cesarean section after prolonged immobilization and pretreatment with magnesium sulfate and a β_2-adrenergic agonist such as ritodrine.

SKELETAL MUSCLE RELAXANTS *(SED-14, 390; SEDA-22, 150; SEDA-23, 152; SEDA-24, 159)*

Carisoprodol

In 104 cases carisoprodol and its metabolite meprobamate were detected in the blood of car drivers who were either involved in accidents or arrested for impaired driving (36[C]). In many of these cases, either alcohol or other CNS depressants were also found. In 21 cases carisoprodol/meprobamate were the only drugs detected. Symptoms and reported driving behavior were similar in all cases. *Impairment of driving ability* appeared to be possible at any concentration of these two drugs. However, the most severe driving impairment and most overt symptoms of intoxication were noted when the combined concentration of carisoprodol and meprobamate exceeded 10 mg/l.

As carisoprodol and its metabolite meprobamate are GABA receptor agonists, the use of the benzodiazepine receptor antagonist flumazenil might be considered in some cases of carisoprodol toxicity (37[A]).

A 51-year-old woman who took 87 tablets of carisoprodol (350 mg each) over 13 days developed lethargy and abnormal speech. She was confused and her Glasgow Coma Score was 9/15. Her pupils were small and reactive. Two naloxone boluses of 2 mg each were administered with no effect. After flumazenil 0.2 mg she became more alert but was still mildly somnolent. After a second dose of flumazenil 0.2 mg all signs of intoxication were reversed within 2 minutes. Her blood concentrations at admission were 7.4 mg/l for carisoprodol and 30.7 mg/l for meprobamate.

This indicates that flumazenil may be an effective therapeutic option if carisoprodol intoxication results in CNS depression. However, carisoprodol overdose may as well produce myoclonic movements or agitation (38[A]), in which case it is questionable if flumazenil should be used.

Cyclobenzaprine

There has so far been only one report linking cyclobenzaprine to activation of manic psychosis (39[A]). Recently, a case of first-onset paranoid *psychosis* has been reported (40[A])

A 36-year-old woman with no past psychiatric problems took 23 tablets of cyclobenzaprine (10 mg each) over 6 weeks to ease back pain resulting from a back injury. She developed insomnia, reduced appetite, poor concentration, irritability, disorganized thoughts, persecutory delusions, and auditory hallucinations. Cyclobenzaprine was withdrawn and a course of loxapine was started, leading to rapid and complete resolution of her agitation and psychotic symptoms within 72 hours. Loxapine was subsequently quickly withdrawn with no ill effects and she recovered fully.

The authors thought that this psychotic episode was related to cyclobenzaprine, in view of the temporal relation of the symptoms to the administration of cyclobenzaprine and their rapid resolution after withdrawal.

Tizanidine

In an open-label study of tizanidine for neuropathic pain several adverse effects were noted, such as *dizziness*, *drowsiness*, *fatigue/weakness*, *dry mouth*, *gastrointestinal upset*, and *sleep difficulty* (41[c]). One patient developed *abnormal liver function tests* accompanied by nausea and vomiting, fatigue, confusion, weakness, and muscle aches. Within 3 weeks after withdrawal of tizanidine, the liver function tests returned to baseline and the symptoms resolved. Two other patients had transient asymptomatic rises in liver function tests, which returned to normal despite continuation of tizanidine. Transiently raised liver function tests during tizanidine treatment have occasionally been reported before (42[A], 43[C]–45[C]).

REFERENCES

1. Allen SJ, Gallagher A, Paxton LD. Anaphylaxis to rocuronium. Anaesthesia 2000; 55: 1223–4.
2. Barthelet Y, Ryckwaert Y, Plasse C, Bonnet-Boyer MC, D'Athis F. Accidents anaphylactiques graves après administration de rocuronium. Ann Fr Anesth Réanim 1999; 18: 896–900.
3. Donnelly T. Anaphylaxis to rocuronium. Br J Anaesth 2000; 84: 696.
4. Heier T, Guttormsen AB. Anaphylactic reactions during induction of anaesthesia using rocuronium for muscle relaxation: a report including 3 cases. Acta Anaesthesiol Scand 2000; 44: 775–81.

5. Neal SM, Manthri PR, Gadiyar V, Wildsmith JA. Histaminoid reactions associated with rocuronium. Br J Anaesth 2000; 84: 108–11.
6. Matthey P, Wang P, Finegan BA, Donnelly M. Rocuronium anaphylaxis and multiple neuromuscular blocking drug sensitivities. Can J Anaesth 2000; 47: 890–3.
7. Yee R, Fernandez JA. Anaphylactic reaction to rocuronium bromide. Anaesth Intensive Care 1996; 24: 601–4.
8. Laxenaire M, Gastin I, Moneret-Vautrin D, Widmer S, Guéant J. Cross-reactivity of rocuronium with other neuromuscular blocking agents. Eur J Anaesthesiol 1995; 12 Suppl 11: 55–64.
9. Rose M, Fisher M. Rocuronium: high risk of anaphylaxis? Br J Anaesth 2001; 86: 678–82.
10. Watkins J. Incidence of UK reactions involving rocuronium may simply reflect market use. Br J Anaesth 2001; 87: 522.
11. Laxenaire MC. Epidemiologie des reactions anaphylactoides peranesthesiques. Quatrieme enquete multicentrique (juillet 1994–decembre 1996). Le Groupe d'Etudes des Reactions Anaphylactoides Peranesthesiques. Ann Fr Anesth Réanim 1999; 18: 796–809.
12. Weston A, Assem ES. Possible link between anaphylactoid reactions to anaesthetics and chemicals in cosmetics and biocides. Agents Actions 1994; 41: C138–9.
13. Laake JH, Rottingen JA. Rocuronium and anaphylaxis – a statistical challenge. Acta Anaesthesiol Scand 2001; 25: 1196–203.
14. Ostergaard D, Rasmussen SN, Viby-Mogensen J, Pedersen NA, Boysen R. The influence of drug-induced low plasma cholinesterase activity on the pharmacokinetics and pharmacodynamics of mivacurium. Anesthesiology 2000; 92: 1581–7.
15. Pace SA, Fuller FP. Out-of-hospital succinylcholine-assisted endotracheal intubation by paramedics. Ann Emerg Med 2000; 35: 568–72.
16. Menegazzi JJ, Wayne MA. Succinylcholine-assisted endotracheal intubation by paramedics. Ann Emerg Med 2001; 37: 360–1.
17. Katz SH, Falk JL. Misplaced endotracheal tubes by paramedics in an urban emergency medical services system. Ann Emerg Med 2001; 37: 32–7.
18. Zink BJ, Snyder HS, Raccio Robak N. Lack of a hyperkalemic response in emergency department patients receiving succinylcholine. Acad Emerg Med 1995; 2: 974–8.
19. Dronen SC, Merigian KS, Hedges JR, Hoekstra JW, Borron SW. A comparison of blind nasotracheal and succinylcholine-assisted intubation in the poisoned patient. Ann Emerg Med 1987; 16: 650–2.
20. Berkahn JM, Sleigh JW. Hyperkalaemic cardiac arrest following succinylcholine in a long-term intensive care patient. Anaesth Intensive Care 1997; 25: 588–9.
21. Biccard BM, Grant IS, Wright DJ, Nimmo SR, Hughes M. Suxamethonium and critical illness polyneuropathy. Anaesth Intensive Care 1998; 26: 590–1.
22. Dornan RI, Royston D. Suxamethonium-related hyperkalaemic cardiac arrest in intensive care. Anaesthesia 1995; 50: 1006.
23. Hansen D. Suxamethonium-induced cardiac arrest and death following 5 days of immobilization. Eur J Anaesthesiol 1998; 15: 240–1.
24. Hemming A, Charlton S, Kelly P. Hyperkalaemia, cardiac arrest, suxamethonium and intensive care. Anaesthesia 1990; 45: 990–1.
25. Horton WA, Fergusson NV. Hyperkalaemia and cardiac arrest after the use of suxamethonium in intensive care. Anaesthesia 1988; 43: 890–1.
26. Lee YM, Fountain SW. Suxamethonium and cardiac arrest. Singapore Med J 1997; 38: 300–1.
27. Markewitz BA, Elstad MR. Succinylcholine-induced hyperkalemia following prolonged pharmacologic neuromuscular blockade. Chest 1997; 111: 248–50.
28. Matthews JM. Succinylcholine-induced hyperkalemia and rhabdomyolysis in a patient with necrotizing pancreatitis. Anesth Analg 2000; 91: 1552–4.
29. Chakravarty EF, Kirsch CM, Jensen WA, Kagawa FT. Cardiac arrest due to succinylcholine-induced hyperkalemia in a patient with wound botulism. J Clin Anesth 2000; 12: 80–2.
30. Passaro DJ, Werner SB, McGee J, Mac Kenzie WR, Vugia DJ. Wound botulism associated with black tar heroin among injecting drug users. J Am Med Assoc 1998; 279: 859–63.
31. Simpson LL. The effects of acute and chronic botulinum toxin treatment on receptor number, receptor distribution and tissue sensitivity in rat diaphragm. J Pharmacol Exp Ther 1977; 200: 343–51.
32. Koltgen D, Ceballos-Baumann AO, Franke C. Botulinum toxin converts muscle acetylcholine receptors from adult to embryonic type. Muscle Nerve 1994; 17: 779–84.
33. Sato K, Nishiwaki K, Kuno N, Kumagai K, Kitamura H, Yano K, Okamoto S, Ishikawa K, Shimada Y. Unexpected hyperkalemia following succinylcholine administration in prolonged immobilized parturients treated with magnesium and ritodrine. Anesthesiology 2000; 93: 1539–41.
34. Pascuzzi RM. Drugs and toxins associated with myopathies. Curr Opin Rheumatol 1998; 10: 511–20.
35. Sholl JS, Hughey MJ, Hirschmann RA. Myotonic muscular dystrophy associated with ritodrine tocolysis. Am J Obstet Gynecol 1985; 151: 83–6.
36. Logan BK, Case GA, Gordon AM. Carisoprodol, meprobamate, and driving impairment. J Forensic Sci 2000; 45: 619–23.
37. Roberge RJ, Lin E, Krenzelok EP. Flumazenil reversal of carisoprodol (Soma) intoxication. J Emerg Med 2000; 18: 61–4.
38. Roth BA, Vinson DR, Kim S. Carisoprodol-induced myoclonic encephalopathy. J Toxicol Clin Toxicol 1998; 36: 609–12.

39. Beeber AR, Manring JM. Psychosis following cyclobenzaprine use. J Clin Psychiatry 1983; 44: 151.
40. O'Neil BA, Knudson GA, Bhaskara SM. First episode psychosis following cyclobenzaprine use. Can J Psychiatry 2000; 45: 763–4.
41. Semenchuk MR, Sherman S. Effectiveness of tizanidine in neuropathic pain: An open-label study. J Pain 2000; 1: 285–92.
42. De Graaf EM, Oosterveld M, Tjabbes T, Stricker BH. A case of tizanidine-induced hepatic injury. J Hepatol 1996; 25: 772–3.
43. Saper JR, Winner PK, Lake AE, 3rd. An open-label dose-titration study of the efficacy and tolerability of tizanidine hydrochloride tablets in the prophylaxis of chronic daily headache. Headache 2001; 41: 357–68.
44. Wallace JD. Summary of combined clinical analysis of controlled clinical trials with tizanidine. Neurology 1994; 44: S60–8.
45. Lapierre Y, Bouchard S, Tansey C, Gendron D, Barkas WJ, Francis GS. Treatment of spasticity with tizanidine in multiple sclerosis. Can J Neurol Sci 1987; 14: 513–17.

Michael Schachter

13 Drugs affecting autonomic functions or the extrapyramidal system

DRUGS THAT STIMULATE BOTH α- AND β-ADRENOCEPTORS

(SED-14, 414; SEDA-22, 154; SEDA-23, 155; SEDA-24, 163)

Adrenaline (epinephrine)

The vasoconstrictor action of adrenaline continues to cause problems. When adrenaline 0.4 ml of a 1 mg/ml solution was inadvertently injected into the penile skin of a 12-hour-old neonate the skin blanched and the error was immediately understood (1[A]). After repeated doses of phentolamine (total 0.65 mg) the skin regained its normal color. There were no sequelae.

Central retinal vein thrombosis occurred in a 75-year-old man 20 minutes after the ipsilateral insertion of a 1% adrenaline-soaked cotton wool stick (2[A]). Unfortunately, his visual acuity did not improve.

Ephedrine and pseudoephedrine

Cardiovascular *Ischemic colitis* has been attributed to pseudoephedrine (3[A]).

A 33-year-old man took pseudoephedrine 240 mg/day for 5 days. His mesenteric vasculature was normal on subsequent magnetic resonance angiography and no other abnormalities were found, leading to the presumption that the drug had caused mesenteric vasoconstriction. He made a full recovery.

Cardiac dysrhythmias have also been attributed to ephedrine (4[A]).

A 25-year-old woman became hypotensive after the administration of epidural anesthesia for an elective cesarean section. She was given intravenous ephedrine 9 mg, after which she complained of nausea. For an unexplained reason this was taken as an indication to give a further 9 mg of ephedrine. She immediately developed sinus tachycardia with atrial and multifocal ventricular extra beats, followed by short runs of ventricular tachycardia. She remained asymptomatic and recovered after about 5 minutes.

One must have some concerns about the high dose used here, for a relatively modest level of hypotension with a systolic blood pressure of 100 mmHg.

Psychiatric After many years, even centuries, of use, ephedrine and its modern synthetic analogue pseudoephedrine continue to cause a wide variety of problems. Some of these are very serious. Ma-huang is a Chinese herbal preparation, which contains ephedrine and which has been used since ancient times as a stimulant and in the treatment of asthma. It can cause psychiatric complications, which can last several weeks. These have been reviewed in the context of two cases of *psychotic reactions* (5[AR]).

A 27-year-old US Marine presented with depressed affect, irritability, and poor concentration and eventually admitted 2 years self-medication with Ma-Huang to improve workout performance. Another 27-year-old US Marine developed a frank psychosis with ideas of reference and some paranoid ideation. He had been taking two preparations containing Ma-Huang, although the duration of use was unclear. After discontinuing the drug both made a full recovery.

The authors emphasized the importance of recognizing possible abuse of such "natural" medications, widely perceived to be harmless

Side Effects of Drugs, Annual 25
J.K. Aronson, ed.

despite warnings and attempted restrictions by regulatory authorities. Treatment is supportive while awaiting spontaneous recovery after drug withdrawal.

Skin A hypersensitivity reaction was confirmed by patch testing in a 73-year-old woman who had taken a single (unspecified) dose of a compound formulation containing pseudoephedrine (6^A). This caused the memorably named *baboon syndrome*, a widespread symmetrical erythematous rash with papules and pustules.

Drug interactions Ephedrine has reportedly interacted with *entacapone* (7^A).

A 76-year-old woman with a long history of Parkinson's disease was given a general anesthetic for ophthalmic surgery. She was taking levodopa/carbidopa together with entacapone. On induction her blood pressure dropped and she was given intravenous ephedrine 3 mg. Her blood pressure rose immediately, reaching a peak of 240/130 mmHg. It was eventually controlled with several intravenous doses of hydralazine.

The authors concluded that entacapone had inhibited the metabolism of ephedrine and of the catecholamines that it had released.

DRUGS THAT PRE-DOMINANTLY STIMULATE α-ADRENOCEPTORS

(SED-14, 417; SEDA-22, 154; SEDA-23, 155; SEDA-24, 164)

Phenylpropanolamine

Cardiovascular In November 2000 the US FDA asked that manufacturers should voluntarily stop marketing products containing phenylpropanolamine. It also began the process of formally banning such products, whether used as nasal decongestants or appetite suppressants. This was prompted by the imminent publication by a group from Yale of a 5-year case-control study of 702 patients who had suffered *intracerebral or subarachnoid hemorrhages* and 1376 control subjects aged 18–49 years (8^C). In women taking phenylpropanolamine as an appetite suppressant the odds ratio for increased risk of hemorrhagic stroke was 16.6 (95% CI = 1.5, 182), while with "first use" of the drug as a cold remedy the corresponding figures were 3.1 (0.9, 12). There was no increased risk in men taking the drug as a cold remedy and none used it as an appetite suppressant. This was consistent with numerous case reports over at least 20 years. The most recent, and one hopes the last, of these concerned a 7-week-old baby who suffered a brain stem hemorrhage within 30 minutes of a single dose of phenylpropanolamine 6.25 mg (9^A). The baby made what appeared to be a full recovery.

Psychiatric A 31-year-old woman with a history of metamphetamine abuse developed *depression, hallucinations*, and *paranoid delusions*. She recovered after 3 weeks but was readmitted with similar symptoms 6 months later. She tested negative for amphetamines but had been taking a phenylpropanolamine-containing decongestant together with cimetidine (10^A). Her symptoms abated within 3 days of drug withdrawal. Clearly this woman was at high risk of drug-induced psychosis, and the problem was possibly aggravated by inhibition of phenylpropanolamine metabolism by the cytochrome P450 inhibitor cimetidine.

DRUGS THAT PRE-DOMINANTLY STIMULATE β_1-ADRENOCEPTORS

(SED-14, 420; SEDA-22, 155; SEDA-23, 156; SEDA-24, 165)

Dobutamine

Cardiovascular Dobutamine stress testing, particularly combined with echocardiography, is a very widely used tool in cardiological investigation, and its safety continues to be examined in great detail. In a review of 37 publications, each reporting on 100 or more patients, with a total of over 26 000 tests, 79 life-threatening complications were described, including *acute myocardial infarction*, a variety of *cardiac dysrhythmias*, and severe *hypotension* (11^M). The authors also referred to 29 isolated case reports of severe complications, including two deaths. They concluded that there must be a clear indication for the procedure, informed consent must be obtained, a physician should be present during the test, and patients should be carefully followed as out-patients in case of delayed problems.

Individual cases of fatal dysrhythmias have also been reported (12[A]).

A 55-year-old man with stable angina was admitted for dobutamine stress testing. He had been taking metoprolol, but this was withdrawn 2 days before the test. During the lowest dose of the dobutamine infusion (5 μg/kg/min) his heart rate rose to 143/min and he developed chest pain and ST segment depression in the lateral chest leads of the electrocardiogram. The drug was stopped and metoprolol and glyceryl trinitrate were given immediately, but a few minutes later he developed torsade de pointes followed by ventricular fibrillation. Resuscitation was unsuccessful. There was no evidence of acute myocardial infarction at autopsy.

Myocardial ischemia has also been reported in susceptible patients. A Japanese group carried out dobutamine stress echocardiography in 51 patients with a presumptive diagnosis of variant angina (13[C]). All had coronary vasospasm in response to intracoronary acetylcholine and seven also had chest pain and reversible ST segment elevation. One must incidentally wonder whether this procedure was entirely advisable.

Acute subaortic left ventricular outflow tract obstruction has been described during dobutamine infusion in a patient who had no evidence of this at rest but developed severe obstruction when his pulse rate exceeded 105 beats/min (14[A]). The subaortic gradient eventually reached the very high figure of 182 mmHg, even though the patient remained asymptomatic and there was no clear reason why this occurred in this particular patient.

There are variants of the standard procedure that do not appear to be associated with increased risk. An accelerated high-dose protocol, in which a constant infusion of 50 μg/kg/min was given for up to 10 minutes in 100 patients has been compared with the standard stepwise procedure in a similar number (15[C]). The cumulative dose was somewhat lower in the accelerated protocol, while the duration of the test was halved. Dysrhythmic adverse effects occurred in 28 patients on the accelerated protocol and in 39 of those tested by the standard method: this difference was said to be non-significant. In another study transesophageal was compared with transthoracic dobutamine stress echocardiography in 63 and 100 patients respectively (16[C]). Baseline pulse and blood pressure were higher in the transesophageal group. The authors noted that there were no cases of ventricular tachycardia or fibrillation in either group, or of myocardial infarction. They also stated that the incidence of less serious dysrhythmias was similar in the two groups: however, no figures were quoted.

DRUGS THAT ACT ON DOPAMINE RECEPTORS *(SED-14, 421; SEDA-22, 156; SEDA-23, 156; SEDA-24, 165)*

Levodopa and dopamine receptor agonists

The tolerability of the newer anti-Parkinsonian agents has been reviewed (17[R]). The authors concluded that there is no conclusive evidence that selegiline is associated with increased mortality, although its symptomatic benefits are limited and neuroprotective properties of uncertain relevance. They suggested that pramipexole and ropinirole are suitable in early disease, largely because they delay the onset of levodopa-induced motor fluctuations. They may also be equally effective in advanced disease, and comparable to bromocriptine and pergolide. They recommended starting at very low doses, followed by slow titration to minimize adverse effects. They noted that entacapone appears to be safe and effective, without the liver toxicity associated with tolcapone, but it appears to have lower efficacy than the older drug, which had been withdrawn because of this problem.

Cardiovascular Many clinicians regard the cardiovascular adverse effects of dopamine receptor agonists as rare and not very significant. A group from Chicago tested the responses of 29 consecutive patients (aged 38–83 years, mean 62 years) starting treatment for Parkinson's disease (18[C]). They were given test doses of pergolide (0.025, 0.05, 0.125, or 0.25 mg), pramipexole (0.125 mg), or ropinirole (0.125 or 0.25 mg), apparently according to the clinicians' judgement. They defined *orthostatic hypotension* as either a drop in systolic pressure of more than 25 mmHg or in diastolic pressure of more than 10 mmHg. By these criteria ten subjects had orthostatic hypotension but only three were symptomatic. There was no greater likelihood with any particular agent, although the sample number was relatively small. The authors commented that measurement of such responses may help in managing titration schedules, although given that the effects are transient and most patients are asymptomatic one rather doubts if this advice will be widely adopted.

Myocardial infarction occurred post-partum in two women taking bromocriptine (19[A]).

A 33-year-old woman taking bromocriptine 5 mg/day for suppression of lactation was given ergotamine 2.25 mg for acute migraine, having taken ergotamine intermittently for over 20 years. She had a myocardial infarction involving the left anterior descending coronary artery, without apparent pre-existing atherosclerosis. She made a good recovery following thrombolysis.

A 29-year-old woman taking bromocriptine 5 mg/day post-partum had a dissection of the left anterior descending coronary artery and needed emergency bypass grafting. She made a good recovery.

These cases emphasize the potential danger of these drugs, even in young and apparently healthy individuals, although in the first case the use of two ergot derivatives simultaneously may have been ill-advised.

Peripheral edema has occasionally been described as an adverse effect of dopamine agonist therapy and has been reported in 17 of 300 patients treated with pramipexole (20[C]). The mean dose at onset of edema was 1.7 mg/day and the time after initiation of therapy was 2.6 months. In all cases the edema disappeared after the drug was withdrawn but reappeared on rechallenge. Although the condition was dose-dependent in affected individuals its occurrence was idiosyncratic with no obvious predisposing features. Response to diuretics was minimal.

Respiratory A 73-year-old man taking pergolide 1.5 mg/day for 4 months developed *dyspnea, bilateral pleural effusions*, and *severe edema of the legs* up to the scrotum (21[A]). There was no pleural thickening or any evidence of cardiac failure or nephrotic syndrome. These clinical features were resistant to diuretic therapy but resolved completely within a month of withdrawal of pergolide. The mechanism of this type of very rare reaction is totally unknown.

Nervous system The effect of using a reduced dosage of levodopa (by a mean of 64%) has been studied in 12 patients receiving high-frequency stimulation of the subthalamic nucleus (22[c]). The patients underwent a challenge with a levodopa dose that was 50 mg greater than the normal preoperative dose before electrode implantation and after 8–9 months of continuous stimulation. However, stimulation was interrupted 2 hours before the challenge. Overall motor disability during on and off periods was not altered, but the dyskinesia/dystonia scores were reduced by 54 and 62% respectively in the two periods. The authors suggested that levodopa-induced *sensitization of dopamine receptors* may be partially reversible if dosage can be reduced.

Sleep episodes associated with the newer drugs have been discussed in detail. Doubt has been cast on the existence of *sleep attacks*, that is acute episodes of sleep that occur without warning (23[R]). In the view of the authors of this review underlying somnolence is always present even if the patient is not aware of it. They did not attempt to differentiate the risk associated with different agents but noted that pramipexole doses below 1.5 mg/day are usually adequate and much less likely to cause this problem than higher doses. In general they stressed the importance of keeping doses of all the agents as low as possible and of warning patients about the risk, particularly when driving. They also commented that the possibility of an underlying sleep disorder should be considered in these circumstances.

A study of the effects of pramipexole was generally in agreement with these conclusions (24[C]). In a double-blind study 22 patients were randomized to pramipexole monotherapy (mean 4.4, range 1.5–6, mg/day) and 18 to placebo. Six patients taking pramipexole reported *somnolence* (one moderate, five mild), compared with two patients taking placebo (one moderate, one mild). In an open-label extension of the study, 21 of 37 patients reported somnolence, including 11 with moderate and three with severe symptoms. The onset of symptoms occurred at a mean dosage of 4 mg/day and patients had been taking treatment for 10 months on average at the time of the worst symptoms. Of the 14 patients with moderate to severe symptoms, 12 were interviewed in detail; seven reported falling asleep while driving and two had been involved in minor accidents. Most of the patients reported continuous drowsiness as a background, but three said that they experienced sudden waves of irresistible sleepiness, although with some prodromal symptoms. The symptoms resolved on drug withdrawal or dosage reduction (though details of this were not given), and the comments on dosage from the previous paper are surely relevant. In patients taking pramipexole patient education is clearly of vital importance.

These problems can occur with longer-established dopamine receptor agonists. A 57-year-old woman and a 61-year-old man taking pergolide 4.5 and 5 mg/day respectively both suffered sleep disorders; the woman did not suffer from sleepiness but had abrupt sleep episodes, while the man was sleepy for much of the day (25[A]). These were high doses and a reduction to 3 mg/day led to cessation of sleepiness in both patients.

Psychiatric Drug-induced *hallucinations* are a more familiar aspect of the treatment of Parkinson's disease. Susceptibility to these shows great interindividual variation and it is hardly surprising that researchers are seeking genetic bases for these. Polymorphisms of dopamine receptor genes seem obvious candidates, and this has been studied by a group in Sheffield (26[C]). They found an association between late-onset hallucinations and a polymorphism close to the D2 receptor. However, the effect is not overwhelming: the abnormal allele of the Taq IA polymorphism was found in 82% of those who hallucinated and 59% of those who did not. This is statistically significant but, as often in this type of study, the biological and clinical relevance is far from certain.

There may be more subtle neuropsychiatric adverse effects of dopaminergic medication. The syndrome of *hedonistic homeostatic dysregulation*, generally associated with substance abuse, has been described in 15 patients with Parkinson's disease (27[c]). Four patients were described in detail. The authors noted that 12 of the 15 patients were men (three of the four described in the paper) and had early onset of Parkinson's disease: those described were aged only 36–42 years. Characteristically, these patients were taking large and increasing doses of levodopa (or other dopamine agonists, including apomorphine) despite worsening dyskinesias; they had impaired social functioning, including absence from work, belligerent behavior and hypersexuality; they had a hypomanic or bipolar affect; they underwent a withdrawal reaction on reducing levodopa dosage, with depression, dysphoria, and anxiety; and they had a disorder with the above features lasting at least 6 months. All of the four patients described in detail had taken apomorphine at some time (75–170 mg/day) and tended to use higher than prescribed doses by intermittent injection. All were also taking levodopa (maximum dose 1875–5500 mg/day). The authors noted that the long-term management of this condition can be very difficult. They suggested management of acute psychosis with atypical neuroleptic drugs, such as olanzapine or risperidone, the use of antidepressants if needed, and careful supervision of patient self-medication. They conceded that this may be extremely difficult.

Skin A 28-year-old woman taking bromocriptine 5 mg/day for a microprolactinoma developed numerous nodular skin lesions (28[A]). Skin biopsy showed a polyclonal proliferation of both B and T lymphocytes in a follicular pattern, and a diagnosis of *cutaneous pseudolymphoma* was made. The lesions disappeared within 8 weeks of withdrawal.

Serosae *Fibrotic reactions* continue to be reported in patients taking ergot derivatives (29[A]).

A 67-year-old man in Germany with Parkinson's disease took co-careldopa and (somewhat unusually) α-dihydroergocryptine 45 mg/day, the latter in order to regulate fluctuations on motor function. After 2 years he developed a dry cough with dyspnea. Chest X-rays showed severe thickening of the pleura bilaterally with associated effusions. Biopsy confirmed fibrosis. The ergot drug was immediately replaced with pramipexole, eventually at a dose of 3 mg/day. Respiratory symptoms improved markedly within weeks, but there was little change radiologically.

Although this is the first description of such a reaction to this particular drug, it has been well documented with several other dopaminergic ergot derivatives.

Retroperitoneal fibrosis is also recognized as an adverse effect of these drugs (30[A]).

A 63-year-old British woman with Parkinson's disease was given pergolide in an attempt to minimize motor fluctuations in response to levodopa. After taking 4.5 mg/day for 8 months she developed shortness of breath and ankle swelling. This gradually deteriorated over the next year, despite diuretic therapy, and by that time her serum creatinine was 807 μmol/l and her hemoglobin was 8 g/dl. She had bilateral hydronephrosis on ultrasound scanning and a CT scan confirmed retroperitoneal fibrosis, which was successfully treated with nephrostomy and stenting, with resolution of the hydronephrosis. Pergolide was discontinued.

Drug formulations When four patients from Argentina experienced deterioration of their Parkinson's disease it was discovered that their medication contained not 250 mg levodopa plus benserazide, as labeled, but only 60 mg of levodopa alone (31[c]). Even more bizarrely, seven patients from Peru developed extrapyramidal symptoms when supposedly taking lincomycin: in fact each capsule contained no less than 500 mg of metoclopramide.

OTHER DRUGS THAT INCREASE DOPAMINE ACTIVITY

(SED-14, 424; SEDA-24, 167)

Catechol-*O*-methyl transferase inhibitors

Liver Despite the withdrawal of tolcapone, the topic of the *hepatotoxicity* of these drugs continues to attract interest (32[R]). While neither drug appeared to cause liver damage in preclinical testing, during clinical trials tolcapone caused significant rises in liver enzymes in 1% of patients taking 100 mg/day and 3% of those taking 200 mg/day. Subsequently there were three deaths from acute liver failure in patients taking the drug during a total exposure of 40 000 patient years, leading to the complete withdrawal of the drug. No serious hepatotoxicity has been attributed to entacapone. An earlier review, predating the withdrawal of the drug, had suggested that tolcapone could be safely used provided liver function was closely monitored in the first 6 months of therapy (33[R]), and some neurologists believe that this course of action may still be reasonable because of what they regard as the superior efficacy of this drug.

Drug interactions An interaction of entacapone with ephedrine is described above.

Selegiline

Drug interactions A rather surprising interaction of selegiline with *dopamine* has been described (34[A]).

A 75-year-old critically ill man taking selegiline 10 mg/day was given intravenous dopamine 3.5 μg/kg/min. Within 50 minutes his systolic pressure had risen from 105 to 228 mmHg. Within 30 minutes of stopping the infusion his systolic blood pressure fell to 121 mmHg. Rather surprisingly, two rechallenges were attempted on that day and the next, at doses of 1.03 and 0.9 μg/kg/min. Severe hypertension occurred on both occasions, with return to normal pressures very soon after the dopamine was discontinued.

As the authors pointed out, the selectivity of selegiline for monoamine oxidase type B may be less than was once thought, and co-administration of the drug with dopamine may be risky.

THE ERGOT ALKALOIDS AND RELATED AGENTS *(SED-14, 431; SEDA-23, 157; SEDA-24, 168)*

Ergot alkaloids are vasoconstrictors and are still sometimes used in the prevention of migraine, despite the availability of more effective compounds (see also Chapter 19). Because of their effects on dopamine receptors they have also occasionally been used to treat Parkinson's disease and to suppress lactation. Ergometrine causes uterine contraction and has been used to prevent and treat postpartum hemorrhage.

Cardiovascular The vasoconstrictor properties of some of the ergot alkaloids continue to cause serious problems. *Myocardial infarction* has been reported in a woman with a history of hyperlipidemia (35[A]).

A 27-year-old woman with familial hypercholesterolemia already treated with lipid-lowering drugs developed acute chest pain after a prophylactic intramuscular injection of 0.5 mg ergometrine, given during the late stages of labor. Angiography showed three-vessel atherosclerotic disease and occlusion of the left anterior descending coronary artery. Angioplasty with stenting was successful and she made an excellent recovery.

Clearly, a history of this kind should be regarded as a contraindication to prophylactic ergometrine administration.

The role of arterial spasm as a cause of angina after angioplasty has been studied in two men, aged 45 and 58 years, who had emergency angioplasties for acute coronary thrombosis (36[A]). Although the primary procedures were successful in both cases, ischemic chest pain returned after 4 and 6 months respectively. Perhaps a little surprisingly, in both cases intravenous ergonovine (0.4 mg) was given during coronary angiography, causing severe arterial spasm, which resolved with intravenous isosorbide dinitrate. There was no evidence of restenosis. The authors noted that recurrence of angina does not necessarily imply restenosis, although it is not clear how many cardiologists will repeat this procedure with their own patients.

The cerebral vasculature can also be vulnerable to ergot-induced vasoconstriction, as a case of *cerebral infarction* shows (37[A]).

A 54-year-old woman with a 20-year history of migraine used a nasal ergotamine spray one evening during an episode of migraine. She used a second dose at 4 p.m. the next day since the migraine had persisted. The following morning she was given subcutaneous sumatriptan 6 mg. Some 30–45 minutes later she developed the symptoms of global amnesia, which resolved by the following morning. Magnetic resonance imaging showed a small infarct in the right thalamus.

It seems likely the co-administration of two cerebral vasoconstrictors increased the likelihood of such an event.

A 36-year-old woman developed a "cerebral angiopathy" within 36 hours after starting to take oral metergoline, an ergot derivative prescribed after delivery to suppress lactation (38[A]). This angiopathy was apparently due to severe narrowing of small and medium cerebral arteries; its main features were sudden hypertension, seizures, and variable reversible neurological deficits.

DRUGS THAT AFFECT THE CHOLINERGIC SYSTEM

(SED-14, 436; SEDA-22, 156; SEDA-23, 158; SEDA-24, 168)

Acetycholinesterase inhibitors

Teratogenicity *Microcephaly* occurred in the child of a woman taking a high dose of pyridostigmine (39[A]).

A 24-year-old woman had suffered from myasthenia gravis from the unusually early age of 10 years. During her first pregnancy pyridostigmine was her sole medication. Because of deterioration in her symptoms during the pregnancy the dose was increased until she was taking 1500–3000 mg/day, or 4–8 times the maximum recommended dose. This still did not produce much clinical improvement but was nevertheless continued throughout the pregnancy. She needed an emergency cesarean section at 36 weeks because of fetal bradycardia. The baby was microcephalic.

The authors failed to find any other cause for this abnormality and concluded that the excessive dose of pyridostigmine had been responsible for the fetal damage.

Anticholinergic drugs

Much of the interest in this area is focused on the use of drugs to treat bladder instability and over-activity. The efficacy, safety, and tolerability of tolterodine and oxybutynin have been compared (40[M]). The authors concluded that the efficacy of tolterodine 2 mg bd is equivalent to that of oxybutynin 5 mg bd, but that tolterodine causes fewer autonomic adverse effects, less need for dosage reduction, and fewer dropouts because of adverse effects.

Means of reducing the adverse effects of oxybutynin have been considered in 226 patients (89% women, mean age 59 years) with urge incontinence and known to be responsive to anticholinergic therapy, who were randomized to take either conventional or modified-release oxybutynin (41[C]). The dosage was titrated up to a maximum of 20 mg/day in both groups. Response rates were similar in both groups, as was the incidence of *dry mouth* (48% in the modified-release group and 59% in the immediate-release group). However, further analysis showed that at any dose significantly fewer patients complaining of dry mouth in the modified-release group, and this was even more apparent in patients with moderate to severe dry mouth.

Another approach is to try to stimulate salivary flow in patients taking oxybutynin. Malic acid pastilles have been used as a salivary stimulant, but the results were not good, although the study has some design problems (42[c]). Of the 67 women enrolled only 32 completed the 8-week study. It is not clear whether there was any attempt to make the trial double-blind.

Nervous system A report of *Parkinsonism* due to propiverine combines a clinical observation with basic pharmacology (43[AE]).

A 72-year-old man had taken propiverine 20 mg/day for nocturia. The exact symptoms are difficult to define, because of the rather curious terminology used in the report, but it appears that he rapidly developed Parkinsonian symptoms soon after the start of treatment and was given levodopa 3 months later, with a limited response. After 1 month it was decided to withdraw propiverine and his symptoms disappeared within 2 weeks.

The authors then studied the effect of propiverine on the induction of catalepsy in mice, comparing it with oxybutynin, pentoxyverine, and etafenone, using haloperidol as a reference. They also examined dopamine receptor binding in the striatum. They concluded that any of these agents could cause catalepsy in mice, and that propiverine had greater potency than oxybutynin but less than the others. It was also noted that all the drugs had submicromolar affinity for striatal D_2 receptors. The authors suggested that any drug, such as these, that has an diethylaminomethyl moiety has the potential for extrapyramidal effects, because of interaction with dopamine receptors in the basal ganglia.

Skin An 83-year-old man developed a generalized pruritic erythematous reaction with a fever after taking flavoxate 200 mg tds for 6 months in combination with tamsulosin hydrochloride and allylestrenol for prostatic hyperplasia (44[A]). Patch tests with these drugs showed a positive reaction on flavoxate 10% on day 3. Rechallenge with flavoxate caused generalized pruritic erythema with fever.

REFERENCES

1. Adams MC, McLaughlin KP, Rink RC. Inadvertent concentrated epinephrine injection at newborn circumcision: effect and treatment. J Urol 2000; 163: 592.
2. Maaranen TH, Mäntyjärvi MI. Central retinal artery occlusion after a local anesthetic with adrenaline on nasal mucosa. J Neuro-Opthalmol 2000; 20: 234–5.
3. Lichtenstein GR, Yee NS. Ischemic colitis associated with decongestant use. Ann Intern Med 2000; 132: 682.
4. Kluger MT. Ephedrine may predispose to arrhythmias in obstetric anaesthesia. Anaesth Intensive Care 2000; 28: 336.
5. Jacobs KM, Kirsch KA. Psychiatric complications of Ma-huang. Psychosomatics 2000; 41: 58–62.
6. Sànchez TS, Sànchez-Pérez J, Aragüés M, Garcïa-Dïez A. Flare-up reaction of pseudoephedrine baboon syndrome after positive patch test. Contact Dermatitis 2000; 42: 312–13.
7. Renfrew C, Dickson R, Schwab C. Severe hypertension following ephedrine administration in a patient receiving entacapone. Anesthesiology 2000; 93: 1562.
8. Kennan WN, Viscoli CM, Brass LM, Broderick JP, Brott T, Feldmann E, Moregenstern LB, Wilterdink JL, Horwitz RI. Phenylpropanolamine and the risk of hemorrhagic stroke. New Engl J Med 2000; 343; 1826–32.
9. Hamilton RF, Sharieff G. Phenylpropanolamine-associated intracranial hemorrhage in an infant. Am J Emerg Med 2000; 18: 343–5.
10. Goodhue A, Bartel RL, Smith NB. Exacerbation of psychosis by phenylpropanolamine. Am J Psychiatry 2000; 157: 1021–2.
11. Lattanzi F, Picano E, Adamo E, Varga A. Dobutamine stress echocardiography. Safety in diagnosing heart disease. Drug Saf 2000; 22: 251–62.
12. Varga A, Picano E, Lakatos F. Fatal ventricular fibrillation during a low-dose dobutamine stress test. Am J Med 2000; 108: 352–3.
13. Kawano H, Fujii H, Motoyama T, Kugiyama K, Ogawa H, Yasue H. Myocardial ischemia due to coronary artery spasm during dobutamine stress echocardiography. Am J Cardiol 2000; 85: 26–30.
14. Roldàn F-J, Vargas-Barrón J, Espinola-Zavaleta N, Keirns C, Romero-Càrdenas A. Severe dynamic obstruction of the left ventricular outflow tract in-

duced by dobutamine. Echocardiography 2000; 17: 37–40.
15. Burger AJ, Notarianni MP, Aronson D. Safety and efficacy of an accelerated dobutamine stress echocardiography protocol in the evaluation of coronary artery disease. Am J Cardiol 2000; 86: 825–9.
16. Garcimartin I, San Román JA, Vilacosta I, Muñoc JC, De la Torre M, Fernández-Avilés F. Complicaciones de la ecocardiografía de estrés transesofàgica con dobutamina. Rev Esp Cardiol 2000; 53: 1136–9.
17. Lambert D, Waters CH. Comparative tolerability of the newer generation antiparkinsonian agents. Drugs Aging 2000; 16: 55–65.
18. Kujawa K, Leurgans S, Raman R, Blasucci L, Goetz CG. Acute orthostatic hypotension when starting dopamine agonists in Parkinson's disease. Arch Neurol 2000; 57: 1461–3.
19. Lindner M, Rosenkranz S, Deutsch HJ, Erdmann E. Ergotamininduzierter postpartaler Myokardinfarct. Herz Kreisl 2000; 32: 65–8.
20. Tan E-K, Ondo W. Clinical characteristics of pramipexole-induced peripheral edema. Arch Neurol 2000; 57: 729–32.
21. Varsano S, Gershman M, Hamaoui E. Pergolide-induced dyspnea, bilateral pleural effusion and peripheral edema. Respiration 2000; 67: 580–2.
22. Bejjani BB, Arnulf I, Demeret S, Damier P, Bonnet A-M, Houeto J-L, Agid Y. Levodopa-induced dyskinesias in Parkinson's disease: is sensitization reversible? Ann Neurol 2000; 47: 655–8.
23. Olanow CW, Schapira AHV, Roth T. Waking up to sleep episodes in Parkinson's disease. Mov Disord 2000; 15: 212–15.
24. Hauser RA, Gauger L, Anderson WM, Zesiewicz TA. Pramipexole-induced somnolence and episodes of daytime sleep. Mov Disord 2000; 15: 658–63.
25. Schapira AHV. Sleep attacks (sleep episodes) with pergolide. Lancet 2000; 355: 1332–3.
26. Makoff AJ, Graham JM, Arranz MJ, Forsyth J, Li, T, Aitchison KJ, Shaikh S, Grünewald RA. Association study of dopamine receptor gene polymorphisms with drug-induced hallucinations in patients with idiopathic Parkinson's disease. Pharmacogenetics 2000; 10: 43–8.
27. Giovannoni G, O'Sullivan JD, Turner K, Manson AJ, Lees AJL. Hedonistic homeostatic dysregulation in patients with Parkinson's disease on dopamine replacement therapies. J Neurol Neurosurg Psychiatry 2000; 68: 423–8.
28. Wiesli P, Joos L, Galeazzi RL, Dummer R. Cutaneous pseudolymphoma associated with bromocriptine therapy. Clin Endocrinol 2000; 53: 655–7.
29. Oechsner M, Groenke L, Mueller D. Pleural fibrosis associated with dihydroergocryptine treatment. Acta Neurol Scand 2000; 101: 283–5.
30. Mondak BK, Suri S. Pergolide-induced retroperitoneal fibrosis. Int J Clin Pract 2000; 54: 403.
31. Consentino C, Torres L, Scorticati MC, Micheli F. Movement disorders secondary to adulterated medication. Neurology 2000; 55: 598–9.
32. Watkins P. COMT inhibitors and liver toxicity. Neurology 2000; 55 Suppl 4: S51–2.
33. Olanow CW. Tolcapone and hepatotoxic effects. Arch Neurol 2000; 57: 263–7.
34. Rose LM, Ohlinger MJ, Mauro VF. A hypertensive reaction induced by concurrent use of selegiline and dopamine. Ann Pharmacother 2000; 34: 1020–4.
35. Mousa HA, McKinkley CA, Thong J. Acute postpartum myocardial infarction after ergometrine administration in a woman with familial hypercholesterolaemia. Br J Obstet Gynaecol 2000; 107: 939–40.
36. Yoshitomi Y, Kojima S, Sugi T, Matsumoto Y, Yano M, Kuramochi M. Coronary artery spasm induced by ergonovine in an infarct related coronary artery late after primary angioplasty. J Intervent Cardiol 2000; 13: 31–4.
37. Pradalier A, Lutz G, Vincent D. Transient global amnesia, migraine, thalamic infarct, dihydroergotamine, and sumatriptan. Headache 2000; 40: 324–7.
38. Cripps G, Sverzelatti E, Pancotti D, Carrara GC. Severe postpartum hypertension and reversible angiopathy associated with ergot derivative (methergoline) administration. Ann Ital Med Interna 2000; 15: 303–5.
39. Niesen CE, Shah NS. Pyridostigmine-induced microcephaly. Neurology 2000; 54: 1873–4.
40. Malone-Lee JG. The efficacy, tolerability and safety profile of tolterodine in the treatment of overactive/unstable bladder. Rev Contemp Pharmacother 2000; 11: 29–42.
41. Versi E, Appell R, Mobley D, Patton W, Saltzstein D. Dry mouth with conventional and controlled-release oxybutynin in urinary incontinence. Obstet Gynecol 2000; 95: 718–21.
42. Tincello DG, Adams EJ, Sutherst ER, Richmond DH. Oxybutynin for detrusor instability with adjuvant salivary stimulant pastilles to improve compliance: results of a multicentre, randomized controlled trial. BJU Int 2000; 85; 416–20.
43. Matsuo H, Matsui A, Nasu R, Takanaga H, Inoue N, Hattori F, Ohtani H, Sawada Y. Propiverine-induced parkinsonism: a case report and a pharmacokinetic/pharmacodynamic study in mice. Pharm Res 2000; 17: 565–71.
44. Enomoto U, Ohnishi Y, Kimura M, Kawada A, Ishibashi A. Drug eruption due to flavoxate hydrochloride. Contact Dermatitis 1999; 40: 337.

W.M.C. Mulder and M.M.H.M. Meinardi

14 Dermatological drugs and topical agents

CONTACT ALLERGY

Miscellaneous reports of contact allergy to ingredients of topical drugs and cosmetics are listed in Table 1 (1[A]–13[A], 14[c], 15[A]–18[A]).

Corticosteroids

Allergic contact dermatitis has again been associated with topical clobetasone (19[A]).

A 36-year-old man, who had a long history of atopic dermatitis of the neck, chest, and arms, developed allergic contact dermatitis after topical administration of clobetasone ointment 0.05% (Kindavate®) and prednisolone ointment 0.3% (Lidomex®). Patch tests with both ointments showed a positive reaction only to Kindavate®. Further testing with the separate ingredients of Kindavate® showed positive reactions to 0.05, 0.01, and 0.005% clobetasone on day 7.

Fragrances

Contact allergic reactions to the fragrance mix in the European patch test standard series are the second most common cause of allergic positive patch tests. A study from Slovenia showed that in 1989–93, 3.9% of 6129 routinely patch tested patients reacted to the fragrance mix; the incidence increased to 7.5% from 1994 to 1998 (20[C]). A Portuguese study with the fragrance mix supplemented with the constituents of the fragrance mix (substances cinnamic alcohol, cinnamic aldehyde, α-amyl cinnamic aldehyde, eugenol, iso-eugenol, geraniol, hydroxycitronellal, and oak moss) and some other fragrance ingredients showed that 10.9% of the 2600 patients tested in 1989–99 reacted to the fragrance mix (21[C]). As expected, under 60% of those patients also reacted to a component of the fragrance mix.

In clinical practice, it is noted that positive reactions to the fragrance mix are not always translated into allergic contact dermatitis on exposure (22[C], 23[C]). However, a Danish study showed that 29% of a group of 1537 randomly sampled adults who were interviewed, confirmed that they had had a rash on exposure to scented products at some point in their life. Indicating the perceived importance of the problem, the authors found higher rates in the last 15 years compared with the preceding period (24[C]).

A study in 25 545 patients who were patch tested with the European standard series from 1980 to 1996, showed that the mean frequency of allergic patch test reactions remained stable (8.5% in women, 6.7% in men) (25[C]). On the level of the individual constituents of the fragrance mix, the authors found an increase in the frequency of allergic reactions to oak moss, iso-eugenol, and α-amyl cinnamic aldehyde. The frequencies with eugenol and geraniol remained stable, while there was a fall with citronellal, cinnamic aldehyde, and cinnamic alcohol. The incidence with sorbitan sesquioleate, an emulsifier added to the fragrance mix in 1985, remained low. Similar results were found in an English study (26[C]). Of 23 660 patients patch tested in 1984–98, 1811 showed a positive patch test to the fragrance mix, while the most frequent positive reactions to the individual constituents occurred to oak moss, iso-eugenol, and eugenol.

Several other fragrance materials can cause sensitization, but not always due to their use in cosmetics. In a Japanese study, patients were patch tested with several essential oils. Only lavender oil 20% in petrolatum showed a sharp increase from 0 to 3.8% from 1990 to

Side Effects of Drugs, Annual 25
J.K. Aronson, ed.

Table 1. *Contact allergy to ingredients of topical drugs and cosmetics*

Ingredient	Use	Test conc. & vehicle	Number studied	Comments	Reference
Alkylammonium amidobenzoate (Osmaron®)	Preservative, disinfectant	0.1% and 0.01% petrolatum	1	Used in udder cream, not included in INCI-list (SEDA-17, 188)	(1[A])
Benzophenone	UV absorber for curing acrylates	Not reported	1	Eyelid dermatitis	(2[A])
1,3-Butylene glycol	Humectant, preservative	5% aqua	1	Eleventh case of contact allergy	(3[A])
Carmustine	Alkylating agent	0.1% aqua	1	Fourth case of contact allergy; patch test with lomustine was negative	(4[A])
Cetrimide	Preservative, antiseptic	0.1% aqua	1	Rare and very weak sensitizer; irritant when tested in higher concentrations (6[A])	(5[A])
Cocamidopropyl hydroxysultaine	Amphoteric surfactant, conditioner in shampoos, cleansing agents	1% aqua	1	Negative reaction to cocamidopropyl betaine	(7[A])
Crocein scarlet MOO and solvent yellow 3	Red skin colorant (alta), also textile dye	1% plastibase	1	Both ingredients showed cross-reactivity with para-amino compounds and caused depigmentation	(8[A])
Diethyl sebacate	Emulsifier	5% petroleum	1	Fifth case (SEDA-24, 173)	(9[A])
Doxepin	Monoamine reuptake blocker; topical treatment of itch	0.05–5% petrolatum	1	Further case (SEDA-19, 158)	(10[A])
Eucalyptol (*Malaleuca alternifolia*)	Antifungal; antibacterial; increases transcutaneous penetration	1% petrolatum	1	Second report	(11[A])
Glyceryl trinitrate (Percutol®)	Topical vasodilator	2% petrolatum	1		(12[A])
Melia azadirachata (Psorigon®)	Topical antipsoriasis cream; insect repellent; insecticide; soil fertilizer; dye; wax; lubricant; soap; oral hygiene products	1–10%, vehicle not stated	1	First report of contact allergy	(13[A])
Parabens	Preservative	Paraben-mix European Standard Series	1	Laser-associated contact dermatitis; see also (14[C])	(15[A])
Polyvinylpyrrolidone/ eicosene co-polymer	Antistatic; binder; film former; suspending and viscosity increasing agent in cosmetics	1% petroleum	1	Second report	(16[A])
Tetrahydroxypropyl ethylenediamine	Humectant; plasticizer; emulsifier	10% petroleum	1	First report; no reaction to ethylenediamine	(17[A])
Tosufloxacin tosilate	Quinolone antibiotic	20% petrolatum on previously affected site	1	Third case of fixed drug reaction to tosufloxacin tosilate	(18[A])

1996, to 8.7% in 1997, and to 13.9% in 1998. The authors associated this increase mainly with aroma therapy with dried lavender flowers (27[C]).

Grains – hydrolysed wheat protein and *Avena sativa* (wild oats)

Hydrolysed wheat protein and *Avena sativa* (wild oats) are added to cosmetics as moisturizers. A 64-year-old non-atopic housewife developed itchy, erythematous, edematous lesions on the eyelids, face, and neck after applying a moisturizing cosmetic cream every day for 2 years. A patch test with 10% hydrolysed wheat protein in water gave a positive reaction, while 34 controls were negative. This proved the first allergic contact dermatitis from a cosmetic cream containing 0.06% hydrolysed wheat protein (28[A]). Another first report concerns a 3-year-old girl who had a flare-up of her atopic dermatitis on exposure to a cosmetic cream containing *Avena sativa*. Patch tests with the compound were strongly positive reaction, while 20 volunteers remained negative (29[A])

Para-phenylenediamine

Para-phenylenediamine can be added to strengthen the color of temporary henna tattoos, and a risk of sensitization when it is used in this way is increasingly being reported (30[A]–32[A]).

Polidocanol

Polidocanol is a solvent and non-ionic emulsifier. In medicaments it is used as topical anesthetic, an antipruritic, and a sclerosing agent. Previously, contact allergic reactions have been reported (33[A]). Patch testing with polidocanol may yield irritant reactions. In a retrospective study of 8739 patients tested with a topical drug patch test series, 3186 patients were tested with 0.5% polidocanol in water (34[C]). There was slight irritation in 0.88%, weakly positive reactions in 0.97%, and strongly positive reactions in 0.25%. In 6202 patients tested with polidocanol 3% in petrolatum, there was slight skin irritation in 0.48%, weakly positive reactions in 1.77%, and strongly positive reactions in 0.34%. Among the 649 patients tested with both preparations, concurrence was moderate.

Polyhexamethylenebiguanide

Polyhexamethylenebiguanide, a biocide structurally related to hexamidine, has recently been added to cosmetics as a preservative. Hexamidine (0.15% petrolatum) (SEDA-10, 128) has rarely been reported to cause a contact allergic reaction (35[A], 36[A]). Of 1554 patients tested with polyhexamethylenebiguanide 2.5% in aqua, six (0.4%) showed a positive reaction, indicating a very low sensitization rate (37[C]).

Tea tree oil *(SEDA-18, 170; SEDA-23, 165)*

Tea tree oil is distilled from the leaves of *Melaleuca alternifolia*, an Australian native plant. Tea tree oil is considered to have antibacterial properties, including an effect on methicillin-resistant *Staphylococcus aureus* (MRSA), while the commensal flora of the skin seem to be less susceptible (38[E]). In addition, tea tree oil is said to have antifungal, antiviral, anti-inflammatory, and analgesic properties.

Undiluted tea tree oil can cause skin irritation. Safety data on tea tree oil used on open wounds are not available. Its systemic toxicity is comparable to that of eucalyptus oil, and ingestion of 10–25 ml has resulted in ataxia, drowsiness, disorientation, or coma for 2 days; recovery was full without complications (39[A]).

The use of tea tree oil has increased significantly over the past several years. Since 1991, several reports have noted contact allergic reactions to tea tree oil (40[A], 41[A]). Degradation products of monoterpenes are the sensitizing agents; patients who are allergic to tea tree oil do not react to patch tests with freshly distilled tea tree oil (42[E]). Many people who are allergic to tea tree oil may therefore also react to turpentine, colophony, fragrances, balsam of Peru, and plant extracts of compositae (43[A]).

A 46-year-old Chinese man developed an allergic contact dermatitis to tea tree oil, colophony, balsam of Peru, and abitol. He had used the tea tree oil under an occlusive dressing on a superficial abrasion on his left shin for 2 weeks, after which the treated area became red and itchy. During the next week skin lesions appeared on his trunk and extremities, and were diagnosed as an erythema multiforme-like id reaction.

Titanium

Titanium, in spite of its widespread use, is only rarely linked with contact allergic reactions. A contact allergic reaction has been reported in three individuals of a group of 23 volunteers who participated in a study with topically applied ammonium titanium lactate 10% (44[A]).

Toothpastes

In a retrospective study of 202 patients with cheilitis, an allergic cause was identified in 34%. In women, lip cosmetics were the commonest cause (54%), followed by toothpastes 21% and topical medications (7%) (45[C]). The literature on allergic contact cheilitis to toothpastes has been reviewed (46[R]).

PHOTOSENSITIVITY

Calcipotriol in combination with photochemotherapy

Hyperpigmentation due to local application of vitamin D in combination with photochemotherapy has been described. The vitamin D3 analog calcipotriol might have the same potential. A case is reported in which profound hyperpigmentation occurred during UVB 311 nm phototherapy in combination with local calcipotriol, applied after the UVB irradiation (47[A]). Calcipotriol-treated areas, and not the surrounding normal skin, started to show increased pigmentation after six sessions of irradiation, stabilized during therapy, and slightly decreased in intensity during the 6 months after photochemotherapy had ended. No photoallergy tests were performed.

Itraconazole

The first case of possible *photosensitivity* from itraconazole (200 mg qds for 5 days) has been reported, with reduced minimal erythema dose for both UVB (0.12 J/cm^2) and UVA (20.1 J/cm^2), negative photopatch testing, and a positive photochallenge (48[A]). The authors proposed a photoallergic mechanism because earlier exposure to itraconazole had been uneventful. However, details about sun exposure during the first exposure and about the intensity of sun exposure during the oral photochallenge procedure were not given. The eruption responded to oral steroids, which is more typical of photoallergic than phototoxic reactions.

NSAIDs

Photocontact allergy to NSAIDs is not uncommon, but the incidence may differ from NSAID to NSAID. The first case of photoallergy from local piketoprofen has been reported (49[A]). Two cases of prolonged photosensitivity after contact photoallergy from ketoprofen, persisting for more than a year after withdrawal, have also been reported (50[A], 51[A]).

Ranitidine

A case of persistent UVB photosensitivity due to ranitidine (300 mg/day) has been reported (52[A]).

CONTACT URTICARIA

Reports of *contact urticaria* to relatively rare antigens in both cosmetic products and drugs are listed in Table 2 (53[A]–57[A]).

IMMUNOSTIMULANTS

Imiquimod *(SEDA-23, 168)*

The incidence of local adverse events of the response-modifying drug imiquimod (5%, applied three times a week) for the treatment of anogenital warts, seems to be lower in HIV-infected patients than has previously been reported in healthy individuals (58[c]; SEDA-23, 168). In a uncontrolled trial of topical 5% imiquimod for the treatment of common warts and molluscum contagiosum in otherwise healthy patients *fever*, healing with *scarring*, and healing with *hyperpigmentation* were each reported by one participant (59[c]).

Table 2. *Contact urticaria to ingredients of topical drugs and cosmetics*

Allergen	Allergen-containing product	20-min patch test	Skin prick test	Reference
Cyclopentolate hydrochloride	Eye drops (Colircursí Cicloplejico 1%)	Eye drops +	Not performed	(53[A])
Di(2-ethylhexyl) phthalate (DOP)	PVC grip cotton gloves	Rubbing with PVC grip +	Gas chromatography extracts +, DOP +, Di-n-butylmaleate +	(54[A])
Glyceryl thioglycolate	Hair permanent fluid	1% in petrolatum +	Not performed	(55[A])
Panthenol	Hair conditioner –	Hair conditioner – Panthenol 30% in petrolatum –	Hair conditioner + Panthenol +++	(56[A])
Wheat hydrolysate	Body cream	Body cream ++	Wheat hydrolysate ++	(57[A])

MISCELLANEOUS REACTIONS

Diphenylcyclopropenone

Diphenylcyclopropenone is a potent sensitizing chemical used to induce a contact dermatitis of the scalp in the topical immunotherapy of alopecia areata. Pressure-induced urticaria and widespread severe dermographism developed after the first application to the scalp of a 0.003% solution of diphenylcyclopropenone in a 19-year-old Japanese man (60[A]). Diphenylcyclopropenone was withdrawn, but the symptoms persisted for almost 3 months. An IgE-mediated hypersensitivity reaction was suggested by the authors, but skin tests were not performed; nor was specific IgE measured. A similar case has recently been described and the adverse events of diphenylcyclopropenone reviewed (61[Ar]).

Hyaluronic acid

Hyaluronic acid is increasingly being used in cosmetic dermatology to treat wrinkles in patients who are sensitive to bovine collagen. Adverse effects of this dermatological application have not yet been reported.

An *exudative granulomatous reaction* started 2 days after the injection of hyaluronic acid (Hylaform®, dose not stated) for perioral wrinkles (62[A]). The eczematous papular skin changes disappeared completely within 6 weeks, and could be provoked by intracutaneous testing with Hylaform® (dose not stated). Histological examination showed a foreign body granuloma.

RETINOIDS (see also p. 457)

The incidence and time-course of adverse events during a 4-month course of oral isotretinoin (1 mg/kg) for severe acne have been studied prospectively in 189 patients (63[C]). Most known adverse events were most often reported during the first 3 months of treatment. However, only a few patients were seen every month as scheduled and only 50 of 189 filled in the questionnaire at 4 months.

Sensory systems *Corneal opacities* following treatment with oral isotretinoin in general disappear after withdrawal. However, in one case corneal opacities were persistent (64[A]).

A 39-year-old woman developed corneal opacities while taking oral isotretinoin 1 mg/kg for 6 months. The opacities persisted for at least 6 years after discontinuation of the drug. She had worn soft hydrophilic contact lenses for 10 years before, but without signs of corneal opacity 1 month before treatment was started.

Urinary tract *Nephrotic syndrome* developed after 4 months treatment with isotretinoin 40 mg/day (65[A]). No other causes were found and the symptoms disappeared with appropriate treatment within some months.

Musculoskeletal *Adult onset Still's disease* occurred after 3 months of oral isotretinoin (66[A]). No other causes were found and the symptoms disappeared with appropriate treatment within some months.

Teratogenicity There are few data about the safety of topical retinoids during pregnancy. Now a case has been reported (67[A]).

A baby was born missing its right ear and external auditory canal. At 20 months an MRI scan of the brain showed focal atrophy and encephalomalacia of the right parieto-occipital lobe. His mother had used topical tretinoin (Retin A 0.025%) on her face and a large surface of the back before conception and during the first 2–3 months of pregnancy. His father had used oral isotretinoin before conception.

This type of ear abnormality is a typical feature of retinoic acid embryopathy. Given the pattern of malformations in this child the authors thought that maternal use of topical tretinoin had been responsible. Three other cases of fetal malformations after topical tretinoin use have been reported (68[A]–70[A]).

REFERENCES

1. Haapasaari KM, Niinimäki A. Allergic contact dermatitis from alkylammonium amidobenzoate (Osmaron®). Contact Dermatitis 2000; 42: 244–3.
2. Guin JD. Eyelid dermatitis from benzophenone used in nail enhancement. Contact Dermatitis 2000; 43: 308–9.
3. Diegenant C, Constandt L, Goossens A. Allergic contact dermatitis due to 1,3-butylene glycol. Contact Dermatitis 2000; 43: 234–5.
4. Thomson KF, Sheehan-Dare RA, Wilkinson SM. Allergic contact dermatitis from topical carmustine. Contact Dermatitis 2000; 42: 112.
5. Lee JY, Wang BJ. Contact dermatitis caused by cetrimide in antiseptics. Contact Dermatitis 1995; 33: 168.
6. Leow Y-H, Tan CSC. Allergic contact dermatitis from cetrimide and cetearyl alcohol in Burnol-plus® cream. Contact Dermatitis 2000; 43: 174–5.
7. Guin JD. Reaction to cocamidopropyl hydroxysultaine, an amphoteric surfactant and conditioner. Contact Dermatitis 2000; 42: 282.
8. Bajaj AK, Misra A, Misra K, Rastogi S. The azo dye solvent yellow 3 produces depigmentation. Contact Dermatitis 2000; 42: 237–8.
9. Tanaka M, Kobayashi S, Murata T, Tanikawa A, Nishikawa T. Allergic contact dermatitis from diethyl sebacate in lanoconazole cream. Contact Dermatitis 2000; 43: 233.
10. Buckley DA. Contact allergy to doxepin. Contact Dermatitis 2000; 43: 231.
11. Vilaplana J, Romaguera C. Allergic contact dermatitis due to eucalyptol in an anti-inflammatory cream. Contact Dermatitis 2000; 43: 118.
12. McKenna KE. Allergic contact dermatitis from glyceryl trinitrate ointment. Contact Dermatitis 2000; 42: 246.
13. Ahmed I, Charles-Holmes R. Contact allergy to Psorigon®. Contact Dermatitis 2000; 42: 276.
14. Mowad CM. Allergic contact dermatitis caused by parabens: 2 case reports and a review. Am J Contact Dermatitis 2000; 11: 53–6.
15. Shaffer M, Williford PM, Sherertz EF. An old reaction in a new setting: the paraben paradox. Am J Contact Dermatitis 2000; 11: 189.
16. Le Coz C-J, Lefèbvre C, Ludmann F, Grosshans É. Polyvinylpyrrolidone (PVP)/eicosene copolymer: an emerging cosmetic allergen. Contact Dermatitis 2000; 43: 61–2.
17. Kirkup ME, Sansom JE. Contact sensitivity to tetrahydroxypropyl ethylenediamine in a sunscreen, without cross-sensitivity to ethylenediamine. Contact Dermatitis 2000; 43; 121–2.
18. Sangen Y, Kawada A, Asai M, Aragane Y, Yudate Y, Tezuka T. Fixed drug eruption induced by tosufloxacin tosilate. Contact Dermatitis 2000; 42: 285.
19. Murata T, Tanaka M, Dekio I, Tanikawa A, Nishikawa T. Allergic contact dermatitis due to clobetasone butyrate. Contact Dermatitis 2000; 42: 305.
20. Lunder T, Kansky A. Increase in contact allergy to fragrances: patch-test results 1989–1998. Contact Dermatitis 2000; 43: 107–9.
21. Brites MM, Gonçalo M, Figueiredo A. Contact allergy to the fragrance mix – a 10 year study. Contact Dermatitis 2000; 43: 181–2.
22. Frosch PJ, Pilz B, Andersen KE. Patch testing with fragrances: results of a multicenter study of the European Environmental and Contact Dermatitis Research Group with 48 frequently used constituents of perfumes. Contact Dermatitis 1995; 33: 333–42.
23. Bárány E, Lodén M. Content of fragrance mix ingredients and customer complaints of cosmetic products. Am J Contact Dermatitis 2000; 11: 74–9.
24. Johansen JD, Andersen TF, Thomsen LK, Kjøller M, Menné T. Rash related to use of scented products, a questionnaire study in the Danish

population. Is the problem increasing? Contact Dermatitis 2000; 42: 222–6.
25. Buckley DA, Wakelin SH, Seed PT, Holloway D, Rycroft RJG, White IR, McFadden JP. The frequency of fragrance allergy in a patch-test population over a 17-year period. Br J Dermatol 2000; 142: 279–83.
26. Buckley DA, Rycroft RJG, White IR, McFadden JP. Contact allergy to individual fragrance mix constituents in relation to primary site of dermatitis. Contact Dermatitis 2000; 43: 304–5.
27. Sugiura M, Hayaka R, Kato Y, Sugiura K, Hashimoto R. Results of patch testing with lavender oil in Japan. Contact Dermatitis 2000; 43: 157–60.
28. Sanchez-Pérez J, Sanz T, García-Díez A. Allergic contact dermatitis from hydrolyzed wheat protein in cosmetic cream. Contact Dermatitis 2000; 42: 360.
29. Pazzaglia M, Jorizzo M, Parente G, Tosti A. Allergic contact dermatitis due to *Avena* extract. Contact Dermatitis 2000; 42: 364.
30. Tosti A, Pazzaglia M, Corazza M, Virgili A. Allergic contact dermatitis caused by mehindi. Contact Dermatitis 2000; 42: 356.
31. Mohamed M, Nixon R. Severe allergic contact dermatitis induced by paraphenylenediamine in paint-on temporary "tattoos". Australas J Dermatol 2000; 41: 168–71.
32. Lestringant GG, Bener A, Frossard PM. Cutaneous reactions to henna and associated additives. Br J Dermatol 1999; 141: 598–600.
33. Frosch PJ, Schulze-Dirks A. Kontaktallergie durch Polidocanol (Thesis). Hautarzt 1989; 40: 146–9.
34. Uter W, Geier J. Contact allergy to polidocanol, 1992 to 1999. J Allergy Clin Immunol 2000; 106: 1203–4.
35. Revuz J, Poli F, Wechsler J, Dubertret L. Dermite de contact a l'hexamidine. Ann Dermatol Venereol 1984; 111: 805–10.
36. Dooms-Goossens A. Hexamidine isethionate: a sensitizer in topical pharmaceutical products and cosmetics. Contact Dermatitis 1989; 21: 270.
37. Schnuch A, Geier J, Brasch J, Fuchs Th, Pirker C, Schulze-Dirks A, Basketter DA. Polyhexamethylene biguanide: a relevant contact allergen? Contact Dermatitis 2000; 42: 302–3.
38. Carson CF, Riley TV, Cookson BD. Efficacy and safety of tea tree oil as a topical antimicrobial agent. J Hosp Infect 1998; 40: 175–8.
39. Seawright A. Comment: tea tree oil poisoning. Med J Aust 1993; 159: 831.
40. Apted JH, Contact dermatitis associated with the use of tea tree oil. Australas J Dermatol 1991; 32: 177.
41. Varma S, Blackford S, Statham BN, Blackwell A. Combined allergy to tea tree oil and lavender oil complicating chronic vulvovaginitis. Contact Dermatitis 2000; 42: 309.
42. Hausen BM, Reichling J, Harkenthal M. Degradation products of monoterpenes are the sensitizing agents in tea tree oil. Am J Contact Dermatitis 1999; 10: 68–77.
43. De Groot AC, Weyland JW. Systemic contact dermatitis from tea tree oil. Contact Dermatitis 1992; 27: 279–80.
44. Basketter DA, Whittle E, Monk B. Possible allergy to complex titanium salt. Contact Dermatitis 2000; 42: 310–11.
45. Lim SW, Goh CL. Epidemiology of eczematous cheilitis at a tertiary dermatological referral centre in Singapore. Contact Dermatitis 2000; 43: 322–6.
46. Francalanci S, Sertoli A, Giorgini S, Pigatto P, Santucci B, Valsecchi R. Multicentre study of allergic contact cheilitis from toothpastes. Contact Dermatitis 2000; 43: 216–22.
47. Rütter A, Schwarz T. Ausgeprägte Hyperpigmentierung in psoriatischen Plaques als Folge einer Kombinationsbehandlung mit UVB–311 nm und Calcipotriol. Hautarzt 2000; 51: 431–3.
48. Alvarez-Fernández JG, Castaño-Suárez E, Cornejo-Navarro P, Gómez de la Fuente E, Ortiz de Frutos FJ, Iglesias-Diez L. Photosensitivity induced by oral itraconazole. J Eur Acad Dermatol Venereol 2000; 14: 501–3.
49. Goday Buján JJ, Oleaga Morante JM, González Gümez M, Del Pozo Lozada J, Fonseca Capdevila E. Photoallergic contact dermatitis from piketoprofen. Contact Dermatitis 2000; 43: 315.
50. Albès B, Marguery MC, Schwarze HP, Journé F, Loche F, Bazex J. Prolonged photosensitivity following contact photoallergy to ketoprofen. Dermatology 2000; 201: 171–4.
51. Offidani AM, Cellini A, Amerio P, Simonetti O, Bossi G. A case of persistent light reaction phenomenon to ketoprofen? Eur J Dermatol 2000; 10: 153–4.
52. Kondo S, Kagaya M, Yamada Y, Matsusaka H, Jimbow K. UVB photosensitivity due to ranitidine. Dermatology 2000; 201: 71–3.
53. Muñoz-Bellido FJ, Beltrán A, Bellido J. Contact urticaria due to cyclopentolate hydrochloride. Allergy 2000; 55: 198–9.
54. Sugiura K, Sugiura M, Hayakawa R, Sasaki K. Di(2-ethylhexyl)phthalate (DOP) in the dotted polyvinyl-chloride grip of cotton gloves as a cause of contact urticaria syndrome. Contact Dermatitis 2000; 43: 237–8.
55. Engasser P. Type I and Type IV immune responses to glyceryl thioglycolate. Contact Dermatitis 2000; 42: 298.
56. Schalock PC, Storrs FJ, Morrison L. Contact urticaria from panthenol in hair conditioner. Contact Dermatitis 2000; 43: 223.
57. Varjonen E, Petman L, Mäkinen-Kiljunen S. Immediate contact allergy from hydrolyzed wheat in a cosmetic cream. Allergy 2000; 55: 294–6.
58. Gilson RJC, Shupack JL, Friedman-Kien AE, Conant MA, Weber JN, Nayagam AT, Swann RV, Pietig DC, Smith MH, Owens ML, and the Imiquimod Study Group. A randomized, controlled, safety study using imiquimod for the topical treatment of anogenital warts in HIV-infected patients. AIDS 1999; 13: 2397–404.

59. Hengge UR, Esser S, Schultewolter T, Behrendt C, Meyer T, Stockfleth E, Goos M. Self-administered topical 5% imiquimod for the treatment of common warts and molluscum contagiosum. Br J Dermatol 2000; 143: 1026–31.
60. Skrebova N, Nameda Y, Takiwaki H, Arase S. Severe dermographism after topical therapy with diphenylcyclopropenone for alopecia universalis. Contact Dermatitis 2000; 42: 212–15.
61. Alam M, Gross EA, Savin RC. Severe urticarial reaction to diphenylcyclopropenone therapy for alopecia areata. J Am Acad Dermatol 1999; 40: 110–12.
62. Raulin C, Greve B, Hartschuh W, Soegdin K. Exudative granulomatous reaction to hyaluronic acid (Hylaform). Contact Dermatitis 2000; 43: 178.
63. Hull PR, Demkiw-Bartel C. Isotretinoin use in acne: prospective evaluation of adverse events. J Cutaneous Med Surg 2000; 4: 66–70.
64. Ellies P, Dighiero P, Legeais JM, Pouliquen YJM, Renard G. Persistent corneal opacity after oral isotretinoin therapy for acne. Cornea 2000; 19: 238–9.
65. Van Oers JAH, De Leeuw J, Van Bommel EFH. Nephrotic syndrome associated with isotretinoin. Nephrol Dial Transplant 2000; 15: 923–4.
66. Leibovitch I, Amital H, Levy Y, Langevitz P, Shoenfeld Y. Isotretinoin-induced adult onset Still's disease. Clin Exp Rheumatol 2000; 18: 616–18.
67. Selcen D, Seidman S, Nigro MA. Otocerebral anomalies associated with topical tretinoin use. Brain Dev 2000; 22: 218–20.
68. Camera G, Pregliasco P. Ear malformation in baby born to mother using tretinoin cream. Lancet 1992; 339: 687.
69. Lipson AH, Collins F, Webster WS. Multiple congenital defects associated with maternal use of topical tretinoin. Lancet 1993; 341: 1352–3.
70. Navarre-Belhassen C, Blanchet P, Hillaire-Buys D, Sarda P, Blayac JP. Multiple congenital malformations associated with topical tretinoin. Ann Pharmacother 1998; 32: 505–6.

Jean Bousquet and Pascal Demoly

15 Antihistamines (H_1 receptor antagonists)

The H_1 histamine receptor antagonists were discovered by Bovet and Staub at the Institut Pasteur in 1937 (1[E]). Although the first antihistamine was too weak and toxic for clinical use, its discovery resulted in an enormous amount of research and led in 1942 to the development of the first antihistamine to be used in the treatment of allergic diseases phenbenzamine (Antegan®) (2[CE]). Within a few years, three other antihistamines became available and are still in use today: mepyramine (pyrilamine) maleate (3[CE]), diphenhydramine (4[CE]), and tripelennamine (5[E]). Despite their pronounced adverse effects, these were the first really useful drugs for the symptomatic relief of allergic disorders. During the last 25 years several compounds with greater potency, longer durations of action, and minimal sedative effects have emerged, the so-called second-generation H_1 antihistamines, as opposed to the older, or classic antihistamines. Two recent papers have confirmed the safety of the second-generation antihistamines; in particular, loratadine, fexofenadine, norastemizole, and descarboxyloratadine (desloratadine) were shown not to have sedative effects (6[R], 7[C]).

The cardiotoxic effects of antihistamines

During the last 15 years terfenadine and astemizole have been described as having dysrhythmogenic actions, and deaths have been described (8[R], 9[R]). These drugs have dose-dependent cardiotoxic effects and are metabolized by cytochrome P450 isozymes. This means that the concomitant administration of compounds that compete with these enzymes (such as macrolides, antifungal azoles, and grapefruit juice) can reduce the metabolism of the histamine H_1 receptor antagonists and increase their plasma concentrations, increasing the risk of cardiotoxicity.

However, the effect is not mediated via histamine receptors and is not a class effect – several newer antihistamines are not cardiotoxic.

Cetirizine *In a prospective, double-blind, parallel-group study for 18 months in 817 children with atopic dermatitis aged 12–24 months, cetirizine 0.25 mg/kg bd had no effect on the QT_c interval (10[C]).*

Desloratadine *There were only small increases (under 15%) in the mean pharmacokinetics of desloratadine when it was coadministered with azithromycin in a randomized, placebo-controlled, parallel-group study (11[C]). Desloratadine with and without azithromycin was well tolerated, and there were no statistically significant changes in PR interval, QT interval, QRS complex, or heart rate.*

Ebastine *The effects of supratherapeutic doses of ebastine on the QT interval have been tested (12[C]). Ebastine in doses up to five times the recommended therapeutic dose did not cause clinically important changes in the QT_c interval.*

Emedastine *There was a moderate but statistically significant pharmacokinetic interaction between emedastine and ketoconazole (13[C]). However, pharmacodynamic data showed no increase in the QT_c interval during concomitant therapy. This result is consistent with the known multiple pathways for the metabolism of emedastine, including different isoforms of CYP450.*

Side Effects of Drugs, Annual 25
J.K. Aronson, ed.

Fexofenadine *Fexofenadine, an active metabolite of terfenadine, is said to be non-cardiotoxic (14[R]). In a pharmacokinetic study peak fexofenadine concentrations were increased by 69% and the AUC was increased by 67% in the presence of azithromycin (11[C]). However, fexofenadine with and without azithromycin was well tolerated, and there were no statistically significant changes in PR interval, QT interval, QRS complex, or heart rate. There has been a report of ventricular fibrillation during fexofenadine administration in a man with a pre-existing long QT interval (15[A]). However, causality between fexofenadine and the cardiac effects was unclear.*

Loratadine *The pharmacokinetics, electrocardiographic effects, and tolerability of loratadine syrup have been studied in 161 children aged 2–5 years (16[C]). A single-dose open-label study was performed to characterize the pharmacokinetic profiles of loratadine and its metabolite desloratadine, and a randomized, double-blind, placebo-controlled, parallel-group study was performed to assess the tolerability of loratadine syrup 5 mg after multiple doses. Electrocardiographic parameters were not altered by loratadine compared with placebo. There were no clinically important changes in other tolerability assessments. In healthy adults loratadine 10 mg/day had no effects on the electrocardiogram when coadministered for 10 days with therapeutic doses of ketoconazole or cimetidine (17[C]).*

Norastemizole *Norastemizole is a metabolite of astemizole (18[R]). Its major advantage is that it is not cardiotoxic and does not interact with drugs that increase the risk of serious dysrhythmias.*

Nervous system Histamine is both a local hormone and a neurotransmitter in the central nervous system (CNS). It is synthesized by neurons and mast cells. There are H_1, H_2, and H_3 receptors in the CNS, but they differ in their localization, biochemical machinery, functions, and affinities for histamine. The most common adverse effects of first-generation antihistamines are sedation and CNS depression or stimulation, even at the usual therapeutic doses. The new generation of compounds are mostly devoid of CNS adverse effects. A battery of cognitive and psychomotor tests has been used to assess both objective and subjective *sedative effects* of antihistamines. Other symptoms of CNS depression are *disturbed co-ordination, dizziness, lassitude*, and an *inability to concentrate*.

Four prescription-event monitoring studies have been carried out in 43 363 patients in general practice in the UK to investigate the frequency with which sedation was reported in postmarketing surveillance studies of acrivastine, cetirizine, fexofenadine, and loratadine (19[C]). Prescriptions were obtained for each cohort in the immediate postmarketing period. Sedation and drowsiness were the main outcome measures. The odds ratios (adjusted for age and sex) for the incidences of sedation compared with loratadine were: 0.63 (95% CI = 0.36, 1.11) for fexofenadine, 2.79 (1.69, 4.58) for acrivastine, and 3.53 (2.07, 5.42) for cetirizine. There was no increased risk of accident or injury with any of the four drugs.

Antihistamines are effective and safe in preventing the symptoms of mosquito bite; ebastine and loratadine did not cause sedation in such cases (20[C], 21[C]).

Mequitazine has a low propensity to cause drowsiness, comparable to that of cetirizine and loratadine. It therefore differs from truly sedative antihistamines, such as dexchlorpheniramine, which cause drowsiness and fatigue in patients with atopy to a degree that is measurably different from placebo (22[R]).

The effects of diphenhydramine, fexofenadine, and alcohol on driving performance have been studied in a randomized, placebo-controlled trial in the Iowa driving simulator (23[C]). Participants had significantly better coherence after alcohol or fexofenadine than after diphenhydramine. Lane holding (steering instability and crossing the center line) was impaired after alcohol and diphenhydramine compared with fexofenadine. Mean response time to the blocking vehicle was slowest after alcohol (2.21 seconds) compared with fexofenadine (1.95 seconds). Self-reported drowsiness did not predict lack of coherence and was weakly associated with minimum following distance, steering instability, and left-lane excursion. In conclusion, the participants performed similarly when they took fexofenadine or placebo. After alcohol they performed the primary task well but not the secondary tasks, resulting in poorer driving performance.

After diphenhydramine, driving performance was poorest, suggesting that diphenhydramine had a greater impact on driving than alcohol did. Drowsiness ratings were not a good predictor of impairment, suggesting that drivers cannot use drowsiness to indicate when they should not drive. Non-sedating antihistamines should therefore be preferred over sedating antihistamines in patients who drive (24[r]).

Although allergic rhinitis is not usually severe, it affects school learning performance and work productivity (25[R]). The effects of loratadine and cetirizine on somnolence and motivation during the working day have been compared in 60 patients with allergic rhinitis in a parallel-group, double-blind study (26[C]). Somnolence scores were similar in the two groups at baseline and at the time of dosing (0800 hours). However, cetirizine caused significantly more somnolence at 1000, 1200, and 1500 hours. The scores of motivation to perform activities were similar in the two groups at baseline and 0800 hours. The patients taking loratadine were relatively more motivated at 1000, 1200, and 1500 hours.

School performance in 63 children aged 8–10 years was not impaired by short-term diphenhydramine or loratadine (27[C]).

Psychological The effects of cetirizine, loratadine, and promethazine on have been assessed in healthy volunteers; promethazine caused *impaired cognitive function and psychomotor performance* (28[C]). The test battery consisted of critical flicker fusion, choice reaction time, compensatory tracking task, and assessment of subjective sedation. Cetirizine and loratadine at all doses tested were not significantly different from placebo in any of the tests used. However, as expected for a drug with known sedative effects, all measures, with the exception of the compensatory tracking task were significantly altered by promethazine.

Functional neuroimaging of cognition was impaired by a first-generation antihistamine, d-chlorpheniramine (29[E]).

Metabolic In a double-blind, randomized, placebo-controlled study of the effect of cetirizine, clemastine, and loratadine for 7 days on blood glucose concentration in patients with allergic rhinitis, cetirizine produced a *significant increase in postprandial blood glucose* and a small *rise in fasting blood glucose*; clemastine caused a small fall in fasting and a small rise in postprandial blood glucose (30[C]). The mechanisms of these effects are not known.

Liver Severe hepatitis has been reported in a man taking cetirizine (31[A]) and *cholestasis* in a 28-year-old man who had taken cetirizine for 2 years (32[A]). However, a causal relation between these uncommon events and cetirizine was difficult to confirm.

Urinary tract *Bladder irritability* is a common adverse effect of tranilast, and another case has been reported in a 59-year-old man who had been taking tranilast 600 mg/day for 15 weeks (33[A]). Cystoscopy showed extensive mucosal edema, strongly suggestive of drug-induced cystitis. He stopped taking tranilast and the symptoms disappeared within 3 weeks.

Skin A man taking cetirizine developed a *multifocal fixed drug eruption* (34[A]).

Generalized urticaria developed in a woman 2 hours after she took cetirizine (35[A]). Two cases of drug allergy have been reported in a 37-year-old woman and a 66-year-old man, who received hydroxyzine for premedication before anesthesia (36[A], 37[A]). In these three patients immediate skin tests with the implicated drug were positive.

Skin reactions with parenteral pheniramine maleate are uncommon, but a case of relapsing generalized *multiple evanescent pruritic erythematous wheals* after antihistamine and steroid injections has recently been reported in a 29-year-old woman (38[A]).

Teratogenicity The teratogenicity of antihistamines has been reviewed (39[R], 40[M]). The view that the antihistamines as a group, and in particular the combination of doxylamine/pyridoxine with or without dicycloverine, are teratogenic has not been substantiated by these reviews.

Risk factors *Children* H_1 receptor antagonists have not been adequately studied in very young children, although they are widely used and assumed to be safe. The effects of cetirizine 0.25 mg/kg bd for 18 months have been investigated in a prospective, double-blind, parallel-group study in 817 children with atopic dermatitis aged 12–24 months (10[C]). Dropouts and serious events, including hospitalization, were infrequent and were less common in the children who took cetirizine, although the differences were not statistically significant. Most of the adverse events were mild and were not related to medication.

Age and sex Ebastine undergoes extensive first-pass metabolism by CYP3A4 to form an active metabolite, carebastine. The effects of age and sex on the pharmacokinetics of ebastine and carebastine have been studied (41[C]). Ebastine can be safely given to elderly subjects and there are no clinically important age- or sex-related differences in the pharmacokinetics of ebastine/carebastine.

Drug overdose Although the clinical features of diphenhydramine overdose are well known, information about dose-dependent toxicity is still scarce. This has now been investigated in patients with acute diphenhydramine poisoning in retrospective and prospective studies in 232 and 50 patients respectively (42[C]). Mild symptoms (somnolence, anticholinergic signs, tachycardia, nausea/vomiting) occurred in 55–64% of patients, moderate symptoms (isolated and spontaneously resolving agitation, confusion, hallucinations, and electrocardiographic disturbances) in 22–27%, and severe symptoms (delirium/psychosis, seizures, coma) in 14–18%. Moderate symptoms occurred at doses over 0.3 g. For severe symptoms the critical dose limit was 1.0 g. Coma and seizures were significantly more frequent in those who took over 1.5 g compared with those who took 1.0–1.5 g. These data show clear dose-dependent acute toxicity of diphenhydramine. They suggest that only patients who take over 1.0 g are at risk of severe symptoms.

Drug interactions Some second-generation H_1 antihistamines (but not cetirizine, desloratadine, fexofenadine, levocetirizine, or norastemizole) undergo hepatic metabolism via the cytochrome P450 system, and are transformed into active metabolites. Cytochrome P4503A is localized in high amounts both in the small intestinal epithelium and liver and it is a major contributor to presystemic elimination following oral drug administration. Drug interactions involving enzyme inhibition or induction are common following the coadministration of two or more CYP3A substrates (43[R]).

Pooled human liver microsomes have been used to determine whether loratadine, desloratadine, and 3-hydroxydesloratadine are inhibitors of CYP1A2, CYP2C9, CYP2C19, CYP2D6, and CYP3A4 (44[E]). Loratadine did not inhibit CYP1A2 or CYP3A4 at concentrations up to 3829 ng/ml, about 815 times greater than the expected maximal human plasma concentration (mean 4.7 ng/ml) after the recommended dose of 10 mg/day. Loratadine inhibited CYP2C19 and CYP2D6 with IC_{50} values of about 0.76 μmol/l (291 ng/ml) and 8.1 μmol/l (3100 ng/ml) respectively, about 60 and 660 times the expected loratadine therapeutic concentrations. Neither desloratadine nor 3-hydroxydesloratadine inhibited CYP1A2, CYP2C9, CYP2C19, CYP2D6, or CYP3A4 by more than 25% at concentrations of about 3000 ng/ml. These results suggest that loratadine and its active metabolites desloratadine and 3-hydroxydesloratadine are unlikely to affect the pharmacokinetics of coadministered drugs that are metabolized by these five cytochrome P450 enzymes.

The first-generation H_1 antihistamine diphenhydramine interacts with CYP2D6 and can cause clinically important interactions with many CYP2D6 substrates, particularly those with a narrow therapeutic index. Diphenhydramine inhibits the metabolism of metoprolol in extensive metabolizers, thereby prolonging its negative chronotropic and inotropic effects (45[C]). CYP2D6 is the major enzyme involved in the metabolism of venlafaxine, and diphenhydramine alters the disposition of venlafaxine, increasing plasma concentrations and predisposing to cardiovascular adverse effects (46[C]). Thus, clinically significant interactions can occur during concomitant administration of diphenhydramine and other antidepressant or antipsychotic drugs that are substrates of CYP2D6.

REFERENCES

1. Staub A, Bovet D. Actions de la thymoethyldiethylamine (929F) et des éthers phénoliques sur le choc anaphylactique du cobaye. CR Soc Biol 1937; 128: 818–25.
2. Halpern B. Les antihistaminiques de synthèse: essai de chimiothérapie des états allergiques. Arch Int Pharmacodyn Ther 1942; 68: 339–45.
3. Bovet D, Horclois R, Walthert F. Propriétés antihistaminiques de la N-p-méthoxybenzyl-N-diméthylaminoéthyl alpha aminopyridine. CR Soc Biol 1944; 138: 99–108.
4. Lowe E, MacMillan R, Katser M. The antihistamine properties of Benadryl, beta-dimethylaminoethyl benzhydryl ether hydrochloride. J Pharmacol Exp Ther 1946; 86: 229.
5. Yonkman F, Chess D, Mathieson D, Hansen N. Pharmacodynamic studies of a new antihistamine agent, N′-pyridyl-N′-benzyl-N-dimethylethylene diamine HCl, pyribenzamine HCl. I. Effects on salivation, nictitating membrane, lachrymation, pupil and blood pressure. J Pharmacol Exp Ther 1946; 87: 256.
6. Ellis A, Day J. Second- and third-generation antihistamines. Dermatol Rev 2000; 13: 327–36.
7. Van Cauwenberge P, Juniper EF. Comparison of the efficacy, safety and quality of life provided by fexofenadine hydrochloride 120 mg, loratadine 10 mg and placebo administered once daily for the treatment of seasonal allergic rhinitis. Clin Exp Allergy 2000; 30: 891–9.
8. Passalacqua G, Bousquet J, Bachert C, Church MK, Bindsley-Jensen C, Nagy L, Szemere P, Davies RJ, Durham SR, Horak F, Kontou-Fili K, Malling HJ, Van Cauwenberge P, Canonica GW. The clinical safety of H_1-receptor antagonists. An EAACI position paper. Allergy 1996; 51: 666–75.
9. Barbey JT, Anderson M, Ciprandi G, Frew AJ, Morad M, Priori SG, Ongini E, Affrime MB. Cardiovascular safety of second-generation antihistamines. Am J Rhinol 1999; 13: 235–43.
10. Estelle F, Simons R. Prospective, long-term safety evaluation of the H_1-receptor antagonist cetirizine in very young children with atopic dermatitis. Allergologie 2000; 23: 244–55.
11. Gupta S, Banfield C, Kantesaria B, Marino M, Clement R, Affrime M, Batra V. Pharmacokinetic and safety profile of desloratadine and fexofenadine when coadministered with azithromycin: a randomized, placebo-controlled, parallel-group study. Clin Ther 2001; 23: 451–66.
12. Gillen MS, Miller B, Chaikin P, Morganroth J. Effects of supratherapeutic doses of ebastine and terfenadine on the QT interval. Br J Clin Pharmacol 2001; 52: 201–4.
13. Herranz U, Rusca A, Assandri A. Emedastine–ketoconazole: pharmacokinetic and pharmacodynamic interactions in healthy volunteers. Int J Clin Pharmacol Ther 2001; 39: 102–9.
14. Eseverri J. Proyeccion de los nuevos antihistaminicos. Allergol Immunopathol (Madr) 2000; 28: 143–52.
15. Anonymous. Severe cardiac arrhythmia on fexofenadine. Prescrire Int 2000; 9: 45.
16. Salmun LM, Herron JM, Banfield C, Padhi D, Lorber R, Affrime MB. The pharmacokinetics, electrocardiographic effects, and tolerability of loratadine syrup in children aged 2 to 5 years. Clin Ther 2000; 22: 613–21.
17. Kosoglou T, Salfi M, Lim JM, Batra VK, Cayen MN, Affrime MB. Evaluation of the pharmacokinetics and electrocardiographic pharmacodynamics of loratadine with concomitant administration of ketoconazole or cimetidine. Br J Clin Pharmacol 2000; 50: 581–9.
18. Bachmann KA. Norastemizole Sepracor. Curr Opin Investig Drugs 2000; 1: 219–26.
19. Mann RD, Pearce GL, Dunn N, Shakir S. Sedation with "non-sedating" antihistamines: four prescription-event monitoring studies in general practice. Br Med J 2000; 320: 1184–6.
20. Karppinen A, Kautiainen H, Reunala T, Petman L, Brummer-Korvenkontio H. Loratadine in the treatment of mosquito-bite-sensitive children. Allergy 2000; 55: 668–71.
21. Karppinen A, Petman L, Jekunen A, Kautiainen H, Vaalasti A, Reunala T. Treatment of mosquito bites with ebastine: a field trial. Acta Dermatol Venereol 2000; 80: 114–16.
22. Didier A, Doussau-Thuron S, Murris-Espin M. Comparative analysis of the sedative effects of mequitazine and other antihistaminic drugs: review of the literature. Curr Ther Res Clin Exp 2000; 61: 770–80.
23. Weiler JM, Bloomfield JR, Woodworth GG, Grant AR, Layton TA, Brown TL, McKenzie DR, Baker TW, Watson GS. Effects of fexofenadine, diphenhydramine, and alcohol on driving performance. A randomized, placebo-controlled trial in the Iowa driving simulator. Ann Intern Med 2000; 132: 354–63.
24. Hennessy S, Strom BL. Nonsedating antihistamines should be preferred over sedating antihistamines in patients who drive. Ann Intern Med 2000; 132: 405–7.
25. Bousquet J, Van Cauwenberge P, Khaltaev N, editors. Allergic rhinitis and its impact on asthma. ARIA. In collaboration with the World Health Organization. J Allergy Clin Immunol 2001; 118 Suppl 10: S1–315.
26. Salmun LM, Gates D, Scharf M, Greiding L, Ramon F, Heithoff K. Loratadine versus cetirizine: assessment of somnolence and motivation during the workday. Clin Ther 2000; 22: 573–82.
27. Bender BG, McCormick DR, Milgrom H. Children's school performance is not impaired by short-term administration of diphenhydramine or loratadine. J Pediatr 2001; 138: 656–60.
28. Shamsi Z, Kimber S, Hindmarch I. An investigation into the effects of cetirizine on cognitive function and psychomotor performance in healthy volunteers. Eur J Clin Pharmacol 2001; 56: 865–71.

29. Okamura N, Yanai K, Higuchi M, Sakai J, Iwata R, Ido T, Sasaki H, Watanabe T, Itoh M. Functional neuroimaging of cognition impaired by a classical antihistamine, d-chlorpheniramine. Br J Pharmacol 2000; 129: 115–23.
30. Lal A. Effect of a few histamine1-antagonists on blood glucose in patients of allergic rhinitis. Indian J Otolaryngol Head Neck Surg 2000; 52: 193–5.
31. Watanabe M, Kohge N, Kaji T. Severe hepatitis in a patient taking cetirizine. Ann Intern Med 2001; 135: 142–3.
32. Fong DG, Angulo P, Burgart LJ, Lindor KD. Cetirizine-induce cholestasis. J Clin Gastroenterol 2000; 31: 250–3.
33. Saito M, Yoshimura S, Fujii A, Iwai A. Bladder irritability caused by tranilast. Iryo Jpn J Natl Med Serv 2000; 54: 361–4.
34. Kranke B, Kern T. Multilocalized fixed drug eruption to the antihistamine cetirizine. J Allergy Clin Immunol 2000; 106: 988.
35. Demoly P, Messaad D, Benahmed S, Sahla H, Bousquet J. Hypersensitivity to H_1-antihistamines. Allergy 2000; 55: 679–80.
36. Okuda T, Karasawa F, Satoh T. [A case of drug allergy to hydroxyzine used for premedication.] Masui 2000; 49: 759–61.
37. Urabe K, Fujii K, Tezuka M, Okuda Y, Kitajima T, Yamazaki T, Yamakage A. [A case of acute urticaria from hydroxyzine hydrochloride used for preanesthetic medication.] Masui 2000; 49: 890–2.
38. Yeon Jin Kim, Jin Hyouk Choi, Jang Seok Bang, Moo Kyu Suh, Jeong Woo Lee, Tae Hoon Kim. A case of pheniramine maleate-aggravated chronic urticaria. Korean J Dermatol 2000; 38: 1414–16.
39. Bishai R, Mazzotta P, Atanackovic G, Levichek Z, Pole M, Magee LA, Koren G. Critical appraisal of drug therapy for nausea and vomiting of pregnancy: II. Efficacy and safety of Diclectin (doxylamine–B6). Can J Clin Pharmacol 2000; 7: 138–43.
40. Mazzotta P, Magee LA. A risk-benefit assessment of pharmacological and non-pharmacological treatments for nausea and vomiting of pregnancy. Drugs 2000; 59: 781–800.
41. Rohatagi S, Gillen M, Aubeneau M, Jan C, Pandit B, Jensen BK, Rhodes G. Effect of age and gender on the pharmacokinetics of ebastine after single and repeated dosing in healthy subjects. Int J Clin Pharmacol Ther 2001; 39: 126–34.
42. Radovanovic D, Meier PJ, Guirguis M, Lorent JP, Kupferschmidt H. Dose-dependent toxicity of diphenhydramine overdose. Hum Exp Toxicol 2000; 19: 489–95.
43. Renwick AG. The metabolism of antihistamines and drug interactions: the role of cytochrome P450 enzymes. Clin Exp Allergy 1999; 3: 116–24.
44. Barecki ME, Casciano CN, Johnson WW, Clement RP. In vitro characterization of the inhibition profile of loratadine, desloratadine, and 3-OH-desloratadine for five human cytochrome P-450 enzymes. Drug Metab Dispos 2001; 29: 1173–5.
45. Hamelin BA, Bouayad A, Methot J, Jobin J, Desgagnes P, Poirier P, Allaire J, Dumesnil J, Turgeon J. Significant interaction between the nonprescription antihistamine diphenhydramine and the CYP2D6 substrate metoprolol in healthy men with high or low CYP2D6 activity. Clin Pharmacol Ther 2000; 67: 466–77.
46. Lessard E, Yessine MA, Hamelin BA, Gauvin C, Labbe L, O'Hara G, Leblanc J, Turgeon J. Diphenhydramine alters the disposition of venlafaxine through inhibition of CYP2D6 activity in humans. J Clin Psychopharmacol 2001; 21: 175–84.

Tracey D. Robinson, Adrian P. Havryk, and J. Paul Seale

16 Drugs acting on the respiratory tract

Intrapleural drugs for pleurodesis

Intrapleural therapy in humans was first reported by Bethune in 1935, when he described the dusting of pleural surfaces with talc before lobectomy to promote pleurodesis (1[A]). Since this initial description, many different agents have been used intrapleurally to produce pleurodesis, both in patients with pleural effusion and in patients with pneumothorax. Some of these agents, talc in particular, have been associated with potentially serious adverse events. Over the last 20 years the role of intrapleural therapy has expanded and now includes the instillation of thrombolytic agents intrapleurally to hasten the resolution of complicated pleural space infections (empyema); both streptokinase and urokinase have been used for this purpose. Adverse events related to the use of these agents have been rare. However, almost any agent introduced into the pleural space can reach the circulation through inflamed pleural surfaces, with potential adverse effects (2[c]).

Agents used for chemical pleurodesis *The aim of pleurodesis is to produce fusion between the visceral and parietal pleural surfaces and so prevent the accumulation of air or fluid in the pleural space. In a chemical pleurodesis, this fusion is generally achieved by the instillation of agents that induce an inflammatory response on the pleural surfaces. These agents can be introduced into the pleural space through a chest tube at the bedside or during thoracoscopy/thoracotomy.*

Side Effects of Drugs, Annual 25
J.K. Aronson, ed.

Talc *The use of talc, one of the most common agents for chemical pleurodesis, has been documented in more than 3000 patients, largely in the form of case series (3[R]). The intrapleural use of talc has been the subject of a number of recent comprehensive reviews (4[R], 5[M], 6[R]). Talc is a magnesium sheet silicate and is produced in an asbestos-free form for use in pleurodesis. The particle size varies considerably (7[c]) depending on the manufacturing process, and may be an important factor in the development of adverse effects (see below). Talc can be insufflated into the pleural space in a powder form, usually at thoracoscopy or thoracotomy (talc poudrage), or can be mixed with normal saline and instilled through a standard chest tube as talc slurry.*

Minor adverse effects related to talc pleurodesis are common: chest pain occurs in about 7% of patients and fever in 16–69%. Fever characteristically starts within 4–12 hours of pleurodesis and rarely lasts more than 72 hours. Chest pain is usually only mild (3[R], 4[R], 5[M]).

The most serious adverse effect of talc is a possible association between talc pleurodesis and the development of acute respiratory failure (usually in the form of ARDS); about 30 cases have been described (3[R]). Most of these cases have occurred in patients with malignant pleural effusions, not all were clearly talc-related, and there is not enough information in some case reports to be certain of the role of talc. For example, in 1980 respiratory failure/pneumonia in seven of 197 patients who underwent talc poudrage for malignant pleural effusion was described in an abstract, but no further information regarding the clinical course of these patients is available (8[r]). In 1983, Rinaldo et al. were the first to carefully document the development of ARDS after intrapleural talc instillation (9[A]). They described three patients who developed progressive dys-

pnea and acute respiratory failure, characterized by bilateral diffuse pulmonary infiltrates, within 72 hours of the instillation of talc 10 g through a chest tube. All three had underlying malignancies and all required intubation and ventilation for respiratory failure. One patient died after 1 month of intensive care support. No other cause for ARDS was found in these patients and the authors were confident that talc had been responsible, by unknown mechanisms. They recommended that other sclerosant agents be used for chemical pleurodesis. At around the same time, a patient who developed acute pneumonitis after chemical pleurodesis with talc 2 g was described (10[A]). The clinical course of this patient was different to that described above: breathlessness occurred within 3 hours of pleurodesis, but the patient did not require intensive care support until 10 days later, when bilateral pulmonary infiltrates developed. At bronchoalveolar lavage 12 days after pleurodesis, talc particles were seen in the lavage fluid. No other cause for the pulmonary infiltrates was found and the patient recovered with oxygen and corticosteroid therapy alone. The authors suggested that systemic absorption of talc, with subsequent embolization to the lung, had produced this picture and they also suggested that pleural biopsies performed just before pleurodesis might have aided the systemic absorption of talc.

Three large case series were published after these reports. In two (6[r], 11[C]) there were no episodes of respiratory distress after talc pleurodesis in 299 and 360 patients respectively. However, respiratory failure occurred in five of 58 patients treated with talc pleurodesis (12[C]). Excess narcotic analgesia and infective pneumonia were considered causative in two patients, and two other patients recovered with oxygen and corticosteroids. No more information on these two patients was provided. The remaining patient developed bilateral pulmonary infiltrates and severe hypoxia consistent with ARDS, but recovered after intubation and ventilation for 5 days. This patient had undergone simultaneous bilateral talc pleurodesis and the authors thought that the higher dose of talc that this patient had received might have contributed to the development of ARDS. Again, the mechanism by which talc produced ARDS was unknown.

The possibility that talc can cause respiratory failure was explored further in 1997 (13[A]). ARDS occurred in four of 338 patients treated with talc poudrage (2 g) via thoracoscopy. All four had malignant effusions and all developed bilateral pulmonary infiltrates, hypoxia, and hypotension within 24–48 hours of talc insufflation. All four required mechanical ventilation and three died. Bronchoalveolar lavage was performed in all four and talc crystals were recovered from lavage fluid in each case. Furthermore, at autopsy in one patient talc crystals were found in almost every organ, showing that systemic distribution of talc did occur after pleurodesis. However, as the authors acknowledged, it was not possible to definitely attribute the symptoms in these patients to the talc pleurodesis. Studies in animals have shown systemic distribution of talc after pleurodesis (14[E]). However, systemic dissemination may occur in all patients treated with pleurodesis and does not confirm that this is the cause of respiratory failure documented in a small number of patients.

The highest incidence of respiratory complications after talc pleurodesis was reported in 1999 in a retrospective review of 89 procedures in 78 patients (15[C]). ARDS occurred in 9% (i.e. after eight procedures in seven patients). All seven patients had increased oxygen requirements, respiratory distress, and bilateral infiltrates on chest X-ray, and required a mean of 38 hours of mechanical ventilation. Six patients had malignant effusions. The other had AIDS, had undergone bilateral pleurodesis for pneumothoraces secondary to Pneumocystis carinii pneumonia, and died within 24 hours of the procedure. No more clinical information was given about the other six patients, particularly regarding the time-course of symptoms and investigations to exclude other diseases.

The literature on this topic largely comprises case reports and retrospective reviews, raising the possibility that complications may be underreported. In addition, there is marked variability in the reported incidence of respiratory complications from series to series, and there is the additional confounding factor that malignant pleural effusion, a condition with a poor short-term survival and significant associated morbidity, is often the indication for talc pleurodesis. Respiratory complications are common in these patients, and talc pleurodesis may be coincidental rather than causative. Other possible causes for respiratory distress in these patients include re-expansion *pulmonary edema, sepsis related to the chest-tube, and bacterial contamination of talc. The presence of talc crystals in bronchoalveolar lavage fluid indicates systemic distribution but not necessarily causation of ARDS, and is likely to occur in all patients treated with talc. There is significant variability in the talc preparations available for pleurodesis, and it has been suggested that smaller particle size poses a higher risk for ARDS, although this is unproven. It has also been suggested that pleural biopsy before pleurodesis may increase the risk of ARDS (also unproven).*

In summary, talc is the most effective agent available for producing pleurodesis and remains the agent of choice in many centers. There have been reports of ARDS after talc pleurodesis, but there is insufficient information to incriminate talc with any certainty. It would seem prudent to avoid simultaneous bilateral procedures and pleural biopsy before pleurodesis and to await information from current trials.

Tetracycline derivatives *The intravenous formulation of tetracycline was instilled intrapleurally to produce chemical pleurodesis, with good effect, from the 1970s through to the 1990s. The adverse effect most commonly seen with tetracycline was chest pain, which was often severe (16[C], 17[C]). In a comprehensive review of intrapleural therapy published in 1994 (5[M]) the incidence of chest pain was estimated at 14%, and fever occurred in 10% of patients. However, the intravenous form of tetracycline has been withdrawn by the manufacturer and so this agent is no longer available for pleurodesis.*

When intravenous tetracycline became no longer available, many centers began to use doxycycline as a sclerosant. In the 1994 review mentioned above, chest pain was the most frequent adverse event with doxycycline, occurring in about 40% of the 60 patients in whom it had been used, and fever occurred in about 7%. In a more recent controlled trial in 106 patients treated with either doxycycline or bleomycin, there was chest pain in 20% of the patients treated with doxycycline, and nausea in one patient (18[C]).

The use of minocycline as an agent for inducing chemical pleurodesis has been reported in only a few patients and there is little information regarding adverse effects.

Bleomycin *Several antineoplastic agents have been introduced into the pleural space to achieve pleurodesis, but the greatest reported experience is with bleomycin. Intrapleural bleomycin has an efficacy similar to that of tetracycline and doxycycline (17[C]). About 45% of the dose of bleomycin is absorbed systemically, but significant adverse events are uncommon (19[c]). Chest pain is reported in around 28% of patients, fever in 24%, and nausea in about 11% (5[M]). A randomized study, published in 1991, compared bleomycin with tetracycline in 85 patients with malignant pleural effusions, and showed that toxicity, predominantly in the form of chest pain and fever, was similar with both drugs (7–17%) (16[C]). Nearly half the patients (34) died within 90 days, due to disease progression. However, one patient died within 2 days of intrapleural bleomycin, and the investigators could not exclude a contribution from the bleomycin. In another comparison of bleomycin with doxycycline (see above) there was fever in 13%, chest pain in 11%, and chills in 4% of patients treated with bleomycin (18[C]).*

Fibrinolytic drugs *Pleural space infection is an important cause of sepsis, and traditional treatment comprises drainage of the pleural space, either through chest tubes or surgically, combined with antibiotics. Attempts at closed drainage with a chest tube often fail owing to the development of loculations within the fluid and the high viscosity of infected fluid. This clinical problem has led to the use of intrapleural fibrinolytic drugs to improve drainage, hasten resolution of infection, and reduce the need for surgical intervention. Earlier use of intrapleural streptokinase and streptodornase was complicated by frequent allergic reactions, but with the availability of purified forms of streptokinase and urokinase these agents have been widely used for intrapleural fibrinolysis. The use of these agents has been the subject of a number of recent reviews.*

Streptokinase *Several reports over the last 10 years, predominantly in the form of case series, have described the use of intrapleural streptokinase for complicated pleural effusions (20[c]–24[c], 25[R], 26[R]). The dose of streptokinase used varies but is usually around 250 000 IU instilled once or twice daily, with tube clamping for 2–4 hours, repeated over several days.*

Local adverse effects are rare, but transient chest pain at the time of instillation occurs occasionally (21[c]). Similarly, there are occasional reports of fever attributed to the intrapleural instillation of streptokinase (20[c], 22[C]). The most important potential adverse event due to intrapleural streptokinase is systemic fibrinolysis. In many of the case series cited above, simple tests of clotting activity were performed before and after treatment and there were no significant changes. However, in 1984 a case report described major hemorrhage in one patient after the intrapleural use of streptokinase 500 000 IU, with tube clamping for 6 hours (27[A]). Within 12 hours this patient developed a generalized coagulopathy, with features of disseminated intravascular coagulation. Following this report, in a carefully designed study, the systemic fibrinolytic effects of one dose (250 000 IU) and multiple doses of intrapleural streptokinase (250 000 IU bd for 3 days) were examined in healthy subjects (28[C]). There were no physiological or statistical changes in any coagulation indices after intrapleural streptokinase. This suggests that the hemorrhage seen in the 1984 case report was probably not related to streptokinase, but was perhaps a complication of underlying sepsis.

Although intrapleural streptokinase does not cause systemic fibrinolytic effects, there may be local fibrinolytic effects. In a case series describing the use of intrapleural streptokinase or urokinase in 26 patients, one developed major "oozing" from rib fractures sustained 1 month before therapy (23[c]). This local bleeding required two thoracotomies. It is not clear from the report if streptokinase or urokinase was used in this patient, but streptokinase was used in most of the patients in this series. Furthermore, the dose used was also not clear, with streptokinase doses of 100 000–750 000 IU.

In 1998, major local hemorrhage after the use of intrapleural streptokinase was described in two patients (29[A]). One patient had undergone mitral valve replacement 6 weeks before and collapsed after 2 days of standard intrapleural streptokinase, with hemorrhage into the chest. The second had undergone a mitral valve replacement 9 months before intrapleural streptokinase and collapsed with bleeding into the chest after 3 days. Both patients recovered, but the authors felt that recent cardiac surgery presented a contraindication to the use of intrapleural fibrinolytics. It is not clear from this report if these two patients were taking oral anticoagulants, such as aspirin or warfarin, which may have confounded these findings.

One other report of local hemorrhage has recently been published (30[A]). The patient died after the instillation of intrapleural streptokinase for presumed empyema; autopsy showed an unsuspected abdominal aortic dissection with extension of blood clot into the thoracic cavity. These reports suggest that intrapleural streptokinase should be used with caution when there has been prior surgery or trauma involving the thorax.

Another potential adverse event associated with the use of intrapleural streptokinase is the development of antistreptokinase antibodies. These antibodies have been documented following intravenous streptokinase and can cause serious adverse events with re-exposure to streptokinase or can limit the efficacy of streptokinase in myocardial revascularization.

Urokinase *Urokinase has also been widely used intrapleurally for fibrinolysis, in doses of 40 000–250 000 IU and is as effective as streptokinase (31[C], 32[c]–34[c]). Furthermore, urokinase is not antigenic and does not produce febrile reactions. Just as for streptokinase, transient chest pain at the time of instillation has occasionally been reported. These considerations have led some authors to prefer urokinase to streptokinase for intrapleural therapy, but urokinase is about twice as costly as streptokinase. There is also more published experience with the use of streptokinase.*

β-ADRENOCEPTOR AGONISTS

(SED-14, 500; SEDA-22, 188; SEDA-23, 181; SEDA-24, 187)

β-adrenoceptor agonists can produce or worsen *hypoxia* acutely in patients with asthma by increasing ventilation–perfusion inequality. It is not known whether this effect is clinically important in patients with asthma not severe enough to require hospital treatment (where supplementary oxygen is standard therapy).

The systemic vascular changes produced by the combination of hypoxia and inhaled salbutamol in eight healthy men with mild asthma have been briefly reported (35[C]). This study examined forearm blood flow non-invasively to obtain a measure of forearm vascular resistance (FVR) (equating with systemic vascular resistance). This was a randomized, double-blind, placebo-controlled, cross-over trial in which measurements were made after inhalation of placebo or salbutamol 800 μg under normoxic or hypoxic conditions. Both salbutamol alone and hypoxia alone produced small non-significant falls in FVR, but the combination of salbutamol and hypoxia resulted in a dramatic fall (30%). The authors pointed out that this fall in FVR was equivalent to the effects of glyceryl trinitrate 0.6–0.9 mg sublingually or felodipine 10 mg orally. This study emphasizes the marked cardiovascular changes that can occur even with small doses of salbutamol in mild asthmatics when hypoxia is present and confirms the importance of supplementary oxygen in these patients.

Paradoxical *bronchoconstriction* has rarely been reported in asthmatics after the inhalation of β-agonists (36[A]).

A 22-year-old woman with mild asthma developed severe laryngospasm and bronchoconstriction after a fourth and subsequent doses of nebulized salbutamol, given during an acute episode of asthma. Her symptoms responded to adrenaline, but recurred after supervised rechallenge with nebulized orciprenaline (metaproterenol) sulfate. Indirect laryngoscopy excluded vocal cord dysfunction, suggesting that her symptoms of severe wheeze, respiratory distress, and hypoxia were due to bronchoconstriction.

This report serves as a reminder of this rare, but serious complication of nebulized β-agonists. It has been attributed to additives to nebulizer solutions, particularly edetate disodium, which produces dose-dependent bronchoconstriction.

The use of long-acting β-adrenoceptor agonists in the management of asthma in children was recently comprehensively reviewed (37[R]). In children, as in adults, regular long-acting β-adrenoceptor agonists can produce bronchodilator subsensitivity to short-acting β-agonists and tolerance to the bronchoprotective effects of long-acting β-agonists against challenges with exercise and methacholine. The clinical significance of these findings is unclear. Formoterol and salmeterol have similar adverse effects profiles, similar to that of salbutamol. The most common medication-related adverse effects are cardiovascular, such as *increased heart rate* and *palpitation*, or *tremor* and *headache*. Small *changes in serum potassium and glucose* can also be seen, but all changes are minor. The exact role of long-acting β-adrenoceptor agonists in childhood asthma remains to be defined.

Bambuterol

Bambuterol is an oral prodrug of terbutaline. It provides prolonged bronchodilator activity (for up to 24 hours). The comparative safety and efficacy of oral bambuterol given once daily and oral terbutaline given three times daily in children with asthma aged 2–12 years has recently been reported in two large similar trials from the same research group. In the first study they reported results from 3 months of treatment in 155 children aged 2–6 years (38[C]); in the second study they reported results from 12 months of treatment in 130 children aged 2–12 years (39[C]). Both were double-blind studies with a 2:1 bambuterol:terbutaline randomization pattern. In both studies, the bambuterol and terbutaline regimens were similarly efficacious in reducing asthma symptoms and improving peak expiratory flow rate. In the 3-month study, the most commonly reported adverse event was *restlessness*, reported in over 85% of patients in both treatment groups; other adverse events were described as mild to moderate, and overall there was no difference in the safety profile of the two drugs. In the 12-month trial, one subject in each treatment group withdrew because of an adverse event (*urticaria* and *dermatitis*). The most commonly reported adverse events attributable to the drugs were *headache* and *tremor*, which respectively occurred in 9 and 0% with terbutaline and 6 and 2% with bambuterol. Other adverse events were not described in detail. It seems that oral bambuterol has an efficacy and safety profile similar to that of oral terbutaline, with the advantage of once-daily dosing. The caveat is that inhaled therapy has fewer systemic adverse effects and is the route of choice.

Drug interactions Bambuterol has been reported to alter the metabolism of *mivacurium* (40[C]). Bambuterol has a dose-dependent inhibitory effect on plasma cholinesterase activity and prolongs the effects of succinylcholine. Bambuterol 10 mg was given to 28 patients 2 hours before an elective operation requiring general anesthesia. The study was originally designed as a randomized blinded trial, but was converted to an open study. The patients given bambuterol had a 67–97% fall in plasma cholinesterase activity, leading to reduced clearance of mivacurium. This resulted in a shorter onset and a 3- to 4-fold prolongation of action of the neuromuscular blockade produced by standard doses of mivacurium.

Formoterol

The non-pulmonary effects of formoterol have been carefully studied in an uncontrolled observational trial in 10 patients with asthma who were already taking regular inhaled budesonide (400 μg bd) (41[C]). Upper limb tremor was evaluated and a 24-hour Holter recording taken at baseline and after a 2-week treatment period with formoterol 12 μg bd. There were no significant changes in blood pressure, heart rate, cardiac morphology, or the circadian rhythm of autonomic regulation as assessed by measurements taken from the Holter monitor after the treatment period. There was a significant increase in *upper limb tremor* with formoterol and this was assessed as discomfort by one patient. This was considered due to stimulation of the β_2 adrenoceptors in skeletal muscle.

Salmeterol

Experimental studies continue to show that regular treatment with either formoterol or salmeterol in patients with asthma can produce subsensitivity to the bronchodilator effects of salbutamol (42[C], 43[C]). This *bronchodilator subsensitivity* can be partly reversed by a bolus dose of inhaled or systemic corticosteroids. The clinical relevance of these experimental findings remains unclear. In a double-blind multicenter trial in primary care, 911 patients with asthma, who were already receiving maintenance anti-inflammatory therapy, were randomized to treatment with salmeterol (50 μg bd) or placebo for 6 months (44[C]). As expected, the patients treated with salmeterol had higher mean peak expiratory flows, used less rescue salbutamol, and had less disturbed sleep than the patients treated with placebo. The most important result from this study was that the number of severe exacerbations was the same in both groups; in other words, salmeterol did not increase the frequency of severe exacerbations.

INHALED CORTICOSTEROIDS

(SED-14, 508; SEDA-22, 182; SEDA-23, 175; SEDA-24, 185)

Respiratory *Churg–Strauss syndrome*, which is characterized by late-onset asthma, upper airways disease, clinical manifestations of vasculitis, and eosinophilia, is due to an underlying eosinophil-associated small-vessel granulomatous vasculitis. The syndrome has come into prominence with the introduction of the leukotriene receptor antagonists, because these drugs allow steroid-dependent asthmatics to discontinue their oral prednisolone. Five patients developed Churg–Strauss syndrome when their oral corticosteroids were withdrawn (45[A]). The duration of oral corticosteroid therapy was 3–216 months and the dosage of prednisolone was 2.5–25.5 mg/day. The diagnosis of Churg–Strauss syndrome was made from 6 to 83 months after withdrawal of the oral corticosteroids. These case reports support the hypothesis that it is the withdrawal of corticosteroids that unmasks the underlying systemic vasculitis in these patients with asthma, rather than an effect of the new therapeutic agents that permits the reduction (and withdrawal) of prednisolone. Case-control studies are needed to determine the respective roles of the new therapeutic agents, prednisolone withdrawal, or other factors in the emergence of Churg–Strauss syndrome in these asthmatic patients.

Nervous system *Benign intracranial hypertension* with systemic or topical corticosteroids is well recognized and another case has been reported (46[A]).

A 13-year-old boy with Crohn's disease in remission, who had taken fluticasone aqueous nasal spray 50 μg to each nostril od regularly for 5 days, gave a 10-day history of head and back pain. He had a right sixth nerve palsy with bilateral swelling of his optic discs. An unenhanced computer tomogram was normal and magnetic resonance imaging excluded cavernous sinus thrombosis. The cerebrospinal fluid was clear with no cells, and protein and glucose concentrations were normal.

Although there was no clear temporal relation between the onset of the symptoms and the regular use of fluticasone, the authors proposed that the fluticasone was responsible, because the symptoms resolved after drug withdrawal.

The association remains unproven but it does highlight the possibility of an association.

Effects of inhaled corticosteroids on bone mineral density

While biochemical indices, such as calcium, hydroxyproline, and pyridinyline cross-links (as markers of bone resorption), and alkaline phosphatase, osteocalcin, and procollagen peptides (as markers of bone formation), may be sensitive to the effects of corticosteroids in the short term, the relation between changes in these markers and intermediate measures, such as bone mineral density, and the more important clinical outcomes of fractures, remains unknown. In the last year, there have been several further investigations of the effects of inhaled corticosteroids on bone mineral density. In a prospective comparison of the change in bone mineral density over 2 years in adults with mild asthma, who were randomized to receive treatment with inhaled corticosteroids or non-corticosteroid treatment 374 subjects with mild asthma (mean FEV_1 86% predicted) were randomized to receive inhaled budesonide, inhaled beclomethasone, or non-corticosteroid treatment (the control group) for 2 years (47[C]). Bone mineral density was measured after 6, 12, and 20 months. The median daily doses of budesonide (87 subjects) and beclomethasone (74 subjects) were 389 and 499 μg respectively. The mean changes in bone mineral density with budesonide, beclomethasone, and controls were 0.1, –0.4, and 0.4% in the lumbar spine and –0.9, –0.9 and –0.4% in the neck of the femur. The mean daily dose of inhaled corticosteroid was related to the reduction in bone mineral density in the lumbar spine but not the femoral neck. Subjects who took inhaled corticosteroids had better control of their asthma than controls (n = 78).

Dose relation *Current evidence suggests that the changes in bone mineral density in asthmatic patients who take inhaled corticosteroids are dose-related. In patients with mild asthma who are well maintained on low doses of inhaled corticosteroids the benefits derived from good control of the asthma appear to outweigh any concerns about minor changes in bone mineral density. The picture is less clear in patients with other risk factors, such as estrogen deficiency and advancing years.*

In an uncontrolled study, 56 women with asthma taking long-term inhaled corticosteroids had bone mineral density measurements of the lumbar spine and hip (48[C]). Women who had taken more than three short courses of systemic corticosteroids per year over the preceding 3 years were excluded. Data on duration of use and dose of inhaled corticosteroids were obtained from the patients' medical records. Doses of inhaled corticosteroids were arbitrarily classified as low (under 500 μg/day), medium (500–1000 μg/day), and high (over 1000 μg/day). More than half the women (61%) had decreased bone mineral density at either the hip or lumbar spine. Amongst the postmenopausal women in the study, 17% of those aged under 65 years had osteoporosis compared with 43% of those aged over 65 years. These figures exceeded those from a national sample of estrogen-deficient women, in which 5.7% under the age of 65 had osteoporosis and 29% over the age of 65 years had osteoporosis. Bone mineral density loss increased with higher doses of inhaled corticosteroids, from 5% in the low-dose group to 50% in the high-dose group. Whilst this is a potentially important finding in women at risk of osteoporosis because of the menopause, there are some aspects of the design of the study that limit the applicability of the findings. There was no appropriate age- and ethnicity-matched control group and the contribution of nasal corticosteroids was not accurately assessed.

In a large cross-sectional study patients aged 20–40 years with asthma who had taken inhaled corticosteroids for a median of 6 years were studied (49[C]). Patients were excluded if they had taken a course of oral or parenteral corticosteroids in the past 6 months or more than two courses ever, or if they had had more than 10 inhalers of nasal corticosteroids or more than 10 prescriptions of a dermal corticosteroid. Computerized records of general practices were used to identify patients for the study. Bone mineral density was measured at the lumbar spine (L2–L4) and the left femur (neck, Ward's triangle, trochanter). The cumulative dose of inhaled corticosteroid was expressed as a product of the mean daily dose and time. This information was obtained from a patient questionnaire and validated against general practice computer and paper records.

More than half of the patients (119/196) were women and the median cumulative dose of inhaled corticosteroid was 876 (range 88–4380) mg. There was a significant inverse relation between the cumulative dose of inhaled corticosteroid and bone mineral density at the spine and hip in both men and women. A doubling of cumulative dose was associated with a 0.16 SD reduction in bone mineral density. Extrapolation from cross-sectional data such as these requires confirmation in longitudinal studies, since bone loss with oral corticosteroids is more rapid in the first 12–24 months of therapy.

Risk of fracture *Whilst there have been several studies of the effects of inhaled corticosteroids on bone mineral density, there are few data on the effects of inhaled corticosteroids on the risk of fracture. In a recent retrospective cohort study the risk of fracture was established by examining the General Practice Research Database (GPRD), which is run by the Medicines Control Agency in the UK (50[C]). Users of inhaled corticosteroids were defined as permanently registered patients aged 18 years or more who received one or more prescriptions for inhaled corticosteroids during the time from enrollment in the GPRD until the end of data collection. Patients who received a prescription for oral corticosteroids for a period of 6 months before to 91 days after the last prescription for an inhaled corticosteroid were excluded. There were two comparison groups – a bronchodilator group, which included adults who received prescriptions for non-systemic corticosteroid and bronchodilators, and a second control group who received non-systemic corticosteroids but never inhaled or systemic corticosteroids or bronchodilators. The database included over 440 000 patients, and all patients who had fractures were identified from their medical records during the follow-up period, which was 91 days after the last prescription for an inhaled corticosteroid. The relative rates of non-vertebral, hip, and vertebral fractures during inhaled corticosteroid treatment compared with controls were 1.15 (95% CI = 1.10, 1.20), 1.22 (CI = 1.04, 1.43), and 1.51 (CI = 1.22, 1.85) respectively. There were no differences between inhaled corticosteroids and bronchodilators (non-vertebral fracture relative rate = 1). The authors concluded that users of inhaled corticosteroids may have an increased risk of fracture, particularly at the hip and spine, but that this excess risk may be related more to the underlying respiratory disease than to the inhaled corticosteroids.*

There were no major differences between the three groups in baseline fracture history. About 1% in each cohort recorded a history of non-vertebral fractures in the year before baseline. During the follow-up, the incidence of non-vertebral fractures was 1.4 fractures per 100 persons with inhaled corticosteroids, 1.4 with bronchodilators, and 1.1 in the control group. Comparing inhaled corticosteroid users with a control group, there was a dose response for hip and vertebral fractures. For a standardized daily dose of under 300 μg/day of budesonide, hip fracture was 0.95, rising to 1.06 at doses of 300–700 μg/day and 1.77 at doses of 700 μg/day or more. There was no consistent trend in the rate of fractures amongst users of inhaled corticosteroid compared with bronchodilators.

This is a noteworthy study, because it has examined the most important clinical outcome of change in bone mineral density, which is the risk of fracture. The results point to an increased risk of fracture, especially at the hip and vertebral bodies, amongst patients who use inhaled corticosteroids as well as those using bronchodilators, when compared with patients not using these drugs. Fracture risk tended to fall after withdrawal of inhaled corticosteroids or bronchodilators. These findings suggest that low-dose inhaled corticosteroids are not associated with an increased risk of fracture and that patients with chronic respiratory disease who use any inhaled therapy are not at risk compared with a control population. There were no differences in fracture risk between the various types of bronchodilators, suggesting that the underlying lung disease itself was the basis of risk rather than any particular type of bronchodilator. The authors noted that 1.9% of patients were using doses of budesonide equivalents of over 1500 μg/day and that the possibility of a more pronounced increased fracture risk at these high doses cannot be excluded. The age- and sex-specific incidence of fracture in the control group was similar to that of the general population in the GPRD.

Estimates of the important outcome of bone fracture have shown a small increased risk with inhaled corticosteroids, but this may well be a feature of the disease rather than the therapy, because comparisons with treatment with bronchodilator drugs show no difference between risk factors in patients taking corticosteroids or bronchodilators.

Time course *The time course of changes in bone mineral density with inhaled corticosteroids has yet to be determined. Longitudinal studies will be required to determine whether bone loss is most rapid in the first 12–24 months after initiating inhaled corticosteroid therapy, as is the case with oral corticosteroids (51[C]) and whether the risk of fracture falls towards baseline after withdrawal of treatment, as was suggested by the GPRD study (50[C]).*

Infection risk *Invasive aspergillosis* occurred after high-dose inhaled fluticasone (440 μg qds) and zafirlukast 20 mg/day in a 44-year-old man with moderately severe asthma; this is the first report of invasive pulmonary aspergillosis associated with an inhaled corticosteroid (52[A]).

LEUKOTRIENE RECEPTOR ANTAGONISTS *(SEDA-24, 183)*

There has been increasing use of the leukotriene receptor antagonists since their approval by more regulatory agents for the treatment of asthma. Zafirlukast is now one of the 200 most prescribed drugs in the USA. Generally these drugs (montelukast, pranlukast, and zafirlukast) have been well tolerated, with few adverse effects.

The efficacy and tolerability of montelukast, in combination with a selective histamine H_1 receptor antagonist (loratadine), has been investigated in a randomized, double-blind, cross-over study for 2 weeks in 125 asthmatic subjects (mean FEV_1 67% predicted), who took montelukast 10 mg plus loratadine 20 mg or placebo od for 2 weeks (53[C]). The subjects were symptomatic, in that their mean baseline daily use of β_2-adrenoceptor agonists was 5.1 inhaled metered doses. During the study the percentage increase in FEV_1 from baseline was significantly greater with montelukast plus loratadine than with montelukast alone (14% vs 9.7%). The most common adverse events during the trial were *headache* and *upper respiratory tract infection* (each in about 10% of subjects). There were no significant differences in the frequencies of adverse experiences between montelukast plus loratadine and montelukast alone. Ten patients withdrew because of an adverse event; six had exacerbation of asthma requiring steroid administration (three in each of the two arms of the study). One patient taking montelukast plus loratadine and four taking montelukast alone had transient self-limiting laboratory abnormalities.

The acute effects of intravenous and oral montelukast on airway function have been compared in a randomized, double-blind, cross-over study in 51 asthmatic patients (mean FEV_1 63.8% predicted) (54[c]). The intravenous dose (7 mg) was known to produce a comparable AUC to that obtained with an oral dose of 10 mg. FEV_1 was measured at 0.25, 0.5, 1, and 2 hours and then at regular intervals up to 24 hours after dosing. After intravenous and oral montelukast, the FEV_1 AUC_{0-24} was significantly greater than after placebo (mean increases 21, 16, and 7.8% for intravenous, oral and placebo respectively). The mean percentage change in FEV_1 for intravenous montelukast was greater than for oral montelukast in the first hour (18% vs 13%). The most frequently reported adverse events included *headaches*, which occurred in three patients taking placebo, four taking oral montelukast, and one taking intravenous montelukast. *Influenza* was reported in two patients taking placebo. It was noteworthy that there were no local adverse events at the intravenous site of the montelukast administration. This study has raised the possibility that a bolus dose of intravenous montelukast may have a role in the management of acute exacerbations of asthma.

Respiratory The possibility that the leukotriene receptor antagonists could cause *Churg–Strauss syndrome* created a considerable amount of interest at the time that these drugs were released (SEDA 24, 183). However, there have been no further reports in the last 12 months and current evidence suggests that previous cases were due to withdrawal of corticosteroids rather than an effect of the leukotriene receptor antagonists (see above).

Liver Asymptomatic *increases in serum liver enzymes*, to two or three times the upper limit of the reference ranges, were reported in 1.5% of over 4000 patients in the premarketing clinical trials of zafirlukast, but no severe hepatotoxicity was reported. With more extensive use of zafirlukast, some case reports of *severe liver injury* have now appeared. Three patients developed severe liver injury after taking zafirlukast 20 mg bd for several months (55[A]). The evidence that zafirlukast was the probable cause of the hepatic injury was based on the rigorous exclusion of other causes of acute hepatitis, liver biopsies with histological characteristics consistent with toxic injury, the presence of hypersensitivity suggestive of a drug reaction in one patient, and inadvertent rechallenge in one patient. In one case a liver transplant was required. The authors stated that the mechanism of the drug induced hepatotoxicity was not known but they speculated that it may be of immunological origin or, alternatively, that metabolism by CYP2C9 may create toxic metabolites. Whatever the mechanism, hepatotoxicity with zafirlukast is rare. The Acute Liver Failure Study Group, a consortium of 20 academic medical institutions in the USA cooperating in the prospective collection of data on acute liver failure, has not identified any other cases of acute liver injury associated with zafirlukast.

Urinary tract *Glomerulonephritis* has been attributed to montelukast (56[A]).

A 46-year-old woman developed a severe systemic inflammatory reaction characterized by eosinophilia and necrotizing glomerulonephritis. about 4 months after montelukast was added to her existing treatment with budesonide, formoterol, and terbutaline for asthma. At the time of her initial presentation she was treated with azithromycin and amoxicillin, but these drugs were discounted as possible causes as her illness had already begun before she was treated with them. Once the diagnosis was made, montelukast was withdrawn and she improved with corticosteroids over the next 4 months. From the limited detail of this brief case report, it is by no means certain that montelukast was the cause of the systemic illness.

ANTICHOLINERGIC DRUGS

(SED-14, 498; SEDA-22, 193; SEDA-23, 187; SEDA-24, 189)

Clinical trials of tiotropium in chronic obstructive pulmonary disease (COPD) have continued, although the drug has yet to be marketed. In a randomized double-blind study, 470 patients with stable COPD (mean FEV_1 38.6% predicted) received tiotropium 18 μg or placebo as a once-daily medication via a lactose-based dry powder inhaler device (57[C]). Spirometry was measured on days 1 and 8 and at regular intervals for 3 months. Tiotropium produced significant improvements in trough FEV_1 and FVC (measured immediately before the next dose), averaging 12% greater than baseline on day 8. The bronchodilatation resulting from tiotropium did not diminish over the 3 months of the study. *Upper respiratory tract infections* were reported in 15% of the patients in each of the treatment groups and exacerbations of COPD were reported in 22% of patients taking placebo and 16% of patients taking tiotropium. *Dry mouth* was significantly more common with tiotropium (9.3% vs 1.6%). There was a 6.8% incidence of serious adverse events or events leading to withdrawal (2.5% with tiotropium and 5.8% with placebo). A patient with a long history of cardiovascular disease, who was randomized to receive tiotropium, was found dead and was suspected to have died of a *cardiac dysrhythmia*. There were no differences in electrocardiograms between the treatment groups nor changes in laboratory values.

A double-blind, double-dummy, parallel-group study of 144 patients with severe COPD (FEV_1 41% predicted) has been conducted over 12 weeks to determine whether the combination of salmeterol 50 μg bd plus ipratropium 40 μg bd was better than salmeterol alone (58[C]). At the beginning of treatment salmeterol increased FEV_1 (a peak of 7% predicted) for over 12 hours. Salmeterol plus ipratropium produced a greater bronchodilator response (peak of 11% predicted) than salmeterol alone during the first 6 hours after inhalation. There were significant improvements in daytime symptom scores and peak flows with both salmeterol and salmeterol plus ipratropium compared with placebo. Adverse events were similar in the treatment groups; *headache* (six patients with salmeterol plus ipratropium, four with salmeterol, and 11 with placebo) and *cough* were the most common drug-related adverse events. Over the 12 weeks, 35 patients had an *exacerbation of COPD*, 36% with placebo, 23% with salmeterol, and 13% with salmeterol plus ipratropium.

N-ACETYLCYSTEINE

There has been a systematic review of published randomized studies of the use of *N*-acetylcysteine in chronic bronchitis (59[M]). A total of 39 trials were considered, of which only nine were included in the meta-analysis. In all cases oral *N*-acetycysteine had been used in a dosage of 200–300 mg bd for 4–32 weeks. There were gastrointestinal adverse effects (*dyspepsia*, *diarrhea*, and *heartburn*) in 10% of 2011 patients and 6.5% withdrew because of their symptoms. However, the rate of gastrointestinal adverse effects was higher in the placebo group (11% with a withdrawal rate of 7.1%). There was no exacerbation of chronic bronchitis in 49% of patients treated with *N*-acetylcysteine compared with 31% of placebo-treated patients, a relative benefit of 1.56 (95% CI = 1.37, 1.77). There was also symptom improvement with treatment – 61% reported improvement in symptoms with *N*-acetylcysteine compared with 35% with placebo.

NITRIC OXIDE *(SEDA-24, 190)*

Nitric oxide is a short-lived molecule that induces pulmonary vasodilatation on inhalation. Its predominant use has been in hypoxemic respiratory failure, especially in persistent pulmonary hypertension of the newborn and in adults with acute lung injury. Currently its use is being extended to the treatment of preterm infants of less than 34 weeks gestation and to adults in ambulatory settings.

Respiratory In a review of two articles it was noted that nitric oxide does not increase the risk of chronic lung disease of the newborn, despite speculation that it may increase chronic lung disease of prematurity due to the formation of nitrogen dioxide and peroxynitrite, in addition to membrane lipid peroxidation and increased unbound plasma iron in preterm infants (60[r]).

In a randomized, double-blind, placebo-controlled, cross-over study of the use of nitric oxide in chronic obstructive pulmonary disease (COPD) 11 patients with documented severe COPD received 25 ppm of nitric oxide combined with supplementary oxygen at a flow rate of 2 l/min via nasal cannulae (61[C]). Four of the patients reported an increase in *cough* and *a feeling of retrosternal rawness* after breathing nitric oxide for 24 hours; two had an increase in *dyspnea*, and one developed *wheezing* and was unable to perform exercise on a treadmill. There were no significant changes in lung spirometry. The authors noted that one patient had underlying reversible airways obstruction, but did not say if it was this individual who developed the wheezing. Nitric oxide is an irritant and causes inflammatory changes in the airways, so it is possible that nitric oxide could cause bronchoconstriction and aggravate asthmatic inflammation. There was a small but significant beneficial fall in pulmonary vascular resistance (183 to 137 dyne.s/cm^3) with nitric oxide. This is the first study of the prolonged use of nitric oxide (for 24 hours) in non-anesthetized non-ventilated patients with COPD.

The role of nitric oxide as salvage therapy to improve pulmonary gas exchange has been studied in children with life-threatening asthma, unresponsive to other therapies (62[A]). Four consecutive patients with hypercapnia or hypoxemia, despite mechanical ventilation, treatment with β-adrenoceptor agonists, ipratropium bromide, intravenous corticosteroids, magnesium sulfate, and a trial of helium/oxygen mixtures, were treated with incremental concentrations of inhaled nitric oxide up to 80 ppm, after a successful trial in an index case. Four of the five had improvements in gas exchange, with a fall in arterial carbon dioxide tension. Gas exchange was also improved by inhaled nitric oxide 20 ppm, from a baseline PaO_2/FiO_2 ratio of 209 (range 175–276) to 430 (range 139–463). However at the higher dose of inhaled nitric oxide of 40 ppm there was a *deterioration in oxygenation*, with PaO_2/FiO_2 ratios falling to 163 (range 139–463). One patient did not respond to treatment and had a rise in $PaCO_2$ on treatment with inhaled nitric oxide 40 ppm, so treatment was withdrawn. This study has provided some supplementary evidence that nitric oxide may impair pulmonary gas exchange by causing *irritation* and further *bronchoconstriction* in susceptible patients, as noted in the COPD study mentioned above (61[C]). Unfortunately, airways resistance was not measured in this study, but caution should be exercised and close monitoring undertaken when using inhaled nitric oxide in patients with bronchoconstriction.

Nervous system Of major concern in the

treatment of preterm infants is that nitric oxide might increase the incidence or severity of *intraventricular hemorrhage*. Nitric oxide impairs platelet aggregation and agglutination in vitro by activating guanylate cyclase and so increasing cGMP concentration. In a meta-analysis of randomized controlled trials of inhaled nitric oxide for the treatment of preterm infants only three studies were identified (63[M]). In all, 300 infants were included in the analysis and the incidence of intraventricular hemorrhage was comparable between treatment and non-treatment groups, 35 of 111 receiving inhaled nitric oxide compared with 25 of 99 controls (OR = 1.37; 95% CI = 0.69, 2.74). There were no changes in mortality with treatment and no differences in neurological outcomes between nitric oxide and placebo during follow-up. These findings have been supported by a second meta-analysis of the use of nitric oxide in near-term infants with hypoxic respiratory failure, which showed no difference in the rate of neurodevelopmental abnormalities in neonates treated with nitric oxide (64[M]).

In a randomized trial in 248 neonates older than 34 weeks of gestation, 126 of whom received nitric oxide, treatment with nitric oxide afforded no protection against neurodevelopmental abnormalities (65[C]). The only benefits conferred by inhaled nitric oxide treatment in 42 preterm neonates was a reduction in the incidence of chronic lung disease along with improvement in oxygenation (66[C]) and significant reductions in oxygenation index, duration of ventilation, and stay in neonatal ICU (67[C]).

During long-term follow-up of the Neonatal Inhaled Nitric Oxide Study (NINOS), the neurodevelopmental safety of nitric oxide in infants over 34 weeks gestation with hypoxemic respiratory failure was assessed at 18–24 months of age, at which time there was a non-significant increase in disability in infants treated with inhaled nitric oxide (68[C]). Of the 199 surviving infants in the study, 173 were assessed. Sensorineural hearing loss (15% and 13%, controls versus treatment), blindness in one or both eyes (2.2% vs 2.4%), the presence of cerebral palsy (10% vs 12%), and the presence of one or more neurodevelopmental abnormalities (30% vs 35%) were all statistically equivalent between the groups. The only significant difference was a greater rate of seizures after discharge in the control patients (15% vs 4.7% in those given inhaled nitric oxide).

Hematologic As previously noted, the use of nitric oxide can lead to *high methemoglobin concentrations* (SEDA 24, 190), but it continues to be monitored and occurs in only a few patients. The incidence is also reduced by the use of low-dose nitric oxide. In a study (65[C]) in which inhaled nitric oxide was used in a dose of 20 ppm for 24 hours, followed by 5 ppm for up to 96 hours, only two infants of 126 randomized to nitric oxide developed methemoglobinemia. In 11 children aged 2.6–48 months undergoing surgery for congenital heart defects with associated pulmonary hypertension no infant receiving inhaled nitric oxide up to 80 ppm developed a methemoglobin concentration over 5% (69[c]). Nitrogen dioxide concentrations rose to over 5% in some patients, with resolution once the dose was reduced. There were no adverse effects.

One of the biochemical adverse effects of nitric oxide is inactivation of vitamin B_{12}, with subsequent potentiation of folate deficiency (70[r]). This effect is mediated by irreversible oxidation of the cobalt residue in Vitamin B_{12} to its Co^{++} and Co^{+++} forms. This leads to a reduction in methionine synthetase activity, with downstream effects on DNA synthesis. Previous studies have identified five patients with unsuspected vitamin B_{12} deficiency who developed subacute combined degeneration of the spinal cord following inhalation anesthesia with nitrous oxide (71[A]). Nitric oxide has a similar effect on vitamin B_{12}, and its prolonged use could theoretically produce similar disorders in vitamin B_{12} metabolism (70[r]).

Drug withdrawal In recent years acute *rebound of pulmonary hypertension and cardiovascular collapse* associated with abrupt discontinuation of nitric oxide has become well recognized. Since the recognition of this rebound phenomenon and the institution of safety measures to ensure continuity of supply, few adverse effects have been reported with the use of nitric oxide. The risk factors for this adverse effect, or its incidence, have not been fully characterized. The incidence, risk factors, and nature of cardiopulmonary deterioration when patients' nitric oxide supply is abruptly discontinued have been investigated in 56 intubated and mechanically ventilated patients with acute hypoxemic respiratory failure, of whom 39 had improved gas exchange (PaO_2 increased by more than 20 mmHg) during treatment with inhaled nitric oxide (72[C]). After at least 10 hours of treatment (range 10–30 hours) inhaled nitric oxide was abruptly withdrawn and the patients were monitored for the rebound phenomenon and the need for continuing administration of inhaled nitric oxide. The mean dose of inhaled nitric oxide at the time of withdrawal was 22.8 (range 3–80) ppm. There was significant deterioration in gas exchange (decrease in SaO_2 more than 5%) and/or a drop in cardiac output of more than 10% in 23 patients (74%) and 15 (48%) had arterial desaturation within 30 minutes, which responded to reintroduction of inhaled nitric oxide. Eight patients had a rapid fall in cardiac output and/or blood pressure of over 20%, with prompt return to baseline measurements with reintroduction of therapy. Independent predictors of hemodynamic collapse were multiple system organ failure, older age, and an increased initial blood pressure in response to institution of inhaled nitric oxide. Hemodynamic measurements suggested that the acute collapse was primarily due to right ventricular overload. The authors also postulated that nitric oxide therapy causes downregulation of nitric oxide synthase, and that removal of exogenous nitric oxide leaves the pulmonary vasculature with insufficient vasodilatory influences, allowing vasoconstriction to predominate. This downregulation has been demonstrated in a rat model, but not in humans (73[E]).

AEROSOLIZED PROSTAGLANDINS (see also Chapter 39)

Intravenous epoprostenol increases exercise tolerance, improves pulmonary hemodynamics, and improves survival in patients with primary pulmonary hypertension. However, there are limitations to treatment with intravenous prostacyclin, and a significant proportion of patients develop catheter-related problems, such as thrombosis, pump failure, and catheter-related sepsis. In an attempt to improve delivery, several trials of aerosolized prostacyclin have now been undertaken, primarily in patients with primary pulmonary hypertension.

There has been a sequential comparison of inhaled nitric oxide 40 ppm with aerosolized iloprost, about 14–17 μg, in 35 adults with primary pulmonary hypertension (74[C]). Five of the patients had minor *headache* and *facial flushing* during the inhalation of iloprost, but these symptoms were short-lived, and abated a few minutes after the inhalation ended. One patient had mild jaw pain after aerosolized iloprost, but again this was short lived. There was an unexpected increase in pulmonary artery pressure in 10 patients (29%) and vascular resistance in six patients (17%) who received nitric oxide. The authors were uncertain of the cause of this increase, as nitric oxide generally behaves as a vasodilator, but they noted that nitric oxide is a vasoconstrictor in certain conditions such as the presence of hemolysate (75[c]).

There has been a trial of aerosolized iloprost in 24 patients with primary pulmonary hypertension and New York Heart Association class III or IV disability, who were refractory to conventional medical treatment (76[C]). They were given aerosolized iloprost in a total daily dose of 100–150 μg (in 6–8 divided doses, given every 2–3 hours whilst awake) over 12 months. The treatment was generally well tolerated, except for *coughing* during inhalation, which was common initially but resolved spontaneously in all patients within the first 4 weeks. Five patients reported symptoms of *flushing*, *headache*, and *jaw pain* at the end of inhalation, but all rated the symptoms as mild and no patients discontinued treatment because of adverse effects. There was an asymptomatic but significant *fall in systemic arterial pressure* (from 98 to 90 mmHg) and vascular resistance at 3 and 12 months compared with baseline.

The effects of aerosolized iloprost have been reported in three patients with severe pulmonary hypertension (mean pulmonary artery pressure 50 mmHg or more) who were already being treated with intravenous epoprostenol (10–16 ng/kg/min) (77[A]). The aim of the study was to replace continuous intravenous epoprostenol with intermittent aerosolized iloprost (150–300 μg/day in 6–18 divided doses). All three patients had gradual weaning of intravenous epoprostenol (1 ng/kg/min every 3–10 hours) under close supervision and hemodynamic monitoring in intensive care. All three had initial falls in pulmonary arterial pressure and improved right ventricular function with inhaled iloprost. The first could not be fully weaned from epoprostenol because of *right ventricular failure* with dyspnea and hypoxemia, accompanied by a 3-fold increase in serum bilirubin and lactate dehydrogenase and echocardiographically demonstrated right ventricular failure. The second and third patients both tolerated complete withdrawal of epoprostenol. However, one developed right ventricular failure within 2 hours of withdrawal. The third was successfully discharged from hospital taking aerosolized therapy, but presented 2 weeks later with severe right ventricular failure. Thus, caution should be taken in patients who have been previously maintained on intravenous prostacyclin when trying to convert to aerosolized therapy, as there appears to be a high chance of treatment failure, which can occur abruptly.

Hematologic Platelet function after inhaled prostacyclin has been measured in a randomized double-blind study in 28 patients undergoing elective cardiothoracic surgery (78[c]). They were given aerosolized prostacyclin (5 or 10 μg) for 6 hours postoperatively. All the patients, regardless of dose, had a lower rate of platelet aggregation in response to adenosine diphosphate than controls. There were no differences in clinically significant indices, such as chest tube drainage or bleeding time. This study has shown that prostacyclin, given as an aerosol, can cause measurable *alterations in platelet function*, with a possibly higher risk of bleeding.

REFERENCES

1. Bethune N. A new technique for the deliberate production of pleural adhesions as a preliminary to lobectomy. J Thorac Surg 1935; 4: 251–61.
2. Wooten SA, Barbarash RA, Strange C, Sahn SA. Systemic absorption of tetracycline and lidocaine following intrapleural instillation. Chest 1988; 94: 960–3.
3. Sahn SA. Talc should be used for pleurodesis. Am J Respir Crit Care Med 2000; 162: 2023–4; discussion 2026.
4. Kennedy L, Sahn SA. Talc pleurodesis for the treatment of pneumothorax and pleural effusion. Chest 1994; 106: 1215–22.
5. Walker-Renard PB, Vaughan LM, Sahn SA. Chemical pleurodesis for malignant pleural effusions. Ann Intern Med 1994; 120: 56–64.
6. Rodriguez-Panadero F, Antony VB. Pleurodesis: state of the art. Eur Respir J 1997; 10: 1648–54.
7. Ferrer J, Villarino MA, Tura JM, Traveria J, Light RW. Comparison of size and composition of nine different talcs: its relevance for pleurodesis. Am J Respir Crit Care Med 1998; 157: A66.
8. Todd TR, Delarue NC, Ilves R, Pearson FG, Cooper JD. Talc poudrage for malignant pleural effusion. Chest 1980; 78: 542–3.
9. Rinaldo JE, Owens GR, Rogers RM. Adult respiratory distress syndrome following intrapleural instillation of talc. J Thorac Cardiovasc Surg 1983; 85: 523–6.
10. Bouchama A, Chastre J, Gaudichet A, Soler P, Gibert C. Acute pneumonitis with bilateral pleural effusion after talc pleurodesis. Chest 1984; 86: 795–7.
11. Weissberg D, Ben-Zeev I. Talc pleurodesis. Experience with 360 patients. J Thorac Cardiovasc Surg 1993; 106: 689–95.
12. Kennedy L, Rusch VW, Strange C, Ginsberg RJ, Sahn SA. Pleurodesis using talc slurry. Chest 1994; 106: 342–6.
13. Campos JR, Werebe EC, Vargas FS, Jatene FB, Light RW. Respiratory failure due to insufflated talc. Lancet 1997; 349: 251–2.
14. Werebe EC, Pazetti R, Milanez de Campos JR, Fernandez PP, Capelozzi VL, Jatene FB, Vargas FS. Systemic distribution of talc after intrapleural administration in rats. Chest 1999; 115: 190–3.
15. Rehse DH, Aye RW, Florence MG. Respiratory failure following talc pleurodesis. Am J Surg 1999; 177: 437–40.
16. Ruckdeschel JC, Moores D, Lee JY, Einhorn LH, Mandelbaum I, Koeller J, Weiss GR, Losada M, Keller JH. Intrapleural therapy for malignant pleural effusions. A randomized comparison of bleomycin and tetracycline. Chest 1991; 100: 1528–35.
17. Martinez-Moragon E, Aparicio J, Rogado MC, Sanchis J, Sanchis F, Gil-Suay V. Pleurodesis in malignant pleural effusions: a randomized study of tetracycline versus bleomycin. Eur Respir J 1997; 10: 2380–3.
18. Patz EF Jr, McAdams HP, Erasmus JJ, Goodman PC, Culhane DK, Gilkeson RC, Herndon J. Sclerotherapy for malignant pleural effusions: a prospective randomized trial of bleomycin vs doxycycline with small-bore catheter drainage. Chest 1998; 113: 1305–11.
19. Alberts DS, Chen HS, Mayersohn M, Perrier D, Moon TE, Gross JF. Bleomycin pharmacokinetics in man. II. Intracavitary administration. Cancer Chemother Pharmacol 1979; 2: 127–32.
20. Robinson LA, Moulton AL, Fleming WH, Alonso A, Galbraith TA. Intrapleural fibrinolytic treatment of multiloculated thoracic empyemas. Ann Thorac Surg 1994; 57: 803–13; discussion 813–14.
21. Taylor RF, Rubens MB, Pearson MC, Barnes NC. Intrapleural streptokinase in the management of empyema. Thorax 1994; 49: 856–9.
22. Bouros D, Schiza S, Panagou P, Drositis J, Si-

afakas N. Role of streptokinase in the treatment of acute loculated parapneumonic pleural effusions and empyema. Thorax 1994; 49: 852–5.
23. Temes RT, Follis F, Kessler RM, Pett SB Jr, Wernly JA. Intrapleural fibrinolytics in management of empyema thoracis. Chest 1996; 110: 102–6.
24. Davies CW, Traill ZC, Gleeson FV, Davies RJ. Intrapleural streptokinase in the management of malignant multiloculated pleural effusions. Chest 1999; 115: 729–33.
25. Sasse SA. Parapneumonic effusions and empyema. Curr Opin Pulm Med 1996; 2: 320–6.
26. Sahn SA. Use of fibrinolytic agents in the management of complicated parapneumonic effusions and empyemas. Thorax 1998; 53 Suppl 2: S65–72.
27. Godley PJ, Bell RC. Major hemorrhage following administration of intrapleural streptokinase. Chest 1984; 86: 486–7.
28. Davies CW, Lok S, Davies RJ. The systemic fibrinolytic activity of intrapleural streptokinase. Am J Respir Crit Care Med 1998; 157: 328–30.
29. Porter J, Banning AP. Intrapleural streptokinase. Thorax 1998; 53: 720.
30. Srivastava P, Godden DJ, Kerr KM, Legge JS. Fatal haemorrhage from aortic dissection following instillation of intrapleural streptokinase. Scott Med J 2000; 45: 86–7.
31. Moulton JS, Benkert RE, Weisiger KH, Chambers JA. Treatment of complicated pleural fluid collections with image-guided drainage and intracavitary urokinase. Chest 1995; 108: 1252–9.
32. Bouros D, Schiza S, Tzanakis N, Drositis J, Siafakas N. Intrapleural urokinase in the treatment of complicated parapneumonic pleural effusions and empyema. Eur Respir J 1996; 9: 1656–9.
33. Bouros D, Schiza S, Patsourakis G, Chalkiadakis G, Panagou P, Siafakas NM. Intrapleural streptokinase versus urokinase in the treatment of complicated parapneumonic effusions: a prospective, double-blind study. Am J Respir Crit Care Med 1997; 155: 291–5.
34. Krishnan S, Amin N, Dozor AJ, Stringel G. Urokinase in the management of complicated parapneumonic effusions in children. Chest 1997; 112: 1579–83.
35. Burggraaf J, Westendorp RG, In't Veen JC, Schoemaker RC, Sterk PJ, Cohen AF, Blauw GJ. Cardiovascular side effects of inhaled salbutamol in hypoxic asthmatic patients. Thorax 2001; 56: 567–9.
36. Mutlu GM, Moonjelly E, Chan L, Olopade CO. Laryngospasm and paradoxical bronchoconstriction after repeated doses of beta 2-agonists containing edetate disodium. Mayo Clin Proc 2000; 75: 285–7.
37. Bisgaard H. Long-acting beta(2)-agonists in management of childhood asthma: a critical review of the literature. Pediatr Pulmonol 2000; 29: 221–34.
38. Kuusela A-L, Marenk M, Sandahl G, Sanderud J, Nikolajev K, Persson B. Comparative study using oral solutions of bambuterol once daily or terbutaline three times daily in 2–5-year-old children with asthma. Bambuterol Multicentre Study Group. Pediatr Pulmonol 2000; 29: 194–201.
39. Zarkovic JP, Marenk M, Valovirta E, Kuusela A-L, Sandahl G, Persson B, Olsson H. One-year safety study with bambuterol once daily and terbutaline three times daily in 2–12-year-old children with asthma. The Bambuterol Multicentre Study Group. Pediatr Pulmonol 2000; 29: 424–9.
40. Ostergaard D, Rasmussen SN, Viby-Mogensen J, Pedersen NA, Boysen R. The influence of drug-induced low plasma cholinesterase activity on the pharmacokinetics and pharmacodynamics of mivacurium. Anesthesiology 2000; 92: 1581–7.
41. Centanni S, Carlucci P, Santus P, Boveri B, Tarricone D, Fiorentini C, Lombardi F, Cazzola M. Non-pulmonary effects induced by the addition of formoterol to budesonide therapy in patients with mild or moderate persistent asthma. Respiration 2000; 67: 60–4.
42. Lipworth BJ, Aziz I. Bronchodilator response to albuterol after regular formoterol and effects of acute corticosteroid administration. Chest 2000; 117: 156–62.
43. Van der Woude HJ, Winter TH, Aalbers R. Decreased bronchodilating effect of salbutamol in relieving methacholine induced moderate to severe bronchoconstriction during high dose treatment with long acting beta2 agonists. Thorax 2001; 56: 529–35.
44. D'Urzo AD, Chapman KR, Cartier A, Hargreave FE, Fitzgerald M, Tesarowski D. Effectiveness and safety of salmeterol in nonspecialist practice settings. Chest 2001; 119: 714–19.
45. Le Gall C, Pham S, Vignes S, Garcia G, Nunes H. Fichet D, Simonneau G, Duroux P, Humbert M. Inhaled corticosteroids and Churg–Strauss syndrome: a report of five cases. Eur Respir J 2000; 15: 978–81.
46. Bond DW, Charlton CPJ. Benign intracranial hypertension secondary to nasal fluticasone propionate. Br Med J 2001; 322: 897.
47. Tattersfield AE, Town GI, Johnell O, Picado C, Aubier M, Braillon P, Karlstrom R. Bone mineral density in subjects with mild asthma randomised to treatment with inhaled corticosteroids or non-corticosteroid treatment for two years. Thorax 2001; 56: 272–8.
48. Bonala SB, Reddy BM, Silverman BA, Bassett CW, Rao YAK, Amara S, Schneider AT. Bone mineral density in women with asthma on long-term inhaled corticosteroid therapy. Ann Allergy Asthma Immunol 2000; 85: 495–500.
49. Wong CA, Walsh LJ, Smith CJP, Wisniewski AF, Lewis SA. Inhaled corticosteroid use and bone-mineral density in patients with asthma. Lancet 2000; 355: 1399–403.
50. Van Staa TP, Leufkens HGM, Cooper C. Use of inhaled corticosteroids and risk of fractures. J Bone Miner Res 2001; 16: 581–8.
51. Sambrook PN, Kemplar S, Birmingham J, Kelly PJ, Pocock NA, Yeates MG, Eisman JA. Corticos-

teroid effects on proximal femur bone loss. J Bone Miner Res 1990; 5: 1211–16.
52. Leav BA, Fanburg B, Hadley S. Invasive pulmonary aspergillosis associated with high-dose inhaled fluticasone. New Engl J Med; 2000: 586.
53. Reicin A, White R, Weinstein SF, Finn AF, Nguyen H, Peszek I, Geissler L, Seidenberg BC. Montelukast, a leukotriene receptor antagonist, in combination with loratadine, a histamine receptor antagonist in the treatment of chronic asthma. Arch Intern Med 2000; 160: 2481–8.
54. Dockhorn RJ, Baumgartner RA, Leff JA, Nonnan M, Vandormael K, Stricker W, Weinland DE, Riess TF. Comparison of the effects of intravenous and oral montelukast on airway function: a double blind, placebo controlled, three period, crossover study in asthmatic patients. Thorax 2000; 55: 260–5.
55. Reinus JF, Persky S, Burkiewicz JS, Quan D, Bass NM, Davern TJ. Severe liver injury after treatment with the leukotriene receptor antagonist zafirlukast. Ann Intern Med 2000; 133: 964–8.
56. Goransson LG, Omdal R. A severe systemic inflammatory reaction following therapy with montelukast (Singulair®). Nephrol Dial Transplant 2000; 15: 1054–5.
57. Casaburi R, Briggs DD Jr, Donohue JF, Serby CW, Menjoge SS, Witek TJ Jr. The spirometric efficacy of once-daily dosing with tiotropium in stable COPD. Chest 2000; 118: 1294–302.
58. Van Noord JA, De Munck DRAJ, Bantje TA, Hop WCJ. Long-term treatment of chronic obstructive pulmonary disease with salmeterol and the additive effect of ipratropium. Eur Respir J 2000; 15: 878–85.
59. Stey C, Steurer J, Bachmann S, Medici TC, Tramer MR. The effect of oral N-acetylcysteine in chronic bronchitis: a quantitative systematic review. Eur Respir J 2000; 16: 253–62.
60. Smyth RL. Inhaled nitric oxide treatment for preterm infants with hypoxic respiratory failure. Thorax 2000; 55 Suppl 1: S51–5.
61. Ashutosh K, Phadke K, Jackson JF, Steele D. Use of nitric oxide inhalation in chronic obstructive pulmonary disease. Thorax 2000; 55: 109–13.
62. Nakagawa TA, Johnston SJ, Falkos SA, Gomez RJ, Morris A. Life-threatening status asthmaticus treated with inhaled nitric oxide. J Pediatr 2000; 137: 119–22.
63. Hoehn T, Krause MF, Buhrer C. Inhaled nitric oxide in premature infants – a meta-analysis. J Perinat Med 2000; 28: 7–13.
64. Finer NN, Barrington KJ. Nitric oxide therapy for the newborn infant. Semin Perinatol 2000; 24: 59–65.
65. Clark RH, Kueser TJ, Walker MW, Southgate WM, Huckaby JL, Perez JA, Roy BJ, Keszler M, Finsella JP. Low-dose nitric oxide therapy for persistent pulmonary hypertension of the newborn. Clinical Inhaled Nitric Oxide Research Group. New Engl J Med 2000; 342: 469–74.
66. Subhedar NV, Ryan SW, Shaw NJ. Open randomised controlled trial of inhaled nitric oxide and early dexamethasone in high risk preterm infants. Arch Dis Child Fetal Neonatal Ed 1997; 77: F185–90.
67. The Franco–Belgium Collaborative NO Trial Group. Early compared with delayed inhaled nitric oxide in moderately hypoxaemic neonates with respiratory failure: a randomised controlled trial. Lancet 1999; 354: 1066–71.
68. Finer NN, Vohr BR, Robertson CMT, Ehrenkranz RA, Verter J, Wright LL, Hoffman HJ, Walsh-Sukys MC, Dusick AM, Fleisher BE, et al. Inhaled nitric oxide in term and near-term infants: neurodevelopmental follow-up of he Neonatal Inhaled Nitric Oxide Study Group (NINOS). J Pediatr 2000; 136: 611–17.
69. Turanlahti MI, Laitinen PO, Pesonen EJ. Preoperative and postoperative response to inhaled nitric oxide. Scand Cardiovasc J 2000; 34: 46–52.
70. Bratman S, Harkness R. Nitric oxide in neonates. Lancet 2000; 356: 1274.
71. Flippo TS, Holder WD. Neurologic degeneration associated with nitrous oxide anesthesia in patients with vitamin B_{12} deficiency. Arch Surg 1993; 128: 1391–5.
72. Christenson J, Lavoie A, O'Connor M, Bhorade S, Pohlman A, Hall JB. The incidence and pathogenesis of cardiopulmonary deterioration after abrupt withdrawal of inhaled nitric oxide. Am J Respir Crit Care Med 2000; 161: 1443–9.
73. Combes X, Mazmanian M, Gourlain H, Herve P. Effect of 48 hours of nitric oxide inhalation on pulmonary vasoreactivity in rats. Am J Respir Crit Care Med 1997; 156: 473–7.
74. Hoeper MM, Olschewski H, Ghofrani HA, Wilkens H, Winkler J, Borst MM, Niedermeyer J, Fabel H, Seeger W, Grimminger F et al. A comparison of the acute hemodynamic effects of inhaled nitric oxide and aerosolized iloprost in primary pulmonary hypertension. German PPH study group. J Am Coll Cardiol 2000; 35: 176–82.
75. Voelkel NF, Lobel K, Westcott JY, Burke TJ. Nitric oxide-related vasoconstriction in lungs perfused with red cell lysate. FASEB J 1995; 9: 379–86.
76. Hoeper MM, Schwarze M, Ehlerding S, Adler-Schuermeyer A, Spiekerkoetter E, Niedermeyer J, Hamm M, Fabel H. Long-term treatment of primary pulmonary hypertension with aerosolized iloprost, a prostacyclin analogue. New Engl J Med 2000; 342: 1866–70.
77. Schenk P, Petkov V, Madl C, Kramer L, Kneussl M, Ziesche R, Lang I. Aerosolized iloprost therapy could not replace long-term IV epoprostenol (prostacyclin) administration in severe pulmonary hypertension. Chest 2001; 119: 296–300.
78. Haraldsson A, Kieler-Jensen N, Wadenvik H, Ricksten S-E. Inhaled prostacyclin and platelet function after cardiac surgery and cardiopulmonary bypass. Intensive Care Med 2000; 26: 188–94.

J.K. Aronson

17 Positive inotropic drugs and drugs used in dysrhythmias

CARDIAC GLYCOSIDES

(SED-14, 523; SEDA-22, 201; SEDA-23, 193; SEDA-24, 197)

The actions, uses, adverse effects, and interactions of digoxin have again been reviewed (1[R], 2[r]).

Gastrointestinal *Mesenteric infarction* is a rare adverse effect of digitalis toxicity (SEDA-17, 215), but another case has recently been reported in a 79-year-old woman with a serum digoxin concentration of 4.9 ng/ml (3[A]). At post mortem no other causes of mesenteric infarction were discovered.

Death Despite the fact that the prospective study called DIG clearly showed that there was no increase in mortality in patients taking long-term digoxin therapy (SEDA-20, 173), retrospective non-randomized studies continue to be reported (SEDA-24, 201). Another such study has recently appeared (4[c]). In this case the overall mortality in 180 patients with idiopathic dilated cardiomyopathy was 19% in those taking digoxin and 10% in those not taking digoxin. However, when the use of digoxin was adjusted for several predictive variables it no longer predicted cardiac death. This finding is reassuring, but results of studies like this, whatever their results, should be ignored, in view of the evidence that is currently available from the one large prospective randomized study.

When interpreting the evidence presented in other accounts of the association between drug therapy and death it is important to remember that the current evidence suggests that digoxin does not cause excess mortality. For example, digoxin was the second most commonly encountered medication in an investigation of 2233 deaths reported to an American County Medical Examiner's office, with a medication history available in 775 cases (5[C]). Furosemide was mentioned 181 times, digoxin 131 times, and glyceryl trinitrate 103 times. All other drugs were mentioned less than 100 times each. The authors suggested that the presence of digoxin at a death scene should suggest heart failure or a cardiac dysrhythmia, but they did not go further and stress that in such a case digoxin need not necessarily be implicated in the death. Post-mortem diagnosis of digoxin toxicity is exceptionally difficult, since serum digoxin concentrations rise rapidly after death. However, measurement of digoxin in the vitreous fluid may be helpful.

In a survey of 2 312 203 deaths in the USA in 1995, 206 (0.009%) were attributed to adverse drug reactions on death certificates (6[C]). At the same time in the MedWatch program, 6894 deaths were reportedly attributed to adverse drug reactions, representing 6.3% of the 108 735 reports of adverse drug reactions. In the death certificate study 18 deaths were attributed to cardiac glycosides and in the MedWatch survey 15 deaths. This compares with figures of 289 and 782 from antimicrobial drugs, 449 and 280 from hormones, and 947 and 477 from drugs that affect the constituents of the blood (e.g. anticoagulants).

Risk factors The risk of digitalis toxicity is increased in *old people*, partly because they have poor renal function and lower bodyweight, factors that tend to increase the concentration of drug at the active site during steady-state therapy, and partly because they are liable to electrolyte imbalances, such as hypokalemia, which tend to increase the response of the tis-

Side Effects of Drugs, Annual 25
J.K. Aronson, ed.

sues to a given concentration. Other factors, such as altered Na/K pump activity, may also contribute to increased tissue sensitivity. This means that the serum digoxin concentration that is associated with an increased risk of toxicity is slightly lower in elderly people than in younger people, and this has been confirmed in a recent study of 899 patients taking digoxin for heart failure or atrial fibrillation (7[C]). No patients with serum digoxin concentrations below 1.4 ng/ml had evidence of digoxin toxicity. All patients who had a concentration of 3.0 ng/ml or more had severe toxicity. However in the range 1.4–2.9 ng/ml there were patients with and without evidence of toxicity, and the overlap was age dependent. In patients aged 51–60 there was more evidence of toxicity with concentrations of 2.4–2.9 ng/ml; in patients aged 61–70 the range was 1.8–2.9 ng/ml, in patients aged 71–80 it was 1.4–2.7 ng/ml, and in those aged over 80 it was 1.4–2.6 ng/ml. The authors therefore suggested that serum digoxin concentrations should be no greater than 1.4 ng/ml during routine steady-state therapy. The incidences of toxicity were 16% in patients over 70 years of age and 7.3% in the whole group. The risk of toxicity was increased in the presence of renal insufficiency.

Because digitoxin is metabolized rather than being renally eliminated, the effects of renal impairment in elderly patients may not be so important in precipitating digitoxin toxicity. In 80 patients hospitalized 147 times, toxicity with digitoxin occurred in 7.6% of 92 admissions and digoxin toxicity occurred in 18.3% of 55 admissions (8[C]). On the basis of these results the authors suggested that digitoxin is safer in elderly patients than digoxin. This is an old debate, and there are arguments in favor of both digoxin and digitoxin (9[r]). However, there is currently no information on the long-term toxicity of digitoxin, and in particular its effects on mortality in patients with heart failure. Neither the severity of toxicity nor its duration was reported in this study.

Drug overdose Plasma glycoside concentrations have been documented after an overdose with purple foxglove in a 36-year-old woman (10[A]). Apart from gitaloxin, which peaked on the fifth day at 113 ng/ml, all the glycosides detected peaked on the first day (gitoxin 13 ng/ml, digitoxin 113 ng/ml, digitoxigenin 3.3 ng/ml, and digitoxigenin monodigitoxoside 8.9 ng/ml). There was a second peak of digitoxin at about 70 hours, and this is consistent with the known enterohepatic recirculation of digitoxin. For this reason, if antidigoxin antibodies are not available, it is wise to give repeated doses of activated charcoal or a binding resin (see below).

Drug interactions *Antifungal imidazoles* Itraconazole increases steady-state serum digoxin concentrations (SEDA-21, 196). The mechanism is inhibition of P-glycoprotein, which reduces both the renal secretion and the biliary secretion of digoxin (SEDA-24, 203). Digoxin toxicity sometimes accompanies this effect, and another case has been reported in a 62-year-old woman who took itraconazole 400 mg/day (11[A]). After 3 days she developed nausea, anorexia, and lethargy; the symptoms improved within 48 hours after withdrawal of itraconazole. The serum digoxin concentrations were not reported.

This interaction is probably dose-related, and in a 75-year-old man who took itraconazole in a low dose (200 mg/day) the steady-state serum digoxin concentration only rose from 0.8 to 1.1 ng/ml after 8 days (12[A]).

β-blockers The effect of talinolol on the pharmacokinetics of digoxin have been studied in 10 healthy volunteers aged 23–30 years in a cross-over study (13[C]). Oral talinolol 100 mg increased the AUC of digoxin significantly, but the renal clearance and half-life of digoxin were unchanged. Intravenous talinolol 30 mg had no effect on the pharmacokinetics of oral digoxin. The authors concluded that the change in AUC after oral talinolol was due to increased systemic availability of digoxin, through inhibition of intestinal P-glycoprotein. They did not discuss the possibility that talinolol had also reduced the non-renal clearance of digoxin by inhibiting its biliary secretion, and indeed there was a small, albeit non-significant reduction in non-renal clearance of digoxin after both oral and intravenous talinolol. In contrast, digoxin did not affect the kinetics of talinolol.

Dihydroergocriptine The effect of dihydroergocriptine on the pharmacokinetics of a single oral dose of digoxin has been studied in 12 healthy men aged 23–39 years (14[C]). There was no interaction.

Macrolide antibiotics Macrolide antibiotics reduce the metabolism of digoxin in the gut before it is absorbed, by inhibiting the growth of the bacterium *Eubacterium glenum* (SEDA-23, 194). Clarithromycin also inhibits P-glycoprotein. The effect of azithromycin has now been reported in a 31-month-old boy with Down's syndrome and Fallot's tetralogy (15[A]). During a 5-day course of azithromycin 5 mg/kg/day the serum digoxin concentration rose and the child had anorexia, diarrhea, and second-degree atrioventricular block with junctional extra beats. The mechanism was not investigated.

Meglitinides In 12 healthy volunteers aged 19–36 years nateglinide had no effects on the pharmacokinetics of a single dose of digoxin (16[C]). Similarly, in 14 healthy adults, repaglinide 2 mg three times had no effect on the steady-state pharmacokinetics of digoxin (17[C]). These results suggest that the meglitinides do not affect P-glycoprotein.

St John's wort St John's wort has previously been reported to have no effects on the single-dose pharmacokinetics of digoxin but to reduce the AUC during steady-state therapy, an effect that was attributed to induction of P-glycoprotein (SEDA-24, 203). In Japan, according to a recent study, enough patients take St John's wort with a cardiac glycoside to make this interaction potentially important; of 741 out-patients taking St John's wort, 171 had been given a prescription for either digoxin or methyldigoxin (18[C]).

Statins A 52-year-old man developed rhabdomyolysis while taking simvastatin, digoxin, ciclosporin, and verapamil (19[A]). The authors proposed that this had been due in part to inhibition of the biliary secretion of simvastatin by digoxin; however, it is likely that the major mechanism of the interaction was inhibition of CYP3A4 by ciclosporin.

Telmisartan Multiple-dose telmisartan 120 mg od administered with digoxin 0.25 mg od resulted in higher serum digoxin concentrations (20[C]). Digoxin AUC rose by 22% and C_{max} by 50%; the rise in C_{min} (13%) was not significant. These results suggest that telmisartan reduces the clearance of digoxin. The magnitude of this effect is comparable to that observed with calcium channel blockers, carvedilol, captopril, amiodarone, quinidine, and propafenone. Monitoring serum digoxin concentrations should be considered when patients first use telmisartan and when the dosage of telmisartan is changed.

Zaleplon The effects of zaleplon on the pharmacokinetics and pharmacodynamics of steady-state digoxin have been studied in 20 healthy men aged 18–45 years (21[C]). There was no interaction.

Diagnosis of toxicity It has yet again been confirmed that the serum digoxin concentration distinguishes between patients with and without digoxin toxicity, but with considerable overlap (22[C]). Of 99 patients, 41 with toxicity had mean serum digoxin concentrations of 3.1 ng/ml compared with 1.6 ng/ml in 58 non-toxic patients. However the digoxin concentration was below 2 ng/ml in 10 patients with toxicity and higher than 2 ng/ml in 16 patients without. There were no significant differences in serum electrolyte concentrations between the toxic and non-toxic patients, and the authors therefore concluded that such abnormalities are less important than they have usually been considered to be. However, this study does not demonstrate that at all; rather it shows that even if serum electrolyte concentrations are well controlled it may not be possible to avoid digitalis toxicity for other reasons. Indeed, in this study the patients with toxicity had significantly worse renal function, which would have explained their increased risk.

Management of toxicity The definitive treatment of digoxin intoxication is antidigoxin antibody, which is highly effective (23[r]). In a systematic review of 250 publications no controlled, randomized trials were found, and the authors concluded that there was little or no scientific evidence of efficacy (24[M]). However, there is no doubt that antidigoxin antibodies are highly effective in the treatment of digoxin intoxication and of intoxication with other cardiac glycosides. The important question is whether there are cases in which the antibodies need not be used, and guidelines have yet to be developed.

When antidigoxin antibodies are not available, alternative measures can be used (SEDA-5, 172). In one 73-year-old woman who took 12.5 mg of digoxin, gastric lavage and activated charcoal tided the patient over until antibodies became available (25[A]). In another case, cholestyramine enhanced the elimination of digoxin in two elderly patients with congestive heart failure and raised serum digoxin concentrations (26[A]). In one case the half-life of digoxin was 20 hours and in the other 24 hours. This effect of cholestyramine is due to inhibition of the reabsorption of digoxin after its biliary secretion. Repeated doses of activated charcoal have also been used for this purpose (SEDA-24, 201).

Because digoxin has a large apparent volume of distribution, plasma exchange, hemodialysis, and hemoperfusion are generally not effective methods of removing digoxin from the body. However, plasma exchange has been used to enhance the rate of removal of anti-digoxin antibody Fab fragments in 46-year-old man with renal insufficiency (27[A]). Removal of the digoxin–Fab complexes in this case prevented their subsequent dissociation and a further increase in the unbound concentration of digoxin. The authors proposed that plasma exchange is best used in these cases within the first 3 hours after the administration of antidigoxin antibodies.

OTHER POSITIVE INOTROPIC DRUGS *(SED-14, 532; SEDA-22, 203; SEDA-23, 195; SEDA-24, 204)*

Amrinone

Hematologic Thrombocytopenia due to amrinone has been briefly reviewed (28[r]).

Enoximone

Long-term treatment with inhibitors of phosphodiesterase type III is associated with increased mortality in congestive heart failure (SEDA-17, 217). The use of a lower dose of enoximone in 105 patients with heart failure of New York Heart Association classes 2 or 3 has been studied over 12 weeks (29[C]). Enoximone 25–50 mg tds improved exercise capacity and reduced dyspnea. There was no evidence of a dysrhythmic effect. The rates of adverse events were similar with enoximone and placebo, and indeed there were fewer cases of dizziness, vertigo, or hypotension in those who took enoximone. There were two deaths in the 70 patients who took enoximone compared with four of the 35 who took placebo. However, this small short-term study does not rule out the possibility that even this small dose of enoximone may cause increased mortality during long-term administration or in patients with more severe cardiac failure.

Milrinone

The results of OPTIME–CHF, as presented to a meeting of the American College of Cardiology in March 2000, had been briefly reviewed (30[r]). This was a randomized placebo-controlled study of milrinone given by infusion for 48 hours in 951 patients with acute exacerbations of chronic heart failure. There was no benefit of milrinone and a significant increase in the incidence of sustained *hypotension*. Hypotension is a common effect of intravenous milrinone and is the main limitation to its short-term use (SEDA-24, 204).

In six patients with severe congestive heart failure being treated with continuous veno-venous hemofiltration, the pharmacokinetics of milrinone 0.25 mg/kg/min by continuous intravenous infusion were different from those that have been previously reported in patients with normal renal function, with a prolonged half-life and a raised mean steady-state concentration, suggestive of reduced clearance (31[c]). The half-life of milrinone was 20 hours, compared with reported half-lives of around 3 hours.

In seven patients with congestive heart failure who developed hypotension (systolic arterial pressure below 90 mmHg), vasopressin 0.03–0.07 U/min increased the systolic arterial pressure to 127 mmHg (32[c]). This effect was due to peripheral vasoconstriction, since the systemic vascular resistance increased from 1112 to 1460 dyne.s.cm^5 with no change in cardiac index. Urine output also improved significantly.

In three patients in whom milrinone caused hypotension, vasopressin (0.03–0.07 U/min) increased the systolic arterial pressure from 90 to 130 mmHg and reduced the dosages of catecholamines that were being used (33[A]). The authors hypothesized that vasopressin may have inhibited the milrinone-induced accumulation of cyclic AMP in vascular smooth muscle.

Vesnarinone

Although vesnarinone was originally developed for the treatment of cardiac failure, its action on tumor cells has prompted its use in the treatment of cancer. In 26 patients who received combinations of vesnarinone and gemcitabine there was no pharmacokinetic interaction between the two drugs (34[C]). Although there were cases of *neutropenia* and *thrombocytopenia*, those effects could have occurred with gemcitabine alone and could not necessarily be attributed to vesnarinone. Other adverse effects of the combination included nausea and vomiting, anorexia and fatigue, diarrhea, headache, and fever. There were no cases of QT_c prolongation or ventricular dysrhythmias. There were rises in hepatic transaminase activities in up to 25% of cases. Again it was not possible to distinguish between adverse effects of gemcitabine and vesnarinone.

DRUGS USED IN DYSRHYTHMIAS

The adverse effects of antidysrhythmic drugs, both cardiac and non-cardiac, have been reviewed (35[R], 36[R]). The prodysrhythmic effects of antidysrhythmic drugs have also been specifically reviewed, with regard to mechanisms at the cellular level (37[R]) and molecular level (38[R]). As far as the cellular mechanisms are concerned, the antidysrhythmic drugs have been divided into three classes (which do not overlap with the classes specified in the Vaughan–Williams classification).

- Group 1 drugs have fast-onset kinetics and the block saturates at rapid rates (about 300 beats/min).
- Group 2 drugs have slow-onset kinetics and the block saturates at rapid rates.
- Group 3 drugs have slow-onset kinetics and there is saturation of frequency-dependent block at slow heart rates (about 100 beats/min).

The fast-onset kinetics of the group 1 drugs makes them the least likely to cause dysrhythmias. Group 2 drugs, which include encainide, flecainide, procainamide, and quinidine, are the most likely to cause dysrhythmias, because of their slow-onset kinetics. Although this also applies to the group 3 drugs, which include propafenone and disopyramide, block is less likely to occur during faster heart rates and serious dysrhythmias are therefore less likely during exercise.

The most common mechanism of dysrhythmias at the molecular level is by inhibition of the potassium channels known as I_{Kr}, which are encoded by the human ether-a-go-go-related gene (HERG). The antidysrhythmic drugs that affect these channels include almokalant, amiodarone, azimilide, bretylium, dofetilide, ibutilide, sematilide, d-sotalol, and tedisamil (all drugs with class III actions) and bepridil, disopyramide, prenylamine, procainamide, propafenone, quinidine, and terodiline (all drugs with class I actions). Other drugs that affect these channels but are not used to treat cardiac dysrhythmias include astemizole and terfenadine (antihistamines), cisapride, erythromycin, haloperidol, sertindole, and thioridazine.

The management of drug-induced cardiac dysrhythmias includes withdrawal of the drug, the administration of potassium if necessary to maintain the serum potassium concentration at over 4.5 mmol/l, the intravenous administration of magnesium sulfate (1–2 g), and in some cases isoprenaline or overdrive pacing to increase the heart rate (SEDA-23, 196). There is some anecdotal evidence that atrioventricular nodal blockade with verapamil or a β-blocker can also be effective. However, in two recent cases the addition of a β-blocker (either atenolol or metoprolol) to treatment with class I antidysrhythmic drugs (cibenzoline in one case and flecainide in the other) did not prevent the occurrence of atrial flutter with a 1:1 response (39[A]). However, the author suggested that in these cases, although the β-blockers had not suppressed the dysrhythmia, they had at least improved the patient's tolerance of it. In both cases the uses of class I antidysrhythmic drugs was contraindicated by virtue of structural damage, in the first case due to mitral valvular disease and in the second due to an ischemic cardiomyopathy.

Drug interactions Interactions with antidysrhythmic drugs have again been reviewed (40[R]).

Adenosine *(SED-14, 536; SEDA-22, 203; SEDA-23, 197; SEDA-24, 205)*

Exercise reduces both non-cardiac adverse effects and dysrhythmias in patients who are given adenosine for diagnostic purposes in myocardial perfusion imaging (SEDA-21, 197). This has been confirmed in two further studies. In the first of these, 793 patients were given an intravenous infusion of adenosine 140 μg/kg/min while exercising for 6 minutes or for a similar time without exercise (41[C]). The rate of hypotension and dysrhythmias was significantly less in those who exercised (14 of 507) than in those who did not exercise (16 of 286). Overall reactions were more common in women than in men (5.7% vs 1.8%). All the adverse effects were transient and no specific therapy was required. The authors attributed the difference to the increase in sympathetic tone during exercise, which would have partly counteracted the hypotension and the negative chronotropic and negative dromotropic effects of adenosine. However, there was a major difference between the two groups, in that those who did not take exercise were considered unfit for exercise, which may have been associated with an increased risk of adverse effects. Nevertheless, the authors discarded that possibility, because the frequency of adverse reactions in those who did not take exercise was similar to frequencies that have previously been reported.

In the second study 19 patients received an intravenous infusion of adenosine 140 μg/kg/min for 4 minutes during exercise or for 6 minutes without exercise; the patients undertook both protocols (42[C]). Again, there were fewer adverse effects in those who took exercise, but only hypotension, chest pain, and headache were significantly different; there was a reduction in the frequency of flushing, which was almost significant. In addition, adverse effects were experienced for longer and the severity was greater in those who did not take exercise.

Cardiovascular There have been further reports of cardiac *dysrhythmias* in patients given either an intravenous infusion of adenosine or a single bolus dose.

A 38-year-old man was given intravenous adenosine 6 mg for a narrow-complex tachycardia (43[A]). Within about 1 minute his heart rate fell from 230 beats/min to bradycardia and then asystole. Cardiopulmonary resuscitation was ineffective. At autopsy there was a 75% occlusion of one of the coronary arteries (unspecified). The cause of the dysrhythmia in response to adenosine was not clear. He was not known to be taking other drugs (e.g. dipyridamole) that might have potentiated the action of adenosine.

A 56-year-old man was given adenosine 12 mg for a narrow-complex tachycardia on four occasions, and on each occasion developed transient atrial fibrillation for a few minutes thereafter. He had a concealed left-sided accessory pathway, which was successfully ablated (44[A]).

An 86-year-old woman was given adenosine 12 mg intravenously for sustained supraventricular tachycardia, which terminated but was followed by atrial fibrillation and paroxysmal ventricular tachycardia (45[A]). Cardioversion was unsuccessful, but normal sinus rhythm was obtained with procainamide. This followed an anteroseptal myocardial infarction.

A 75-year-old man who had had coronary bypass surgery was given an intravenous infusion of adenosine for stress testing (46[A]). After 1 minute he developed a three-beat run of wide-complex tachycardia, followed by a 20-second run of a regular wide-complex tachycardia at a rate of 115 beats per minute. There was left bundle branch block, and the tachycardia ended spontaneously. Adenosine infusion was continued and some ventricular extra beats with the same configuration occurred. In this case there was impaired perfusion of the left ventricle.

In patients with ischemic heart disease adenosine may prolong the QT_c interval and can increase the frequency of ventricular extra beats when there is myocardial scarring. It also causes increased release of catecholamines, and this may be the mechanism whereby it causes dysrhythmias in susceptible patients. If a dysrhythmia occurs, theophylline or one of its derivatives may be beneficial (43[A]).

Drug administration route Intracoronary adenosine has been compared with intravenous adenosine for the measure of fractional flow reserve in 52 patients with coronary artery lesions (47[C]). The intravenous dose was 140 μg/kg/min and the intracoronary bolus dose was 15–20 μg to the right coronary artery and 18–24 μg to the left coronary artery. The two routes of administration were equally effective in measuring hyperemic flow, and adverse effects were limited to two patients who received intravenous adenosine; one patient had severe nausea and one patient with asthma had an episode of bronchospasm.

The use of intrathecal adenosine in patients with chronic neuropathic pain (48[c], 49[c]) has been briefly reviewed (50[r]).

Ajmaline and derivatives

(SED-14, 537; SEDA-24, 206)

Ajmaline occasionally causes *cardiac dysrhythmias* (SEDA-17, 219), and another case has been reported in a 13-year-old boy with Brugada syndrome (right bundle branch block with persistent ST segment elevation) (51[A]). Shortly after an injection of ajmaline 1 mg/kg there was greater ST segment elevation and the right bundle branch block morphology was more marked. This was followed by short runs of non-sustained polymorphic ventricular tachycardia, gradually increasing until monomorphic ventricular tachycardia occurred. The dysrhythmia eventually resolved without further treatment. It is unwise to give antidysrhythmic drugs to patients with the Brugada syndrome.

Amiodarone *(SED-14, 537; SEDA-22, 204; SEDA-23, 198; SEDA-24, 206)*

The effects of amiodarone in treating tachydysrhythmias

There have been numerous recent reports of the efficacy and adverse effects of amiodarone in patients with various tachydysrhythmias.

Atrial fibrillation *In 186 patients randomized equally to amiodarone 200 mg/day, sotalol 160–480 mg/day, or placebo, the incidence of atrial fibrillation after 6 months was higher in those taking placebo compared with amiodarone and sotalol and higher in those taking sotalol compared with amiodarone (52[C]). Of the 65 patients who took amiodarone, 15 had significant adverse effects after an average of 16 months. There were eight cases of hypothyroidism, four of hyperthyroidism, two of symptomatic bradycardia, and one of ataxia. There were minor adverse effects in 9% of the patients, including gastrointestinal discomfort, nausea, photosensitivity, and eye problems. These patients had recurrent symptomatic atrial fibrillation. In contrast, only two patients using sotalol developed symptomatic bradycardia and one had severe dizziness. On the basis of these results, a reasonable strategy would be start with sotalol and switch to amiodarone if sotalol is ineffective or causes unacceptable adverse effects.*

In 208 patients with atrial fibrillation of various duration, including 50 with chronic atrial fibrillation, randomized to amiodarone or placebo, 80% converted to sinus rhythm after amiodarone compared with 40% of those given placebo (53[C]). Amiodarone was given as an intravenous loading dose of 300 mg for 1 hour and 20 mg/kg for 24 hours, followed by 600 mg/day orally for 1 week and 400 mg/day for 3 weeks. Those who converted to sinus rhythm had had atrial fibrillation for a shorter duration and had small atria than those who did not convert. The shorter the duration of fibrillation and the smaller the atria the sooner conversion occurred. There was significant hypotension in 12 of the 118 patients who received amiodarone during the first hour of intravenous administration, but in all cases this responded to intravenous fluids alone. There was phlebitis at the site of infusion in 17 patients, and the peripheral catheter was replaced by a central catheter. There were no dysrhythmic effects.

In 40 patients with atrial fibrillation, some with severe heart disease (including cardiogenic shock in eight and pulmonary edema in 12) amiodarone 450 mg was given through a peripheral vein within 1 minute, followed by 10 ml of saline; 21 patients converted to sinus rhythm, 13 within 30 minutes and another eight within 24 hours (54[c]). There were two cases of hypotension, but in those that converted to sinus rhythm there was a slight increase in systolic blood pressure. There were no cases of thrombophlebitis. Efficacy is hard to judge from this study, because it was not placebo-controlled.

In 72 patients with paroxysmal atrial fibrillation randomized to either amiodarone 30 mg/kg or placebo, those who received amiodarone converted to sinus rhythm more often than those given placebo (55[C]). The respective conversion rates were about 50% and 20% at 8 hours, and 87% and 35% after 24 hours. The time to conversion in patients who converted did not differ. One patient developed slow atrial fibrillation (35 beats/min) with a blood pressure of 75/55 mmHg. Three other patients who received amiodarone had diarrhea and one had nausea. In the control group two patients had headache, one had diarrhea, one had nausea, and two had episodes of sinus arrest associ-

ated with syncope during conversation to sinus rhythm; the last of these was thought to have sick sinus syndrome.

In a single-blind study 150 patients with acute atrial fibrillation were randomized to intravenous flecainide, propafenone, or amiodarone (56[C]). At 12 hours there was conversion to sinus rhythm in 45 of 50 patients given flecainide, 36 of the 50 given propafenone, and 32 of the 50 given amiodarone. Thus, flecainide and propafenone were both more effective than amiodarone. There were no differences between the groups in the incidences of adverse effects; there was one withdrawal in each group, due to cerebral embolism in a patient given amiodarone, heart failure in a patient given propafenone, and atrial flutter in a patient given flecainide. There were no ventricular dysrhythmias during the study.

Amiodarone and magnesium have been compared in a placebo-controlled study to reduce the occurrence of atrial fibrillation in 147 patients after coronary artery bypass graft surgery (57[C]). Amiodarone was given as a infusion of 900 mg/day for 3 days and magnesium by infusion of 4 g/day for 3 days. The cumulative occurrences of atrial fibrillation with placebo, amiodarone, and magnesium were 27%, 14%, and 23% respectively. These differences were not significant. Amiodarone delayed the onset of the first episode of dysrhythmia significantly, but the slight benefit was associated with a longer period of invasive monitoring and was not considered worth while. Patients who were more likely to develop atrial fibrillation were older and had a plasma magnesium concentration at 24 hours of under 0.95 mmol/l. Patients who were given amiodarone had a slightly higher rate of adverse events, including hypotension, atrioventricular block, and bradycardia; adverse events led to withdrawal in four cases.

Amiodarone, sotalol, and propafenone have been compared for the prevention of atrial fibrillation in 403 patients who had had at least one episode of atrial fibrillation within the previous 6 months; the study was not placebo-controlled (58[c]). The rate of recurrence of atrial fibrillation was significantly higher in those given sotalol or propafenone than in those given amiodarone. During the study nine patients given amiodarone died, compared with eight given sotalol or propafenone. Four deaths were thought to be dysrhythmic, three in patients given amiodarone. There were major non-fatal adverse events in 36 of the 201 patients given amiodarone and in 35 of the 202 patients given propafenone or sotalol. These included one case of torsade de pointes in a patient who received propafenone, and congestive heart failure in 11 patients given amiodarone and nine given sotalol or propafenone. There were strokes and intracranial hemorrhages in one patient given amiodarone and nine patients given sotalol or propafenone, of whom most were taking warfarin at the time. In all, 68 of the patients who were given amiodarone and 93 of those given sotalol or propafenone withdrew from the study; 17 of those taking amiodarone withdrew because of lack of efficacy compared with 56 of those taking sotalol or propafenone; 36 of those who took amiodarone withdrew because of adverse events compared with 23 of those who took sotalol or propafenone, and this was almost statistically significant.

Amiodarone, propafenone, and sotalol have also been compared in the prevention of atrial fibrillation in 214 patients with recurrent symptomatic atrial fibrillation. They were randomized to amiodarone 200 mg/day, propafenone 450 mg/day, or sotalol 320 mg/day. There was recurrence of atrial fibrillation in 25 of the 75 patients who took amiodarone compared with the 51 of 75 who took sotalol and 24 of the 64 who took propafenone. There were adverse effects requiring withdrawal of treatment in 14 patients who took amiodarone, five who took sotalol and one who took propafenone while they were in sinus rhythm. These effects included symptomatic bradycardia in three patients, hyperthyroidism in six, hypothyroidism in four, and ataxia in one patient who took amiodarone. In those taking sotalol the adverse effects were bradycardia in three and severe dizziness in two. In the one patient in whom propafenone was withheld the reason was symptomatic bradycardia. Thus, amiodarone and propafenone were both more effective than sotalol, but amiodarone also caused more adverse effects requiring withdrawal (59[C]).

Atrial flutter Antidysrhythmic drugs have been compared with radiofrequency ablation in 61 patients with atrial flutter (60[c]). Drug treatment was with at least two drugs, one of which was amiodarone. Of the 30 patients who took drug therapy, 19 needed to come into hospital one or more times, whereas after ra-

diofrequency ablation that happened in only seven of 31 cases. In those who took the antidysrhythmic drugs the mean number of drugs was 3.4 and the range of drugs used was very wide. Quality-of-life and symptoms scores improved significantly in those in whom radiofrequency ablation was used, but not in those who took the antidysrhythmic drugs, apart from the symptom of palpitation, which improved in both groups, but to a greater extent in the non-drug group. Adverse effects were not discussed in this study, but it is clear that it suggests that radiofrequency ablation is to be preferred in these patients.

Ventricular tachycardia *The effects of amiodarone in 55 patients with sustained ventricular tachycardia after myocardial infarction have been assessed in a long-term follow-up study (61[C]). The patients underwent programmed ventricular stimulation after having been loaded with amiodarone. They were divided into those in whom ventricular tachydysrhythmias could be induced or not, and all were then given amiodarone 200 mg/day. In 11 cases a cardioverter defibrillator was implanted, because the first episode of ventricular tachycardia had been poorly tolerated or had caused hemodynamic instability. A defibrillator was also implanted in five other cases during follow-up, because of recurrence of dysrhythmias. There was a non-significant trend to a difference between the cumulative rates of dysrhythmias during long-term follow-up, with more events in those in whom a dysrhythmia had been inducible after loading. However, mortality rates in the two groups did not differ, and was around 25% at a mean follow-up of 42 months. Survival was significantly higher in patients with a left ventricular ejection fraction over 0.4, and the lower the left ventricular ejection fractions the higher the mortality. Amiodarone was withdrawn in six patients after a mean of 34 months because of neuropathy (n = 1), hypothyroidism (n = 1), prodysrhythmia with incessant ventricular tachycardia (n = 2), and non-specific adverse effects (n = 2). There was no pulmonary toxicity and no cases of torsade de pointes. In two patients there was evidence of hypothyroidism, mild neuropathy, and skin discoloration, but these events did not lead to withdrawal. In two patients the doses of amiodarone was reduced to 100 mg/day because of sinus bradycardia.*

Prevention of dysrhythmias *In a study of the use of implantable defibrillators or antidysrhythmic drugs in patients resuscitated from cardiac arrest in 288 patients the defibrillator was associated with a slightly lower rate of all-cause mortality compared with the antidysrhythmic drugs (amiodarone or metoprolol) (62[C]). However, the small difference was not significantly significant. There was hyperthyroidism in three of those given amiodarone and drug withdrawal was required in nine of those given amiodarone and 10 of those given metoprolol. Five patients fitted with a defibrillator died perioperatively, and two patients given amiodarone died. Cross-over to the other therapy occurred in 6% in each group, usually because of recurrence of the dysrhythmia. When sudden cardiac death was analyzed, the reduction in mortality with the defibrillator was much larger (61%). There were no differences in all-cause mortality and sudden death rates between those given amiodarone and those given metoprolol.*

Amiodarone and carvedilol have been used in combination in 109 patients with severe heart failure and left ventricular ejection fractions of 0.25 (63[C]). They were given amiodarone 1000 mg/week plus carvedilol titrated to a target dose of 50 mg/day. A dual-chamber pacemaker was inserted and programmed in back-up mode at a basal rate of 40. Significantly more patients were in sinus rhythm after 1 year, and in 47 patients who were studied for at least 1 year the resting heart rate fell from 90 to 59. Ventricular extra beats were suppressed from 1 to 0.1/day and the number of bouts of tachycardia over 167 per minute was reduced from 1.2 to 0.3 episodes per patient per 3 months. The left ventricular ejection fraction increased from 0.26 to 0.39 and New York Heart Association Classification improved from 3.2 to 1.8. The probability of sudden death was significantly reduced by amiodarone plus carvedilol compared with 154 patients treated with amiodarone alone and even more so compared with 283 patients who received no treatment at all. However, the study was not randomized, and this vitiates the results. The main adverse effect was symptomatic bradycardia, which occurred in seven patients; two of those developed atrioventricular block and four had sinoatrial block and/or sinus bradycardia; one patient developed slow atrial fibrillation.

Cardiovascular *Bradycardia* has previously been reported to occur in about 5% of patients taking amiodarone (SEDA-20, 176). Of 2559 patients admitted to an intensive cardiac care unit over 3 years, 64 with major cardiac iatrogenic problems were reviewed (64[c]). Of those, 58 had dysrhythmias, mainly bradydysrhythmias, secondary to amiodarone, β-blockers, calcium channel blockers, electrolyte imbalance, or a combination of those. Amiodarone was implicated in 19 cases, compared with 44 cases attributed to β-blockers and 28 to calcium channel blockers. Of the 56 patients with sinus bradycardia, 10 were taking a combination of amiodarone and a β-blocker, six were taking amiodarone alone, and three were taking amiodarone plus a calcium channel blocker.

Amiodarone has been reported to cause *atrial flutter* in 10 patients who had been given it for paroxysmal atrial fibrillation (65[c]). In nine of those the atrial flutter was successfully treated by catheter ablation. However, during a mean follow-up period of 8 months after ablation atrial fibrillation occurred in two patients, who had continued to take amiodarone; this was a lower rate of recurrence than in patients in whom atrial flutter was not associated with amiodarone. The authors therefore suggested that in patients with atrial flutter secondary to amiodarone given for atrial fibrillation, catheter ablation allows continuation of amiodarone therapy.

Reports of *polymorphous ventricular tachycardia* after amiodarone continue to appear, and there has been a recent report of three boys with congenital cardiac defects who were given intravenous amiodarone; two died (66[A]).

An 8-day-old boy was given intravenous amiodarone 5 mg/kg over 60 minutes followed by 10 mg/kg/day for a postoperative junctional ectopic tachycardia after a cardiac operation. He developed ventricular fibrillation 12 hours later, but recovered with defibrillation and internal cardiac massage. His serum amiodarone concentration was 1–2.5 mg/l, within the usual target range.

A 3-month-old boy underwent a cardiac operation and 6 hours later developed a junctional ectopic tachycardia. He was given amiodarone as a continuous intravenous infusion of 10 mg/kg/day for 3 hours and developed ventricular fibrillation, from which he was not resuscitated. The serum amiodarone concentration was 0.3 mg/l.

A 3-month-old boy developed a postoperative junctional ectopic tachycardia 48 hours after operation and was given a continuous intravenous infusion of amiodarone 10 mg/kg/day. After 2 hours he developed ventricular fibrillation and was not resuscitated. His serum amiodarone concentration was in the target range.

However, it is not clear that the dysrhythmias in these cases were due to amiodarone, particularly since the doses had been very low and the serum concentrations no higher than the usual target range; QT intervals were not reported.

In a 66-year-old woman taking amiodarone 1200 mg/week there was such marked *prolongation of the QT interval*, to 680 ms, that the succeeding P waves fell within the refractory period of the preceding beat and were unable to institute conduction (67[A]). This resulted in 2:1 atrioventricular block. Amiodarone was withdrawn and the QT interval normalized with a time course consistent with the long half-life of amiodarone. A subsequent rechallenge with intravenous amiodarone caused further prolongation of the QT interval. The authors hypothesized that this patient had a silent mutation in one of the genes coding for the two major potassium channel proteins (I_{Kr} or I_{Ks}) that are involved in the mode of action of amiodarone. However, they did not present any genetic studies to support this hypothesis.

Respiratory Another case of bilateral pulmonary infiltrates has been reported (68[A]).

A 77-year-old man who had taken amiodarone 400 mg/day for 11 months developed crackles at the lung bases and scattered respiratory wheeze. His leukocyte count was raised at 13.5×10^9/l and he had progressive reduction in carbon monoxide diffusing capacity, serially measured. A chest X-ray showed bilateral opacities in the upper zones, peripheral in distribution, and a CT scan showed dense bilateral lung parenchymal opacities. The symptoms of dyspnea on exertion, cough with minimal sputum, pleuritic chest pain, and low-grade fever abated after withdrawal, and the upper lobe densities resolved.

In some cases amiodarone can cause more than one adverse respiratory effect (69[A]).

A 62-year-old man took amiodarone 400 mg bd and developed several adverse effects, including bilateral apical opacities with left hilar lymphadenopathy. Amiodarone was withdrawn and he was given corticosteroids, with good effect; there was dramatic radiographic resolution within 3 weeks and he was no longer breathless with 1 week. The lung biopsy showed typical foamy macrophages. He had fibrosis of the bronchioles and interstitium, foci of obliterative bronchiolitis, and thickening of the alveolar walls. He had an accompanying peripheral neuropathy, which improved after withdrawal, and impaired visual acuity, about which no further information was given. Biopsy of the right vastus lateralis muscle showed type II atrophy with vacuolization, which the authors suggested supported the suspicion of amiodarone toxicity.

The sialylated carbohydrate antigen KL-6 has been reported to be a serum marker of the activity of *interstitial pneumonitis*. This has now been studied in seven patients with amiodarone-induced pulmonary toxicity (70[c], 71[c]). The dosages of amiodarone were 200–800 mg as an oral loading dose followed by 75–200 mg/day. Pulmonary complications occurred at 17 days to 48 months of treatment. In two patients with severe dyspnea and interstitial shadows on chest X-ray the KL-6 concentrations were very high (2100 and 3000 u/ml). In one of these the concentration increased from 695 to 2100 u/ml at a time when the interstitial changes on the CT scan worsened. In contrast, in two patients in whom pneumonia resolved with antibiotic treatment and without withdrawal of amiodarone, the serum KL-6 concentrations were lower (120 and 330 u/ml). In a patient in whom congestion of the lungs due to congestive cardiac failure had been confused with interstitial shadows the KL-6 concentration was only 190 u/ml. In two patients with lung cancers the concentrations were 260 and 360 u/ml. The authors proposed that a KL-6 concentration above the reference range (more than 520 u/ml) might be useful in differentiating patients with amiodarone-induced pneumonitis from patients with similar features not associated with amiodarone.

Special senses *Optic neuropathy* is uncommon with amiodarone, but two further cases have recently been reported.

A 51-year-old man developed blurred vision after having taken amiodarone 600 mg/day for 3 months and 400 mg/day for 5 months (72[A]). There was mild optic disc palor and edema on the right side, with a nearby flame-shaped hemorrhage; the optic disc on the left side was normal. There were accompanying corneal opacities in both eyes. Amiodarone was withdrawn and the optic neuropathy and corneal opacities improved.

A 48-year-old man developed bilateral blurred vision and visual field changes after having taken amiodarone 400 mg/day for 2 months; 3 weeks after withdrawal of amiodarone his symptoms improved (73[A]). There was no optic disc edema.

The absence of optic disc edema in the last case is unusual; most cases are accompanied by some form of swelling of the optic disc.

Endocrine *Hyperthyroidism* continues to be reported from time to time in association with amiodarone.

A 72-year-old woman with dilated cardiomyopathy was given amiodarone for fast atrial flutter and 6 months later developed abnormal thyroid function tests, with a suppressed TSH and a raised serum thyroxine. The autoantibody profile was negative and a thyroid uptake scan showed reduced uptake (74[A]).

Despite the fact that she was clinically euthyroid, the authors suggested that this patient had amiodarone-induced hyperthyroidism. However, amiodarone inhibits the peripheral conversion of thyroxine to triiodothyronine; it can therefore increase the serum thyroxine and suppress the serum TSH, as in this case. On the other hand, the reduced uptake by the thyroid gland is consistent with type 2 amiodarone-induced hyperthyroidism. The authors did not report the serum concentrations of free thyroxine and triiodothyronine.

A 67-year-old man took amiodarone 200 mg/day for 20 months, after which it was withdrawn; 8 months later his serum TSH was suppressed and the free thyroxine and free triiodothyronine were both raised; there were no thyroid antibodies and an ultrasound scan showed a diffuse goiter with a nodule in the right lobe and reduced iodine uptake (75[A]). Histological examination of the nodule showed a papillary cancer.

The authors attributed these changes to an effect of amiodarone, but it is not clear that amiodarone-induced changes would have taken so long to become manifest after withdrawal. However, the diagnosis of type 2 amiodarone-induced hyperthyroidism was supported by a poor response to prednisone, potassium perchlorate, and methimazole. Lithium produced temporary benefit, but thyroidectomy was required.

In five patients who presented in Tasmania during 1 year, all of whom were taking amiodarone 200 mg/day, serum TSH was undetectable and the free thyroxine and triiodothyronine concentrations were raised (76[c]). In one case there was a low titer of TSH receptor antibodies and in another a high titer of antithyroid peroxidase antibodies. In all cases the hyperthyroidism was severe and occurred after at least 2 years of treatment with amiodarone. In one of two patients in whom it was measured the serum concentration of interleukin-6 was raised, as has been previously shown (SEDA-19, 193). In two cases the hyperthyroidism was refractory to treatment with propylthiouracil, lithium, and dexamethasone; in these cases thyroidectomy was required. Two patients responded to propylthiouracil, lithium, and dexamethasone, and one responded to carbimazole.

Hematologic Bone-marrow biopsy in a patient taking amiodarone 100 mg/day showed *multiple non-caseating epithelioid granulomata*, which resolved 3 months after the withdrawal of amiodarone in a 67-year-old man (77[A]). Similar granulomas were found in a 77-year-old woman who had taken amiodarone 100 mg/day for many years and had thrombocytopenia; the bone marrow contained an increased number of megakaryocytes. Her platelet count normalized 1 month after amiodarone had been withdrawn, and after 3 months there were fewer granulomata in the bone marrow. Bone-marrow granulomata have only previously been reported in two cases (SEDA-23, 199). The mechanism is unknown.

Liver *Chronic liver damage* of various sorts is an occasional adverse effect of amiodarone.

A 40-year-old man who had taken amiodarone 400 mg/day for 6 weeks developed an acute hepatitis accompanied by clusters of light brown granular cells, which were identified as macrophages (78[A]). There were phospholipid inclusions in the macrophages and hepatocytes.

The authors proposed that the granular macrophages represented an early marker of amiodarone-induced hepatotoxicity. Their unusual color was attributed to the deposition of a combination of phospholipid, lipofuscin, and bile breakdown products.

Skin Another case of *blue-gray discoloration* of the face and other exposed areas has been reported in a 69-year-old white man who had taken amiodarone 400 mg/day for 3 years (79[A]). Areas that had been protected from the sun (the forehead by a broad-brimmed hat and the skin under his wrist watch) were not affected.

Immunologic *Angio-edema* has been reported, apparently for the first time, in a 70-year-old woman who had taken amiodarone 200 mg/day for 8 years (80[A]). The amiodarone was withdrawn and the symptoms disappeared. Rechallenge produced facial flush and facial angio-edema within 20 minutes of a 200 mg dose.

Death The effect of intravenous and oral amiodarone on morbidity and mortality has been studied in 1073 patients during the first hours after the onset of acute myocardial infarction (81[C]). The patients were randomized to receive amiodarone or placebo for 6 months. The interim analysis showed an increased mortality, albeit not significant, with high-dose amiodarone (16% vs 10%) and the dose was therefore reduced from 400 to 200 mg/day. Low-dose amiodarone was associated with a reduced death rate (6.6% vs 9.9%). There were non-fatal adverse events in 108 patients taking amiodarone and 73 taking placebo. The only non-fatal adverse effect that occurred significantly more often with amiodarone was hypotension during the initial intravenous loading phase, a well-known effect. In the context of this study, it should be remembered that in several previous studies amiodarone has been shown to reduce mortality after myocardial infarction (SEDA-23, 198; SEDA-24, 206; 82[r]).

Drug interactions The corticosteroid *budesonide* undergoes a high degree of first-pass elimination in the liver after oral administration, and therefore causes few systemic adverse effects. It was therefore surprising that Cushing's syndrome occurred in an 81-year-old man taking oral budesonide 9 mg/day and amiodarone 100 mg/day (83[A]). When amiodarone was withdrawn the clinical effects of Cushing's syndrome disappeared. The authors suggested that amiodarone had inhibited the metabolism of budesonide by hepatic CYP3A.

Bepridil *(SED-14, 541, 605; SEDA-17, 222)*

Because it prolongs the QT interval, bepridil can cause *torsade de pointes*. Of 75 elderly patients who took bepridil 200 mg/day, 23 had prolongation of the QT interval. The factors that were associated with this were hypokalemia, bradycardia, renal insufficiency, and an increased plasma bepridil concentration (84[c]).

Cibenzoline *(SED-14, 541; SEDA-23, 200; SEDA-24, 210)*

Nervous system Various nervous system complaints have been reported in occasional patients taking cibenzoline, including *disturbances of visual accommodation, tremulousness, dizziness, lightheadedness, anticholinergic effects*, and a *myasthenia-like syndrome*. Now *choreiform movements* associated with persistent orofacial dystonia have been attributed to cibenzoline in a 77-year-old woman who took 260 mg/day for 1 week (85[A]). When cibenzoline was eventually withdrawn the effects resolved with 1 month. The authors proposed that the effect was due to inhibition of potassium channels.

Metabolic Cibenzoline has previously been reported to cause *hypoglycemia* (SEDA-18, 204). In a case-control study of 14 156 outpatients, 91 had hypoglycemia, and each was matched with five controls (86[C]). Eight of those with hypoglycemia were taking cibenzoline and three were taking disopyramide. In contrast, only seven of the controls were taking cibenzoline, a significant difference. However, 20 of the controls were taking disopyramide, which was not significant from the patients with hypoglycemia, although disopyramide is known to cause hypoglycemia. Insulin was also associated with hypoglycemia, but sulfonylureas were not. Furthermore, there was a positive association with what were termed "thyroid agents". All of these features cast some doubt on the validity of these results in relation to cibenzoline.

Liver *Hepatotoxicity* with cibenzoline has been rarely reported, but another case has emerged, in a 67-year-old woman, who also had mild thrombocytopenia (87[A]). The liver function tests, which were markedly abnormal, normalized with 3 months of withdrawal.

Disopyramide *(SED-14, 543; SEDA-22, 207; SEDA-23, 200; SEDA-24, 211)*

Disopyramide (by intravenous infusion of 2 mg/kg/min up to a maximum total dose of 100 mg) has been compared with pilsicainide (in a single oral dose of 100–150 mg) in the treatment of paroxysmal atrial fibrillation in 72 patients (88[C]). Conversion to sinus rhythm occurred in 29 of the 40 patients given pilsicainide and 18 of 32 patients given disopyramide, a non-significant difference. However, the mean time to conversion was faster with disopyramide (23 vs 60 minutes). No adverse effects were observed with either drug.

Drug interactions The *macrolide antibiotics* have previously been reported to inhibit the clearance of disopyramide (SEDA-24, 211), presumably by inhibition of dealkylation of disopyramide to its major metabolite, mono-*N*-dealkyldisopyramide. For example, in human liver microsomes the macrolide antibiotic troleandomycin significantly inhibited the mono-*N*-dealkylation of disopyramide enantiomers by inhibition of CYP3A4 (89[E]). This interaction can result in serious dysrhythmias or other adverse effects of disopyramide. Interactions have again been reported with azithromycin (90[A]) and clarithromycin (91[A]).

A 35-year-old woman taking disopyramide phosphate modified-release capsules 150 mg qds was given azithromycin 500 mg initially and 250 mg/day thereafter. In 11 days she developed malaise, lightheadedness, and urinary retention. After the insertion of a urinary catheter she developed a monomorphic ventricular tachycardia with left bundle branch block. She was successfully cardioverted and the electrocardiogram showed a markedly prolonged QT interval of 560 ms and T wave inversion in the anterolateral leads. Her serum disopyramide concentration, which had previously been 2.6 mg/l, was 11 mg/l.

An 86-year-old woman presented with severe hypoglycemia after clarithromycin 500 mg/day had been added for 3 days to her other therapy, which included disopyramide 500 mg/day. The hypoglycemia resolved completely after withdrawal of disopyramide.

Flecainide *(SED-14, 545; SEDA-22, 207; SEDA-24, 211)*

Cardiovascular *Cardiac dysrhythmias* are less common with flecainide than with other antidysrhythmic drugs of class I. When dysrhythmias occur, prolongation of the QT interval is an important mechanism, but in a recent case it was suggested that tachycardia was due to re-entry within the His–Purkinje system (92[A]). In another case flecainide reportedly caused a wide-complex tachycardia due to atypical atrial flutter with 1:1 conduction and aberrant QRS complexes (93[A]). Although drugs of class IC, such as flecainide, can slow atrial and atrioventricular nodal conduction in patients with atrial fibrillation or atrial flutter, they do not alter the refractoriness of the atrioventricular node, and this allows 1:1 atrioventricular conduction as the atrial rate slows. This happens despite prolongation of the PR interval.

Respiratory *Interstitial pneumonitis* with acute respiratory failure was attributed to flecainide in a 59-year-old man with congenital heart disease related to the LEOPARD syndrome, in which there are multiple freckles (Lentigines), Electrocardiographic abnormalities, Ocular hypertelorism, Pulmonic stenosis, Abnormalities of the genitalia, Retarded growth, and sensorineural Deafness (94[A]). A CT scan showed diffuse interstitial injury characterized by thickening of the intralobular septa, with areas of ground-glass pattern. Flecainide was withdrawn and within 2 weeks the changes on CT scan had almost completely disappeared.

Fetotoxicity A pregnant woman was given digoxin and flecainide at 29 weeks of gestation for fetal tachycardia and hydrops fetalis (95[A]). The child was delivered spontaneously at 33 weeks and had mild respiratory distress. His electrocardiogram showed bifid P waves, a prolonged PR interval, deep wide Q waves, and raised ST segments. The QT interval was not prolonged. The serum digoxin concentration in the neonate was 1.2 mg/ml and the authors attributed the electrocardiographic abnormalities to the maternal use of flecainide. The abnormalities resolved within 3 weeks of birth, despite continued digoxin therapy.

Lidocaine (lignocaine) *(SED-14, 546; SEDA-22, 208; SEDA-23, 200; SEDA-24, 212)*

Intravenous lidocaine has been used to treat severe chronic daily headache in 19 patients (median age 37 years, three men) (96[c]). There were adverse effects during four infusions of lidocaine: hyperkalemia (6.4 mmol/l), which did not resolve after withdrawal of lidocaine; transient *hypotension* (75/50 mmHg), which was attributed to concomitant droperidol; an unspecified *abnormality of cardiac rhythm* and on another occasion a transient *bradycardia*; and *chest pain* with a normal electrocardiogram, fever, and intractable nausea. The study was neither randomized nor placebo-controlled, and in no case was the adverse event strongly associated with the administration of lidocaine.

In a double-blind, placebo-controlled study of the use of intravenous lidocaine for neuropathic pain, 16 patients were given 5 ml/kg intravenously over 30 minutes (97[C]). Lidocaine was better than placebo in relieving pain. The major adverse effect was *lightheadedness*, which occurred in seven patients given lidocaine and none given saline. Other adverse effects included *somnolence*, *nausea* and *vomiting*, *dysarthria or garbled speech*, *blurred vision*, and *malaise*. In two patients the rate of infusion had to be reduced because of adverse effects.

Cardiovascular Lidocaine does not usually cause *conduction disturbances*, but recently two cases have been reported in the presence of hyperkalemia (98[A]).

- A 57-year-old man with a wide-complex tachycardia was given lidocaine 100 mg intravenously and immediately became asystolic. Resuscitation was unsuccessful.
- A 31-year-old woman had a cardiac arrest and was resuscitated to a wide-complex tachycardia, which was treated with intravenous lidocaine 100 mg. She immediately became asystolic but responded to calcium chloride.

In both cases there was severe hyperkalemia, and the authors suggested that hyperkalemia-induced resting membrane depolarization had increased the number of inactivated sodium channels, thus increasing the binding of lidocaine and potentiating its effects.

Liver *Liver damage* due to lidocaine has rarely been reported. However, severe liver damage has recently been reported shortly after the withdrawal of mexiletine 300 mg/day and the introduction of lidocaine 1000 mg/day, although lidocaine in the same dose had been used during the previous week (99[A]). The lidocaine was withdrawn and the liver enzymes normalized after treatment with prednisolone.

Risk factors A low dose of lidocaine (1 mg/kg intravenously) has been used to test liver function, by measuring the extent of production of one of its major metabolites, monoethylglycinexylidide. When 200 patients with different liver diseases and 23 organ donors were given lidocaine for this test, 38 had transient adverse effects, such as *dizziness and paresthesia of the tongue*; these effects resolved spontaneously within a few minutes (100[C]). In another study of 30 patients with cirrhosis and 20 with chronic hepatitis, lidocaine (mean dose about 75 mg) did not affect performance on a simple psychometric test, based on the Symbol Digit Test (101[C]). Adverse effects of lidocaine were more common in patients with chronic hepatitis than in those with cirrhosis; they included *tinnitus*, *disorientation*, *paresthesia*, *a metallic taste*, and *vertigo*. Of these, tinnitus was the most common (22 patients) followed by disorientation (13 patients), which was the only adverse effect to occur more commonly in patients with cirrhosis.

Mexiletine *(SED-14, 547; SEDA-22, 208; SEDA-23, 200; SEDA-24, 212)*

In addition to its use as an antidysrhythmic drug, mexiletine has also been used in the treatment of various types of neuropathic pain and dystonias (50[r], 102[c]). The adverse effects in these circumstances have been reported (103[c], 104[C], 105[C]) and reviewed (106[r]).

In an open-label study of the antidystonic effect of mexiletine (200 mg/day increasing to a maximum of 800 mg/day) in spasmodic torticollis in six patients, mexiletine produced significant improvement and there were no adverse effects in five of the six patients; in the other patient *dizziness* occurred at the highest dose and required a reduction in dosage (103[c]).

In a double-blind, placebo-controlled, cross-over study of the use of mexiletine in 20 patients with neuropathic pain with prominent allodynia the dosage was titrated to a maximum of 900 mg/day or until dose-limiting adverse effects occurred. Mexiletine had little beneficial effect and the two most common adverse effects were *nausea* and *sedation* (104[C]). Other adverse effects that occurred in one or two patients each included *insomnia*, *trismus*, *headache*, *agitation*, *nightmares*, and *tremor*.

In a double-blind, placebo-controlled, cross-over study in 12 healthy volunteers mexiletine, in a dose that was titrated to a maximum of 1350 mg/day or until there were dose-limiting adverse effects, was used to alleviate capsaicin-induced allodynia and hyperalgesia (105[C]). Mexiletine had no significant effect on any of the major measures of pain or neurosensory thresholds after intradermal capsaicin; however, it did reduce the flare response. All 12 subjects had dose-limiting adverse effects and the mean maximum tolerable daily dose was 850 mg. The adverse effects included *nausea*, *lightheadedness*, *muscle twitching and weakness*, *blurred vision*, *headache*, *tremor*, *difficulty in concentrating*, *dysphoria*, *sedation*, *pruritus*, and *rash*. These adverse effects occurred at an average daily dose of 993 mg. The three most common adverse effects were nausea, dizziness, and tremor in 10, nine, and four of the subjects respectively.

In previous studies in patients with diabetic peripheral neuropathy, adverse effects included *nausea*, *hiccups*, *tremor*, *headache*, *weakness and dizziness*, *tachycardia*, and *allergic reactions* (106[r]).

The adverse effects reported in all of these studies are typical of those caused by mexiletine when it is used as an antidysrhythmic drug, i.e. mostly gastrointestinal and central nervous system adverse effects (SED-14, 547).

Skin Mexiletine rarely causes skin reactions, but another case of *exfoliative dermatitis* has recently been reported in a 68-year-old man who had taken mexiletine and diltiazem for 3 weeks (107[A]). Patch tests with 1, 10, and 30% mexiletine and diltiazem in petrolatum were positive, but a lymphocyte stimulation test was negative.

There has also been a report of three cases of drug eruption in a 56-year-old woman, a 50-year-old man, and a 66-year-old woman, who developed disseminated maculopapular eruptions with high fever after oral mexiletine (108[A]). In all cases the liver transaminase activities were raised and there was an eosinophilia with atypical lymphocytes; in two cases there was a lymphadenopathy. In all cases patch tests were positive.

In addition to these cases, 37 cases of drug eruption due to mexiletine have been reported in Japan, with several common clinical features (107^A). The interval between initial drug therapy and the start of the eruption was relatively long (48–88 days); there was a high proportion of positive patch tests (86–97%) but a low incidence of positive lymphocyte stimulation tests (23–27%); there were frequent systemic symptoms, such as *fever* (93–94%) and *liver dysfunction* (43–78%); finally, some patients had *multiple drug eruptions*.

Drug overdose *Status epilepticus* was the chief presenting feature in a 17-year-old boy who took an unspecified amount of mexiletine (109^A). The seizures responded to intravenous diazepam and phenytoin, but he also had agitation and hallucinations, which took 24 hours to abate. A urine specimen was positive for both benzodiazepines and amphetamines, but this was subsequently found to be a false positive result, because of the presence of large amounts of mexiletine, confirmed by thin-layer chromatography. The serum mexiletine concentration was 44 μmol/l, the usual target range being about 4–11 μmol/l.

Drug interactions Mexiletine and *propafenone* are metabolized by the same enzymes, CYP2D6, CYP1A2, and CYP3A4. In 15 healthy volunteers, eight of whom were extensive metabolizers of CYP2D6, coadministration of oral mexiletine 100 mg bd on days 1–8, oral propafenone 1 mg bd on days 5–12 significantly reduced the clearance of R^- mexiletine from 41 to 28 l/hour and of S^+ mexiletine from 43 to 29 l/hour in the extensive metabolizers (110^C). The new values were no different from the clearance values in the poor metabolizers. Propafenone also reduced the partial metabolic clearances of mexiletine to hydroxymethylmexiletine, parahydroxymexiletine, and metahydroxymexiletine by about 70% in the extensive metabolizers. Propafenone had no effect on the kinetics of mexiletine in the poor metabolizers. There was no change in the electrocardiogram during this interaction. Smokers had higher clearance rates than non-smokers but the effects of propafenone were similar in the two groups. In contrast, mexiletine had little effect on the disposition of propafenone. The authors proposed that these effects could explain at least in part the increased efficacy that sometimes occurs when mexiletine and propafenone are combined in patients in whom a single drug was not effective. They also recommended that the dosages of the drugs should be titrated slowly when they are used together, in order to reduce the risk of adverse effects.

Propafenone *(SED-14, 551; SEDA-22, 209; SEDA-23, 202; SEDA-24, 214)*

Propafenone has often been used to treat atrial fibrillation (SEDA-23, 202), and this has been the subject of another recent randomized, double-blind, placebo-controlled study in 55 patients (111^C). The dose of propafenone was chosen according to bodyweight: 450 mg, 600 mg, and 750 mg for those weighing 50–64 kg, 65–80 kg, and over 80 kg respectively. Propafenone converted atrial fibrillation to sinus rhythm significantly more quickly than placebo, and most patients given propafenone had converted by 6 hours. However, by 24 hours there was no significant difference between the two groups. Four patients had *hypotension* after propafenone, in three cases transiently. The patient with sustained hypotension had poor left ventricular systolic function, but it responded promptly to the administration of fluids and electrical cardioversion. In one patient with transient hypotension there was a brief episode of sinus bradycardia and in another an isolated sinus pause.

In another study quinidine was added to propafenone with the intention of inhibiting propafenone metabolism via CYP2D6 (112^C). Of 60 patients with paroxysmal atrial fibrillation given propafenone 300–450 mg/day for 8 weeks there were 19 refractory cases, who were then randomized double-blind to receive either a higher dose of propafenone (450–675 mg/day) or the standard dose of propafenone with extra low-dose quinidine (150 mg/day), each for 8 weeks, with subsequent cross-over to the alternative. Patients who even then were not adequately controlled were given the standard dose of propafenone plus a standard dose of quinidine (600 mg/day) for a further 8 weeks. The plasma propafenone concentrations during the four phases were as follows:

- standard-dose propafenone alone 128 ng/ml;
- standard-dose propafenone plus low-dose quinidine 259 ng/ml;

- high-dose propafenone alone 336 ng/ml;
- standard-dose propafenone plus standard-dose quinidine 490 ng/ml.

The beneficial effects were related to these plasma concentrations, as were the time to the first bout of atrial fibrillation, the frequency of bouts of atrial fibrillation, and the time between episodes. However, when atrial fibrillation occurred there was no difference in the ventricular rate in the different groups. Adverse effects necessitated drug withdrawal in four patients; one had heart failure and two had gastrointestinal symptoms. These effects were not dose-related, although there were too few occurrences for a definitive conclusion. The authors suggested that this stepwise approach, with increasing doses of propafenone and increasing doses of quinidine could be beneficial in the treatment of paroxysmal atrial fibrillation.

Cardiovascular There have been two reports of *wide-complex tachycardias* in elderly patients (a 74-year-old man and an 80-year-old woman) who had taken propafenone for atrial fibrillation (93[A]). In the first case the dysrhythmia was due to atrial flutter with 1:1 conduction. Although drugs of class IC, such as propafenone, can slow atrial and atrioventricular nodal conduction in patients with atrial fibrillation or atrial flutter, they do not alter the refractoriness of the atrioventricular node, and this allows 1:1 atrioventricular conduction as the atrial rate slows. This happens despite prolongation of the PR interval.

Nervous system Propafenone often causes mild central nervous system adverse effects (SEDA-20, 179). There has now been a report of three cases of ataxia in patients taking propafenone (113[A]).

An 80-year-old man taking propafenone 150 mg tds for paroxysmal atrial fibrillation developed progressive generalized ataxia and weakness 4 days after starting treatment. He had a bilateral symmetrical ataxia, unclear speech, impairment of gait, altered hand coordination, and tremor. The ataxia resolved completely within 3 days of withdrawal.

A 73-year-old woman taking propafenone 150 mg tds for paroxysmal atrial tachycardia underwent cardioversion during an attack, and the dose of propafenone was increased to 300 mg tds. After 5 days she developed severe ataxia and progressive weakness. The ataxia was symmetrical and there was severe impairment of gait, altered hand coordination, and tremor. The dose of propafenone was reduced to 600 mg/day and the ataxia resolved completely within 6 days. A year later, when the dose of propafenone was increased to 900 mg/day, progressive ataxia again developed after 2 days and became severe within 1 week. Propafenone was withdrawn and the ataxia resolved within a few days.

An 85-year-old woman took propafenone 150 mg tds for paroxysmal atrial fibrillation and 2 months later developed a progressive ataxia and recurrent falls. The ataxia was symmetrical and there was altered hand coordination, impairment of gait, and tremor. The propafenone was withdrawn and the ataxia resolved completely within 4 days.

Quinidine *(SED-14, 552; SEDA-22, 209; SEDA-23, 202; SEDA-24, 214)*

Cardiovascular Quinidine commonly causes *cardiac dysrhythmias* by prolongation of the QT interval. It has recently been reported that this effect is greater in women than in men at equivalent serum concentrations (114[c]). In 12 men and 12 women who received a single intravenous dose of quinidine (4 mg/kg) in a randomized, single-blind, placebo-controlled, cross-over study, total and unbound serum concentrations of quinidine and 3-hydroxyquinidine were measured and QT intervals were corrected for differences in heart rate using Bazett's method. The QT interval at baseline was longer in women than in men (407 vs 395 ms). The slope of the relation between the serum concentration of quinidine and the change in the QT_c interval from baseline was 44% greater in the women than in the men. However, there were no significant differences between the men and the women in the disposition of quinidine, apart from a small reduction in the unbound fraction of 3-hydroxyquinidine in the men (0.47 vs 0.53). The authors proposed that estrogens and androgens differentially affect the expression and activity of potassium channels in the heart, and that a lower density of potassium channels could contribute to a larger effect of quinidine in the women. They suggested that women are at greater risk of quinidine-induced cardiac dysrhythmias and that altering dosages according to weight would not correct for this difference. They also pointed to the fact that in the SWORD study the risk of excess mortality in those taking d-sotalol was greater in the women than in the men.

Gastrointestinal The quinidine derivative

hydroquinidine had some beneficial effects in 10 patients with myotonic dystrophy with slow saccadic eye movements, apathy, and hypersomnia (115^C, 116^C). However, two patients had *nausea* and *epigastric pain* and withdrew while taking the active treatment. Although there were no cases of cardiac abnormalities, the authors raised the concern that in patients with myotonic dystrophy, who have a high frequency of cardiac disturbances, the risk of cardiac dysrhythmias with quinidine derivatives may be too high to take.

REFERENCES

1. Haji SA, Movahed A. Update on digoxin therapy in congestive heart failure. Am Fam Phys 2000; 62: 409–16.
2. Gibbs CR, Davies MK, Lip GYH. ABC of heart failure. Management: digoxin and other inotropes, beta-blockers, and antiarrhythmic and antithrombotic treatment. Br Med J 2000; 320: 495–8.
3. Guglielminotti J, Tremey B, Maury E, Alzieu M, Offenstadt G. Fatal non-occlusive mesenteric infarction following digoxin intoxication. Intensive Care Med 2000; 26: 829.
4. Fauchier L, Babuty D, Cosnay P, Fauchier JP. Digoxin and mortality in idiopathic dilated cardiomyopathy. Eur Heart J 2000; 21: 858–9.
5. Heninger MM. Commonly encountered prescription medications in medical-legal death investigation: a guide for death investigators and medical examiners. Am J Forensic Med Pathol 2000; 21: 287–99.
6. Chyka PA. How many deaths occur annually from adverse drug reactions in the United States? Am J Med 2000; 109: 122–30.
7. Miura T, Kojima R, Sugiura Y, Mizutani M, Takatsu F, Suzuki Y. Effect of aging on the incidence of digoxin toxicity. Ann Pharmacother 2000; 34: 427–32.
8. Roever C, Ferrante J, Gonzalez EC, Pal N, Roetzheim RG. Comparing the toxicity of digoxin and digitoxin in a geriatric population: should an old drug be rediscovered? South Med J 2000; 93: 199–202.
9. Aronson JK. [Book review: Handbook of renal-independent cardiac glycosides: pharmacology and clinical pharmacology, by N Rietbrock and BG Woodcock]. Lancet 1989; 2: 1130–1.
10. Lacassie E, Marquet P, Martin-Dupont S, Gaulier J-M, Lachâtre G. A non-fatal case of intoxication with foxglove, documented by means of liquid chromatography–electrospray–mass spectrometry. J Forensic Sci 2000; 45: 1154–8.
11. Brodell RT, Elewski B. Antifungal drug interactions. Postgrad Med 2000; 107: 41–3.
12. Mochizuki M, Murase S, Takahashi K, Shimada S, Kume H, Iizuka T, Fukuda M. Serum intraconazole and hydroxyitraconazole concentrations and interaction with digoxin in a case of chronic hypertrophic pachymeningitis caused by *Aspergillus flavus*. Jpn J Med Mycol 2000; 41: 33–9.
13. Westphal K, Weinbrenner A, Giessmann T, Stuhr M, Franke G, Zschiesche M, Oertel R, Terhaag B, Kroemer HK, Siegmund W. Oral bioavailability of digoxin is enhanced by talinolol: evidence for involvement of intestinal P-glycoprotein. Clin Pharmacol Ther 2000; 68: 6–12.
14. Retzow A, Althaus M, De Mey C, Mazur D, Vens-Cappell B. Study on the interaction of the dopamine agonist alpha-dihydroergocryptine with the pharmacokinetics of digoxin. Arzneim-Forsch Drug Res 2000; 50: 591–6.
15. Ten Eick AP, Sallee D, Preminger T, Weiss A, Reed MD. Possible drug interaction between digoxin and azithromycin in a young child. Clin Drug Invest 2000; 20: 61–4.
16. Zhou H, Walter YH, Smith H, Devineni D, McLeod JF. Nateglinide, a new mealtime glucose regulator. Lack of pharmacokinetic interaction with digoxin in healthy volunteers. Clin Drug Invest 2000; 19: 465–71.
17. Hatorp V. Thomsen MS. Drug interaction studies with repaglinide: repaglinide on digoxin or theophylline pharmacokinetics and cimetidine on repaglinide pharmacokinetics. J Clin Pharmacol 2000; 40: 184–92.
18. Homma M, Takeda M, Yamamoto Y, Suga H, Horiuchi M, Satoh S, Kohda Y. Consultation and survey for drug interaction in outpatients taking the medicines potentially interact with St John's wort. Yakugaku Zasshi 2000; 120: 1435–40.
19. Kusus M, Stapleton DD, Lertora JJL, Simon EE, Dreisbach AW. Rhabdomyolysis and acute renal failure in a cardiac transplant recipient due to multiple drug interactions. Am J Med Sci 2000; 320: 394–7.
20. Stangier J, Su C-APF, Hendriks MGC, Van Lier JJ, Sollie FAE, Oosterhuis B, Jonkman JHG. The effect of telmisartan on the steady-state pharmacokinetics of digoxin in healthy male volunteers. J Clin Pharmacol 2000; 40: 1373–9.
21. Sanchez Garcia P, Paty I, Leister CA, Guerra P, Frías J, Garcia Pérez LE, Darwish M. Effect of zaleplon on digoxin pharmacokinetics and pharmacodynamics. Am J Health-Syst Pharm 2000; 57: 2267–70.
22. Abad-Santos F, Carcas AJ, Ibáñez C, Frías J. Digoxin level and clinical manifestations as determinants in the diagnosis of digoxin toxicity. Ther Drug Monit 2000; 22: 163–8.

23. Lapostolle F, Adnet F, Baud F, Lapandry C. Intoxications digitaliques: l'antidote existe. Rev Prat Méd Gén 2000; 14: 345–7.
24. González Andrés VL. Revisión sistemática sobre la efectividad e indicaciones de los anticuerpos antidigoxina en la intoxicación digitálica. Rev Esp Cardiol 2000: 53: 49–58.
25. López-Gómez D, Valdovinos P, Comin-Colet J, Esteve F, Sabaté X, Esplugas E. Intoxicación grave por digoxina. Utilización exitosa del tratamiento clásico. Rev Esp Cardiol 2000; 53: 471–2.
26. Roberge RJ, Sorensen T. Congestive heart failure and toxic digoxin levels: role of cholestyramine. Vet Hum Toxicol 2000; 42: 172–3.
27. Zdunek M, Mitra A, Mokrzycki MH. Plasma exchange for the removal of digoxin-specific antibody fragments in renal failure: Timing is important for maximizing clearance. Am J Kidney Dis 2000; 36: 177–83.
28. Patnode NM, Gandhi PJ. Drug-induced thrombocytopenia in the coronary care unit. J Thromb Thrombolysis 2000; 10: 155–67.
29. Lowes BD, Higginbotham M, Petrovich L, DeWood MA, Greenberg M A, Rahko PS, Dec GW, LeJemtel TH, Roden RL, Schleman MM, Robertson AD, Gorczynski RJ, Bristow MR, for the Enoximone Study Group. Low-dose enoximone improves exercise capacity in chronic heart failure. J Am Coll Cardiol 2000; 36: 501–8.
30. Thackray S, Witte K, Clark AL, Cleland JGF. Clinical trials update: OPTIME-CHF, PRAISE–2, ALL-HAT. Eur J Heart Fail 2000; 2: 209–12.
31. Taniguchi T, Shibata K, Saito S, Matsumoto H, Okeie K. Pharmacokinetics of milrinone in patients with congestive heart failure during continuous venovenous hemofiltration. Int Care Med 2000; 26: 1089–93.
32. Gold J, Cullinane S, Chen J, Seo S, Oz MC, Oliver JA, Landry DW. Vasopressin in the treatment of milrinone-induced hypotension in severe heart failure. Am J Cardiol 2000; 85: 506–8.
33. Gold JA, Cullinane S, Chen J, Oz MC, Oliver JA, Landry DW. Vasopressin as an alternative to norepinephrine in the treatment of milrinone-induced hypotension. Crit Care Med 2000; 28: 249–52.
34. Patnaik A, Rowinsky EK, Tammara BK, Hidalgo M, Drengler RL, Garner AM, Siu LL, Hammond LA, Felton SA, Mallikaarjun S, Von Hoff DD, Eckhardt SG. Phase I and pharmacokinetic study of the differentiating agent vesnarinone in combination with gemcitabine in patients with advanced cancer. J Clin Oncol 2000; 18: 3974–85.
35. Lip GYH, Kamath S. Adverse reactions of drugs used to treat arrhythmia. Adverse Drug React Bull 2000; 201: 767–70.
36. Wooten JM, Earnest J, Reyes J. Review of common adverse effects of selected antiarrhythmic drugs. Crit Care Nurs Q 2000; 22: 23–38.
37. Chaudhry GM, Haffajee CI. Antiarrhythmic agents and proarrhythmia. Crit Care Med 2000; 28 Suppl: N158–64.
38. Witchel HJ, Hancox JC. Familial and acquired long QT syndrome and the cardiac rapid delayed rectifier potassium current. Clin Exp Pharmacol Physiol 2000; 27: 753–66.
39. Brembilla-Perrot B, Houriez P, Claudon O, Yassine M, Suty-Selton C, Vancon AC, Abo El Makarem Y, Courtelour JM. Les effets proarythmiques supraventricularires des antiarythmiques de classe IC sont-ils prévenus par l'association avec des bêtabloquants? Ann Cardiol Angeiol 2000; 49: 439–43.
40. Trujillo TC, Nolan PE. Antiarrhythmic agents: drug interactions of clinical significance. Drug Saf 2000; 23: 509–32.
41. Thomas GS, Prill NV, Majmundar H, Fabrizi RR, Thomas JJ, Hayashida C, Kothapalli S, Payne JL, Payne MM, Miyamoto MI. Treadmill exercise during adenosine infusion is safe, results in fewer adverse reactions, and improves myocardial perfusion image quality. J Nucl Cardiol 2000; 7: 439–46.
42. Elliott MD, Holly TA, Leonard SM, Hendel RC. Impact of an abbreviated adenosine protocol incorporating adjunctive treadmill exercise on adverse effects and image quality in patients undergoing stress myocardial perfusion imaging. J Nucl Cardiol 2000; 7: 584–9.
43. Christopher M, Key CB, Persse DE. Refractory asystole and death following the prehospital administration of adenosine. Prehosp Emerg Care 2000; 4: 196–8.
44. Israel C, Klingenheben T, Grönefeld G, Hohnloser SH. Adenosine-induced atrial fibrillation. J Cardiovasc Electrophysiol 2000; 11: 825.
45. Kaplan IV, Kaplan AV, Fisher JD. Adenosine induced atrial fibrillation precipitating polymorphic ventricular tachycardia. PACE Pacing Clin Electrophysiol 2000; 23: 140–1.
46. Misra D, Van Tosh A, Schweitzer P. Adenosine induced monomorphic ventricular tachycardia. PACE Pacing Clin Electrophysiol 2000; 23: 1044–6.
47. Jeremias A, Whitbourn RJ, Filardo SD, Fitzgerald PJ, Cohen DJ, Tuzcu EM, Anderson WD, Abizaid AA, Mintz GS, Yeung AC, Kern MJ, Yock PG. Adequacy of intracoronary versus intravenous adenosine-induced maximal coronary hyperemia for fractional flow reserve measurements. Am Heart J 2000; 140: 651–7.
48. Belfrage M, Segerdahl M, Arner S, Sollevi A. The safety and efficacy of intrathecal adenosine in patients with chronic neuropathic pain. Anesth Analg 1999; 89: 136–42.
49. Sjolund KF, Segerdahl M, Sollevi A. Adenosine reduces secondary hyperalgesia in two human models of cutaneous inflammatory pain. Anesth Analg 1999; 88: 605–10.
50. Kopf A, Ruf W. Novel drugs for neuropathic pain. Curr Opin Anaesthesiol 2000; 13: 577–83.
51. Bermúdez EP, García-Alberola A, Martínez Sánchez J, Sánchez Munoz JJ, Valdés Chávarri

MV. Spontaneous sustained monomorphic ventricular tachycardia after administration of ajmaline in a patient with Brugada syndrome. PACE Pacing Clin Electrophysiol 2000; 23: 407–9.
52. Kochiadakis GE, Igoumenidis NE, Marketou ME, Kaleboubas MD, Simantirakis EN, Vardas PE. Low dose amiodarone and sotalol in the treatment of recurrent, symptomatic atrial fibrillation: a comparative, placebo controlled study. Heart 2000; 84: 251–7.
53. Vardas PE, Kochiadakis GE, Igoumenidis NE, Tsatsakis AM, Simantirakis EN, Chlouverakis GI. Amiodarone as a first-choice drug for restoring sinus rhythm in patients with atrial fibrillation: a randomized, controlled study. Chest 2000; 117: 1538–45.
54. Hofmann R, Wimmer G, Leisch F. Intravenous amiodarone bolus immediately controls heart rate in patients with atrial fibrillation accompanied by severe congestive heart failure. Heart 2000; 84: 635.
55. Peuhkurinen K, Niemelä M, Ylitalo A, Linnaluoto M, Lilja M, Juvonen J. Effectiveness of amiodarone as a single oral dose for recent-onset atrial fibrillation. Am J Cardiol 2000; 85: 462–5.
56. Martínez-Marcos FJ, Garcia-Garmendia JL, Ortega-Carpio A, Fernández-Gómez JM, Santos JM, Camacho C. Comparison of intravenous flecainide, propafenone, and amiodarone for conversion of acute atrial fibrillation to sinus rhythm. Am J Cardiol 2000; 86: 950–3.
57. Treggiari-Venzi MM, Waeber J-L, Perneger TV, Suter PM, Adamec R, Romand J-A. Intravenous amiodarone or magnesium sulphate is not cost-beneficial prophylaxis for atrial fibrillation after coronary artery bypass surgery. Br J Anaesth 2000; 85: 690–5.
58. Roy D, Talajic M, Dorian P, Connolly S, Eisenberg MJ, Green M, Kus T, Lambert J, Dubuc M, Gagné P, Nattel S, Thibault B, for the Canadian Trial of Atrial Fibrillation investigators. Amiodarone to prevent recurrence of atrial fibrillation. New Engl J Med 2000; 342: 913–20.
59. Kochiadakis GE, Marketou ME, Igoumenidis NE, Chrysostomakis SI, Mavrakis HE, Kaleboubas MD, Vardas PE. Amiodarone, sotalol, or propafenone in atrial fibrillation: which is preferred to maintain normal sinus rhythm? PACE Pacing Clin Electrophysiol 2000; 23: 1883–7.
60. Natale A, Newby K H, Pisanó E, Leonelli F, Fanelli R, Potenza D, Beheiry S, Tomassoni G. Prospective randomized comparison of antiarrhythmic therapy versus first-line radiofrequency ablation in patients with atrial flutter. J Am Coll Cardiol 2000; 35: 1898–904.
61. Maury P, Zimmermann M, Metzger J, Reynard C, Dorsaz P-A, Adamec R. Amiodarone therapy for sustained ventricular tachycardia after myocardial infarction: long-term follow-up, risk assessment and predictive value of programmed ventricular stimulation. Int J Cardiol 2000; 76: 199–210.
62. Kuck K-H, Cappato R, Siebels J, Rüppel R, for the CASH investigators. Randomized comparison of antiarrhythmic drug therapy with implantable defibrillators in patients resuscitated from cardiac arrest. The Cardiac Arrest Study Hamburg (CASH). Circulation 2000; 102: 748–54.
63. Nägele H, Bohlmann M, Eck U, Petersen B, Rödiger W. Combination therapy with carvedilol and amiodarone in patients with severe heart failure. Eur J Heart Fail 2000; 2: 71–9.
64. Hammerman H. Kapeliovich M. Drug-related cardiac iatrogenic illness as the cause for admission to the intensive cardiac care unit. Isr Med Assoc J 2000; 2: 577–9.
65. Reithmann C, Hoffmann E, Spitzlberger G, Dorwarth U, Gerth A, Remp T, Steinbeck G. Catheter ablation of atrial flutter due to amiodarone therapy for paroxysmal atrial fibrillation. Eur Heart J 2000; 21: 565–72.
66. Yap S-C, Hoomtje T, Sreeram N. Polymorphic ventricular tachycardia after use of intravenous amiodarone for postoperative junctional ectopic tachycardia. Int J Cardiol 2000; 76: 245–7.
67. Raviña T, Gutierrez J. Amiodarone-induced AV block and ventricular standstill: a forme fruste of an idiopathic long QT syndrome. Int J Cardiol 2000; 75: 105–8.
68. Kagawa FT, Kirsch CM, Jensen WA, Wehner JH. A 77-year-old man with bilateral pulmonary infiltrates and shortness of breath. Semin Respir Infect 2000; 15: 90–2.
69. Burns KEA, Piliotis E, Garcia BM, Ferguson KA. Amiodarone pulmonary, neuromuscular and ophthalmological toxicity. Can Respir J 2000; 7: 193–7.
70. Endoh Y, Hanai R, Uto K, Uno M, Nagashima H, Takizawa T, Narimatsu A, Ohnishi S, Kasanuki H. Diagnostic usefulness of KL-6 measurements in patients with pulmonary complications after administration of amiodarone. J Cardiol 2000; 35: 121–7.
71. Endoh Y, Hanai R, Uto K, Uno M, Nagashima H, Narimatsu A, Takizawa T, Onishi S, Kasanuki H. KL-6 as a potential new marker for amiodarone-induced pulmonary toxicity. Am J Cardiol 2000; 86: 229–31.
72. Eryilmaz T, Atilla H, Batioglu F, Günalp I. Amiodarone-related optic neuropathy. Jpn J Ophthalmol 2000; 44: 565–8.
73. Speicher MA, Goldman MH, Chrousos GA. Amiodarone optic neuropathy without disc edema. J Neuro-Ophthalmol 2000; 20: 171–2.
74. Findlay PF, Seymour DG. Hyperthyroidism in an elderly patient. Postgrad Med J 2000; 76: 173–5.
75. Cattaneo F. Type II amiodarone-induced thyrotoxicosis and concomitant papillary cancer of the thyroid. Eur J Endocrinol 2000; 143: 823–4.
76. Claxton S, Sinha SN, Donovan S, Greenaway TM, Hoffman L, Loughhead M, Burgess JR. Refractory amiodarone-associated thyrotoxicosis: an indication for thyroidectomy. Aust NZ J Surg 2000; 70: 174–8.

77. Boutros NYZ, Dilly S, Bevan DH. Amiodarone-induced bone marrow granulomas. Clin Lab Haematol 2000; 22: 167–70.
78. Jain D, Bowlus CL, Anderson JM, Robert ME. Granular cells as a marker of early amiodarone hepatotoxicity. J Clin Gastroenterol 2000; 31: 241–3.
79. Rogers KC, Wolfe DA. Amiodarone-induced blue-gray syndrome. Ann Pharmacother 2000; 34: 1075.
80. Burches E, Garcia-Verdegay F, Ferrer M, Pelaez A. Amiodarone-induced angioedema. Allergy Eur J Allergy Clin Immunol 2000; 55: 1199–200.
81. Elizari MV, Martinez JM, Belziti C, Ciruzzi M, Pérez De La Hoz R, Sinisi A, Carbajales J, Scapin O, Garguichevich J, Girotti L, Cagide A, on behalf of the GEMICA study investigators, GEMA Group, Buenos Aires, Argentina. Morbidity and mortality following early administration of amiodarone in acute myocardial infarction. Eur Heart J 2000; 21: 198–205.
82. Scheinman MM. Amiodarone after acute myocardial infarction. Eur Heart J 2000; 21: 177–8.
83. Ahle GB, Blum AL, Martinek J, Oneta CM, Dorta G. Cushing's syndrome in an 81-year-old patient treated with budesonide and amiodarone. Eur J Gastroenterol Hepatol 2000; 12: 1041–2.
84. Viallon A, Laporte-Simitsidis S, Pouzet V, Venet C, Tardy B, Zéni F, Bertrand JC. Bépridil: intérêt du dosage sérique dans la surveillance du traitement. Presse Méd 2000; 29: 645–7.
85. Devos D, Defebvre L, Destée A, Caron J. Choreic movements induced by cibenzoline: an Ic class antiarrhythmic effect? Mov Disord 2000; 15: 1030–1.
86. Takada M, Fujita S, Katayama Y, Harano Y, Shibakawa M. The relationship between risk of hypoglycemia and use of cibenzoline and disopyramide. Eur J Clin Pharmacol 2000; 56: 335–42.
87. Binois F, Guiserix J, Kilian D. Hépatite aiguë au cours d'un traitement par la cibenzoline. Presse Méd 2000; 29: 703.
88. Kumagai K, Abe H, Hiraki T, Nakashima H, Oginosawa Y, Ikeda H, Nakashima Y, Imaizumi T, Saku K. Single oral administration of pilsicainide versus infusion of disopyramide for termination of paroxysmal atrial fibrillation: a multicenter trial. PACE Pacing Clin Electrophysiol 2000; 23: 1880–2.
89. Echizen H, Tanizaki M, Tatsuno J, Chiba K, Berwick T, Tani M, Gonzalez FJ, Ishizaki T. Identification of CYP3A4 as the enzyme involved in the mono-N-dealkylation of disopyramide enantiomers in humans. Drug Metab Dispos 2000; 28: 937–44.
90. Granowitz EV, Tabor KJ, Kirchhoffer JB. Potentially fatal interaction between azithromycin and disopyramide. PACE Pacing Clin Electrophysiol 2000; 23: 1433–5.
91. Morlet-Barla N, Narbonne H, Vialettes B. Hypoglycëmie grave et rëcidivante secondaire à l'interaction disopyramide–clarithromicine. Presse Mëd 2000; 29: 1351.
92. Chalvidan T, Cellarier G, Deharo JC, Colin R, Savon N, Barra N, Peyre JP, Djiane P. His–Purkinje system reentry as a proarrhythmic effect of flecainide. PACE Pacing Clin Electrophysiol 2000; 23: 530–3.
93. Mackstaller LL, Marcus FI. Rapid ventricular response due to treatment of atrial flutter or fibrillation with Class I antiarrhythmic drugs. Ann Noninvasive Electrocardiol 2000; 5: 101–4.
94. Robain A, Perchet H, Fuhrman C. Flecainide-associated pneumonitis with acute respiratory failure in a patient with the LEOPARD syndrome. Acta Cardiol 2000; 55: 45–7.
95. Trotter A, Kaestner M, Pohlandt F, Lang D. Unusual electrocardiogram findings in a preterm infant after fetal tachycardia with hydrops fetalis treated with flecainide. Pediatr Cardiol 2000; 21: 259–62.
96. Hand PJ, Stark RJ. Intravenous lignocaine infusions for severe chronic daily headache. Med J Aust 2000; 172: 157–9.
97. Attal N, Gaudë V, Brasseur L, Dupuy M, Guirimand F, Parker F, Bouhassira D. Intravenous lidocaine in central pain. A double-blind, placebo-controlled, psychophysical study. Neurology 2000; 54: 564–74.
98. McLean SA, Paul ID, Spector PS. Lidocaine-induced conduction disturbance in patients with systemic hyperkalemia. Ann Emerg Med 2000; 36: 615–18.
99. Kakinoki K, Tachibana Y, Yonejima H, Ogino H, Satomura Y, Unoura M. A case of mexiletine and lidocaine induced severe liver injury. Acta Hepatol Jpn 2000; 41: 812–16.
100. Ercolani G, Grazi GL, Callivà R, Pierangeli F, Cescon M, Cavallari A, Mazziotti A. The lidocaine (MEGX) test as an index of hepatic function: its clinical usefulness in liver surgery. Surgery 2000; 127: 464–71.
101. Botta F, Giannini E, Fasoli A, Romagnoli P, Risso D, Testa R. The monoethylglycinexylidide test does not impair psychometric performance in patients with chronic hepatitis or cirrhosis. Ther Drug Monit 2000; 22: 371–4.
102. Sloan P, Basta M, Storey P, Von Gunten C. Mexiletine as an adjuvant analgesic for the management of neuropathic cancer pain. Anesth Analg 1999; 89: 760–1.
103. Lucetti C, Nuti A, Gambaccini G, Bernardini S, Brotini S, Manca ML, Bonuccelli U. Mexiletine in the treatment of torticollis and generalized dystonia. Clin Neuropharmacol 2000; 23: 186–9.
104. Wallace MS, Magnuson S, Ridgeway B. Efficacy of oral mexiletine for neuropathic pain with allodynia: a double-blind, placebo-controlled, crossover study. Reg Anesth Pain Med 2000; 25: 459–67.
105. Ando K, Wallace MS, Braun J, Schulteis G. Effect of oral mexiletine on capsaicin-induced allodynia and hyperalgesia: a double-blind, placebo-controlled, crossover study. Reg Anesth Pain Med 2000; 25: 468–74.

106. Nabulsi LH, McLendon BM, Vondracek TG. Mexiletine for diabetic peripheral neuropathy. J Pharm Technol 2000; 16: 8–11.
107. Umebayashi Y. Drug eruption due to mexiletine and diltiazem. Nishinihon J Dermatol 2000; 62: 80–2.
108. Kayaba M, Tanaka T, Misago N, Narisawa Y. Three cases of hypersensitivity syndrome due to mexiletine hydrochloride. Nishinihon J Dermatol 2000; 62: 338–42.
109. Kozer E, Verjee Z, Koren G. Misdiagnosis of a mexiletine overdose because of a nonspecific result of urinary toxicologic screening. New Engl J Med 2000; 343: 1971.
110. Labbë L, O'Hara G, Lefebvre M, Lessard E, Gilbert M, Adedoyin A, Champagne J, Hamelin B, Turgeon J. Pharmacokinetic and pharmacodynamic interaction be mexiletine and propafenone in human beings. Clin Pharmacol Ther 2000; 68: 44–57.
111. Azpitarte J, Alvarez M, Baün O, García R, Moreno E, Navarrete A, Fernández R. Using propafenone to convert recent-onset atrial fibrillation. Cardiol Rev 2000; 17: 37–43.
112. Lau C-P, Chow MSS, Tse H-F, Tang M-O, Fan C. Control of paroxysmal atrial fibrillation recurrence using combined administration of propafenone and quinidine. Am J Cardiol 2000; 86: 1327–32.
113. Odeh M, Seligmann H, Oliven A. Propafenone-induced ataxia: report of three cases. Am J Med Sci 2000; 320: 151–3.
114. Benton RE, Sale M, Flockhart DA, Woosley RL. Greater quinidine-induced QT_c interval prolongation in women. Clin Pharmacol Ther 2000; 67: 413–18.
115. Di Costanzo A, Mottola A, Toriello A, Di Iorio G, Tedeschi G, Bonavita V. Does abnormal neuronal excitability exist in myotonic dystrophy? I. Effects of the antiarrhythmic drug hydroquinidine on slow saccadic eye movements. Neurol Sci 2000; 21: 73–80.
116. Di Costanzo A, Mottola A, Toriello A, Di Iorio G, Tedeschi G, Bonavita V. Does abnormal neuronal excitability exist in myotonic dystrophy? II. Effects of the antiarrhythmic drug hydroquinidine on apathy and hypersomnia. Neurol Sci 2000; 21: 81–6.

A.P. Maggioni, M.G. Franzosi, and R. Latini

18 β-adrenoceptor antagonists and antianginal drugs

β-ADRENOCEPTOR ANTAGONISTS *(SED-14, 579; SEDA-22, 213; SEDA-23, 206; SEDA-24, 220)*

Nervous system Propranolol and gabapentin are both effective in essential tremor. Gabapentin can occasionally cause reversible *movement disorders*. A patient who developed dystonic movements after the combined use of gabapentin and propranolol has now been described (1[A]).

A 68-year-old man with a 10-year history of essential tremor was initially treated with propranolol (120 mg/day), which was only slightly effective. Propranolol was replaced by gabapentin (900 mg/day). The tremor did not improve and propranolol (80 mg/day) was added. Two days later he developed paroxysmal dystonic movements in both hands. Between episodes neurological examination was normal. When propranolol was reduced to 40 mg/day the abnormal movements progressively disappeared.

This case suggests that there is a synergistic effect between propranolol and gabapentin.

Sensory systems The effects of topical brimonidine and timolol have been compared in two trials in 926 subjects with glaucoma or ocular hypertension already using systemic β-blockers (2[C]). Concurrent systemic β-blocker therapy had no deleterious effects on ocular hypotensive efficacy and no impact on safety with topical brimonidine, but the combination of timolol and brimonidine significantly *reduced systolic and diastolic blood pressures and heart rate* compared with brimonidine alone. This observation suggests that ocular hypotensive agents other than β-blockers, such as brimonidine, may be appropriate as a first-choice therapy for glaucoma in patients concurrently taking systemic β-blockers.

A 60-year-old man with open-angle glaucoma developed an *allergic contact conjunctivitis and dermatitis* from carteolol, a topical non-cardioselective β-blocker (3[A]). He had extensive cross-reactivity to other topical β-blockers, such as timolol and levobunolol. Cross-reactivity among different β-blockers is possibly due to a common lateral aliphatic chain.

Psychological In a placebo-controlled trial of propranolol in 312 patients with diastolic hypertension, 13 tests of cognitive function were assessed at baseline, 3 months, and 12 months (4[C]). Propranolol had no significant effects on 11 of the 13 tests. Compared with placebo, patients taking propranolol had fewer correct responses at 3 months and made more errors of commission.

Drug overdose Two regional poison centers in the USA have recently reviewed 280 cases of β-blocker overdose (5[C]). All patients with symptoms developed them within 6 hours of ingestion. Four patients died as a result of overdosage. There was cardiovascular morbidity in 41 patients (15%), requiring treatment with cardioactive drugs. Propranolol, atenolol, and metoprolol were responsible for 87% of the cases and 84% of cardiovascular morbidity. β-blockers with membrane stabilizing activity (propranolol, metoprolol, labetalol, acebutolol, and pindolol) accounted for 62% of β-blocker exposures and 73% of cardiovascular morbidity. Symptomatic bradycardia (heart rate less than 60 bpm) or hypotension (systolic blood pressure less than 90 mmHg) were observed

Side Effects of Drugs, Annual 25
J.K. Aronson, ed.

in all cases classified as having cardiovascular morbidity.

β-blocker exposure was complicated by a history of at least one co-ingestant in 73% of the cases, benzodiazepines and ethanol being the most frequent. Cardioactive co-ingestants were reported in 26% of cases: calcium channel blockers, cyclic antidepressants, neuroleptic drugs, and ACE inhibitors were the most common.

Multivariate analysis showed that the only independent variable significantly associated with cardiovascular morbidity was the presence of another cardioactive drug. When patients who took another cardioactive drug were excluded, the only variable associated with cardiovascular morbidity was the ingestion of a β-blocker with membrane stabilizing activity.

Two fatal cases of acebutolol intoxication (6 and 4.0 g) have been reported (6^A). In both cases, the onset of symptoms was sudden (within 2 hours of ingestion), with diminished consciousness, PR, QRS, and QT_c prolongation, and hypotension unresponsive to inotropic drugs. In both cases there were episodes of repetitive polymorphous ventricular tachycardia.

These cases have confirmed the potential toxicity of β-blockers with membrane stabilizing activity; they predispose the patient to changes in ventricular repolarization, which can cause QT_c prolongation and serious ventricular dysrhythmias. This is generally not seen in cases of propranolol intoxication.

Fetotoxicity The adverse effects of β-adrenoceptor antagonists on the fetus have been reviewed (7^R).

β-blockers cross the placenta, and can have adverse maternal and fetal effects. Studies of β-blockers during pregnancy have generally been small, and the gestational age at the start of the study was generally 29–33 weeks, leaving substantially unanswered the possibility that treatment of more patients and/or longer treatment durations may reveal unrecognized adverse events. These observations underline the fact that the safety of β-blockers remains uncertain and that they are therefore better not given before the third trimester.

Non-cardioselective β-adrenoceptor antagonists Observations derived from uncontrolled studies have shown an association between maternal use of propranolol and intrauterine growth retardation, neonatal respiratory depression, bradycardia, hypoglycemia, and increased perinatal mortality. However, in randomized, placebo-controlled studies of metoprolol and oxprenolol, there was no evidence of effects on birthweight.

Cardioselective β-adrenoceptor antagonists There is reluctance to use atenolol in pregnancy, especially if treatment starts early. In placebo-controlled studies, birthweight was significantly lower with atenolol groups. The same was true when atenolol was compared with other non-cardioselective agents: the weight of infants born to women taking atenolol was significantly lower. When atenolol was started later there was no difference in birthweight between infants born to women treated with atenolol or other β-blockers, suggesting the relevance of the time of initiation of atenolol. Atenolol should therefore be avoided in the early stages of pregnancy and given with caution in the later stages.

NITRATE DERIVATIVES

(SED-14, 594; SEDA-22, 218; SEDA-23, 207; SEDA-24, 222)

Glyceryl trinitrate (nitroglycerin)

Surgery is the standard treatment of anal fissures, the most common and painful anal disease. Local application of glyceryl trinitrate improves symptoms by relaxing the internal anal sphincter (SEDA-24, 222). In a multicenter, randomized, placebo-controlled, double-blind study of 0.2% glyceryl trinitrate ointment in 132 patients over at least 4 weeks healing rates were similar with glyceryl trinitrate and placebo, but adverse events were more frequent in those who used glyceryl trinitrate: 34% complained of *headache* and 5.9% had *orthostatic hypotension* (8^C).

The results of this study have been confirmed and extended by another trial, in which 90 patients were randomly assigned to surgery (internal sphinterectomy) or topical glyceryl trinitrate (9^{Cr}). Surgery led to a higher rate of healing than glyceryl trinitrate, with fewer adverse events: 29% of surgical patients versus 84% of glyceryl trinitrate patients.

In conclusion, glyceryl trinitrate should not be used to treat anal fissure.

Intravenous glyceryl trinitrate (starting rate 50 μg/min uptitrated with blood pressure monitoring) for an average of 63 hours was very effective in preventing adverse ischemic events in 200 patients with unstable angina secondary to restenosis after coronary artery angioplasty, while heparin had no effect (10[Cr]). In this acute setting, complications and adverse effects were not frequent, even if there was an excess of cases with *headache* or *hypotension* with glyceryl trinitrate, never leading to premature discontinuation. This study has shown that glyceryl trinitrate is safe and effective in reducing the need for invasive procedures in these patients.

Besides its usual indications, glyceryl trinitrate has been used to prevent intravenous infusion failure because of phlebitis and extravasation, which occur in 30–60% of patients and can cause discomfort and harm, such as pulmonary embolism, septicemia, and increased mortality. Local application of glyceryl trinitrate patches has been found efficacious in several studies, recently reviewed (11[MR]); the mechanism is probably vasodilatation and increased capillary flow. Glyceryl trinitrate is safe, since it causes only *skin rashes* and transient *headache*.

Nervous system Glyceryl trinitrate can reduce cerebral blood flow, and this might explain occasional reports of impaired cognitive function and neurological disturbances in patients with coronary heart disease treated with glyceryl trinitrate. Continuous intravenous infusion of glyceryl trinitrate in 12 healthy volunteers reduced blood flow velocity in the middle cerebral artery and increased slow-wave power during electroencephalography (12[cr]). Patients with cognitive disturbances receiving glyceryl trinitrate should be carefully monitored.

Drug tolerance There is progressive attenuation of the effects of nitrates within the first 24 hours of continuous exposure. Although its causes are still poorly understood, several remedies have been proposed, including the concurrent administration of vitamin C. Three published controlled trials in 77 subjects overall have been reviewed (13[MR]). Vitamin C (3–6 g/day orally or by intravenous infusion) reduced nitrate tolerance for up to 3 days, without causing adverse reactions. However, before making definitive recommendations, studies of longer duration should be done in a larger number of patients.

Isosorbide-5-mononitrate

Variceal bleeding is a frequent and serious event in cirrhosis, and it carries an increased risk of death (SEDA-22, 218). Therapy to prevent bleeding is therefore essential in these patients. Propranolol alone has been compared with propranolol plus isosorbide-5-mononitrate in a randomized, double-blind study in 95 patients (14[C]). The combined treatment reduced the incidence of variceal bleeding compared with propranolol alone, but without any improvement in survival. Isosorbide-5-mononitrate added to propranolol appeared to be less well tolerated than propranolol alone, since seven patients had to be withdrawn from treatment because of adverse effects (four with feelings of *faintness*, two with *headache*, one with *angina-like chest pain*), compared with one with atrioventricular block taking propranolol alone.

CALCIUM CHANNEL BLOCKERS *(SED-14, 578; SEDA-22, 215; SEDA-23, 208; SEDA-24, 222)*

Liver *Hepatic damage* due to calcium channel blockers has rarely been reported.

A 69-year-old hypertensive man who had taken amlodipine for 10 months abruptly developed jaundice, choluria, raised serum bilirubin, and increased transaminases (15[Ar]). After amlodipine withdrawal he progressively recovered in a few weeks without sequelae or relapses. However, after several months he presented again with jaundice and an enlarged liver, having started to take diltiazem 5 months before. He recovered completely in a few weeks after drug withdrawal.

The authors hypothesized an idiosyncratic mechanism.

Amlodipine

Vasodilatory calcium channel blockers have been reported to improve exercise tolerance in some preliminary studies. A multicenter, randomized, placebo-controlled trial was therefore performed in 437 patients with mild to moderate heart failure to assess the effects of amlodipine 10 mg/day in addition to standard therapy (16[C]). Over 12 weeks amlodipine did not improve exercise time and did not increase the incidence of adverse events.

Mental stress is a risk factor for cardiovascular disease. In 24 patients with mild to moderate hypertension amlodipine reduced the blood pressure rise during mental stress compared with placebo, but increased plasma noradrenaline concentrations (17[C]).

Hypertension leading to cardiac dysfunction is very frequent in patients with the inherited syndrome called Ribbing's disease, which is characterized by multiple epiphyseal dystrophy. In a randomized double-blind comparison of amlodipine (10 mg/day) and enalapril (20 mg/day) in 50 patients for 6 months, both drugs significantly reduced blood pressure, but amlodipine increased heart rate and plasma concentrations of noradrenaline and angiotensin II (18[Cr]). These undesired effects make ACE inhibitors a better choice for prevention of cardiac dysfunction.

Skin *Photosensitivity* presenting with telangiectasia induced by calcium channel blockers has previously been described.

A 57-year-old hypertensive man developed telangiectasia, initially on the forehead and rapidly extending to the upper back, shoulders, and chest, particularly during the summer (19[Ar]). The eruption began 1 month after starting amlodipine and diminished considerably 3 months after withdrawal.

Diltiazem

Cardiovascular *Atrioventricular block* has been reported in three patients taking therapeutic doses of diltiazem; one died (20[A]).

A 47-year-old man taking furosemide for hypertension was given diltiazem 300 mg/day to achieve better blood pressure control; 1 month later he developed atrioventricular block, resolved by atropine.

A 62-year-old hypertensive man with renal artery stenosis, an adrenal adenoma, peripheral artery disease, and an abdominal aortic aneurysm developed a hypertensive crisis with chest pain. He was treated with nitrates, heparin, aspirin, and nicardipine, which was afterwards replaced by diltiazem 200 mg/day, because of persistent chest pain. He developed atrioventricular block 2 hours after the second dose of diltiazem, and was successfully treated with a pacemaker.

A 59-year-old woman with a previous myocardial infarction, hypertension, diabetes, and uterine cancer developed angina. She was treated with nitrates, aspirin, and heparin; diltiazem 200 mg/day was then added because of persistent chest pain. She developed atrioventricular block 72 hours later, and despite resuscitative efforts died in electromechanical dissociation

Skin *Exfoliative dermatitis with fever* occurred in a 69-year-old man with ischemic heart disease treated with mexiletine and diltiazem for 3 weeks; the rash resolved after withdrawal of both drugs and systemic corticosteroid therapy. Patch tests with mexiletine and diltiazem were positive. In addition to this case, 39 cases of drug eruption due to diltiazem have been reported in Japan (21[Ar]).

Drug overdose A potentially fatal case of diltiazem overdose caused by inappropriate self-treatment has been reported (22[Ar]).

A 54-year-old man with severe triple vessel coronary artery disease took six modified-release diltiazem tablets 180 mg following an episode of severe angina, and 10 hours later developed bradycardia, hypotension, and severe pulmonary edema, but was free of chest pain. After intensive hemodynamic monitoring and noradrenaline treatment, his renal, respiratory, and cardiac problems recovered to baseline over the next 48 hours. Diltiazem overdose was confirmed by a diltiazem serum concentration of 1230 ng/ml (usual target range 40–160 ng/ml).

Drug interactions *Sildenafil* is metabolized predominantly by CYP3A4, which diltiazem inhibits. An interaction of diltiazem with sildenafil has been reported (23[Ar]).

A 72-year-old man, who regularly took aspirin, metoprolol, diltiazem, and sublingual glyceryl trinitrate for stable angina, reported chest pain during elective prognostic coronary angiography, which resolved with half of a sublingual tablet of glyceryl trinitrate. Within 2 minutes he developed severe hypotension, with an unchanged electrocardiogram and no evidence of anaphylaxis. He had taken sildenafil 50 mg 48 hours before angiography.

The interval after which even short-acting nitrates can be safely given after the use of sildenafil is likely to be substantially longer than 24 hours when elderly patients are concurrently taking a CYP3A4 inhibitor, such as diltiazem.

Statins Uncertain results have been reported concerning the possible interaction of diltiazem with simvastatin (SEDA-24, 224). Ten healthy volunteers were randomized in a two-way, cross-over study either to oral lovastatin or to intravenous diltiazem followed by oral lovastatin. Intravenous diltiazem did not significantly affect the pharmacokinetics of lovastatin (oral AUC, C_{max}, t_{max}, or $t_{1/2}$), suggesting that the interaction does not occur systemically and is primarily a first-pass effect (24[c]). Drug interactions with diltiazem may become evident when a patient is changed from intravenous to oral dosing.

Coadministration of diltiazem with *methylprednisolone* increased plasma concentrations of methylprednisolone and its adrenal suppressant effects in nine healthy volunteers (25[Cr]). Care should be taken when these two drugs are coadministered for a long period, even if the clinical relevance of this pharmacokinetic interaction still needs to be evaluated.

Felodipine

Drug interactions Some components of grapefruit irreversibly inactivate enteric CYP3A4 and can increase the systemic availability of drugs that undergo extensive presystemic metabolism. In the first study of this interaction in 12 elderly people (70 years of age and over), *grapefruit juice* increased the AUC of felodipine 3-fold and its peak concentration 4-fold (26[C]). Blood pressure was lower with grapefruit juice after a single dose of felodipine, but not at steady state. Heart rate was higher with grapefruit juice after both single and multiple doses. Elderly patients should avoid taking grapefruit juice during treatment with felodipine because of this marked and unpredictable interaction.

Lercanidipine

Lercanidipine, a third-generation dihydropyridine for once-daily dosing in hypertension, has similar antihypertensive efficacy and tolerability to other calcium antagonists (27[R]).

Mibefradil

Drug interactions Mibefradil, a selective blocker of T-type calcium channels, has been studied in a placebo-controlled mortality trial in 2590 patients with moderate to severe congestive heart failure, the MACH-1 (Mortality Assessment in Congestive Heart Failure) Trial (28[C]). Mibefradil given for a maximum of 3 years did not affect mortality or morbidity. However, a subgroup analysis by concomitant drugs showed that *digoxin*, *class I antidysrhythmic drugs*, *amiodarone*, and other *drugs associated with torsade de pointes* increased the risk of death with mibefradil. These worrisome drug–drug interactions are consistent with the results of postmarketing surveillance, which prompted withdrawal of mibefradil from the market by its manufacturers in June 1998, even before complete results of the trial became available (SEDA-23, 210).

Nifedipine

Cardiovascular The long-term safety of dihydropyridine calcium channel blockers has been extensively debated since 1995, with reports of conflicting results from observational and randomized clinical studies about possible *increases in cardiovascular mortality, myocardial infarction, and neoplastic diseases* (SEDA 22, 214). Two recent studies have contributed to this controversy. In the INSIGHT (Intervention as a Goal in Hypertension Treatment) study, a prospective, multicenter, double-blind study in 6321 hypertensive patients aged 55–80 years, long-acting nifedipine 30 mg was compared with co-amilozide (hydrochlorothiazide 25 mg plus amiloride 2.5 mg) (29[C]). There were no differences between the two treatments in the primary endpoints of cardiovascular death, myocardial infarction, heart failure, or stroke during follow-up for 4 years.

In the Canadian Study of Health and Aging, a population-based prospective study of people aged 65 years or more, 5-year follow-up of 837 subjects who reportedly used at least one antihypertensive or diuretic agent showed that the risk of all-cause and cardiac mortality was significantly higher among nifedipine users than β-blocker users (30[C]). Compared with β-blockers, the hazard ratios (95% CI) were:

- loop diuretics 1.84 (1.21, 2.82);
- nifedipine 1.82 (1.09, 3.04);
- ACE inhibitors 0.98 (0.54, 1.78);
- diltiazem/verapamil 0.96 (0.58, 1.60).

Among nifedipine users, the risk of death

increased with the average daily dose and with recent initiation of therapy and remained significant for long-acting formulations.

Gastrointestinal Two patients developed severe *gastric mucosal damage* probably due to nifedipine (31[A]).

A 62-year-old man with gastric hemorrhage had a deep fundal ulcer in which a tablet of nifedipine was firmly embedded. The tablet was removed endoscopically and he was given cimetidine and recovered.

A 67-year-old man with diabetes and hypertension, taking glibenclamide and nifedipine, developed dysphagia. Gastroscopy showed severe damage to the mid-esophagus. He did not respond to omeprazole and sucralfate, but gradually improved after nifedipine withdrawal, and the lesion disappeared.

Modified-release formulations of nifedipine have been associated in case reports with the formation of bezoars, concretions of undigested material within the gastrointestinal tract, mostly in the stomach. An unusual case of *tablet impaction in the duodenum*, with gastric outlet obstruction, was discovered 1 year after the patient stopped taking a modified-release formulation of nifedipine (32[A]).

A 77-year-old woman developed constipation and weight loss. Esophagogastroduodenoscopy showed a deformed pylorus and an elongated duodenal bulb, with numerous impacted tablets and ulceration in the outlet. Since only a few tablets could be recovered by endoscopy, she underwent partial duodenal resection to remove the contents, 25 intact tablets that were confirmed to be modified-release nifedipine.

Skin Bullous eruptions secondary to nifedipine include bullous fixed drug eruptions, phototoxic bullous eruptions, erythema multiforme, and pemphigus foliaceus. Probable nifedipine-induced *pemphigoid* has now also been reported (33[A]).

A 70-year-old man with hypertension took nifedipine 10 mg bd and 3 months later developed a pruritic eruption on his back, which spread to cover his trunk, limbs, face, and scalp, with involvement of the mouth. His skin deteriorated after the dosage of nifedipine was increased to 20 mg bd 1 year later. Antibodies to the 230 kDa pemphigoid antigen were detected in his serum. His skin improved considerably after withdrawal of nifedipine and the use of topical steroids and oral minocycline.

The findings supported a diagnosis of pemphigoid.

Fetotoxicity The use of nifedipine during pregnancy and labor has been widely debated, although its effects on child development have not been well evaluated. In a recent study nifedipine did not affect the development and health of 190 children, aged 18 months, born to women with mild to moderate hypertension who had been randomized to nifedipine, given for 12–34 gestational weeks before delivery, or expectant management (34[C]).

Drug overdose Unlike verapamil and diltiazem, overdose with nifedipine is not usually fatal. Multiple case series of pediatric nifedipine ingestion have been published, and none has reported any deaths. However, two fatal cases of ingestion of long-acting nifedipine in children have now been reported: a 24-month-old girl who took 20 tablets of nifedipine 10 mg and a 14-month-old girl who took a single tablet of nifedipine 10 mg; neither responded to aggressive supportive care (35[A]).

Drug interactions *Melatonin* has a hypotensive effect in both normotensive and hypertensive subjects. In a double-blind, randomized, cross-over study designed to evaluate whether evening ingestion of melatonin potentiates the antihypertensive effect of nifedipine monotherapy in 50 patients with well-controlled mild to moderate hypertension aged 38–65 years (28 men, 22 women) there was a surprising significant increase in blood pressure and heart rate throughout 24 hours (36[C]). The authors suggested that there was competition between melatonin and nifedipine, with impairment of the antihypertensive efficacy of the calcium channel blocker.

Verapamil

Cardiovascular Verapamil can cause *cardiac failure*, because it has a potent negative inotropic effect and causes increased capillary filtration pressure by vasodilatation (37[A]).

A 16-year-old boy who took long-term verapamil after a Mustard operation for transposition of the great arteries developed severe congestive heart failure, which did not respond to diuretics. Systemic vascular resistance was increased by 75% and pulmonary vascular resistance by 150%; the cardiac index was reduced from 3.0 to 1.8 l/min/m^2. Ejection fraction and atrial pressure were unchanged and neurohormonal causes were excluded. The heart failure resolved after withdrawal of verapamil.

Risk factors In therapeutic doses verapamil has a negative dromotropic effect, reflected in plasma concentration-dependent prolongation of the PR interval and AV nodal block. PR interval prolongation is detectable even after small single doses. The effects of *rheumatoid arthritis* on the pharmacokinetics and pharmacodynamics of verapamil have been studied in eight patients and eight age- and sex-matched healthy volunteers (38[c]). Verapamil and norverapamil concentrations were substantially increased in the patients with rheumatoid arthritis, accompanied by significantly less dromotropic activity. Regardless of the mechanism involved in the altered pharmacokinetics of verapamil, the rise in drug concentrations was accompanied by a significant reduction in dromotropic activity. Therefore, administration of verapamil to patients with rheumatoid arthritis may require close attention to prevent therapeutic failure.

Drug overdose Several cases of verapamil poisoning have been reported; it generally causes cardiac toxicity and is often fatal.

A 28-year-old man developed rhabdomyolysis and acute renal insufficiency 10 hours after taking four capsules containing verapamil 180 mg plus trandolapril 2 mg. He survived with gastric lavage and activated charcoal 70 g. By 4 hours after admission he was awake and complained of diffuse muscle cramps and myalgia. Creatinine and creatine kinase reached 565 μmol/l (6.7 mg/dl) and 10 700 U/l respectively. After 6 days the laboratory tests were all within the reference ranges.

The authors suggested that *rhabdomyolysis* should be considered in patients with myalgia and muscle cramps taking verapamil plus trandolapril, and that routine serum creatinine kinase should be checked (39[A]).

Drug interactions The addition of low doses of verapamil to *ACE inhibitor* therapy reversed ACE inhibitor-induced increases in creatinine concentrations in eight elderly hypertensive patients (40[c]). During an average of 25 weeks, ACE inhibitors significantly reduced blood pressure, but serum creatinine concentrations rose. During an average of 10 weeks, the addition of verapamil did not reduce the blood pressure further, but the serum creatinine concentrations were normalized. Verapamil appears to have a beneficial effect, through dilatation of constricted afferent and efferent arterioles and reduction of the mesangial cell contraction induced by endothelin-1, factors that have been implicated in the increase in intraglomerular pressure and proteinuria due to ACE inhibitors.

Calcium channel blockers are given to transplant patients for their protective effect against *ciclosporin*-induced nephrotoxicity. Verapamil has been particularly preferred, as it causes a significant increase in plasma ciclosporin concentrations and also seems to have a direct immunosuppressive action. However, in a recent study in 152 kidney transplant recipients verapamil increased the incidence of postoperative infections (41[c]). The patients, all of whom were taking ciclosporin, were assigned either to verapamil 240 mg/day or to no verapamil; during a postoperative period of 2–14 months, the incidence of infections was 22% (17/77) of those given verapamil compared with 5% (4/75) of the others. However, since the study was not randomized, it is not possible to draw reliable conclusions.

REFERENCES

1. Palomeras E, Sanz P, Cano A, Fossas P. Dystonia in a patient treated with propranolol and gabapentin. Arch Neurol 2000; 57: 570–1.
2. Schuman JS. Effects of systemic beta-blocker therapy on the efficacy and safety of topical brimonidine and timolol. Ophthalmology 2000; 107: 1171–7.
3. Quiralte J, Florido F, De San Pedro BS. Allergic contact dermatitis from carteolol and timolol in eyedrops. Contact Dermatitis 2000; 42: 245.
4. Pèrez-Stable EJ, Halliday R, Gardiner PS, Baron RB, Hauck WW, Acree M, Coates TJ. The effects of propranolol on cognitive function and quality of life: a randomized trial among patients with diastolic hypertension. Am J Med 2000; 108: 359–65.
5. Love JN, Howell JM, Litovitz TL, Klein-Schwartz W. Acute beta blocker overdose: factors associated with the development of cardiovascular morbidity. Clin Toxicol 2000; 38: 275–81.

6. Love JN. Acebutolol overdose resulting in fatalities. J Emerg Med 2000; 18: 341–4.
7. Khedun SM, Maharaj B, Moodley J. Effects of antihypertensive drugs on the unborn child. Paediatr Drugs 2000; 2: 419–36.
8. Richard CS, Gregoire R, Plewes EA, Silverman R, Burul C, Buie D, Reznick R, Ross T, Burnstein M, O'Connor BI, Mukraj D, McLeod RS. Internal sphincterotomy is superior to topical nitroglycerin in the treatment of chronic anal fissure. Results of a randomized, controlled trial by the Canadian Colorectal Surgical Trials Group. Dis Colon Rectum 2000; 43: 1048–58.
9. Altomare DF, Rinaldi M, Milito G, Arcana F, Spinelli F, Nardelli N, Scardigno D, Pulvirenti G, D'Urso A, Bottini C, Pescatori M, Lovreglio R. Glyceryl trinitrate for chronic anal fissure-healing or headache? Results of a multicenter, randomized, placebo-controlled, double-blind trial. Dis Colon Rectum 2000; 43: 174–81.
10. Doucet S, Malekianpour M, Thèroux P, Bilodeau L, Cote G, De Guise P, Dupuis J, Joyal M, Gosselin G, Tanguay J-F, Juneau M, Harel F, Nattel S, Tardif JC, Lesperance J. Randomized trial comparing intravenous nitroglycerin and heparin for treatment of unstable angina secondary to restenosis after coronary artery angioplasty. Circulation 2000; 101: 955–61.
11. Tjon JA, Ansani NT. Transdermal nitroglycerin for the prevention of intravenous infusion failure due to phlebitis and extravasation. Ann Pharmacother 2000; 34: 1189–92.
12. Siepmann M, Kirch W. Effects of nitroglycerine on cerebral blood flow velocity, quantitative electroencephalogram and cognitive performance. Eur J Clin Invest 2000; 30: 832–7.
13. Daniel TA, Nawarskas JJ. Vitamin C in the prevention of nitrate tolerance. Ann Pharmacother 2000; 34: 1193–7.
14. Gournay J, Masliah C, Martin T, Perrin D, Galmiche JP. Isosorbide mononitrate and propranolol compared with propranolol alone for the prevention of variceal rebleeding. Hepatology 2000; 31: 1239–45.
15. Lafuente NG, Egea AM. Calcium channel blockers and hepatotoxicity. Am J Gastroenterol 2000; 95: 2145.
16. Udelson JE, DeAbate CA, Berk M, Neuberg G, Packer M, Vijay NK, Gorwitt J, Smith WB, Kukin ML, LeJemtel T, Levine Barry, Konstam MA, for the Amlodipine Exercise Trial Investigators. Effects of amlodipine on exercise tolerance, quality of life, and left ventricular function in patients with heart failure from left ventricular systolic dysfunction. Am Heart J 2000; 139: 503–10.
17. Spence JD, Munoz C, Huff MW, Tokmakjian S. Effect of amlodipine on hemodynamic and endocrine responses to mental stress. Am J Hypertens 2000; 13: 518–22.
18. Cocco G, Ettlin T, Baumeler HR. The effect of amlodipine and enalapril on pressure and neurohumoral activation in hypertensive patients with Ribbing's disease (multiple epiphyseal dystrophy). Clin Cardiol 2000; 23: 109–14.
19. Grabczynska SA, Cowley N. Amlodipine-induced photosensitivity presenting as telangiectasia. Br J Dermatol 2000; 142: 1255–6.
20. Boujnah MR, Jaafari A, Boukhris B, Boussabah I, Thameur M. Bloc sino-auriculaire induit par le diltiazem aux doses therapeutiques. A propos de trois observations. Tunis Med 2000; 78: 735–7.
21. Umebayashi Y. Drug eruption due to mexiletine and diltiazem. Nishinihon J Dermatol 2000; 62: 80–2.
22. Satchithananda DK, Stone DL, Chauhan A, Ritchie AJ. Unrecognised accidental overdose with diltiazem. Br Med J 2000; 321: 160–1.
23. Khoury V, Kritharides L. Diltiazem-mediated inhibition of sildenafil metabolism may promote nitrate-induced hypotension. Aust NZ J Med 2000; 30: 641–2.
24. Masica AL, Azie NE, Brater DC, Hall SD, Jones DR. Intravenous diltiazem and CYP3A-mediated metabolism. Br J Clin Pharmacol 2000; 50: 273–6.
25. Varis T, Backman JT, Kivistö KT, Neuvonen PJ. Dilitazem and mibefradil increase the plasma concentrations and greatly enhance the adrenal-suppressant effect of oral methylprednisolone. Clin Pharmacol Ther 2000; 67: 215–21.
26. Dresser GK, Bailey DG, Carruthers SG. Grapefruit juice–felodipine interaction in the elderly. Clin Pharmacol Ther 2000; 68: 28–34.
27. McClellan KJ, Jarvis B. Lercanidipine: a review of its use in hypertension. Drugs 2000; 60: 1123–40.
28. Levine TB, Bernink PJLM, Caspi A, Elkayam U, Geltman EM, Greenberg B, McKenna WJ, Ghali JK, Giles TD, Marmor A, Reisin LH, Ammon S, Lindberg E. Effect of mibefradil, a T-type calcium channel blocker, on morbidity and mortality in moderate to severe congestive heart failure: The MACH-1 Study. Circulation 2000; 101: 758–64.
29. Brown MJ, Palmer CR, Castaigne A, De Leeuw PW, Mancia G, Rosenthal T, Ruilope LM. Morbidity and mortality in patients randomised to double-blind treatment with a long-acting calcium-channel blocker or diuretic in the international nifedipine GITS study: intervention as a goal in hypertension treatment (INSIGHT). Lancet 2000; 356: 366–72.
30. Maxwell CJ, Hogan DB, Campbell NRC, Ebly EM. Nifedipine and mortality risk in the elderly: relevance of drug formulation, dose and duration. Pharmacoepidemiol Drug Saf 2000; 9: 11–23.
31. Lavy A. Corrosive effect of nifedipine in the upper gastrointestinal tract. Diagn Ther Endosc 2000; 6: 39–41.
32. Niezabitowski LM, Nguyen BN, Gums JG. Extended-release nifedipine bezoar identified one year after discontinuation. Ann Pharmacother 2000; 34: 862–4.
33. Ameen M, Harman KE, Black MM. Pemphigoid nodularis associated with nifedipine. Br J Dermatol 2000; 142: 575–7.
34. Bortulus R, Ricci E, Chatenoud L, Parazzini F. Nifedipine administered in pregnancy: effect on the

development of children at 18 months. Br J Obstet Gynaecol 2000; 107: 792–4.
35. Lee DC, Greene T, Dougherty T, Pearigen P. Fatal nifedipine ingestions in children. J Emerg Med 2000; 9: 359–61.
36. Lusardi P, Piazza E, Fogari R. Cardiovascular effects of melatonin in hypertensive patients well controlled by nifedipine: a 24-hour study. Br J Clin Pharmacol 2000; 49: 423–7.
37. Buchhorn R, Motz R, Bursch J. Hemodynamic and neurohormonal causes of a severe verapamil induced cardiac decompensation in a child after mustard operation. Herz Kreisl 2000; 32: 74–7.
38. Mayo PR, Skeith K, Russell AS, Jamali F. Decreased dromotropic response to verapamil despite pronounced increased drug concentration in rheumatoid arthritis. Br J Clin Pharmacol 2000; 50: 605–13.
39. Gokel Y, Paydas S, Duru M. High-dose verapamil–trandolapril induced rhabdomyolysis and acute renal failure. Am J Emerg Med 2000; 18: 738–9.
40. Bitar R, Flores O, Reverte M, Lòpez-Novoa JM, Macìas JF. Beneficial effect of verapamil added to chronic ACE inhibitor treatment on renal function in hypertensive elderly patients. Int Urol Nephrol 2000; 32: 165–9.
41. Nanni G, Panocchia N, Tacchino R, Foco M, Piccioni E, Castagneto M. Increased incidence of infection in verapamil-treated kidney transplant recipients. Transplant Proc 2000; 32: 551–3.

R. Verhaeghe

19 Drugs acting on the cerebral and peripheral circulations

Buflomedil *(SED-14, 630; SEDA-24, 229)*

Drug overdose Direct central *neurotoxicity* and *cardiotoxicity* are the main hallmarks of acute buflomedil overdose. Two new cases of self-poisoning with buflomedil have been reported (1[A], 2[A]).

A young girl took a single dose of buflomedil 7.5 g and a young man 18 g. Coma with convulsions occurred in both, soon followed by rhythm and conduction disturbances. Intensive resuscitation attempts could not prevent a fatal outcome in the girl.

Chronic overdose can also lead to *convulsions* (3[A]).

A 75-year-old woman had fever and convulsions. She had diabetes mellitus and angina pectoris and took buflomedil for peripheral arterial disease. No cause for her symptoms was found, but she had a high plasma concentration of buflomedil (6.3 mg/l, usual target range 4–4.5 mg/l). The drug was withdrawn and the symptoms did not recur. On questioning, it appeared that she had mistakenly forgot to abandon her old commercial formulation when her pharmacist proposed a cheaper new generic brand but took both, each at the correctly prescribed dose.

Cilostazol *(SED-14, 630; SEDA-22, 221; SEDA-24, 229)*

Cilostazol was approved by the US FDA in January 1999 for the treatment of symptoms of intermittent claudication. From 1984 to 1999, pentoxifylline was the only drug approved in the USA for this indication. The two drugs have now been compared with placebo in a large randomized double-blind trial (4[C]). After 24 weeks of treatment the mean increase in maximal walking distance was 54% with cilostazol and only 30 and 34% with pentoxifylline and placebo respectively. *Headache*, *diarrhea*, *abnormal stools*, and bouts of *palpitation* were significantly more common with cilostazol. They were reported as generally mild to moderate and self-limiting and have been previously recognized as related to cilostazol.

The efficacy of antithrombotic prophylaxis with cilostazol for the secondary prevention of cerebral infarction has been studied in a Japanese trial in 1095 patients (5[C]). There was a 42% relative risk reduction in comparison with placebo. As in the trials in patients with peripheral arterial disease, mild to moderate *headache* and *palpitation* were the most commonly observed symptomatic adverse events attributed to cilostazol; they respectively occurred in 13% and 5.3%. Headache with cilostazol is attributed to cerebral vasodilatation induced by the relaxation of vascular smooth muscle.

Defibrotide

Defibrotide is a polydeoxyribonucleotide extracted from mammalian organs. It is being developed as a drug in Italy. The antithrombotic activity of defibrotide is partly ascribed to enhancement of eicosanoid metabolism, in particular increased release of prostacyclin with ensuing vasodilatation and inhibition of platelet aggregation. An additional mechanism is activation of the fibrinolytic system, primarily increased activation of tissue plasminogen in the vessel wall.

The antithrombotic potential of this drug has previously been reported in patients with hepatic veno-occlusive disease after stem cell transplantation. In a randomized placebo-controlled trial in 310 patients with claudication there was significant improvement in walking distance with defibrotide, but no difference in

Side Effects of Drugs, Annual 25
J.K. Aronson, ed.

efficacy between the two doses of the drug tested (800 and 1200 mg/day) (6[C]). Twenty patients stopped taking the drug because of cardiovascular events, preset endpoints of the study. Seven others stopped because of adverse drug reactions, mainly *gastrointestinal intolerance* and *skin reactions*. They were equally distributed among the placebo and the two defibrotide groups.

DRUGS USED IN THE TREATMENT OF MIGRAINE

Ergotamine *(SED-14, 431, 635; SEDA-23, 214; SEDA-24, 168)*

Ergotamine has being used in the management of migraine for many decades, despite a lack of agreement on its value and exact place in daily practice. An expert European group has re-evaluated the preclinical and clinical data on ergotamine as they relate to treatment of migraine and have tried to reach a consensus on how to use it prudently (7[S]).

Cardiovascular Many of the adverse effects of ergotamine, commonly referred to as "ergotism", are explained by its sustained contractile action on smooth muscle in blood vessels (and occasionally in the uterus). *Organ ischemia* (and *uterine contracture*) are the feared consequences. Some recent cases with complications of ergotamine abuse are examples of the same mechanism.

Rupture of a splenic artery aneurysm in a 46-year-old woman was ascribed to excessive ergotamine ingestion for migraine (8[A]). The authors thought that significant vasospasm may have led to damage and weakening of the vessel wall and consequently to the development of a false aneurysm. It should be noted that splanchnic aneurysms are occasionally discovered in otherwise healthy people and carry a 5% risk of spontaneous rupture.

A necrotic small intestine was resected in a 65-year-old man with ergotamine abuse (9[A]). Histological examination showed hypertrophy of the smooth muscle of the mesenteric arteries resulting from chronic vasospasm. The patient developed postoperatively limb ischemia and tongue gangrene before he died.

The cerebral vasculature can also be vulnerable to ergotamine-induced vasoconstriction; *global amnesia* has been reported as a result (10[A]).

A 54-year-old woman with a 20-year history of migraine used a nasal ergotamine spray one evening during an episode of migraine. She used a second dose at 16.00 hours the next day, since the migraine had persisted. The following morning she was given subcutaneous sumatriptan 6 mg. Some 30–45 minutes later she developed the symptoms of global amnesia, which resolved by the following morning. Magnetic resonance imaging showed a small infarct in the right thalamus.

It seems likely the coadministration of two cerebral vasoconstrictors increased the likelihood of such an event.

Triptans *(SED-14, 635; SEDA-22, 222; SEDA-23, 215; SEDA-24, 229)*

Rizatriptan

Four randomized double-blind clinical trials in which rizatriptan was compared with sumatriptan have been reviewed (11[M]). The two drugs have similar safety profiles, but the frequency of adverse effects depends largely on the dose, which varied from trial to trial. Adverse events reported in over 5% of patients were *somnolence*, *dizziness*, *weakness/fatigue*, *nausea and vomiting*, *abdominal pain*, and *chest pain*.

Sumatriptan

Cardiovascular *Chest tightness and pain* are reported in up to 15% of patients taking sumatriptan and are presumed to be due to vasoconstriction of the coronary arteries. *Myocardial infarction* has been reported and as a consequence sumatriptan should not be used in patients with coronary disease. *Cardiac dysrhythmias* are uncommonly associated with sumatriptan (12[A]).

A 34-year-old man with migraine had palpitation after taking sumatriptan by nasal spray for a severe headache. A similar episode had occurred after he had previously taken sumatriptan. He had atrial fibrillation with a rapid ventricular rate. Sinus rhythm returned spontaneously within a few hours. No structural cardiac abnormality could be detected.

Myocardial ischemia secondary to coronary spasm was the putative trigger of atrial fibrillation in this case.

Ischemia in other vascular beds is rarely reported. A few cases of *ischemic colitis* have been described without many details and to these can now be added two reports of patients with several episodes of mesenteric ischemia (13[A]).

Two women were investigated for cramping abdominal pain and bloody diarrhea. In only one did the episodes completely disappear after withdrawal of sumatriptan. The other underwent an exploratory laparotomy and right hemicolectomy for transmural bowel necrosis.

Drug interactions Since ergot derivatives and triptans share the same propensity to induce vasoconstriction, a day-long interval is frequently recommended in patients in whom consecutive use of the two classes of drugs is considered for persisting migraine. Failure to respect this interval may increase the risk of adverse effects. An interaction of sumatriptan with ergotamine is described above under Ergotamine (10[A]).

Zolmitriptan

Cardiovascular A *spinal cord infarct* temporally related to zolmitriptan use has been reported after the use of zolmitriptan in a 50-year-old woman with a history of migraine (14[A]).

OTHER PERIPHERAL VASODILATORS

Sildenafil *(SED-14, 636; SEDA-22, 222; SEDA-23, 215; SEDA-24, 231)*

Cardiovascular Debate continues on the risk of death after taking sildenafil: can it entirely be attributed to co-existing cardiovascular disease with an inherent high risk of mortality, particularly during sexual activity, or does the drug contribute (15[R], 16[r])? The publication of a second case of a 44-year-old man who developed an *acute myocardial infarction* after taking sildenafil but before sexual intercourse appears to point to the drug as a potential trigger in people with unknown critical coronary lesions (17[A]).

Sildenafil has weak inhibitory effects on the isoenzyme phosphodiesterase type V in the retina, leading to temporary *changes in the perception of color hue and brightness*. In addition, asymptomatic electroretinographic abnormalities have been reported. Two new reports describe a temporal association between vascular events in the eye and sildenafil dosage.

A fit, healthy 69-year-old man presented with sudden painless loss of vision in the left eye, a few hours after taking sildenafil 100 mg (18[A]). Fundus examination showed occlusion of a branch of the retinal artery. No cardiovascular abnormality was detected.

A 52-year-old man developed sweating, headache, and blurred vision in his left eye 1 hour after a first dose of sildenafil 50 mg (19[A]). The same symptoms recurred on the next night, after a second dose of sildenafil. Fundoscopy a few days later showed an ischemic optic neuropathy.

Whereas *priapism* has not been reported with sildenafil in controlled clinical trials, this adverse effect is being mentioned in postmarketing drug surveillance programs and the first two case reports have now appeared in a healthy young man and in a patient with sickle cell trait (20[A], 21[A]).

Drug interactions Sildenafil potentiates the hypotensive effects of *glyceryl trinitrate* and combined use of the two drugs is therefore best avoided. On the other hand, drugs that are metabolized by the same cytochrome P450 isozymes (CYP3A4, the major pathway, and CYP2C9) may reinforce and prolong the effects of sildenafil. The antihypertensive agent diltiazem is metabolized by CYP3A4 and was held responsible for unanticipated prolonged hypotension after sublingual glyceryl trinitrate in a patient who underwent coronary angiography 2 days after last using sildenafil (22[A]).

REFERENCES

1. Perrot C, Rifler J-P, Freysz M. Intoxication volontaire fatale au buflomedil: à propos d'un cas. JEUR 2000; 13: 135–8.
2. Vandemergel X, Biston P, Lelearts L, Marécaux G, Daune M. Buflomedil poisoning: a potentially life-threatening intoxication. Intensive Care Med 2000; 26: 1713.
3. Chiffoleau A, Yatim D, Garrec F, Veyrac

G, Raoult P, Larousse C, Bourin M. Warning! One buflomedil may hide another one. Thérapie 2000; 55: 221–3.
4. Dawson DL, Cutler BS, Hiatt WR, Hobson RW II, Martin JD, Bortey EB, Forbes WP, Strandness DE. A comparison of cilostazol and pentoxifylline for treating intermittent claudication. Am J Med 2000; 109: 523–30.
5. Gotoh F, Tohgi H, Hirai S, Terashi A, Fukuuchi Y, Otomo E, Shinohara Y, Itoh E, Matsuda T, Sawada T, Yamaguchi T, Nishimaru K, Ohashi Y. Cilostazol stroke prevention study: a placebo-controlled double-blind trial for secondary prevention of cerebral infarction. J Stroke Cerebrovasc Dis 2000; 9: 147–57.
6. Violi F, Marubini E, Coccheri S, Nenci GG. Improvement of walking distance by defibrotide in patients with intermittent claudication. Results of a randomized, placebo-controlled study (the DICLIS study). Thromb Haemostasis 2000; 83: 672–7.
7. Tfelt-Hansen P, Saxena PR, Dahlöf C, Pascual J, Làinez M, Henry P, Diener H-C, Schoenen J, Ferrari MD, Goadsby PJ. Ergotamine in the acute treatment of migraine. A review and European consensus. Brain 2000; 123: 9–18.
8. Vaz FM, Edwards C, Owen ERTC. False aneurysm of the splenic artery as a complication of ergotamine overdose. J Ir Coll Phys Surg 2000; 29: 201–3.
9. Payne B, Sasse B, Franzen D, Hailemariam S, Gemsenjäger E. Manifold manifestations of ergotism. Schweiz Med Wochenschr 2000; 130: 1152–6.
10. Pradalier A, Lutz G, Vincent D. Transient global amnesia, migraine, thalamic infarct, dihydroergotamine and sumatriptan. Headache 2000; 40: 324–7.
11. Tfelt-Hansen P, Ryan RE. Oral therapy for migraine: comparisons between rizatriptan and sumatriptan. A review of four randomized, double-blind clinical trials. Neurology 2000; 55 Suppl 2: S19–24.
12. Morgan DR, Trimble M, McVeigh GE. Atrial fibrillation associated with sumatriptan. Br Med J 2000; 321: 275.
13. Liu JJ, Brandhagen DJ, Ardolf JC. Sumatriptan-associated mesenteric ischemia. Ann Intern Med 2000; 132: 597.
14. Vijayan N, Peacock JH. Spinal cord infarction during use of zolmitriptan: a case report. Headache 2000; 40: 57–60.
15. Kloner RA. Cardiovascular risk and sildenafil. Am J Cardiol 2000; 86 Suppl 1: 57F–61F.
16. Mitka M. Some men who take Viagra die. Why? J Am Med Assoc 2000; 283: 590–1.
17. Muniz AE, Holstege CP. Acute myocardial infarction associated with sildenafil (Viagra) ingestion. Am J Emerg Med 2000; 18: 353–5.
18. Tripathi A, O'Donnell NP. Branch retinal artery occlusion; another complication of sildenafil. Br J Ophthalmol 2000; 84: 934–5.
19. Egan R, Pomeranz H. Sildenafil (Viagra) associated anterior ischemic optic neuropathy. Arch Ophthalmol 2000; 118: 291–2.
20. Sur RL, Kane CJ. Sildenafil citrate-associated priapism. Urology 2000; 55: 950.
21. Kassim AA, Fabry ME, Nagel RL. Acute priapism associated with the use of sildenafil in a patient with sickle cell trait. Blood 2000; 95: 1878–9.
22. Khoury V, Kritharides L. Diltiazem-mediated inhibition of sildenafil metabolism may promote nitrate-induced hypotension. Aust NZ J Med 2000; 30: 641–2.

Faiez Zannad

20 Antihypertensive drugs

ANGIOTENSIN CONVERTING ENZYME INHIBITORS

(SED-14, 638; SEDA-22, 225; SEDA-23, 217; SEDA-24, 233)

The saga of the angiotensin converting enzyme (ACE) inhibitors continues with the publication of the HOPE (Heart Outcomes Prevention Evaluation) mega-trial results (1[C]). This was a placebo-controlled trial of ramipril in 9279 patients over the age of 55 with a high risk of cardiovascular events. Eligible patients included those with coronary artery disease or a history of diabetes mellitus plus another cardiovascular risk factor. Exclusion criteria included congestive heart failure or a history of myocardial infarction or stroke within 4 weeks of the study. The primary outcome was myocardial infarction, stroke, or death from any cardiovascular event. The study was designed to continue for 5 years, but it was stopped early because of the beneficial effects of ramipril on the primary outcome (14% vs 18%). The results were consistent among subgroups and benefit extended to a number of secondary outcomes. The reduction in the incidence of diabetes among patients on ramipril is an important observation. Ramipril was well tolerated; *cough* resulted in drug withdrawal in 7.3% of patients.

Respiratory Chinese patients experience more *cough* from ACE inhibitors than Caucasians. A review of the pharmacokinetics and blood pressure-lowering efficacy of ACE inhibitors as well as of ACE and angiotensinogen gene polymorphism did not find significant differences between Chinese and Caucasians to account for the difference in cough incidence (2[R]).

Skin Two new cases of *pemphigus* have been attributed to ACE inhibitors (fosinopril and quinapril) and the authors reviewed ACE inhibitor-related pemphigus (3[AR]). Drug-related pemphigus can be classified into two major types, based on the clinical course: induced pemphigus and triggered pemphigus, in which endogenous factors are more important and the drug plays a secondary role. The first type is usually related to thiol drugs. It is impossible to distinguish drug-related pemphigus reliably from idiopathic pemphigus on the basis of clinical findings, histopathology, or immunofluorescence. Captopril tends to be associated with pemphigus foliaceus, whereas the non-thiol ACE inhibitors are more often associated with pemphigus vulgaris, although there are exceptions. A transition from pemphigus vulgaris to pemphigus foliaceus is more common than the reverse. Several mechanisms have been proposed to be involved in the induction of pemphigus: interaction of the thiol group with sulfur-containing groups on the keratinocyte membrane, leading to acantholysis by biochemical interference with adhesion mechanisms; antigen modification resulting in antibody formation; inhibition of suppressor T cells, resulting in pathogenic autoantibody formation by B cells clones; or enzyme activation or inhibition.

The maximum latency to the development of pemphigus reported for ACE inhibitors is 2 years. It may take up to 17 months for lesions to resolve after drug withdrawal. A significant proportion of cases will not improve or resolve spontaneously on drug withdrawal alone. It is important to withdraw the offending drug, treat the bullous reaction appropriately, and advise avoidance of ACE inhibitors, although substitution of enalapril for captopril or vice versa has been successful in some cases.

Metabolism About 10–20% of 307 unselected consecutive out-patients with type 1 dia-

Side Effects of Drugs, Annual 25
J.K. Aronson, ed.

betes mellitus have a high risk of severe *hypoglycemia*. Diabetics with the ACE DD genotype have a relative risk of severe hypoglycemia of 3.2 (95% CI = 1.4, 7.4) compared with those who have the II genotype (4[C]). There is a significant relation between serum ACE activity and the risk of severe hypoglycemia. The authors therefore suggested that the protective effect of ACE inhibitors against severe hypoglycemia should be tested in high-risk patients with high ACE activity.

Immunologic Two new cases of *anaphylactoid reactions* induced by extracorporeal therapy with AN69 membranes in combination with ACE inhibition have been reported (5[A]). This combination should be avoided, since well-established alternatives are available.

Two patients presented with isolated *visceral angio-edema* with episodes of recurrent abdominal symptoms (6[A]). Each had undergone surgical procedures for symptoms that persisted after surgery and were ultimately relieved by withdrawal of their ACE inhibitors. These cases call attention to what may be an underappreciated cause of abdominal pain. Another similar case was diagnosed as *angioedema* of the small bowel after an abdominal CT scan (7[Ar]). The authors reviewed nine other previously reported similar cases and made the intriguing and as yet unexplained observation that all cases, including theirs, occurred in women.

Drug interactions *Aspirin* The issue of whether aspirin interferes with the beneficial effects of ACE inhibitors, or vice versa, is still unresolved. A systematic overview (8[M]) and two additional post hoc analyses of clinical trials (9[C]) have merely added to the confusion.

The overview of major ACE inhibitor trials (CONSENSUS II, AIRE, TRACE, SMILE) found a trend toward less benefit from ACE inhibitors among aspirin users. Although the interaction was not statistically significant, the authors concluded that the data did not "refute the hypothesis of a major aspirin interaction with ACE inhibitors", especially because patients taking aspirin had only 60% of the benefit seen in patients not taking it.

GUSTO-1 and EPILOG, two different antithrombotic trials, the first in acute myocardial infarction and the second during coronary stenting, compared the event rates in patients taking aspirin, an ACE inhibitor, or both (9[C]). In each of these trials, events were more frequent in patients taking the combination than in those taking aspirin alone. The authors interpreted these findings as suggesting that ACE inhibitors may reduce the benefit of aspirin in these patients, whereas the results of the ACE inhibitor trials suggested that aspirin may interfere with the effect of ACE inhibitors.

None of the analysed trials that suggested that there is an interaction between aspirin and ACE inhibitors was designed to examine this question. Post hoc and subgroup analyses may be heavily biased, and multivariate adjustment may not have been able to account fully for confounding factors. Aspirin in itself may be harmful in certain patients, such as those with heart failure, because of its antiprostaglandin activity, rather than because it interferes with the actions of ACE inhibitors, a phenomenon that would also manifest as an aspirin–ACE inhibitor interaction.

The Warfarin–Antiplatelet Trial in Chronic Heart Failure (WATCH) is indirectly addressing the issue. It is based on the hypothesis that warfarin, or clopidogrel (an antiplatelet agent that acts by a cyclooxygenase-independent pathway) may be preferred to aspirin as antithrombotic therapy in patients with heart failure. It will randomize 4500 patients, most of whom will be taking ACE inhibitors. Meanwhile, it may be advisable to avoid aspirin in patients with heart failure and no clear indication for aspirin (no evidence of atherosclerosis), and to consider substituting warfarin or clopidogrel for aspirin in patients with refractory or rapidly progressive heart failure (10[r]). In all other cases, because each drug is clearly associated with a substantial clinical benefit, it would be excessive to deny patients aspirin or ACE inhibitors.

Selective cyclooxygenase-2 (COX-2) inhibitors Because COX-2 inhibitors have become available only recently, their interaction with ACE inhibitors has been much less well investigated than aspirin. In a review of Phase II/III studies of COX-2 inhibitors, it was reported that the coadministration of rofecoxib 25 mg/day and benazepril 10–40 mg/day for 4 weeks was associated with an average increase in mean arterial pressure of about 3 mmHg compared with ACE inhibitor monotherapy (11[R]).

One report has described a case of *increased blood pressure* in a patient taking rofecoxib and lisinopril (12[A]).

The blood pressure of a 59-year-old man with hypertension and normal renal function rose when rofecoxib 25 mg/day was added to lisinopril 10 mg/day (from an average of 135/80–85 to 168/98 mmHg within 5 weeks). Four days after rofecoxib was withdrawn the blood pressure was 127/78 mmHg. Rechallenge with the same dose of rofecoxib produced the same effect and the blood pressure fell when the dosage of lisinopril was increased to 20 mg/day on continuous rofecoxib. The authors did not report on the course of renal function.

The increase in blood pressure with COX-2 inhibitors from interaction with ACE inhibitors may be greater in some patients than has previously been reported.

Captopril *(SED-14, 642; SEDA-22, 226; SEDA-24, 237)*

Urinary tract *Acute renal insufficiency* with *tubular necrosis* has been described (13[A]). It occurred within 24 hours of first dose of captopril and required 8 weeks hemodialysis. The diagnosis of ischemic tubular necrosis was confirmed by renal biopsy. Few previous cases of ACE inhibitor-induced nephropathy have been documented by renal biopsy.

Cilazapril *(SEDA-23, 219)*

Skin and appendages A case of *pemphigus vulgaris* possibly triggered by cilazapril has been reported (14[A]). It falls within the general description of ACE inhibitor-related pemphigus described above.

Enalapril *(SED-14, 643; SEDA-22, 227; SEDA-23, 219; SEDA-24, 237)*

Liver Another case of *hepatitis*, rather unusual and unconvincing, has been reported (15[A]).

A 46-year-old man had taken enalapril for hypertension for 3 years before he presented with jaundice and progressive liver failure. He was taking no other drugs and had a moderate daily consumption of alcohol. All known causes of acute liver failure were excluded by careful and extensive investigation. Analysis of liver biopsies showed a pathological pattern comparable to that observed in severe halothane hepatitis. Serological studies, including T-cell stimulation with enalapril and a broad spectrum of tests for autoimmunity, were negative. The hepatitis persisted despite enalapril withdrawal and finally led to orthotopic liver transplantation and subsequently to death.

The mechanism of enalapril-induced liver injury in this case was obscure. The causal relation was unconvincing.

Lisinopril *(SEDA-22, 228; SEDA-23, 220; SEDA-24, 238)*

An updated and comprehensive review of the use of lisinopril in congestive heart failure has been published (16[R]), including a section on tolerability and details of the ATLAS (Assessment with Treatment with Lisinopril and Survival) trial. The tolerance of high doses of lisinopril (32.5–35 mg od) in heart failure, one of the issues addressed by this trial, was not significantly different from that of low doses (2.5–5 mg od). Since high doses were more effective than low doses, the authors recommended that more aggressive use of ACE inhibitors is warranted (17[C]). However, this conclusion is valid only in the conditions of the trial, with careful and slow dose escalation. With such a strategy, most patients with heart failure can be titrated successfully to high maintenance doses.

Cardiovascular *Shock* after myocardial infarction has been attributed to an ACE inhibitor (18[A]).

A 42-year-old woman suffered an acute anterior myocardial infarction, initially associated with pulmonary edema. After hemodynamic stabilization she was given lisinopril 10 mg orally. Two hours later she developed circulatory failure in conjunction with acute renal insufficiency. Right heart catheterization showed markedly reduced systemic vascular resistance but a normal cardiac index. After the usual causes of cardiogenic shock had been ruled out, repeated fluid challenges and intravenous noradrenaline failed to improve her hemodynamic status. She was therefore given angiotensin II intravenously (5–7.5 μg/min), which immediately and markedly raised the systematic vascular resistance and resulted in subsequent regression of shock. She was discharged after an otherwise uneventful course.

Endocrine The *syndrome of inappropriate antidiuretic hormone secretion* (SIADH) has been attributed to lisinopril (19[A]).

A 76-year-old woman taking lisinopril 20 mg/day and metoprolol for hypertension developed headaches, nausea, and a tingling sensation in her arms. Her serum sodium was 109 mmol/l, with a serum osmolality of 225 mOsm/kg, urine osmolality of 414 mOsm/kg, and urine sodium of 122 mmol/l. She had taken and diclofenac 75 mg/day for arthritic pain for 6 years, but about 1 month before naproxen then propoxyphene napsylate and paracetamol had been substituted and zolpidem had been started. A diagnosis of SIADH was postulated and thyroid and adrenal causes were excluded. Lisinopril was withdrawn and fluid was restricted to 100 ml/day. The serum sodium gradually corrected to 143 mmol/l.

The authors referred to three other similar cases, in two of which the diagnosis may have been confused by the concomitant use of diuretics in patients with heart failure. However the present and one other case had occurred without co-existing risk factors for hyponatremia. They discussed a synergistic effect of zolpidem and/or diclofenac, and suggested a potential mechanism involving non-inhibition of brain ACE, which leaves brain angiotensin II receptors exposed to high circulating concentrations of angiotensin, which would strongly stimulate thirst and the release of antidiuretic hormone.

Drug interactions Hypotension followed the addition of *tizanidine* to lisinopril (20[A]).

A 10-year-old boy developed hypotension and reduced alertness. His blood pressure was 56/24 mmHg and his heart rate was 88/min. He had a history of a hypoxic ischemic insult to the central nervous system, subsequent hypertension, and spastic quadriplegia. His blood pressure had been controlled for the last 10 months with lisinopril (dose not stated). Tizanidine had been added 1 week before admission for spasticity. Lisinopril and tizanidine were withdrawn and his blood pressure rose to 149/89 mmHg over the next day. He was discharged and lisinopril was restarted but not tizanidine. He had no further problems with hypotension.

The authors interpreted the finding as a consequence of limited ability of the patient to respond to hypotension because of simultaneous blockade of the sympathetic system with the centrally acting α_2 adrenoceptor agonist tizanidine.

Perindopril *(SED-14, 643; SEDA-22, 228; SEDA-23, 220)*

An updated review of the use of perindopril in hypertension has appeared (21[R])

Quinapril *(SED-14, 643; SEDA-24, 238)*

Psychiatric *Acute psychosis* has been attributed to quinapril (22[A]).

A 93-year-old woman with heart failure was given quinapril 2.5 mg bd. Two hours after the first dose she became confused, disoriented, and anxious. During the night, she made many frantic telephone calls to her daughter and other family members, complaining that she was being assaulted. Her anxiety, disorientation, and visual hallucinations continued for 5 days. She had had an episode of hallucinations 2 years before, while taking a β-blocker. Quinapril was withdrawn. She recovered over the next day.

The authors commented on three previous cases of visual hallucination with other ACE inhibitors.

Zofenopril

Zofenopril is a prodrug that, once absorbed, undergoes rapid and complete hydrolysis to the sulfhydryl-containing active metabolite zofenoprilat. Its use in hypertension and in acute myocardial infarction has been extensively reviewed (23[R]).

ANGIOTENSIN II RECEPTOR ANTAGONISTS *(SED-14, 644; SEDA-22, 229; SEDA-23, 220; SEDA-24, 239)*

Six angiotensin II receptor antagonists are now available commercially. They share the same mechanism of action but have different pharmacokinetic profiles and different binding characteristics to AII receptors. These differences can result in non-comparable degrees of blockade of the renin–angiotensin system and therefore different antihypertensive efficacy. Some have longer durations of action (candesartan, irbesartan, and telmisartan). Their comparative pharmacology, safety, and therapeutic uses have been discussed in a brief review (24[R]).

Several clinical trials are currently proceeding in a variety of cardiovascular and renal diseases and cardiovascular risk conditions. The results of some of these have been presented at meetings and are still unpublished (PRIME, IDNT, RENAAL in diabetic nephropathy). ELITE II (the Losartan Heart Failure Survival Study) was conducted in order to confirm, in 3152 patients, the unexpected survival benefit of losartan 50 mg/day, compared with captopril 50 mg tds, in elderly patients with heart failure. Median follow up was 555 days. Losartan was not superior to captopril in improving survival, but was significantly better tolerated. Fewer patients discontinued treatment because of adverse effects (10% vs 15%), including effects attributed to the study drug (3% vs 8%) or because of *cough* (0.4% vs 2.8%) (25[C]).

SPICE (The Study of Patients Intolerant of Converting Enzyme Inhibitors) was a smaller trial (270 patients, 12 weeks follow-up) which evaluated the use of candesartan versus placebo in patients with heart failure and a history of intolerance of ACE inhibitors (most commonly because of *cough*, symptomatic *hypotension*, or *renal insufficiency*). Titration to the highest dose of candesartan 16 mg was possible in 69% of the patients (84% in the placebo group). Death and cardiovascular events tended to be lower with candesartan (26[C]).

The results of SPICE and of the previously published RESOLVD (Randomized Evaluation of Strategies for Left Ventricular Dysfunction) led to the design of the current CHARM trial, which is investigating the effect of candesartan in 6600 patients with heart failure in three different ways: versus an ACE inhibitor in patients with preserved left ventricular function; versus placebo in patients intolerant of ACE inhibitors; and in addition to ACE inhibitors in all other patients. While waiting for the results of this trial it is advisable to continue to use ACE inhibitors as the initial therapy for heart failure. In patients with documented intolerance of ACE inhibitors (which may represent 10–20% of patients with heart failure) angiotensin receptor antagonists may be useful as a substitute to block the renin–angiotensin–aldosterone system.

The results of another trial in heart failure with another angiotensin receptor antagonist (valsartan) are now available but are still to be published. In the VAL-HeFT (Valsartan in Heart Failure Trial) valsartan 160 mg bd was compared with placebo in 5010 patients with heart failure and left ventricular systolic dysfunction receiving optimal conventional therapy, including ACE inhibitors. The results showed a non-significant effect on mortality (19% on placebo, 20% on valsartan), but a highly significant effect on the primary endpoint of all-cause mortality and morbidity (32% on placebo, 29% on valsartan). A subgroup analysis suggested that the combination of valsartan, an ACE inhibitor, and a β-blocker was not beneficial and might even be harmful, whereas the combination of valsartan and an ACE inhibitor caused a reduction of 45% (27[C]).

Irbesartan *(SEDA-24, 240)*

An updated review of the pharmacology and therapeutic use of irbesartan in cardiovascular disorders has been published, including a brief section on drug tolerability, which referred to an unpublished postmarketing surveillance study in which 14% of the patients (1232 of 9009) had mostly mild adverse events (28[R]). No further details were given on the nature of the adverse events.

Urinary system *Renal insufficiency* has been attributed to irbesartan .

A 78-year-old Caucasian man with type II diabetes had switched to insulin within the last 2 years, hypertension and stable mild renal insufficiency took captopril 25 mg/day and torasemide 150 mg/day. His general physician substituted irbesartan 150 mg/day for the captopril. The basal average serum creatinine rose from 220 to 294 μmol/l 10 days after beginning irbesartan, and to 752 μmol/l 3 weeks later, at which stage he was admitted with acute renal insufficiency, oliguria, and edema with a 6 kg weight gain. Two days after withdrawal of irbesartan his creatinine reached a maximum of 907 μmol/l and then fell progressively to 570 μmol/l and never returned to basal values. The patient was started on chronic hemodialysis. Renal Doppler and MRI scans showed no renal artery stenosis, but there were signs of chronic renal ischemia, which may have contributed to the adverse drug reaction.

It is possible that irbesartan 150 mg/day produced abrupt and more pronounced inhibition of the renin–angiotensin system than the basal stable small dose of captopril 25 mg/day (29[A]).

Liver The first case of *cholestasis* with irbesartan has been reported (30[A]).

A 62-year-old woman developed deep icterus and hepatomegaly 1 month after starting to take irbesartan 300 mg/day. She had been hypertensive for 15 years and had no history of liver disease or risk factors for liver disease. Her bilirubin was 403 μmol/l, alkaline phosphatase 3193 IU/l, and AsT 177 IU/l. Serology and autoimmune screens were negative, as were liver ultrasonography and computerized tomography. Cholangiopancreatography was normal. Irbesartan was replaced by amlodipine and metoprolol, and 2 months later she remained jaundiced (bilirubin 324 μmol/l). Liver biopsy showed portal tract expansion, minimal inflammation, ectatic ductules, and cholestatic rosettes. Within 16 weeks she fully recovered and continued to be anicteric more than 1 year later.

The temporal profile in this case and the lack of an alternative cause for liver dysfunction suggested a drug reaction.

Drug interactions A small well-designed study in 14 healthy subjects showed no significant effect of irbesartan on the single-dose pharmacokinetics of total simvastatin acid (31[c]).

Losartan *(SED-14, 645; SEDA-22, 229; SEDA-23, 221; SEDA-24, 240)*

An extensive review of the use of losartan, with special focus on elderly patients, has included an update on the tolerability profile, mainly in clinical trials, but with no significant new information (32[R]).

Sensory systems Because it has been suggested that there is a local renin-angiotensin system in the eye, losartan may be useful in treating glaucoma. In a small, well-designed, placebo-controlled, cross-over study in four groups of subjects (controls, hypertensive patients with normal intraocular pressure, and patients with primary open-angle glaucoma with and without hypertension), a single oral dose of losartan 50 mg produced a drop in intraocular pressure in all subjects within 2–6 hours after drug intake, proportional to baseline eye pressure (33[C]). Blood pressure fell only in the hypertensive subjects. Thus, the fall in intraocular pressure was independent of the systemic effect on blood pressure. Beyond the potential for using losartan as a therapy for glaucoma, ophthalmologists should take into account concomitant therapy with losartan (and possibly other angiotensin receptor antagonists) when measuring intraocular pressure.

Telmisartan

Drug interactions The single-dose pharmacokinetics of telmisartan 120 mg were not affected by a concurrent single dose of *paracetamol* 1 g or *ibuprofen* 400 mg tds for 7 days (34[c]).

Multiple-dose telmisartan 120 mg od administered with *digoxin* 0.25 mg od resulted in higher serum digoxin concentrations (35[C]). Digoxin AUC and C_{max} rose by 22% and 50% respectively; the rise in C_{min} (13%) was not significant. These results suggest that telmisartan reduces the clearance of digoxin. The magnitude of this effect is comparable to that observed with calcium channel blockers, carvedilol, captopril, amiodarone, quinidine, and propafenone. Monitoring serum digoxin concentrations should be considered when patients first receive telmisartan and in the event of any changes in the dosage of telmisartan.

DRUGS THAT ACT ON THE SYMPATHETIC NERVOUS SYSTEM *(SED-14, 646; SEDA-22, 230; SEDA-23, 222; SEDA-24, 242)*

PRESYNAPTIC α-ADRENOCEPTOR AGONISTS

Clonidine *(SED-14, 646; SEDA-24, 242)*

Drug interactions Hypertension has been reported with *mirtazipine* plus clonidine (36[A]).

A 20-year-old man who had had Goodpasture's syndrome for 2.5 years, end-stage renal disease on chronic hemodialysis for 15 months, and hypertension controlled with metoprolol, losartan, and clonidine, developed dyspnea and hypertension (blood pressure 178/115 mmHg) 2 weeks after his psychiatrist first gave on mirtazipine 15 mg at bedtime to treat depression. His blood pressure did not fall significantly, despite the addition of losartan and minoxidil and the use of intravenous glyceryl trinitrate and labetalol. Only after emergency dialysis and intravenous nitroprusside did his blood pressure fall to 150–180/80–100 mmHg. When mirtazipine was withdrawn, his blood pressure was controllable with minoxidil 5 mg, clonidine 0.1 mg, and metoprolol 10 mg, all bd.

The authors recognized that mirtazipine alone could have caused the hypertensive event. In postmarketing surveillance of mirtazipine, hypertension occurred in at least 1% of patients. However, it is likely that the patient lost antihypertensive control because mirtazipine antagonized the antihypertensive effect of clonidine. Mirtazipine, a tetracyclic antidepressant, stimulates the noradrenergic system through antagonism at central α_2 inhibitory receptors, which is precisely opposite to the effect of clonidine.

Drug overdose A *hypertensive crisis and myocardial infarction* occurred in a 62-year-old woman after a combined injection of hydromorphone 48 mg and clonidine 12 mg subcutaneously in an attempt to refill an implanted epidural infusion pump (37[A]). She was immediately treated with naloxone, but she subsequently had accelerated hypertension, a brief tonic–clonic seizure, and an anteroseptal myocardial infarction. Cardiac catheterization showed no coronary narrowing or blockage, but an anterior infarct was confirmed. It is believed that the reaction was secondary to the vasoconstricting effects of high-dose clonidine through stimulation of peripheral α-adrenoceptors.

POSTSYNAPTIC ADRENOCEPTOR ANTAGONISTS *(SED-14, 648; SEDA-22, 231; SEDA-23, 222; SEDA-24, 242)*

Alfuzosin *(SEDA-22, 231; SEDA-23, 222)*

In a large database of 7093 patients with lower urinary tract symptoms related to benign prostatic hyperplasia treated for up to 3 years with alfuzosin in general practice, adverse events were reported in a very complex and uninformative way (38[C]). In another paper, the same authors reported on a subcohort of 2829 patients, with special focus on effects on quality of life. Adverse events occurred in 15% of the patients, 1.7% died during the study, and 5.2% had serious effects, which the authors did not detail, but which they stated were not related to treatment. Most adverse effects occurred during the first 3 months of treatment (39[C]). In another database of 3095 Spanish patients taking alfuzosin 5 mg bd for 60 days, adverse events were reported in 3.3% of the patients, and led to drug withdrawal in 1.6%; *postural hypotension* occurred in 1.8% (40[R]).

Liver What seems to be the first case of *hepatitis* potentially related to alfuzosin has been reported (41[A]).

A 63-year-old man, who had taken amiloride and alfuzosin for 9 months for hypertension and benign prostatic hyperplasia, became jaundiced. His AsT was 3013 IU/l, AlT 2711 IU/l, alkaline phosphatase 500 IU/l, and total bilirubin 415 μmol/l. Viral causes, autoimmune hepatitis, and biliary obstruction were excluded. After withdrawal of alfuzosin, his liver function tests gradually returned to normal within 6 months.

Immunologic A second case of *dermatomyositis*, with typical clinical effects, biochemical tests, electromyography, and muscle biopsy, has been reported in a 75-year-old man who had taken alfuzosin for 1 year (42[A]). There was no malignancy and the patient recovered fully after alfuzosin withdrawal (timing not given).

Doxazosin *(SED-14, 649; SEDA-22, 231; SEDA-23, 222; SEDA-24, 242)*

The Antihypertensive and Lipid Lowering Treatment to Prevent Heart Attack Trial (ALLHAT) was designed to see if the effects of doxazosin, amlodipine, and lisinopril were superior to those of chlortalidone on the incidence of cardiovascular disease in high-risk hypertensive patients (43[C]). Following an interim analysis of 24 335 patients, the doxazosin treatment arm was stopped because of an increased incidence of secondary cardiovascular endpoints relative to chlortalidone. While there were no differences between the groups in the only composite primary endpoint of fatal coronary heart disease or non-fatal myocardial infarction, or in all-cause mortality, patients randomized to treatment with doxazosin had a higher incidence of combined cardiovascular morbidity (relative risk (RR) = 1.25; 95% CI = 1.17, 1.33), driven by an approximate doubling in the risk of *congestive heart failure* with doxazosin relative to chlortalidone (RR = 2.04; 95%CI = 1.79, 2.32). *Coronary heart disease* (RR = 1.10; 95% CI = 1.00, 1.12) and *stroke* (RR = 1.19; 95% CI = 1.01, 1.40) were also significantly higher in the doxazosin arm.

Because of these results, it is expected that national and international guidelines for the treatment of hypertension will have to be amended. Doxazosin, and perhaps the whole class of α-blockers, should no longer be considered as first-line antihypertensive therapy.

Doxazosin can still be used for symptom relief in patients with nocturia secondary to prostatic hyperplasia, although it should probably be avoided in patients with manifest or latent congestive heart failure (44[r]). This issue is currently under intense debate (45[r]).

Drug overdose Hypotension, bradycardia, and ST segment elevation on the electrocardiogram occurred in a patient admitted who doxazosin 40 mg (46[A]). His blood pressure was 90/60 mmHg and his heart rate fell to 50/min. Eight hours after aggressive saline infusion and orogastric lavage the patient was awake, but his hypotension and bradycardia were corrected only after 96 hours and the administration of intravenous atropine 0.5 mg.

Prazosin *(SED-14, 649)*

Drug interactions In a well-controlled study in 10 Japanese patients with mild hypertension, the blood pressure reduction caused by *alcohol* 1 ml/kg was significantly increased by concurrent treatment with prazosin 1 mg tds (47[c]). At 2–4 hours after ingestion the blood pressure fell by 18/12 mmHg without prazosin and by 24/18 mmHg with prazosin. These results raise the possibility that heavy drinking may cause symptomatic hypotension in patients taking prazosin.

Terazosin *(SED-14, 649)*

In order to investigate the mechanisms of adverse events associated with α_1 adrenoceptor antagonists, the Veterans Affairs Cooperative Study database was analysed with respect to the relation between adverse events and hypotension in 1229 men with benign prostate hyperplasia. Treatment with terazosin produced the following rates of adverse events: *dizziness* 19%, *weakness* 6%, *postural hypotension* 6%, and *syncope* 1%. Of these adverse events only postural hypotension was associated with orthostatic blood pressure changes. Weakness, dizziness, and postural hypotension occurred to the same extent in patients with falls in systolic blood pressure of 5 mmHg or more or less than 5 mmHg. Thus, dizziness and weakness do not seem to be associated with changes in blood pressure, suggesting that these adverse events associated with α-blockers are not related to vascular effects. Designing a subtype selective α_1-antagonist that has less effect on blood pressure may not result in marked improvement in tolerability over currently available α_1-antagonists (48[R]).

DIRECT VASODILATORS

(SED-14, 649; SEDA-22, 231; SEDA-24, 243)

Hydralazine *(SED-14, 650; SEDA-21, 223)*

Immunologic A variety of vasculitic diseases, including Wegener's granulomatosis, microscopic polyangiitis, Churg–Strauss syndrome, and crescentic glomerulonephritis, are associated with antineutrophil cytoplasmic antibodies (ANCA) or leukocytoclastic vasculitis. In drug-induced ANCA-positive vasculitis antimyeloperoxidase antibodies are most often found; they produce a perinuclear pattern of staining by indirect immunofluorescence (pANCA), but antiproteinase 3 (anti-PR3) antibodies can also occur (cANCA).

The possible drug causes of *ANCA-positive vasculitis* with high titers of antimyeloperoxidase antibodies in 30 new patients have been reviewed (49[CR]). The findings illustrate that this type of vasculitis is a predominantly drug-induced disorder. Only 12 of the 30 cases were not related to a drug. The most frequently implicated drug was hydralazine (10 cases); the remainder involved propylthiouracil (three cases), penicillamine (two cases), allopurinol (two cases), and sulfasalazine.

Minoxidil *(SED-14, 650; SEDA-22, 231; SEDA-24, 243)*

Skin *Leukoderma* has been reported in two men from India who used 2% minoxidil lotion for 2–3 months to treat baldness (50[A]). The depigmentation was localized to the scalp. Other possibilities of leukoderma were ruled out, as was vitiligo. There was repigmentation of the leukodermic area within 3 months of minoxidil withdrawal in both cases.

REFERENCES

1. Yusuf S, Sleight P, for the Heart Outcomes Prevention Evaluation Study Investigators. Effects of an angiotensin-converting-enzyme inhibitor, ramipril, on cardiovascular events in high-risk patients. New Engl J Med 2000; 342: 145–53.
2. Ding PYA, Hu OYP, Pool PE, Liao W-C. Does Chinese ethnicity affect the pharmacokinetics and pharmacodynamics of angiotensin-converting enzyme inhibitors? J Hum Hypertens 2000; 14: 163–70.
3. Ong CS, Cook N, Lee S. Drug-related pemphigus and angiotensin converting enzyme inhibitors. Australas J Dermatol 2000; 41: 242–6.
4. Pedersen-Bjergaard U, Agerholm-Larsen B, Pramming S, Hougaard P, Thorsteinsson B. Activity of angiotensin-converting enzyme and risk of severe hypoglycaemia in type 1 diabetes mellitus. Lancet 2001; 357: 1248–53.
5. Kammerl MC, Schaefer RM, Schweda F, Schreiber M, Riegger GAJ, Kramer BK. Extracorporal therapy with AN69 membranes in combination with ACE inhibition causing severe anaphylactoid reactions: still a current problem? Clin Nephrol 2000; 53: 486–8.
6. Byrne TJ, Douglas DD, Landis ME, Heppell JP. Isolated visceral angioedema: an underdiagnosed complication of ACE inhibitors? Mayo Clin Proc 2000; 75: 1201–4.
7. Chase MP, Fiarman GS, Scholz FJ, MacDermott RP. Angioedema of the small bowel due to an angiotensin-converting enzyme inhibitor. J Clin Gastroenterol 2000; 31: 254–7.
8. Flather MD, Yusuf S, Kober L, Pfeffer M, Hall A, Murray G, Torp-Pedersen C, Ball S, Pogue J, Moye L, Braunwald E. Long-term ACE-inhibitor therapy in patients with heart failure or left ventricular dysfunction: a systematic overview of data from individual patients. Lancet 2000; 355: 1575–81.
9. Peterson JG, Topol EJ, Sapp SK, Young JB, Lincoff AM, Lauer MS. Evaluation of the effects of aspirin combined with angiotensin-converting enzyme inhibitors in patients with coronary artery disease. Am J Med 2000; 109: 371–7.
10. Massie BM, Teerlink JR. Interaction between aspirin and angiotensin-converting enzyme inhibitors: real or imagined. Am J Med 2000; 109: 431–3.
11. Kaplan-Machlis B, Klostermeyer BS. The cyclooxygenase-2 inhibitors: safety and effectiveness. Ann Pharmacother 1999; 33: 979–88.
12. Brown CH. Effect of rofecoxib on the antihypertensive activity of lisinopril. Ann Pharmacother 2000; 34: 1486.
13. Al Shohaib S, Raweily E. Acute tubular necrosis due to captopril. Am J Nephrol 2000; 20: 149–52.
14. Orion E, Gazit E, Brenner S. Pemphigus vulgaris possibly triggered by cilazapril. Acta Derm Venereol 2000; 80: 220.
15. Jeserich M, Ihling C, Allgaier HP, Berg PA, Heilmann C. Acute liver failure due to enalapril. Herz 2000; 25: 689–93.
16. Simpson K, Jarvis B. Lisinopril: a review of its use in congestive heart failure. Drugs 2000; 59: 1149–67.
17. Massie BM, Armstrong PW, Cleland JGF, Horowitz JD, Packer M, Poole-Wilson PA, Ryden L. Toleration of high doses of angiotensin-converting enzyme inhibitors in patients with chronic heart failure. Results from the ATLAS trial. Arch Intern Med 2001; 161: 165–71.
18. Desachy A, Normand S, Francois B, Cassat C, Gastinne H, Vignon P. Refractory shock after converting enzyme administration: usefulness of angiotensin II. Presse Med 2000; 29: 696–8.
19. Shaikh ZHA, Taylor HC, Maroo PV, Llerena LA. Syndrome of inappropriate antidiuretic hormone secretion associated with lisinopril. Ann Pharmacother 2000; 34: 176–9.
20. Johnson TR, Tobias JD. Hypotension following the initiation of tizanidine in a patient treated with an angiotensin converting enzyme inhibitor for chronic hypertension. J Child Neurol 2000; 15: 818–19.
21. Hurst M, Jarvis B. Perindopril: an updated review of its use in hypertension. Drugs 2001; 61: 867–96.
22. Tarlow MM, Sakaris A, Scoyni R, Wolf-Klein G. Quinapril-associated acute psychosis in an older woman. J Am Geriatr Soc 2000; 48: 1533.
23. Borghi C, Ambrosioni E. Zofenopril: a review of the evidence of its benefits in hypertension and acute myocardial infarction. Clin Drug Invest 2000; 20: 371–84.
24. Burnier M. Angiotensin II type 1 receptor blockers. Circulation 2001; 103: 904–12.
25. Pitt B, Poole-Wilson PA, Segal R, Martinez FA, Dickstein K, Camm AJ, Konstam MA, Riegger G, Klinger GH, Neaton J, Sharma D, Thiyagarajan B. Effect of losartan compared with captopril on mortality in patients with symptomatic heart failure: randomised trial – the Losartan Heart Failure Survival Study ELITE II. Lancet 2000; 355: 1582–7.
26. Granger CB, Ertl G, Kuch J, Maggioni AP, McMurray J, Rouleau JL, Stevenson LW, Swedberg K, Young J, Yusuf S, Califf RM, Bart BA, Held P, Michelson EL, Sellers MA, Ohlin G, Sparapani R, Pfeffer MA. Randomized trial of candesartan cilexetil in the treatment of patients with congestive heart failure and a history of intolerance to angiotensin-converting enzyme inhibitors. Am Heart J 2000; 139: 609–17.
27. Cohn JN, Tognoni G, Glazer RD, Spormann D, Hester A. Rationale and design of the Valsartan Heart Failure Trial: a large multinational trial to assess the effects of valsartan, an angiotensin-receptor blocker, on morbidity and mortality in chronic congestive heart failure. J Card Fail 1999; 5: 155–60.
28. Markham A, Spencer CM, Jarvis B. Irbesartan:

an updated review of its use in cardiovascular disorders. Drugs 2000; 59: 1187–206.

29. Descombes E, Fellay G. End-stage renal failure after irbesartan prescription in a diabetic patient with previously stable chronic renal insufficiency. Renal Fail 2000; 22: 815–21.
30. Hariraj R, Stoner E, Jader S, Preston DM. Drug points. Prolonged cholestasis associated with irbesartan. Br Med J 2000; 321: 547.
31. Marino MR, Vachharajani NN, Hadjilambris OW. Irbesartan does not affect the pharmacokinetics of simvastatin in healthy subjects. J Clin Pharmacol 2000; 40: 875–9.
32. Simpson KL, McClellan KJ. Losartan. A review of its use, with special focus on elderly patients. Drugs Aging 2000; 16: 227–50.
33. Costagliola C, Verolino M, De Rosa ML, Iaccarino G, Ciancaglini M, Mastropasqua L. Effect of oral losartan potassium administration on intraocular pressure in normotensive and glaucomatous human subjects. Exp Eye Res 2000; 71: 167–71.
34. Stangier J, Su C-APF, Fraunhofer A, Tetzloff W. Pharmacokinetics of acetaminophen and ibuprofen when coadministered with telmisartan in healthy volunteers. J Clin Pharmacol 2000; 40: 1338–46.
35. Stangier J, Su C-APF, Hendriks MGC, Van Lier JJ, Sollie FAE, Oosterhuis B, Jonkman JHG. The effect of telmisartan on the steady-state pharmacokinetics of digoxin in healthy male volunteers. J Clin Pharmacol 2000; 40: 1373–9.
36. Abo-Zena RA, Bobek MB, Dweik RA. Hypertensive urgency induced by an interaction of mirtazapine and clonidine. Pharmacotherapy 2000; 20: 476–8.
37. Frye CB, Vance MA. Hypertensive crisis and myocardial infarction following massive clonidine overdose. Ann Pharmacother 2000; 34: 611–15.
38. Lukacs B, Grange JC, Comet D, McCarthy C. History of 7093 patients with lower urinary tract symptoms related to benign prostatic hyperplasia treated with alfuzosin in general practice up to 3 years. Eur Urol 2000; 37: 183–90.
39. Lukacs B, Grange JC, Comet D. One-year follow-up of 2829 patients with moderate to severe lower urinary tract symptoms treated with alfuzosin in general practice according to IPSS and a health-related quality-of-life questionnaire. Urology 2000; 55: 540–6.
40. Sanchez-Chapado M, Guil M, Alfaro V, Badiella L, Fernandez-Hernando N. Safety and efficacy of sustained-release alfuzosin on lower urinary tract symptoms suggestive of benign prostatic hyperplasia in 3095 Spanish patients evaluated during general practice. Eur Urol 2000; 37: 421–7.
41. Zabala S, Thomson C, Valdearcos S, Gascon A, Pina MA. Alfuzosin-induced hepatotoxicity. J Clin Pharm Ther 2000; 25: 73–4.
42. Schmutz JL, Barbaud A, Trechot P. Alfuzosine-induced dermatomyositis. Ann Dermatol Venereol 2000; 127: 449.
43. Davis BR, Furberg CD, Wright JT, for the ALLHAT Collaborative Research Group. Major cardiovascular events in hypertensive patients randomized to doxazosin vs chlorthalidone : the antihypertensive and lipid-lowering, treatment to prevent heart attack trial (ALLHAT). J Am Med Assoc 2000; 283: 1967–75.
44. Messerli FH. Implications of discontinuation of doxazosin arm of ALLHAT. Lancet 2000; 355: 863–4.
45. Beevers DG, Lip GYH. Do alpha blockers cause heart failure and stroke? Observations from ALLHAT. J Hum Hypertens. 2000; 14: 287–9.
46. Gokel Y, Dokur M, Paydas S. Doxazosin overdosage. Am J Emerg Med 2000; 18: 638–9.
47. Kawano Y, Abe H, Kojima S, Takishita S, Omae T. Interaction of alcohol and an $alpha_1$-blocker on ambulatory blood pressure in patients with essential hypertension. Am J Hypertens 2000; 13 307–12.
48. Lepor H, Jones K, Williford W. The mechanism of adverse events associated with terazosin: an analysis of the Veterans Affairs Cooperative Study. J Urol 2000; 163: 1134–7.
49. Choi HK, Merkel PA, Walker AM, Niles JL. Drug-associated antineutrophil cytoplasmic antibody-positive vasculitis: prevalence among patients with high titers of antimyeloperoxidase antibodies. Arthritis Rheum 2000; 43: 405–13.
50. Malakar S, Dhar S. Leucoderma associated with the use of topical minoxidil: a report of two cases. Dermatology 2000; 201: 184–5.

Domenic A. Sica

21 Diuretics

R
Diuretics in renal insufficiency

Diuretics remain a mainstay in the therapy of hypertension, particularly in the presence of renal insufficiency or the nephrotic syndrome. For example, about 84% of the patients in the Reduction of Endpoints in NIDDM with the Angiotensin II Antagonist Losartan Study (RENAAL) required diuretic therapy to effect blood pressure control (1[C]). Although not specifically reported, a similarly high proportion of patients were likely to have required diuretic therapy to reach the target blood pressure in the Irbesartan Diabetic Nephropathy Trial (IDNT) (2[C]). These studies remind us once again of the importance of targeting volume control in order to reduce blood pressure in patients with chronic renal insufficiency.

Thiazide and loop diuretics *Various factors influence the choice of a diuretic in patients with renal insufficiency. First, it is widely believed that thiazide diuretics are ineffective once renal function falls below a creatinine clearance of 40–50 ml/min. Diuretics need to enter the renal tubule to reach their luminal sites of action. In renal insufficiency, higher diuretic doses are required to overcome disease-related impediments to drug delivery to their sites of action. In the case of the loop diuretics the common practice is to titrate the dose of the diuretic until the desired response occurs (3[R]). No such titration generally occurs with thiazide-type diuretics; consequently they are likely to fail, although for no reason other than their not being titrated to a truly effective dose. The true basis for "failure" of thiazide-type diuretics in patients with renal insufficiency resides in the fact that these diuretics are not of sufficient maximal efficacy to produce adequate volume control in these typically volume-expanded patients (4[R]).*

However, resistance to loop diuretics can occur, by various mechanisms (5[R]). These include poor compliance, poor absorption, progressive worsening of heart failure, excess volume loss, renal insufficiency, secondary hyperaldosteronism, and hypertrophy of the tubular cells of the distal nephron. Resistance due to inadequate drug absorption – either its speed or extent – is common with furosemide, which is poorly absorbed (3[R]). Once recognized, this hurdle to response can be overcome by using loop diuretics that are predictably well absorbed, such as bumetanide and torasemide, or by giving intravenous furosemide (6[R]).

If loop diuretics fail to produce the desired diuretic response, combination diuretic therapy can be considered., by adding a thiazide or a thiazide-like diuretic, such as metolazone. Such combinations are generally quite successful in both advanced congestive heart failure and late-stage chronic renal insufficiency, although excessive diuresis is a constant risk with such combinations. An excess diuresis with combination loop plus thiazide diuretic therapy is best managed by temporarily withdrawing both diuretics. Generally, diuretic doses are reduced when therapy is resumed (7[R]).

An alternative in the diuretic-resistant patient is the use of continuous infusions of loop diuretics rather than bolus diuretic therapy. Such infusions can also be given with a small volume of hypertonic saline, with good effect (8[C]). The reasons why continuous infusions of loop diuretics work when bolus doses have failed may relate to a more efficient time-course of diuretic delivery and/or less activation of the renin–angiotensin system (9[R]). Furosemide and torasemide may be the safest loop diuretics to be given as infusions, in that infusion of bumetanide has been associated with severe musculoskeletal symptoms (10[A]).

The importance of volume control in patients with renal insufficiency extends beyond its

Side Effects of Drugs, Annual 25
J.K. Aronson, ed.

effect on blood pressure. Accordingly, the addition of hydrochlorothiazide can overcome the blunting by a high sodium intake of the therapeutic efficacy of ACE inhibition on proteinuria (11[c]). This presumably relates to volume-related activation of the renin–angiotensin system.

Finally, loop diuretics reduce the metabolic demand of tubular cells, reducing oxygen requirements and thereby, in theory, increasing resistance to ischemic insults and perhaps other toxic circumstances. This property has been advanced as the basis for using diuretics in acute renal insufficiency. Although an attractive hypothesis to date, there is no compelling evidence to suggest any benefit from loop diuretics in established acute renal insufficiency. Alternatively, loop diuretics can convert oliguric to non-oliguric acute renal insufficiency, thereby easing the fluid restriction that would otherwise be necessary in such patients (12[R]).

Aldosterone receptor antagonists *Recent observations have suggested that it is no longer appropriate to consider the endocrine or paracrine properties of aldosterone as being restricted to the classical target cells. Hemodynamic and humoral actions of aldosterone have important clinical implications for the pathogenesis of progressive renal disease, and may therefore affect future antihypertensive strategies. Initially, one might anticipate that the adverse effects of aldosterone could be attenuated merely by blocking aldosterone release with either an ACE inhibitor or angiotensin-II receptor antagonists. However, this appears not to be the case. Several investigators have now shown that ACE inhibitors acutely reduce aldosterone concentrations, but that with continued use this suppression fades. Thus, the presumption that ACE inhibitors would suppress the production of both aldosterone and angiotensin-II was incorrect. So, although ACE inhibitors and angiotensin-II receptor antagonists are individually very effective in retarding disease progression, additional benefit may be realized with a concurrent aldosterone receptor antagonist. As observed in clinical studies of congestive heart failure, as well as in animals with renal disease, antagonism of aldosterone receptors protects against end-organ damage through a combination of both hemodynamic and direct cellular actions (13[R]).*

An important consideration regarding the feasibility of aldosterone receptor antagonist therapy in chronic renal insufficiency is the risk of provoking hyperkalemia. Many patients with chronic renal insufficiency are already taking an ACE inhibitor or an angiotensin-II receptor antagonist, with the attendant risk of hyperkalemia. Despite such concerns, the results of the RALES trial have been reassuring (14[C]). In that study, patients taking an ACE inhibitor who were randomized to spironolactone 25–50 mg/day had only a 0.3 mmol/l increase in median potassium concentration. Although the difference between the spironolactone and placebo groups was statistically significant, the mean increase was not clinically important, and the incidence of serious hyperkalemia was minimal in both groups of patients.

Although it is an effective aldosterone receptor antagonist, spironolactone is limited by its tendency to cause undesirable sexual adverse effects. At standard doses, impotence and gynecomastia can occur in men, whereas premenopausal women can have menstrual disturbances. These adverse effects, caused by the binding of spironolactone to progesterone and androgen receptors, are substantial causes of drug discontinuation. In the RALES study there was a 10% incidence of gynecomastia or breast pain in men, compared with 1% with placebo, and significantly more patients discontinued treatment (2% vs 0.2%). Although troublesome, these adverse effects are reversible and dose-related. The advent of selective aldosterone receptor antagonists, such as eplerenone, should reduce these adverse effects and thereby improve patient compliance.

CARBONIC ANHYDRASE INHIBITORS *(SED-14, 669; SEDA-22, 236; SEDA-23, 229; SEDA-24, 249)*

Hematologic Recommendations for hematological monitoring of patients taking oral carbonic anhydrase inhibitors are a source of conflict and debate. *Aplastic anemia* as an adverse effect of oral carbonic anhydrase inhibitors occurs in about 1 in 18 000 patient-years of exposure. Most cases occur within the first 6 months, and peak at 2–3 months. The National Registry of Drug-Induced Ocular Side Effects has not received a report of blood dyscrasias in patients who have taken oral carbonic anhydrase inhibitors for less than 2 weeks (15[M]). Since there is generally some time before abnormal blood counts progress to bone-marrow failure, seeking a symptomless "early window" is precisely the point of routine hematological screening; thus, patients taking long-term oral carbonic anhydrase inhibitors should have erythrocyte, leukocyte, and platelet counts bimonthly during the first 6 months of therapy and then every 6 months thereafter. Routine hematological surveillance should always be accompanied by patient education about warning signs and symptoms of progressive marrow failure.

Acetazolamide

Acid-base balance Acetazolamide can cause a *metabolic acidosis* by inhibiting bicarbonate reabsorption. This effect is of particular use in treating patients with chronic respiratory acidosis with superimposed metabolic alkalosis. Life-threatening metabolic acidosis is rarely observed in the absence of renal insufficiency and/or diabetes mellitus. In three patients with central nervous system pathology alone conventional doses of acetazolamide resulted in severe metabolic acidosis (16[A]). After withdrawal it took up to 48 hours for the metabolic acidosis and accompanying hyperventilation to resolve.

Immunologic *Fatal anaphylactic shock* with massive pulmonary edema has been reported in a 66-year-old woman who was using acetazolamide for glaucoma (17[A]). She had a history of sulfonamide allergy, and acetazolamide is a sulfonamide derivative. Sulfonamide allergy should be regarded as a contraindication to acetazolamide.

Dorzolamide

Sensory systems A 68-year-old woman developed bilateral *marginal keratitis* 2 weeks after starting to use dorzolamide eye-drops (18[A]). One week after withdrawal she was asymptomatic with complete resolution of her corneal infiltrates. In this case the allergic reaction was caused by dorzolamide hydrochloride and not the preservative, benzalkonium chloride, since therapy was uneventfully continued with timolol maleate, which also contains benzalkonium chloride as a preservative. This is the first report of this phenomenon with a carbonic anhydrase inhibitor.

THIAZIDE-LIKE AND LOOP DIURETICS *(SED-14, 656; SEDA-23, 228; SEDA-24, 250)*

Sensory systems Transient *myopia* associated with diffuse choroidal thickening has been described in a 38-year-old white man who had taken indapamide for hypertension; it resolved after withdrawal (19[A]).

Sensorineural hearing loss occurs in a small proportion of very premature babies. Various causative mechanisms have been suggested, including bilirubin, drugs, infection, and/or hypoxic brainstem injury. In a case-control study of 15 children and 30 controls born before 33 weeks of gestation, renal insufficiency and/or aminoglycoside use in conjunction with furosemide was associated with sensorineural hearing loss (20[c]).

Metabolism It has been stated that indapamide has fewer adverse metabolic effects than hydrochlorothiazide. If that were true it might justify the substantial difference in the costs of the two drugs. The metabolic effects of hydrochlorothiazide 25 mg/day and indapamide 2.5 mg/day for 6 months have been compared in a randomized, double-blind study in 44 patients with mild to moderate hypertension (21[C]). There was little difference between the effects of the drugs on a wide range of lipid parameters, glucose, and potassium. The purported metabolic differences with indapamide are unlikely to be of sufficient magnitude to warrant its preferential use in hyperlipidemia.

Nutrition Patients with congestive heart failure taking high doses of furosemide can develop *thiamine deficiency*, which is improved by thiamine supplementation, but it is unclear whether thiamine supplementation has a role in the management of congestive cardiac failure. More precise analytical methods have now suggested that there is whole-blood thiamine phosphate deficiency, but no reduction in the storage form of thiamine, thiamine diphosphate. These observations suggest that thiamine supplementation may not be necessary in elderly patients taking furosemide for congestive heart failure (22[M]).

Electrolyte balance *Hyponatremia* is the most common electrolyte abnormality in the general hospital population and is associated with a wide range of diseases and a variety of drugs. Acute hyponatremic encephalopathy can develop rapidly with diuretics, particularly thiazides. Women, patients with hypokalemia, and those with a low sodium and/or solute intake are particularly susceptible to diuretic-induced hyponatremia. Severe hyponatremia (115 mmol/l) occurred in a 69-year-old woman who took only two doses of hydrochlorothiazide 25 mg (23[A]).

Metal metabolism *Hypomagnesemia* is common with both loop and thiazide diuretics and occurred in 19.4% of 242 patients (24[c]). It was corrected with potassium–magnesium citrate, whereas potassium citrate or potassium chloride alone had little corrective effect.

Diuretic-induced hypomagnesemia is of particular relevance to patients with congestive heart failure (25[R]). There is a reduced rate of sudden cardiac death in patients who take long-term diuretic therapy when potassium- and magnesium-sparing diuretics and/or magnesium supplements are also used. All potassium-sparing diuretics are also magnesium-sparing, and diuretic-induced hypokalemia is difficult to correct unless underlying magnesium deficiency is also addressed (26[c]).

Urinary tract There is an association between diuretic use and *renal cell carcinoma* (27[M]). Some of the studies that support this association can be dismissed, since the epidemiological data on which they were based were not suitably adjusted for confounding variables, including obesity, hypertension, age, and cigarette smoking. However, other case-control studies have shown a small risk of renal cell carcinoma in patients taking long-term diuretics after adjustment of the data for potentially confounding variables. The carcinogenic mechanism of diuretics is not know, but could be related to a carcinogenic action of *N*-nitroso metabolic derivatives of thiazide and loop diuretics or structural changes in the transporting tubular epithelia, which provoke different stages of apoptosis. The available information does not support a change in current prescription practices for diuretics in the treatment of hypertension and cardiac failure. Physicians should be more concerned about controlling blood pressure rather than concerning themselves with what at best might be a small risk of renal cell carcinoma.

Four children with the nephrotic syndrome developed transient *hypercalciuria* and *intraluminal calcification* in renal histopathological specimens without radiological evidence of renal calcification. These children were resistant to corticosteroids and were receiving furosemide plus albumin for the management of edema (28[A]). This result stresses the pervasive effect of furosemide, and probably all loop diuretics, in increasing urinary calcium excretion, with resultant nephrocalcinosis. Whenever possible, steps should be taken to limit the hypercalciuric effect of loop diuretics. Such maneuvers could include limiting the sodium content of the diet and/or combining the loop diuretic with a thiazide diuretic.

Skin A 60-year-old man with a history of renal insufficiency and hypertension, treated with hydrochlorothiazide, furosemide, and amiloride, developed *pellagroid dermatitis* involving light-exposed areas (29[A]). The pigmentation disappeared slowly after withdrawal of hydrochlorothiazide and amiloride. There has also been a report of hydrochlorothiazide-related allergic photodermatitis, just one of many cases that have been reported with hydrochlorothiazide, which is a well-known photoallergen (30[A]).

A man developed acute generalized exanthematous pustulosis while taking furosemide (31[A]). A positive lymphocyte transformation test suggested an immunological mechanism.

Furosemide has also been associated with *disseminated superficial porokeratosis*, a heritable disorder of cornification, in a man (32[A]).

Immunologic Thiazides and some loop diuretics are often avoided in patients with a prior history of sulfonamide allergy. It has long been thought that loop and thiazide diuretics pose a theoretical risk of cross-sensitivity in patients with sulfonamide allergy because of their common structures. However, the available literature does not provide sufficient numbers of well-documented cases to support this impression (33[A]). It seems that careful administration of loop diuretics is permissible in patients with documented sulfonamide allergy, but as always such a drug challenge should not be attempted without careful follow-up.

Torasemide is loop diuretic with few adverse effects. Two possible cases of *vasculitis* with renal insufficiency have been reported (34[A], 35[A]). Drugs cause 10% of all cases of hypersensitivity vasculitis. Although this adverse reaction has not been previously reported with torasemide, it is not surprising, since its chemical structure is similar to that of other sulfa drugs, which can cause vasculitis.

Drug interactions The value of low doses of thiazide diuretics in the management of hypertension is well attested, and low doses of diuretics have synergistic actions with other antihypertensive drug classes, including the *angiotensin-II receptor antagonists* (36[c]–38[c]). It still is unclear what represents the optimal dose of a thiazide diuretic in combination with either an ACE inhibitor or an angiotensin-II receptor antagonist. The addition of an angiotensin-II receptor antagonist to diuretic therapy also seems to blunt the associated electrolyte disturbances. In particular, hydrochlorothiazide-induced hyperuricemia is specifically attenuated by losartan (39[c]).

ALDOSTERONE RECEPTOR ANTAGONISTS *(SED-14, 674; SEDA-22, 229; SEDA-23, 239; SEDA-24, 251)*

Spironolactone

Electrolyte balance The beneficial effects of spironolactone in congestive cardiac failure and hypertension are additive to those of ACE inhibitors. In the RALES trial patients taking an ACE inhibitor who were randomized to spironolactone 25–50 mg/day had only a 0.3 mmol/l increase in median potassium concentration (14[C]). Although the difference between the spironolactone and placebo groups was statistically significant, the mean increase was not clinically important, and the incidence of serious *hyperkalemia* was minimal in both groups of patients.

However, it is essential to identify patients who are likely to develop serious hyperkalemia during combined treatment and to evaluate the associated morbidity and mortality. The effects of ACE inhibitors plus spironolactone have been evaluated in 25 patients (11 men, 14 women, mean age 74 years, five with diabetes mellitus) with a mean serum potassium concentration of 7.7 mmol/l (40[R]). The mean serum creatinine was 336 μmol/l, the mean arterial pH 7.3, and the mean plasma bicarbonate 18 mmol/l. The main causes of acute renal insufficiency were dehydration ($n = 12$) and worsening heart failure ($n = 9$). The mean dose of spironolactone was 57 mg/day and 12 patients were also taking other drugs that can cause hyperkalemia. Two patients died and two were resuscitated and survived. Hemodialysis was necessary in 17 patients. The mean duration of hospitalization was 12 days. The combination of ACE inhibitors and spironolactone should be used cautiously in patients with chronic renal insufficiency, diabetes, older age, worsening cardiac failure, a risk of dehydration (e.g. diarrhea), and in those who are taking other drugs that can cause hyperkalemia (41[A]). A dose of spironolactone of 25 mg/day should be exceeded only with caution. In four similar elderly patients with underlying renal insufficiency taking spironolactone there was an increased risk of hyperkalemia associated with diarrhea (42[c]).

Hematologic *Agranulocytosis* has been reported in an 87-year-old man with congestive heart failure who took spironolactone 25 mg/day for 3 weeks (43[A]). The agranulocytosis rapidly reversed after withdrawal of spironolactone and a short course of granulocyte-colony-stimulating-factor. In general, the onset of agranulocytosis with spironolactone ranges from 4 days to 5 weeks and it takes 5–7 days to resolve without the aid of a growth factor. With the renewed interest in spironolactone an increased awareness of this rare adverse effect is needed, because it is potentially reversible if identified early.

REFERENCES

1. Brenner BM, Cooper ME, De Zeeuw D, Keane WF, Mitch WE, Parving HH, Remuzzi G, Snapinn SM, Zhang Z, Shahinfar S. Effects of losartan on renal and cardiovascular outcomes in patients with type 2 diabetes and nephropathy. New Engl J Med 2001; 345: 861–9.
2. Lewis EJ, Hunsicker LG, Clarke WR, Berl T, Pohl MA, Lewis JB, Ritz E, Atkins RC, Rohde R, Raz I. Renoprotective effect of the angiotensin-receptor antagonist irbesartan in patients with nephropathy due to type 2 diabetes. New Engl J Med 2001; 345: 851–60.
3. Brater DC. Diuretic therapy. New Engl J Med 1998; 339: 387-95.
4. Schwenger V, Zeier M, Ritz E. Antihypertensive therapy in renal patients–benefits and difficulties. Nephron 1999; 83: 202–13.
5. Grahame-Smith DG. The Lilly Prize Lecture 1996. "Keep on taking the tablets": pharmacological adaptation during long-term drug therapy. Br J Clin Pharmacol 1997; 44: 227–38.
6. Knauf H, Mutschler E. Clinical pharmacokinetics and pharmacodynamics of torasemide. Clin Pharmacokinet 1998; 34: 1–24.
7. Sica DA, Gehr TW. Diuretic combinations in refractory oedema states: pharmacokinetic–pharmacodynamic relationships. Clin Pharmacokinet 1996; 30: 229–49.
8. Paterna S, Di Pasquale P, Parrinello G, Amato P, Cardinale A, Follone G, Giubilato A, Licata G. Effects of high-dose furosemide and small-volume hypertonic saline solution infusion in comparison with a high dose of furosemide as a bolus, in refractory congestive heart failure. Eur J Heart Fail 2000; 2: 305–13.
9. Ravnan SL, Ravnan MC. Management of adult heart failure: bolus versus continuous infusion loop diuretics, a review of the literature. Hosp Pharm 2000; 35: 832–6.
10. Howard PA, Dunn MI. Severe musculoskeletal symptoms during continuous infusion of bumetanide. Chest 1997; 111: 359–64.
11. Buter H, Hemmelder MH, Navis G, De Jong PE, De Zeeuw D. The blunting of the antiproteinuric efficacy of ACE inhibition by high sodium intake can be restored by hydrochlorothiazide. Nephrol Dial Transplant 1998; 13: 1682–5.
12. Dishart MK, Kellum JA. An evaluation of pharmacological strategies for the prevention and treatment of acute renal failure. Drugs 2000; 59: 79–91.
13. Epstein M. Aldosterone as a mediator of progressive renal disease: pathogenetic and clinical implications. Am J Kidney Dis 2001; 37: 677–88.
14. Pitt B, Zannad F, Remme WJ, Cody R, Castaigne A, Perez A, Palensky J, Wittes J. The effect of spironolactone on morbidity and mortality in patients with severe heart failure. New Engl J Med 1999; 341: 709–17.
15. Fraunfelder FT, Bagby GC. Monitoring patients taking oral carbonic anhydrase inhibitors. Am J Ophthalmol 2000; 130: 221–3.
16. Venkatesha SL, Umamaheswara Rao GS. Metabolic acidosis and hyperventilation induced by acetazolamide in patients with central nervous system pathology. Anesthesiology 2000; 93: 1546–8.
17. Gerhards LJ, Van Arnhem AC, Holman ND, Nossent GD. Fatal anaphylactic reaction after oral acetazolamide (Diamox) for glaucoma. Ned Tijdschr Geneeskd 2000; 144: 1228–30.
18. Taguri AH, Khan MA, Sanders R. Marginal keratitis: an uncommon form of topical dorzolamide allergy. Am J Ophthalmol 2000; 130: 120–2.
19. Blain P, Paques M, Massin P, Erginay A, Santiago P, Gaudric A. Acute transient myopia induced by indapamide. Am J Ophthalmol 2000; 129: 538–40.
20. Marlow ES, Hunt LP, Marlow N. Sensorineural hearing loss and prematurity. Arch Dis Child Fetal Neonatal Ed 2000; 82: F141–4.
21. Spence JD, Huff M, Barnett PA. Effects of indapamide versus hydrochlorothiazide on plasma lipids and lipoproteins in hypertensive patients: a direct comparison. Can J Clin Pharmacol 2000; 7: 32–7.
22. Hardig L, Daae C, Dellborg M, Kontny F, Bohmer T. Reduced thiamine phosphate, but not thiamine diphosphate, in erythrocytes in elderly patients with congestive heart failure treated with furosemide. J Intern Med 2000; 247: 597–600.
23. Al-Salman J, Pursell R. Hyponatremic encephalopathy induced by thiazides. West J Med 2001; 175: 87.
24. Pak CY. Correction of thiazide-induced hypomagnesemia by potassium-magnesium citrate from review of prior trials. Clin Nephrol 2000; 54: 271–5.
25. Seelig MS. Interrelationship of magnesium and congestive heart failure. Wien Med Wochenschr 2000; 150: 335–41.
26. Cohen N, Alon I, Almoznino-Sarafian D, Zaidenstein R, Weissgarten J, Gorelik O, Berman S, Modai D, Golik A. Metabolic and clinical effects of oral magnesium supplementation in furosemide-treated patients with severe congestive heart failure. Clin Cardiol 2000; 23: 433–6.
27. Schmieder RE, Delles C, Messerli FH. Diuretic therapy and the risk for renal cell carcinoma. J Nephrol 2000; 13: 343–6.
28. Mocan H, Yildiran A, Camlibel T, Kuzey GM. Microscopic nephrocalcinosis and hypercalciuria in nephrotic syndrome. Hum Pathol 2000; 31: 1363–7.
29. Stingeni L, Hansel K, Lisi P. Pellagroid allergic photodermatitis induced by hydrochlorothiazide. Ann Ital Dermatol Clin Sper 2000; 54: 36–8.
30. Wagner SN, Welke F, Goos M. Occupational UVA-induced allergic photodermatitis in a welder due to hydrochlorothiazide and ramipril. Contact Dermatitis 2000; 43: 245–6.
31. Noce R, Paredes BE, Pichler WJ, Krahen-

buhl S. Acute generalized exanthematic pustulosis (AGEP) in a patient treated with furosemide. Am J Med Sci 2000; 320: 331–3.
32. Kroiss MM, Stolz W, Hohenleutner U, Landthaler M. Disseminated superficial porokeratosis induced by furosemide. Acta Derm Venereol 2000; 80: 52–3.
33. Phipatanakul W, Adkinson NF Jr. Cross-reactivity between sulfonamides and loop or thiazide diuretics: a theoretical or actual risk? Allergy Clin Immunol Int 2000; 12: 26–8.
34. Palop-Larrea V, Sancho-Calabuig A, Gorriz-Teruel JL, Martinez-Mir I, Pallardo-Mateu LM. Vasculitis with acute kidney failure and torasemide. Lancet 1998; 352: 1909–10.
35. Sanfelix-Genoves J, Benlloch-Nieto H, Verdu-Tarraga R, Costa-Alcaraz AM. Erupcion purpurica compatible con vasculitis y torasemida. Aten Primaria 1998; 21: 252–3.
36. Ohman KP, Milon H, Valnes K. Efficacy and tolerability of a combination tablet of candesartan cilexetil and hydrochlorothiazide in insufficiently controlled primary hypertension–comparison with a combination of losartan and hydrochlorothiazide. Blood Press 2000; 9: 214–20.
37. Scholze J, Probst G, Bertsch K. Valsartan alone and in combination with hydrochlorothiazide in general practice. Clin Drug Invest 2000; 20: 1–7.
38. Koenig W. Comparison of the efficacy and tolerability of combination tablets containing candesartan cilexetil or losartan and hydrochlorothiazide in patients with moderate to severe hypertension. Results of the CARLOS-Study. Clin Drug Invest 2000; 19: 239–46.
39. Manolis AJ, Grossman E, Jelakovic B, Jacovides A, Bernhardi DC, Cabrera WJ, Watanabe LA, Barragan J, Matadamas N, Mendiola A, Woo KS, Zhu JR, Mejia AD, Bunt T, Dumortier T, Smith RD. Effects of losartan and candesartan monotherapy and losartan/hydrochlorothiazide combination therapy in patients with mild to moderate hypertension. Losartan Trial Investigators. Clin Ther 2000; 22: 1186–203.
40. Schepkens H, Vanholder R, Billiouw JM, Lameire N. Life-threatening hyperkalemia during combined therapy with angiotensin-converting enzyme inhibitors and spironolactone: an analysis of 25 cases. Am J Med 2001; 110: 438–41.
41. Vanpee D, Swine CH. Elderly heart failure patients with drug-induced serious hyperkalemia. Aging (Milano) 2000; 12: 315–19.
42. Berry C, McMurray JJ. Serious adverse events experienced by patients with chronic heart failure taking spironolactone. Heart 2001; 85: E8.
43. Hui CH, Das PK, Horvath N. Spironolactone and agranulocytosis. Aust NZ J Med 2000; 30: 515.

Gijsbert B. van der Voet and Frederik A. de Wolff

22 Metals

ALUMINIUM *(SED-14, 683; SEDA-22, 242; SEDA-23, 231; SEDA-24, 253)*

Aluminium is found in medications for antacid therapy and phosphate depletion; alternatives are under investigation (1[R]). It is also still used as a vaccine adjuvant (2[R]).

Many aluminium salts, including aluminium hydroxide gel, aluminium carbonate, aluminium glycinate, and aluminosilicate, are used therapeutically, and the absorption rate depends on the chemical species. Aluminium citrate is well absorbed (3[r]), but aluminium hydroxide gel antacid is poorly absorbed (0.003%) (4[r]). Aluminium glycinate is well absorbed and excreted in the urine. Poorly absorbed aluminium-containing formulations should be preferred in elderly people, who have poor renal function.

Respiratory Aluminium is also increasingly widely used in modern consumer products. It is obtained from bauxite ores by the production of alumina, which is then smelted to produce aluminium. A syndrome known as *pot-room asthma* occurs in around 2% of new aluminium smelters each year, with a wide range of incidence around the world (5[R]).

In 1529 men in two smelting factories, work-related respiratory symptoms were reported significantly more often among the ingot mill, anode, and pot-room groups in factory A after adjusting for age and smoking, while in factory B ingot employees were more likely to report work-related wheeze and pot-room employees were more likely to report work-related rhinitis (6[C]). Symptoms tended to increase with increasing time in the pot-rooms, but were more likely to occur in new employees in the ingot mill and anode process groups.

Side Effects of Drugs, Annual 25
J.K. Aronson, ed.

Nervous system The toxicology of aluminium in the brain has recently been reviewed (7[R]).

The relation between aluminium and *Alzheimer's disease* continues to be discussed. According to Munoz and Feldman (8[R]) the theory that aluminium plays a role in the pathogenesis of Alzheimer's disease has been largely discarded as our understanding of the pathogenic mechanisms of Alzheimer's disease has advanced.

However, the relation between different chemical forms of aluminium in drinking water and Alzheimer's disease has been studied in 68 patients with Alzheimer's disease diagnosed according to recognized criteria and paired for age and sex with non-demented controls (9[C]). Aluminium speciation was assessed using established standard analytical protocols along with quality control procedures (total aluminium, total dissolved aluminium, monomeric organic aluminium, monomeric inorganic aluminium, polymeric aluminium, Al^{3+}, AlOH, AlF, $AlH_3SiO_4{}^{2+}$, $AlSO_4$). The results suggested a possible association between monomeric aluminium exposition and Alzheimer's disease. In contrast to the results of earlier studies, this association was observed in a geographical environment characterized by low aluminium concentrations and a high pH.

Risk factors Aluminium slowly accumulates in patients on long-term *hemodialysis* and can cause various clinical effects, including osteomalacia (10[c]), bone and joint pain and muscular weakness (11[c]), iron-resistant microcytic anemia (12[c]), and neurological disorders (13[c]).

In 33 patients on hemodialysis, who were exposed to moderately high serum aluminium concentrations for less than 4 months, even moderately high aluminium concentrations produced significant hematological alterations and depletion of body iron stores before clinical manifestations were evident (14[C]).

ANTIMONY *(SED-14, 685; SEDA-24, 254)*

Urinary tract *Septic shock with oliguria* developed soon after the first intramuscular administration of meglumine antimoniate 20 mg/kg (equivalent to 510 mg of antimony) to a patient with visceral leishmaniasis and normal renal function (15[A]). Creatinine clearance fell to 23 ml/min. Treatment was withdrawn, and antimony urinary excretion was measured. After the initial dose, 500 mg of antimony was recovered in the urine over 8 days (98% of the dose); 66% was eliminated within the first 48 hours. Nine days after the dose, meglumine antimoniate was reintroduced in a dosage of 11.7 mg/kg (equivalent to 300 mg of antimony) every 48 hours, with good tolerance. At that time creatinine clearance had returned to 88 ml/min. By day 14 of therapy the dosage interval was reduced to 24 hours and from day 17 to day 31 the dosage was increased to 16.6 mg/kg/day (equivalent to 425 mg of antimony). The patient eventually completely recovered, with normal renal function. Although there are no specific guidelines for dosage adjustment in renal insufficiency, monitoring antimony urinary excretion indicates that the kidneys are the almost exclusive route of elimination.

ARSENIC *(SED-14, 686; SEDA-22, 243; SEDA-23, 232; SEDA-24, 254)*

Arsenic is sometimes used in the treatment of leukemia (16[R]) and is increasingly found as a contaminant in herbal medicine formulations (17[R]).

Hematologic Arsenic trioxide is a new investigational agent for the treatment of relapsed or refractory acute promyelocytic leukemia. *Leukocytosis* has been commonly noted, but this adverse effect usually resolves spontaneously and is generally not treated; to date, no deaths have been reported.

A 27-year-old woman (18[A]) with acute promyelocytic leukemia was given arsenic trioxide 0.15 mg/kg/day intravenously. Her white cell count was 8.2×10^9/l; after two doses it rose to 15×10^9/l and after three doses to 21×10^9/l. The white blood cell count continued to rise to 101×10^9/l on day 7 and 213×10^9/l on day 8; the platelet count was 61×10^9/l. Arsenic trioxide was withdrawn. Later that day she became confused with slurred speech and right-sided weakness. A CT scan showed a left middle cerebral artery infarct. Twelve hours later she had a generalized seizure. The white blood cell count was now 292×10^9/l and chemotherapy with idarubicin and cytarabine was started. She continued to deteriorate and died on day 15.

Liver *Liver damage* has been attributed to arsenic (19[A]).

A 50-year-old man developed upper gastrointestinal bleeding, with no history of alcohol abuse, viral hepatitis, hepatotoxic drugs, or any family history of liver disease. He had thalassemia minor and psoriasis, for which he had taken Fowler's solution, 2 ml/day for 5 years. Fowler's solution is a solution of potassium arsenite that contains 10 mg of arsenic trioxide. He had palmar and plantar hyperkeratosis, splenomegaly, and signs of hypovolemia, normal liver function tests, negative viral serological markers and autoantibodies, and high arsenic excretion in the urine. Abdominal ultrasonography and color Doppler showed marked wall thickening of the portal vein and its intrahepatic branches, with signs of portal hypertension and partial splenic vein thrombosis. Endoscopy showed grade III esophageal varices, with signs of recent bleeding. Liver biopsy showed venous wall hyperplasia, with signs of cellular regeneration tending toward a focal nodular pattern and terminal hepatic vein fibrosis. The wedge hepatic pressure was 12 mmHg and the free hepatic venous pressure 5 mmHg; splenoportography confirmed partial obstruction of the splenic vein.

Skin Human papillomavirus has been implicated as a co-factor in the pathogenesis of arsenic-induced *skin tumors* (20[A]).

A 38-year-old Pakistani woman developed verrucose papules on her palms and soles 3 years after she had been treated orally with a herbal solution by a travelling Indian doctor for a period of 12 months for "white spot disease". She had widespread depigmented macules on the trunk and limbs, suggestive of vitiligo, and multiple hyperkeratotic papules on her palms and soles, some of which were coalescing into large leathery plaques. Histological examination showed compact hyperkeratosis, intermittent columns of parakeratosis, and an akanthotic epidermis with minor nuclear atypicality. Polymerase chain reaction analysis with degenerate primers identified an atypical human papillomavirus; sequencing showed an RX-variant of HPV, type 23. There were no other signs of chronic arsenic intoxication, and clinical, radiographic, and laboratory investigations showed no evidence of an internal malignancy.

BISMUTH *(SED-14, 686; SEDA-22, 243; SEDA-23, 232; SEDA-24, 255)*

Bismuth compounds, such as ranitidine bismuth citrate, are sometimes used to treat *Helicobacter pylori* infection (21[R]). Bismuth subsalicylate is used to treat collagenous colitis (22[A]). Bismuth compounds are also used as hemostatic compounds (23[A]).

Respiratory Two cases of *respiratory complications* following the use of bismuth gallate have been reported (23[A]).

A 19-month-old boy with reactive airways disease had a tonsillectomy and adenoidectomy, and bismuth-coated sponges were used for hemostasis. Excessive bleeding was not reported. In the recovery room he developed difficulty in breathing, and required oxygen followed by bronchodilators and deep suctioning. A chest X-ray showed speckled opacities throughout the lung fields and in the oropharynx and nasopharynx, probably due to aspiration of bismuth particles. He went on to develop a pneumonitis.

An 8-year-old girl with asthma underwent tonsillectomy and adenoidectomy; hemostasis was performed with bismuth–adrenaline paste. A small amount of bismuth was noted in the endotracheal tube before extubation, and in the recovery room she developed respiratory difficulty associated with nasal flaring and sternal retraction. A chest X-ray showed aspirated radiopaque material outlining the tracheobronchial tree and early pulmonary infiltrates.

Both patients had a history of refractory airway disease that put them at risk of respiratory complications after bismuth aspiration. Fortunately neither developed any serious respiratory compromise immediately after aspiration or required intubation.

CHROMIUM *(SED-14, 683; SEDA-22, 242; SEDA-23, 231; SEDA-24, 255)*

The essentiality of chromium continues to be discussed (24[R]). The biochemistry of chromium has recently been reviewed (25[R]). Chromium picolinate may aid muscle insulin sensitivity, and initial reports suggest that it is an effective therapy for non-insulin-dependent diabetes (26[R]). Chromium picolinate supplementation alone does not improve insulin sensitivity (27[R]).

Psychiatric There have been three reports of the efficacy of chromium in depression, with adverse effects, including *dizzy spells* and *vivid dreams* (28[A]).

A 50-year-old man developed bipolar II disorder with the onset of a major depressive episode in his late twenties. His mood stabilized with lithium, but he continued to have periods of irritability and breakthrough depression. He took chromium picolinate 400 μg/day and within 2 days felt more relaxed and stable than he had since the onset of his disorder. He discontinued the lithium. Several months later he forgot to take his chromium, and within a few days his symptoms returned. In order to catch up he took 800 μg/day and developed sweating each morning and a mild hand tremor. After reducing the dosage to 600 μg/day he again went into complete remission. After more than 1 year of chromium treatment he developed uric acid kidney stones. One year after switching to a different chromium salt (polynicotinate), there was no recurrence of kidney stones.

A 38-year-old man with bipolar II disorder took chromium polynicotinate 400 μg/day. Shortly after the first dose his mood started to improve, but he had unusually vivid intense dreams. The dose of chromium was increased to 600 μg/day. He then developed intermittent brief dizzy spells due to orthostatic hypotension. After switching to chromium picolinate his dizzy spells did not recur.

A 47-year-old man with a dysthymic disorder and intermittent panic attacks and rage outbursts took chromium 400 μg/day, and after 1 day had strikingly vivid dreams. Over the next several days there was a dramatic improvement in his mood and behavior. The efficacy of chromium was later confirmed by a double-blind, placebo-controlled, n-of-1 trial.

Immunologic Chromium has been reported to cause *dermatitis* when ingested (29[A]).

A 35-year-old man developed a subacute dermatitis with scattered patches of erythema and scaling on the lower legs, ankles, hands, and wrists. He had no history of atopy but a prior history of allergy to a leather watch-strap. He had taken various oral vitamin and mineral formulations for several weeks. Patch testing showed reactions to potassium dichromate at 48 and 96 hours.

COPPER *(SED-14, 688; SEDA-22, 244; SEDA-23, 233; SEDA-24, 256)*

Developments in copper research continue (30[R]), including developments in the study of Menkes' disease and Wilson's disease (31[R]). The medical uses of copper are limited to oral or parenteral nutrition and copper-containing intrauterine contraceptive devices.

GALLIUM *(SED-14, 690; SEDA-22, 244; SEDA-23, 234; SEDA-24, 256)*

Gallium compounds (^{67}Ga) are used in biomedical imaging (32[R]) and in the treatment of cancer (gallium nitrate). Gallium is also used in dental prostheses and is a source of increased sensitivity to postoperative dental pain (33[R]).

GOLD *(SED-14, 690; SEDA-22, 245; SEDA-23, 234; SEDA-24, 257)*

Dental gold alloys continue to be used and remain a source of *contact hypersensitivity* (34[C]). Gold compounds are commonly used in the treatment of rheumatoid arthritis. *Leukopenia* and *liver damage* has been reported (35[A]).

A 62-year-old woman with rheumatoid arthritis developed swelling and pain of both knees. Aurothiomalate was given in a test dose of 12.5 mg, followed the next day by a dose of 25 mg, and then 50 mg twice weekly (total cumulative dose 137.5 mg). She had a leukocyte count of 2.2×10^9/l, a normochromic anemia, and a normal platelet count. Her liver enzyme activities were raised. Aurothiomalate was withdrawn and about 6 weeks later her liver function tests returned to normal and her white cell count rose to 6.9×10^9/l.

IRON *(SED-14, 697; SEDA-22, 246; SEDA-23, 235; SEDA-24, 257)*

Respiratory *Acute respiratory distress syndrome* has been attributed to iron (36[A]).

A 3.5-year-old girl was admitted after accidental ingesting 50–60 tablets of ferrous sulfate 200 mg. She was unresponsive and her serum iron concentration was 138 μmol/l. She required resuscitation and ventilation and an intravenous infusion of deferoxamine was started at a rate of 15 mg/kg/hour, reducing to 5 mg/kg/hour 20 hours later, when the iron concentration was 27 μmol/l. At that time, her liver function deteriorated, with raised aminotransferase activity (AlT 57 IU/L), bilirubin (56 μmol/l), and a coagulopathy with an INR of 2.7. She was given an infusion of *N*-acetylcysteine 12.5 mg/kg/hour and her hepatic function stabilized. After about 40 hours she had acute respiratory deterioration with tachypnea and hypoxemia. A chest X-ray showed widespread bilateral infiltrates. A diagnosis of acute respiratory distress syndrome was made.

Hematologic *Thrombocytopenia* has been attributed to intramuscular iron (37[A]).

A 30-year-old woman had a hemoglobin concentration of 3.1 g/daily, a mean cell volume of 77 fl, a reticulocyte count of 2.13%, a platelet count of 426×10^9/l, a serum iron concentration of 5 μg/l, a transferrin saturation of 1%, and a ferritin concentration of 8 μg/l. She was intolerant of oral iron and was given intramuscular iron dextran, 100 mg/day for 8 days, when she developed asymptomatic thrombocytopenia (platelet count 20×10^9/l). Iron dextran was withdrawn, and she took oral ferrous fumarate, 200 mg/day plus ascorbic acid 120 mg/day. Within 2 days her platelet count improved.

Liver *Chronic liver disease* has been attributed to oral iron.

A healthy 5-year-old girl, who had taken large doses of oral ferrous sulfate 300 mg five times a day (300 mg of elemental iron/day) for 5 years, developed severe hemosiderosis (38[A]). Liver biopsy showed preserved lobular architecture, but the portal tracts were expanded by fibrosis and there was mild septal fibrosis. There was siderosis of the hepatic parenchymal cells and hemosiderin deposition in the Kupffer cells. She had no underlying hematological disease and her iron absorption was normal. HLA phenotypes and DNA analysis for the most common mutations associated with hemochromatosis excluded homozygous and heterozygous hereditary hemochromatosis. She was successfully treated by phlebotomy. Iron studies 10 years later were normal.

A 22-year-old woman with adult-onset Still's disease and massive hyperferritinemia became progressively more anemic, with a fall in hemoglobin to 8.2 g/daily, and was given oral ferrous fumarate, 300 mg bd (39[A]). She developed acute florid hepatitis with an intraparenchymatous histiocytic infiltration, which settled on withdrawal of the iron.

In the latter case iron may have exacerbated the macrophage hyperactivity that is presumed to be present in adult-onset Still's disease. Oral iron may be inadvisable in the acute phase of this disease.

Immunologic *Skin reactions* to oral iron are extremely rare. Another case has recently been reported (40[A]).

A 40-year-old woman with iron deficiency anemia due to menstrual blood loss took oral iron for 3 months without any adverse effects. Nine months later she became anemic again and 2 hours after an oral dose of ferrous sulfate 525 mg (105 mg of elemental iron) she developed generalized pruritus and an erythematous maculopapular rash. This recurred 1 week later, when she took ferrous protein succinilate 800 mg (40 mg of iron). Desensitization with oral iron was carried out. Skin prick tests and patch tests with iron formulations were negative. Two single-blind placebo-controlled oral challenges were performed and she began to have similar cutaneous symptoms. A slow desensitization protocol, using increasing doses, was tolerated without adverse effects. Chronic oral iron therapy once a day for 9 months sustained the desensitized state and the anemia disappeared.

LEAD *(SED-14, 701; SEDA-24, 258)*

Nervous system Lead toxicity has been reported in a child who was exposed to lead in a Tibetan herbal remedy (41[A]).

A 5-year-old Indian boy had static encephalopathy, seizures, and developmental delay from neonatal asphyxia and was referred to a hematologist for persistent anemia (hemoglobin 9.2 g/dl) without basophilic stippling, refractory to iron therapy. He was alert and active but non-verbal, able to stand with support but not able to walk, and had no focal neurological defects. Skeletal and abdominal X-rays showed no lead lines and no gastric lead particles. He had normal iron stores and normal hemoglobin electrophoresis. The blood lead concentration was 860 μg/l. He was given EDTA and dimercaprol (BAL), and his lead concentration fell to 256 μg/l. His mother had been giving him a Tibetan herbal vitamin, in the form of tablets, three times a day for the previous 5 years. A traditional medicine healer had told her that the tablets were pure medicinal herbs and plants prepared according to ancient Tibetan pharmacological traditions. They were said to be free from harmful or toxic substances and would actually promote brain growth and improve his mental capabilities. The tablets were produced in India and each was individually wrapped. They were analysed for lead, arsenic, cadmium, and mercury, and it was estimated that he had ingested about 63 g of lead over 4 years. Seven months later his blood lead concentration was 760 μg/l and he was given EDTA and BAL. On day 2 he had a tonic–clonic seizure lasting 1 minute and his urinary lead concentration was 2310 μg/l. On discharge his blood lead concentration was 413 μg/l. During the next 4 years he had a further six chelations with succimer when his lead concentration was over 450 μg/l. After 4 years his lead concentration was 245 μg/l.

MAGNESIUM *(SED-14, 702)*

Drug overdose Magnesium was administered in high doses to a child as part of an alternative regimen of megavitamin/megamineral therapy (42[A]). The treatment was prescribed by an alternative nutritionist without the knowledge of the pediatrician in charge. The child died of *hypermagnesemia*.

MANGANESE *(SED-14, 702; SEDA-22, 246; SEDA-23, 235; SEDA-24, 259)*

Nervous system Workers who have been exposed to manganese, patients with hepatic pathology, and patients undergoing total parenteral nutrition with excessive amounts of manganese (43[R], 44[C]) can accumulate manganese selectively in the globus pallidus of the basal ganglia without immediate neurological effects. Because of its paramagnetic properties manganese can be visualized by MRI, and produces high-intensity, bilateral, symmetrical signals, visible in T1-weighted images. Two indicators of exposure and hyperintensity should be considered: the concentration of manganese in total blood and the pallidal index.

In patients on home patenteral nutrition, sustained inflammation may facilitate *hypermanganesemia* through (1) cholestatic liver disease and thereby reduced manganese biliary excretion, (2) high nutritional requirements (responsible for increased manganese supply), and/or (3) modified manganese metabolism or body distribution (44[C]).

Progressive *myelopathy* is a rare complication of chronic hepatic disease that has never before been reported in children.

A 14-year-old boy presented with progressive hepatic myelopathy caused by cryptogenic micronodular cirrhosis, associated with persistent polycythemia and large increases in whole blood manganese concentration (45[A]). An MRI scan showed manganese deposition in the basal ganglia and other regions of the brain. The liver manganese concentration was raised. Environmental exposure to manganese was investigated and excluded.

Apparently the liver disorder initiated altered manganese metabolism. However, the patient developed neither liver failure nor parkinsonism.

MERCURY *(SED-14, 702; SEDA-22, 247; SEDA-23, 235; SEDA-24, 260)*

Nervous system Mercury poisoning has been reported in a child who took a Chinese herbal medicine (46[A]).

A 5-year-old Chinese boy developed oral ulceration, mainly affecting the left lateral aspect of his tongue, and 5 weeks later motor and vocal tics. Herpetic ulceration was diagnosed and confirmed by the isolation of *Herpes simplex* virus type 1 from a tongue swab. The lesion improved with oral aciclovir (200 mg five times a day for 5 days), but relapsed a few days later. A local pharmacist prescribed a Chinese medicinal herb mouth spray called "Watermelon Frost", said to be useful in controlling pain and healing difficult mucosal wounds. Over the following weeks his oral symptoms improved but he became irritable and cleared his throat frequently. He developed a transient skin rash on his trunk and motor tics (eye blinking, head turning, and shoulder shrugging). His blood lead concentrations was 0.31 μmol/l (normal below 1.5) and his blood manganese concentration was 246 nmol/l (normal 70–280); his urine arsenic concentration was 10 nmol/mmol creatinine (normal <68). His blood mercury concentration was 83 nmol/l (normal for adults <50). The mercury content of the spray was 878 ppm (2% methylmercury and 98% inorganic mercury). There was a significant difference in mercury content between different brands and between batches of the same brand of the Chinese medicinal herb. The spray was withdrawn and his tics completely resolved within 4 weeks.

Immunologic *Allergic reactions* to mercury compounds such as thimerosal seem to be on the increase. Merthiolate was tested as a matter of routine in an extended standard series of skin tests in patients with different subtypes of eczema and varicose complex (47[C]). Of 880 patients 53% responded positively to one or more allergens, 3.9% to merthiolate. The latest results of skin tests in adults have confirmed the persistence of contact allergy to merthiolate and justify further follow up and systematic screening.

There have also been more reports of allergic reactions to dental amalgam.

A 32-year-old male dentist had multiple exudative erythematous pruritic plaques on his limbs and trunk for 3 years (48[A]). Although the eruptions were seen almost throughout the year, his symptoms tended to be worse in the summer. Topical corticosteroids, white petrolatum, and oral antihistamines had given slight relief and an oral corticosteroid gave him transient relief from the itchy eruptions. Patch tests showed that he reacted to 1% ammoniated mercuric chloride in petrolatum and to 0.05% mercuric chloride in water. It was suggested that his dental amalgam should be removed and that he avoid contact with amalgam during his work. Two weeks later his skin symptoms had dramatically improved, leaving pigmentation. Thereafter he was free of symptoms for several months. However, when he handled amalgam again, similar but less severe eruptions appeared on his legs the next day. Subsequent strict avoidance of amalgam improved his eruptions.

A 70-year-old man had multiple coin-sized exudative eczematous plaques on his legs and trunk for several months (48[A]). Various kinds of corticosteroid ointments and white petrolatum as an emollient gave him little relief. Patch tests showed that he reacted to 1% ammoniated mercuric chloride in petrolatum and 0.05% mercuric chloride in water. He had all his dental amalgam removed, and 1 month later his eruption had subsided, leaving pigmentation.

A 50-year-old man complained of soreness of the left buccal mucosa and the right side of his tongue, made worse by consuming spicy foods and acidic drinks (49[A]). He had a heavily restored dentition, with asymmetrically distributed white striated and red atrophic lesions on the left buccal mucosa and the right and left borders of the tongue. The lesions were in direct contact with the buccal and palatal surfaces of an old corroding and amalgam restoration and the lingual surface of an amalgam restoration. A provisional diagnosis of a lichenoid reaction to amalgam was made and patch tests showed a strong positive response to mercury and a slightly weaker response to amalgam after 72 hours. One amalgam filling was covered with a bonded porcelain crown and the other was replaced with glass ionomer cement. Within 2 months he was asymptomatic and after 12 months the lichenoid lesions had completely resolved.

A 57-year-old woman (49[A]) had a recurrent urticarial rash on the skin of her face, scalp, and neck precipitated by restorative dental treatment. The reactions were fully established within 12 hours and would resolve over 2–3 days and be completely gone within 1 week. Patch tests showed a strong reaction to mercury. She was advised that alternative dental materials should be used and that existing amalgam should be removed.

NICKEL *(SED-14, 704; SEDA-22, 248; SEDA-23, 235; SEDA-24, 260)*

Immunologic *Nickel allergy* and *contact dermatitis* with nickel-based appliances have been reviewed (50[R]). The use of nickel is not limited to jewellery; it is also incorporated into orthodontic appliances and medical surgical appliances.

A 79-year-old woman had an abdominal aortic aneurysm repaired with a straight Vanguard R stent, mainly composed of nickel (about 55%) and titanium (about 21%) with a reinforcing thread of platinum (51[A]). Three weeks later she developed severe erythema and eczema on the legs with continuous pruritus and excoriated papules. Patch tests were positive to nickel sulfate and cobalt chloride.

The need for preoperative patch testing for metals is controversial. Enquiry about metal allergy is recommended before endoluminal surgical procedures.

The mobile-phone culture is spreading so rapidly that possible effects connected with its use may still be underestimated (52[A]).

A 36-year-old dermatologist with a history of jewellery intolerance developed dermatitis on the right side of the chin, with red pruritic papules. The dermatitis had worsened after prolonged use of her mobile phone. Patch tests were positive to nickel sulfate. She solved the problem by covering the phone with a plastic case.

A 32-year-old woman developed dermatitis on her left cheek and suggested that it might have been caused or worsened by her mobile phone. Patch tests showed only positive reaction to nickel sulfate. The dimethylglyoxime test for nickel on the side of her phone was positive. The skin lesion resolved rapidly after she covered the phone with a plastic case.

SELENIUM *(SED-14, 704; SEDA-22, 249; SEDA-23, 236; SEDA-24, 260)*

Selenium is important as a nutritional factor. It has functions in many selenoproteins and also in relation to the immune response and cancer prevention. It has recently been reviewed, and no specific adverse effects have been reported (53[R]).

SILVER *(SED-14, 705; SEDA-22, 250; SEDA-23, 236; SEDA-24, 261)*

Silver is used to treat burns and in various medical devices. Its adverse effects are not new, but the circumstances in which they occur vary. The use of silver compounds in the treatment of burns has recently been reviewed (54[R], 55[R]).

Sensory systems Argyrosis should be considered in the differential diagnosis of focal *pigmented conjunctival lesions* (56[A]).

An 82-year-old woman with strabismus amblyopia, for which she had had surgery as a child, developed an asymptomatic pigmented conjunctival lesion in the right eye, mainly involving the underlying subconjunctival connective tissue and the insertion of the lateral rectus muscle; there was no scleral thinning. Biopsy of the conjunctiva and lateral rectus muscle showed numerous extracellular black pigment granules, many of which were aligned in a linear array along the muscle fibers. Energy dispersive X-ray microanalysis showed the pigmentation to be due to silver deposits. During strabismus surgery a silver clip had probably been used to shorten the lateral rectus muscle.

Skin *Argyria* has followed the use of dietary supplements containing colloidal silver protein (57[A]).

A 56-year-old man developed blue color changes of his fingernails. His face had a dusky appearance, and there was no scleral or conjunctival discoloration, or hyperpigmentation of the gums. His fingernails had a blue–gray proximal band of discoloration, as did the lunulae of both thumbnails. His toenails were not involved and the rest of his skin showed no discoloration. His serum silver concentration was 85 μg/l (normal <5.0). He had taken colloidal silver for the previous 3 years as an allergy and cold medication, following the recommended regimen of 1 teaspoon of a 200 ppm silver solution tds.

TITANIUM *(SED-14, 706; SEDA-22, 250; SEDA-23, 237; SEDA-24, 261)*

Titanium and its alloys are in use as implant material bone surgery (58[R], 59[R]) and dental restoration (60[R]).

Immunologic A *hypersensitivity reaction* has been attributed to titanium in a pacemaker (61[A]).

An 86-year-old Japanese man received a pacemaker for atrioventricular block, and 2 months later developed a scaly erythema over the implantation site and later widespread nummular eczema. Histologically, the lesions showed slight spongiosis, intracellular edema, moderate acanthosis in the epidermis, and perivascular infiltration with thickened capillary walls in the dermis. The pacemaker contained titanium and a variety of other metals, but patch tests were all negative. However, titanium sensitivity was demonstrated by intracutaneous and lymphocyte stimulation tests.

Titanium is so widely used that the risk of contact sensitivity to it must be very small. If a patient shows contact sensitivity to titanium, a replacement pacemaker should be completely encased in patch-tested non-allergenic material.

Carcinogenicity A *rhabdomyosarcoma* has been reported near the site of a pacemaker (62[A]).

An 85-year-old man developed a voluminous, rapidly evolving tumor beneath the right clavicle where a titanium pacemaker had been implanted 5 years before. Immunohistochemistry showed that it was a rhabdomyosarcoma.

The role of the pacemaker and especially of titanium in the development of this tumor was not clear.

ZINC *(SED-14, 706; SEDA-22, 251; SEDA-23, 237; SEDA-24, 261)*

Zinc supplementation reduces the incidence of infection and increases the survival rate after infections in elderly people, in whom its use is encouraged (63[R]).

Hematologic *Hypocupremia* and *sideroblastic anemia* can result from long-term or excessive exposure to zinc (64[A]).

A 17-year-old man with anemia, leukopenia, and neutropenia had been self-medicating with over-the-counter zinc formulations for acne for almost 2 years at doses of up to 300 mg/day. Serum copper and serum ceruloplasmin concentrations were less than 100 μg/l (reference range 70–155) and 20 mg/l (23–49) respectively. His serum zinc concentration was 2 mg/l (0.6–1.3). Within 1 month of withdrawal, and without copper supplementation, the ceruloplasmin concentration had risen to 90 mg/l. By 2 months his complete blood count was normal.

Liver *Liver damage* has been attributed to zinc in a patient with Wilson's disease (65[A]).

A 25-year-old woman with Wilson's disease took oral zinc acetate 50 mg tds and 21 days later developed right hypochondrial pain, nausea, vomiting, fever, arthralgia, and tender hepatomegaly. Her hemoglobin was at 10.5 g/daily, AsT 393 U/l and AlT 911 U/l. Oral zinc was withdrawn and oral D-penicillamine (250 mg qds) was prescribed. One week later she was asymptomatic, and her liver enzymes returned to normal within 4 months.

REFERENCES

1. Burke SK. Renagel: reducing serum phosphorus in haemodialysis patients. Hosp Med 2000; 61: 622–7.
2. White JL, Hem SL. Characterization of aluminium-containing adjuvants. Dev Biol 2000; 103: 217–28.
3. Fairweather-Tait S, Hickson K, McGaw B, Reid M. Orange juice enhances aluminium absorption from antacid preparation. Eur J Clin Nutr 1994; 48: 71–3.
4. Meshitsuka S. Inoue M. Urinary excretion of aluminum from antacid ingestion and estimation of its apparent biological half-time. Trace Elem Electrolytes 1998; 15: 132–5.
5. Abramson MJ, Wlodarczyk JH, Saunders NA, Hensley MJ. State of the art: does aluminum smelting cause lung disease? Am Rev Respir Dis. 1982; 139: 1042–57.
6. Fritschi L, Beach J, Sim M, Abramson M, Benke G, Musk AW, De Klerk N, McNeil J. Respiratory symptoms and lung function in two prebake aluminum smelters. Am J Ind Med 1999; 35: 491–8.
7. Yokel RA. The toxicology of aluminium in the brain: a review. Neurotoxicology 2000; 21: 813–28.
8. Munoz DG, Feldman H. Causes of Alzheimer's disease. Can Med Assoc J 2000; 162: 65–72.
9. Gauthier E, Fortier I, Courchesne F, Pepin P, Mortimer J, Gauvreau D. Aluminum forms in drinking water and risk of Alzheimer's disease. Environ Res 2000; 84: 234–46.
10. Andress DL, Maloney NA, Coburn JW, Endres DB, Sherrard DJ. Osteomalacia and aplastic bone disease in aluminum-related osteodystrophy. J Clin Endocrinol Metab 1987; 65: 11–16.
11. Netter P, Kessler M, Burnel D, Hutin MF, Delones S, Benoit J. Aluminium in the joint tissues of chronic renal failure patients treated with regular hemodialysis and aluminum compounds. J Rheumatol 1984; 11: 66–70.
12. Bia MJ, Cooper K, Schnall S, Duffy T, Hendler E, Malluche H, Solomon L. Aluminum induced anemia: pathogenesis and treatment in patients on chronic hemodialysis. Kidney Int 1989; 36: 852–8.
13. Alfrey AC, Mishell HM, Burks J, Contigulia SR, Rudolph H, Lewin E. Syndrome of dyspraxia and multifocal seizures associated with chronic hemodialysis, Trans Am Soc Artif Intern Organs 1972; 18: 257–61.
14. Gonzales Revalderia J, Casares M, De Paula M, Pascual T, Giner V, Miravalles E. Biochemical

and hematological changes in low-level aluminum intoxication. Clin Chem Lab Med 2000; 38: 221–5.
15. Hantson P, Luyasu S, Haufroid V, Lambert M. Antimony excretion in a patient with renal impairment during meglumine antimoniate therapy. Pharmacotherapy 2000; 20: 1141–3.
16. Novick SC, Warrell RP. Arsenicals in hematologic cancers. Semin Oncol 2000; 27: 495–501.
17. Ernst E. Adverse effects of herbal drugs in dermatology. Br J Dermatol 2000; 143: 923–9.
18. Roberts TF, Sprague K, Schenkein D, Miller KB, Relias V. Hyperleukocytosis during induction therapy with arsenic trioxide for relapsed acute promyelocytic leukemia associated with central nervous system infarction. Blood 2000; 96: 4000–1.
19. Viudez P, Castano G, Sookoian S, Frider B, Alvarez E. Arsenic and portal hypertension. Am J Gastroenterol 2000; 95: 1602–3.
20. Gerdsen R, Stockfleth E, Uerlich M, Fartasch M, Steen KH, Bieber T. Papular palmoplantar hyperkeratosis following chronic medical exposure to arsenic: human papillomavirus as a co-factor in the pathogenesis of arsenical keratosis? Acta Derm Venereol 2000; 80: 292–3.
21. Van Oijen AH, Verbeek AL, Jansen JB, De Boer WA. Treatment of *Helicobacter pylori* infection with ranitidine bismuth citrate- or proton pump inhibitor-based triple therapies. Aliment Pharmacol Ther 2000; 14: 991–9.
22. Amaro R, Poniecka A, Rogers AI. Collagenous colitis treated successfully with bismuth subsalicylate. Dig Dis Sci 2000; 45: 1447–50.
23. Murray AD, Gibbs SR, Billings KR, Biavati MJ. Respiratory difficulty following bismuth subgallate aspiration. Arch Otolaryngol Head Neck Surg 2000; 126: 79–81.
24. Stearns DM. Is chromium a trace essential metal? Biofactors 2000; 11: 149–62.
25. Vincent JB. The biochemistry of chromium. J Nutr 2000; 130: 715–18.
26. McCarthy MF. Toward practical prevention of type 2 diabetes. Med Hypotheses 2000; 54: 786–93.
27. Amato P, Morales AJ, Yen SSC. Effects of chromium picolinate supplementation on insulin sensitivity, serum lipids, and body composition in healthy, nonobese, older men and woman. J Gerontol Med Sci 2000; 55A: M260-3.
28. McLeod MN, Golden RN. Chromium treatment of depression. Int J Neuropsychopharmacol 2000; 3: 311–14.
29. Fowler JF. Systemic contact dermatitis caused by oral chromium picolinate. Cutis 2000; 65: 116.
30. Harris ED. Cellular copper transport and metabolism. Annu Rev Nutr 2000; 20: 291–310.
31. Loudianos G, Gitlin JD. Wilson's disease. Semin Liver Dis 2000; 20: 353–64.
32. Delcambre C, Reman O, Henry-Amar M, Peny AM, Macro M, Che Genot JY, Tanguy A, Switsers O, Van HL, Couette JE, Leporrier S. Clinical relevance of gallium-67 scintigraphy in lymphoma during and after therapy. Eur J Nucl Med 2000; 27: 176–84.
33. Dunne SM, Abraham R. Dental post-operative sensitivity associated with a gallium-restorative material. Br Dent J 2000; 189: 310–13.
34. Vamnes JS, Morken T, Helland S, Gjerdet NR. Dental gold alloys and contact hypersensitivity. Contact Dermatitis 2000; 42: 128–33.
35. Uhm WS, Yoo DH, Lee JH, Kim TH, Jun JB, Lee IH, Bae SC, Kim SY. Injectable gold-induced hepatitis and neutropenia in rheumatoid arthritis. Korean J Intern Med 2000; 15: 156–9.
36. Ioannides AS, Panisello JM. Acute respiratory distress syndrome in children with acute poisoning: the role of intravenous desferrioxamine. Eur J Pediatr 2000; 159: 158–9.
37. Go RS, Porrata LF, Call TG. Trombocytopenia after iron dextran administration in a patient with severe iron deficiency anemia. Ann Intern Med 2000; 132: 925.
38. Pearson HA, Ehrenkranz RA, Rinder HM, Riely CA. Hemosiderosis in a normal child secondary to oral iron medication. Pediatrics 2000; 105: 429–31.
39. Maclachlan D, Tyndall A. Acute hepatitis in adult Still's disease apparently resulting from oral iron substitution: a case report. Clin Rheumatol 2000; 19: 222–5.
40. Ortega N, Castillo R, Blanco C, Alvarez M, Carillo T. Oral iron cutaneous adverse reaction and successful desensitization. Ann Allergy Asthma Immunol 2000; 84: 43–5.
41. Moore C, Adler R. Herbal vitamins: lead toxicity and developmental delay. Pediatrics 2000; 106: 600–12.
42. McGuire JK, Kulkarni MS, Baden HP. Fatal hypermagnesemia in a child treated with megavitamin/megamineral therapy. Pediatrics 2000; 105: E18.
43. Lucchini R, Albini E, Placidi D, Gasparotti R, Pigozzi MG, Montani G, Alessio L. Brain magnetic resonance imaging and manganese exposure. Neurotoxicology 2000; 21: 769–75.
44. Reimund JM, Dietemann JL, Warter JM, Baumann R, Duclos B. Factors associated to hypermanganesemia in patients receiving home parenteral nutrition. Clin Nutr 2000; 19: 343–8.
45. Gospe SM, Caruso RD, Clegg MS, Keen CL, Pimstone NR, Ducore JM, Gettner SS, Kreuzer RA. Paraparesis, hypermanganesaemia, and polycythaemia: a novel presentation of cirrhosis. Arch Dis Child 2000; 83: 439–42.
46. Li AM, Chan MHM, Leung TF, Cheung RCK, Lam CWK, Fok TF. Mercury intoxication presenting with tics. Arch Dis Child 2000; 83; 174–5.
47. Novak M, Klezlova V. Allergy to merthiolate (Thimerosalum) in a set of standard epicutaneous tests in patients with eczematous diseases and leg ulcer during three periods between 1979 and 1999 [in Czech]. Cesko-Slov Dermatol 2000; 75: 3–10.

48. Adachi A, Horikawa T, Takashima T, Ichihashi M. Mercury-induced nummular dermatitis. J Am Acad Dermatol 2000; 43: 383–5.
49. McGivern B, Pemberton M, Theaker ED, Buchanan JA, Thornhill MH. Delayed and immediate hypersensitivity reactions associated with the use of amalgam. Br Dent J 2000; 188: 73–6.
50. Budinger L, Hertl M. Immunologic mechanisms in hypersensitivity reactions to metal ions: an overview. Allergy 2000; 55: 108–15.
51. Giménez-Arnau A, Riambau V, Serra-Baldrich E, Camarasa JG. Metal-induced generalized pruriginous dermatitis and endovascular surgery. Contact Dermatitis 2000; 43: 35–40.
52. Pazzaglia M, Lucente P, Vincenzi C, Tosti A. Contact dermatitis from nickel in mobile phones. Contact Dermatitis 2000; 42: 362–3.
53. Rayman MP. The importance of selenium to human health. Lancet 2000; 356: 233–41.
54. Klasen HJ. Historical review of the use of silver in the treatment of burns. I. Early uses. Burns 2000; 26: 117–30.
55. Klasen HJ. A historical review of the use of silver in the treatment of burns. II. Renewed interest for silver. Burns 2000; 26: 131–8.
56. Holck DEE, Klintworth GK, Dutton JJ, Foulks GN, Manning FJ. Localized conjunctival argyrosis: a late sequelae of strabismus surgery. Ophthalmic Surg Lasers 2000: 31: 495–8.
57. Gulbranson SH, Hud JA, Hansen RC. Argyria following the use of dietary supplements containing colloidal silver protein. Cutis 2000; 66: 373–4.
58. Disegi JA. Titanium alloys for fracture fixation implants. Injury 2000; 31 Suppl 4: D14–17.
59. Pohler OEM. Unalloyed titanium for implants in bone surgery. Injury 2000; 31 Suppl 4: D7–13.
60. Thompson SA. An overview of nickel–titanium alloys used in dentistry. Int Endod J 2000; 33: 297–310.
61. Yamauchi R, Morita A, Tsuji T. Pacemaker dermatitis from titanium. Contact Dermatitis 2000; 42: 52–3.
62. Carpentier O, Dubost-Brama A, Martin De Lassalle E, Piette F, Delaporte E. Rhabdomyosarcoma at site of pacemaker implantation. Ann Dermatol Venereol 2000; 127: 837–40.
63. Mocchegiani E, Muzzioli M, Giacconi R. Zinc and immunoresistance to infection in aging: new biological tools. Trends Pharmacol Sci 2000; 21: 205–8.
64. Porea TJ, Belmont JW, Mahoney DH. Zinc-induced anemia and neutropenia in an adolescent. J Pediatr 2000; 136; 688–90.
65. Castilla-Higuero L, Romero-Gomez M, Suarez E, Castro M. Acute hepatitis after starting zinc therapy in a patient with presymptomatic Wilson's disease. Hepatology 2000; 32: 877.

R.H.B. Meyboom

23 Metal antagonists

Deferoxamine *(SED-14, 714; SEDA-22, 254; SEDA-23, 240; SEDA-24, 265)*

Special senses Of 75 adults with thalassemia major (age range 17–32 years) 50 had normal audiography (1[CR]). Of the other 25, 13 had a *sensorineural deficit* of 35 dB or less, with high frequency losses, and two had a deficit of 35–75 dB. There was no association between age, ferritin concentration, therapeutic index, and hearing loss. The authors concluded that their findings were not different from those in a healthy population of the same age and were not suggestive of an ototoxic effect of deferoxamine.

Musculoskeletal Two Chinese studies in 35 consecutive thalassemic patients on a hypertransfusion scheme and chelation therapy have confirmed that deferoxamine-induced *bone dysplasia* was associated with *height reduction* and occurred at doses below 50 mg/kg/day (2[CR], 3[CR]). Prompt dosage reduction may improve bone growth.

In the first study, the patients had radiography of the left hand for bone age determination, and 12 had deferoxamine-induced long bone dysplasia (2[CR]). There was irregularity at the physeal–metaphyseal junction of the distal ulna (the site most frequently affected) and radius; metaphyseal sclerosis was also common, especially of the ulna, but also of the radius, metacarpals, and phalanges. Radiolucent lesions occasionally accompanied metaphyseal sclerosis. In six patients with relatively mild lesions, the dysplastic changes had been missed or not mentioned.

In another study, probably in the same 35 patients, coronal T_1-weighted MRI scanning of the femur was performed, and in 11 patients also of the patella (3[CR]). In the distal but not proximal femurs of 11 of the 35 patients the following abnormalities were seen (in decreasing frequency): blurred physeal–methaphyseal junction, distal metaphyseal areas of hyperintensity, physeal widening, metadiaphyseal lesions, and (in only two) patellar lesions. Patients with MRI evidence of bone dysplasia had a significantly greater reduction in height than patients without.

Of 180 thalassemic patients receiving chelation therapy with subcutaneous deferoxamine, five had deferoxamine-induced serious rickets-like lesions of the long bones; two more had vertebral compression without long bone involvement (4[CR]). A microstructural analysis was made of tibia biopsy specimens taken in six patients during orthopedic surgery and a biopsy of the iliac crest in one. With microradiography and X-ray diffraction there was irregular and reduced mineralization in all seven patients, compared with autopsy bone tissue. Apparently the osteochondrodystrophic lesions in deferoxamine osteopathy are areas with poor mineralization. The bone tissue does not reach maturity, and reduced microhardness leads to an increased risk of microfractures.

In a separate study, apparently in the same seven patients, the histological findings were presented (5[CR]). All the bone specimens showed a similar pathological pattern, with irregular columnar cartilage, lacunae in the cartilaginous tissue, abnormal chondrocytes, and impaired mineralization. Microfractures were common and were a likely explanation for the pain experienced by the patients.

A change to deferiprone lead to general improvement in a 14-year-old boy with deferoxamine-induced osteochondropathy (6[Ar]). Unfortunately, the patient's sitting height had deteriorated, illustrating the irreversibility of platyspondylosis.

The issue of deferoxamine osteochondropathy is even more complex, because thalassemia itself is also associated with growth

Side Effects of Drugs, Annual 25
J.K. Aronson, ed.

impairment and body disproportionality with truncal shortening, whether puberty is induced or spontaneous (7[cr]).

Drug administration route Intravenous deferoxamine can be indicated in gross iron overload, serious cardiomyopathy, or intolerance of or non-compliance with subcutaneous administration. The results of continuous 24-hour deferoxamine infusion via indwelling intravenous catheters in 17 patients (25 intravenous lines) have been presented (8[CR]). The doses of deferoxamine were calculated with reference to the serum ferritin concentration, with a view to maintaining the therapeutic index (mean daily dose in mg/kg divided by the serum ferritin concentration in μg/l) below 0.025. The usual regimen was 6 or 7 days of continuous treatment. Only eight patients received mean daily deferoxamine doses exceeding 50 mg/kg at any time. The mean number of catheter days per patient was 697 and the median follow-up was 54 months (the longest study reported to date). The main catheter-related complications were *infection* (1.15 events per 1000 catheter days) and *thromboembolism* (0.48 events per 1000 catheter days). There were 10 episodes of bacteremic infection (with a variety of species) and 11 of port or exit-site infections (mainly coagulase-negative staphylococci). Line thrombosis occurred in four instances, pulmonary embolism in two, superior vena cava thrombosis in one, and internal jugular thrombosis in one. Since deferoxamine is a risk factor for acquiring bacterial and fungal infections (SED-14, 717), it is noteworthy that the observed rate of infection was similar to that in other patient groups. During this study audiometric abnormalities were not observed. Only one of the 17 patients, while the therapeutic index was briefly exceeded (mean daily dose 80 mg/kg deferoxamine), had manifestations of deferoxamine toxicity, with *visual field and acuity defects* (*retinopathy*). In this patient full resolution occurred over a period of 9 months after dosage reduction.

The local tolerability of subcutaneous bolus injections of deferoxamine has been studied in 27 patients; deferoxamine was given 12-hourly into the abdominal wall on 5 days per week (30 mg/kg/day) (9[cr]). The patients had iron overload due to multiple transfusions and were treated for a mean period of 20 months. All had mild transient painless swelling during injection, disappearing within 10–15 minutes. Two also had *pain at the injection site*, with *redness* in one case.

Deferiprone *(SED-14, 719; SEDA-22, 254; SEDA-23, 240; SEDA-24, 265)*

A *joint effusion* developed in one of 14 children using deferiprone; another had *gastric intolerance* (10[cr]). In a Greek study in 11 patients, using 75–100 mg/kg/day deferiprone for 6 months, there were no serious adverse events of any kind (11[cr]).

Liver In view of the suspicion that deferiprone can cause *hepatic fibrosis*, experience at the Sydney Children's Hospital in Australia has been reviewed, encompassing two liver biopsies in 14 patients taking deferiprone and 22 receiving deferoxamine (10[cr]; SEDA-23, 240). The liver iron concentrations in the two groups, both at initial biopsy and subsequent biopsy, were not significantly different. Fibrosis progressed in five of 14 deferiprone users and in eight of 22 deferoxamine users. Progression greater than one unit occurred in four of 14 deferiprone users and two of 22 deferoxamine users. In those with positive hepatitis C serology, fibrosis showed progression in one of three patients using deferiprone and two of nine deferoxamine users; these findings were not significantly different. Pericellular fibrosis and Councilman bodies were seen in some patients: four of 11 deferiprone users and one of 20 deferoxamine users, a significant difference. However, errors of presentation of the data hindered interpretation of the findings.

Edetate *(SED-14, 721; SEDA-22, 255; SEDA-23, 242)*

Preservatives and other excipients can cause unexpected responses to generic formulations (SEDA-23, 242). There has been a case of paradoxical *bronchoconstriction* and *laryngospasm* necessitating emergency admission after the use of salbutamol in a metered-dose inhaler, which also contained edetate disodium as a preservative (12[Ar]). Although there was prompt relapse on re-exposure, there were no positive findings demonstrating the role of edetate disodium.

Penicillamine *(SED-14, 723; SEDA-22, 256; SEDA-23, 242; SEDA-24, 266)*

In considering the adverse effects of penicillamine, sooner or later one returns to question of what has been achieved in the treatment of rheumatoid arthritis and what the current balance of benefit and harm is of the various drugs, combinations, and regimens used. Recent "state of the art" papers have stood firm and are confident that early, aggressive, and continuous use of disease-modifying antirheumatic drugs (DMARDs) and of combinations thereof slows joint destruction, modifies the natural course of the disease, and improves outcome (13[R], 14[R]). On closer inspection, however, the evidence still seems thin. Schemes for treatment and monitoring are variable and complex, and none is demonstrably superior to any other. It is in any case always important to tailor treatment to the needs of the individual patient rather than following rigid guidelines.

In other update reviews of the literature the conclusion has again been reached that the long-term use of DMARDs, including penicillamine, is limited by both frequent loss of response and serious adverse reactions, and that the advantages of combination DMARDs treatments remain controversial (15[R], 16[R]; SEDA-19, 229; SEDA-20, 219; SEDA-25, 266). In particular the treatment of juvenile rheumatoid arthritis is difficult, since DMARDs are often poorly active in children and some (gold compounds, sulfasalazine) cause special adverse reactions, such as the macrophage activation syndrome (which in turn can lead to severe infections) (17[R]). There is still much to be achieved and improved. As Fries has put it (16[R]): "Determining the most clinically useful DMARD combinations and the optimal sequence of DMARD use requires effectiveness studies, Bayesian approaches and analyses of long-term outcomes. Such approaches will allow optimization of multiple drug therapies in rheumatoid arthritis, and should substantially improve the long-term outcome for many patients". In the same paper it is emphasized that patients taking penicillamine should have blood cell counts and urine protein measurements every 2 weeks during drug titration and then about monthly for as long as treatment lasts.

Special senses *Ocular pseudotumor* has been described in one patient as part of an ANCA-positive vasculitis (18[AR]).

In a helpful review of drug-induced olfactory disorders penicillamine was mentioned as a cause of abnormal smell (19[r]). However, there may have been confusion with the well-established effect of penicillamine on taste.

Endocrine *Macromastia* (enlargement of the female breast), a remarkable adverse effect of penicillamine (SED-14, 733), has been reviewed in the context of two idiopathic cases (20[R]).

Liver In a Chinese study of 29 patients there was evidence in one patient that DMARDs and chronic viral hepatitis have synergistic hepatotoxic effects (21[CR]). However, the relevance of this anecdotal observation is uncertain.

Skin A further case of *pemphigus* attributed to penicillamine has been reported (22[Ar]). The case had some unusual features.

A 71-year-old woman taking penicillamine (dosage not specified) developed pemphigus vulgaris rather than pemphigus foliaceus, which is the usual form of pemphigus that penicillamine causes. She presented with pustular bullae (due to secondary infection with *Pseudomonas aeruginosa*), and the indication for penicillamine was not rheumatoid arthritis but systemic sclerosis.

When taken for a long time in high doses, penicillamine can cause deterioration of collagen fibers; rare and peculiar disorders such as *elastosis perforans serpiginosa* and *cutis laxa* can develop. In one patient the characteristic features of both of these diseases developed (23[AR]).

A 36-year-old man, who had had Wilson's disease since the age of 4 years, had used penicillamine for about 13 years in a dosage of 2–3 g/day. He developed an itching papular eruption, initially resolving after withdrawal of the drug but recurring and progressing 6 months later. Generalized cutis laxa developed, with perforating elastolytic nodules on the neck and elastosis perforans serpiginosa over the shoulders. A biopsy showed perforating channels from the dermis through the epidermis, with a surrounding inflammatory infiltrate and horseshoe-shaped multinuclear giant cells phagocytosing abnormal elastic fibers. Van Giesen staining showed a lumpy–bumpy appearance of elastin fibers, typical of penicillamine dermopathy, as originally described by Bardach et al. (SED-14, 730).

Presumably the mechanism underlying penicillamine dermopathy is inhibition by penicillamine of cross-linkage of collagen fibers. In addition, the enzyme lysyl oxidase, required for the cross-linking of collagen fibers, is copper-dependent and may be inhibited by copper chelation by penicillamine. Another argument for a possible role of copper deficiency is the fact that cutis laxa is common in Menke's disease, a rare genetically determined disturbance of copper metabolism. Perforating elastoma occurs when abnormal elastic fibers accumulate, cause a foreign body reaction, and are transepidermally eliminated. Although the patient was also thought to have elastolytic involvement of the lining of the upper respiratory tract, there was no objective evidence of this.

There were no serious adverse reactions in 55 children who received 66 courses of low-dose penicillamine (about 15 mg/kg/day for a mean period of 77 days) for mild to moderate lead poisoning (24[Cr]). However, in three children penicillamine was withdrawn because of a transient rash.

Musculoskeletal In a prospective analysis of 74 women with systemic sclerosis, a low bone mineral density and densitometric osteoporosis were related to the menopause and not to the previous use of penicillamine or other drugs (25[c]).

Immunologic A further case of *lupus-like syndrome* has been attributed to penicillamine (26[A]).

A 6-year-old Taiwanese girl, who had taken penicillamine (dosage not specified) for Wilson's disease for 17 months, developed arthralgia, fever, and oral ulcers. She had antinuclear antibodies with a homogeneous pattern at a dilution of 1/5120, and a direct Coombs' test was positive. On the other hand, anti-DNA antibodies were within the reference range and antibodies against non-histone nuclear antigens (Sm, RNP, SS-A/Ro, SS-B/La, Scl-70) were all negative. She improved with prednisolone, and penicillamine was continued in a lower dosage.

A variety of vasculitic diseases, including Wegener's granulomatosis, microscopic polyangiitis, Churg–Strauss syndrome, and crescentic glomerulonephritis, are associated with antineutrophil cytoplasmic antibodies (ANCA) or leukocytoclastic vasculitis. In drug-induced ANCA-positive vasculitis antimyeloperoxidase antibodies are most often found; they produce a perinuclear pattern of staining by indirect immunofluorescence (pANCA), but antiproteinase 3 (anti-PR3) antibodies can also occur (cANCA).

The possible drug causes of ANCA-positive vasculitis with high titers of antimyeloperoxidase antibodies in 30 new patients have been reviewed (18[CR]). The findings illustrate that this type of vasculitis is a predominantly drug-induced disorder. Only 12 of the 30 cases were not related to a drug. The most frequently implicated drug was hydralazine (10 cases); the remainder involved propylthiouracil (three cases), penicillamine (two cases), allopurinol (two cases), and sulfasalazine.

A 49-year-old woman with systemic sclerosis, taking penicillamine 750 mg/day, developed a vasculitis, with an *orbital pseudotumor* and 2 months later fatal *alveolar hemorrhage*. She had also antinuclear antibodies with a homogeneous pattern.

A 56-year-old woman with systemic sclerosis taking penicillamine 750 mg/day had homogeneous antinuclear antibodies and antinative DNA antibodies. Her manifestations of vasculitis were glomerulonephritis with *renal insufficiency*, *pulmonary hemorrhage*, and bilateral *hemothorax* (i.e. similar to *Goodpasture's syndrome*).

As the authors pointed out, practically all drugs known to cause *ANCA-positive vasculitis* (including penicillamine) have also been associated with a lupus-like syndrome, suggesting the possibility of a similar underlying mechanism. However, the presence of discriminating markers (such as antielastase and antilactoferrin antibodies) in drug-induced ANCA-positive vasculitis, but not in idiopathic cases, is suggestive of different pathways in these conditions.

In three Japanese patients with penicillamine-associated *glomerulonephritis*, antimyeloperoxidase ANCA assays were strongly positive (27[AR]). These patients had been taking penicillamine for rheumatoid arthritis in daily doses of 100, 200, and 300 mg for 32, 42, and 39 months respectively. All three had proteinuria, hematuria, anemia, and rapidly progressive renal insufficiency. Histological examination showed crescentic glomerulonephritis with granular deposits of IgG, IgM, IgA, C1q, and C3 in the mesangium. Penicillamine was withdrawn and the patients were given steroid pulse therapy, warfarin, and in two cases cyclophosphamide. Renal function gradually improved and the antineutrophil cytoplasmic antibodies disappeared.

In a further detailed case report of a 69-year-old man with penicillamine-induced *crescentic glomerulonephritis* ANCA tests were repeatedly negative (28[CR]). He had been taking penicillamine up to 750 mg/day for systemic sclerosis.

Polystyrene sulfonates

Polystyrene sulfonic acid has been used as sodium, potassium, and calcium salts. Sodium polystyrene sulfonate has been used to treat hyperkalemia in patients with renal insufficiency and as an adjuvant during hemodialysis. It can be given orally or rectally in all age groups (29[R]). It has also been added to feeding formulae and nutritional supplements to reduce their potassium contents and so prevent hyperkalemia; however, the reduction in potassium content was more than balanced by a concomitant increase in sodium content, presumably because of exchange of the sodium with calcium and magnesium (30[E], 31[E]). The uses and adverse effects of sodium polystyrene sulfonate have been reviewed (32[R], 33[R]).

Potassium polystyrene sulfonate has been used to treat hypercalciuria and renal calculi. Calcium polystyrene sulfonate has been used to treat hyperkalemia, particularly in patients who cannot tolerate the extra sodium that would be provided by the sodium salt.

A confection containing sodium polystyrene sulfonate resin 5.0 g per piece was used to treat six chronic dialysis patients with predialysis serum potassium concentrations of 5.2 mmol/l or more (34[c]). Over 2 weeks the mean serum potassium fell by 0.7 mmol/l. However, the effectiveness of sodium polystyrene sulfonate in lowering serum potassium concentrations in patients with renal insufficiency has been questioned (35[C]). A cathartic alone (phenolphthalein) in six patients caused an average fecal potassium output of 54 mmol. The addition of sodium polystyrene sulfonate had no further significant effect on total potassium output. With placebo the average serum potassium concentration increased slightly (0.4 mmol/l) during 12 hours. This rise was attenuated by sodium polystyrene sulfonate, perhaps in part because of extracellular volume expansion caused by the absorption of sodium. Phenolphthalein was associated with a slight rise in serum potassium concentration (similar to placebo), perhaps because of extracellular volume contraction produced by a sodium-rich diarrhea and acidosis secondary to bicarbonate loss. None of the regimens reduced the serum potassium concentration, compared with baseline.

Respiratory *Pneumonitis has been reported in a woman taking sodium polystyrene sulfonate (36[A]).*

Electrolyte and mineral balance *Sodium polystyrene sulfonate can cause hypokalemia, hypocalcemia, and hypernatremia. Calcium polystyrene sulfonate can cause hypokalemia and hypercalcemia.*

Acid–base balance *Cation-containing antacids and laxatives (e.g. magnesium hydroxide, calcium carbonate) can reduce the effect of polystyrene sulfonate and metabolic acidosis can develop. This has been reported in both children (37[A]) and adults (38[A]).*

A patient with end-stage renal disease undergoing long-term maintenance hemodialysis developed moderately severe metabolic alkalosis in the absence of vomiting or gastric drainage (38[A]). The cause of the acid–base disorder was the oral administration of exogenous alkali, in the form of "non-absorbable" antacids (aluminum hydroxide and magnesium hydroxide), neutral phosphate, and sodium polystyrene sulfonate.

In a patient with chronic renal insufficiency, chronic hypocalcemia plus severe metabolic alkalosis due to combined administration of sodium polystyrene sulfonate and magnesium hydroxide caused a generalized tonic–clonic seizure (39[A]).

Hematologic *Thrombocytopenia has been attributed to sodium polystyrene sulfonate (Kayexalate) (40[A]).*

An 84-year-old man with diabetes mellitus and hypertension had gradually worsening renal insufficiency with hyperkalemia and was given oral sodium polystyrene sulfonate (Kayexalate). After 7 days he developed gradually worsening thrombocytopenia, and 12 days later his platelet count, which had initially been 207 × 10^9/l, fell to 86 × 10^9/l. The thrombocytopenia rapidly improved after withdrawal of the sodium polystyrene sulfonate. At a later date readministration of sodium polystyrene sulfonate for *the treatment of hyperkalemia again caused thrombocytopenia. Bone-marrow aspiration biopsy showed normal numbers of nucleated cells and megakaryocytes with no increase in blast count. No other disorders which could have caused thrombocytopenia were seen in this patient.*

Gastrointestinal *After oral administration the polystyrene sulfonates commonly cause anorexia, nausea, vomiting, and constipation.*

Upper gastrointestinal damage associated with sodium polystyrene sulfonate in sorbitol is reported far less often than colonic damage. However, endoscopic appearances were markedly abnormal in 11 patients with crystals of sodium polystyrene sulfonate in biopsies from the esophagus (n = 7), stomach (n = 6), and duodenum (n = 2) (41[C]). There was histological and/or endoscopic evidence of mucosal injury in the form of an ulcer or erosion in nine patients, and in four patients with mucosal injury, no other cause could be identified.

After rectal and oral administration intestinal ulcers and necrosis have occurred (42[AR]). Several cases affecting the large bowel have been reported.

A 67-year-old man underwent laparotomy for a ruptured abdominal aortic aneurysm (43[A]). Postoperatively he was treated with hemodialysis because of acute renal insufficiency. Hyperkalemia was treated with sodium polystyrene sulfonate, after which he developed ulceration of the colon and required a hemicolectomy because of intractable blood loss.

Two patients, who had died after cardiac surgery, were in renal insufficiency, and had received sodium polystyrene sulfonate in sorbitol, had colonic luminal crystals of sodium polystyrene sulfonate associated with underlying mucosal necrosis, submucosal edema, and transmural inflammation (44[A]).

In a patient who developed near total colonic necrosis shortly after renal transplantation the onset of symptoms was temporally related to the administration of sodium polystyrene sulfonate plus sorbitol enemas (Kayexalate) for hyperkalemia (45[Ar]).

In another case colonic necrosis presented as an acute abdomen within 24 hours of administration of sodium polystyrene sulfonate in sorbitol (46[A]). After prompt surgical resection of the necrotic transverse colon there was rapid recovery of bowel function.

In 15 patients who were given sodium polystyrene sulfonate (Kayexalate) in sorbitol as an enema or orally to treat hyperkalemia, sodium polystyrene sulfonate crystals were observed in specimens from gastrointestinal surgical resections (n = 9) or endoscopic biopsies (n = 7) (47[C]). There was necrosis in seven of eight surgical resection specimens and three of five endoscopic biopsy specimens; four also had necrosis of the small intestine. Four patients with colonic necrosis in the initial resection specimen developed progressive necrosis of the small intestine or rectum, and five died within 1 day to 6 weeks. There were sodium polystyrene sulfonate crystals in upper gastrointestinal tract specimens from four patients, including one with hemorrhagic gastritis.

The incidence of intestinal necrosis has been estimated in 752 hospitalized patients who had received sodium polystyrene sulfonate, of whom 117 were exposed within 1 week of surgery (48[C]). There were two cases of intestinal necrosis, both in patients who had received oral sodium polystyrene sulfonate in sorbitol. Based on these two cases, the postoperative incidence of intestinal necrosis associated with sodium polystyrene sulfonate was 1.8%. In 862 patients, who had undergone hemodialysis, renal transplantation, or cardiac transplantation, but had not received sodium polystyrene sulfonate, there were no cases of idiopathic intestinal necrosis.

Because uremia and the concomitant use of sorbitol appear to be common denominators in the pathophysiology of this complication, some have suggested that Kayexalate enemas be avoided in renal transplant patients (45[Ar]).

In five infants of extremely low birthweights, who were given either sodium polystyrene sulfonate or calcium polystyrene sulfonate orally for hyperkalemia, masses were palpable in the left upper quadrant of the abdomen and visible radiographically as opaque masses in the stomach (49[C]). At autopsy the palpable mass was identified as a solid chalk-like concretion and X-ray diffraction showed that the material was Brushite. The authors suggested that oral exchange resins should not be used in critically ill, extremely low-birthweight infants.

Two other cases of neonatal bowel opacification secondary to oral and rectal sodium polystyrene sulfonate have been reported (50[A]). Abdominal radiography showed a faint homogeneous increase in density within the bowel lumen.

With high doses impaction can occur and this has been associated with perforation (51[A]).

A 650-g, 24-week-old neonate with hyperkalemia was given sodium polystyrene sulfonate enemas and developed cecal impaction and perforation. Abdominal radiographs showed radiodense impacted resin outlining the bowel. Pathological examination showed sodium polystyrene sulfonate crystals in a cecal abscess.

Hematochezia in a neonate who had been given sodium polystyrene sulfonate enemas prompted a review of the use of such enemas in 20 of 2317 patients (52[C]). Of these 20 patients, four had evidence of hematochezia temporally related to the use of the enemas. There were no episodes of bleeding in infants who were older than 29 weeks or over 1250 g birthweight. In one case an autopsy performed within 2 days of the enema showed extensive vascular congestion in the mucosa and submucosa, with focal areas of hemorrhage. Sorbitol 20% (1098 mosm/l) was the vehicle for suspension of the sodium polystyrene sulfonate, and the authors thought that the hyperosmolarity of sorbitol had contributed to the colonic damage in these children.

Drug interactions *Sodium polystyrene sulfonate binds lithium in vitro (53[E]); it is more effective than charcoal, but has a higher affinity for potassium (54[E]). In healthy volunteers who took a single dose of lithium carbonate 600 mg, sodium polystyrene sulfonate 30 g reduced the area under the lithium serum concentration-time curve by 11%, reduced the mean* C_{max} *by 0.07 mmol/l, and delayed the* t_{max} *by 2.04 hours (55[C]). In six young healthy volunteers who took lithium carbonate 0.5 mmol/kg (18.5 mg/kg), sodium polystyrene sulfonate 857 mg/kg in 4 ml of water/g sodium polystyrene sulfonate taken 1 hour later reduced the mean AUC by 15% and the* C_{max} *by 0.20 mmol/l (56[C]). There was no significant difference in 24-hour urine lithium excretion or in serum sodium and potassium concentrations. Both of these results suggest that sodium polystyrene sulfonate reduces the absorption of lithium. Furthermore, sodium polystyrene sulfonate increased the clearance of oral lithium in a volunteer when given 30 min after each dose of lithium (57[c]). For these reasons it has been used to treat lithium overdose (58[A], 59[A]). However, it can cause hypokalemia and is not currently recommended as routine therapy (60[R]).*

It has also been suggested that sodium polystyrene sulfonate might be useful in treating iron overdose, since it binds iron in vitro with high affinity (61[E]). However, in a placebo-controlled cross-over study in six healthy adults sodium polystyrene sulfonate 30 g had no significant effect on the kinetics of an oral dose of elemental iron 10 mg/kg (62[C]).

Since calcium salts can bind tetracyclines, leading to reduced absorption (SED-14, 910), an interaction of this kind might be expected with calcium polystyrene sulfonate, but it does not seem to have been reported.

REFERENCES

1. Ambrosetti U, Donde E, Piatti G, Cappellini MD. Audiological evaluation in adult beta-thalassemia major patients under regular chelation treatment. Pharmacol Res 2000; 42: 485–7.
2. Chan Y-I, Li C-K, Chu WC-W, Pang L-M, Cheng JC-Y, Chik K-W. Deferoxamine-induced bone dysplasia in the distal femur and patella of pediatric patients and young adults: MR imaging appearance. Am J Roentgenol 2000; 175: 1561–6.
3. Chan YL, Li CK, Pang LM, Chik KW. Desferrioxamine-induced long bone changes in thalassaemic patients – radiographic features, prevalence and relations with growth. Clin Radiol 2000; 55: 610–14.
4. De Sanctis V, Savarino L, Stea S, Cervellati M, Ciapetti G, Tassinari L, Pizzoferrato A. Microstructural analysis of severe bone lesions in seven thalassemic patients treated with deferoxamine. Calcif Tissue Int 2000; 67: 128–33.
5. De Sanctis V, Stea S, Savarino L, Granchi D, Visentin M, Sprocati M, Govoni R, Pizzoferrato A. Osteochondrodystrophic lesions in chelated thalassemic patients: an histological analysis. Calcif Tissue Int 2000; 67: 134–40.
6. Mangiagli A, De Sanctis V, Campisi S, Di Silvestro G, Urso L. Treatment with deferiprone (L1) in a thalassemic patient with bone lesions due to desferrioxamine. J Pediatr Endocrinol Metab 2000; 13: 677–80.
7. Filosa A, Di Maio S, Baron I, Esposito G, Galati MG. Final height and body disproportion in thalassaemic boys and girls with spontaneous or induced puberty. Acta Paediatr Int J Paediatr 2000; 89: 1295–301.
8. Davis BA, Porter JB. Long-term outcome of continuous 24-hour deferoxamine infusion via indwelling intravenous catheters in high-risk beta-thalassemia. Blood 2000; 95: 1229–36.

9. Franchini M, Gandini G, De Gironcoli M, Vassanelli A, Borgna-Pignatti C, Aprili G. Safety and efficacy of subcutaneous bolus injection of deferoxamine in adult patients with iron overload. Blood 2000; 95: 2776–9.
10. Berdoukas V, Bohane T, Eagle C, Lindeman R, DeSilva K, Tobias V, Painter D, Fraser I. The Sydney Children's Hospital experience with the oral iron chelator deferiprone (L1). Transfus Sci 2000; 23: 239–40.
11. Rombos Y, Tzanetea R, Konstantopoulos K, Simitzis S, Zervas C, Kyriaki P, Kavouklis M, Aessopos A, Sakellaropoulos N, Karagiorga M, Kalotychou V, Loukopoulos D. Chelation therapy in patients with thalassemia using the orally active iron chelator deferiprone (L1). Haematologica 2000; 85: 115–17.
12. Mutlu GM, Moonjelly E, Chan L, Olopade CO. Laryngospasm and paradoxical bronchoconstriction after repeated doses of beta2-agonists containing edetate disodium. Mayo Clin Proc 2000; 75: 285–7.
13. Lacaille D. Rheumatology: 8. Advanced therapy. Can Med Assoc J 2000; 163: 721–8.
14. Madhok R, Kerr H, Capell HA. Recent advances: rheumatology. Br Med J 2000; 321: 882–5.
15. Simon LS. DMARDs in the treatment of rheumatoid arthritis: current agents and future developments. Int J Clin Pract 2000; 54: 243–9.
16. Fries JF. Current treatment paradigms in rheumatoid arthritis. Rheumatology (UK) 2000; 39 Suppl 1: 30–5.
17. Prieur A-M, Quartier P. Comparative tolerability of treatments for juvenile idiopathic arthritis. Biodrugs 2000; 14: 159–83.
18. Choi HK, Merkel PA, Walker AM, Niles JL. Drug-associated antineutrophil cytoplasmic antibody-positive vasculitis: prevalence among patients with high titers of antimyeloperoxidase antibodies. Arthritis Rheum 2000; 43: 405–13.
19. Nores JM, Biacabe B, Bonfils P. Olfactory disorders due to medicinal drugs: an analysis and review of the literature. Rev Med Interne 2000; 21: 972–7.
20. O'Hare PM, Frieden IJ. Virginal breast hypertrophy. Pediatr Dermatol 2000; 17: 277–81.
21. Mok MY, Ng WL, Yuen MF, Wong RWS, Lau CS. Safety of disease modifying anti-rheumatic agents in rheumatoid arthritis patients with chronic viral hepatitis. Clin Exp Rheumatol 2000; 18: 363–8.
22. Shapiro M, Jimenez S, Werth VP. Pemphigus vulgaris induced by D-penicillamine therapy in a patient with systemic sclerosis. J Am Acad Dermatol 2000; 42: 297–9.
23. Hill VA, Seymour CA, Mortimer PS. Penicillamine-induced elastosis perforans serpiginosa and cutis laxa in Wilson's disease. Br J Dermatol 2000; 142: 560–1.
24. Shannon MW, Townsend MK. Adverse effects of reduced-dose d-penicillamine in children with mild to moderate lead poisoning. Ann Pharmacother 2000; 34: 15–18.
25. Sampaio-Barros PD, De Paiva Magalhaes E, Sachetto Z, Samara AM, Marques Neto JF. Bone mineral density in systemic sclerosis. Rev Bras Reumatol 2000; 40: 153–8.
26. Lin HC, Hwang KC, Lee HJ, Tsai MJ, Ni YH, Chiang BL. Penicillamine induced lupus-like syndrome: a case report. J Microbiol Immunol Infect 2000; 33: 202–4.
27. Nanke Y, Akama H, Terai C, Kamatani N. Rapidly progressive glomerulonephritis with D-penicillamine. Am J Med Sci 2000; 320: 398–402.
28. Garcia-Porrua C, Gonzalez-Gay MA, Bouza P. D-Penicillamine-induced crescentic glomerulonephritis in a patient with scleroderma. Nephron 2000; 84: 101–2.
29. Meyer I. Sodium polystyrene sulfonate: a cation exchange resin used in treating hyperkalemia. ANNA J 1993; 20: 93–5.
30. Bunchman TE, Wood EG, Schenck MH, Weaver KA, Klein BL, Lynch RE. Pretreatment of formula with sodium polystyrene sulfonate to reduce dietary potassium intake. Pediatr Nephrol 1991; 5: 29–32.
31. Fassinger N, Dabbagh S, Mukhopadhyay S, Lee DY. Mineral content of infant formula after treatment with sodium polystyrene sulfonate or calcium polystyrene sulfonate. Adv Perit Dial 1998; 14: 274–7.
32. Takasu T. [Treatment of hyperkalemia associated with renal insufficiency – clinical effects and side reactions of positive-ion-exchange resins, sodium polystyrene sulfonate (Kayexalate).] Nippon Rinsho 1970; 28: 1941–6.
33. Osawa A, Okoshi M, Higuchi J, Yamayoshi W. [Treatment of hyperkalemia in renal insufficiency with cation exchange resin. Experience with use of sodium polystyrene sulfonate.] Hinyokika Kiyo 1969; 15: 645–51.
34. Johnson K, Cazee C, Gutch C, Ogden D. Sodium polystyrene sulfonate resin candy for control of potassium in chronic dialysis patients. Clin Nephrol 1976; 5: 266–8.
35. Gruy-Kapral C, Emmett M, Santa-Ana CA, Porter JL, Fordtran JS, Fine KD. Effect of single dose resin-cathartic therapy on serum potassium concentration in patients with end-stage renal disease. J Am Soc Nephrol 1998; 9: 1924–30.
36. Haupt HM, Hutchins GM. Sodium polystyrene sulfonate pneumonitis. Arch Intern Med 1982; 142: 379–81.
37. Nassif F, Sinnassamy P, Bensman A. Une cause d'alcalose chez l'enfant hemodialyse: la coadministration d'hydroxyde de magnesium et de polystyrene sulfonate de sodium. Presse Med 1987; 16: 1003.
38. Metabolic alkalosis due to absorption of "non-absorbable" antacids. Madias NE, Levey AS. Am J Med 1983; 74: 155–8.
39. Ziessman HA. Alkalosis and seizure due to a cation-exchange resin and magnesium hydroxide. South Med J 1976; 69: 497–9.
40. Mogi Y, Kura T, Takimoto R, Muto F, Maeda T,

Muramatsu H, Niitsu Y. [Thrombocytopenia associated with sodium polystyrene sulfonate.] Rinsho Ketsueki 1997; 38: 1224–8.
41. Abraham SC, Bhagavan BS, Lee LA, Rashid A, Wu TT. Upper gastrointestinal tract injury in patients receiving Kayexalate (sodium polystyrene sulfonate) in sorbitol: clinical, endoscopic, and histopathologic findings. Am J Surg Pathol 2001; 25: 637–44.
42. Rogers FB, Li SC. Acute colonic necrosis associated with sodium polystyrene sulfonate (Kayexalate) enemas in a critically ill patient: case report and review of the literature. J Trauma 2001; 51: 395–7.
43. Schiere S, Karrenbeld A, Tulleken JE, Van der Werf TS, Zijlstra JG. Natriumpolystyreensulfonaat (Resonium A) als mogelijke oorzaak van rectaal bloedverlies. Ned Tijdschr Geneeskd 1997; 141: 2127–9.
44. Gardiner GW. Kayexalate (sodium polystyrene sulphonate) in sorbitol associated with intestinal necrosis in uremic patients. Can J Gastroenterol 1997; 11: 573–7.
45. Scott TR, Graham SM, Schweitzer EJ, Bartlett ST. Colonic necrosis following sodium polystyrene sulfonate (Kayexalate)-sorbitol enema in a renal transplant patient. Report of a case and review of the literature. Dis Colon Rectum 1993; 36: 607–9.
46. Dardik A, Moesinger RC, Efron G, Barbul A, Harrison MG. Acute abdomen with colonic necrosis induced by Kayexalate-sorbitol. South Med J 2000; 93: 511–13.
47. Rashid A, Hamilton SR. Necrosis of the gastrointestinal tract in uremic patients as a result of sodium polystyrene sulfonate (Kayexalate) in sorbitol: an underrecognized condition. Am J Surg Pathol 1997; 21: 60–9.
48. Gerstman BB, Kirkman R, Platt R. Intestinal necrosis associated with postoperative orally administered sodium polystyrene sulfonate in sorbitol. Am J Kidney Dis 1992; 20: 159–61.
49. Ohlsson A, Hosking M. Complications following oral administration of exchange resins in extremely low-birth-weight infants. Eur J Pediatr 1987; 146: 571–4.
50. Sherman S, Friedman AP, Berdon WE, Haller JO. Kayexalate: a new cause of neonatal bowel opacification. Radiology 1981; 138: 63–4.
51. Bennett LN, Myers TF, Lambert GH. Cecal perforation associated with sodium polystyrene sulfonate-sorbitol enemas in a 650 gram infant with hyperkalemia. Am J Perinatol 1996; 13: 167–70.
52. Milley JR, Jung AL. Hematochezia associated with the use of hypertonic sodium polystyrene sulfonate enemas in premature infants. J Perinatol 1995; 15: 139–42.
53. Linakis JG, Savitt DL, Lockhart GR, Trainor B, Lacouture PG, Lewander WJ. In vitro binding of lithium using the cation exchange resin sodium polystyrene sulfonate. Am J Emerg Med 1995; 13: 669–70.
54. Watling SM, Gehrke JC, Gehrke CW, Zumwalt R, Pribble J. In vitro binding of lithium using the cation exchange resin sodium polystyrene sulfonate. Am J Emerg Med 1995; 13: 294–6.
55. Belanger DR, Tierney MG, Dickinson G. Effect of sodium polystyrene sulfonate on lithium bioavailability. Ann Emerg Med 1992; 21: 1312–15.
56. Tomaszewski C, Musso C, Pearson JR, Kulig K, Marx JA. Lithium absorption prevented by sodium polystyrene sulfonate in volunteers. Ann Emerg Med 1992; 21: 1308–11.
57. Gehrke JC, Watling SM, Gehrke CW, Zumwalt R. In-vivo binding of lithium using the cation exchange resin sodium polystyrene sulfonate. Am J Emerg Med 1996; 14: 37–8.
58. Dupuis RE, Cooper AA, Rosamond LJ, Campbell Bright S. Multiple delayed peak lithium concentrations following acute intoxication with an extended-release product. Ann Pharmacother 1996; 30: 356–60.
59. Roberge RJ, Martin TG, Schneider SM. Use of sodium polystyrene sulfonate in a lithium overdose. Ann Emerg Med 1993; 22: 1911–15.
60. Scharman EJ. Methods used to decrease lithium absorption or enhance elimination. J Toxicol Clin Toxicol 1997; 35: 601–8.
61. O'Connor TA, Gruner BA, Gehrke JC, Watling SM, Gehrke CW. In vitro binding of iron with the cation-exchange resin sodium polystyrene sulfonate. Ann Emerg Med 1996; 28: 504–7.
62. Shepherd G, Klein-Schwartz W, Burstein AH. Efficacy of the cation exchange resin, sodium polystyrene sulfonate, to decrease iron absorption. J Toxicol Clin Toxicol 2000; 38: 389–94.

Pam Magee

24 Antiseptic drugs and disinfectants

BISBIGUANIDES

Chlorhexidine *(SED-14, 764; SEDA-23, 247; SEDA-24, 270)*

The risks and benefits of using catheters impregnated with chlorhexidine continue to be studied. In a randomized clinical study of the efficacy of catheters impregnated with antiseptics for the prevention of central venous catheter-related infections in intensive care units in 204 patients with 235 central venous catheters between November 1998 and June 1999 a standard triple-lumen polyurethane catheter and a catheter impregnated with chlorhexidine and silver sulfadiazine were indistinguishable from each other (1^C). Compared with standard polyurethane catheters, antiseptic catheters were less likely to be *colonized by microorganisms* when they were cultured at removal (8 vs 20 colonized catheters per 100 catheters; relative risk 0.34 (95% CI = 0.15, 0.74). There was no significant difference between the groups in *catheter-related infections* (0.9 vs 4.9 infections per 100 catheters; relative risk 0.17 (95% CI = 0.03, 1.15). Gram-positive cocci and fungi were more likely to colonize the standard polyurethane catheters than antiseptic catheters. Two of the cases in the control group died because of catheter-related candidemia. There were no adverse reactions such as hypersensitivity or leukopenia with the antiseptic catheters. The authors concluded that central venous catheters with antiseptic coating are safe and carry less risk of colonization of bacteria and fungi than standard catheters in critically ill patients.

Side Effects of Drugs, Annual 25
J.K. Aronson, ed.

Immunologic There have been many reports of *hypersensitivity* of both the immediate and delayed types after exposure to chlorhexidine. Anaphylaxis has been reported after application to the skin, eyes, and other mucous membranes, and with catheters treated with the antiseptic (SEDA-23, 248; SEDA-24, 270). The molecular basis of the recognition of chlorhexidine in a sensitive patient has been examined (2^{AE}).

A 75-year-old man was referred following three anaphylactic events. The first occurred in September 1995 during general anesthesia for coronary artery bypass grafts. Ten minutes after induction he developed a marked drop in blood pressure, bronchospasm, tachycardia, and increased pulmonary artery pressure. In July 1996 a transurethral resection of prostate was performed under spinal anesthetic. At cystoscopy he developed a headache, a rash, and bronchospasm, which settled after treatment. He had a further cystoscopy in February 1998, during which he became flushed, wheezy, and hypotensive, and had a cardiac arrest. He was successfully resuscitated. He had raised serum tryptase activities (60.4 and 26.6 μg/l at 3.5 and 9.5 hours after the event), indicating a true anaphylactic reaction. Since the only pharmacological agent common to all three procedures was urethral jelly containing lidocaine 2% and chlorhexidine 0.05%, he subsequently had skin prick tests, intradermal tests, and sequential subcutaneous challenges to lidocaine without any positive or adverse effects. Because he had developed profound anaphylaxis with cardiac arrest after the topical administration of chlorhexidine, skin tests were deemed unethical, and an in vitro method for detecting sensitivity to chlorhexidine was pursued. Detailed quantitative hapten inhibition studies were carried out with chlorhexidine-reactive IgE antibodies identified in the serum of the patient.

The authors concluded that unlike most drug allergic determinants the whole chlorhexidine molecule is complementary to the IgE antibody combining sites and that the 4-chlorophenol, biguanide, and hexamethylene structures together comprise the allergenic component.

ETHYLENE OXIDE *(SED-14, 761; SEDA-21, 254; SEDA-23, 248; SEDA-24, 271)*

Hematologic Epidemiological studies have associated ethylene oxide with hematological diseases (mainly *anemia*, *leukopenia*, and *leukemia*) (SEDA-24, 271). To determine whether occupational exposure to low concentrations of ethylene oxide can cause hematological abnormalities and whether blood monitoring could be used as health surveillance, a cross-sectional study was undertaken (3^C). Blood samples were collected from 47 hospital workers who were exposed to ethylene oxide during a mean period of 6.6 years. Ethylene oxide concentrations were in the range <0.01 to 0.06 ppm. The control group, individually matched by age, sex, and smoking habits, consisted of 88 workers from the administrative sector who had never been occupationally exposed to ethylene oxide. There were significant differences between the exposed and the control groups in the frequency of workers with low white blood cell counts. There was no significant difference in the absolute mean number of white blood cells, but there was an increase in the mean number of monocytes and eosinophils and a reduction in the absolute mean number of lymphocytes in the exposed group compared with the control group. There was an increase in the percentage hematocrit and the mean absolute number of erythrocytes and a fall in the mean absolute number of platelets in the exposed group compared with the controls. The mean absolute numbers of eosinophils and erythrocytes were significantly higher as was the hematocrit, and the mean absolute numbers of lymphocytes and platelets were significantly lower in the subgroups with a higher cumulative dose of exposure. There was a dose relation between cumulative exposure and the absolute mean number of eosinophils.

The results of this study suggest that the total white blood cell count and the eosinophil count could be used to monitor for early detection of health problems in ethylene oxide workers.

Mutagenicity Ethylene oxide has been used to sterilize heat-sensitive medical supplies since the 1950s, and its mutagenicity and toxicity in workers in sterile supply departments has been a major concern. Although the volume of ethylene oxide used for sterilization is relatively small, many workers are involved. Exposure control through monitoring ethylene oxide in the workplace air is the occupational health method commonly used to assess risk (SEDA-21, 254; SEDA-23, 248). Health surveillance of the mutagenicity of ethylene oxide is not undertaken, as there is no recognized biological marker.

IODOPHORS *(SED-14, 768; SEDA-22, 263; SEDA-24, 271)*

Iodine

Endocrine Severe transient postnatal *hypothyroidism* has been reported in infants whose mothers have received high doses of iodine during pregnancy or multiple local applications of povidone iodine during pregnancy and for delivery (SED-14, 472). Transient neonatal hypothyroidism during breastfeeding after postnatal maternal topical iodine treatment has also been reported (4^A).

A baby girl was born prematurely at 29 weeks. Her weight, length, and head circumference were appropriate to her gestational age. Parenteral feeding was stopped at 20 days, and breastfeeding was gradually increased. TSH screening for congenital hypothyroidism on day 5 was negative (<1 μU/ml), but a second screening on day 23 was high at 23 μU/ml. There were no signs of hypothyroidism and no palpable goiter. A confirmatory laboratory test on day 29 showed a high serum TSH concentration (288 μU/ml, reference range 0.45–10.0) and reduced concentrations of free T4 (2.8 ng/l, reference range 19–23) and free T3 (1.52 pg/ml, reference range 2.2–5.4). The mother had developed an abscess of the abdominal wall 1 week after cesarean section and had been treated with intravenous antibiotics and iodine tampons, 60 cm^2 daily to the abscess wound, containing about 10.5 mg of iodine. Maternal thyroid function was normal (TSH 1.59 μU/ml and free T4 12 ng/l). Thyroid antibodies to thyroglobulin, TSH receptors, and thyroperoxidase were negative. Iodine concentrations in the maternal milk and infant urine were extremely high: 4410 (reference range 29-490) μg/l and 3932 (reference range <185) μg/l respectively. Treatment with levothyroxine (25 μg/day) was started on day 32, breastfeeding was discontinued, and disinfection with iodine was stopped. Thyroid function normalized after 6 days, levothyroxine was withdrawn, and breastfeeding was restarted. Thyroid function remained normal over a follow-up period of 4 months.

Antiseptics with iodine should be avoided not only during pregnancy and delivery but also after the delivery during breastfeeding.

Skin A complication of the use of alcoholic iodine solution has been described in three women undergoing cesarean section, who developed *painful, superficial, inflammatory reactions* on their buttocks after skin preparation for surgery with 10% iodine in alcohol (5[A]). These lesions were believed to have been caused by pooling of the solution underneath the patients, topical skin damage being exacerbated by heat and occlusive drapes.

ORGANIC MERCURY COMPOUNDS *(SED-14, 771; SEDA-22, 263; SEDA-23, 248)*

Thiomersal

Thiomersal is a mercury-containing preservative that has been used as an additive in some blood products and in vaccines since the 1930s to prevent bacterial and fungal contamination. In an effort to reduce exposure to mercury the FDA have recommended that vaccine manufacturers phase out its use. In response to this, some blood products are also being manufactured free of thiomersal (6[S]).

REFERENCES

1. Sheng W-H, Ko W-J, Wang J-T, Chang S-C, Hsueh P-R, Luh K-T. Evaluation of antiseptic-impregnated central venous catheters for prevention of catheter related infection in intensive care unit patients. Diagn Microbiol Infect Dis 2000; 38: 1–5.
2. Pham NH, Weiner JM, Reisner GS, Baldo BA. Anaphylaxis to chlorhexidine. Case report. Implication of immunoglobulin E antibodies and identification of an allergenic determinant. Clin Exp Allergy 2000; 30: 1001–7.
3. Shaham J, Levi Z, Gurvich R, Shain R, Ribak J. Haematological changes in hospital workers due to chronic exposure to low levels of ethylene oxide. J Occup Environ Med 2000; 42: 843–50.
4. Casteels K, Punt S, Bramswig J. Transient neonatal hypothyroidism during breast feeding after post-natal maternal topical iodine treatment. Eur J Pediatr 2000; 159: 716–17.
5. Chilvers RJ, Weisz MT. Side-effects of alcoholic iodine solution (10%). Br J Anaesth 2000; 85: 178.
6. Sawyer LA. Antibodies for the prevention and treatment of viral diseases. Antiviral Res 2000; 47: 57–77.

T. Midtvedt

25 Penicillins, cephalosporins, other β-lactam antibiotics, and tetracyclines

The prudent use of antibiotics

The development of resistance *Over the years, the increasing rate of antibiotic resistance in an increasing number of microbial species worldwide has been addressed almost yearly in SEDA, and has been pointed out as the most serious adverse effect of these drugs. As early as in 1988 it was stated that "The time has come to tell the World Health Organization that increasing worldwide microbial resistance is an acute and serious threat to public health; it is not the sort of matter which can be left for leisurely evaluations by slow-working committees working with the pharmaceutical industry" (SEDA-12; 208).*

Now the topic is very well recognized by the WHO, and the Director-General wrote on the front page of WHO's Report on Infectious Diseases 2000 (1[S]): "Now, at the dawn of a new millennium, humanity is faced with another crisis. Formerly curable diseases such as gonorrhea and typhoid are rapidly becoming difficult to treat, while old killers such as tuberculosis and malaria are now arrayed in the increasingly impenetrable armor of antimicrobial resistance.

"This phenomenon is potentially containable. It is a deepening and complex problem accelerated by the overuse of antibiotics in developed countries and the paradoxical underuse of quality antimicrobials in developed nations owing to poverty and a resultant dearth of effective healthcare …

"This year's report focuses on the issue of drug resistance and how this disturbing development is closing the windows of opportunity to treat infectious diseases. By developing a global strategy to contain resistance and building alliances involving all healthcare providers – countries, governments, international organizations, non-governmental organizations and both the private and public healthcare sectors – we have an opportunity to launch a massive effort against infectious diseases that perpetuate poverty. Used wisely and widely, the drugs we have today can be made available to the world's poorest to prevent the healthcare catastrophes of tomorrow.

"This is our challenge and must be our goal".

Amen!

New indications? *The prudent use of antibiotics might be challenged from another angle. Tetracyclines have many effects on cells involved in inflammatory reactions (SEDA-24, 278), and it is well documented that they might be of value in the treatment of rheumatoid arthritis and periodontal disease. The hottest theory for the mechanism of this action is that they inhibit collagenolytic activity in the host. It has been suggested that tetracyclines and fluoroquinolones may protect against myocardial infarction (2[r]), and that a more liberal use of antibiotics in patients with mild gastric disorders may be of some benefit (3[M]). In all the disorders mentioned, the proposed mechanisms are on the host side rather than on the microbial side. Therefore, microbial sensitivity tests will have no meaning. However, one thing is certain: the microbial empire will strike back.*

Taken together, these new indications will involve some tens of millions patients. It goes

Side Effects of Drugs, Annual 25
J.K. Aronson, ed.

without saying that antimicrobials should be used against microbes and not against host factors.

Another new indication for antibiotics is the treatment of filariasis – a disease that has caused an estimated minimum all-time worldwide total of 150 million infections (4[C]). The world community had made it a goal to eliminate these diseases (5[S]). However, with current therapy, this goal may be difficult to achieve (6[S]).

Based on observations in animals that filariae live in close symbiosis with some bacteria (Wolbachia spp.) and that depletion of these bacteria leads to degeneration and sterility of adult worms, a group of patients with onchocerciasis in Ghana were given either doxycycline (21 patients, 100 mg/day) or placebo (14 patients) for 6 weeks (4[C]). Four months later, onchocercomata (cutaneous nodules containing female worms) were excised and investigated in a blinded fashion. None of the nodules from patients taking doxycycline contained live female worms with intact embryogenesis, whereas such worms were present in all the control patients. This is very exciting and challenging, and the authors (4[C]) opened up an even wider view: "endobacterial targeting could be developed as a treatment not only for onchocerciasis, but also for lymphatic filariasis, in view of the presence of endobacteria in the respective species". If so, we are talking about some hundreds of millions of patients to treat.

As stated above, antimicrobial sensitivity testing will be of no use. However, the development of resistance is not uncommon in endosymbiotic microorganisms as well as in the intestinal microflora.

Taken together, all these new uses of antibiotics represent a major challenge for a future prudent use of these life-saving drugs in the infections for which they were created. There is no reason to believe that the industry is not interested in entering these new fields. Nor is there reason to believe that uses for new indications not will be followed by reduced antibiotic sensitivity in pathogens, if the right strategy is not established.

En garde, Director-General of the WHO.

β-lactams, tetracyclines, and pregnancy

Since the days of the thalidomide disaster about 40 years ago – resulting in the birth of some thousands of malformed babies – it has been well recognized that drugs taken by pregnant mothers can have severe adverse effects on their unborn children. A consequence of the thalidomide disaster was worldwide awareness that drugs can cause congenital malformations and the necessity to investigate this possibility in animals. Since thalidomide, around 30 drugs have been proven to be teratogenic, not all of which are currently in clinical use (7[R]). For most drugs, however, safety in pregnancy has still to be established. With the risk of teratogenicity and dysmorphogenesis ever present, clinicians are in general very cautious in prescribing drugs for pregnant women. Despite this, over 60% of pregnant women consume therapeutic agents not directly related to their pregnancy, and it has been estimated that about 5% of birth defects are caused by maternal drug therapy (8[R]).

Even if a drug is "generally recognized as safe" after animal experiments, it is wise to be suspicious when giving it to a pregnant woman. One major obstacle in evaluating safety in humans is the sample size required to reach sound conclusions. For example, in Europe neural tube defects and cleft lips both occur with a prevalence of around 7 per 10 000 live births (9[R]). It has been calculated that for an uncommon drug exposure (i.e. a frequency of less than 1 per 1000 pregnant women and a background malformation prevalence of 0.001) detection of teratogenic effects would require that more than 1 000 000 births should be monitored, even though the relative risk associated with the drug might be as high as 20 (i.e. a 20-fold increased risk of a particular malformation). In contrast, for formulations that are commonly used in pregnancy (e.g. by 2% of women, as was the case with thalidomide), and that are associated with an extremely high relative risk (such as 175), 1000 births would be sufficient to detect the teratogenic potential, even when the background malformation prevalence was as low as 0.0024 (10[R]).

Another issue that has to be taken into consideration is the temporal relation between drug exposure and the effect on the embryo/fetus (11[R]). Exposure to harmful drugs in the 2 weeks after conception usually leads to abortion, which may not be noticed by the woman. In the next 6–7 weeks the embryo is assumed to be extremely sensitive to teratogens (12[R]). However, different organs or systems may be susceptible to teratogens at different times during this period. Therefore, in order 'to postulate a meaningful relationship between drug use during pregnancy – and a congenital malformation – drug intake must have taken place during a gestation period in which the organ or organ system is sensitive to harmful agents" (11[R]). It goes without saying that exact information on the timing of exposure is crucial.

In an ideal world, no drug would become available before it had been thoroughly tested for safety and effectiveness in a randomized, double-blind, placebo-controlled trial in pregnant women (13[R]). However, because of ethical concerns about the welfare of the mother and fetus, pregnant women are traditionally excluded from drug trials. Therefore, usage is most often based on indirect measures of safety, such as in vitro studies and animal models. However, the thalidomide disaster still has something to tell us about the inadequacy of relying too much on animal models.

In reality, most information about the safety of antimicrobials in pregnancy comes from a history of long-term use with no reported adverse outcomes. As underlined by Weller and Rees (13[R]) "most practitioners are happy to prescribe penicillin and its derivatives, for instance, although there are no data from formal trials". Now data have appeared that show that penicillin V is safe during pregnancy (14[R]). The study took place in Hungary between 1980 and 1996. The case group consisted of 22 865 malformed infants or fetuses, of whom 173 (0.8%) had mothers who had taken penicillin V during pregnancy. As a population control, two newborn infants without malformation were matched with every case according to sex, week of birth, and the district of the parent's residence. In the control group (38 151 infants) 218 been treated with penicillin V. This difference was explained mainly by recall bias and confounders, because there was no difference in the adjusted odds ratio for medically documented phenoxymethylpenicillin treatment during the second and third months of gestation, i.e. during the critical period for most major congenital abnormalities in case-matched control pairs. Thus, treatment with oral phenoxymethylpenicillin during pregnancy presents very little if any teratogenic risk to the fetus. The authors also underlined the need to examine the teratogenic potential of different penicillins separately, and two such reports have recently appeared.

In the first study, 791 women who had redeemed a prescription for pivampicillin during their first pregnancy, birth outcomes (malformations, preterm delivery, and low birthweight) were matched with similar outcomes in 7472 reference pregnancies in which the mother had not redeemed any prescription for pivampicillin during pregnancy (15[C]). There were no significant differences in any of the three parameters mentioned. The authors thought that their data showed that pivampicillin had no teratogenic or fetotoxic risk, "but further studies are need to permit non-specific risk assessment".

In the second study, of 78 women who took cefuroxime axetil during pregnancy, none of the 13 women who were treated in the first trimester gave birth to any malformed child, but one baby with hip dysplasia was found among 20 babies from mothers treated in their second trimester, and there was one case of hypospadias and one of imperforate anus in 47 children of mothers treated in the third trimester (16[C]). The authors correctly concluded that the number of patients who had taken cefuroxime in the first trimester of pregnancy was small, and that the drug "should be used with caution in the early months of pregnancy".

The same group that investigated the possible effects of penicillin V has also studied the teratogenic potential of tetracyclines (17[R]), which was suggested early on in some animal and human studies (18[r], 19[c], 20[c]). However, the authors listed a similar number of investigations in which no teratogenic effects have been shown. Of 38 151 pregnant women who had babies without any defects (controls), 214 (0.6%) had taken oral oxytetracycline; in contrast, of 22 865 pregnant women who had offspring with congenital abnormalities, 216 (0.9%) had taken oxytetracycline (OR = 1.7; 95% CI = 1.4, 2.0). More women whose babies had congenital abnormalities had taken oxytetracycline in the second month of pregnancy: neural-tube defects (OR = 9.7; CI = 2.0, 47), cleft palate (OR = 17; CI = 3.5, 84), and multiple congenital abnormalities (particularly the combination of neural-tube defects and cardiovascular malformations) (OR = 13; CI = 3.8, 44). The *authors mentioned that their previous study had not shown a teratogenic potential of doxycycline (21[R]), but concluded, far more rigorously, that "all tetracyclines are contraindicated during pregnancy". That seems to be a prudent statement.*

PENICILLINS *(SED-14, 810; SEDA-22, 266; SEDA-23, 252; SEDA-24, 276)*

Amoxicillin

Metabolism *Lipoatrophy* can occur after the injection of some drugs, including penicillin (22[A]).

A 2-year-old boy developed a non-tender, hypopigmented, atrophic patch measuring around 2 × 6 cm on his right buttock. He had been well until 5 months before, when he had received an injection of penicillin into the right buttock.

The incidence of this adverse effect is unknown, as is the mechanism.

Urinary tract Drug-induced *nephrolithiasis* was often seen during the sulfonamide era, but is nowadays rare, especially in patients taking β-lactams. However, it should not be forgotten (23[A]).

A 48-year-old woman with pneumococcal meningitis developed acute oliguric renal insufficiency after taking high-dose amoxicillin (320 mg/kg/day) for 4 days. Amoxicillin crystallization was documented by infrared spectrometry. The outcome was favorable after dosage reduction, a single hemodialysis, and adequate hydration.

As was true for the sulfonamides, "crystalluria [due to amoxicillin] is increased by low urinary pH, low urine output, and high dose".

Skin *Palmar exfoliation* Although several reports have described fixed rashes due to amoxicillin, palmar exfoliation has rarely been described (24[A]).

Five patients (1 man, 4 women, aged 30–72 year) developed intense palmar rashes and itching during treatment with amoxicillin (doses not given). All the episodes began after several days of treatment with amoxicillin, either alone or in combination with clavulanic acid. Three of the patients had repeated episodes, and the interval between treatment and onset was shorter each time (down to 5 hours on the third occasion). In all cases the rash was followed by exfoliation and cleared in 7–10 days without residual lesions. Skin prick tests, intradermal tests, and patch tests were performed with several β-lactams, including amoxicillin, and were all negative. A challenge test with amoxicillin was performed in one patient, and the erythema recurred in 3–4 hours. All five patient tolerated cefuroxime and ceftazidime. Cefalexin was given to one patient only, and palmar exfoliative erythema developed a few days later.

Nicolau syndrome Tissue damage supposedly caused by intramuscular injection of various drugs, especially long-acting derivatives, occurred more often in the past (SEDA-11, 224). However, there is still a risk of that complication. A recent review covered 102 patients, of whom 80 were under 12 years of age (25[C]). Injection of other drugs may cause similar symptoms (26[A]). In addition to skin damage, severe complications, such as limb gangrene, paraplegia, and even death, can occur. Whether the mechanisms are intra-arterial injection or spasm after a para-arterial injection, and whether crystals in the injected suspension play an important role or not, is of minor importance for the patient. The key point is that special emphasis should be put on "the precautionary measures to be taken in intramuscular injection of long-acting penicillin or other drugs in crystalline suspensions".

Co-amoxiclav

Liver *Hepatotoxic reactions* in patients taking co-amoxiclav were reported last year (SEDA-24, 276), but new reports and new theories continue to appear.

A 33-month-old boy was treated with co-amoxiclav (dose not stated) for 10 days for otitis media (27[A]). He had taken it twice before. One day after completing the course he developed a rash over his entire body, followed 3 days later by lethargy, jaundice, pale stools, and pruritus. The jaundice persisted, the liver was markedly enlarged, and all liver function tests were abnormal. Tests for known viral and metabolic causes of cholestasis were negative. A percutaneous liver biopsy showed centrilobular cholestasis "consistent with a drug reaction". He was given ursodeoxycholic acid (30 mg/kg/day) and vitamins A, D, and K; later prednisolone was added. However, his jaundice persisted, as did severe pruritus. He also developed extensive xanthomatosis and failure to grow. A liver transplantation was successfully performed 8 months after the onset of symptoms. His explanted liver had features of biliary cirrhosis, with ductular proliferation and ductopenia.

Pediatric cases of hepatotoxicity associated with co-amoxiclav are supposed to be rare, but they can be overlooked if they start some time after the end of therapy. The authors stated that co-amoxiclav "should be considered in the differential diagnosis of progressive, severe cholestatic disease in children".

The recently described association (SEDA-24, 276) between the HLA haplotype DRB1*1501-DQB1*0602 and liver disease associated with co-amoxiclav has been confirmed (28[C]). There was an increased frequency of homozygous status for this haplotype. This might reflect population differences and the small sample size in both studies (29[C]). The authors proposed two theories. One explanation was based on the formation through metabolism of neoantigens, and subsequent recognition of these antigens as foreign by the immune system. This "immune allergic hypothesis" is supported by the strong association with an HLA class II haplotype. The authors argued that "HLA class II molecules are required for antigen presentation to CD4 positive T cells. HLA alleles may differ by as little as a single codon, and one amino acid residue difference at a critical site in the resulting polypeptide may be functionally significant, determining not only the affinity with which a given antigen is presented but also the interaction of the HLA peptide complex with the T cell receptor".

Their other theory was that the liver disease may arise through linkage with another gene on chromosome 6p. This "linked-gene" hypothesis, they proposed, may explain why jaundice is rare after treatment with co-amoxiclav, although this particular HLA haplotype is common in Northern Europe, where co-amoxiclav is commonly prescribed.

Whatever the mechanisms might be, at present it is reasonable to look on clavulanate as the "driving force" in the development of hepatotoxicity with co-amoxiclav. Hepatotoxicity has also been reported with clavulanate plus ticarcillin (30[A]). So far, however, there has been no genetic evaluation of patients with hepatotoxic reactions after therapy with clavulanate and ticarcillin.

In a retrospective cohort study of family practitioners' records, with a high proportion of mild cases, there was a rate of 1 per 4449 prescriptions (31[C]). If this is the case, it is wise to reserve co-amoxiclav (and maybe also clavulanate/ticarcillin) for use in infections caused by strains producing β-lactamases that can destroy amoxicillin (or ticarcillin).

CEPHALOSPORINS *(SED-14, 821; SEDA-22, 267; SEDA-23, 254; SEDA-24, 277)*

Skin *Rashes* are very common after the use of antibiotics, especially β-lactams. However, there may be differences in the frequencies of rashes, and this has recently been retrospectively investigated in 5923 children (32[C]). All the children who developed a rash after treatment with one or more of the commonly used oral antibiotics were identified – a total of 472. Significantly more rashes were documented for cefaclor (4.79%) compared with penicillins (2.72%), sulfonamides (3.46%), and other cephalosporins (1.04%). Based on the numbers of patients for whom the antibiotics were prescribed, the frequencies of rashes were 12.3% for cefaclor, 7.4% for penicillins, 8.5% for sulfonamides, and 2.6% for other cephalosporins. The authors concluded that "physicians considering the use of oral cefaclor need to be aware of its relatively high association with rashes".

Cefepime

Nervous system Among antibiotics that can cause *seizures*, the β-lactams are most commonly implicated (SEDA-18, 261) and cefepime is no exception (33[c]). However, status epilepticus seems to be rare. Now there is a report of two patients with status epilepticus during treatment with cefepime for *Pseudomonas aeruginosa* sepsis (34[A]).

A 44-year-old man, who had previously had a bilateral lung transplantation and who was on hemodialysis for chronic renal insufficiency, was given cefepime 2 g/day. Within 24 hours he started to become confused and developed diffuse hyper-reflexia. Two days later an electroencephalogram showed "nearly continuous, generalized sharp-wave/slow-wave activity". After lorazepam 2 mg the status epilepticus resolved, but he remained confused. A follow-up electroencephalogram showed recurrence of generalized sharp-wave activity. Cefepime was withdrawn, and within hours he rapidly recovered his mental status. An electroencephalogram showed absence of epileptiform discharges.

A 28-year-old woman with a thoracic spina bifida was given cefepime 1 g bd for an infection with *Ps. aeruginosa*. After a time (not stated) an electroencephalogram showed a continuous generalized spike and wave pattern. She was given lorazepam 2 mg, which resulted in resolution. Cefepime was withdrawn and she promptly recovered.

In the first case the dose was inappropriate for the degree of renal impairment and in the second case the dose was inappropriate for the patient's bodyweight. The authors underlined the importance of giving cefepime with great care, especially to patients with renal impairment and low bodyweight.

Cefotaxime

Skin *Telangiectasiae* in a light-exposed distribution have rarely, if ever, been reported with cephalosporins.

An otherwise healthy 57-year-old man developed telangiectatic skin lesions after receiving intramuscular cefotaxime 1 g bd for 7 days for a urinary tract infection (35[A]). He had used no other medications, and there was no history of photosensitivity or rosacea. He had several asymptomatic telangiectasiae widely distributed on the forehead and on the backs of both hands. Antinuclear antibodies and antineutrophil cytoplasmic antibodies were negative. Skin biopsy showed dilated capillaries without signs of vasculitis. A light provocation test produced telangiectatic lesions at 36 hours. Because of the relation between the administration of cefotaxime and the onset of the telangiectasia, confirmed by light testing, cefotaxime was withdrawn, with progressive improvement and complete resolution after 2 months; rechallenge was not performed.

Iatrogenic telangiectasis is a poorly understood dermatological adverse effect of several drugs, including cephalosporins (36[A], 37[A]). Telangiectasiae localized to light-exposed areas, as in this case, have been described with some calcium channel blockers (38[A], 39[A])

TETRACYCLINES *(SED-14, 906; SEDA-22, 268; SEDA-23, 255; SEDA-24, 278)*

Doxycycline

Gastrointestinal *Esophageal ulceration* occurred in two adults taking doxycycline as malaria chemoprophylaxis (40[A]).

A 20-year-old woman, who had been taking doxycycline malaria prophylaxis, took a doxycycline capsule (dose not given) before going to bed and awoke hours later with the feeling that the capsule was stuck in her esophagus. Over the next 4 days she developed worsening dysphagia. Esophagoscopy showed an esophageal ulcer over 20% of the esophageal surface. She was treated with ranitidine and sucralfate and improved over the next 2 days.

A 27-year-old man with an 8-day history of dysphagia and retrosternal pain was taking doxycycline prophylaxis and occasional terfenadine (doses not stated). He recalled no problems with taking any of his doxycycline prophylaxis. He had an esophagoscopy, which showed a 1 cm esophageal ulcer. He improved with ranitidine.

Metabolic Although other tetracyclines have been associated with *hypoglycemia*, the first reported case of doxycycline-induced hypoglycemia has been reported (41[A]).

A 70-year-old man with type 2 diabetes mellitus presented with sudden confusion, which rapidly progressed to loss of consciousness. The only drug he had taken during the previous 2 months was doxycycline (100 mg/day), which he had taken for 5 days for an upper respiratory tract infection. Urine tests for sulfonylureas were negative. Routine hematological and biochemical tests and an electrocardiogram were normal. He improved with intravenous glucose and withdrawal of doxycycline and had no further episodes of hypoglycemia over the next 3 months.

Plasma insulin was not measured in this case, so the mechanism of hypoglycemia is unclear.

Minocycline

Liver *Hepatotoxicity* associated with minocycline recently has been reviewed, covering data reported to a WHO Center for International Drug Monitoring, which had recorded 8025 reactions to minocycline, of which 493 were reactions involving the liver (42[M]). The authors stated that "fields available to define indications for use, time of treatment and outcome subsequent to the reactions were seldom completed". They therefore concentrated on more complete records in patients known to have used minocycline for acne. Patients taking minocycline for reasons other than acne or those given intravenous minocycline were excluded. Altogether, 65 patients were then commented on; 58% were women and 94% were aged under 40 years. Briefly, two types of hepatic reactions were recognized: autoimmune hepatitis associated with lupus-like symptoms occurring after 1 year of more of exposure to minocycline, and hypersensitivity reactions associated with eosinophilia and exfoliative dermatitis occurring within 35 days of therapy.

The authors stated that "we do not have any clear information about the absolute and relative risks of hepatitis, whether hypersensitivity reaction or autoimmune hepatitis, in patients receiving minocycline therapy for varying lengths of time", and that a "study of the comparative rates of hepatitis in people exposed to minocycline compared with those not exposed is required". In the meantime, new reports of severe hepatic reactions to minocycline continue to appear (43^A–45^A), including one case of autoimmune hepatitis requiring liver transplantation in a woman who had used minocycline 50–200 mg/day for 3 years (45^A). Another case of liver transplantation has previously been reported in patients with hepatic failure after minocycline therapy (46^C).

Some patients consider the use of drugs to treat a common dermatological disease such as acne vulgaris to be cosmetics rather than medications. Safer alternatives than minocycline should be considered in the treatment of acne.

Skin A *generalized pustular eruption* was reported in a patient with acne treated with minocycline (47^A). Skin prick tests with minocycline were positive at 48 hours.

REFERENCES

1. Brundtland GH. Overcoming Antimicrobial Resistance. World Health Organization Report on Infectious Diseases 2000. www.who.int./infectious-disease-report/2000/intro.htm.
2. Herings RMC, Leufkens HGM, Vandenbroucke JP. Acute myocardial infarction and prior antibiotic use. J Am Med Assoc 2000; 284: 2998–9.
3. Moayyedi P, Soo S, Deeks J, Forman D, Mason J, Innes M, Delaney B. Systematic review and economic evaluation of *Helicobacter pylori* eradication treatment for non-ulcer dyspepsia. Dyspepsia Review Group. Br Med J 2000; 321: 659–64.
4. Hoerauf A, Volkmann L, Hamelmann C, Ajei O, Autenrieth IB, Fleischer B, Büttner DW. Endosymbiotic bacteria in worms as targets for a novel chemotherapy in filariasis. Lancet 2000; 355: 1242–3.
5. WHO. Chagas disease, leprosy, lymphatic filariasis, onchocerciasis: prospect for elimination. Geneva: WHO, TDR/Gen 97-1. 1997: 1–35.
6. Plaister AP, Alley ES, Van Oortmarssen GJ, Boatin BA, Habbema JD. Required duration of combined annual ivermectin treatment and vector control in the Onchocerciasis Control Programme in West Africa. Bull WHO 1997; 75: 237–45.
7. Koren G, Pastuszak A, Ito S. Drugs in pregnancy. New Engl J Med 1998; 338: 1128–37.
8. Rao JM, Arulappu R. Drug use in pregnancy. How to avoid problems. Drugs 1981; 22: 409–14.
9. EUROCAT Working Group. EUROCAT Report 7: 15 years of surveillance of congenital anomalies in Europe 1980–1994. Brussels: Scientific Institute of Public Health – Louis Pasteur, 1997.
10. Khoury MJ, Holtzman NA. On the ability of birth defects monitoring to detect new teratogens. Am J Epidemiol 1987; 126: 136–43.
11. Irl C, Hasford J. Assessing the safety of drugs in pregnancy. The role of prospective cohort studies. Drug Saf 2000; 22: 169–77.
12. Lenz W. Kindliche Missbildungen nach Medikamenten wärhend der Gravidität. Dtsch Med Wochenschr 1961; 86: 2555–6.
13. Weller TMA, Rees N. Antibacterial use in pregnancy. Drug Saf 2000; 22: 335–8.
14. Czeizel AE, Rockenbauer M, Olsen J, Sorensen HT. Oral phenoxymethylpenicillin treatment during pregnancy. Results of a population-based Hungarian case-control study. Arch Gynecol Obstet 2000; 263: 178–81.
15. Larsen H, Nielsen GL, Sorensen HT, Molle M, Olsen J, Schonheyder HC. A follow-up study of birth outcome in users of pivampicillin during pregnancy. Acta Obstet Gynecol Scand 2000; 70: 379–83.
16. Manka W, Solowiow R, Okrzeja D. Assessment of infant development during an 18-month follow-up after treatment of infections in pregnant women with cefuroxime axetil. Drug Saf 2000; 22: 83–8.
17. Czeizel AE, Rockenbauer M. A population-based case-control teratologic study of oral oxytetracycline treatment during pregnancy. Eur J Obstet Gynecol Reprod Biol 2000; 88: 27–33.
18. McColl JD, Globus M, Robinson S. Effect of some therapeutic agents on the developing rat fetus. Toxicol Appl Pharmacol 1965; 7: 409–17.
19. Krejci L, Brettschneider I. Congenital cataract due to tetracycline. Animal experiments and clinical observation. Ophthalmic Paediatr Genet 1983; 3: 59–60.
20. Mennie AT. Tetracycline and congenital limb abnormalities. Br Med J 1962; 2: 480.

21. Czeizel AE, Rockenbauer M. Teratogenic study of doxycycline. Obstet Gynecol 1997; 89: 524–8.
22. Kuperman-Beade M, Laude TA. Partial lipoatrophy in a child. Pediatr Dermatol 2000; 17: 302–3.
23. Boffa JJ, De Preuneuf H, Bouadma L, Daudon M, Pallot JL. Insuffisance renale aiguë par cristallisation d'amoxicilline. Presse Med 2000; 29: 699–701.
24. Gastaminza G, Audicana MT, Fernandez E, Anda M, Ansotegui IJ. Palmar exfoliative exanthema to amoxicillin. Allergy Eur J Allergy Clin Immunol 2000; 55: 510–11.
25. Saputo V, Bruni G. La sindrome di Nicolau da preparati di penicillina: analisi della letteratura alla ricercá di potenziali fattori di rischio. Pediatr Med Chir 1998; 20: 105–23.
26. Beissert S, Presser D, Rütter A, Metze D, Luger TA, Schwarz T. Embolia cutis medicamentosa (Nicolau-Syndrom) nach intraartikulärer injektion. Hautarzt 1999; 50: 214–16.
27. Chawla A, Kahn E, Yunis E, Daum F. Rapidly progressive cholestasis: an unusual reaction to amoxicillin/clavulanic acid therapy in a child. J Pediatr 2000; 136: 121–3.
28. O'Donohue J, Oien KA, Donaldson P, Underhill J, Clare M, MacSween RNM, Mills PR. Co-amoxiclav jaundice: clinical and histological features and HLA class II association. Gut 2000; 47: 717–20.
29. Hautekeete ML, Horsmans Y, Van Wayenberge C, Demanet C, Henrion J, Verbist L, Brenard J, Sempoux C, Michielsen PP, Yap PS, et al. HLA association of amoxicillin–clavulanate-induced hepatitis. Gastroenterology 1999; 117: 1181–6.
30. Sweet JM, Jones MP. Intrahepatic cholestasis due to ticarcillin–clavulanate. Am J Gastroenterol 1995; 90: 675–6.
31. Garcia Rodriguez LA, Stricker BH, Zimmermann HJ. Risk of acute liver injury associated with the combination of amoxicillin and clavulanic acid. Arch Intern Med 1996; 156: 1327–32.
32. Ibia EO, Schwartz RH, Wiedermann BL. Antibiotic rashes in children. Arch Dermatol 2000; 136: 849–54.
33. Chetaille E, Hary L, De Cagny B, Gras-Champel V, Decocq G, Andrejak M. Crises convulsives associées à un surdosage en cefepime. Therapie 1998; 53: 167–8.
34. Dixit S, Kurle P, Buyan-Dent L, Sheth RD. Status epilepticus associated with cefepime. Neurology 2000; 54: 2153–5.
35. Borgia F, Vaccaro M, Guarneri F, Cannavo SP. Photodistributed telangiectasia following use of cefotaxime. Br J Dermatol 2000; 143: 674–5.
36. Vinks SAT, Heijerman HGM, De Jonge P, Bakker W. Photosensitivity due to ambulatory intravenous ceftazidime in cystic fibrosis patient. Lancet 1993; 341: 1221–2.
37. Flax SH, Uhle P. Photo recall-like phenomenon following the use of cefazolin and gentamicin sulfate. Cutis 1990; 46: 59–61.
38. Collins P, Ferguson J. Photodistributed nifedipine-induced facial telangiectasis. Br J Dermatol. 1993; 129: 630–3.
39. Basarab T, Yu R, Jones RR. Calcium antagonist-induced photoexposed telangiectasia. Br J Dermatol 1997; 136: 974–5.
40. Morris TJ, Davis TP. Doxycycline-induced esophageal ulceration in the US Military Service. Mil Med 2000; 165: 316–19.
41. Odeh M, Oliven A. Doxycycline-induced hypoglycemia. J Clin Pharmacol 2000; 40: 1173–4.
42. Lawrenson RA, Seaman HE, Sunström A, Williams TJ, Farmer RDT. Liver damage associated with minocycline use in acne: a systematic review of the published literature and pharmacovigilance data. Drug Saf 2000; 23: 333–49.
43. Kettaneh A, Fain O, Ziol M, Thomas M, Lejeune F, Eclache-Saudreau V, Biaggi A, Guettier-Bouttier C. Minocycline-induced systemic adverse reaction with liver and bone marrow granulomas and Sezary-like cells. Am J Med 2000; 108: 353–4.
44. Nietsch HH, Libman BS, Pansze TW, Eicher JN, Reeves JRT, Krawitt EL. Minocycline-induced hepatitis. Am J Gastroenterol 2000; 95: 2993–5.
45. Pohle T, Menzel J, Domschke W. Minocycline and fulminant hepatic failure necessitating liver transplantation. Am J Gastroenterol 2000; 95: 560–1.
46. Boudreaux JP, Hayes DH, Mizrahi S, Hussey J, Regenstein F, Balart L. Fulminant hepatic failure, hepatorenal syndrome, and necrotizing pancreatitis after minocycline hepatotoxicity. Transplant Proc 1993; 25: 1873.
47. Antunes A, Davril A, Trechot P, Grandidier M, Truchetet F, Cuny JF. Minocycline hypersensitivity syndrome. Ann Dermatol Venereol 1999; 126: 518–21.

Alexander Imhof and Roland Walter

26 Miscellaneous antibacterial drugs

AMINOGLYCOSIDES *(SED-14, 837; SEDA-22, 274; SEDA-23, 264; SEDA-24. 283)*

Sensory systems The incidence of aminoglycoside associated *hearing loss* is 2–45%. A review of nearly 10 000 adults suggested rates of 8.6% for gentamicin, 14% for amikacin, and 2.4% for netilmicin. Aminoglycoside toxicity is markedly lower in infants and children, with an incidence of 0–2%. A long duration of treatment and repeated courses or high cumulative doses appear to be critical for ototoxicity, which occurs in high frequency hearing beyond the range of normal speech.

Gentamicin also damages the vestibular apparatus at a rate of 1.4–3.7%, resulting in *vertigo* and *impaired balance*. This effect is reversible in only about 50% from 1 week to 6 months after administration. The coadministration of aminoglycosides with ototoxic drugs (e.g. ethacrynic acid) can worsen toxicity (1[R]).

In 40 patients tobramycin had little effect on audiometric thresholds, but produced a change in the amplitude of the distortion products, currently considered an objective method for rapidly evaluating the functional status of the cochlea (2[C]). In one case, tobramycin caused bilateral high-frequency vestibular toxicity, which subsequently showed clinical and objective evidence of functional recovery (3[A]).

In a quantitative assessment of vestibular hair cells and Scarpa's ganglion cells in 17 temporal bones from 10 individuals with aminoglycoside ototoxicity, streptomycin caused a significant loss of both type I and type II hair cells in all five vestibular sense organs (4[C]). The vestibular ototoxic effects of kanamycin appeared to be similar to those of streptomycin, whereas neomycin did not cause loss of vestibular hair cells. There was no significant loss of Scarpa's ganglion cells.

Of 20 patients with Dandy's syndrome, 15 had previously been treated with aminoglycosides (13 with gentamicin and two with streptomycin), of whom 10 had symptoms of pre-existing chronic nephrosis or transitory renal insufficiency. In all 13 patients who had gentamicin, peripheral vestibular function was destroyed or severely damaged, whereas there was no hearing loss (5[c]).

In a case-control study in 15 children under 33 weeks' gestation with significant sensorineural hearing loss and 30 matched controls, the children with sensorineural hearing loss had longer periods of intubation, ventilation, oxygen treatment, and acidosis, and more frequent treatment with dopamine or furosemide (6[C]). However, neither peak nor trough aminoglycoside concentrations, nor duration of jaundice or bilirubin concentration varied between the groups. At 12 months of age, seven of the children with sensorineural hearing loss had evidence of cerebral palsy compared with two of the 30 controls. Therefore, preterm children with sensorineural hearing loss required more intensive care in the perinatal period and developed more neurological complications than controls, and the coexistence of risk factors for hearing loss may be more important than the individual factors themselves.

Intratympanic gentamicin therapy has gained some popularity in the treatment of vertigo associated with Menière's disease, as it offers some advantages over traditional surgical treatment. However, although the vestibulotoxic effect of gentamicin is well documented, there is no general agreement about the dose needed to control attacks of vertigo without affecting hearing. In 27 patients treated

Side Effects of Drugs, Annual 25
J.K. Aronson, ed.

with small doses of gentamicin delivered via a microcatheter in the round window niche and administered by an electronic micropump, vertigo was effectively controlled; however, the negative effect on hearing was unacceptable (7[C], 8[R]).

Using lymphoblastoid cell lines derived from five deaf and five hearing individuals from an Arab–Israeli family carrying the A1555G mutation, the first direct evidence has been provided that the mitochondrial 12S rRNA carrying the A1555G mutation is the main target of the aminoglycosides (9[E]). This suggests that they exert their detrimental effect through altering mitochondrial protein synthesis, which exacerbates the inherent defect caused by the mutation and reduces the overall translation rate below the minimal level required for normal cellular function.

In hatched chicks repeatedly injected with kanamycin, afferent innervation of the regenerated hair cells was related more to the recovery of hearing than efferent innervation (10[E]).

In rats, ototoxicity caused by gentamicin or tobramycin was ameliorated by melatonin, which did not interfere with the antibiotic action of the aminoglycosides (11[E]). The free radical scavenging agent α-lipoic acid has previously been shown to protect against the cochlear adverse effects of systemically administered aminoglycoside antibiotics, and in a recent animal study it also prevented cochlear toxicity after the administration of neomycin 5% directly to the round window membrane over 7 days (12[E]).

Loss of spiral ganglion neurons can be prevented by neurotrophin 3, whereas hair cell damage can be prevented by *N*-methyl-D-aspartate (NMDA) receptor antagonists. In a recent animal study, an NMDA receptor antagonist (MK801) protected against noise-induced excitotoxicity in the cochlea; in addition, combined treatment with neurotrophin 3 and MK801 had a potent effect in preserving both auditory physiology and morphology against aminoglycoside toxicity induced by amikacin (13[E]).

Electrolyte balance Aminoglycoside-induced proximal tubular dysfunction, which causes some manifestations of *Fanconi's syndrome*, is rare.

A 72-year-old man was treated with ceftriaxone (2 g bd) and gentamicin (80 mg tds) for a severe urinary tract infection (14[A]). On day 5 his serum potassium concentration was 3 mmol/l with a normal serum creatinine and urine examination. Despite treatment with oral potassium chloride plus a high potassium diet, his serum potassium fell to 2.3 mmol/l 4 days later, accompanied by inappropriate kaliuresis, hypouricemia with inappropriate uricosuria, and hypophosphatemia with inappropriate phosphaturia. There was no bicarbonate wasting, but there was proteinuria 1.2 g/day, with a predominance of low molecular weight proteins; in contrast, serum creatinine was normal and creatinine clearance was 78 ml/min. The aminoglycoside was withdrawn with subsequent progressive improvement in renal proximal tubular function, which normalized 9 days later.

Metal metabolism Aminoglycosides can cause renal magnesium wasting and *hypomagnesemia*, usually associated with acute renal insufficiency. However, animal studies have shown frequent renal magnesium wasting, even in the absence of renal insufficiency and abnormalities of renal tubular morphology. In 24 patients with cystic fibrosis, treatment with amikacin plus ceftazidime for exacerbation of pulmonary symptoms by *Pseudomonas aeruginosa* resulted in mild hypomagnesemia due to renal magnesium wasting, even in the absence of a significant rise in circulating creatinine and urea concentrations (15[C]).

In five healthy volunteers gentamicin 5 mg/kg caused immediate but transient renal calcium and magnesium wasting (16[C]).

Reversible hypokalemic metabolic alkalosis and hypomagnesemia can occur with gentamicin, and routine monitoring has been recommended (17[A]).

The results of an in vitro study on immortalized mouse distal convoluted tubule cells have suggested that aminoglycosides act through an extracellular polyvalent cation-sensing receptor and that they inhibit hormone-stimulated magnesium absorption in the distal convoluted tubule (18[E]).

Hematologic In an in vitro study both gentamicin sulfate and netilmicin sulfate showed competitive *inhibition of glucose-6-phosphate dehydrogenase* from human erythrocytes, whereas streptomycin sulfate showed non-competitive inhibition (19[E]).

Urinary tract In a survey of the use of antibiotics in a surgical service, aminoglycosides were given to 26 patients, of whom four developed *nephrotoxicity* (20[c]).

Pregnancy Using the population-based dataset of the Hungarian Case–Control Surveillance of Congenital Abnormalities (1980–96), which includes 38 151 pregnant women who had newborn infants without any defects and 22 865 pregnant women who had fetuses or newborns with congenital abnormalities, no teratogenic risk of parenteral gentamicin, streptomycin, tobramycin, or oral neomycin was discovered when restricted to structural developmental disturbances (21[C]).

Drug dosage regimens Once-daily dosing regimens of aminoglycosides are routinely used in critically ill patients with trauma, although there is a marked variability in pharmacokinetics in these patients, eventually leading to prolonged drug-free intervals, and individualized dosing on the basis of at least two serum aminoglycoside concentrations may be recommended when once-daily dosing regimens are chosen (22[C]).

Drug administration route Bolus *intraperitoneal* gentamicin or tobramycin (5 mg/kg ideal bodyweight) is safe, achieves therapeutic blood concentrations for extended intervals, causes no clinical ototoxicity or vestibular toxicity, is cost-effective, and is convenient for patients and nurses (23[C]).

Drug interactions Combinations of *meropenem* and aminoglycosides may be effective against *Pseudomonas aeruginosa* strains that are resistant to meropenem at clinically relevant concentrations; synergistic effects were observed in combinations that included arbekacin or amikacin (24[C]).

Diagnosis and management of adverse drug reactions In a 10-year follow-up survey of aminoglycoside treatment in 2022 patients in Saudi Arabia, 8.8%, 18%, and 12% had trough concentrations considered toxic for amikacin, gentamicin, and tobramycin respectively, whereas there were peak serum drug concentrations in the subtherapeutic range in 53%, 50%, and 57% respectively (25[C]). Toxic concentrations were noticed mainly in patients aged over 60 years and in patients in the intensive care unit, coronary care unit, and burn unit.

Amikacin

Nervous system Amikacin may have been the causative agent in an *apneic episode* in an infant on peritoneal dialysis (26[A]).

Drug administration route Amikacin has been tested for compatibility with a new chlorhexidine-bearing central venous catheter, the ARROWg+ard Blue Plus, and did not cause a substantial increase in chlorhexidine delivery (27[C]). The amount of amikacin sulfate that was delivered was slightly less than the amount in the infusion solution (92%), but this was considered acceptable.

Arbekacin

Drug interactions In in vitro susceptibility studies on 99 clinical *Staphylococcus aureus* isolates, 68 of 73 methicillin-resistant *S. aureus* (MRSA) and two of 26 methicillin-susceptible *S. aureus* were gentamicin-resistant (28[E]). However, the combination of arbekacin plus vancomycin produced synergistic killing against 12 of 13 gentamicin-resistant MRSA isolates. Synergy of meropenem with arbekacin is mentioned above.

Gentamicin

Urinary tract After a full course of gentamicin 1–55% of patients have *nephrotoxicity*. The increased serum creatinine concentration peaks on day 6 of therapy and is reversible in most cases within 30 days. Nephrotoxicity appears to be more common among patients with pre-existing renal impairment, longer treatment duration (over 7 days), repeated courses of aminoglycosides, and after the coadministration of other nephrotoxic drugs (e.g. amphotericin, cisplatin, daunorubicin, furosemide, and vancomycin). Animal studies have suggested that hydrocortisone, angiotensin converting enzyme inhibitors, and hypercalcemia can also increase aminoglycoside nephrotoxicity, whereas acetazolamide, bicarbonate, ceftriaxone, lithium, magnesium, melatonin, piperacillin, polyaspartic acid, pyridoxal-5′-phosphate, and a high protein diet may be protective (1[R], 29[E]).

In 87 patients with intertrochanteric hip fractures, preoperative antibiotic prophylaxis (gentamicin 240 mg and dicloxacillin 2 g) had no significant effect on wound infections; however, there were 16 reversible cases of nephrotoxicity and one irreversible case among patients who received antibiotic prophylaxis, compared with only four cases of reversible kidney damage among 76 patients who did not receive antibiotics (30[C]).

Since serum creatinine does not accurately reflect renal function in patients with spinal cord injury, dosage regimens of gentamicin should be individualized, based on age, sex, weight, height, the level of spinal cord injury, and renal function (31[c]).

Body temperature Of 155 patients (38% men, mean age 41 years) with *pyrogenic reactions* due to gentamicin, 81% received once-daily dosing (70% in a dose of 5–7 mg/kg) and 10% received a conventional dose (3 mg/kg in three divided doses) (32[c]). Reactions typically occurred within 3 hours after infusion (98%) and lasted for less than 3 hours (96%). Patients reported *chills, shaking, or shivering* (75%), *rigors* (23%), *fever* (68%), *tachycardia* (17%), *hypertension or hypotension* (17%), and *respiratory symptoms* (47%). More serious reactions also occurred, including *cyanosis* (4%), *oxygen saturation below 80%* (7%), and *pulmonary edema* (one patient); 8% had severe reactions leading to hospitalization (with intubation, resuscitation, or admission to the intensive care unit in five cases), but none died. An FDA investigation showed that 10% of gentamicin lots tested had raised endotoxin concentrations, and an additional 4% of the lots would have exposed a patient to concentrations above the acceptable threshold with once-daily dosing. The two products implicated in these clusters involved the same supplier of bulk gentamicin; inadequacies in manufacturing practices had led to an increase in overall impurities (33[C], 34[C]).

Risk factors In *premature neonates*, gentamicin clearance depends on gestational age, with a cut-off at 30 weeks: younger neonates have lower gentamicin clearance, a slightly higher volume of distribution, and a longer half-life compared with the older neonates. Loading doses of 3.7 and 3.5 mg/kg followed by maintenance doses of 2.8 mg/kg/24 hours and 2.6 mg/kg/18 hours have been recommended for younger and older neonates respectively (35[C]).

Drug dosage regimens In febrile neutropenic episodes after intensive chemotherapy, once-daily gentamicin (7 mg/kg/day) in combination with azlocillin was more effective than a multiple-daily dosing regimen, but the incidence of toxicity was low overall and was slightly but not significantly higher in the once-daily group (36[C]).

Once-daily dosing is appealing for cost savings and may have a therapeutic advantage and possibly cause less toxicity. However, these latter effects have been modest. Although once-daily dosing appears to be effective in limited studies in children, its role in Gram-positive coccal endocarditis, in individuals with neutropenia or cystic fibrosis, and in individuals with altered volumes of distribution remains uncertain (37[R]).

For external otitis, therapeutic local antibiotic concentrations can be achieved by giving gentamicin ear drops twice daily; more frequent administration is not needed (38[C]).

Drug interactions Gentamicin and other aminoglycosides have increased activity when they are combined with *β-lactams*, resulting in increased bacterial aminoglycoside uptake (1[R]). The proposed mechanism of synergism is damage to the cell membrane by the β-lactam, followed by improved diffusion of gentamicin across the outer bacterial membrane. A second type of synergism, pharmacodynamic synergism, occurs when high serum concentrations of aminoglycosides cause efficient bacterial killing, resulting in reduced bacterial concentrations, which are more effectively eliminated by β-lactams, as they work more efficiently against lower bacterial concentrations. The action of gentamicin is inhibited by some antimicrobials, which are bacteriostatic rather than bactericidal; e.g. antagonism occurs with macrolides, tetracycline and doxycycline, and chloramphenicol. The clinical significance of this antagonism is unknown.

Gentamicin is synergistic with *methylene blue* in vitro against *Pseudomonas aeruginosa* (39[E]).

Diagnosis and management of adverse drug reactions Salivary sampling is of potential interest in monitoring drug therapy, especially in children. Although there was no correlation between serum gentamicin concentrations and salivary concentrations when gentamicin was given two or three times daily in children with uncomplicated infections, there was a good correlation after once-daily dosing (40[C]).

Isepamicin

Isepamicin is similar to amikacin but has better activity against strains that produce type I 6′-acetyltransferase. It can cause nephrotoxicity, vestibular toxicity, and ototoxicity. However, it is one of the less toxic of the aminoglycosides (41[R]). The antibacterial spectrum of isepamicin includes *Enterobacteriaceae* and staphylococci; anerobes, *Neisseriae*, and streptococci are resistant (41[R]). Isepamicin was as effective and safe as amikacin in the treatment of acute pyelonephritis in children and might prove an advantageous alternative in areas with a high incidence of resistance to other aminoglycosides (42[C]).

Isepamicin is given intravenously or intramuscularly in a dosage of 15 mg/kg od or 7.5 mg/kg bd. It is not bound to plasma proteins, it distributes in extracellular fluids, and it enters some cells (outer hair cells, kidney cortex) by an active transport mechanism (41[R]); the transference of isepamicin to the bone marrow is excellent (43[C]). Isepamicin is not metabolized and is renally excreted with a half-life of 2–3 hours in adults with normal renal function. Its clearance is reduced in neonates, and a dose of 7.5 mg/kg od is recommended in children younger than 16 days. Its clearance is also reduced in elderly people, but no dosage adjustment is required. In patients with chronic renal impairment, isepamicin clearance is proportional to creatinine clearance.

Neomycin

Skin In a randomized study of the effects of bacitracin-containing triple-antibiotic ointment (polymyxin B + bacitracin + neomycin) and simple gauze-type dressings on scarring of dermabrasion wounds, the ointment was superior to the simple dressing in minimizing scarring; the beneficial effect on pigmentary changes was especially pronounced (44[C]).

Immunologic In 145 patients with eczema of the external ear canal, *allergic contact dermatitis* was diagnosed in one-third; topical therapeutic agents, especially neomycin sulfate and probably polymyxin B, were the dominating allergens (45[C]).

Netilmicin

Risk factors In 186 *neonates* and 95 *infants* receiving netilmicin, postnatal age, bodyweight, and plasma creatinine reduced the expected variance in the plasma clearance of netilmicin by more than 10% in the neonates, as did plasma urea and creatinine in the infants (46[C]). Variations in bodyweight and sex explained the variability in the volume of distribution.

Drug administration route In a study of the compatibility of 82 commonly used parenteral medications with a chlorhexidine-bearing central venous catheter (ARROWg+ard BluePlus), the effluent sample concentration of netilmicin sulfate was slightly lower than the initial drug concentration, but this was considered acceptable (27[C]).

Paromomycin

In patients with visceral leishmaniasis, paromomycin (12 or 18 mg/kg/day) plus a standard dose of sodium stibogluconate for 21 days was statistically more effective than sodium stibogluconate alone in producing a final cure (47[C]). There were no serious adverse events in 100 patients given paromomycin; however, only 19 of those patients had a complete audiogram series conducted, making assessment of ototoxicity difficult.

The early bactericidal activity of paromomycin in doses of 7.5 and 15 mg/kg was measured in 22 patients with previously untreated smear-positive pulmonary tuberculosis (48[E]). The fall in the number of colony-forming units per ml of sputum per day during the first 2 days of treatment in seven patients who received paromomycin 7.5 or 15 mg/kg/day was dose-related. Since paromomycin is no more toxic than other aminoglycosides and since there is no known cross-resistance with streptomycin, paromomycin may be valuable for the management of multidrug-resistant tuberculosis.

Streptomycin

It has previously been hypothesized that stretch-activated ion channels and not calcium channels contribute to stretch-related alterations in cell membrane repolarization, and that these effects can be neutralized by blocking stretch-activated channels. In isolated retrogradely perfused rabbit hearts, in which the left ventricular size was modified by abruptly changing the volume of a fluid-filled balloon placed in the left ventricle, the stretch-activated channel blocker streptomycin, but not the specific calcium channel blocker verapamil, inhibited the stretch-related shortening of repolarization (49[E]). Acute ventricular dilatation led to a rate-dependent decrease in repolarization and nearly completely suppressed stretch-related extra ventricular beats; this may have important implications for the development of new antidysrhythmic drugs.

Tobramycin

Respiratory Nebulized antipseudomonal antibiotic treatment improves lung function and reduces the frequency of exacerbations of infection in patients with cystic fibrosis, but the significance of development of antibiotic-resistant organisms remains to be determined (50[R]). In 10 healthy adults, the inhalation of tobramycin 80 mg resulted in the deposition of 11.8 mg in the lungs (51[C]). In a double-blind, randomized, placebo-controlled study inhaled tobramycin significantly reduced sputum *Pseudomonas aeruginosa* density. More patients in the treatment group reported increased *cough*, *dyspnea*, *wheezing*, and *non-cardiac chest pain*, but the symptoms did not limit therapy (52[C]).

Inhalation of the intravenous formulation of tobramycin can cause *bronchoconstriction*, as has now been confirmed in 26 children with mild to moderate cystic fibrosis (53[C]). Nevertheless, while bronchoconstriction did occur, many patients did not have bronchoconstriction in response to the standard intravenous formulation. The risk of bronchoconstriction may further be reduced by pretreatment with salbutamol.

Drug dosage regimens The addition of tobramycin reduced the amount of cefuroxime-induced endotoxin released per killed *Escherichia coli* to a level that was even lower than that of tobramycin alone, despite an increased killing rate (54[C]). Increasing concentrations of tobramycin led to reduction in endotoxin release, pointing to a possible benefit of once-daily dosing regimens.

In an analysis of sera from 60 adults with cystic fibrosis, it was suggested that the potential benefit of achieving a greater peak/MIC with once-daily aminoglycoside administration may be offset by the significantly greater time that the concentration was below the MIC, compared with that achieved with multiple-daily dosing regimens (55[C]).

Based on a study of 10 patients with automated peritoneal dialysis, it was recommended that for empirical treatment of dialysis-related peritonitis, the dosage of intermittent intraperitoneal tobramycin must be 1.5 mg/kg for one exchange during the first day and then 0.5 mg/kg thereafter, to reduce the risk of adverse effects (56[C]).

Drug administration route With combined inhalational and intravenous tobramycin, toxic serum drug concentrations may occur (57[c]).

CHLORAMPHENICOL AND RELATED DRUGS *(SED-14, 848; (SEDA-23, 268; SEDA-24, 287)*

Chloramphenicol

Sensory systems The neurotoxicity of chloramphenicol has been well documented; recently, a Spanish case of bilateral *optic neuritis* associated with chloramphenicol has been added (58[A]).

Hematologic Chloramphenicol has adverse effects on the bone marrow, the most serious of which is *aplastic anemia*. It has been confirmed that chloramphenicol can induce apoptosis in purified human bone marrow $CD34^+$ cells; however, there was no protection from a variety of antioxidants on chloramphenicol-induced suppression of burst-forming unit erythroid and colony-forming unit granulocyte/monocyte in vitro (59[E]). In contrast, a caspase inhibitor ameliorated the apoptotic-inducing effects of chloramphenicol.

Drug tolerance (antibacterial resistance) The flo gene that confers resistance to chloramphenicol and the veterinary antibiotic florfenicol has previously been identified in *Photobacterium piscicida* and *Salmonella enterica* serovar typhimurium DT104 (60[C]). Florfenicol-resistant *E. coli* isolates were tested and found to contain large flo-positive plasmids, suggesting that several *E. coli* isolates may have a chromosomal flo gene. The *E. coli* flo gene also specifies non-enzymatic cross-resistance to both florfenicol and chloramphenicol (61[C]). Florfenicol resistance has recently emerged among veterinary *E. coli* isolates incriminated in bovine diarrhea.

Pregnancy In the large population-based dataset of the Hungarian Case Control Surveillance of Congenital Abnormalities, of 38 151 pregnant women who had babies without any defects and 22 865 pregnant women who had neonates or fetuses with congenital abnormalities, 51 and 52 had been treated with oral chloramphenicol respectively. Treatment during early pregnancy presented little, if any, teratogenic risk to the fetus (62[C]). However, chloramphenicol may be safe to use in pregnancy only if it is not circulating at the time of delivery, since it can cause *gray syndrome* in neonates (63[R]).

Risk factors In a retrospective study of 30 consecutive *children with sepsis* treated with oral chloramphenicol, weight, albumin, and white blood cell count were the most important determinants for chloramphenicol distribution volume, whereas age, white blood cell count, and serum creatinine were most important for drug clearance (64[C]).

Drug interactions The first report of an interaction of chloramphenicol with *tacrolimus* was published in 1998 in a pediatric renal transplant recipient. Now a significant interaction has been reported in an adult (65[A]).

A 47-year-old white man with a cadaveric liver transplant took chloramphenicol for a urinary tract infection due to a vancomycin-resistant *Enterococcus* and inadvertently received 1850 mg qds (roughly twice the maximum recommended dose). On day 4 he had a 12-hour trough tacrolimus concentration of over 60 ng/ml, and complained of fatigue, lethargy, headache, and tremor, symptoms consistent with tacrolimus toxicity.

It was suggested that the underlying mechanism might be inhibition of CYP3A4 by chloramphenicol.

Thiamphenicol

Thiamphenicol, an amine derivative of hydrocarbylsulfonylpropandiol, has been used to treat 1171 patients with chancroid (66[C]). Each patient was given granulated thiamphenicol 5.0 g orally in a single dose. Only 0.89% did not respond. A few patients had adverse effects, including *epigastric pain, headache, nausea*, and *skin rashes*; all were mild and of short duration.

FLUOROQUINOLONES

(SED-14, 852; SEDA-22, 279; SEDA-23, 277)

Following the introduction of the first quinolone (nalidixic acid), structural modifications to the basic quinolone and naphthyridone nucleus and to the side-chains produced improvements in the coverage of bacterial pathogens, with high activity against Gram-negative species and a number of atypical pathogens, and good-to-moderate activity against Gram-positive species. However, despite the broad spectrum and clinical success, defects became evident, and compounds developed in recent years have targeted improvements in pharmacokinetic properties (improved systemic availability, once-daily dosing), greater activity against Gram-positive cocci and anerobes, activity against fluoroquinolone-resistant strains, and better coverage of non-fermenting Gram-negative species (68[R]–71[R]).

Fluoroquinolones are becoming accepted in the treatment of community-acquired pneumonia and are established choices for acute exacerbations of chronic bronchitis. However, owing to their adverse effects (including severe *anaphylaxis*, *QT interval prolongation*, and potential *cardiotoxicity*), several fluoroquinolones have had to be withdrawn (e.g. temafloxacin and grepafloxacin) or strictly limited in their use (e.g. trovafloxacin) after marketing (72[R]). A serious idiosyncratic reaction profile may be related to the immunologically reactive 1-difluorophenyl substituent that characterizes temafloxacin, trovafloxacin, and tosufloxacin (68[R]).

Cardiovascular Some quinolones can prolong the QT interval, with a risk of *cardiac dysrhythmias*. In an in vitro study in isolated canine cardiac Purkinje fibers the rank order of potency in prolonging action potential duration was sparfloxacin > grepafloxacin = moxifloxacin > ciprofloxacin (73[C]).

Urinary tract In a Medline search to investigate the incidence and features of fluoroquinolone *nephrotoxicity* only primarily case reports and temporally related events could be identified (74[R]). Ciprofloxacin was associated with an increased risk of renal insufficiency, probably because it has been in use longer and more widely than the newer agents.

Skin A combination of primary ear swelling analysis and cell counting of ear-draining lymph nodes after UV irradiation in mice was fast and highly predictive of the risks of *photosensitization* and *photoirritancy* of fluoroquinolones, depending on the route of exposure (oral or dermal) and may therefore be good tools for preclinical risk assessment in terms of discriminating photoreactions (75[E]).

Musculoskeletal In 42 spontaneous reports of fluoroquinolone-associated tendon disorders, 32 patients had *tendinitis*, 24 bilaterally, and 10 patients had a *tendon rupture*; most affected the Achilles tendon (76[C]). The median age was 68 years and there was a male predominance. In 16 cases ofloxacin was implicated, in 13 ciprofloxacin, in eight norfloxacin, and in five pefloxacin. The delay between the start of treatment and the appearance of the first symptoms was 1–510 (median 6) days. Most patients recovered within 2 months after withdrawal, but 26% had not yet recovered at follow-up.

Drug tolerance (antibacterial resistance) From 8419 worldwide clinical isolates of *Streptococcus pneumoniae* associated with lower respiratory tract or blood infections obtained from 519 geographically distinct hospital laboratories during 1997–8, 69 had reduced susceptibility or resistance to fluoroquinolones. Only mutations in parC and gyrA (especially in combination), but not in gyrB or parE, contributed significantly to resistance. Efflux is probably crucial in reduced susceptibility for new hydrophilic fluoroquinolones (77[E]).

In an *in vitro* study, ciprofloxacin, grepafloxacin, levofloxacin, moxifloxacin, ofloxacin, and sparfloxacin had similar good activity against *Hemophilus influenzae* and *Moraxella catarrhalis* (78[E]). Against *S. pneumoniae* (irrespective of the strain's susceptibility to penicillin), grepafloxacin, levofloxacin, moxifloxacin, and sparfloxacin had better activity than ciprofloxacin and ofloxacin.

Clinafloxacin, moxifloxacin, sparfloxacin, and trovafloxacin were significantly more active *in vitro* than ciprofloxacin and levofloxacin against *Stenotrophomonas maltophilia*, a microorganism with inherent resistance to many antibiotics; new-generation quinolones may become very useful in the treatment of certain severe or life-threatening infectious conditions due to this bacterium (79[C]).

Alatrofloxacin and trovafloxacin

Alatrofloxacin is a fluoronaphthyridone that is hydrolysed to the active moiety, trovafloxacin, following intravenous administration. This fourth-generation broad-spectrum fluoroquinolone has activity against Gram-positive, Gram-negative, anerobic, and atypical respiratory pathogens.

Because trovafloxacin is hepatotoxic, the list of appropriate indications has been limited to patients who have at least one of several specified infections, such as nosocomial pneumonia or complicated intra-abdominal infections that are serious and life- or limb-threatening in the physician's judgement.

Trovafloxacin may downregulate cytokine mRNA transcription in human peripheral blood mononuclear cells stimulated with lipopolysaccharide or lipoteichoic acid (80[E]). Likewise, trovafloxacin inhibited *Salmonella typhimurium*-induced TNF-α production, HIV-1 replication, and reactivation of latent HIV-1 in promonocytic U1 cells at concentrations comparable to the plasma and tissue concentrations achieved by therapeutic dosages (81[E]).

Cardiovascular *Phlebitis* can occur during parenteral administration of trovafloxacin. High concentrations of trovafloxacin (2 mg/ml) significantly reduced intracellular ATP content in cultured endothelial cells and reduced ADP, GTP, and GDP concentrations (82[E]). These in vitro data suggest that high doses of trovafloxacin are not compatible with maintenance of endothelial cell function and may explain the occurrence of phlebitis. Commercial formulations should be diluted and given into large veins.

Nervous system Alatrofloxacin can cause *seizures* (83[A]).

A 37-year-old Asian man received several antibiotics (including intravenous ceftazidime, gentamicin, meropenem, metronidazole, and vancomycin) postoperatively. After 3 weeks he was given alatrofloxacin 75 mg in 25 ml of dextrose 5% (1.875 mg/ml) and developed generalized clonus. On rechallenge, infusing at half the initial rate, the seizure recurred. A CT scan of the brain was normal.

Seizures are rare but have occurred during treatment with other fluoroquinolones. This is the first report of a case of seizures associated with slow infusion of alatrofloxacin. However, as of 21 June 2000, the manufacturers have received 53 reports of seizures through worldwide postmarketing surveillance. In rat hippocampus slices, trovafloxacin had significant convulsive potential; the underlying mechanism is hitherto incompletely understood.

Trovafloxacin has been associated with diffuse weakness due to a *demyelinating polyneuropathy* in a patient without an underlying neurological disorder (84[A]).

Hematologic Alatrofloxacin has been associated with severe *thrombocytopenia* (85[A]).

A 54-year-old woman was given alatrofloxacin 300 mg iv qds and on day 4 developed epistaxis. Her platelet count was 7×10^9/l, with normal hemoglobin and white blood cell counts. Direct antiglobulin testing showed coating of erythrocytes with polyspecific immunoproteins, and platelet-associated antibody testing was positive for IgM and IgG antibodies. Alatrofloxacin was withdrawn and azithromycin was given instead. She was given methylprednisolone 125 mg intravenously bd and the platelet count fell to 2×10^9/l and then rose, reaching 60×10^9/l on day 8.

During clinical trials, thrombocytopenia occurred in under 1% of more than 7000 patients who received alatrofloxacin or trovafloxacin.

Liver More than 100 cases of hepatotoxicity associated with trovafloxacin have been reported to the FDA. A case of severe *acute hepatitis* during trovafloxacin therapy has now been added (86[A]).

A 66-year-old man had taken trovafloxacin 100 mg/day for 4 weeks for refractory chronic sinusitis. For several years he had also taken allopurinol, doxepin, hydrochlorothiazide, losartan, metoprolol, and nabumetone. He developed nausea, vomiting, malaise, and abdominal distention. His white cell count was 8000×10^9/l with 16% eosinophils; his serum AsT was 537 IU/l, AlT 841 IU/l, direct bilirubin 17 μmol/l; total bilirubin 27 μmol/l, alkaline phosphatase 111 IU/l; blood urea nitrogen 5 μmol/l; and creatinine 190 μmol/l. Tests for hepatitis A, B, and C were negative. A biopsy of the liver showed centrilobular and focal periportal necrosis and eosinophilic infiltration; the sinusoids were dilated and contained lymphocytes and eosinophils; many hepatocytes were undergoing mitosis. After withdrawal of trovafloxacin and treatment with prednisone, his hepatic and renal function returned to normal, and the eosinophilia gradually resolved.

Skin The photosensitizing potential of trovafloxacin 200 mg od has been compared with that of ciprofloxacin 500 mg bd, lomefloxacin 400 mg od, and placebo in 48 healthy men (aged 19–45 years) (87[C]). Trovafloxacin had significantly less photosensitizing potential than either ciprofloxacin or lomefloxacin. *Photosensitivity* seemed to be induced only by wavelengths in the UVA region, was maximal at 24 hours, and had a short-term effect.

Musculoskeletal Trovafloxacin inhibited growth and extracellular matrix mineralization in MC3T3-E1 osteoblast-like cell cultures (88[E]). The IC_{50} was 0.5 μg/ml, which is below clinically achievable serum concentrations. The authors suggested that the clinical relevance of this observation to bone healing in orthopedic patients should be evaluated.

Pregnancy In an *ex vivo* study, trovafloxacin crossed the human placenta by simple diffusion and neither accumulated in the media nor bound to tissues or accumulated in the placenta (89[E]). This implies that it should have no effects on the fetus if given during pregnancy.

Risk factors The pharmacokinetics of a single intravenous dose of alatrofloxacin have been determined in six *infants aged 3–12 months* and in 14 *children aged 2–12 years* (90[C]). The peak trovafloxacin concentration at the end of the infusion was 4.3 μg/ml; the volume of distribution at steady-state was 1.6 l/kg, clearance 2.5 ml/min/kg, and the half-life 9.8 hours, with no age-related differences. Less than 5% of the administered dose was excreted in the urine over 24 hours.

The pharmacokinetics of trovafloxacin after the administration of alatrofloxacin were not substantially altered in seven *critically ill patients* (three men, four women) with APACHE II scores of 27 (range 15–32) and normal or mildly impaired hepatic function (91[C]).

Diagnosis and management of adverse drug reactions In 17 patients aged over 18 years with severe acute community-acquired pneumonia trovafloxacin concentrations were persistently high in the sputum, bronchial secretions, bronchoalveolar lavage fluid, and epithelial lining fluid, with no significant difference between these compartments (92[C]). The authors proposed that measurement of sputum concentrations could be used to monitor the outcome of treatment.

Ciprofloxacin

Using electron spin resonance spectroscopy and spin trapping, ciprofloxacin has been shown to cause free radical production in a dose- and time-dependent manner; the authors suggested that this effect may contribute to drug-related adverse effects, including phototoxicity and cartilage defects (93[E]).

The imaging of inflammation/infection with ^{99m}Tm-labeled ciprofloxacin in 96 patients had a sensitivity of 81% and specificity of 87%. The positive and negative predictive values were 90% and 75% respectively. No adverse effects were reported (94[C]).

Nervous system Ciprofloxacin can cause *facial dyskinesia* or *hypoactive delirium* (95[A], 96[A]).

Sensory systems Topical 0.2% ciprofloxacin solution was effective and well tolerated in 232 patients with chronic suppurative otitis media; the most frequently reported adverse events were *pruritus*, *stinging*, and *earache*. Audiometric tests did not show changes attributable to ciprofloxacin (97[C]).

In children with tympanic membrane perforation, topical ciprofloxacin caused no signs of local intolerance or ototoxicity and did not result in significant serum concentrations (98[C]).

Hematologic Ciprofloxacin has been associated with *hemolysis* in combination with a severe skin reaction in a young adult (99[A]).

Gastrointestinal Ciprofloxacin can cause *diarrhea* due to *Clostridium difficile* (100[A]).

Pancreas A report has suggested that ciprofloxacin can cause *pancreatitis* (101[A]).

Urinary tract *Acute renal insufficiency* is a rare adverse effect of ciprofloxacin in young patients. An 18-year-old woman with cystic fibrosis had a pronounced reduction in renal function after taking oral ciprofloxacin for 3 weeks; withdrawal of the drug led to normalization of renal function within 10 days (102[A]).

Experimental studies in humans and animals have suggested that *crystalluria* may be associated with fluoroquinolones. Bilateral hydronephrosis and acute renal insufficiency due to urinary tract stones predominantly composed of ciprofloxacin has now been reported (103[A]).

Skin Ciprofloxacin can cause *purpuric skin lesions* (104[A], 105[A]), *bullous pemphigoid* (106[A]), and *cutaneous vasculitis* (107[A]).

Musculoskeletal Ciprofloxacin can cause partial or complete *tendon rupture*, as corroborated by three new case reports (108[A], 109[A]). In a study of fibroblast metabolism in vitro, ciprofloxacin stimulated matrix-degrading protease activity and inhibited fibroblast metabolism; these effects may both contribute to the tendinopathy that is associated with ciprofloxacin (110[E]).

The use of ciprofloxacin in children is limited, because quinolone damages cartilage in young experimental animals. Recent reports have shown that ciprofloxacin is usually well tolerated in children, although photosensitivity and joint pain can occur. For example, in 75 children with typhoid fever, aged under 6 years (mean age 32 months), ciprofloxacin had no adverse effects on growth or joints (111[C]). In another study only two of 219 children treated with ciprofloxacin developed *arthropathy*, in one case transiently (112[C]). In a necropsy study on children treated with ciprofloxacin 20–40 mg/kg/day for an average of 148 days, there were no chondrotoxic effects; however, synovial membranes showed signs of subacute synovitis, which had not been noted in life (113[C]).

In Wistar rats treated with ciprofloxacin, there was poor healing of experimental fractures during the early stages of repair, suggesting that ciprofloxacin may compromise the clinical course of fracture healing (114[E]).

Immunologic *Anaphylactoid reactions* occurred in three of about 3200 students who took ciprofloxacin 500 mg for chemoprophylaxis of meningococcal meningitis; two had no history of atopic illness (115[C]). All three recovered. Additional adverse reactions were mild skin rashes in three students and nausea and vomiting in two.

Risk factors *Children* In 36 premature infants, delivered at 25–35 weeks and with birthweights of 750–2050 g, ciprofloxacin (13.8 mg/kg/day in two or three divided doses for 3–20 days) had good efficacy in 66% of cases (116[C]). Thrombocytopenia (five cases), raised transaminases (three cases), hyperbilirubinemia (three cases), and raised creatinine concentration (two patients) were reported as adverse events; one child developed femoral osteitis.

In a Russian study of children with cystic fibrosis, the adverse effects of ciprofloxacin were chiefly gastrointestinal (nausea, stomach pain, diarrhea) and increased transaminase activity (117[C]). One episode of arthrotoxicity was transient. There were no negative effects on growth and no chondrotoxicity.

Oral ciprofloxacin (10 mg/kg bd) was as safe and effective as intramuscular ceftriaxone (50 mg/kg/day) in the treatment of acute invasive diarrhea in 201 children (ages 6 months to 10 years) (118[C]). Possible drug-related adverse events occurred in 8% and were mild and transient. Joints were normal during and after the completion of therapy in all patients.

Elderly patients In a retrospective analysis there were no clinically important differences in the safety profile of ciprofloxacin in patients aged under or over 65 years. The incidence of drug-related adverse events was higher in those under 65 years (25%) than in those aged 65 years or more (17%); the most common adverse events affected the gastrointestinal and central nervous systems (119[C]).

Drug interactions The most common drug interactions with ciprofloxacin include the malabsorption interactions associated with multivalent cations and CYP450 interactions (120[R]).

Didanosine Didanosine, one enteric-coated capsule/day (400 mg/day), did not affect the absorption of ciprofloxacin in 16 patients. (121[C]).

Glibenclamide Hypoglycemia and raised serum concentrations of glibenclamide, which is metabolized by CYP2C9, occurred after treatment with ciprofloxacin for 1 week in a patient taking long-term glibenclamide (122[A]).

Methadone Ciprofloxacin, given to a patient who had been successfully treated with methadone for more than 6 years, caused profound sedation, confusion, and respiratory depression (123[A]). This may have been due to inhibition of CYP1A2 and CYP3A4, two of the isozymes involved in the metabolism of methadone.

Rifampicin Rifampicin-induced lupus-like syndrome is associated with combination therapy with ciprofloxacin, since rifampicin is metabolized by (among others) CYP3A4, which is inhibited by ciprofloxacin, and combined usage may lead to higher rifampicin blood concentrations (124[C]).

Ropinirole During coadministration of ciprofloxacin with ropinirole in 12 patients there was an increase in the plasma ropinirole concentration, which is metabolized by CYP1A2 (125[C]).

Warfarin Ciprofloxacin can occasionally cause an exaggerated hypoprothombinemic response and bleeding in patients taking warfarin. In 66 patients (median age 72 years, range 36–94), the mean time to detection of the coagulopathy after ciprofloxacin challenge was 5.5 days (126[C]). Hospitalization was reported in 15 cases, bleeding in 25, and death in one. The median INR was 10.0. Patients in their seventh decade and those requiring polypharmacy were most at risk.

Enoxacin

Sensory systems In unmedicated young and elderly volunteers and unmedicated HIV-infected patients, enoxacin applied to the tongue was described as metallic by young subjects, but bitter by elderly subjects (127[C]).

Drug interactions CYP1A2 participates in the metabolism of both enoxacin and *caffeine*, and inhibition of caffeine metabolism by enoxacin can cause adverse effects (128[C]).

Fleroxacin

Risk factors *Race* The pharmacokinetics of fleroxacin (200 mg intravenously or 200 mg orally) have been studied in 19 Nigerian men. Maximum serum concentration and AUC were 3- to 4-fold lower than previously reported after identical doses, but the systemic availability profile was as previously reported (129[C]).

Gatifloxacin

Gatifloxacin is a an 8-methoxyfluoroquinolone with enhanced activity against Gram-positive and atypical agents and broad-spectrum activity against Gram-negative bacteria. It is bactericidal and produces a postantibiotic effect in Gram-positive and Gram-negative bacteria. The standard dose is 400 mg od and both oral and intravenous formulations are available (130[R], 131[R]).

Since gatifloxacin has a high oral systemic availability (96%), oral and intravenous formulations are bioequivalent and interchangeable (132[C]). It has a large volume of distribution (about 1.8 l/kg), low protein binding (about 20%), broad tissue distribution, and is primarily excreted unchanged in the urine (over 80%) (131[R]). After daily repeated administration, there was predictable modest accumulation; steady-state concentrations were reached after the third dose (133[C]).

The in vitro antibacterial spectrum of gatifloxacin has been tested against a variety of clinically important microorganisms (134[E]). It is two to four times more potent than ciprofloxacin and ofloxacin against staphylococci, streptococci, pneumococci, and enterococci. However, it is two times less potent than ciprofloxacin, but the same as or two times more potent than ofloxacin against *Enterobacteriaceae*. Gatifloxacin and ofloxacin have similar antipseudomonal activity, while ciprofloxacin is two to eight times more potent. Gatifloxacin is highly potent against *Hemophilus influenzae*, *Legionella* spp., and *Helicobacter pylori*, and also has activity against *Bacteroides fragilis* and *Clostridium difficile*. Like other quinolones, it has poor activity against *Mycobacterium avium-intracellulare*, but is 8–16 times more potent against *M. tuberculosis*.

Cardiovascular Gatifloxacin has little effect on the QT interval of the electrocardiogram (131[R]).

Endocrine Gatifloxacin was well tolerated in patients with non-insulin-dependent diabetes mellitus maintained with diet and exercise (135[C]). It had no significant effect on glucose homeostasis, β-cell function, or long-term fasting serum glucose concentrations, but it caused a brief increase in serum insulin concentrations.

Risk factors Gatifloxacin can be administered without dose modification in patients with hepatic impairment (136[C]), in women, and in the elderly (137[C]).

Drug administration route Intravenous gatifloxacin can cause dose-related local reactions (132[C]).

Drug interactions Gatifloxacin does not interact with drugs metabolized by the CYP450 enzyme family, as assessed in 14 healthy adult men using midazolam as a probe (138[C]).

Gemifloxacin

Gemifloxacin is a fluoroquinolone that has enhanced affinity for topoisomerase. Compared with other fluoroquinolones, gemifloxacin was the most potent against penicillin-intermediate and -resistant pneumococci, methicillin-susceptible and -resistant *Staphylococcus epidermidis* isolates, and coagulase-negative staphylococci (139[C], 140[C]). It has excellent activity against *Hemophilus influenzae* and *Moraxella catarrhalis* and is unaffected by β-lactamases. It is generally 2-fold less active than ciprofloxacin against most *Enterobacteriaceae* (141[C]). Atypical respiratory pathogens (*Legionella*, *Mycoplasma*, and *Chlamydia* spp.) and *Neisseria gonorrheae* are highly susceptible (142[C]).

In phase II trials oral gemifloxacin 320 mg/day produced bacteriological responses in 94% of patients with acute exacerbations of chronic bronchitis (143[C]) and in 95% of patients with uncomplicated urinary tract infections. Adverse events included *nausea*, *abdominal pain*, *headache*, and a mild *rash* in both patients and healthy volunteers.

After a single dose of 20–800 mg of gemifloxacin, there were no significant changes in clinical chemistry, hematology, or urinalysis, vital signs, or 12-lead electrocardiograms in healthy men, irrespective of dose (144[C]).

Hematologic Gemifloxacin reached intracellular concentrations in human polymorphonuclear leukocytes eight times higher than extracellular concentrations. Uptake was rapid, reversible, and non-saturable and was affected by environmental temperature, cell viability, and membrane stimuli (145[E]).

Skin Gemifloxacin has a low potential for mild *phototoxicity* (146[R]).

Drug interactions In an open, randomized, single-dose, five-way, cross-over study of the effects of *sucralfate* and *ferrous sulfate* on the systemic availability of gemifloxacin there were no changes when gemifloxacin was given at least 2 hours before sucralfate or ferrous sulfate, or at least 3 hours after ferrous sulfate (144[C]).

Food had a minor and clinically insignificant effect on the systemic availability of gemifloxacin (320 and 640 mg) (147[C]).

Grepafloxacin

Grepafloxacin is a synthetic quinolone that has extensive tissue distribution and strong antibacterial activity in vivo. However, it was withdrawn from the market in 1999 because of its adverse cardiovascular events, which included *dysrhythmias* (148[R]).

Immunologic Like other fluoroquinolones, grepafloxacin has some immunomodulatory effects, at least partly at the gene transcription level, demonstrated by inhibition of cytokine (IL-1α, TNF-α, IL-6, and IL-8) mRNA and cytokine (IL-1α and IL-1β) concentrations by grepafloxacin (1–30 mg/l) in vitro (149[E]).

Levofloxacin

Levofloxacin, the (–)-(S)-enantiomer of the racemate ofloxacin, is an oral and parenteral fluoroquinolone that has bactericidal activity against a wide spectrum of Gram-negative and Gram-positive bacilli (including *Streptococcus pneunomiae*), as well as atypical respiratory pathogens.

In 10 patients who took levofloxacin 500 mg/day and rifampicin 600 mg/day for 2–6 months, there were no adverse reactions in 46% of patients, occasional *digestive symptoms* in 40%, and mild *diarrhea* in 13%; these patients also took unspecified anti-inflammatory drugs (150[c]). There was *sleeplessness* in 6%. Neither tendinitis nor changes in liver function were observed.

Cardiovascular *Phlebitis* can occur during parenteral administration of levofloxacin. High concentrations of levofloxacin (5 mg/ml) significantly reduced intracellular ATP content in cultured endothelial cells and reduced ADP, GTP, and GDP concentrations (82[E]). These in vitro data suggest that high doses of levofloxacin are not compatible with maintenance of endothelial cell function and may explain the occurrence of phlebitis. Commercial formulations should be diluted and given into large veins.

Respiratory *Eosinophilic pneumonia* complicated by bronchial asthma has been attributed to levofloxacin (151[A]).

A 76-year-old woman took levofloxacin for a productive cough with non-segmental infiltration in both lung fields. She developed eosinophilia in both the peripheral blood (24%) and sputum (10%), airflow limitation, hypoxemia, and increased airway responsiveness to methacholine. Bronchoalveolar lavage fluid showed increased total cells and a 55% increase in eosinophils, and the CD4/CD8 ratio was reduced to 0.8. Histological features included increased infiltration of eosinophils in the alveolar and interstitial compartments and goblet cell metaplasia. Levofloxacin was withdrawn, and her symptoms improved without steroid therapy. A leukocyte migration test for levofloxacin was weakly positive.

Skin In a double-blind randomized study in 30 healthy adults oral levofloxacin (500 mg/day for 5 days) had a low photosensitizing potential (152[C]).

Levofloxacin can cause a *rash* similar to the ampicillin rash in patients with infectious mononucleosis (153[A]).

Musculoskeletal *Tendinopathy* is a class-related adverse effect of the fluoroquinolones;

old age, renal dysfunction, and concomitant corticosteroid therapy are predisposing risk factors (154[A], 155[A]).

Immunologic *Anaphylactic and anaphylactoid reactions* are rare adverse events after the administration of fluoroquinolones (about 0.46–1.2 per 100 000 patients). On two occasions a 49-year-old asthmatic woman who took levofloxacin for a chest infection developed worse respiratory distress, requiring intubation (156[A]). The second reaction was accompanied by a marked skin reaction.

An in vitro study in rat peritoneal mast cells showed that levofloxacin-mediated release of histamine may be closely linked to activation of pertussis toxin-sensitive G proteins (157[E]).

Drug interactions Coadministration with levofloxacin can cause severe *lithium* toxicity; the authors did not discuss the mechanism (158[A]).

Lomefloxacin

Sensory systems In a study in unmedicated young and elderly volunteers and unmedicated HIV-infected patients, lomefloxacin applied to the tongue was described as bitter (127[C]).

Skin In eight patients (mean age 69 years) with eczematous or acute sunburn-like lesions in photo-exposed areas, who took lomefloxacin for 1 week to several months, *phototoxicity* appeared to be the main mechanism of photosensitivity, particularly in older patients with concomitant diseases and long-term use of the drug (159[c]).

Carcinogenicity In vitro lomefloxacin photochemically produced oxidative DNA damage, an effect known to be of mutagenic potential (160[E]). This may be the basis of the photochemical mutagenicity and photochemical carcinogenicity of lomefloxacin.

Moxifloxacin

Moxifloxacin is an 8-methoxyquinolone with enhanced potency against important Gram-positive pathogens, notably *Streptococcus pneumoniae* (penicillin-resistant and -susceptible strains), and class activity against Gram-negative bacteria. Its activity is not affected by β-lactamases. Moxifloxacin may therefore represent a promising alternative for treatment of respiratory tract infections (78[C]). In a prospective, uncontrolled, unblinded, phase III trial in 254 patients with community-acquired pneumonia diagnosed by culture or serologically, moxifloxacin (400 mg orally od for 10 days) produced a bacteriological response of 91% (161[c]). Drug-related adverse events were reported in 33% of patients; *nausea* (9%), *diarrhea* (6%), and *dizziness* (4%) were the most common adverse events.

Moxifloxacin (400 mg/day orally od for 7 days) in 12 healthy men significantly reduced the normal oropharyngeal microflora (α-hemolytic streptococci and *Neisseriae*), whereas the number of Gram-negative anerobic bacteria increased markedly; however, no new colonizing moxifloxacin-resistant strains were isolated (162[c]). Moxifloxacin caused a significant reduction in enterococci and enterobacteria, while the numbers of staphylococci, streptococci, *Bacillus* spp., and *Candida albicans* were unaffected. There was no impact on peptostreptococci, lactobacilli, *Veillonella, Bacteroides*, or fusobacteria, but bifidobacteria and *Clostridia* decreased during moxifloxacin administration. The microflora normalized after 35 days (163[C]).

Cardiovascular Moxifloxacin can prolong the QT interval; however, the effect is small, and the risk of moxifloxacin-induced *torsade de pointes* is expected to be minimal when the drug is given in the recommended dosage (400 mg/day) (164[C]).

Nervous system *Syncope* after the use of moxifloxacin has been reported (165[A]).

Skin Moxifloxacin has a low propensity for causing *phototoxic reactions* relative to other fluoroquinolones (166[R]).

Risk factors Dosage adjustment is not required for patients of advanced age or those with renal or mild hepatic impairment (166[R]).

Nalidixic acid

Second generation effects The *genotoxic effects* of nalidixic acid (400 mg bd for 10 days) and metronidazole (250 mg tds for 10 days) have been investigated in a prospective randomized study in 20 patients with *Trichomonas* *vaginalis* infections (167[C]). Evaluation was by the sister-chromatid exchange test, in which an increased number of exchanges in lymphocytes reflects mutagenic action. Metronidazole had no effect but there was a significant increase with nalidixic acid.

Norfloxacin

Psychiatric There has been only one previous report of *hallucinations* with norfloxacin. Now a second case has been reported (168[A]).

Gastrointestinal *Eosinophilic necrotizing granulomatous hepatitis* associated with norfloxacin has been reported (169[A]).

Urinary tract The newer fluoroquinolones have only rarely been associated with nephrotoxicity, with an estimated incidence of 0.4–0.8%. *Acute interstitial nephritis*, probably related to norfloxacin, has now been reported (170[A]).

A 38-year-old woman took norfloxacin (300 mg/day) and tiaramide hydrochloride (300 mg tds) for an infection with *Mycoplasma pneumoniae*. One day after the start of treatment, her symptoms of cough and fever worsened and she developed lumbago and hematuria. The diagnosis was confirmed by percutaneous renal biopsy. She slowly improved without specific treatment. Lymphocyte stimulation tests were negative, but rechallenge with norfloxacin was followed by bilateral lumbago.

The authors identified two previous reports of acute interstitial nephritis associated with norfloxacin.

Drug tolerance (antibacterial resistance) In over 90 000 routine samples of *E. coli* in five Dutch laboratories during 1989–98 resistance to norfloxacin increased from 1.3% to 5.8% (171[E]). In addition, multiresistance, defined as resistance to norfloxacin and at least two other antibiotics (from a group consisting of amoxicillin, trimethoprim, and nitrofurantoin), increased from 0.5% to 4.0%.

Drug formulations The stability of norfloxacin in suspensions prepared from two brands of film-coated tablets has been studied (172[C]). The vehicle consisted of tragacanth, saccharin sodium, sorbitol solution, glycerin, paraben concentrate, peppermint spirit, purified water, and syrup USP, yielding a final concentration of norfloxacin of 20 mg/ml. The resulting suspensions were chemically stable for 28 days when stored in amber glass bottles at room temperature.

Drug interactions Norfloxacin can interact with *antacids* containing aluminium or magnesium salts, by complexation, reducing its solubility and therefore its absorption; this can result in therapeutic failure. In an in vitro study, dissolution rates were markedly reduced in the presence of all antacids studied; however, this phenomenon was practically avoided when a disintegrant (sodium starch glycolate or crospovidone) was included in the tablet (173[E]).

Ofloxacin

Sensory systems In 135 unmedicated young volunteers, 13 elderly volunteers and 14 unmedicated HIV-infected patients, ofloxacin applied to the tongue was primarily described as bitter (127[C]).

Hematologic Antimicrobial chemotherapy against diseases caused by *E. coli* producing Shiga toxin has previously been implicated as a risk factor for progression to the *hemolytic–uremic syndrome*. This has been corroborated by the report of a further case in a 75-year-old woman who took ofloxacin (174[A]), and is in agreement with the results of an in vitro study that showed that the addition of ofloxacin to a cell culture increased toxin activity by more than 200-fold (175[E]).

Liver Ofloxacin can cause *fatal hepatic failure* (176[A]).

Skin *Photosensitivity* reactions to ofloxacin may be initiated by oxygen radicals and/or by ofloxacin radicals acting as haptens (177[C]).

Pefloxacin

There was a significant reduction in proteinuria in 10 children with idiopathic nephrotic syndrome after pefloxacin therapy (mean dose 2–4.6 mg/kg/day for 4–8 weeks) (178[C]). All had received a course of cyclophosphamide at least 6 months before. One patient discontinued pefloxacin within 2 weeks because of *nausea and vomiting*, one complained of *arthralgia*, and one developed *nail discoloration*.

Musculoskeletal The efficacy and safety of pefloxacin, 15–20 mg/kg bd for 14–28 days in combination with ceftazidime and amikacin, have been investigated in 21 children (aged 7–16 years) with mucoviscidosis or aplastic anemia (179[C]). Combined therapy had good clinical efficacy. *Arthropathy* developed frequently and children at risk were over 10 years old and had a history of allergies.

In rodents, pefloxacin (400 mg/kg for several days) caused oxidative damage to the type I collagen in the Achilles' tendon; these alterations were identical to those observed in experimental tendinous ischemia and a reperfusion model (180[E]). Oxidative damage was prevented by the coadministration of *N*-acetylcysteine (150 mg/kg).

Sitafloxacin

Skin Data obtained in albino mice have suggested that the phototoxic potential of sitafloxacin is milder than that of lomefloxacin or sparfloxacin (181[E]).

Sparfloxacin

Sparfloxacin has activity against the major respiratory pathogens and atypical pathogens that cause pneumonia. *Photosensitivity*, *nausea*, and *diarrhea* have been the most common adverse events reported in trials, and sparfloxacin is contraindicated in patients with QT interval prolongation (182[R]).

The efficacy and safety of sparfloxacin (400 mg loading dose followed by 200 mg/day for 10 days) in the treatment of acute bacterial maxillary sinusitis has been evaluated in 253 patients (183[C]). The overall success rate was 92%. The majority of adverse events were mild or moderate and the most frequent were *photosensitivity reactions*, *headache*, *nausea*, and *diarrhea*.

Cardiovascular In an in vitro comparison of sparfloxacin, grepafloxacin, moxifloxacin, and ciprofloxacin, sparfloxacin caused the greatest prolongation of the action potential duration (73[E]). In an in vivo study in conscious dogs with stable idioventricular automaticity and chronic complete atrioventricular block, oral sparfloxacin 60 mg/kg caused *torsade de pointes*, leading to ventricular fibrillation within 24 hours, while 6 mg/kg did not (184[E]). In halothane-anesthetized dogs, intravenous sparfloxacin 0.3 mg/kg prolonged the effective refractory period, and an extra 3.0 mg/kg reduced the heart rate and prolonged the effective refractory period and ventricular repolarization phase to a similar extent, suggesting that a backward shift of the relative repolarization period during the cardiac cycle may be the mechanism responsible for the *dysrhythmogenic effect* of sparfloxacin.

Skin During the first 9 months of marketing of sparfloxacin, 371 severe *phototoxic reactions* were reported to the French pharmacovigilance system or the manufacturers, reporting rate of 0.4 per thousand treated patients (about 4–25 times that reported with other fluoroquinolones) (185[C]).

Mutagenicity DNA damage produced by sparfloxacin and UVA in retinal pigment epithelial cells in vitro was remedied by antioxidants, suggesting a possible in vivo strategy for preventing or minimizing retinal damage in humans (186[E]).

Drug interactions In eight healthy Japanese, the absorption of sparfloxacin (300 mg orally) was reduced when *sucralfate* (1.5 g orally) was administered concurrently or 2 hours after sparfloxacin, but not 4 hours after sparfloxacin (187[C]).

Tosufloxacin

In 58 Japanese patients with typhoid fever, 42 with paratyphoid fever, and one with both typhoid fever and paratyphoid fever, almost 80% of whom were treated with tosufloxacin, there were adverse effects (*nausea*, *urticaria*, *aphthous stomatitis*) in 3.6% and *raised serum amylase* in 8.3% (188[C]). All the adverse reactions resolved with or without a change in drug therapy.

Skin Tosufloxacin has been associated with a *fixed drug eruption* (189[A]).

FUSIDIC ACID *(SED-14, 912; SEDA-24, 288)*

Fusidic acid is usually bacteriostatic but it may be bactericidal at higher concentrations. It exerts its antibacterial effect by inhibiting protein synthesis, but the exact mechanism by which this inhibition occurs has not yet been elucidated.

Gastrointestinal Oral fusidic acid can cause *Klebsiella oxytoca-associated colitis* (190[A]).

Skin Sensitization to sodium fusidate is rare, and most often found in patients with stasis dermatitis or atopic dermatitis. An *allergic contact dermatitis* has now been reported in a 26-year-old Korean woman after treatment of an abrasion on the left knee with Fucidin ointment and Betadine (191[A]). The diagnosis was confirmed by a strongly positive patch test for sodium fusidate.

Drug tolerance (antibacterial resistance) In a prospective randomized trial, oral fusidic acid alone (500 mg tds for 7 days) failed to eradicate methicillin-resistant *Staphylococcus aureus* colonization but resulted in the emergence of fusidic acid-resistant strains (192[C]).

Drug interactions In a 32-year-old man infected with HIV plasma concentrations of *ritonavir*, *saquinavir*, and fusidic acid were significantly raised when these drugs were administered in combination, possibly from mutual inhibition of metabolism (193[C]).

Acute rhabdomyolysis has been attributed to an interaction of fusidic acid with *atorvastatin* (194[A]).

A 66-year-old kidney transplant recipient developed a gangrenous lesion on the left foot infected with *Staphylococcus aureus* and *Escherichia coli*. He was given ciprofloxacin and clindamycin for 6 weeks and then fusidic acid 1500 mg/day for 2 weeks. He became ill, with myalgia and no active movement of his legs, and rhabdomyolysis was established by laboratory tests. He had also taken atorvastatin 10 mg/day and he slowly recovered after withdrawal of both atorvastatin and fusidic acid.

The authors identified only one previous report of a patient with rhabdomyolysis who had taken simvastatin and fusidic acid.

GLYCOPEPTIDES *(SED-14, 858; SEDA-22, 276; SEDA-23, 269; SEDA-24, 288)*

Urinary tract In children with febrile neutropenia and Gram-positive bacteremia associated with antineoplastic drug therapy, teicoplanin was significantly less *nephrotoxic* than vancomycin (195[C]).

Skin Teicoplanin may be safely administered to patients with a history of red man syndrome due to vancomycin, as has been confirmed in six children treated with teicoplanin for febrile neutropenia and Gram-positive bacteremia (195[c]).

Immunologic Vancomycin reportedly caused a severe *delayed skin reaction* with allergic cross-reactivity between vancomycin and teicoplanin requiring steroid therapy (196[A]).

A 68-year-old woman who was being treated with vancomycin for *Staphylococcus epidermidis* bacteremia developed pruritus and a generalized maculopapular skin rash after 2 weeks. After a short course of prednisolone, she was given teicoplanin and developed general malaise, fever, conjunctival injection, an extensive rash, and later blisters on the legs, again requiring treatment with steroids.

Drug tolerance (antibacterial resistance) In a study of antibiotic resistance in enterococci from raw meat, there was a high prevalence of glycopeptide-resistant strains (197[E]). Resistance to vancomycin was significantly associated with resistance to teicoplanin, erythromycin, tetracycline, and chloramphenicol.

Teicoplanin

Teicoplanin is more effectively administered once daily than vancomycin and it may be given intramuscularly or intravenously; it is not absorbed after oral administration. It is 90% bound to plasma proteins and its elimination is primarily by renal excretion, allowing dosage adjustments to be made on the basis of the measured creatinine clearance. A dosing regimen of 12 mg/kg on day 1 followed by 6 mg/kg/day most often results in efficacious serum concentrations, but premature neonates and children require higher dosages. However, doses of 10 mg/kg/day are required to achieve adequate bone concentrations, and there is little penetration into cerebrospinal fluid or aqueous or vitreous humors. In fat, concentrations may be subtherapeutic after a dose of 400 mg. Unlike vancomycin, routine drug monitoring is not required, although it may sometimes be useful for predicting the therapeutic effect of the drug. The most common adverse events associated with teicoplanin are *hypersensitivity*, *fever*, *rash*, *diarrhea*, *nephrotoxicity*, and *thrombocytopenia* (198[R], 199[R]).

In 76 patients receiving long-term teicoplanin for chronic osteomyelitis due to oxacillin-resistant *Staphylococcus aureus*, teicoplanin had to be withdrawn in only one subject because of *low-grade fever*, *muscular pain*, and *sleeplessness*; these adverse effects abated after withdrawal (200[C]).

Hematologic In trials in the USA, *thrombocytopenia* occurred more commonly with teicoplanin than with vancomycin, but this was almost exclusively in patients who received much larger doses than are now recommended. Severe thrombocytopenia has now been reported in a 46-year-old white man treated with teicoplanin 6 mg/kg/day for methicillin-resistant *Staphylococcus aureus* bacteremia (201[A]). The platelet count fell to 25 $\times 10^9$/l on day 8 (baseline 110). After drug withdrawal the platelet count improved within 4 days. The trough teicoplanin concentrations were 17 mg/l on day 4 and 15.4 mg/l on day 9.

Urinary tract In two of 76 patients receiving long-term teicoplanin a reduction in dosage was required because of *reduced renal function*, which recovered within 30 days (200[C]).

Vancomycin

Psychiatric Many parents of children with regressive-onset autism have noted antecedent antibiotic exposure followed by chronic diarrhea. In a subgroup of children, disruption of indigenous gut flora might promote colonization by one or more neurotoxin-producing bacteria, contributing at least in part to their autistic symptoms. In 11 children with regressive-onset autism who had broad-spectrum antimicrobial exposure followed by chronic persistent diarrhea, oral vancomycin resulted in short-term improvement; however, these gains had largely waned at follow-up (202[c]).

Hematologic *Neutropenia* is an uncommon adverse effect associated with prolonged vancomycin therapy; it normally recovers after drug withdrawal. The neutrophil count may recover when vancomycin is replaced by teicoplanin, as has recently been reported (203[c]).

A 35-year-old man was given vancomycin (1.5 g bd) for a wound infection with a coagulase-negative staphylococcus, a peptostreptococcus, and a coryneform Gram-positive bacillus. On day 37 his white blood cell count was 2.8 $\times 10^9$/l (baseline 5.2) with a low neutrophil count (0.5 $\times 10^9$/l). Vancomycin was withdrawn and 2 days later he was given teicoplanin 400 mg/day, by which time the cell count had increased to 3.5 $\times 10^9$/l. neutrophils 0.9 10^9/l. On day 45, the total white cell count was 4.9 $\times 10^9$/l, neutrophils 2.3 $\times 10^9$/l. Teicoplanin was continued for 1 month, and the white cell count remained normal.

Treatment with vancomycin can rarely cause reversible pancytopenia, as outlined in two case reports (204[A], 205[A]).

A 43-year-old white woman was given vancomycin for a suspected methicillin-resistant *Staphylococcus aureus* infection. On day 10 she developed a fever, chills, and a disseminated lacy macular rash. Vancomycin was withdrawn but reinstituted 48 hours later. Another 24 hours later, she again developed a fever, chills, and a confluent erythematous rash. Sepsis developed, and ceftazidime was added. There was thrombocytopenia (118 $\times 10^9$/l), and a fall in the white blood count (from 7.6 to 3.5 $\times 10^9$/l) and hemoglobin (from 13.8 to 12.2 g/daily). One day later the leukocyte count was 2.6 $\times 10^9$/l and the hemoglobin fell to 10 g/daily. Both drugs were withdrawn. The rash disappeared, the temperature returned to normal, and the blood cell counts completely recovered 4 days later.

An 87-year-old white woman was treated with vancomycin for an abscess due to methicillin-resistant *Staphylococcus epidermidis*. On day 30, her white blood cell count fell to 0.5 $\times 10^9$/l after a total dose of 55 g of vancomycin. Vancomycin was withdrawn, and the white blood cell count returned to normal within 5 days. After 6 weeks vancomycin was reintroduced, and the white blood cell count fell to 0.325 $\times 10^9$/l after a total dose of 14 g of vancomycin on day 9, but resolved rapidly after vancomycin was withdrawn.

Skin An 87-year-old white woman treated with vancomycin and phenytoin and a 65-year-old white man with renal insufficiency developed *linear immunoglobulin A bullous disease* (206[A], 207[A]).

Erythema multiforme has been attributed to vancomycin (196[A]).

A 70-year-old woman was given vancomycin postoperatively developed fever on day 5 and vancomycin was withdrawn. She then developed a generalized urticarial rash with oral and vaginal erosive lesions on day 6, requiring treatment with steroids and antihistamines. The diagnosis was confirmed by skin biopsy.

Vancomycin can cause either *Stevens–Johnson syndrome* (involvement of less than 30% of the skin surface) or *toxic epidermal necrolysis* (more than 30% of the skin surface involved); both conditions include mucosal involvement.

A 53-year-old white woman with liver cirrhosis took vancomycin (1 g bd) for sepsis due to methicillin-resistant *Staphylococcus aureus* and a catheter-associated infection due to *Enterococcus fecalis*, developed oral and vaginal mucositis and conjunctivitis followed by a maculopapular rash (208^{A}). The diagnosis was confirmed by skin biopsy. Vancomycin was replaced by teicoplanin and corticosteroids; the symptoms disappeared within 7 days.

A 36-year-old white woman with relapsing acute myeloid leukemia took ceftazidime (2 g tds) and aciclovir for febrile neutropenia and *Herpes labialis*. She developed an itchy rash and treatment was changed to imipenem (500 mg qds for 5 days), vancomycin (1 g bd for 3 days), and gentamicin (2 mg/kg for 3 days); chemotherapy included idarubicin, cytarabine, etoposide, ondansetron, and dexamethasone for 3 days. Within a few days the rash developed into blisters and erosions, affecting more than 80% of the skin. The diagnosis was confirmed histologically, and she subsequently died from shock (209^{A}).

Immunologic Vancomycin can cause *anaphylactoid reactions* by histamine release. In rat peritoneal mast cells it provoked histamine release dose-dependently; fosfomycin inhibited this effect (210^{E}).

Vancomycin *anaphylaxis* is a major management problem in patients with methicillin-resistant *Staphylococcus aureus* sepsis. However, desensitization in patients with previous anaphylaxis is possible (211^{A}).

Drug tolerance (antibacterial resistance) The prevalence of vancomycin-resistant enterococci (VRE) has been investigated in 49 laboratories from 27 European countries, which collected 4208 clinical isolates; 18 vanA and 5 vanB isolates of VRE were identified (212^{E}). The prevalence of vanA VRE was highest in the UK (2.7%), while the prevalence of vanB VRE was highest in Slovenia (2%). Most vanA and vanB vancomycin-resistant enterococci were identified as *Enterococcus fecium*. A total of 71 isolates containing the vanC gene were identified. The prevalence of vanC VRE was highest in Latvia and Turkey, where rates were 14% and 12% respectively. Two-thirds of these isolates were identified as *Enterococcus gallinarum* and one-third as *Enterococcus casseliflavus*.

Drug overdose Accidental 10-fold vancomycin overdose in a 6-month-old girl resulted in flushing and a transient rise in serum creatinine concentration, but she recovered completely without specific therapeutic intervention (213^{A}).

Drug interactions In critically ill patients, coadministration with *dopamine* and/or *dobutamine* can enhance vancomycin clearance by increasing cardiac output and renal blood flow and by interacting with the renal anion transport system, increasing glomerular filtration rate and renal tubular secretion (214^{C}).

Vancomycin and *ceftazidime* are incompatible in vitro because of precipitation due to the alkaline pH of vancomycin relative to ceftazidime. This phenomenon was encountered in two cases of post-traumatic endophthalmitis (215^{A}). Immediately on local administration of the antibiotics, which were injected using different needles and syringes for each drug, dense yellow-white precipitates were observed along the needle tract in the vitreous cavity. During follow-up the vitreous opacities gradually disappeared over a period of 2 months, with complete resolution.

Vancomycin is incompatible with *gelatin fluids*, resulting in precipitation (216^{A}).

KETOLIDES *(SEDA-24, 294)*

Telithromycin (HMR 3647) is the first member of a new family of the macrolide–lincosamide–streptogramin-B (MLS(B)) class of antimicrobials, the ketolides. It has a good spectrum of activity against respiratory pathogens, including penicillin- and erythromycin-resistant pneumococci, intracellular bacteria, and atypical bacteria. It penetrates rapidly into bronchopulmonary, tonsillar, sinus, and middle ear tissues/fluids, achieves high concentrations at sites of infection, and concentrates within polymorphonuclear neutrophils. Telithromycin is well tolerated across all patient populations, and adverse events, most commonly diarrhea, nausea, dizziness, and vomiting, are generally mild to moderate in intensity and seldom lead to treatment withdrawal (217[R], 218[C]).

Drug tolerance (antibacterial resistance) In subjects receiving oral telithromycin (800 mg/day for 10 days), high drug concentrations were detected in the saliva indicating a good therapeutic profile for throat infections. Quantitative ecological disturbances in the normal microflora during administration of telithromycin were moderate, and no overgrowth of yeasts or *Clostridium difficile* occurred. However, resistant bacterial strains emerged (219[C]).

The in vitro activity of the new ketolide ABT773 was very similar to that of telithromycin, with an MIC_{90} of 0.5 mg/l or less for all bacteria examined, except methicillin-resistant *Staphylococcus aureus*, *Enterococcus fecalis*, *Enterococcus fecium*, *Hemophilus influenzae*, and *Bacteroides* spp. However, the antichlamydial activity of ABT773 was greater than that of telithromycin (220[A]).

Drug interactions Cytokines modify phagocyte activity and may interfere with the immunomodulating properties of antibacterial agents. In an in vitro study, TNF-α and GM-CSF reduced the inhibitory effect of telithromycin on oxidant production by polymorphonuclear neutrophils, suggesting an effect of telithromycin downstream of the priming effect of cytokines. In addition, TNF-α and GM-CSF moderately impaired the uptake of telithromycin by polymorphonuclear neutrophils; the inhibitory effect of these two cytokines seemed to be related to activation of the p38 mitogen-activated protein kinase (221[E]).

LINCOSAMIDES *(SED-14, 871; SEDA-22, 278; SEDA-23, 273; SEDA-24, 293)*

Clindamycin

In a prospective, open, randomized trial clindamycin (600 mg tds) and quinine (650 mg tds) were compared with atovaquone (750 mg bd) plus azithromycin (500 mg on day 1 followed by 250 mg/day) in 58 patients with non-life-threatening babesiosis (222[C]). Bacterial response was complete 3 months after the end of treatment. Adverse effects were reported by 72% of those who received clindamycin and quinine compared with 15% of those who received atovaquone and azithromycin. The most common adverse effects with clindamycin and quinine were *tinnitus* (39%), *diarrhea* (33%), and *impaired hearing* (28%); the symptoms had resolved in 73% of the patients assigned to clindamycin/quinine 3 months after the start of therapy and in 100% after 6 months.

In 233 women with bacterial vaginosis, a 3-day regimen of clindamycin (intravaginal ovules, 100 mg/day) was as effective as a 7-day regimen of oral metronidazole (500 mg bd) and better tolerated (223[C]). Treatment-related adverse events were reported more often with metronidazole, and systemic symptoms, such as nausea and taste disturbance, accounted for most of the difference between the groups.

Gastrointestinal Clindamycin can cause *esophagitis* (224[R]).

Clindamycin can cause *pseudomembranous colitis*, and a new report has appeared (225[A]).

A young otherwise healthy nurse developed severe diarrhea and vomiting, profuse ascites, pleural effusion, abdominal tenderness, peritoneal irritation, and systemic toxicity 10 days after taking oral clindamycin for a dental infection. Although the assay for *Clostridium difficile* was repeatedly negative, features compatible with pseudomembranous colitis were seen at sigmoidoscopy, and the diagnosis was confirmed histologically.

Skin The first report of acute *generalized exanthematous pustulosis* associated with clindamycin has been published (226[A]).

MACROLIDES *(SED-14, 873; SEDA-23, 273; SEDA-24, 295)*

Cardiovascular In a comparative pharmacodynamic analysis of QT interval prolongation induced by macrolide antibiotics in rats, the rank order of clinical *dysrhythmogenicity* was estimated to be erythromycin > clarithromycin > roxithromycin > azithromycin (227[E]).

Immunologic *Allergy* to macrolides is uncommon, occurring in 0.4–3% of treatments (228[R]). Of 21 patients with assumed allergy to macrolides, principally urticaria, only three had a positive provocation test (positive prick and intradermal tests with injectable forms of spiramycin and erythromycin), suggesting that provocation tests for diagnosis of hypersensitivity reactions to macrolides are not useful (229[C]). In a patient with a non-immediate skin reaction to spiramycin plus metronidazole, peripheral blood T cells expressing the cutaneous lymphocyte-associated antigen, the skin-homing receptor, were increased after drug exposure, supporting the immunological nature of delayed skin reactions to these drugs (230[C]).

In vitro, some macrolide antibiotics have anti-inflammatory activity, which probably depends on their ability to prevent the production of proinflammatory mediators and cytokines, suggesting that these agents can have therapeutic effects independent of their antibacterial activity (231[E]).

Drug tolerance (antibacterial resistance) In 1050 clinical isolates of *Streptococcus pyogenes*, overall resistance rates to azithromycin, clarithromycin, and erythromycin were 16%, 15%, and 16%, respectively (232[E]). Erythromycin resistance rates were highest in Italy (31%) and Spain (27%), with lower rates in Turkey (4.8%), France (3.8%), and Sweden (3.7%).

In mouse leukemia cells, macrolide antibiotics overcame drug resistance by inhibiting the binding of vinblastine or ciclosporin to P-glycoprotein (233[E]).

Drug interactions Pharmacokinetic interactions with the macrolides clarithromycin, erythromycin, and troleandomycin often result from an inhibition of cytochrome P450, especially CYP3A4. Torsade de pointes can occur when these inhibitors are coadministered with *terfenadine*, *astemizole*, *cisapride*, or *pimozide* (234[R]).

Other interactions of this sort can cause rhabdomyolysis (associated with the coadministration of some 3-hydroxy-3-methylglutaryl-coenzyme A reductase inhibitors, e.g. *lovastatin* or *simvastatin*), hypoprothrombinemia (associated with *warfarin*), excessive sedation (associated with certain benzodiazepines, e.g. *midazolam*, *triazolam*, *alprazolam*, or *diazepam*), ataxia (associated with *carbamazepine*), and ergotism (associated with ergotamine).

Beneficial drug interactions can also occur. For example, coadministration of macrolides with *ciclosporin* may allow reduction of the dosage and cost of the immunosuppressant (235[R], 236[R]).

Azithromycin

In a prospective, randomized, multicenter trial in community-acquired pneumonia in 145 patients, azithromycin monotherapy was associated with adverse events (*intravenous catheter site reactions*, *gastrointestinal tract disturbances*) in 12% of treated patients (237[C]).

Sensory systems Azithromycin rarely causes ototoxicity, mostly after prolonged high-dose therapy in patients with acquired immunodeficiency syndrome, and results in a reversible *sensorineural hearing loss*; however, low-dose exposure to azithromycin can also be associated with irreversible sensorineural hearing loss in otherwise healthy subjects (238[A]).

Hematologic *Angioimmunoblastic lymphadenopathy with dysproteinemia* is a rare benign reactive process that often follows exposure to certain drugs, such as penicillin. Although treatment with corticosteroids usually reverses the process, a significant number of cases evolve into non-Hodgkin's lymphoma. Now, angioimmunoblastic lymphadenopathy with dysproteinemia and resultant lymphoma has been reported after treatment with azithromycin in a woman with a history of various drug hypersensitivities (239[A]).

Gastrointestinal In an open study of azithromycin (1 g on day 1 followed by 500 mg/day for 8 days) in early syphilis, two of 14 patients had *gastrointestinal adverse effects*, which did not require interruption of treatment (240[C]).

Liver Azithromycin has been suggested to cause acute *pseudoangiocholitic hepatitis* (241[A]).

Skin The first case of a *skin reaction* in a patient with infectious mononucleosis treated with azithromycin has been reported, and an immune-based hypothesis to explain the transient sensitivity has been proposed (242[A]).

Pregnancy In 21 term placentas the mean transplacental transfer of azithromycin was 2.6%, calculated as the ratio between the steady-state concentrations in fetal venous and maternal arterial sides (243[E]). Thus, the placenta seems to produce an effective barrier to azithromycin, reducing fetal exposure.

Drug interactions In a two-way, open-label, cross-over study in 12 subjects, azithromycin caused a statistically, but not clinically, significant reduction in *nelfinavir* concentrations (244[C]). In contrast, nelfinavir caused large increases in azithromycin C_{max} and AUC. Inhibition of P-glycoprotein by nelfinavir may have been the mechanism of this interaction.

Azithromycin can cause *disopyramide* toxicity, presumably by inhibition of dealkylation of disopyramide to its major metabolite, mono-*N*-dealkyldisopyramide, as in a patient who developed ventricular tachycardia requiring cardioversion (245[A]).

Clarithromycin

Respiratory Clarithromycin can cause acute *bronchospasm*, the speed and clinical characteristics of which suggest immediate-type hypersensitivity (246[A]).

Immunologic *Allergy* to tacrolimus has been reported in a patient who was allergic to clarithromycin (247[A]).

A 45-year-old woman received a haploid allogenic bone-marrow transplant for acute myelogenous leukemia. She had a history of allergy to allopurinol, ciprofloxacin, clarithromycin, and vancomycin, all of which caused a rash, except vancomycin, which caused itching. For prophylaxis of graft–versus–host disease, she was given tacrolimus 0.03 mg/kg/day as a continuous infusion on the day before transplantation. After 3 days she developed an erythematous follicular rash and the next day had diffuse generalized erythema. Because of the escalating skin problems, tacrolimus was stopped and replaced with ciclosporin. The erythema abated after 24 hours and resolved after 3 days.

Dirithromycin

In a double-blind, randomized, multicenter study in 439 patients dirithromycin (500 mg/day for 5 days) caused significantly less *nausea* than erythromycin (250 mg qds for 7 days) but was comparable in efficacy for the treatment of skin and soft tissue infections (248[C]).

Erythromycin

Hematologic Erythromycin shortens the survival of peripheral human neutrophils by *accelerating apoptosis* (249[E]).

Gastrointestinal The prokinetic effect of erythromycin at subantimicrobial doses has been investigated in infants and children with a variety of gastrointestinal dysmotility disorders. Most studies have shown beneficial effects in either promoting tolerance of enteral feeds or enhancing gastrointestinal motility. Erythromycin appears to be equally effective orally or intravenously, and no serious adverse effects have been reported in studies in which it has been used for its prokinetic effects (250[R], 251[C]).

Pregnancy In 21 term placentas the mean transplacental transfer of erythromycin was 3%, calculated as the ratio between the steady-state concentrations in fetal venous and maternal arterial sides (243[E]). Thus, the placenta seems to produce an effective barrier to erythromycin, reducing fetal exposure.

Drug interactions Rhabdomyolysis occurs in about 0.1% of patients who take 3-hydroxy-3-methylglutaryl coenzyme A (HMG-CoA) reductase inhibitors (statins). The incidence is increased when HMG-CoA reductase inhibitors are used in combination with agents that share a common metabolic pathway, such as erythromycin (252[R]).

Josamycin

Teratogenicity In a case-control study, the dataset of the Hungarian Case-Control Surveillance of Congenital Abnormalities 1980–96 (22 865 cases, 38 151 controls) was used to investigate the teratogenic potential of josamycin (253[C]). The authors did not detect any teratogenic risk, but the power of the study was low.

Miocamycin

Drug tolerance (antibacterial resistance) Of 486 clinical isolates of *Streptococcus pyogenes* obtained from 20 geographically distinct Spanish hospital laboratories during 1998, 24% were resistant to erythromycin and 1% were resistant to miocamycin; of the erythromycin-resistant strains, 96% were susceptible to miocamycin (254[E]).

The in vitro activity of miocamycin against erythromycin-resistant *Streptococcus pneumoniae*, *S. pyogenes* (50% erythromycin-resistant), and *Streptococcus agalactiae* (50% erythromycin-resistant) has been determined (255[E]). The M phenotype was found in 85%, 6.3%, and 1.9% of *S. pyogenes*, *S. agalactiae*, and *S. pneumoniae* respectively, and these strains were susceptible to both miocamycin and clindamycin. In contrast, all of the strains with the inducible phenotype, which accounted for 27% of *S. agalactiae* and 9.4% each of *S. pyogenes* and *S. pneumoniae*, were also resistant to miocamycin.

Drug interactions CYP3A4 is mainly responsible for the hydroxylation of miocamycin. Some macrolide antibiotics alter the metabolism of concomitantly administered drugs by forming a metabolic intermediate complex with CYP3A4 or by competitive inhibition. However, in an in vitro study miocamycin did not inhibit CYP3A4 by forming a metabolic intermediate complex (256[E]).

Oleandomycin

Teratogenicity In a case-control study, the dataset of the Hungarian Case-Control Surveillance of Congenital Abnormalities 1980–96 (22 865 cases, 38 151 controls) was used to investigate the teratogenic potential of oleandomycin (253[C]). The authors did not detect any teratogenic risk, but the power of the study was low.

Roxithromycin

Cardiovascular The dysrhythmogenic potency of macrolide antibiotics is well known. In male Sprague–Dawley rats, roxithromycin was less potent at provoking dysrhythmias than erythromycin and clarithromycin (227[E]). However, *dysrhythmias* can occur (257[A]).

A 72-year-old patient with congestive heart failure due to coronary artery disease developed severe prolongation of the QT interval after taking roxithromycin (150 mg bd) for 3 days. Concomitant medications included amiodarone, aspirin, digoxin, captopril, and furosemide. An electrocardiogram showed sinus rhythm and incomplete left bundle branch block; the QT interval was normal. After 3 days the QT_c interval was 660 ms. Serum concentrations of potassium, calcium, amiodarone, and digoxin were unremarkable. Digoxin, roxithromycin, and amiodarone were withdrawn and the QT_c interval slowly shortened to 430 ms.

The authors concluded that the prolongation of the QT interval had been due to the concomitant use of roxithromycin and amiodarone, which also prolongs the QT interval.

Musculoskeletal Roxithromycin inhibited TNF-α-induced vascular endothelial growth factor expression in cultured human periodontal ligament cells (258[E]).

Immunologic Roxithromycin has an anti-inflammatory activity by preventing the production of proinflammatory mediators, cytokines, and co-stimulatory molecules (231[E], 259[E]).

Roxithromycin has an immunomodulatory action in human peripheral blood mononuclear cells (260[E]). It suppressed both the proliferation of cells stimulated with phytohemagglutinin and the production of cytokines from lipopolysaccharide-stimulated cells, whereas it increased adherent cells. Roxithromycin also augmented apoptosis of human peripheral neutrophils (249[E]).

Pregnancy In 21 term placentas the mean transplacental transfer of roxithromycin was 4.3%, calculated as the ratio between the steady-state concentrations on the fetal venous and maternal arterial sides (243[E]). Thus, the placenta seems to produce an effective barrier to roxithromycin, reducing fetal exposure.

Teratogenicity In a case-control study, the dataset of the Hungarian Case-Control Surveillance of Congenital Abnormalities 1980–96 (22 865 cases, 38 151 controls) was used to investigate the teratogenic potential of roxithromycin (253[C]). The authors did not detect any teratogenic risk, but the power of the study was low.

Drug interactions In two cross-over studies

with *omeprazole* (20 mg bd), *lansoprazole* (30 mg bd), and roxithromycin (300 mg bd) in 12 healthy volunteers over 6 days, proton pump inhibitors increased the local concentration of roxithromycin in the stomach but did not alter its systemic availability (261[C]).

Interference with diagnostic tests Colorimetry can not be used for the determination and assay of roxithromycin in acidic solution, as the metabolite of roxithromycin interferes.

Spiramycin

Teratogenicity In a case-control study, the dataset of the Hungarian Case-Control Surveillance of Congenital Abnormalities 1980–96 (22 865 cases, 38 151 controls) was used to investigate the teratogenic potential of spiramycin (253[E]). The authors did not detect any teratogenic risk, but the power of the study was low.

Troleandomycin

Drug interactions Troleandomycin inhibits CYP3A4 and is often used to investigate the involvement of this isoform in the biotransformation of other xenobiotics. In human liver microsomes troleandomycin significantly inhibited:

- the primary metabolism of the novel immunomodulator *roquinimex* (over 90% inhibition) (262[E]);
- the 4-hydroxylation of highly embryotoxic and teratogenic retinoic acids catalyzed by human fetal liver microsomes (CYP3A7), a catalysis that might play an important role in protecting the human fetus against embryotoxicity induced by retinoic acids (70–75% inhibition) (263[E]);
- the metabolism of *cisapride*, an interaction that was considered to be of probable clinical relevance (236[R], 264[E]);
- the degradation of *bupivacaine* to its major metabolite pipecolylxylidine (95% at 50 μmol/l) (265[E]);
- the metabolism of the 5-HT_{1D} receptor agonist *L-775 606* to its principal metabolites (hydroxylated M1 and *N*-dealkylated M2; over 80% inhibition) (266[E]);
- the metabolism of the non-peptidic substance P receptor antagonist *ezlopitant* to CJ-12,764, a benzyl alcohol analog, and a dehydrogenated metabolite (CJ-12,458) (267[E]);
- the biotransformation of rifalazil to 32-*hydroxyrifalazil*, one of the major metabolites besides 25-deacetylrifalazil that is generated through a B-esterase (268[E]);
- the mono-*N*-dealkylation of *disopyramide* enantiomers (269[E]);
- the alternative *N*-dechloroethylation of the anticancer alkylating agents *cyclophosphamide* and, to a lesser extent, *ifosfamide*; these *N*-dechloroethylated metabolites are inactive but neurotoxic (270[E]).
- the *N*-de-ethylation of *lidocaine* to monoethylglycinexylidide and 3-hydroxylation preferentially at high lidocaine concentrations, suggesting that CYP3A4 may be of importance at these concentrations, whereas at low concentrations CYP1A2 is the major isoform responsible for lidocaine metabolism (271[E]).

NITROFURANTOIN *(SED-14, 884)*

Respiratory Acute respiratory reactions to nitrofurantoin include *dyspnea*, *cough*, *interstitial pneumonitis*, and *pleural effusion*, while *interstitial pneumonitis and fibrosis* are common chronic reactions (272[R]).

In nitrofurantoin-induced pulmonary toxicity, in which high-resolution computed tomography initially showed a widespread reticular pattern and associated distortion of the lung parenchyma, thought to represent established and irreversible fibrosis, follow-up scans after drug withdrawal nevertheless showed resolution of pulmonary changes (273[A]). These findings have been corroborated by a report of two middle-aged women who developed respiratory symptoms after prolonged treatment with nitrofurantoin (274[A]). Both had impaired lung function and abnormal CT scans, and lung biopsies showed features compatible with *bronchiolitis obliterans organizing pneumonia*. Their condition improved when nitrofurantoin was withdrawn and corticosteroid treatment was given.

Nervous system While taking nitrofurantoin after urinary tract surgery, a 10-year-old girl developed *diplopia and ptosis*. A sleep test confirmed ocular myasthenia. Her signs and symptoms resolved after drug withdrawal (275[A]).

Drug tolerance (antibacterial resistance) Nitrofurantoin is effective against enterobacteriaceae; the rates of resistance were below 2% in a single-center study (276[E]) and 3.5% in a multicenter study (277[E]).

Teratogenicity No teratogenic effects have been associated with nitrofurantoin in Denmark, Finland, Norway, and Sweden (278[C]).

Fetotoxicity *Hemolytic anemia* occurred during the first hours of life in a full-term neonate whose mother had taken nitrofurantoin during the last month of pregnancy (279[A]). It may therefore be wise not to prescribe nitrofurantoin at the end of pregnancy.

POLYMYXINS *(SED-14, 887; SEDA-24, 300)*

Skin Topical polymyxin B was the predominant allergen in patients who underwent patch testing for evaluation of eczema of the external ear canal (45[C]).

In a randomized study of the effects of an antibiotic ointment and simple gauze dressings on scarring of dermabrasion wounds, each of three uniform dermabrasion wounds was treated concurrently with a triple-antibiotic ointment (polymyxin B + bacitracin + neomycin), a double antibiotic (polymyxin B + bacitracin), or a simple non-occlusive gauze dressing. The triple antibiotic ointment was superior to the simple gauze dressing alone in minimizing scarring, and this benefit was more pronounced in its effect on pigmentary changes (44[C]).

Drug tolerance (antibacterial resistance) Resistance to colistin has been analysed in 44 adults with cystic fibrosis treated with inhaled colistin. Five developed polymyxin resistance (280[C]). After therapy *Pseudomonas aeruginosa* became sensitive to polymyxin within a few months, enabling the reintroduction of colistin for antibacterial treatment.

Drug administration route Bolus intravenous colistin (160 mg in 10 ml of saline tds) has been studied in a phase I open-label study during acute respiratory exacerbations in adults with cystic fibrosis and chronic *Pseudomonas aeruginosa* infection; patients without total indwelling venous access systems had mild to moderate injection pain (281[C]).

In a study of the intrathecal administration of colistin adverse events were not reported (282[A]). This may be an effective alternative treatment of bacterial meningitis caused by multiresistant Gram-negative rods.

During sepsis, toxins (e.g. released from bacteria) can cause shock, disseminated intravascular coagulation, multiorgan dysfunction, and death. Apheresis may be a way of reducing the amounts of toxins and other harmful compounds in the circulation, and polymyxin B may serve as an adsorber. In three patients with septic shock, direct hemoperfusion using a polymyxin B-immobilized fiber column was carried out after antibacterial and antishock therapy. As a result, cardiovascular instabilities improved without increasing the supply of catecholamines (283[C]). Furthermore, in seven patients with endotoxic shock after laparotomy undergoing hemoperfusion with the polymyxin B-immobilized fiber, there was an early increase in urine volume, attributable to increased glomerular filtration independent of systemic hemodynamic factors (284[C]).

STREPTOGRAMINS *(SEDA-24, 300)*

Pristinamycin

Skin Mean antibiotic concentrations of pristinamycin in dermal interstitial fluid (from suction bullae) are low; nevertheless, the concentrations achieved should theoretically inhibit the growth of group A streptococci (285[C]).

Drug tolerance (antibacterial resistance) The in vitro activity of pristinamycin has been evaluated in 200 isolates of *Streptococcus pneumoniae* strains with various degrees of susceptibility to penicillin G and erythromycin (286[E]). All the strains were susceptible to pristinamycin, irrespective of their susceptibility to penicillin G or erythromycin.

Quinupristin/dalfopristin

Quinupristin/dalfopristin can be used to treat macrolide-resistant streptococci, staphylococcal infections after failure of conventional therapy, or vancomycin-resistant *E. fecium* (and probably *E. raffinosus*), but not vancomycin-resistant *E. fecalis*, *E. avium*, *E. casseliflavus*, or *E. gallinarum* (255[C], 287[C], 288[C], 289[R]–298[R]). Its adverse effects of include *arthralgia*, *myalgia*, and *pain at the infusion site* (299[R]).

Electrolyte balance Quinupristin/dalfopristin has been associated with *hyponatremia*, probably secondary to inappropriate secretion of antidiuretic hormone (300[A]).

A 67-year-old woman with peripheral neuropathy, IgM paraproteinemia, and chronic obstructive pulmonary disease developed dyspnea and hyponatremia, and a small-cell lung cancer was diagnosed. She was given 3 cycles of chemotherapy (etoposide, cyclophosphamide, and adriamycin). Her serum sodium concentrations normalized. On day 103, she was given quinupristin/dalfopristin (7.5 mg/kg every 8 hours) because of septicemia with vancomycin-resistant *E. fecium*. The serum sodium concentration thereafter fell (day 110: 117 mmol/l; serum osmolarity 268 mosm/l; urine osmolarity 426 mosm/l). Therapy was withdrawn on day 111, and the sodium concentration gradually returned to normal.

Immunologic Quinupristin/dalfopristin reduces cytokine production in stimulated monocytes from healthy volunteers, suggesting significant immunomodulatory activity (301[E]).

Risk factors The pharmacokinetics of a single intravenous injection of quinupristin/dalfopristin (7.5 mg/kg over 1 hour) have been assessed in 13 patients with severe *chronic renal insufficiency* (creatinine clearance 6–28 ml/min/1.73 m^2) (302[C]). Although the mean peak plasma drug concentration and AUC of quinupristin plus its active derivatives and of both unchanged dalfopristin and dalfopristin plus its active derivatives were about 1.3–1.4 times higher than in healthy volunteers, the authors concluded that no formal reduction in the dosage of quinupristin/dalfopristin is necessary in patients with chronic renal insufficiency.

Drug tolerance (antibacterial resistance) The use of the growth-promoting streptogramin virginiamycin has been associated with the high rate of resistance to quinupristin/dalfopristin (see below).

SULFONAMIDES, TRIMETHOPRIM, AND CO-TRIMOXAZOLE *(SED-14, 896; SEDA-22, 279; SEDA-23, 280)*

Sulfonamides

In an open trial in 25 patients treated with sulfamethoxypyridazine (1 g/day) for mucous membrane pemphigoid unresponsive to topical steroid treatment, 12% of patients were withdrawn, 4% because of *allergic reactions*, the others because of significant *hemolysis* (303[C]).

Cardiovascular Of 98 patients with drug-induced *long QT interval*, one taking sulfamethoxazole carried a single-nucleotide polymorphism (SNP; found in about 1.6% of the general population) in KCNE2, which encodes MinK-related peptide 1 (MiRP1), a subunit of the cardiac potassium channel IK_r (304[C]). Channels with the SNP were normal at baseline but were inhibited by sulfamethoxazole at therapeutic concentrations, which did not affect wild-type channels.

Sensory systems In unmedicated young and elderly volunteers and HIV-infected patients, sulfamethoxazole applied to the tongue was described as sour by young subjects, whereas it was described as bitter by elderly subjects (127[C]).

Urinary tract Sulfadiazine can be nephrotoxic due to *crystalluria* and can cause oliguric renal insufficiency and radiolucent renal calculi, even in previously healthy people. The course is typically benign and adequate hydration and alkalinization may be required (305[A]).

Skin In a survey of 5923 pediatric records, 3.46% prescriptions for sulfonamides were followed by the development of a *skin rash*, but none was severe enough to require hospitalization (306[C]).

In a study from Cameroon, eight of 10 patients with *toxic epidermal necrolysis* had taken sulfonamides (five sulfadoxine, three sulfamethoxazole); two patients died after taking sulfadoxine (307[C]).

Generalized *cutaneous depigmentation* after sulfamide therapy occurred in a 41-year-old man (308[A]). Melanocytes were not seen on electron microscopy, but there were clear cells with the characteristics of Langerhans cells along the basal layer.

There has been a case report of *toxic epidermal necrolysis* caused by co-trimoxazole, improving with high-dose methylprednisolone (309[A]). However, previous studies of the use of steroids in toxic epidermal necrolysis have given contradictory results.

Immunologic *Sulfa allergy* refers to a specific hypersensitivity response to a group of chemicals containing a sulfonamide moiety covalently bound to a benzene ring; drugs structurally similar to sulfonamides may cross-react, e.g. sulfonylureas, thiazides, and furosemide (310[r]).

In an in vitro study, plasma from HIV-positive patients was less able to detoxify nitrososulfamethoxazole than control plasma, suggesting that a disturbance in redox balance in HIV-positive patients may alter metabolic detoxification capacity, thereby predisposing to sulfamethoxazole hypersensitivity (311[E]).

Risk factors In *children* with acute uncomplicated *Plasmodium falciparum* malaria, pyrimethamine + sulfadoxine (25 mg/500 mg) and artesunate (4 mg/kg) were well tolerated, and no adverse reactions attributable to treatment were recorded (312[C]).

Drug interactions The inhibitory effect of sulfonamides on *tolbutamide* metabolism is mediated by CYP2C9, and therefore other drugs with narrow therapeutic ranges that are metabolized by CYP2C9, such as *phenytoin* and *warfarin*, deserve attention when certain sulfonamides (e.g. sulfaphenazole, sulfadiazine, sulfamethizole, and sulfisoxazole) are coadministered (313[C]).

Trimethoprim

Sensory systems In unmedicated young and elderly volunteers and unmedicated HIV-infected patients, trimethoprim applied to the tongue was primarily described as bitter and medicinal (127[C]).

Electrolyte balance *Hyperkalemia* is a relatively common complication of trimethoprim therapy and occurs at both standard and high dosages. Trimethoprim reduces renal potassium excretion by competitively inhibiting epithelial sodium channels in the distal nephron like triamterene does. Higher dosages and pre-existing renal dysfunction are associated with an increased risk of hyperkalemia, as are probably other disturbances in potassium homeostasis, such as hypoaldosteronism and treatment with other drugs that impair renal potassium excretion. Withdrawal of trimethoprim is often required; in addition, alkalinization of the urine and the induction of high urinary flow rates with intravenous fluids and loop diuretics block the antikaliuretic effect of trimethoprim on distal nephron cells (314[R], 315[C]).

Teratogenicity The relative risks of *cardiovascular defects and oral clefts* in infants whose mothers have been exposed to dihydrofolate reductase inhibitors, such as trimethoprim, during the second or third month after the last menstrual period, compared with infants whose mothers have had no such exposure, are 3.4 (95% CI = 1.8, 6.4) and 2.6 (1.1, 6.1) respectively; multivitamin supplements containing folic acid reduce the adverse effects of dihydrofolate reductase inhibitors (316[C]).

Drug interactions The antihistaminic phenothiazine *trimeprazine* has significant antibacterial activity in vitro and in vivo, and a combination with trimethoprim is highly synergistic, as shown in vivo in Swiss white mice using *Salmonella typhimurium* as the challenge bacterium (317[E]).

Trimethoprim inhibits the active tubular secretion of *procainamide* (318[R]).

Co-trimoxazole

Nervous system Co-trimoxazole can cause *tremor* (319[A]).

A 66-year-old man with pulmonary fibrosis and cor pulmonale was given intravenous co-trimoxazole for 3 weeks followed by oral treatment for an infection with *Nocardia farcinica*. On day 3 of oral treatment he developed a tremor in both arms and legs, exacerbated by trying to stay calm. The symptoms resolved 3 days after drug withdrawal.

Delirium occurred after treatment with co-trimoxazole in a patient with AIDS; the episode completely resolved within 72 hours of drug withdrawal (320[A]).

Aseptic meningitis is a rare adverse effect

of co-trimoxazole. The pathogenetic mechanism is still uncertain. Immune complex deposition, immediate hypersensitivity, direct drug toxicity, and induction of antitissue antibodies have all been suggested. Interleukin-6 may be an important mediator of trimethoprim-induced aseptic meningitis in some patients. Some recent reports have again illustrated this adverse effect (321[AR], 322[A], 323[A], 324[Ar]).

Electrolyte balance Trimethoprim-induced *hyperkalemia* has been increasingly recognized in recent years, especially in patients with AIDS. Life-threatening hyperkalemia secondary to the use of standard doses of co-trimoxazole has now been reported in two renal transplant recipients who developed end-stage renal disease secondary to familial Mediterranean fever, who may be at increased risk of hyperkalemia because of concurrent renal insufficiency, concomitant use of ciclosporin, and associated tubulointerstitial disease (325[A]). In one patient, underlying adrenal insufficiency might have contributed to the hyperkalemia.

Endocrine Co-trimoxazole can cause reversible *hypoglycemia*, which may be prolonged, particularly in patients with risk factors for hypoglycemia. Common risk factors include compromised renal function, prolonged fasting, malnutrition, and the use of excessive doses. It has been postulated that the sulfonamide mimics the action of sulfonylureas, stimulating pancreatic islet cells to secrete insulin. In elderly people, co-trimoxazole-induced hypoglycemia can cause altered mental state (326[A], 327[A]).

Hematologic Treatment with co-trimoxazole can *impair the function of mobilized autologous peripheral blood stem cells* (328[A]).

Liver A mild rise in serum transaminases or cholestatic hepatotoxicity are well reported with co-trimoxazole, usually starting after a latent period of several weeks, and associated with a rash. There have been very few case reports of *fulminant hepatic failure* associated with co-trimoxazole, but recently a report of a fatal case has appeared (329[A]).

A 32-year-old woman developed a pruritic maculopapular rash and fever. She had taken a 12-day course of co-trimoxazole that had finished 5 days before and was taking no other drugs. She had normal hematological indices but a raised alkaline phosphatase and AsT. Serological testing for Epstein–Barr virus, hepatitis A, B, and C, cytomegalovirus, echo virus, rubella, and measles showed no evidence of recent infection. Her rash improved but her general condition worsened and steroids were started. An abdominal CT scan showed a large liver with a moderate amount of ascites. The AsT rose to 1330 IU/l and the prothrombin time increased. She developed progressive liver failure and died while awaiting liver transplant. At autopsy the liver showed signs of massive hepatic necrosis with no other abnormalities.

Hepatorenal insufficiency combined with pancytopenia followed the administration of co-trimoxazole for 10 days for suspected pyelonephritis in a 48-year-old man (330[A]). Hemodialysis was temporarily required, and renal and liver function and blood counts returned to normal afterwards.

Urinary tract Treatment with co-trimoxazole (or other antibiotics) can increase the risk of the *hemolytic–uremic syndrome* in children with gastrointestinal infections caused by *Escherichia coli* O157:H7 compared with children with no antibiotic treatment (331[C]).

Skin Methotrexate, a folic acid antagonist, is used in the treatment of several disorders. Its major action is inhibition of dihydrofolate reductase, a critical enzyme in intracellular folate metabolism. Co-trimoxazole competes with methotrexate in inhibiting dihydrofolate reductase and further impairs DNA synthesis. A fatal case of *toxic epidermal necrolysis* that involved 90% of the total body surface has been described in a 15-year-old boy with T-cell acute lymphoblastic leukemia treated concomitantly with co-trimoxazole and methotrexate (332[A]). The authors suggested that methotrexate toxicity was precipitated by co-trimoxazole.

Another case of toxic epidermal necrolysis, associated with co-trimoxazole for sinusitis in a 16-year-old woman, was successfully treated with intravenous immunoglobulins (0.4 g/kg for 5 days) (333[A]).

Co-trimoxazole was the offender in 75% of 64 cases of *fixed drug eruption*. The eruption was mainly located on male genitalia, but unusual findings included familial occurrence, symmetrical and asymmetrical non-pigmented lesions, linear lesions, a solitary plaque on the cheek, and wandering lesions (334[C]).

In 20 Indian patients (of whom 70% were women) with *Stevens–Johnson syndrome* and ocular involvement, co-trimoxazole was the commonest identifiable risk factor (335[C]). Conjunctival involvement and its sequelae were the major ocular manifestations.

Hair, nails, and sweat glands Co-trimoxazole was suggested to have caused *loss of fingernails and toenails* in a 3-year-old boy (336[A]). He was initially treated with gentamicin 2 mg/kg intravenously every 8 hours for *E. coli* urinary tract infection, and co-trimoxazole was given once daily in a prophylactic dose. After 2 weeks his fingernails and toenails began to slough. Co-trimoxazole was withdrawn, and within 2 weeks his nails had returned to normal.

Immunologic *Sulfonamide hypersensitivity syndrome* is most consistent with an immune-mediated reaction with delayed onset, characterized by fever, rash, and eosinophilia. IgG antibodies may be present and directed against proteins in the endoplasmic reticulum (about 80% of patients) or against the drug covalently bound to protein (about 5% of patients). High-dose methylprednisolone sodium succinate (250 mg every 6 hours for 48 hours) may not only alleviate the signs but also markedly attenuate the antibody response, as reported in a 19-year-old man (337[A]).

Infection risk There have been rare reports of an association between sulfonamide antibiotics and *increased severity of rickettsial* infections. Sulfonamides do not increase the pathogenicity of *Ehrlichia* species, but a case of human monocytic ehrlichiosis complicated by ARDS has previously been reported in a patient who had taken oral co-trimoxazole. Now it has been speculated that oral co-trimoxazole, given for acne, may have contributed to the unusual severity of *Ehrlichia chaffeensis* infection that progressed to respiratory failure in a previously healthy 16-year-old boy (338[A]).

Drug tolerance (antibacterial resistance) From a total of 31 319 Shigella strains isolated in Israel between 1990 and 1996, the rates of resistance of *Shigella sonnei*, *Shigella flexneri*, and *Shigella boydii* to co-trimoxazole were 94%, 51%, and 62% respectively; the proportion of strains that exhibited multiple drug resistance was higher for *Shigella sonnei* than for the other serotypes studied (339[E]).

Among 12 045 isolates of *Streptococcus pneumoniae* collected between 1995 and 1998, resistance to co-trimoxazole increased slightly, from 25% to 29% (340[E]).

Teratogenicity There have been two reports of severe *spinal malformations* in the fetuses of HIV-positive women treated with combination antiretroviral therapy and co-trimoxazole (341[A]).

Risk factors The use of co-trimoxazole in *HIV-positive patients* has been associated with a high rate of hypersensitivity reactions (40–80%), attributed to the bioactivation of the sulfonamide component, sulfamethoxazole, to its toxic hydroxylamine and nitroso metabolites. In a study of HIV-positive patients with (n = 56) and without (n = 89) hypersensitivity to co-trimoxazole, functionally significant polymorphisms in the genes coding for enzymes involved in co-trimoxazole metabolism were unlikely to have been major predisposing factors in determining individual susceptibility to co-trimoxazole hypersensitivity (342[C]).

In a randomized double-blind study in 372 HIV-positive patients with CD4+ counts below 250×10^6/l, gradual initiation of co-trimoxazole treatment was associated with significantly fewer adverse drug reactions compared with standard initiation (343[C]).

Drug interactions Massive hepatic necrosis after exposure to *phenytoin* and co-trimoxazole is rare. Acute liver failure has recently been reported in a 60-year-old woman after concomitant ingestion of these drugs over 9 days (344[A]). Autopsy showed acute fulminant hepatic failure. Drug–drug interactions can potentiate the hepatotoxicity of single agents; withdrawal of co-trimoxazole may be needed in the presence of early liver injury.

A hypoprothrombinemic effect can occur when co-trimoxazole is given with *warfarin* (345[A]).

Prolonged treatment with co-trimoxazole can reduce *cyclophosphamide* and *glucocorticoid* requirements in patients with Wegener's granulomatosis (346[A]).

Management of adverse drug reactions *Desensitization* may be efficient in a large proportion of patients (88%) using a 5-day protocol, in which co-trimoxazole is administered orally in a granular formulation in increasing doses, beginning with trimethoprim 0.4 mg and sulfamethoxazole 2 mg and doubling the dose every 12 hours until the therapeutic dose is achieved (347[C]). Another dosage regimen (12 doses of increasing amounts of co-trimoxazole at half-hour intervals) resulted in an overall success rate of 91% at 1 month in 44 patients (348[C]). Such tolerance induction protocols can be adopted, even during pregnancy without risk to the mother or to the fetus (349[C]).

Another uncontrolled trial of a 6-day desensitization procedure in 33 cases has been reported (350[C]). The protocol started with a dose of 0.2 mg rising to 800 mg over 6 days and 32 of the subjects successfully completed the course. In addition, 12 of 14 cases were successfully rechallenged with co-trimoxazole. However, this study lacked a clear description of follow-up or the reasons for the selection of subjects for desensitization or rechallenge, and cannot be used as a basis for recommending this desensitization technique.

In a randomized study of desensitization with rechallenge in HIV-positive patients with previous adverse effects of co-trimoxazole 73 patients were given a 14-day course of trimethoprim 200 mg/day (351[C]). Fourteen had adverse reactions to trimethoprim. The remaining 59 subjects were randomized to a 2-day desensitization technique (34 subjects) or rechallenge (25 subjects). There were seven hypersensitivity reactions in both groups. Clearly there is no advantage of this 2-day desensitization technique over rechallenge with co-trimoxazole in HIV-positive individuals.

Overall it appears that desensitization to co-trimoxazole is safe in the absence of previous serious adverse events, although it is not yet certain whether desensitization is better than rechallenge or indeed what the ideal desensitization method should be.

OTHER ANTIMICROBIAL DRUGS

Bacitracin *(SED-14, 911; SEDA-22, 279; SEDA-23, 268; SEDA-24, 301)*

Sensory systems Inadvertent injection of bacitracin ointment into the orbit can cause a postoperative orbital *compartment syndrome*. Acute proptosis, chemosis, reduced vision, and ophthalmoplegia occurred after endoscopic sinus surgery in a 73-year-old woman (352[A]). The orbit was tense and the intraocular pressure was 54 mmHg. The presence of bacitracin ointment was established by computed tomography.

Skin The effects of a bacitracin-containing antibiotic ointment and simple gauze dressings on scarring of dermabrasion wounds have been studied (44[C]). Each of three uniform dermabrasion wounds was treated concurrently with polymyxin B + bacitracin + neomycin), polymyxin B + bacitracin, or a simple non-occlusive gauze dressing. The triple-antibiotic ointment was superior to the gauze dressing alone in minimizing scarring, and this benefit was more pronounced than its effect on pigmentary changes.

Successful eradication of colonization by methicillin-resistant *Staphylococcus aureus* with an ointment containing bacitracin, polymyxin B, and gramicidin was achieved in 82% of 11 patients who had previously failed a 1-week course of topical mupirocin (353[c]).

Immunologic There have been many reports of allergic reactions to topical bacitracin ointment, but very few cases of intraoperative *anaphylaxis* due to bacitracin irrigation. Cases of anaphylaxis have now been reported (354[A], 355[c]).

A 65-year-old man undergoing elective sternal debridement and rewiring was given a prophylactic infusion of vancomycin 1 g preoperatively. Anesthesia was induced with thiopental, succinylcholine, and fentanyl, and maintained with fentanyl, vecuronium, and isoflurane. A few minutes after wound irrigation with bacitracin (about 25 U/ml), his blood pressure fell precipitously, necessitating intravenous fluids and adrenaline. His face and arms were flushed. Afterwards, he reported having had a rash several years before after the use of an over-the-counter ointment composed of polymyxin B, bacitracin, and neomycin.

A 9-year-old child with a repaired myelomeningocele and congenital hydrocephalus who had undergone four previous shunt revisions in the past had two episodes of anaphylaxis during insertion of the ventriculoperitoneal shunt. The shunt tubing had been soaked in a solution of bacitracin 2500 U/ml. A skin-prick test was positive for bacitracin.

Drug formulations Commercial bacitracin comprises more than 30 different substances, but the major antibiotic isoforms A and B account for about 60% of the mixture. Recently, an impurity has been identified in some but not all bacitracin lots (356[E]). The impurity is a powerful subtilisin-type protease capable of cleaving many proteins, including protein disulfide isomerase, myosin, and a variety of artificial substrates. Investigators using bacitracin are therefore reminded to determine whether their bacitracin is contaminated by a protease. If it is, careful reinterpretation of the results or retesting with an enzyme-free bacitracin reagent may be warranted.

Daptomycin

Daptomycin is a novel lipopeptide antibiotic, an inhibitor of lipoteichoic acid synthesis, with potent bactericidal activity against most clinically important Gram-positive bacteria, including resistant strains.

Musculoskeletal Daptomycin may have adverse effects on skeletal muscle, since it *increases serum creatine kinase activity*. To find the dosing regimen that has the least effects on skeletal muscle, dogs were given repeated intravenous daptomycin every 24 hours or every 8 hours for 20 days (357[E]). The results suggested that adverse effects on skeletal muscle are primarily related to dosing frequency but not peak plasma concentrations, and once-daily administration appeared to minimize the potential for daptomycin-related skeletal-muscle effects, possibly by allowing more time between doses for repair of subclinical effects.

Drug tolerance (antibacterial resistance) The activity of daptomycin against both vancomycin-sensitive and vancomycin-resistant *E. fecalis* was greater than that of quinupristin–dalfopristin (358[E]). Daptomycin was as active as quinupristin–dalfopristin but more active than linezolid. At concentrations four times the MIC, daptomycin and vancomycin achieved 99.9% killing of methicillin-resistant *S. aureus* after 8 hours, which was greater than the killing seen with linezolid and quinupristin–dalfopristin. However, the antibacterial activity of daptomycin strongly depended on the calcium concentration of the medium.

Fosfomycin *(SED-14, 911; SEDA-24, 302)*

Fosfomycin is a broad-spectrum antibiotic used to treat uncomplicated lower urinary tract infections. It penetrates interstitial space fluids of soft tissues well and reaches concentrations sufficient to substantially inhibit the growth of relevant bacteria at the target site (359[C]).

Drug tolerance (antibacterial resistance) There is a serious reduction in the susceptibility of *E. coli* strains to amoxicillin (due to R-TEM enzymes), to co-trimoxazole, and to trimethoprim. However, fosfomycin–trometamol remains highly active against urinary Enterobacteriaceae, and over 90% of *E. coli* are susceptible (360[E]). Fosfomycin is as active as fluoroquinolones or better for treating intestinal infections caused by *Salmonella* spp., pathogenic *E. coli*, *Campylobacter* spp., and *Shigella* spp. (361[C]).

Infection risk Bacterial biofilms develop on a number of living and inert surfaces within the urinary tract, producing chronic *intractable urinary tract infections*. Combination therapy with fosfomycin and a fluoroquinolone (or a fluoroquinolone and a macrolide) may be the most effective regimen available at present. Nevertheless, management of the local urinary condition and removal of the local underlying disease are the most effective approaches for treating urinary biofilm infection (362[C]).

Drug interactions Fosfomycin is both otoprotective and nephroprotective against *cisplatin*-induced toxicity, without inhibiting the tumoricidal activity of cisplatin (363[C]). Mice treated with cisplatin and fosfomycin also survived longer than animals treated with cisplatin alone, probably owing to lessening of immediate cisplatin systemic toxicity (364[E]).

Novobiocin *(SEDA-24, 302)*

Drug interactions Novobiocin potentiates the activity of *etoposide* in vitro by increasing intracellular accumulation of etoposide. A phase I trial showed that the maximum tolerated dose of novobiocin was 7 g/m^2/day when it was given in combination with etoposide; dose-limiting adverse effects consisted of neutropenic fever and reversible hyperbilirubinemia. Novobiocin did not augment the toxic effects of etoposide on the bone marrow or the gastrointestinal mucosa, and nausea, a dose limiting adverse effect in other trials of novobiocin, was well controlled by $5HT_3$ receptor antagonists (365[C]). However, in a phase II study of the combination of novobiocin and high-dose cyclophosphamide and thiotepa, followed by autologous bone-marrow support in women with chemosensitive advanced breast cancer, there was no significant increase in progression-free survival and overall survival compared with historical controls treated with high-dose alkylating drugs alone (366^C).

REFERENCES

1. Santucci RA, Krieger JN. Gentamicin for the practicing urologist: review of efficacy, single daily dosing and "switch" therapy. J Urol 2000; 163: 1076–84.
2. Orts Alborch M, Morant Ventura A, Garcia Callejo J, Ferrer Baixauli F, Martinez Beneito MP, Marco Algarra J. Monitorizacion de la ototoxicidad por farmacos con productos de distorsion. Acta Otorrinolaringol Esp 2000; 51: 387–95.
3. Walsh RM, Bath AP, Bance ML. Reversible tobramycin-induced bilateral high-frequency vestibular toxicity. ORL J Otorhinolaryngol Relat Spec 2000; 62: 156–9.
4. Tsuji K, Velazquez-Villasenor L, Rauch SD, Glynn RJ, Wall C, Merchant SN. Temporal bone studies of the human peripheral vestibular system. Aminoglycoside ototoxicity. Ann Otol Rhinol Laryngol Suppl 2000; 181: 20–5.
5. Lange G, Keller R. Bilateral malfunction of peripheral vestibular organs. Observations of 20 cases of Dandy syndrome. Laryngo Rhino Otol 2000; 79: 77–80.
6. Marlow ES, Hunt LP, Marlow N. Sensorineural hearing loss and prematurity. Arch Dis Child Fetal Neonatal Ed 2000; 82: F141–4.
7. Thomsen J, Charabi S, Tos M. Preliminary results of a new delivery system for gentamicin to the inner ear in patients with Menière's disease. Eur Arch Otorhinolaryngol 2000; 257: 362–5.
8. Quaranta A, Piazza F. Menière's disease: diagnosis and new treatment perspectives. Recenti Prog Med 2000; 91: 33–7.
9. Guan M-X, Fischel-Ghodsian N, Attardi G. A biochemical basis for the inherited susceptibility to aminoglycoside ototoxicity. Hum Mol Genet 2000; 9: 1787–93.
10. Xiang ML, Mu MY, Pao X, Chi FL. The reinnervation of regenerated hair cells in the basilar papilla of chicks after kanamycin ototoxicity. Acta Otolaryngol 2000; 120: 912–21.
11. Lopez-Gonzalez MA, Guerrero JM, Torronteras R, Osuna C, Delgado F. Ototoxicity caused by aminoglycosides is ameliorated by melatonin without interfering with the antibiotic capacity of the drugs. J Pineal Res 2000; 28: 26–33.
12. Conlon BJ, Smith DW. Topical aminoglycoside ototoxicity: attempting to protect the cochlea. Acta Otolaryngol 2000; 120: 596–9.
13. Duan M, Agerman K, Ernfors P, Canlon B. Complementary roles of neurotrophin 3 and a N-methyl-D-aspartate antagonist in the protection of noise and aminoglycoside-induced ototoxicity. Proc Natl Acad Sci USA 2000; 97: 7597–602.
14. Liamis G, Alexandridis G, Bairaktari ETh, Elisaf MS. Aminoglycoside-induced metabolic abnormalities. Ann Clin Biochem 2000; 37: 543–4.
15. Von Vigier RO, Truttmann AC, Zindler-Schmocker K, Bettinelli A, Aebischer CC, Wermuth B, Bianchetti MG. Aminoglycosides and renal magnesium homeostasis in humans. Nephrol Dial Transplant 2000; 15: 822–6.
16. Elliott C, Newman N, Madan A. Gentamicin effects on urinary electrolyte excretion in healthy subjects. Clin Pharmacol Ther 2000; 67: 16–21.
17. Shetty AK, Rogers NL, Mannick EE, Aviles DH. Syndrome of hypokalemic metabolic alkalosis and hypomagnesemia associated with gentamicin therapy: case reports. Clin Pediatr 2000; 39: 529–33.
18. Kang HS, Kerstan D, Dai L-E, Ritchie G, Quamme GA. Aminoglycosides inhibit hormone-stimulated Mg2+ uptake in mouse distal convoluted tubule cells. Can J Physiol Pharmacol 2000; 78: 595–602.
19. Ciftci M, Kufrevioglu OI, Gundogdu M, Ozmen I. Effects of some antibiotics on enzyme activity of glucose-6-phosphate dehydrogenase from human erythrocytes. Pharmacol Res 2000; 41: 107–11.
20. English WP, Williams MD. Should aminoglycoside antibiotics be abandoned? Am J Surg 2000; 180: 512–16.
21. Czeizel AE, Rockenbauer M, Olsen J, Sorensen HT. A teratological study of aminoglycoside antibiotic treatment during pregnancy. Scand J Infect Dis 2000; 32: 309–13.
22. Barletta JF, Johnson SB, Nix DE, Nix LC, Erstad BL. Population pharmacokinetics of aminoglycosides in critically ill trauma patients on once-daily regimens. J Trauma Inj Infect Crit Care 2000; 49: 869–72.
23. Mars R-L, Moles K, Pope K, Hargrove P. Use of bolus intraperitoneal aminoglycosides for treating peritonitis in end-stage renal disease patients receiving continuous ambulatory peritoneal dialysis and continuous cycling peritoneal dialysis. Adv Perit Dial 2000; 16: 280–4.
24. Nakamura A, Hosoda M, Kato T, Yamada Y, Itoh M, Kanazawa K, Nouda H. Combined effects of meropenem and aminoglycosides on *Pseudomonas aeruginosa* in vitro. J Antimicrob Chemother 2000; 46: 901–4.
25. Adjepon-Yamoah KK, Al-Homrany M, Bahar Y, Ahmed ME. Aminoglycoside usage and monitoring in a Saudi Arabian teaching hospital: a ten-year laboratory audit. J Clin Pharmacol Ther 2000; 25: 303–7.

26. Cano F, Morales M, Delucchi A. Amikacin-related apneic episode in an infant on peritoneal dialysis. Pediatr Nephrol 2000; 14: 357.
27. Xu QA, Zhang Y, Trissel LA, Gilbert DL. Adequacy of a new chlorhexidine-bearing polyurethane central venous catheter for administration of 82 selected parenteral drugs. Ann Pharmacother 2000; 34: 1109–16.
28. You I, Kariyama R, Zervos MJ, Kumon H, Chow JW. In-vitro activity of arbekacin alone and in combination with vancomycin against gentamicin- and methicillin-resistant *Staphylococcus aureus*. Diagn Microbiol Infect Dis 2000; 36: 37–41.
29. Ozbek E, Turkoz Y, Sahna E, Ozugurlu F, Mizrak B, Ozbek M. Melatonin administration prevents the nephrotoxicity induced by gentamicin. BJU Int 2000; 85: 742–6.
30. Solgaard L, Tuxoe JI, Mafi M, Due Olsen S, Toftgaard Jensen T. Nephrotoxicity by dicloxacillin and gentamicin in 163 patients with intertrochanteric hip fractures. Int Orthop 2000; 24: 155–7.
31. Vaidyanathan S, Watt JW, Singh G, Soni BM, Sett P. Dosage of once-daily gentamicin in spinal cord injury patients. Spinal Cord 2000; 38: 197–8.
32. Fanning MM, Wassel R, Piazza-Hepp T. Pyrogenic reactions to gentamicin therapy. New Engl J Med 2000; 343: 1658–9.
33. Chuck SK, Raber SR, Rodvold KA, Areff D. National survey of extended-interval aminoglycoside dosing. Clin Infect Dis 2000; 30: 433–9.
34. Buchholz U, Richards C, Murthy R, Arduino M, Pon D, Schwartz W, Fontanilla E, Pegues C, Boghossian N, Peterson C, Kool J, Mascola L, Jarvis WR. Pyrogenic reactions associated with single daily dosing of intravenous gentamicin. Infect Control Hosp Epidemiol 2000; 21: 771–4.
35. Rocha MJ, Almeida AM, Afonso E, Martins V, Santos J, Leitao F, Falcao AC. The kinetic profile of gentamicin in premature neonates. J Pharm Pharmacol 2000; 52: 1091–7.
36. Bakri FE, Pallett A, Smith AG, Duncombe AS. Once-daily versus multiple-daily gentamicin in empirical antibiotic therapy of febrile neutropenia following intensive chemotherapy. J Antimicrob Chemother 2000; 45: 383–6.
37. Fishman DN, Kaye KM. Once-daily dosing of aminoglycoside antibiotics. Infect Dis Clin North Am 2000; 14: 475–87.
38. Rakover Y, Smuskovitz A, Colodner R, Keness Y, Rosen G. Duration of antibacterial effectiveness of gentamicin ear drops in external otitis. J Laryngol Otol 2000; 114: 827–9.
39. Gunics G, Motohashi N, Amaral L, Farkas S, Molnar J. Interaction between antibiotics and non-conventional antibiotics on bacteria. Int J Antimicrob Agents 2000; 14: 239–42.
40. Berkovitch M, Goldman M, Silverman R, Chen-Levi Z, Greenberg R, Marcus O, Lahat E. Therapeutic drug monitoring of once daily gentamicin in serum and saliva of children. Eur J Pediatr 2000; 159: 697–8.
41. Tod M, Padoin C, Petitjean O. Clinical pharmacokinetics and pharmacodynamics of isepamicin. Clin Pharmacokinet 2000; 38: 205–23.
42. Kafetzis DA, Maltezou HC, Mavrikou M, Siafas C, Paraskakis I, Delis D, Bartsokas C. Isepamicin versus amikacin for the treatment of acute pyelonephritis in children. Int J Antimicrob Agents 2000; 14: 51–5.
43. Shibata Y, Midorikawa K, Naito M, Yatsunami M, Hamada K. Concentration of isepamicin sulfate in bone marrow blood. Jpn J Antibiot 2000; 53: 609–13.
44. Berger RS, Pappert AS, Van Zile PS, Cetnarowski WE. A newly formulated topical triple-antibiotic ointment minimizes scarring. Cutis 2000; 65: 401–4.
45. Hillen U, Geier J, Goos M. Kontaktallergien bei Patienten mit Ekzemen des ausseren Gehorgangs. Ergebnisse des Informationsverbundes Dermatologischer Kliniken und der Deutschen Kontaktallergie-Gruppe. Hautarzt 2000; 51: 239–43.
46. Treluyer JM, Merle Y, Semlali A, Pons G. Population pharmacokinetic analysis of netilmicin in neonates and infants with use of a nonparametric method. Clin Pharmacol Ther 2000; 67: 600–9.
47. Thakur CP, Kanyok TP, Pandey AK, Sinha GP, Zaniewski AE, Houlihan HH, Olliaro P. A prospective randomized, comparative, open-label trial of the safety and efficacy of paromomycin (aminosidine) plus sodium stibogluconate versus sodium stibogluconate alone for the treatment of visceral leishmaniasis. Trans R Soc Trop Med Hyg 2000; 94: 429–31.
48. Donald PR, Sirgel FA, Kanyok TP, Danziger LH, Venter A, Botha FJ, Parkin DP, Seifart HI, Van De Wal BW, Maritz JS, Mitchison DA. Early bactericidal activity of paromomycin (aminosidine) in patients with smear-positive pulmonary tuberculosis. Antimicrob Agents Chemother 2000; 44: 3285–7.
49. Eckhardt L, Kirchhof P, Monning G, Breithardt G, Borggrefe M, Haverkamp W. Modification of stretch-induced shortening of repolarization by streptomycin in the isolated rabbit heart. J Cardiovasc Pharmacol 2000; 36: 711–21.
50. Ryan G, Mukhopadhyay S, Singh M. Nebulised anti-pseudomonal antibiotics for cystic fibrosis (Cochrane Review). In: The Cochrane Library, Issue 2, 2000. Oxford: Update Software.
51. Coates AL, Dinh L, MacNeish CF, Rollin T, Gagnon S, Ho SL, Lands LC. Accounting for radioactivity before and after nebulization of tobramycin to insure accuracy of quantification of lung deposition. J Aerosol Med Deposition Clear Eff Lung 2000; 13: 169–78.
52. Barker AF, Couch L, Fiel SB, Gotfried MH, Ilowite J, Meyer KC, O'Donnell A, Sahn SA, Smith LJ, Stewart JO, Abuan T, Tully H, Van Dalfsen J, Wells CD, Quan J. Tobramycin solution for inhalation reduces sputum *Pseudomonas aeruginosa* density in bronchiectasis. Am J Respir Crit Care Med 2000; 162: 481–5.

53. Ramagopal M, Lands LC. Inhaled tobramycin and bronchial hyperactivity in cystic fibrosis. Pediatr Pulmonol 2000; 29: 366–70.
54. Sjolin J, Goscinski G, Lundholm M, Bring J, Odenholt I. Endotoxin release from *Escherichia coli* after exposure to tobramycin: dose-dependency and reduction in cefuroxime-induced endotoxin release. Clin Microbiol Infect 2000; 6: 74–81.
55. Beringer PM, Vinks AA, Jelliffe RW, Shapiro BJ. Pharmacokinetics of tobramycin in adults with cystic fibrosis: implications for once-daily administration. Antimicrob Agents Chemother 2000; 44: 809–13.
56. Manley HJ, Bailie GR, Frye R, Hess LD, McGoldrick MD. Pharmacokinetics of intermittent intravenous cefazolin and tobramycin in patients treated with automated peritoneal dialysis. J Am Soc Nephrol 2000; 11: 1310–16.
57. Elidemir O, Maciejewski SR, Oermann CM. Falsely elevated serum tobramycin concentrations in cystic fibrosis patients treated with concurrent intravenous and inhaled tobramycin. Pediatr Pulmonol 2000; 29: 43–5.
58. Venegas-Francke P, Fruns-Quintana M, Oporto-Caroca M. Neuritis optica bilateral por cloranfenicol. Rev Neurol 2000; 31: 699–700.
59. Kong CT, Holt DE, Ma SK, Lie AK, Chan LC. Effects of antioxidants and a caspase inhibitor on chloramphenicol-induced toxicity of human bone marrow and HL-60 cells. Hum Exp Toxicol 2000; 19: 503–10.
60. Cloeckaert A, Sidi Boumedine K, Flaujac G, Imberechts H, D'Hooghe I, Chaslus-Dancla E. Occurrence of a *Salmonella enterica serovar typhimurium* DT104-like antibiotic resistance gene cluster including the floR gene in *S. enterica serovar agona*. Antimicrob Agents Chemother 2000; 44: 1359–61.
61. White DG, Hudson C, Maurer JJ, Ayers S, Zhao S, Lee MD, Bolton L, Foley T, Sherwood J. Characterization of chloramphenicol and florfenicol resistance in *Escherichia coli* associated with bovine diarrhea. J Clin Microbiol 2000; 38: 4593–8.
62. Czeizel AE, Rockenbauer M, Sorensen HT, Olsen J. A population-based case-control teratologic study of oral chloramphenicol treatment during pregnancy. Eur J Epidemiol 2000; 16: 323–7.
63. Amstey MS. Chloramphenicol therapy in pregnancy. Clin Infect Dis 2000; 30: 237.
64. Lugo Goytia G, Lares-Asseff I, Perez Guille MG, Perez AG, Mejia CL. Relationship between clinical and biologic variables and chloramphenicol pharmacokinetic parameters in pediatric patients with sepsis. Ann Pharmacother 2000; 34: 393–7.
65. Taber DJ, Dupuis RE, Hollar KD, Strzalka AL, Johnson MW. Drug–drug interaction between chloramphenicol and tacrolimus in a liver transplant recipient. Transplant Proc 2000; 32: 660–2.
66. Belda W Jr, De Goes Siqueira LF, Fagundes LJ. Thiamphenicol in the treatment of chancroid. A study of 1,128 cases. Rev Inst Med Trop São Paulo 2000; 42: 133–5.
67. Appelbaum PC, Hunter PA. The fluoroquinolone antibacterials: past, present and future perspectives. Int J Antimicrob Agents 2000; 16: 5–15.
68. Ball P. New antibiotics for community-acquired lower respiratory tract infections: improved activity at a cost? Int J Antimicrob Agents 2000; 16: 263–72.
69. Hooper DC. The fluoroquinolones after ciprofloxacin and ofloxacin. Curr Clin Top Infect Dis 2000; 20: 63–91.
70. O'Donnell JA, Gelone SP. Fluoroquinolones. Infect Dis Clin North Am 2000; 14: 489–513.
71. King DE, Malone R, Lilley SH. New classification and update on the quinolone antibiotics. Am Fam Phys 2000; 61: 2741–8.
72. Bertino J, Fish D. The safety profile of the fluoroquinolones. Clin Ther 2000; 22: 798–817.
73. Patmore L, Fraser S, Mair D, Templeton A. Effects of sparfloxacin, grepafloxacin, moxifloxacin, and ciprofloxacin on cardiac action potential duration. Eur J Pharmacol 2000; 406: 449–52.
74. Lomaestro BM. Fluoroquinolone-induced renal failure. Drug Saf 2000; 22: 479–85.
75. Blotz A, Michel L, Moysan A, Blumel J, Dubertret L, Ahr HJ, Vohr H-W. Analyses of cutaneous fluoroquinolones photoreactivity using the integrated model for the differentiation of skin reactions. J Photochem Photobiol B Biol 2000; 58: 46–53.
76. Van der Linden PD, Van Puijenbroek EP, Feenstra J, Veld BA, Sturkenboom MC, Herings RM, Leufkens HG, Stricker BH. Tendon disorders attributed to fluoroquinolones: a study on 42 spontaneous reports in the period 1988 to 1998. Arthritis Rheum 2001; 45: 235–9.
77. Jones ME, Sahm DF, Martin N, Scheuring S, Heisig P, Thornsberry C, Köhrer K, Schmitz F-J. Prevalence of gyrA, gyrB, parC, and parE mutations in clinical isolates of *Streptococcus pneumoniae* with decreased susceptibilities to different fluoroquinolones and originating from worldwide surveillance studies during the 1997–1998 respiratory season. Antimicrob Agents Chemother 2000; 44: 462–6.
78. Esposito S, Noviello S, Ianniello F. Comparative in vitro activity of older and newer fluoroquinolones against respiratory tract pathogens. Chemotherapy 2000; 46: 309–14.
79. Weiss K, Restieri C, De Carolis E, Laverdiere M, Guay H. Comparative activity of new quinolones against 326 clinical isolates of *Stenotrophomonas maltophilia*. J Antimicrob Chemother 2000; 45: 363–5.
80. Purswani M, Eckert S, Arora H, Johann-Liang R, Noel GJ. The effect of three broad-spectrum antimicrobials on mononuclear cell responses to encapsulated bacteria: evidence for down-regulation of cytokine mRNA transcription by trovafloxacin. J Antimicrob Chemother 2000; 46: 921–9.
81. Gollapudi S, Gupta S, Thadepalli H. *Salmonella typhimurium*-induced reactivation of latent HIV-1

in promonocytic U1 cells is inhibited by trovafloxacin. Int J Mol Med 2000; 5: 615–18.
82. Armbruster C, Robibaro B, Griesmacher A, Vorbach H. Endothelial cell compatibility of trovafloxacin and levofloxacin for intravenous use. J Antimicrob Chemother 2000; 45: 533–5.
83. Melvani S, Speed BR. Alatrofloxacin-induced seizures during slow intravenous infusion. Ann Pharmacother 2000; 34: 1017–19.
84. Murray CK, Wortmann GW. Trovafloxacin-induced weakness due to a demyelinating polyneuropathy. South Med J 2000; 93: 514–15.
85. Gales BJ, Sulak LB. Severe thrombocytopenia associated with alatrofloxacin. Ann Pharmacother 2000; 34: 330–4.
86. Chen HJL, Bloch KJ, Maclean JA. Acute eosinophilic hepatitis from trovafloxacin. New Engl J Med 2000; 342: 359–60.
87. Ferguson J, McEwen J, Al-Ajmi H, Purkins L, Colman PJ, Willvize SA. A comparison of the photosensitizing potential of trovafloxacin with that of other quinolones in healthy subjects. J Antimicrob Chemother 2000; 45: 503–9.
88. Holtom PD, Pavkovic SA, Bravos PD, Patzakis MJ, Shepherd LE, Frenkel B. Inhibitory effects of the quinolone antibiotics trovafloxacin, ciprofloxacin, and levofloxacin on osteoblastic cells in vitro. J Orthop Res 2000; 18: 721–7.
89. Casey B, Bawdon RE. Ex vivo human placental transfer of trovafloxacin. Infect Dis Obstet Gynecol 2000; 8: 228–9.
90. Bradley JS, Kearns GL, Reed MD, Capparelli EV, Vincent J. Pharmacokinetics of a fluoronaphthyridone, trovafloxacin (CP 99,219), in infants and children following administration of a single intravenous dose of alatrofloxacin. Antimicrob Agents Chemother 2000; 44: 1195–9.
91. Olsen KM, Rebuck JA, Weidenbach T, Fish DN. Pharmacokinetics of intravenous trovafloxacin in critically ill adults. Pharmacotherapy 2000; 20: 400–4.
92. Peleman RA, Van De Velde V, Germonpré PR, Fleurinck C, Rosseel MT, Pauwels RS. Trovafloxacin concentrations in airway fluids of patients with severe community-acquired pneumonia. Antimicrob Agents Chemother 2000; 44: 178–80.
93. Gurbay A, Gonthier B, Daveloose D, Favier A, Hincal F. Microsomal metabolism of ciprofloxacin generates free radicals. Free Radic Biol Med 2001; 30: 1118–21.
94. Sundram FX, Wong WY, Ang ES, Goh AS, Ng DC, Yu S. Evaluation of technetium-99m ciprofloxacin (Infecton) in the imaging of infection. Ann Acad Med Singapore 2000; 29: 699–703.
95. Lee CH, Cheung RT, Chan TM. Ciprofloxacin-induced oral facial dyskinesia in a patient with normal liver and renal function. Hosp Med 2000; 61: 142–3.
96. Grassi L, Biancosino B, Pavanati M, Agostini M, Manfredini R. Depression or hypoactive delirium? A report of ciprofloxacin-induced mental disorder in a patient with chronic obstructive pulmonary disease. Psychother Psychosom 2001; 70: 58–9.
97. Miro N. Controlled multicenter study on chronic suppurative otitis media treated with topical applications of ciprofloxacin 0.2% solution in single-dose containers or combination of polymyxin B, neomycin, and hydrocortisone suspension. Otolaryngol Head Neck Surg 2000; 123: 617–23.
98. Claros P, Sabater F, Claros AJ, Claros A. Determinacion de niveles plasmaticos de ciprofloxacino en ninos tratados con ciprofloxacino topico al 0,2% en presencia de perforacion timpanica. Acta Otorrinolaringol Esp 2000; 51: 97–9.
99. Kundu AK. Ciprofloxacin-induced severe cutaneous reaction and haemolysis in a young adult. J Assoc Physicians India 2000; 48: 649–50.
100. Zabala Lopez S, Iglesias Quiros E, Gonzalez Heras S, Martinez Navarro C, Gambaro Royo B. Diarrea asociada a Clostridium difficile secundaria al uso de ciprofloxacino, complicando un primer brote de enfermedad inflamatoria intestinal. Rev Esp Enferm Dig 2000; 92: 539–40.
101. Mann S, Thillainayagam S. Is ciprofloxacin a new cause of acute pancreatitis? J Clin Gastroenterol 2000; 31: 336.
102. Bald M, Ratjen F, Nikolaizik W, Wingen AM. Ciprofloxacin-induced acute renal failure in a patient with cystic fibrosis. Pediatr Infect Dis J 2001; 20: 320–1.
103. Chopra N, Fine PL, Price B, Atlas I. Bilateral hydronephrosis from ciprofloxacin induced crystalluria and stone formation. J Urol 2000; 164: 438.
104. Pons R, Escutia B. Vasculitis por ciprofloxacino con afectacion cutanea y renal. Nefrologia 2001; 21: 209–12.
105. Rodriguez-Morales A, Llamazares AA, Benito RP, Cocera CM. Fixed drug eruption from quinolones with a positive lesional patch test to ciprofloxacin. Contact Dermatitis 2001; 44: 255.
106. Kimyai-Asadi A, Usman A, Nousari HC. Ciprofloxacin-induced bullous pemphigoid. J Am Acad Dermatol 2000; 42: 847.
107. Perez Vazquez A, Gutierrez Perez B, Carreter de Granda E, Zuniga Perez-Lemaur M, Conde Yague R. Vasculitis cutanea por ciprofloxacino. An Med Interna 2000; 17: 225.
108. Casparian JM, Luchi M, Moffat RE, Hinthorn D. Quinolones and tendon ruptures. South Med J 2000; 93: 488–91.
109. Saint F, Gueguen G, Biserte J, Fontaine C, Mazeman E. Rupture du ligament patellaire un mois apres traitement par fluoroquinolone. Rev Chir Orthop Repar Appar Mot 2000; 86: 495–7.
110. Williams RJI, Attia E, Wickiewicz TL, Hannafin JA. The effect of ciprofloxacin on tendon, paratenon, and capsular fibroblast metabolism. Am J Sports Med 2000; 28: 364–9.
111. Doherty CP, Saha SK, Cutting WA. Typhoid fever, ciprofloxacin and growth in young children. Ann Trop Paediatr 2000; 20: 297–303.
112. Singh UK, Sinha RK, Prasad B, Chakrabati B, Sharma SK. Ciprofloxacin in children: is arth-

ropathy a limitation? Indian J Pediatr 2000; 67: 386–7.

113. Postnikov SS, Nazhimov VP, Semykin SI, Kapranov NI. Comparative morphological analysis of the articular cartilage, epiphyseal plate, spongy bone, and synovial membrane of the knee joint in children treated and not treated with ciprofloxacin [in Russian]. Antibiot Khimioter 2000; 45: 9–13.

114. Huddleston PM, Steckelberg JM, Hanssen AD, Rouse MS, Bolander ME, Patel R. Ciprofloxacin inhibition of experimental fracture healing. J Bone Joint Surg Ser A 2000; 82: 161–73.

115. Burke P, Burne SR. Allergy associated with ciprofloxacin. Br Med J 2000; 320: 679.

116. Wlazlowski J, Krzyzanska-Oberbek A, Sikora JP, Chlebna-Sokol D. Use of the quinolones in treatment of severe bacterial infections in premature infants. Acta Pol Pharm Drug Res 2000; 57 Suppl: 28–31.

117. Postnikov SS, Semykin SI, Kapranov NI, Perederko LV, Polikarpova SV. The efficacy and safety of ciprofloxacin in treating children with mucoviscidosis [in Russian]. Antibiot Khimioter 2000; 45: 14–17.

118. Leibovitz E, Janco J, Piglansky L, Press J, Yagupsky P, Reinhart H, Yaniv I, Dagan R. Oral ciprofloxacin vs. intramuscular ceftriaxone as empiric treatment of acute invasive diarrhea in children. Pediatr Infect Dis J 2000; 19: 1060–7.

119. Heyd A, Haverstock D. Retrospective analysis of the safety profile of oral and intravenous ciprofloxacin in a geriatric population. Clin Ther 2000; 22: 1239–50.

120. Berning SE. The role of fluoroquinolones in tuberculosis today. Drugs 2001; 61: 9–18.

121. Jablonowski H. Didanosin als Kapsel. Bewahrtes Medikament in neuer Form. MMW Fortschr Med 2001; 143 Suppl 1: 92–5.

122. Roberge RJ, Kaplan R, Frank R, Fore C. Glyburide–ciprofloxacin interaction with resistant hypoglycemia. Ann Emerg Med 2000; 36: 160–3.

123. Herrlin K, Segerdahl M, Gustafsson LL, Kalso E. Methadone, ciprofloxacin, and adverse drug reactions. Lancet 2000; 356: 2069–70.

124. Patel GK, Anstey AV. Rifampicin-induced lupus erythematosus. Clin Exp Dermatol 2001; 26: 260–2.

125. Kaye CM, Nicholls B. Clinical pharmacokinetics of ropinirole. Clin Pharmacokinet 2000; 39: 243–54.

126. Ellis RJ, Mayo MS, Bodensteiner DM. Ciprofloxacin–warfarin coagulopathy: a case series. Am J Hematol 2000; 63: 28–31.

127. Schiffman SS, Zervakis J, Westall HL, Graham BG, Metz A, Bennett JL, Heald AE. Effect of antimicrobial and anti-inflammatory medications on the sense of taste. Physiol Behav 2000; 69: 413–24.

128. Carillo JA, Benitez J. Clinically significant pharmacokinetic interactions between dietary caffeine and medications. Clin Pharmacokinet 2000; 39: 127–53.

129. Chukwuani CM, Coker HA, Oduola AM, Sowunmi A, Ifudu ND. Bioavailability of ciprofloxacin and fleroxacin: results of a preliminary investigation in healthy adult Nigerian male volunteers. Biol Pharm Bull 2000; 23: 968–72.

130. Blondeau JM. Gatifloxacin: a new fluoroquinolone. Expert Opin Investig Drugs 2000; 9: 1877–95.

131. Grasela DM. Clinical pharmacology of gatifloxacin, a new fluoroquinolone. Clin Infect Dis 2000; 31 Suppl 2: S51–8.

132. LaCreta FP, Kaul S, Kollia GD, Duncan G, Randall DM, Grasela DM. Interchangeability of 400-mg intravenous and oral gatifloxacin in healthy adults. Pharmacotherapy 2000; 20: 59S–66S.

133. Gajjar DA, LaCreta FP, Uderman HD, Kollia GD, Duncan G, Birkhofer MJ, Grasela DM. A dose-escalation study of the safety, tolerability, and pharmacokinetics of intravenous gatifloxacin in healthy adult men. Pharmacotherapy 2000; 20: 49S–58S.

134. Fung-Tomc J, Minassian B, Kolek B, Washo T, Huczko E, Bonner D. In vitro antibacterial spectrum of a new broad-spectrum 8-methoxyfluoroquinolone, gatifloxacin. J Antimicrob Chemother 2000; 45: 437–46.

135. Gajjar DA, LaCreta FP, Kollia GD, Stolz RR, Berger S, Smith WB, Swingle M, Grasela DM. Effect of multiple-dose gatifloxacin or ciprofloxacin on glucose homeostasis and insulin production in patients with noninsulin-dependent diabetes mellitus maintained with diet and exercise. Pharmacotherapy 2000; 20: 76S–86S.

136. Grasela DM, Christofalo B, Kollia GD, Duncan G, Noveck R, Manning JA, LaCreta FP. Safety and pharmacokinetics of a single oral dose of gatifloxacin in patients with moderate to severe hepatic impairment. Pharmacotherapy 2000; 20: 87S–94S.

137. LaCreta FP, Kollia GD, Duncan G, Behr D, Grasela DM. Age and gender effects on the pharmacokinetics of gatifloxacin. Pharmacotherapy 2000; 20: 67S–75S.

138. Grasela DM, LaCreta FP, Kollia GD, Randall DM, Uderman HD. Open-label, nonrandomized study of the effects of gatifloxacin on the pharmacokinetics of midazolam in healthy male volunteers. Pharmacotherapy 2000; 20: 330–5.

139. Hardy D, Amsterdam D, Mandell LA, Rotstein C. Comparative in vitro activities of ciprofloxacin, gemifloxacin, grepafloxacin, moxifloxacin, ofloxacin, sparfloxacin, trovafloxacin, and other antimicrobial agents against bloodstream isolates of Gram-positive cocci. Antimicrob Agents Chemother 2000; 44: 802–5.

140. Jones RN, Pfaller MA, Erwin ME. Evaluation of gemifloxacin (SB-265805, LB20304a): in vitro activity against over 6000 gram-positive pathogens from diverse geographic areas. Int J Antimicrob Agents 2000; 15: 227–30.

141. Marchese A, Debbia EA, Schito GC. Comparative in vitro potency of gemifloxacin against European respiratory tract pathogens isolated in the

Alexander Project. J Antimicrob Chemother 2000; 46 Suppl T1: 11–15.
142. Berron S, Vazquez JA, Gimenez MJ, De la Fuente L, Aguilar L. In vitro susceptibilities of 400 Spanish isolates of *Neisseria gonorrhoeae* to gemifloxacin and 11 other antimicrobial agents. Antimicrob Agents Chemother 2000; 44: 2543–4.
143. File T, Schlemmer B, Garau J, Lode H, Lynch S, Young C. Gemifloxacin versus amoxicillin/clavulanate in the treatment of acute exacerbations of chronic bronchitis. The 070 Clinical Study group. J Chemother 2000; 12: 314–25.
144. Allen A, Bygate E, Oliver S, Johnson M, Ward C, Cheon AJ, Choo YS, Kim IC. Pharmacokinetics and tolerability of gemifloxacin (SB-265805) after administration of single oral doses to healthy volunteers. Antimicrob Agents Chemother 2000; 44: 1604–8.
145. Garcia I, Pascual A, Ballesta S, Joyanes P, Perea EJ. Intracellular penetration and activity of gemifloxacin in human polymorphonuclear leukocytes. Antimicrob Agents Chemother 2000; 44: 3193–5.
146. Lowe MN, Lamb HM. Gemifloxacin. Drugs 2000; 59: 1137–47.
147. Allen A, Bygate E, Clark D, Lewis A, Pay V. The effect of food on the bioavailability of oral gemifloxacin in healthy volunteers. Int J Antimicrob Agents 2000; 16: 45–50.
148. Gibaldi M. Grepafloxacin withdrawn from market. Drug Ther Topics Suppl 2000; 29: 6.
149. Ono Y, Ohmoto Y, Ono K, Sakata Y, Murata K. Effect of grepafloxacin on cytokine production in vitro. J Antimicrob Chemother 2000; 46: 91–4.
150. Ortega M, Soriano A, Garcia S, Almela M, Alvarez JL, Tomas X, Mensa J, Soriano E. Perfil de tolerabilidad y seguridad de levofloxacinoen tratamientos prolongados. Rev Esp Quimioter 2000; 13: 263–6.
151. Fujimori K, Shimatsu Y, Suzuki E, Arakawa M, Gejyo F. Levofloxacin-induced eosinophilic pneumonia complicated by bronchial asthma [in Japanese]. Nihon Kokyuki Gakkai Zasshi 2000; 38: 385–90.
152. Boccumini LE, Fowler CL, Campbell TA, Puertolas LF, Kaidbey KH. Photoreaction potential of orally administered levofloxacin in healthy subjects. Ann Pharmacother 2000; 34: 453–8.
153. Paily R. Quinolone drug rash in a patient with infectious mononucleosis. J Dermatol 2000; 27: 405–6.
154. Fleisch F, Hartmann K, Kuhn M. Fluoroquinolone-induced tendinopathy: also occurring with levofloxacin. Infection 2000; 28: 256–7.
155. Casado Burgos E, Vinas Ponce G, Lauzurica Valdemoros R, Olive Marques A. Tendinitis por levofloxacino. Med Clin 2000; 114: 319.
156. Smythe MA, Cappelletty DM. Anaphylactoid reaction to levofloxacin. Pharmacotherapy 2000; 20: 1520–3.
157. Mori K, Maru C, Takasuna K, Furuhama K. Mechanism of histamine release induced by levofloxacin, a fluoroquinolone antibacterial agent. Eur J Pharmacol 2000; 394: 51–5.
158. Takahashi H, Higuchi H, Shimizu T. Severe lithium toxicity induced by combined levofloxacin administration. J Clin Psychiatry 2000; 61: 949–50.
159. Oliviera HS, Goncalo M, Figueiredo AC. Photosensitivity to lomefloxacin. A clinical and photobiological study. Photodermatol Photoimmunol Photomed 2000; 16: 116–20.
160. Jeffrey AM, Shao L, Brendler-Schwaab SY, Schluter G, Williams GM. Photochemical mutagenicity of phototoxic and photochemically carcinogenic fluoroquinolones in comparison with the photostable moxifloxacin. Arch Toxicol 2000; 74: 555–9.
161. Patel T, Pearl J, Williams J, Haverstock D, Church D. Efficacy and safety of ten day moxifloxacin 400 mg once daily in the treatment of patients with community-acquired pneumonia. Community Acquired Pneumonia Study Group. Respir Med 2000; 94: 97–105.
162. Beyer G, Hiemer-Bau M, Ziege S, Edlund C, Lode H, Nord CE. Impact of moxifloxacin versus clarithromycin on normal oropharyngeal microflora. Eur J Clin Microbiol Infect Dis 2000; 19: 548–50.
163. Edlund C, Beyer G, Hiemer-Bau M, Ziege S, Lode H, Nord CE. Comparative effects of moxifloxacin and clarithromycin on the normal intestinal microflora. Scand J Infect Dis 2000; 32: 81–5.
164. Demolis JL, Kubitza D, Tenneze L, Funck-Brentano C. Effect of a single oral dose of moxifloxacin (400 mg and 800 mg) on ventricular repolarization in healthy subjects. Clin Pharmacol Ther 2000; 68: 658–66.
165. Carrion Valero F, Facila Rubio L, Marin Pardo J. Sincope tras la administracion de moxifloxacino. Arch Bronconeumol 2000; 36: 603–4.
166. Balfour JA, Lamb HM. Moxifloxacin: a review of its clinical potential in the management of community-acquired respiratory tract infections. Drugs 2000; 59: 115–39.
167. Akyol D, Mungan T, Baltaci V. A comparative study of genotoxic effects in the treatment of *Trichomonas vaginalis* infection: metronidazole or nalidixic acid. Arch Gynecol Obstet 2000; 264: 20–3.
168. Kundu AK. Norfloxacin-induced hallucination – an unusual CNS toxicity of 4-fluoroquinolones. J Assoc Phys India 2000; 48: 944.
169. Björnsson E, Olsson R, Remotti H. Norfloxacin-induced eosinophilic necrotizing granulomatous hepatitis. Am J Gastroenterol 2000; 95: 3662–4.
170. Nakamura M, Ohishi A, Aosaki N, Hamaguchi K. Norfloxacin-induced acute interstitial nephritis. Nephron 2000; 86: 204–5.
171. Goettsch W, Van Pelt W, Nagelkerke N, Hendrix MG, Buiting AG, Petit PL, Sabbe LJ, van Griethuysen AJ, de Neeling AJ. Increasing resistance to fluoroquinolones in *Escherichia coli*

from urinary tract infections in the Netherlands. J Antimicrob Chemother 2000; 46: 223–8.
172. Boonme P, Phadoongsombut N, Phoomborplub P, Viriyasom S. Stability of extemporaneous norfloxacin suspension. Drug Dev Ind Pharm 2000; 26: 777–9.
173. Cordoba-Diaz M, Cordoba-Borrego M, Cordoba-Diaz D. Influence of pharmacotechnical design on the interaction and availability of norfloxacin in directly compressed tablets with certain antacids. Drug Dev Ind Pharm 2000; 26: 159–66.
174. Miedouge M, Hacini J, Grimont F, Watine J. Shiga toxin-producing *Escherichia coli* urinary tract infection associated with hemolytic-uremic syndrome in an adult and possible adverse effect of ofloxacin therapy. Clin Infect Dis 2000; 30: 395–6.
175. Kimmitt PT, Harwood CR, Barer MR. Induction of type 2 Shiga toxin synthesis in *Escherichia coli* O157 by 4-quinolones. Lancet 1999; 353: 1588–9.
176. Gonzalez Carro P, Huidobro ML, Zabala AP, Vicente EM. Fatal subfulminant hepatic failure with ofloxacin. Am J Gastroenterol 2000; 95: 1606.
177. Navaratnam S, Claridge J. Primary photophysical properties of ofloxacin. Photochem Photobiol 2000; 72: 283–90.
178. Sharma RK, Sahu KM, Gulati S, Gupta A. Pefloxacin in steroid dependent and resistant idiopathic nephrotic syndrome. J Nephrol 2000; 13: 271–4.
179. Postnikov SS, Semykin SI, Kapranov NI, Perederko LV, Polikarpova SV, Khamidullina KF. Evaluation of tolerance and efficacy of pefloxacin in the treatment and prevention of severe infections in children with mucoviscidosis and aplastic anemia [in Russian]. Antibiot Khimioter 2000; 45: 25–30.
180. Simonin MA, Gegout-Pottie P, Minn A, Gillet P, Netter P, Terlain B. Pefloxacin-induced Achilles tendon toxicity in rodents: biochemical changes in proteoglycan synthesis and oxidative damage to collagen. Antimicrob Agents Chemother 2000; 44: 867–72.
181. Shimoda K, Ikeda T, Okawara S, Kato M. Possible relationship between phototoxicity and photodegradation of sitafloxacin, a quinolone antibacterial agent, in the auricular skin of albino mice. Toxicol Sci 2000; 56: 290–6.
182. Schentag JJ. Sparfloxacin: a review. Clin Ther 2000; 22: 372–87.
183. Garrison N, Spector S, Buffington D, Stafford C, Granito K, Zhang H, Talbot GH. Sparfloxacin for the treatment of acute bacterial maxillary sinusitis documented by sinus puncture. Ann Allergy Asthma Immunol 2000; 84: 63–71.
184. Chiba K, Sugiyama A, Satoh Y, Shiina H, Hashimoto K. Proarrhythmic effects of fluoroquinolone antibacterial agents: in vivo effects as physiologic substrate for torsades. Toxicol Appl Pharmacol 2000; 169: 8–16.
185. Pierfitte C, Royer RJ, Moore N, Begaud B. The link between sunshine and phototoxicity of sparfloxacin. Br J Clin Pharmacol 2000; 49: 609–12.
186. Verna LK, Holman SA, Lee VC, Hoh J. UVA-induced oxidative damage in retinal pigment epithelial cells after H2O2 or sparfloxacin exposure. Cell Biol Toxicol 2000; 16: 303–12.
187. Kamberi M, Nakashima H, Ogawa K, Oda N, Nakano S. The effect of staggered dosing of sucralfate on oral bioavailability of sparfloxacin. Br J Pharmacol 2000; 49: 98–103.
188. Ohnishi K, Kimura K, Masuda G, Tsunoda T, Obana M, Yoshida H, Goto T, Sakaue Y, Kim YK, Sakamoto M, Sagara H. Oral administration of fluoroquinolones in the treatment of typhoid fever and paratyphoid fever in Japan. Intern Med 2000; 39: 1044–8.
189. Sangen Y, Kawada A, Asai M, Aragane Y, Yudate T, Tezuka T. Fixed drug eruption induced by tosufloxacin tosilate. Contact Dermatitis 2000; 42: 285.
190. Seksik P, Galula G, Maury E, Levy VG, Offenstadt G. *Klebsiella oxytoca*-associated colitis after oral administration of fusidic acid. Gastroenterol Clin Biol 2000; 24: 587–8.
191. Lee AY, Joo HJ, Oh JG, Kim YG. Allergic contact dermatitis from sodium fusidate with no underlying dermatosis. Contact Dermatitis 2000; 42: 53.
192. Chang SC, Hsieh SM, Chen ML, Sheng WH, Chen YC. Oral fusidic acid fails to eradicate methicillin-resistant *Staphylococcus aureus* colonization and results in emergence of fusidic acid-resistant strains. Diagn Microbiol Infect Dis 2000; 36: 131–6.
193. Khaliq Y, Gallicano K, Leger R, Foster B, Badley A. A drug interaction between fusidic acid and a combination of ritonavir and saquinavir. Br J Clin Pharmacol 2000; 50: 82–3.
194. Wenisch C, Krause R, Fladerer P, El Menjawi I, Pohanka E. Acute rhabdomyolysis after atorvastatin and fusidic acid therapy. Am J Med 2000; 109: 78.
195. Sidi V, Roilides E, Bibashi E, Gompakis N, Tsakiri A, Koliouskas D. Comparison of efficacy and safety of teicoplanin and vancomycin in children with antineoplastic therapy-associated febrile neutropenia and Gram-positive bacteremia. J Chemother 2000; 12: 326–31.
196. Padial MA, Barranco P, Lopez-Serrano C. Erythema multiforme to vancomycin. Allergy Eur J Allergy Clin Immunol 2000; 55: 1201.
197. Pavia M, Nobile CG, Salpietro L, Angelillo IF. Vancomycin resistance and antibiotic susceptibility of enterococci in raw meat. J Food Prot 2000; 63: 912–15.
198. Harding I, Sorgel F. Comparative pharmacokinetics of teicoplanin and vancomycin. J Chemother 2000; 12 Suppl 5: 15–20.
199. Wilson AP. Clinical pharmacokinetics of teicoplanin. Clin Pharmacokinet 2000; 39: 167–83.
200. Testore GP, Uccella I, Sarrecchia C, Mattei A, Impagliazzo A, Sordillo P, Andreoni M. Long-term intramuscular teicoplanin treatment of chronic

osteomyelitis due to oxacillin-resistant *Staphylococcus aureus* in outpatients. J Chemother 2000; 12: 412–15.
201. Lambiotte F, Miczek S, Bierent S, Socolovsky C, Chagnon JL. Thrombopénie acquise sous teicoplanine. Med Mal Infect 2000; 30: 481–2.
202. Sandler RH, Finegold SM, Bolte ER, Buchanan CP, Maxwell AP, Vaisanen ML, Nelson MN, Wexler HM. Short-term benefit from oral vancomycin treatment of regressive-onset autism. J Child Neurol 2000; 15: 429–35.
203. Sanche SE, Dust WN, Shevchuk YM. Vancomycin-induced neutropenia resolves after substitution with teicoplanin. Clin Infect Dis 2000; 31: 824–5.
204. Shahar A, Berner Y, Levi S. Fever, rash, and pancytopenia following vancomycin rechallenge in the presence of ceftazidime. Ann Pharmacother 2000; 34: 263–4.
205. Petit N, Rohrbach P, Mathieu P, Cronier B. Neutropénie a la vancomycine confirmée par une épreuve de réintroduction positive. Med Mal Infect 2000; 20: 665–6.
206. Mofid MZ, Costarangos C, Bernstein B, Wong L, Munster A, Nousari HC. Drug-induced linear immunoglobulin A bullous disease that clinically mimics toxic epidermal necrolysis. J Burn Care Rehabil 2000; 21: 246–7.
207. Klein PA, Callen JP. Drug-induced linear IgA bullous dermatosis after vancomycin discontinuance in a patient with renal insufficiency. J Am Acad Dermatol 2000; 42: 316–23.
208. Santaeugenia S, Pedro Botet ML, Sabat M, Sobena N, Sadria M. Stevens–Johnson syndrome associated with vancomycin. Rev Esp Quimioter 2000; 13: 425–6.
209. Thestrup-Pedersen K, Hainau B, Al'Eisa A, Al'Fadley A, Hamadah I. Fatal toxic epidermal necrolysis associated with ceftazidine and vancomycin therapy: a report of two cases. Acta Derm Venereol 2000; 80: 316–17.
210. Toyoguchi T, Ebihara M, Ojima F, Hosoya J, Shoji T, Nakagawa Y. Histamine release induced by antimicrobial agents and effects of antimicrobial agents on vancomycin-induced histamine release from rat peritoneal mast cells. J Pharm Pharmacol 2000; 52: 327–31.
211. Chopra N, Oppenheimer J, Derimanov GS, Fine PL. Vancomycin anaphylaxis and successful desensitization in a patient with end stage renal disease on hemodialysis by maintaining steady antibiotic levels. Ann Allergy Asthma Immunol 2000; 84: 633–5.
212. Schouten MA, Hoogkamp-Korstanje JA, Meis JF, Voss A. Prevalence of vancomycin-resistant enterococci in Europe. European VRE Study Group. Eur J Clin Microbiol Infect Dis 2000; 19: 816–22.
213. Balen RM, Betts T, Ensom MHH. Vancomycin overdose in 6-month-old girl. Can J Hosp Pharm 2000; 53: 32–5.
214. Pea F, Porreca L, Baraldo M, Furlanut M. High vancomycin dosage regimens required by intensive care unit patients cotreated with drugs to improve haemodyndamics following cardiac surgical procedures. J Antimicrob Chemother 2000; 45: 329–35.
215. Lifshitz T, Lapid-Gortzak R, Finkelman Y, Klemperer I. Vancomycin and ceftazidime incompatibility upon intravitreal injection. Br J Ophthalmol 2000; 84: 117–18.
216. Ng HP, Koh KF, Tham LS. Vancomycin causes dangerous precipitation when infused with gelatin fluid. Anaesthesia 2000; 55: 1039–40.
217. Balfour JA, Figgitt DP. Telithromycin. Drugs 2001; 61: 815–29.
218. Baltch AL, Smith RP, Ritz WJ, Franke MA, Michelsen PB. Antibacterial effect of telithromycin (HMR 3647) and comparative antibiotics against intracellular *Legionella pneumophila*. J Antimicrob Chemother 2000; 46: 51–5.
219. Edlund C, Alvan G, Barkholt L, Vacheron F, Nord CE. Pharmacokinetics and comparative effects of telithromycin (HMR 3647) and clarithromycin on the oropharyngeal and intestinal microflora. J Antimicrob Chemother 2000; 46: 741–9.
220. Andrews JM, Weller TM, Ashby JP, Walker RM, Wise R. The in vitro activity of ABT773, a new ketolide antimicrobial agent. J Antimicrob Chemother 2000; 46: 1017–22.
221. Vazifeh D, Bryskier A, Labro MT. Effect of proinflammatory cytokines on the interplay between roxithromycin, HMR 3647, or HMR 3004 and human polymorphonuclear neutrophils. Antimicrob Agents Chemother 2000; 44: 511–21.
222. Krause PJ, Lepore T, Sikand VK, Gadbaw J, Burke G, Telford SR, Brassard P, Pearl D, Azlanzadeh J, Christianson D, McGrath D, Spielman A. Atovaquone and azithromycin for the treatment of babesiosis. New Engl J Med 2000; 343: 1454–8.
223. Paavonen J, Mangioni C, Martin MA, Wajszczuk CP. Vaginal clindamycin and oral metronidazole for bacterial vaginosis: a randomized trial. Obstet Gynecol 2000; 96: 256–60.
224. Boaz A, Dan M, Charuzi I, Landau O, Aloni Y, Kyzer S. Pseudomembranous colitis: report of a severe case with unusual clinical signs in a young nurse. Dis Colon Rectum 2000; 43: 264–6.
225. Jaspersen D. Drug-induced oesophageal disorders: pathogenesis, incidence, prevention and management. Drug Saf 2000; 22: 237–49.
226. Schwab RA, Vogel PS, Warschaw KE. Clindamycin-induced acute generalized exanthematous pustulosis. Cutis 2000; 65: 391–3.
227. Ohtani H, Taninaka C, Hanada E, Kotaki H, Sato H, Sawada Y, Iga T. Comparative pharmacodynamic analysis of Q-T interval prolongation induced by the macrolides clarithromycin, roxithromycin, and azithromycin in rats. Antimicrob Agents Chemother 2000; 44: 2630–7.
228. Demoly P, Benahmed S, Valembois M, Sahla H, Messaad D, Godard P, Michel FB, Bousquet J. L'allergie aux macrolides. Revue de la litterature. Presse Med 2000; 29: 321–6.
229. Demoly P, Benahmed S, Sahla H, Messaad D, Valembois M, Godard P, Michel FB, Bousquet J.

L'allergie aux macrolides. 21 observations. Presse Med 2000; 29: 294–8.
230. Blanca M, Posadas S, Torres MJ, Leyva L, Mayorga C, Gonzalez L, Juarez C, Fernandez J, Santamaria LF. Expression of the skin-homing receptor in peripheral blood lymphocytes from subjects with nonimmediate cutaneous allergic drug reactions. Allergy Eur J Allergy Clin Immunol 2000; 55: 998–1004.
231. Ianaro A, Ialenti A, Maffia P, Sautebin L, Rombola L, Carnuccio R, Iuvone T, D'Acquisto F, Di Rosa M. Anti-inflammatory activity of macrolide antibiotics. J Pharmacol Exp Ther 2000; 292: 156–63.
232. Bandak SI, Turnak MR, Allen BS, Bolzon LD, Preston DA. Oral antimicrobial susceptibilities of *Streptococcus pyogenes* recently isolated from five countries. J Clin Pract 2000; 54: 585–8.
233. Wang L, Kitaichi K, Hui CS, Takagi K, Takagi K, Sakai M, Yokogawa K, Miyamoto KI, Hasegawa T. Reversal of anticancer drug resistance by macrolide antibiotics in vitro and in vivo. Clin Exp Pharmacol Physiol 2000; 27: 587–93.
234. Dresser GK, Spence JD, Bailey DG. Pharmacokinetic–pharmacodynamic consequences and clinical relevance of cytochrome P450 3A4 inhibition. Clin Pharmacokinet 2000; 38: 41–57.
235. Westphal JF. Macrolide-induced clinically relevant drug interactions with cytochrome P-450A (CYP) 3A4: an update focused on clarithromycin, azithromycin and dirithromycin. Br J Clin Pharmacol 2000; 50: 285–95.
236. Michalets EL, Williams CR. Drug interactions with cisapride: clinical implications. Clin Pharmacokinet 2000; 39: 49–75.
237. Vergis EN, Indorf A, File TM, Phillips J, Bates J, Tan J, Sarosi GA, Grayston JT, Summersgill J, Yu VL. Azithromycin vs cefuroxime plus erythromycin for empirical treatment of community-acquired pneumonia in hospitalized patients: a prospective, randomized, multicenter trial. Arch Intern Med 2000; 160: 1294–300.
238. Ress BD, Gross EM. Irreversible sensorineural hearing loss as a result of azithromycin ototoxicity. A case report. Ann Otol Rhinol Laryngol 2000; 109: 435–7.
239. Sasaki TY, Sumida KN. Angioimmunoblastic T-cell lymphoma (AIL-TCL) following macrolide administration. Hawaii Med J 2000; 59: 44–7, 56.
240. Gruber F, Kastelan M, Cabrijan L, Simonic E, Brajac I. Treatment of early syphilis with azithromycin. J Chemother 2000; 12: 240–3.
241. Macaigne G, Mokbel M, Marty O, De La Lande P, Mallet L. Hépatite aiguë pseudo-angiocholitique probablement induite par l'azithromycine. Gastroenterol Clin Biol 2000; 24: 969–70.
242. Schissel DJ, Singer D, David-Bajar K. Azithromycin eruption in infectious mononucleosis: a proposed mechanism of interaction. Cutis 2000; 65: 163–6.
243. Heikkinen T, Laine K, Neuvonen PJ, Ekblad U. The transplacental transfer of the macrolide antibiotics erythromycin, roxithromycin and azithromycin. Br J Obstet Gynaecol 2000; 107: 770–5.
244. Amsden GW, Nafziger AN, Foulds G, Cabelus LJ. A study of the pharmacokinetics of azithromycin and nelfinavir when coadministered in healthy volunteers. J Clin Pharmacol 2000; 40: 1522–7.
245. Granowitz EV, Tabor KJ, Kirchhoffer JB. Potentially fatal interaction between azithromycin and disopyramide. Pacing Clin Electrophysiol 2000; 23: 1433–5.
246. Gangemi S, Ricciardi L, Fedele R, Isola S, Purello-D'Ambrosio F. Immediate reaction to clarithromycin. Allergol Immunopathol 2001; 29: 31–2.
247. Riley L, Mudd L, Baize T, Herzig R. Cross-sensitivity reaction between tacrolimus and macrolide antibiotics. Bone Marrow Transplant 2000; 25: 907–8.
248. Wasilewski MM, Wilson MG, Sides GD, Stotka JL. Comparative efficacy of 5 days of dirithromycin and 7 days of erythromycin in skin and soft tissue infections. J Antimicrob Chemother 2000; 46: 255–62.
249. Inamura K, Ohta N, Fukase S, Kasajima N, Aoyagi M. The effects of erythromycin on human peripheral neutrophil apoptosis. Rhinology 2000; 38: 124–9.
250. Curry JI, Lander TD, Stringer MD. Erythromycin as a prokinetic agent in infants and children. Aliment Pharmacol Ther 2001; 15: 595–603.
251. Ng PC, So KW, Fung KS, Lee CH, Fok TF, Wong E, Cheung KL, Cheng AF. Randomised controlled study of oral erythromycin for treatment of gastrointestinal dysmotility in preterm infants. Arch Dis Child Fetal Neonatal Ed 2001; 84: F177–82.
252. Farmer JA, Torre-Amione G. Comparative tolerability of the HMG-CoA reductase inhibitors. Drug Saf 2000; 23: 197–213.
253. Czeizel AE, Rockenbauer M, Olsen J, Sorensen HT. A case-control teratological study of spiramycin, roxithromycin, oleandomycin and josamycin. Acta Obstet Gynecol Scand 2000; 79: 234–7.
254. Alos JI, Aracil B, Oteo J, Torres C, Gomez-Garces JL. High prevalence of erythromycin-resistant, clindamycin/miocamycin-susceptible (M phenotype) *Streptococcus pyogenes*: results of a Spanish multicentre study in 1998. Spanish Group for the Study of Infection in the Primary Health Care Setting. J Antimicrob Chemother 2000; 45: 605–9.
255. Betriu C, Redondo M, Palau ML, Sanchez A, Gomez M, Culebras E, Boloix A, Picazo JJ. Comparative in vitro activities of linezolid, quinupristin–dalfopristin, moxifloxacin, and trovafloxacin against erythromycin-susceptible and -resistant streptococci. Antimicrob Agents Chemother 2000; 44: 1838–41.
256. Kasahara M, Suzuki H, Komiya I. Studies on the cytochrome P450 (CYP)-mediated metabolic properties of miocamycin: evaluation of the possibility of a metabolic intermediate complex formation

with CYP, and identification of the human CYP isoforms. Drug Metab Dispos 2000; 28: 409–17.
257. Woywodt A, Grommas U, Buth W, Rafflenbeul W. QT prolongation due to roxithromycin. Postgrad Med J 2000; 76: 651–3.
258. Oyama T, Sakuta T, Matsushita K, Maruyama I, Nagaoka S, Torii M. Effects of roxithromycin on tumor necrosis factor-alpha-induced vascular endothelial growth factor expression in human periodontal ligament cells in culture. J Periodontol 2000; 71: 1546–53.
259. Kawazu K, Kurokawa M, Asano K, Mita A, Adachi M. Suppressive activity of a macrolide antibiotic, roxithromycin on co-stimulatory molecule expression on mouse splenocytes in vivo. Mediators Inflamm 2000; 9: 39–43.
260. Yoshimura T. Modulation of cytokine production from human mononuclear cells by several agents [in Japanese]. Yakugaku Zasshi 2000; 120: 1277–90.
261. Kees F, Holstege A, Ittner KP, Zimmermann M, Lock G, Scholmerich J, Grobecker H. Pharmacokinetic interaction between proton pump inhibitors and roxithromycin in volunteers. Aliment Pharmacol Ther 2000; 14: 407–12.
262. Tuvesson H, Wienkers LC, Gunnarsson PO, Seidegard J, Persson R. Identification of cytochrome P4503A as the major subfamily responsible for the metabolism of roquinimex in man. Xenobiotica 2000; 30: 905–14.
263. Chen H, Fantel AG, Juchau MR. Catalysis of the 4-hydroxylation of retinoic acids by CYP3A7 in human fetal hepatic tissues. Drug Metab Dispos 2000; 28: 1051–7.
264. Bohets H, Lavrijsen K, Hendrickx J, Van Houdt J, Van Genechten V, Verboven P, Meuldermans W, Heykants J. Identification of the cytochrome P450 enzymes involved in the metabolism of cisapride: in vitro studies of potential co-medication interactions. Br J Pharmacol 2000; 129: 1655–67.
265. Gantenbein M, Attolini L, Bruguerolle B, Villard PH, Puyoou F, Durand A, Lacarelle B, Hardwigsen J, Le-Treut YP. Oxidative metabolism of bupivacaine into pipecolylxylidine in humans is mainly catalyzed by CYP3A. Drug Metab Dispos 2000; 28: 383–5.
266. Prueksaritanont T, Lu P, Gorham L, Sternfeld F, Vyas KP. Interspecies comparison and role of human cytochrome P450 and flavin-containing monooxygenase in hepatic metabolism of L-775,606, a potent 5-HT(1D) receptor agonist. Xenobiotica 2000; 30: 47–59.
267. Obach RS. Metabolism of ezlopitant, a non-peptidic substance P receptor antagonist, in liver microsomes: enzyme kinetics, cytochrome P450 isoform identity, and in vitro-in vivo correlation. Drug Metab Dispos 2000; 28: 1069–76.
268. Mae T, Inaba T, Konishi E, Hosoe K, Hidaka T. Identification of enzymes responsible for rifalazil metabolism in human liver microsomes. Xenobiotica 2000; 30: 565–74.
269. Echizen H, Tanizaki M, Tatsuno J, Chiba K, Berwick T, Tani M, Gonzalez FJ, Ishizaki T. Identification of CYP3A4 as the enzyme involved in the mono-N-dealkylation of disopyramide enantiomers in humans. Drug Metab Dispos 2000; 28: 937–44.
270. Huang Z, Roy P, Waxman DJ. Role of human liver microsomal CYP3A4 and CYP2B6 in catalyzing N-dechloroethylation of cyclophosphamide and ifosfamide. Biochem Pharmacol 2000; 59: 961–72.
271. Wang JS, Backman JT, Taavitsainen P, Neuvonen PJ, Kivisto KT. Involvement of CYP1A2 and CYP3A4 in lidocaine N-deethylation and 3-hydroxylation in humans. Drug Metab Dispos 2000; 28: 959–65.
272. Ben-Noun L. Drug-induced respiratory disorders: incidence, prevention and management. Drug Saf 2000; 23: 143–64.
273. Sheehan RE, Wells AU, Milne DG, Hansell DM. Nitrofurantoin-induced lung disease: two cases demonstrating resolution of apparently irreversible CT abnormalities. J Comput Assist Tomogr 2000; 24: 259–61.
274. Cameron RJ, Kolbe J, Wilsher ML, Lambie N. Bronchiolitis obliterans organising pneumonia associated with the use of nitrofurantoin. Thorax 2000; 55: 249–51.
275. Wasserman BN, Chronister TE, Stark BI, Saran BR. Ocular myasthenia and nitrofurantoin. Am J Ophthalmol 2000; 130: 531–3.
276. Kahlmeter G. The ECO.SENS Project: a prospective, multinational, multicentre epidemiological survey of the prevalence and antimicrobial susceptibility of urinary tract pathogens – interim report. J Antimicrob Chemother 2000; 46 Suppl 1: 15–22.
277. Newell A, Riley P, Rodgers M. Resistance patterns of urinary tract infections diagnosed in a genitourinary medicine clinic. Int J STD AIDS 2000; 11: 499–500.
278. Christensen B. Which antibiotics are appropriate for treating bacteriuria in pregnancy? J Antimicrob Chemother 2000; 46 Suppl 1: 29–34.
279. Bruel H, Guillemant V, Saladin-Thiron C, Chabrolle JP, Lahary A, Poinsot J. Hemolytic anemia in a newborn after maternal treatment with nitrofurantoin at the end of pregnancy. Arch Pediatr 2000; 7: 745–7.
280. Tamm M, Eich C, Frei R, Gilgen S, Breitenbucher A, Mordasini C. Inhaled colistin in cystic fibrosis. Schweiz Med Wochenschr 2000; 130: 1366–72.
281. Conway SP, Etherington C, Munday J, Goldman MH, Strong JJ, Wootton M. Safety and tolerability of bolus intravenous colistin in acute respiratory exacerbations in adults with cystic fibrosis. Ann Pharmacother 2000; 34: 1238–42.
282. Vasen W, Desmery P, Ilutovich S, Di Martino A. Intrathecal use of colistin. J Clin Microbiol 2000; 38: 3523.
283. Yuasa J, Naya Y, Tanaka M, Amakasu M, Yamaguchi K. Clinical experiences of endotoxin removal columns in septic shock due to urosepsis: report of three cases [in Japanese]. Hinyokika Kiyo 2000; 46: 819–22.

284. Terawaki H, Kasai K, Kobayashi H, Hirano K, Hamaguchi A, Kase Y, Horiguchi T, Yokoyama K, Yamamoto H, Nakayama M, Kawaguchi Y, Hosoya T. A study on the mechanism of enhanced diuresis following direct hemoperfusion with polymyxin B-immobilized fiber [in Japanese]. Nippon Jinzo Gakkai Shi 2000; 42: 359–64.

285. Vaillant L, Le Guellec C, Jehl F, Barruet R, Sorensen H, Roiron R, Autret-Leca E, Lorette G. Comparative diffusion of fusidic acid, oxacillin, and pristinamycin in dermal interstitial fluid after repeated oral administration. Ann Dermatol Venereol 2000; 127: 33–9.

286. Lozniewski A, Lion C, Mory F, Weber M. Comparison of the in vitro activity of pristinamycin and quinupristin/dalfopristin against *Streptococcus pneumoniae*. Pathol Biol 2000; 48: 463–6.

287. Elsner HA, Sobottka I, Feucht HH, Harps E, Haun C, Mack D, Ganschow R, Laufs R, Kaulfers PM. Nosocomial outbreak of vancomycin-resistant *Enterococcus faecium* at a German university pediatric hospital. Int J Hyg Environ Health 2000; 203: 147–52.

288. Von Eiff C, Reinert RR, Kresken M, Brauers J, Hafner D, Peters G. Nationwide German multicenter study on prevalence of antibiotic resistance in staphylococcal bloodstream isolates and comparative in vitro activities of quinupristin–dalfopristin. J Clin Microbiol 2000; 38: 2819–23.

289. Johnson AP, Warner M, Hallas G, Livermore DM. Susceptibility to quinupristin/dalfopristin and other antibiotics of vancomycin-resistant enterococci from the UK, 1997 to mid-1999. J Antimicrob Chemother 2000; 46: 125–8.

290. McGeer AJ, Low DE. Vancomycin-resistant enterococci. Semin Respir Infect 2000; 15: 314–26.

291. Levison ME, Mallela S. Increasing Antimicrobial Resistance: Therapeutic implications for enterococcal infections. Curr Infect Dis Rep 2000; 2: 417–23.

292. Bergogne-Berezin E. Resistances et nouvelles stratégies antibiotiques. Nouveaux antibiotiques antistaphylococciques. Presse Med 2000; 29: 2025–7.

293. Livermore DM. Antibiotic resistance in staphylococci. Int J Antimicrob Agents 2000; 16 Suppl 1: S3–10.

294. Bhavnani SM, Ballow CH. New agents for Gram-positive bacteria. Curr Opin Microbiol 2000; 3: 528–34.

295. Bush K, Macielag M. New approaches in the treatment of bacterial infections. Curr Opin Chem Biol 2000; 4: 433–9.

296. Jones RN. Perspectives on the development of new antimicrobial agents for resistant Gram-positive pathogens. Braz J Infect Dis 2000; 4: 1–8.

297. Murray BE. Problems and perils of vancomycin resistant enterococci. Braz J Infect Dis 2000; 4: 9–14.

298. Lundstrom TS, Sobel JD. Antibiotics for Gram-positive bacterial infections. Vancomycin, teicoplanin, quinupristin/dalfopristin, and linezolid. Infect Dis Clin North Am 2000; 14: 463–74.

299. Delgado G, Neuhauser MM, Bearden DT, Danziger LH. Quinupristin-dalfopristin: an overview. Pharmacotherapy 2000; 20: 1469–85.

300. Cole RP, Roberts WD, Cheng MD. Hyponatremia associated with quinupristin–dalfopristin. Ann Intern Med 2000; 133: 485.

301. Khan AA, Slifer TR, Araujo FG, Remington JS. Effect of quinupristin/dalfopristin on production of cytokines by human monocytes. J Infect Dis 2000; 182: 356–8.

302. Chevalier P, Rey J, Pasquier O, Leclerc V, Baguet JC, Meyrier A, Harding N, Montay G. Pharmacokinetics of quinupristin/dalfopristin in patients with severe chronic renal insufficiency. Clin Pharmacokinet 2000; 39: 77–84.

303. Thornhill M, Pemberton M, Buchanan J, Theaker E. An open clinical trial of sulphamethoxypyridazine in the treatment of mucous membrane pemphigoid. Br J Dermatol 2000; 143: 117–26.

304. Sesti F, Abbott GW, Wei J, Murray KT, Saksena S, Schwartz PJ, Priori SG, Roden DM, George AL Jr, Goldstein SA. A common polymorphism associated with antibiotic-induced cardiac arrhythmia. Proc Natl Acad Sci USA 2000; 97: 10613–18.

305. Crespo M, Quereda C, Pascual J, Rivera M, Clemente L, Cano T. Patterns of sulfadiazine acute nephrotoxicity. Clin Nephrol 2000; 54: 68–72.

306. Ibia EO, Schwartz RH, Wiedermann BL. Antibiotic rashes in children: a survey in a private practice setting. Arch Dermatol 2000; 136: 849–54.

307. Moussala M, Beharcohen F, Dighiero P, Renard G. Le syndrome de Lyell et ses manifestations ophtalmologiques en milieu camerounais. J Fr Ophtalmol 2000; 23: 229–37.

308. Martinez-Ruiz E, Ortega C, Calduch L, Molina I, Montesinos E, Revert A, Carda C, Navarro V, Jorda E. Generalized cutaneous depigmentation following sulfamide-induced drug eruption. Dermatology 2000; 201: 252–4.

309. Soylu H, Akkol N, Erduran E, Aslan Y, Gunes Z, Yildiran A. Co-trimoxazole-induced toxic epidermal necrolysis treated with high dose methylprednisolone. Ann Med Sci 2000; 9: 38–40.

310. Dwenger CS. 'Sulpha' hypersensitivity. Anaesthesia 2000; 55: 200–1.

311. Naisbitt DJ, Vilar FJ, Stalford AC, Wilkins EG, Primohamed M, Park BK. Plasma cysteine deficiency and decreased reduction of nitrososulfamethoxazolewith HIV infection. AIDS Res Hum Retroviruses 2000; 16: 1929–8.

312. Von Seidlein L, Milligan P, Pinder M, Bojang K, Anyalebechi C, Gosling R, Coleman R, Ude JI, Sadiq A, Duraisingh M, Warhurst D, Alloueche A, Targett G, McAdam K, Greenwood B, Walraven G, Olliaro P, Doherty T. Efficacy of artesunate plus pyrimethamine–sulphadoxine for uncomplic-

ated malaria in Gambian children: a double-blind, randomised, controlled trial. Lancet 2000; 355: 352–7.
313. Komatsu K, Ito K, Nakajima Y, Kanamitsu S, Imaoka S, Funae Y, Green CE, Tyson CA, Shimada N, Sugiyama Y. Prediction of in vivo drug–drug interactions between tolbutamide and various sulfonamides in humans based on in vitro experiments. Drug Metab Dispos 2000; 28: 475–81.
314. Perazella MA. Trimethoprim-induced hyperkalaemia: clinical data, mechanism, prevention and management. Drug Saf 2000; 22: 227–36.
315. Gabriels G, Stockem E, Greven J. Potassium-sparing renal effects of trimethoprim and structural analogues. Nephron 2000; 86: 70–8.
316. Hernandez-Diaz S, Werler MM, Walker AM, Mitchell AA. Folic acid antagonists during pregnancy and the risk of birth defects. New Engl J Med 2000; 343: 1608–14.
317. Guha Thakurta A, Mandal SK, Ganguly K, Dastidar SG, Chakrabarty AN. A new powerful antibacterial synergistic combination of trimethoprim and trimeprazine. Acta Microbiol Immunol Hung 2000; 47: 21–8.
318. Trujillo TC, Nolan PE. Antiarrhythmic agents: drug interactions of clinical significance. Drug Saf 2000; 23: 509–32.
319. De Arce Borda AM, Goenaga Sanchez MA. Tremor produced by trimethoprim–sulfamethoxazole. Neurologia 2000; 15: 264–5.
320. Salkind AR. Acute delirium induced by intravenous trimethoprim-sulfamethoxazole therapy in a patient with the acquired immunodeficiency syndrome. Hum Exp Toxicol 2000; 19: 149–51.
321. Capra C, Monza GM, Meazza G, Ramella G. Trimethoprim-sulfamethoxazole-induced aseptic meningitis: case report and literature review. Intensive Care Med 2000; 26: 212–14.
322. Meng MV, St Lezin M. Trimethoprim–sulfamethoxazole induced recurrent aseptic meningitis. J Urol 2000; 164: 1664–5.
323. Antonen J, Hulkkonen J, Pasternack A, Hurme M. Interleukin 6 may be an important mediator of trimethoprim-induced systemic adverse reaction resembling aseptic meningitis. Arch Intern Med 2000; 160: 2066–7.
324. Andrade A, Hilmas E, Walter C. A rare occurrence of trimethoprim/sulfamethoxazole (TMP/SMX)-induced aseptic meningitis in an older woman. J Am Geriatr Soc 2000; 48: 1537–8.
325. Koc M, Bihorac A, Ozener CI, Kantarci G, Akoglu E. Severe hyperkalemia in two renal transplant recipients treated with standard dose of trimethoprim-sulfamethoxazole. Am J Kidney Dis 2000; 36: E18.
326. Fox GN. Trimethoprim–sulfamethoxazole-induced hypoglycemia. J Am Board Fam Pract 2000; 13: 386.
327. Mathews WA, Manint JE, Kleiss J. Trimethoprim–sulfamethoxazole-induced hypoglycemia as a cause of altered mental status in an elderly patient. J Am Board Fam Pract 2000; 13: 211–12.
328. Fuchs M, Scheid C, Schulz A, Diehl V, Sohngen D. Trimethoprim/sulfamethoxazole prophylaxis impairs function of mobilised autologous peripheral blood stem cells. Bone Marrow Transplant 2000; 26: 815–16.
329. Tse W, Singer C, Dominick D. Acute fulminant hepatic failure caused by trimethoprim–sulfamethoxazole. Infect Dis Clin Pract 2000; 9: 302–3.
330. Windecker R, Steffen J, Cascorbi I, Thurmann PA. Co-trimoxazole-induced liver and renal failure. Case report. Eur J Clin Pharmacol 2000; 56: 191–3.
331. Wong CS, Jelacic S, Habeeb RL, Watkins SL, Tarr PI. The risk of the hemolytic–uremic syndrome after antibiotic treatment of *Escherichia coli* O157:H7 infections. New Engl J Med 2000; 342: 1930–6.
332. Yang CH, Yang LJ, Jaing TH, Chan HL. Toxic epidermal necrolysis following combination of methotrexate and trimethoprim–sulfamethoxazole. Int J Dermatol 2000; 39: 621–3.
333. Magina S, Lisboa C, Goncalves E, Conceicao F, Leal V, Mesquita-Guimaraes J. A case of toxic epidermal necrolysis treated with intravenous immunoglobin. Br J Dermatol 2000; 142: 191–2.
334. Ozkaya-Bayazit E, Bayazit H, Ozarmagan G. Drug related clinical pattern in fixed drug eruption. Eur J Dermatol 2000; 10: 288–91.
335. Pushker N, Tandon R, Vajpayee RB. Stevens–Johnson syndrome in India – risk factors, ocular manifestations and management. Ophthalmologica 2000; 214: 285–8.
336. Canning DA. A suspected case of trimethoprim–sulfamethoxazole-induced loss of fingernails and toenails. J Urol 2000; 163: 1386–7.
337. Bedard K, Smith S, Cribb A. Sequential assessment of an antidrug antibody response in a patient with asystemic delayed-onset sulphonamide hypersensitivity syndrome reaction. Br J Dermatol 2000; 142: 253–8.
338. Peters TR, Edwards KM, Standaert SM. Severe erlichiosis in an adolescent taking trimethoprim–sulfamethoxazole. Pediatr Infect Dis J 2000; 19: 170–2.
339. Mates A, Eyny D, Philo S. Antimicrobial resistance trends in *Shigella* serogroups isolated in Israel, 1990–1995. Eur J Clin Microbiol Infect Dis 2000; 19: 108–11.
340. Whitney CG, Farley MM, Hadler J, Harrison LH, Lexau C, Reingold A, Lefkowitz L, Cieslak PR, Cetron M, Zell ER, Jorgensen JH, Schuchat A. Increasing prevalence of multidrug-resistant *Streptococcus pneumoniae* in the United States. New Engl J Med 2000; 343: 1917–24.
341. Richardson MP, Osrin D, Donaghy S, Brown NA, Hay P, Sharland M. Spinal malformations in the fetuses of HIV infected women receiving combination antiretroviral therapy and co-trimoxazole. Eur J Obstet Gynecol Reprod Biol 2000; 93: 215–17.
342. Pirmohamed M, Alfirevic A, Vilar J, Stalford A, Wilkins EG, Sim E, Park BK. Association analysis of drug metabolizing enzyme gene poly-

morphisms in HIV-positive patients with co-trimoxazole hypersensitivity. Pharmacogenetics 2000; 10: 705–13.
343. Para MF, Finkelstein D, Becker S, Dohn M, Walawander A, Black JR. Reduced toxicity with gradual initiation of trimethoprim-sulfamethoxazole as primary prophylaxis for *Pneumocystis carinii* pneumonia: AIDS Clinical Trials Group 268. J Acquired Immune Defic Syndr 2000; 24: 337–43.
344. Ilario MJ, Ruiz JE, Axiotis CA. Acute fulminant hepatic failure in a woman treated with phenytoin and trimethoprim–sulfamethoxazole. Arch Pathol Lab Med 2000; 124: 1800–3.
345. Chafin CC, Ritter BA, James A, Self TH. Hospital admission due to warfarin potentiation by TMP–SMX. Nurse Pract 2000; 25: 73–5.
346. Rusterholz D, Schlegel C. Infectious aspects of Wegener's granulomatosis. Schweiz Med Wochenschr 2000; 125 Suppl: 41S–43S.
347. Yoshizawa S, Yasuoka A, Kikuchi Y, Honda M, Gatanaga H, Tachikawa N, Hirabayashi Y. A 5-day course of oral desensitization to trimethoprim/sulfamethoxazole (T/S) in patients with human immunodeficiency virus type-1 infection who were previously intolerant to T/S. Ann Allergy Asthma Immunol 2001; 85: 241–4.
348. Demoly P, Messaad D, Reynes J, Faucherre V, Bousquet J. Trimethoprim–sulfamethoxazole-graded challenge in HIV-infected patients: long-term follow-up regarding efficacy and safety. J Allergy Clin Immunol 2000; 105: 588–9.
349. Nucera E, Schiavino D, Buonomo A, Del Ninno M, Sun JY, Patriarca G. Tolerance induction to cotrimoxazole. Allergy 2000; 55: 681–2.
350. Lopez-Serrano MC, Moreno-Ancillo A. Drug hypersensitivity reactions in HIV-infected patients. Induction of cotrimoxazole tolerance. Allergol Immunol Clin 2000; 15: 347–51.
351. Bonfanti P, Pusterla L, Parazzini F, Libanore M, Cagni AE, Franzetti M, Faggion I, Landonio S, Quirino T. The effectiveness of desensitization versus rechallenge treatment in HIV-positive patients with previous hypersensitivity to TMP-SMX: a randomized multicentric study. Biomed Pharmacother 2000; 54: 45–9.
352. Castro E, Seeley M, Kosmorsky G, Foster JA. Orbital compartment syndrome caused by intraorbital bacitracin ointment after endoscopic sinus surgery. Am J Ophthalmol 2000; 130: 376–8.
353. Fung S, O'Grady S, Kennedy C, Dedier H, Campbell I, Conly J. The utility of polysporin ointment in the eradication of methicillin-resistant *Staphylococcus aureus* colonization: a pilot study. Infect Control Hosp Epidemiol 2000; 21: 653–5.
354. Blas M, Briesacher KS, Lobato EB. Bacitracin irrigation: a cause of anaphylaxis in the operating room. Anesth Analg 2000; 91: 1027–8.
355. Carver ED, Braude E, Atkinson AR, Gold M. Anaphylaxis during insertion of a ventriculoperitoneal shunt. Anesthesiology 2000; 93: 578–9.
356. Rogelj S, Reiter KJ, Kesner L, Li M, Essex D. Enzyme destruction by a protease contaminant in bacitracin. Biochem Biophys Res Commun 2000; 273: 829–32.
357. Oleson FB, Berman CL, Kirkpatrick JB, Regan KS, Lai JJ, Tally FP. Once-daily dosing in dogs optimizes daptomycin safety. Antimicrob Agents Chemother 2000; 44: 2948–53.
358. Rybak MJ, Hershberger E, Moldovan T, Grucz RG. In vitro activities of daptomycin, vancomycin, linezolid, and quinupristin–dalfopristin against staphylococci and enterococci, including vancomycin-intermediate and -resistant strains. Antimicrob Agents Chemother 2000; 44: 1062–6.
359. Frossard M, Joukhadar C, Erovic BM, Dittrich P, Mrass PE, Van Houte M, Burgmann H, Georgopoulos A, Muller M. Distribution and antimicrobial activity of fosfomycin in the interstitial fluid of human soft tissues. Antimicrob Agents Chemother 2000; 44: 2728–32.
360. Chomarat M. Resistance of bacteria in urinary tract infections. Int J Antimicrob Agents 2000; 16: 483–7.
361. Fukuyama M, Furuhata K, Oonaka K, Hara T, Sunakawa K. Antibacterial activity of fosfomycin against the causative bacteria isolated from bacterial enteritis. Jpn J Antibiot 2000; 53: 522–31.
362. Kumon H. Management of biofilm infections in the urinary tract. World J Surg 2000; 24: 1193–6.
363. Sakamoto M, Kaga K, Kamio T. Extended high-frequency ototoxicity induced by the first administration of cisplatin. Otolaryngol Head Neck Surg 2000; 122: 828–33.
364. Tandy JR, Tandy RD, Farris P, Truelson JM. In vivo interaction of cis-platinum and fosfomycin on squamous cell carcinoma. Laryngoscope 2000; 110: 1222–4.
365. Murren JR, DiStasio SA, McKeon A, Zuhowski EG, Egorin MJ, Sartorelli AC, Rappa G. Phase I and pharmacokinetic study of novobiocin in combination with VP-16 in patients with refractory malignancies. Cancer J 2000; 6: 256–65.
366. Hahm HA, Armstrong DK, Chen TL, Grochow L, Passos-Coelho J, Goodman SN, Davidson NE, Kennedy MJ. Novobiocin in combination with high-dose chemotherapy for the treatment of advanced breast cancer: a phase 2 study. Biol Blood Marrow Transplant 2000; 6: 335–43.

Andreas H. Groll and Thomas J. Walsh

27 Antifungal drugs

ALLYLAMINES *(SED-14, 937; SEDA-22, 290; SEDA-23, 298; SEDA-24, 314)*

Terbinafine

Sensory systems A second case of persistent taste disturbance associated with terbinafine has been described (1[A]).

A 51-year-old woman had altered taste sensation and recurrent ulceration affecting the lateral borders of her tongue during a 2-month course of terbinafine prescribed for toe nail mycosis. Initially, she had complete loss of taste, followed by partial recovery to a persistent bitter taste. Concurrent long-term medications included propranolol and tetracycline; her past medical history was non-contributory, and there were no laboratory abnormalities.

Impairment of taste has been reported in association with terbinafine and is believed to be associated with taste receptor dysfunction through inhibition of CYP450-dependent enzymes. A postmarketing surveillance study in more than 10 000 patients showed that all patients with taste loss recovered fully, and there was no evidence to suggest that the effect was irreversible. However, recovery times varied between 2 and 186 days; about 5% of patients with taste loss had loss of taste for 12 weeks or longer (1[C]).

Risk factors *Children* Terbinafine and griseofulvin have been compared in a double-blind randomized study in 50 Peruvian children and adolescents (1–14 years of age) with tinea capitis (2[c]). Terbinafine and micronized griseofulvin were given once a day in weight-related doses for 4 or 8 weeks followed by 4 or 8 weeks of placebo. In both groups, one patient had mild symptoms of gastric upset and nausea; none of the 50 patients withdrew because of adverse events. Clinical and mycological cure rates were similar at end of treatment (72% vs 76%); however, at 12-weeks follow-up only 44% of the patients who had taken griseofulvin were still disease free, compared with 76% of the patients who had taken terbinafine. This was probably related to accumulation of terbinafine in the skin and its appendages.

Elderly patients The safety of terbinafine in individuals over 60 years of age has been analysed in 30 Caucasian non-immunocompromised patients with onychomycosis of the feet (3[R]). They took oral terbinafine 250 mg qds for 12 weeks, and follow-up evaluations were performed for the next 60 weeks. None of the patients withdrew because of adverse events; no serious adverse events were reported at any time during treatment or within 6 weeks after. Thirteen patients had mild to moderate reversible adverse events that were possibly, probably, or definitely related to drug administration. Efficacy analysis included 15 patients; at the end of the study, 47% of the patients were considered clinically and microbiologically cured.

AMPHOTERICIN B FORMULATIONS *(SED-14, 922; SEDA-22, 285; SEDA-23, 289; SEDA-24, 315)*

Amphotericin remains the cornerstone of therapy of invasive mycoses and serves as a comparator in the laboratory and clinical evaluation of new antifungal azoles and the novel class of echinocandin lipopeptides. Newer lipid-based formulations are less nephrotoxic than conventional amphotericin B deoxycholate. Data on their safety and tolerance continue to accrue with their increased clinical use.

Side Effects of Drugs, Annual 25
J.K. Aronson, ed.

Amphotericin B Colloidal Dispersion (ABCD)

Safety data have been reported from a randomized comparison of intravenous amphotericin B colloidal dispersion (ABCD; Amphocil) 2 mg/kg and oral fluconazole 200 mg/day for the prevention of fungal infections in 24 neutropenic patients with hematological malignancies (4[C]). Twelve patients were assigned to receive prophylactic ABCD, which was given for a mean of 12 (range 1–27) days, and four patients were switched from fluconazole to ABCD 4 mg/kg for unresolved fever after 4 days. Of these 16 patients, 15 developed *chills* and 14 a *rise in temperature* of at least 1° C. Other adverse events were *hypotension* (4), *nausea with vomiting* (5), *tachycardia* (7), *headache* (3), and *dyspnea* (3). ABCD was discontinued in eight patients because of *infusion-related adverse effects*, which ultimately dictated early termination of the study. There was no nephrotoxicity. One patient with concurrent veno-occlusive disease developed an *increased bilirubin concentration*, leading to early withdrawal of ABCD. These data are consistent with tolerance data from a randomized double-blind study in patients with fever and neutropenia, in whom probable or possible infusion-related hypoxia and chills were more common with ABCD than with conventional amphotericin (5[C]).

Musculoskeletal *Malignant hyperthermia with rhabdomyolysis* has been attributed to ABCD (6[A]).

A 16-year-old boy who had received a matched sibling bone-marrow transplant for recurrent T cell lymphoblastic leukemia was given ABCD 1 mg/kg. Immediately after the 90-minute infusion he developed severe chills, hyperthermia (41.6° C), trismus, generalized muscular hypertonicity, hypotension (95/30 mmHg), tachycardia (205 beats/min), and tachypnea (50/min). Intravenous hydrocortisone 750 mg, diazepam 10 mg, paracetamol 1 g, dopamine 5 mg/kg/min, and hydration produced mild improvement, but 30 minutes later he had another episode of severe chills and trismus with loss of consciousness and 5 hours later developed profuse sweating, cyanosis, dyspnea, anuria, severe muscle pains, and shock. He had myoglobinuria and a raised creatine phosphokinase activity (21 730 U/l). He was ventilated for 10 days and recovered. There were no signs of muscle damage or neuropathy 180 days later.

Since they could identify no other known causes, the authors attributed this acute episode to ABCD.

Risk factors *Children* The safety of ABCD has been analysed in 119 children with fever and neutropenia ($n = 49$; randomized comparative design) or with presumed or documented invasive fungal infections refractory to or intolerant of conventional amphotericin ($n = 90$; open non-comparative design) (7[R]). In the randomized trial, the children who received ABCD (4 mg/kg qds for a mean of 9.6 days) had significantly less nephrotoxicity than those who received amphotericin B deoxycholate (0.8 mg/kg qds for a mean of 8.5 days) (12% vs 42%). Other adverse events were not significantly different. In the open study 80% of those who received ABCD (median dosage 4.4 mg/kg qds; range 0.8–7.5; mean duration 30 days) reported some adverse symptoms. Most of these were infusion-related, and nephrotoxicity was reported in only 12%. These data suggest similar safety profiles of ABCD in children and adults.

Amphotericin B Lipid Complex (ABLC)

Risk factors *Solid organ transplant patients* The safety and efficacy of Amphotericin B Lipid Complex (ABLC; Abelcet) have been analyzed in 79 solid-organ transplant patients with invasive mycoses refractory to or intolerant of standard therapies (8[R]). The median duration of ABLC therapy was 28 (range 1–178) days and the daily dose was 1.6–7.4 (median, 4.6) mg/kg. Overall, 39 of 67 evaluable patients had a clinical response. At the end of treatment, 64 patients had stable ($n = 37$) or improved ($n = 27$) serum creatinine concentrations. Of the 12 patients whose serum creatinine increased during therapy, one had an increase from below 132 μmol/l (1.5 mg/dl) to above 132 μmol/l at the end of therapy, and 11 had an increase of over 20% from a baseline value of below 1.5 mg/dl. Three patients had insufficient serum creatinine data. The mean baseline serum creatinine concentration in the 45 patients with a baseline serum creatinine of less than 2.5 mg/dl fell significantly each week, and this fall was statistically significant from week 1 to week 5. Seven patients had infusion-related chills. Nine discontinued ABLC because of adverse events.

Ethnic background The safety of ABLC had been studied in a retrospective analysis of 21 Swedish patients (9[c]) in response to a previous Scandinavian publication that had reported a discontinuation rate of over 70% because of adverse events, and had posed the question of whether Scandinavians might be more sensitive to ABLC than the British or Americans (10[c]). Most of the patients had been pretreated with conventional amphotericin B, and were given ABLC 1.1–5.1 (mean 4.1) mg/kg of for 3–77 (median 20) days for presumed or documented invasive fungal infections. There was nephrotoxicity, defined as an increase of 100% or more from baseline serum creatinine, in two patients. The bilirubin concentration increased by more than 100% from baseline in four patients. There were infusion-related reactions in nine patients. ABLC was withdrawn because of adverse events in one patient. These data do not support the hypothesis that Scandinavians have more adverse effects with ABLC than people from other countries.

Liposomal Amphotericin B (L-AmB)

The safety of two lipid formulations of amphotericin B in neutropenic patients with unresolved fever after 3 days of antibacterial therapy has been reported in a randomized double-blind study (11[C]). Patients were randomized to amphotericin B lipid complex (ABLC) 5 mg/kg/day ($n = 78$) or liposomal amphotericin B either 3 mg/kg/day ($n = 85$) or 5 mg/kg/day ($n = 81$). The median duration of therapy was 7.5–8.6 days. Therapeutic success was similar in all three groups. The following adverse effects were significantly less common with both doses of liposomal amphotericin: *fever* on day 1 (24% and 20% vs 58%), *chills/rigors* on day 1 (19% and 24% vs 80%), *nephrotoxicity* (defined as a serum creatinine of twice the baseline value; 14% and 15% vs 42%), and toxicity-related withdrawal of therapy (13% and 12% vs 32%). After day 1, infusion reactions were less frequent with ABLC, but chills/rigors were still significantly more common (21% and 24% vs 51%). Hepatotoxicity occurred in 12% of patients, with no differences between the three groups. While the higher rate of infusion-related reactions with ABLC is supported by cumulative data from non-comparative clinical studies, the differences in nephrotoxicity are more difficult to interpret. For example, the peak creatinine concentration was over 2 mg/dl in 24% of those given ABLC and in 17% of those given liposomal amphotericin 3 mg/kg, but in only 5% of those given liposomal amphotericin 5 mg/kg; and the peak creatinine concentration was over 3 mg/dl in 13% of those given ABLC and 7.1% of those given liposomal amphotericin 3 mg/kg, but in only 1.2% of those given liposomal amphotericin 5 mg/kg. The rationale for selection of the dosages investigated in this study is unclear, but it may have created a bias in the interpretation of the comparative nephrotoxicity data.

Risk factors *Children* The safety and antifungal efficacy of unilamellar liposomal amphotericin B (LAMB; AmBisome) has been prospectively evaluated in 24 infants of very low birthweights (mean 847 g, mean gestational age 26 weeks) with invasive candidiasis (12[c]). LAMB was given as a 1-hour infusion in dosages of 2.5–7 (mean 5.22) mg/kg/day for a mean of 21 (range 2–31) days. Twenty infants were considered cured at the end of treatment. There were no major adverse effects. One patient developed an increased bilirubin concentration and increased activities of hepatic transaminases. Renal function returned to normal in three infants who had developed renal insufficiency during previous amphotericin B treatment. Hypokalemia (serum potassium below 3.0 mmol/l) and infusion-related reactions were not observed. These data document excellent safety and efficacy of LAMB in the treatment of invasive candidiasis in the vulnerable population of very low birthweight infants.

AZOLE DERIVATIVES *(SED-14, 928; SEDA-22, 293; SEDA-23, 295; SEDA-24, 318)*

Fluconazole

Fluconazole and amphotericin as empirical antifungal drugs in febrile neutropenic patients have been investigated in a prospective, randomized, multicenter study in 317 patients randomized to either fluconazole (400 mg qds) or amphotericin B deoxycholate (0.5 mg/kg qds) (13[C]). Adverse events (*fever*, *chills*, *renal insufficiency*, *electrolyte disturbances*, and *res-*

piratory distress) occurred significantly more often in patients who were given amphotericin (128/151 patients, 81%) than in those given fluconazole (20/158 patients, 13%). Eleven patients treated with amphotericin, but only one treated with fluconazole, were withdrawn because of an adverse event. Overall mortality and mortality from fungal infections were similar in both groups. There was a satisfactory response in 68% of the patients treated with fluconazole and 67% of those treated with amphotericin. Thus, fluconazole may be a safe and effective alternative to amphotericin for empirical therapy of febrile neutropenic patients; however, since fluconazole is ineffective against opportunistic molds, the possibility of an invasive infection by a filamentous fungus should be excluded before starting empirical therapy. Similarly, patients who take azoles for prophylaxis are not candidates for empirical therapy with fluconazole.

Conventional amphotericin (0.2 mg/kg qds) and fluconazole (400 mg qds) have been compared in a prospective randomized study in 355 patients with allogeneic and autologous bone-marrow transplantation (14[C]). The drugs were given prophylactically from day –1 until engraftment. There was no difference in the occurrence of invasive fungal infections, but amphotericin was significantly more toxic than fluconazole, especially in related allogeneic transplantation, after which 19% of patients developed toxicity compared with none of those who received fluconazole.

Nervous system Central nervous system abnormalities constitute the major dose-limiting adverse effects of fluconazole and are observed at dosages over 1200 mg/day (15[c]). Two Japanese patients developed *clonic convulsions* while taking fluconazole 800 mg/day (16[A]).

A 66-year-old woman with complicated invasive *Candida tropicalis* infection but no renal impairment took fluconazole 800 mg/day. On the 21st day she developed clonic convulsions. The fluconazole trough concentration at the time of the event was 82 μg/ml.

A 62-year-old man with deteriorating renal and hepatic function after coronary artery bypass surgery was given fluconazole 400 mg bd for a fungal sternal wound infection. On the 15th day he developed seizures. His trough plasma fluconazole concentration was 88 μg/ml. Nineteen days after dosage adjustment to 400 mg qds, he had another seizure. The trough fluconazole concentration was 103 μg/ml, probably because of deteriorating renal function.

In both cases, the seizures abated after dosage reduction. These case reports suggest an association between trough plasma fluconazole concentrations of 80 μg/ml and central nervous system toxicity; they re-emphasize the need for careful monitoring and dosage adjustment in patients with reduced renal function.

Hematologic *Leukopenia with eosinophilia* has been attributed to fluconazole (17[A]).

A 75-year-old man with non-Hodgkin's lymphoma and cryptococcal meningoencephalitis developed neutropenia with eosinophilia associated with fluconazole. After 1 week of fluconazole 400 mg/day his total white blood cell count began to fall and his eosinophils increased. Concurrent medications included levothyroxine, famotidine, and co-trimoxazole. The last two drugs were stopped and he was given G-CSF. However, his white blood cell count continued to fall and 4 days later reached a nadir of 700×10^6/l; the platelet count remained normal. The leukopenia and eosinophilia resolved promptly after withdrawal of fluconazole.

Since the leukopenia and eosinophilia did not resolve until fluconazole was withdrawn, an effect of the compound was plausible. This case and two other reported cases (18[A], 19[A]) emphasize the importance of recognizing fluconazole as a rare but potential cause of bone-marrow suppression in patients in whom drug-induced agranulocytosis is suspected.

Skin A case of *fixed drug eruption* caused by systemic fluconazole has been reported (20[A]).

A 36-year-old woman with a history of atopy and recurrent *Candida* vaginitis developed a fixed drug eruption while taking fluconazole 150 mg/day. Local provocation with 10% fluconazole in petrolatum applied at the site of a previous site of fixed drug eruption reproduced the eruption clinically and histopathologically.

Drug interactions The effects of fluconazole on plasma *fluvastatin* and *pravastatin* concentrations have been studied in two separate, randomized, double blind, two-phase, cross-over studies (21[c]). Healthy volunteers were given oral fluconazole (400 mg on day 1 and 200 mg on days 2–4) or placebo. On day 4, they took a single oral dose of fluvastatin 40 mg or pravastatin 40 mg. Fluconazole increased the plasma AUC and the half-life of fluvastatin by 80% but had no significant effects on the pharmacokinetics of pravastatin. The mechanism of the prolonged elimination of fluvastatin was probably inhibition of CYP2C9. Pravastatin, in contrast, appears not to be susceptible to interactions with fluconazole and other CYP2C9 inhibitors.

The effects of fluconazole and clarithromycin on the pharmacokinetics of *rifabutin* and 25-*O*-desacetylrifabutin have been studied in ten HIV-infected patients who were given rifabutin 300 mg qds in addition to fluconazole 200 mg qds and clarithromycin 500 mg qds (22[c]). There was a 76% increase in the plasma AUC of rifabutin when either fluconazole or clarithromycin was given alone and a 152% increase when both drugs were given together. The authors concluded that patients should be monitored for adverse effects of rifabutin when it is coadministered with fluconazole or clarithromycin.

The effect of fluconazole on the plasma pharmacokinetics of *doxorubicin* has been investigated in a randomized cross-over study in non-human primates (23[E]). Fluconazole (10 mg/kg/day) was given intravenously for 4 days before doxorubicin (2.0 mg/kg intravenously). Pretreatment with fluconazole had no effect on the pharmacokinetics of doxorubicin, and the incidence of severe neutropenia (absolute neutrophil count below 0.5×10^9/l) was higher with doxorubicin alone than with the combination of doxorubicin and fluconazole. Thus, fluconazole does not appear to contribute to the marrow suppressive effects of doxorubicin.

An interaction of fluconazole with *amitriptyline* has been reported (24[A]).

A 12-year-old boy with prostatic rhabdomyosarcoma had episodes of syncope periodically over 7 months while taking fluconazole for chemotherapy-induced mucositis. He had taken fluconazole in the past without problems but had also taken a stable dose of amitriptyline for neuropathic pain. On withdrawal of amitriptyline he had no further episodes. The effect was confirmed by readministration.

Concurrent administration of fluconazole probably causes increased exposure to amitriptyline. Three reports of adults have shown increased amitriptyline plasma concentrations with concurrent administration of fluconazole; in one patient, a 57-year-old woman, the *QT interval was prolonged* and *torsade de pointes* occurred (25[A]).

Itraconazole

Itraconazole elixir 2.5 mg/kg bd has been compared with amphotericin capsules 500 mg qds for the prophylaxis of systemic and superficial fungal infections in a double-blind, randomized, placebo-controlled, multicenter trial (26[C]). The drugs were given for 1–59 days. While itraconazole significantly reduced the frequency of superficial fungal infections, it was not superior in reducing invasive fungal infections or in improving mortality. Adverse events were reported in 222 patients taking itraconazole (79%) and in 205 patients taking amphotericin (74%). The commonest adverse events were *gastrointestinal*, followed by rash and *hypokalemia*, with no differences between the two regimens. In both groups, 5% of the adverse events were considered to be definitely drug-related. Comparable numbers of patients in the two groups permanently stopped treatment because of adverse events (including death), 75 (27%) in the itraconazole group and 78 (28%) in the amphotericin group. *Nausea* (9 and 11%) and *vomiting* (8% and 7%) were the most frequently reported adverse events that led to withdrawal. Biochemical changes were comparable in the two groups.

Oral fluconazole 400 mg qds and oral itraconazole 200 mg bd have been compared in a randomized, double blind, placebo-controlled trial in 198 patients with progressive non-meningeal coccidioidomycosis (27[C]). Overall, 57% and 72% of patients responded to 12 months of therapy with fluconazole and itraconazole respectively. Relapse rates after withdrawal did not differ significantly. Both drugs were well tolerated. Serious adverse events occurred in eight of 97 fluconazole-treated patients and six of 101 itraconazole-treated patients. They included *raised liver enzymes*, *gastrointestinal disturbances*, *hypokalemia*, and *skin rash*. Alopecia was reported in 15 of 97 patients taking fluconazole and in only four of 101 patients taking itraconazole. Similarly, *dry lips* were reported in 11 of 97 patients taking fluconazole and in none of 101 patients taking itraconazole. Both adverse events have previously been reported with fluconazole.

Skin *Skin reactions* are infrequent with itraconazole.

A 29-year-old man developed an infiltrative maculopapular eruption after 1 week of itraconazole 100 mg bd for tinea corporis (28[A]). Itraconazole was withdrawn, and the lesions disappeared within 7 days. Scratch tests, patch tests, scratch–patch tests, and drug-induced lymphocyte stimulation tests for itraconazole were negative; however, rechallenge with systemic itraconazole induced a maculopapular eruption on the face, hands, and the dorsa of the feet. Empty itraconazole capsules had no cutaneous effects, suggesting an allergic reaction to a metabolite of the compound.

Drug interactions Itraconazole markedly increases both systemic exposure to *dexamethasone* and its effects. This interaction has been investigated in a randomized, double-blind, placebo-controlled, cross-over study (29[c]). Eight healthy volunteers took either oral itraconazole 200 mg od or placebo for 4 days. On day 4, each subject was given oral dexamethasone 4.5 mg or intravenous dexamethasone sodium phosphate 5.0 mg. Itraconazole reduced the systemic clearance of intravenous dexamethasone by 68%, and increased its AUC and prolonged its half-life more than 3-fold; the AUC of oral dexamethasone was increased nearly 4-fold and its half-life nearly 3-fold. Morning plasma cortisol concentrations at 47 and 71 hours after dexamethasone were significantly lower after itraconazole than placebo.

The effects of itraconazole on the pharmacokinetics and pharmacodynamics of oral *prednisolone* have been investigated in a double-blind, randomized, cross-over study (30[c]). Ten healthy subjects took either oral itraconazole 200 mg od or placebo for 4 days. On day 4 they took oral prednisolone 20 mg. Itraconazole increased the plasma AUC of prednisolone by 24% and its half-life by 29% compared with placebo. The peak plasma concentration and time to the peak of prednisolone were not affected. Itraconazole reduced the mean morning plasma cortisol concentration, measured 23 hours after prednisolone, by 27%. The minor interaction of itraconazole with oral prednisolone is probably of limited clinical significance. The susceptibility of prednisolone to interact with CYP3A4 inhibitors is considerably smaller than that of methylprednisolone, and itraconazole and probably also other inhibitors of CYP3A4 can be used concomitantly with prednisolone without marked interaction.

Statins (3-hydroxy-3-methylglutaryl coenzyme A reductase inhibitors) are metabolized by distinct oxidative pathways. In a randomized, open, three-way, cross-over study, 18 healthy subjects took single doses of cerivastatin 0.8 mg, atorvastatin 20 mg, or pravastatin 40 mg without or with itraconazole 200 mg (31[c]). Concomitant cerivastatin/itraconazole and pravastatin/itraconazole produced small increases in AUC, C_{max}, and half-life (up to 51%, 25%, and 23% respectively). However, itraconazole markedly increased atorvastatin AUC (150%), C_{max} (38%), and half-life (30%). Thus, itraconazole markedly increases systemic exposure to atorvastatin, but results in only modest increases in the plasma concentrations of cerivastatin and pravastatin.

The HIV protease inhibitor *saquinavir* has limited and variable oral systemic availability and ritonavir, an inhibitor of CYP450 and P-glycoprotein, is widely used to increase its systemic exposure. A small pilot study in three HIV-infected patients has suggested that oral itraconazole can have similar effects on the oral availability of saquinavir (32[A]). Concomitant use of itraconazole 200 mg/day with a combination of saquinavir and two nucleoside reverse transcriptase inhibitors led to a 2.5- to 6.9-fold increase in the AUC of saquinavir, a 2.0- to 5.4-fold increase in peak plasma concentrations, and a 1.6- to 17-fold increase in trough plasma concentrations. The effect of itraconazole on saquinavir was comparable to that of ritonavir.

Apart from its well-known effects on ciclosporin blood concentrations, itraconazole can also increase exposure to *tacrolimus*, which may have negative effects on renal function, as a recent case has illustrated (33[A]).

A 30-year-old man with a renal transplant had a more than 2-fold increase in blood tacrolimus concentrations after starting to take itraconazole 200 mg/day, accompanied by a reduced glomerular filtration rate and biopsy-proven tacrolimus-associated tubulopathy.

Because of the narrow therapeutic index of tacrolimus, blood concentrations should be monitored particularly carefully when itraconazole is coadministered, and the dosage of tacrolimus may have to be altered (34[A]).

The effect of the combination of itraconazole with *amphotericin* on liver enzyme activities has been studied retrospectively in 20 patients with hematological malignancies or chronic lung disease complicated by fungal infection or colonization (35[c]). They took itraconazole 200–600 mg/day for a median of 143 (range 44–455) days. Nine had no abnormal liver function tests, including periods of high concentrations of itraconazole (over 5000 ng/ml) and its active hydroxylated metabolite; only one had received concomitant amphotericin. All of the 11 patients with liver function abnormalities had received concomitant amphotericin. For each patient, liver function abnormalities were greatest during the time of concomitant therapy with both antifungal drugs. Although liver enzyme abnormalities are uncommon with amphotericin (36[R]), and although this retrospective analysis was subject to several flaws and potential biases, it nevertheless suggests that hepatotoxicity should be carefully monitored if itraconazole and amphotericin are coadministered.

Ketoconazole

The efficacy of ketoconazole 400 mg qds in the early treatment of acute lung injury and acute respiratory distress syndrome has been investigated in a randomized, double-blind, placebo-controlled trial in 234 patients (37[C]). Ketoconazole was safe but had no effects on mortality, lung function, or the duration of mechanical ventilation.

Because of its potent inhibitory effects on adrenal steroidogenesis by interference with cytochrome CYP450, ketoconazole controls hypercortisolism when surgery is contraindicated or unsuccessful. The effects of oral ketoconazole 200–1200 mg qds for 65–83 months in three patients who had residual or recurrent Cushing's disease after surgical treatment have been reported (38[A]). The dosage of ketoconazole was adjusted according to the clinical response and 24-hour urinary excretion of free cortisol. All three patients had good clinical and biochemical responses to therapy with ketoconazole and had no adverse effects.

Drug interactions The effect of ketoconazole (200 and 400 mg qds) on plasma and cerebrospinal fluid concentrations of *ritonavir* (400 mg bd) and *saquinavir* (400 mg bd) have been investigated in a two-period, two-group, longitudinal pharmacokinetic study in 12 HIV-infected patients (39[c]). Ketoconazole significantly increased the AUC and trough concentrations of ritonavir and prolonged its half-life (by 29%, 62%, and 31% respectively). It produced similar changes (37%, 94%, and 38% respectively) in the kinetics of saquinavir. Ketoconazole significantly increased the ritonavir CSF concentration at 4–5 hours after the dose by 178% (from 2.4 to 6.6 ng/ml), with no change in the paired unbound plasma concentration (26 ng/ml). The changes were not related to ketoconazole dose or plasma exposure. The corresponding changes in saquinavir CSF concentrations were not significant. The authors concluded that ketoconazole inhibited the systemic clearance of ritonavir and, because of the disproportionate increase in CSF concentrations compared with the increase in plasma concentrations, that there was greater inhibition of drug efflux from the CSF.

A study in seven HIV-infected men who took *saquinavir* 600 mg tds in addition to two other antiretroviral drugs and concomitant ketoconazole (200 mg qds for 7 days, followed by 400 mg qds for another 7 days) showed no significant differences in peak and trough concentrations of saquinavir after the addition of ketoconazole (40[c]). There was substantial intersubject variability in the study, and the authors concluded that saquinavir concentrations may be unpredictable in individual patients and that drug monitoring may be required for optimizing saquinavir treatment.

Ketoconazole affects plasma concentrations of *loratadine*, a non-sedating antihistamine, but appears to be devoid of any electrocardiographic effects (41[c]). In a randomized, single-blind, multiple-dose, three-way, cross-over study concomitant administration of loratadine 10 mg qds and ketoconazole 200 mg bd significantly increased mean loratadine (307%) and desloratadine (73%) plasma concentrations; ketoconazole plasma concentrations were unaffected by loratadine. Despite increased concentrations of loratadine and its metabolite, there were no statistically significant differences in the electrocardiographic QT_c interval.

Ziprasidone is oxidatively metabolized by CYP3A4, but it does not inhibit CYP3A4 or other isoenzymes at clinically relevant concentrations. The effect of ketoconazole (400 mg qds for 6 days) on ziprasidone single-dose pharmacokinetics (40 mg on day 5 of ketoconazole/placebo) has been evaluated in an open, placebo-controlled, cross-over study in healthy volunteers (42[c]). Ketoconazole caused a modest increase in the mean AUC (33%) and the mean C_{max} (34%) of ziprasidone. This effect was not considered clinically relevant and suggests that other inhibitors of CYP3A4 are unlikely to affect the pharmacokinetics of ziprasidone significantly. Most of the reported adverse events were mild. The adverse events that were most commonly reported in subjects who took the drugs concomitantly were dizziness, weakness, and somnolence. There were no treatment-related laboratory abnormalities or abnormal vital signs during the study and at the 6-day follow-up evaluation.

ECHINOCANDINS

The echinocandins are a class of semisynthetic antifungal lipopeptides that are structurally characterized by a cyclic hexapeptide core linked to a variably configured lipid side chain. The echinocandins act by non-competitive inhibition of the synthesis of 1,3-β-D-glucan, a major polysaccharide component of the cell wall of many pathogenic fungi, absent from mammalian cells. In concert with chitin, the rope-like glucan fibrils are important in maintaining the osmotic integrity of the fungal cell and play a key role in cell division and cell growth.

The current echinocandins, anidulafungin (Versicor Inc, Freemont, CA), caspofungin (Merck & Co, Inc, Rahway, NJ), and micafungin (Fujisawa Inc, Deerfield, IL) have relatively similar pharmacological properties. All three compounds have potent and broad-spectrum antifungal activity against *Candida* spp. and *Aspergillus* spp. without cross-resistance to existing agents. They have prolonged postantifungal effects and fungicidal activity against *Candida* and cause severe damage of *Aspergillus* at the sites of hyphal growth. Their efficacy against these organisms in vivo has been demonstrated in animals (43[R], 44[R]).

The echinocandins are currently available only for intravenous administration. They have dose-proportional plasma pharmacokinetics, with half-lives of 10–15 hours, which allows once-daily dosing. All echinocandins are highly protein bound (over 95%) and distribute into all major tissues, including the brain; concentrations in non-inflammatory CSF are low. The echinocandins are metabolized by the liver and are slowly excreted as inactive metabolites in the urine and feces; only small fractions are excreted unchanged in the urine. They lack significant potential for drug interactions mediated by the CYP450 enzyme system and are generally well tolerated (43[R], 44[R]).

The clinical efficacy of anidulafungin, caspofungin, and micafungin against *Candida* spp. has been documented in phase II or phase III studies in immunocompromised patients with esophageal candidiasis. All achieved therapeutic efficacy at least comparable with standard agents. Phase III efficacy studies of echinocandins for invasive candidiasis and for empirical antifungal therapy in persistently febrile neutropenic patients are under way. Caspofungin has recently been approved by the FDA for definite or probable invasive aspergillosis in patients refractory to or intolerant of conventional therapies.

Caspofungin

Caspofungin (Cancidas; 50 and 70 mg/day for 14 days; $n = 74$) has been compared with conventional amphotericin (0.5 mg/kg/day for 14 days; $n = 54$) in the treatment of esophageal candidiasis in a randomized, double-blind, multicenter trial in South America (45[C]). Most of the patients (over 75%) were HIV-infected and about half of them had CD4+ lymphocyte counts of under 50×10^6/l. Caspofungin was well tolerated: eight patients in the amphotericin group and one patient in the combined caspofungin group developed a *raised serum creatinine* of over 176 μmol/l (2 mg/dl) during treatment. Of the patients who received caspofungin 4.1% withdrew prematurely owing to drug-associated adverse effects, compared with 22% in the amphotericin arm. There was a clinical response (symptoms plus endoscopy) in 85% of the patients in the combined caspofungin group versus 67% in the amphotericin group.

Caspofungin has been studied in a multicenter, open, non-comparative phase II trial in 63 patients with definite or probable invasive aspergillosis refractory to or intolerant of standard therapies (46[C]). Caspofungin was administered in a dose of 70 mg on day 1, followed by 50 mg od for a mean duration of 34 (range 1–162) days. Most of these patients (42/63) had hematological malignancies as underlying diseases or had undergone bone-marrow transplantation. Caspofungin was generally well tolerated. One serious adverse event was reported as possibly drug-related. *Infusion-related reactions* and *nephrotoxicity* were uncommon. Three patients discontinued caspofungin because of adverse events. An independent expert panel judged that there were favorable responses in 26 patients who received at least one dose of caspofungin; of 52 patients who received caspofungin for over 7 days, there was a good response in 26.

Drug interactions In vitro biotransformation studies of caspofungin have shown that it is not a substrate of P-glycoprotein and is a poor substrate and a weak inhibitor of cytochrome P450 enzymes.

In rats, caspofungin did not alter the plasma pharmacokinetics of *indinavir*, a substrate and competitive inhibitor of CYP3A2, or *ketoconazole*, a potent CYP3A4 inhibitor (47[R]).

Consistent with these findings, the coadministration of caspofungin 50 mg/day and *itraconazole* 200 mg/day to healthy subjects for 14 days did not alter the pharmacokinetics of either drug (48[c]).

There were no pharmacokinetic interactions of caspofungin with *amphotericin B deoxycholate* or of caspofungin with the immunosuppressant *mycophenolate* in healthy volunteers (47[R]).

While *tacrolimus* had no effect on the plasma pharmacokinetics of caspofungin, chronic caspofungin reduced the AUC of tacrolimus by about 20% (47[R]).

Ciclosporin increased the AUC of caspofungin by about 35% but caspofungin did not increase the plasma concentrations of ciclosporin. Because of transient rises in hepatic transaminases not exceeding 2–3 times the upper limit of the reference range in single-dose interaction studies, the concomitant use of caspofungin with ciclosporin is not recommended until multiple-dose use in patients has been studied (47[R]).

Regression analysis of pharmacokinetic data from patients have suggested that coadministration of inducers of drug clearance and/or mixed inducer/inhibitors, namely *carbamazepine*, *dexamethasone*, *efavirenz*, *nelfinavir*, *nevirapine*, *phenytoin*, and *rifampicin*, with caspofungin can cause clinically important reductions in caspofungin concentrations. However, no data are currently available from formal interaction studies, and it is not known which clearance mechanisms of caspofungin are inducible. The manufacturer currently recommends considering an increase in the daily dose of caspofungin to 70 mg in patients taking these drugs concurrently who are not clinically responding (47[R]).

PYRIMIDINE ANALOGUES

(SED-14, 926; SEDA-23, 295)

Fluorocytosine (5-fluorocytosine)

The toxicity and drug interactions of fluorocytosine have been reviewed (49[R]). The most common adverse effects include *gastrointestinal disturbances*, *increases in hepatic transaminases and alkaline phosphatase*, and *bone-marrow depression*. Hepatic and hematological adverse events are concentration dependent and are usually reversible with drug withdrawal or dosage reduction; they are potentially avoidable by close monitoring to maintain plasma fluorocytosine concentrations below 100 mg/l.

The mechanism of toxicity of fluorocytosine is not fully understood; conversion of fluorocytosine to certain metabolites, in particular 5-fluorouracil, in the liver or by the intestinal microflora after oral administration have been proposed. Toxicity may also occur through impurities in the raw material and the formation of fluorouracil from fluorocytosine after sterilization and storage. To avoid serious toxicity, plasma concentration monitoring is recommended, with target trough and peak concentrations of 25–50 mg/l and 50–100 mg/l respectively. In patients receiving a continuous infusion of fluorocytosine, a plasma concentration of 50 mg/l is recommended. Pharmacokinetic drug interactions involving fluorocytosine can arise with the concomitant use of compounds that impair glomerular filtration, in particular amphotericin.

Cardiovascular Life-threatening fluorouracil-like *cardiotoxicity* has been attributed to fluorocytosine (50[A]).

A 34-year-old woman took fluorocytosine, 500 mg 12 times a day for 2 days, for vaginal candidiasis. After the last dose she complained of chest pain, which persisted for a week and was associated with ST segment elevation during exercise. Coronary angiography showed normal coronary arteries. One month later she was rechallenged with 500 mg 12 times a day for 2 days. The day after completion of this regimen, she developed severe chest pain. Electrocardiography showed widespread ST segment elevation and echocardiography showed apicolateral septal hypokinesia with a left ventricular ejection fraction of less than 15%. Her fluorocytosine plasma concentration 48 hours after the last dose was not high, but the fluorouracil concentration was similar to that found during a 5-day continuous infusion of 5-fluorouracil. Her lymphocytes showed no abnormalities of intracellular fluorocytosine clearance, and cytosine deaminase, the enzyme that converts fluorocytosine to fluorouracil, was not detectable.

Similar cardiotoxicity has been reported with 5-fluorouracil. The reported events were generally consistent with a drug- or metabolite-induced increase in coronary vasomotor tone and spasm, leading to myocardial ischemia. The authors concluded that more attention should be given to the conversion of fluorocytosine to fluorouracil in patients who receive fluorocytosine; however, it is not clear whether fluorocytosine should be contraindicated in patients with vasospastic or exertional angina.

Hematologic The relation between toxicity and the pharmacokinetics of fluorocytosine has been investigated in a retrospective study in 53 patients in an intensive care unit (51[c]). *Thrombocytopenia*, as a marker of bone-marrow depression, was associated with a reduced clearance of fluorocytosine; the lowest thrombocyte count was linearly related to the clearance of fluorocytosine. Patients with fluorocytosine concentrations over 100 mg/l were at higher risk of thrombocytopenia and raised hepatic transaminases than those who did not exceed this threshold. In a second study, the authors corroborated their earlier findings and showed a significant relation between the lowest thrombocyte counts and thrombocyte counts predicted on the basis of the creatinine clearance in a new set of patients admitted to the intensive care unit (52[c]).

REFERENCES

1. Duxbury AJ, Oliver RJ, Pemberton MN. Persistent impairment of taste associated with terbinafine. Br Dent J 2000; 188: 295–6.
2. Caceres-Rios H, Rueda M, Ballona R, Bustamante B. Comparison of terbinafine and griseofulvin in the treatment of tinea capitis. J Am Acad Dermatol 2000; 42: 80–4.
3. Smith EB, Stein LF, Fivenson DP, Atillasoy ES. Clinical trial: the safety of terbinafine in patients over the age of 60 years: a multicenter trial in onychomycosis of the feet. Int J Dermatol 2000; 39: 861–4.
4. Timmers GJ, Zweegman S, Simoons-Smit AM, Van Loenen AC, Touw D, Huijgens PC. Amphotericin B colloidal dispersion (Amphocil) vs fluconazole for the prevention of fungal infections in neutropenic patients: data of a prematurely stopped clinical trial. Bone Marrow Transplant 2000; 25: 879–84.
5. White MH, Bowden RA, Sandler ES, Graham ML, Noskin GA, Wingard JR, Goldman M, Van Burik JA, McCabe A, Lin JS, Gurwith M, Miller CB. Randomized, double-blind clinical trial of amphotericin B colloidal dispersion vs. amphotericin B in the empirical treatment of fever and neutropenia. Clin Infect Dis 1998; 27: 296–302.
6. Rossi MR, Longoni DV, Rovelli AM, Uderzo C. Severe rhabdomyolysis, hyperthermia and shock after amphotericin B colloidal dispersion in an allogeneic bone marrow transplant recipient. Pediatr Infect Dis J 2000; 19: 172–3.
7. Sandler ES, Mustafa MM, Tkaczewski I, Graham ML, Morrison VA, Green M, Trigg M, Abboud M, Aquino VM, Gurwith M, Pietrelli L. Use of amphotericin B colloidal dispersion in children. J Pediatr Hematol Oncol 2000; 22: 242–6.
8. Linden P, Williams P, Chan KM. Efficacy and safety of amphotericin B lipid complex injection (ABLC) in solid-organ transplant recipients with invasive fungal infections. Clin Transplant 2000; 14: 329–39.
9. Furebring M, Oberg G, Sjolin J. Side-effects of amphotericin B lipid complex (Abelcet) in the Scandinavian population. Bone Marrow Transplant 2000; 25: 341–3.
10. Ringden O, Jonsson V, Hansen M, Tollemar J, Jacobsen N. Severe and common side-effects of amphotericin B lipid complex (Abelcet). Bone Marrow Transplant 1998; 22: 733–4.
11. Wingard JR, White MH, Anaissie E, Raffalli J, Goodman J, Arrieta A. A randomized, double-blind comparative trial evaluating the safety of liposomal amphotericin B versus amphotericin B lipid complex in the empirical treatment of febrile neutropenia. L Amph/ABLC Collaborative Study Group. Clin Infect Dis 2000; 31: 1155–63.
12. Juster-Reicher A, Leibovitz E, Linder N, Amitay M, Flidel-Rimon O, Even-Tov S, Mogilner B, Barzilai A. Liposomal amphotericin B (AmBisome) in the treatment of neonatal candidiasis in very low birth weight infants. Infection 2000; 28: 223–6.

13. Winston DJ, Hathorn JW, Schuster MG, Schiller GJ, Territo MC. A multicenter, randomized trial of fluconazole versus amphotericin B for empiric antifungal therapy of febrile neutropenic patients with cancer. Am J Med 2000; 108: 282–9.
14. Wolff SN, Fay J, Stevens D, Herzig RH, Pohlman B, Bolwell B, Lynch J, Ericson S, Freytes CO, LeMaistre F, Collins R, Pineiro L, Greer J, Stein R, Goodman SA, Dummer S. Fluconazole vs low-dose amphotericin B for the prevention of fungal infections in patients undergoing bone marrow transplantation: a study of the North American Marrow Transplant Group. Bone Marrow Transplant 2000; 25: 853–9.
15. Anaissie EJ, Kontoyiannis DP, Huls C, Vartivarian SE, Karl C, Prince RA, Bosso J, Bodey GP. Safety, plasma concentrations, and efficacy of high-dose fluconazole in invasive mold infections. J Infect Dis 1995; 172: 599–602.
16. Matsumoto K, Ueno K, Yoshimura H, Morii M, Takada M, Sawai T, Mitsutake K, Shibakawa M. Fluconazole-induced convulsions at serum trough concentrations of approximately 80 microg/ml. Ther Drug Monit 2000; 22: 635–6.
17. Wong-Beringer A, Shriner K. Fluconazole-induced agranulocytosis with eosinophilia. Pharmacotherapy 2000; 20: 484–6.
18. Chuncharunee S, Sathapatayavongs B, Singhasivanon P, Singhasivanon V. Fluconazole-induced agranulocytosis. Therapie 1994; 49: 517–18.
19. Murakami H, Katahira H, Matsushima T, Sakura T, Tamura J, Sawamura M, Tsuchiya J. Agranulocytosis during treatment with fluconazole. J Int Med Res 1992; 20: 492–4.
20. Heikkila H, Timonen K, Stubb S. Fixed drug eruption due to fluconazole. J Am Acad Dermatol 2000; 42: 883–4.
21. Kantola T, Backman JT, Niemi M, Kivisto KT, Neuvonen PJ. Effect of fluconazole on plasma fluvastatin and pravastatin concentrations. Eur J Clin Pharmacol 2000; 56: 225–9.
22. Jordan MK, Polis MA, Kelly G, Narang PK, Masur H, Piscitelli SC. Effects of fluconazole and clarithromycin on rifabutin and 25-O-desacetylrifabutin pharmacokinetics. Antimicrob Agents Chemother 2000; 44: 2170–2.
23. Warren KE, McCully CM, Walsh TJ, Balis FM. Effect of fluconazole on the pharmacokinetics of doxorubicin in nonhuman primates. Antimicrob Agents Chemother 2000; 44: 1100–1.
24. Robinson RF, Nahata MC, Olshefski RS. Syncope associated with concurrent amitriptyline and fluconazole therapy. Ann Pharmacother 2000; 34: 1406–9.
25. Dorsey ST, Biblo LA. Prolonged QT interval and torsades de pointes caused by the combination of fluconazole and amitriptyline. Am J Emerg Med 2000; 18: 227–9.
26. Harousseau JL, Dekker AW, Stamatoullas-Bastard A, Fassas A, Linkesch W, Gouveia J, De Bock R, Rovira M, Seifert WF, Joosen H, Peeters M, De Beule K. Itraconazole oral solution for primary prophylaxis of fungal infections in patients with hematological malignancy and profound neutropenia: a randomized, double-blind, double-placebo, multicenter trial comparing itraconazole and amphotericin B. Antimicrob Agents Chemother 2000; 44: 1887–93.
27. Galgiani JN, Catanzaro A, Cloud GA, Johnson RH, Williams PL, Mirels LF, Nassar F, Lutz JE, Stevens DA, Sharkey PK, Singh VR, Larsen RA, Delgado KL, Flanigan C, Rinaldi MG. Comparison of oral fluconazole and itraconazole for progressive, nonmeningeal coccidioidomycosis. A randomized, double-blind trial. Mycoses Study Group. Ann Intern Med 2000; 133: 676–86.
28. Goto Y, Kono T, Teramae K, Ishii M. Itraconazole-induced drug eruption confirmed by challenge test. Acta Derm Venereol 2000; 80: 72.
29. Varis T, Kivisto KT, Backman JT, Neuvonen PJ. The cytochrome P450 3A4 inhibitor itraconazole markedly increases the plasma concentrations of dexamethasone and enhances its adrenal-suppressant effect. Clin Pharmacol Ther 2000; 68: 487–94.
30. Varis T, Kivisto KT, Neuvonen PJ. The effect of itraconazole on the pharmacokinetics and pharmacodynamics of oral prednisolone. Eur J Clin Pharmacol 2000; 56: 57–60.
31. Mazzu AL, Lasseter KC, Shamblen EC, Agarwal V, Lettieri J, Sundaresen P. Itraconazole alters the pharmacokinetics of atorvastatin to a greater extent than either cerivastatin or pravastatin. Clin Pharmacol Ther 2000; 8: 391–400.
32. Koks CH, Van Heeswijk RP, Veldkamp AI, Meenhorst PL, Mulder JW, Van der Meer JT, Beijnen JH, Hoetelmans RM. Itraconazole as an alternative for ritonavir liquid formulation when combined with saquinavir. AIDS 2000; 14: 89–90.
33. Ideura T, Muramatsu T, Higuchi M, Tachibana N, Hora K, Kiyosawa K. Tacrolimus/itraconazole interactions: a case report of ABO-incompatible living-related renal transplantation. Nephrol Dial Transplant 2000; 15: 1721–3.
34. Outeda Macias M, Salvador P, Hurtado JL, Martin I. Tacrolimus–itraconazole interaction in a kidney transplant patient. Ann Pharmacother 2000; 34: 536.
35. Persat F, Schwartzbrod PE, Troncy J, Timour Q, Maul A, Piens MA, Picot S. Abnormalities in liver enzymes during simultaneous therapy with itraconazole and amphotericin B in leukaemic patients. J Antimicrob Chemother 2000; 45: 928–9.
36. Groll AH, Piscitelli SC, Walsh TJ. Clinical pharmacology of systemic antifungal agents: a comprehensive review of agents in clinical use, current investigational compounds, and putative targets for antifungal drug development. Adv Pharmacol 1998; 44: 343–500.
37. The ARDS Network. Ketoconazole for early treatment of acute lung injury and acute respiratory distress syndrome: a randomized controlled trial. J Am Med Assoc 2000; 283: 1995–2002.
38. Chou SC, Lin JD. Long-term effects of ketoconazole in the treatment of residual or recurrent Cushing's disease. Endocr J 2000; 47: 401–6.

39. Khaliq Y, Gallicano K, Venance S, Kravcik S, Cameron DW. Effect of ketoconazole on ritonavir and saquinavir concentrations in plasma and cerebrospinal fluid from patients infected with human immunodeficiency virus. Clin Pharmacol Ther 2000; 68: 637–46.
40. Collazos J, Martinez E, Mayo J, Blanco MS. Effect of ketoconazole on plasma concentrations of saquinavir. J Antimicrob Chemother 2000; 46: 151–2.
41. Kosoglou T, Salfi M, Lim JM, Batra VK, Cayen MN, Affrime MB. Evaluation of the pharmacokinetics and electrocardiographic pharmacodynamics of loratadine with concomitant administration of ketoconazole or cimetidine. Br J Clin Pharmacol 2000; 50: 581–9.
42. Miceli JJ, Smith M, Robarge L, Morse T, Laurent A. The effects of ketoconazole on ziprasidone pharmacokinetics – a placebo-controlled crossover study in healthy volunteers. Br J Clin Pharmacol 2000; 49 Suppl 1: 71S–76S.
43. Kurtz MB, Douglas CM. Lipopeptide inhibitors of fungal glucan synthase. J Med Vet Mycol 1997; 35: 79–86.
44. Georgopapadakou NH. Update on antifungals targeted to the cell wall: focus on beta-1,3-glucan synthase inhibitors. Expert Opin Investig Drugs 2001; 10: 269–80.
45. Sable CA, Villanueva A, Arathon E, Gotuzzo E, Turcato G, Uip D, Noriega L, Rivera C, Rojas E, Taylor V, Berman R, Calandra GB, Chodakewitz J. A randomized, double-blind, multicenter trial of MK-991 (L-743,872) vs. amphotericin B (AMB) in the treatment of Candida esophagitis in adults. Abstracts of the 37th Interscience Conference on Antimicrobial Agents and Chemotherapy, 1997: LB-33.
46. Maertens J, Raad I, Sable CA, Ngui A, Berman R, Patterson TF, Denning D, Walsh TJ. Multicenter, noncomparative study to evaluate safety and efficacy of caspofungin in adults with invasive aspergillosis refractory or intolerant to amphotericin B, amphotericin B lipid formulations, or azoles. Abstracts of the 40th International Conference on Antimicrobial Agents and Chemotherapy, 2000: 1103.
47. Groll AH, Walsh TJ. Caspofungin: pharmacology, safety, and therapeutic potential in superficial and invasive fungal infections. Expert Opin Invest Drugs 2001; 10: 1545–58.
48. Stone JA, McCrea J, Wickersham P, Holland S, Deutsch P, Bi S, Cicero T, Greenberg H, Waldman SA. Phase I study of caspofungin evaluating the potential for drug interactions with itraconazole, the effect of gender and the use of a loading dose. Abstracts of the 40th Interscience Conference on Antimicrobial Agents and Chemotherapy, 2000: 854.
49. Vermes A, Guchelaar HJ, Dankert J. Flucytosine: a review of its pharmacology, clinical indications, pharmacokinetics, toxicity and drug interactions. J Antimicrob Chemother 2000; 46: 171–9.
50. Isetta C, Garaffo R, Bastian G, Jourdan J, Baudouy M, Milano G. Life-threatening 5-fluorouracil-like cardiac toxicity after treatment with 5-fluorocytosine. Clin Pharmacol Ther 2000; 67: 323–5.
51. Vermes A, Van der Sijs H, Guchelaar HJ. Flucytosine: correlation between toxicity and pharmacokinetic parameters. Chemotherapy 2000; 46: 86–94.
52. Vermes A, Guchelaar HJ, Dankert J. Prediction of flucytosine-induced thrombocytopenia using creatinine clearance. Chemotherapy 2000; 46: 335–41.

Tim Planche and Sanjeev Krishna

28 Antiprotozoal drugs

ANTIMALARIAL DRUGS

(SED-14, 799; SEDA-22, 302; SEDA-23, 304; SEDA 24, 330)

Recommendations for the prophylaxis of malaria vary greatly between geographical regions and are constantly under revision. Recommendations for avoidance of malaria also include the use of physical antimosquito measures and are particularly important, as some studies have shown limited adherence to chemoprophylaxis regimens (1[C]).

4-AMINOQUINOLINES (CHLOROQUINE AND CONGENERS) *(SED-14, 950; SEDA-22, 303; SEDA-23, 305; SEDA-24, 331)*

Chloroquine is still effective in non-falciparum malaria, but is of very limited use against falciparum malaria, owing to the spread of chloroquine resistance. Most information on adverse events with chloroquine and its use in pregnancy comes from its use in rheumatological conditions, in which higher doses are used for longer periods of time.

Nervous system Chloroquine and desethylchloroquine concentrations have been studied in 109 Kenyan children during the first 24 hours of admission to hospital with cerebral malaria (2[C]). Of the 109 children 100 had received chloroquine before admission. Blood chloroquine and desethylchloroquine concentrations were no higher in children who had seizures than in those who did not, suggesting that chloroquine does not play an important role in the development of seizures in malaria.

Side Effects of Drugs, Annual 25
J.K. Aronson, ed.

Special senses Chloroquine-induced *retinopathy* is well described. Three patients with chloroquine retinopathy have been studied with multifocal electroretinography (3[Ar]). All three had been taking chloroquine for rheumatological diseases and all had electroretinographic changes that were more sensitive than full field electroretinography. It may be that multifocal electroretinography will be a useful technique in the assessment of suspected cases of subtle chloroquine retinopathy.

Respiratory *Acute pneumonitis* probably due to chloroquine has been described (4[Ar]).

A 41-year-old man with chronic discoid lupus erythematosus was given chloroquine 150 mg bd for 10 days followed by 150 mg od. After 2 weeks he developed fever, a diffuse papular rash, dyspnea, and sputum. A chest X-ray showed peripheral pulmonary infiltrates. He improved on withdrawal of chloroquine and treatment with cefpiramide and roxithromycin. No organism was isolated. A subsequent oral challenge with chloroquine provoked a similar reaction.

Drug overdose Deaths from chloroquine overdose have been reported with doses as low as 2–3 g in adults, and the death rate is as high as 25%. The effects of chloroquine overdose include cardiac effects (such as *dysrhythmias*, *reduced myocardial contractility*, and *hypotension*) and central nervous system complications (such as *confusion*, *coma*, and *seizures*). There have been three more reports of chloroquine overdose, two from Oman (5[A]) and one from the Netherlands (6[A]). The two reports from Oman were similar to previously published reports of chloroquine overdose associated with cardiac dysfunction, confusion, and coma; both patients had standard treatment with activated charcoal, diazepam infusions, and positive inotropic drugs, and both survived. The single case report from Holland gave pharmacokinetic measurements performed before, during, and after hemoperfusion. This showed that hemoperfusion extracted very little chloroquine and was unlikely to be of any use in chloroquine overdose, as would be expected from the high protein binding and large volume of distribution of chloroquine.

Halofantrine *(SED-14, 968; SEDA-22, 304; SEDA-23, 305; SEDA-24, 331)*

Halofantrine has long been associated with *prolongation of the QT interval* and has fallen out of use in many parts of the world. There have already been several case reports of cardiac deaths related to its use and a further case of possible death due to a dysrhythmia has been reported in a woman who had taken halofantrine for malaria (7[A]). She had a normal electrocardiogram before treatment and no family history of heart disease.

Mefloquine *(SED-13, 808; SEDA-22, 304; SEDA-23, 303; SEDA-24, 332)*

Neuropsychiatric The use of mefloquine for the prophylaxis of malaria has been extensively reviewed, particularly with regard to the severe *neuropsychiatric disturbances* that occur in a minority of travelers. Two retrospective non-randomized postal studies of the use of mefloquine for prophylaxis against malaria have recently been published. Both included groups with no prophylaxis. Up to 25% of these travelers reported neuropsychiatric adverse events attributable to mefloquine.

A postal survey of 5446 returning Danish travelers examined the adverse effects of unstated doses of mefloquine, chloroquine, and chloroquine plus proguanil for malaria prophylaxis (8[C]). There were 4158 responders (76%); 1223 travelers took chloroquine, 1827 took chloroquine plus proguanil, and 809 took mefloquine. Overall, although chloroquine plus proguanil and chloroquine were associated with a large number of mild (mainly gastrointestinal) adverse effects, 30–50% had *diarrhea* and about 20% had *nausea* or *abdominal pain*. There was a significantly larger number of reported "unacceptable symptoms" (not defined): 2.7%, 1.0%, and 0.6% for mefloquine, chloroquine, and chloroquine plus proguanil respectively. Most of the more serious adverse events were in those who took mefloquine. Compared with chloroquine alone the relative risks (95%CI) of *"depression"*, *experiencing "strange thoughts"*, or *having altered spatial perception* were 5.1 (2.7, 9.5), 6.4 (2.5, 16.1), and 3.0 (1.4, 6.2) respectively. There was also a higher incidence of depression in women than in men. The relative risk of hospital admission or early termination of travel possibly related to prophylaxis was higher with mefloquine than with either chloroquine or chloroquine plus proguanil.

A postal survey of the incidence of neuropsychiatric disturbances in 2500 returning Israeli travelers (9[C]) showed that travelers with this class of adverse effects were more likely to have taken mefloquine than other antimalarials. Of 117 travelers with neuropsychiatric adverse effects, 115 had taken mefloquine compared with 948/1340 for the entire cohort. This was a retrospective postal study with a response rate of 54% (1340 out of 2500), and of those who responded 71% had taken mefloquine, 5% had taken chloroquine, and 24% had taken no prophylaxis. In this study 11% (117) of the respondents reported neuropsychiatric disturbances, mainly *sleep disturbance*, *fatigue*, *vivid dreams*, or *"lack of mood"*. Only 16 of the respondents had symptoms lasting 2 months or more. Those who had had a neuropsychiatric disturbance were also more likely to have been female and to have taken recreational drug use.

Although the above studies were limited by retrospective design, their results are in broad agreement with the results of other studies over the past few years that indicate that women have a higher incidence of neuropsychiatric adverse effects from mefloquine than men (10[Cr], 11[C]–13[C]).

There have been further case reports of neuropsychiatric problems with mefloquine.

> A 7-year-old Indian boy was diagnosed as having "cerebral malaria" and received quinine followed by mefloquine (dose not given) (14[A]). He developed hallucinations and removed his clothes and danced. His symptoms resolved within 24 hours of stopping mefloquine. This case highlights the fact that mefloquine should not be given after quinine in cases of severe malaria.

Liver *Raised transaminases* (up to 20 times normal activities) have been seen in a 68-year-old man taking mefloquine prophylaxis; they resolved after withdrawal of mefloquine (15[A]).

Skin Skin reactions to mefloquine have been reviewed, in relation to 74 case reports published between 1983 and 1997 (16[R]). *Pruritus* and *maculopapular rash* were the most common skin reactions associated with mefloquine: in some studies their approximate frequency was 4–10% for pruritus and up to 30% for non-specific maculopapular rashes. Adverse effects less commonly associated with mefloquine included urticaria, facial lesions, and cutaneous vasculitis. There was one case of *Stevens–Johnson syndrome* and one fatal case of *toxic epidermal necrolysis*.

Risk factors A recent study of the pharmacokinetics of oral mefloquine in 12 healthy adults (6 men, 6 women) over 10 weeks has given insights into *sex differences* in mefloquine pharmacokinetics (17[C]). Five weekly doses of mefloquine 250 mg were given to healthy volunteers. After this, half the subjects took 5 weekly doses of mefloquine 125 mg and half continued to have 250 mg per week. By the second week, all the subjects had plasma mefloquine concentrations over 1.5 μmol/l (the effective prophylactic threshold), but it was only after the fourth dose that the trough concentrations reached this threshold. The women had significantly higher values of C_{max} and $C_{min\,ss}$ than the men. Although the dose of mefloquine was reduced to 125 mg, the plasma mefloquine concentration was maintained above 1.5 μmol/l in all subjects. In this small study the most commonly reported adverse events were headache, insomnia, and vertigo, with most adverse events occurring between weeks 5 and 8, when plasma mefloquine concentrations were highest. Women had significantly more adverse events (number of days with adverse events/total number of days exposed 149/420) than men (43/420).

Women probably suffer more adverse events with mefloquine than men because of sex differences in mefloquine pharmacokinetics, which may explain why earlier studies in male military personnel failed to detect a higher proportion of neuropsychiatric problems with mefloquine compared with other prophylactic regimens.

Use in pregnancy A 7-day quinine regimen (10 mg/kg salt, 8-hourly for 7 days) has been compared with oral mefloquine 25 mg/kg plus artesunate 4 mg/kg/day for 3 days in 108 women on the Thai–Burmese border (18[C]). The mefloquine plus artesunate regimen was significantly more effective than quinine (day 63 cure rate 98% vs 67%). There were more episodes of *dizziness* (RR = 1.93; 95% CI = 1.14, 3.25) or *tinnitus* (RR = 3.93; 95% CI = 1.98, 7.80) with quinine, but no serious adverse events were attributable to either drug. There were also two *mid-trimester abortions* in the mefloquine plus artesunate group and none in the quinine treated group. There were no birth defects in either group. Although the numbers were very small, the authors concluded that despite a better parasitological cure rate the increased risk of abortion associated with mefloquine in pregnancy precluded its routine use. Larger studies are needed to confirm this observation.

Proguanil plus atovaquone

(SEDA 24, 333)

Proguanil plus atovaquone (Malarone™) has been studied for chemoprophylaxis of malaria in African children (19[C]) and in travelers (20[C]) and is formulated as a combination of proguanil 100 mg plus atovaquone 250 mg for daily dosing. Atovaquone is a hydroxynaphthoquinone that inhibits the electron transport system (bc_1 system) of parasites. Proguanil plus atovaquone is active against hepatic stages of *P. falciparum*, making it unnecessary to continue 4 weeks of prophylaxis after return from an endemic region. Current recommendations are that proguanil plus atovaquone should be continued for 1 week after returning from a malaria endemic region.

In a recent comparison of proguanil plus atovaquone with proguanil (100 mg/day) plus chloroquine (155 mg base weekly) in travelers, proguanil plus atovaquone was 100% effective in the prevention of malaria [20[C]). Those who received proguanil plus atovaquone (n = 540) had significantly fewer adverse events than those who received proguanil plus chloroquine (n = 543) (22% vs 28% respectively), particularly less *diarrhea*, *abdominal pain*, and *vomiting*. Only one person who took proguanil plus atovaquone had to discontinue prophylaxis owing to adverse events, as opposed to 10 who had to discontinue proguanil plus chloroquine. There have been no other studies of similar size on the use of proguanil plus atovaquone. This combination is becoming established for the prophylaxis of malaria and the results of further phase IV studies are awaited.

8-AMINOQUINOLINES (PRIMAQUINE AND CONGENERS) *(SED-14, 958; SEDA-22, 305; SEDA-23, 306; SEDA-24, 332)*

Tafenoquine

Tafenoquine (WR 238605) is an 8-aminoquinoline and a synthetic analogue of primaquine, proposed to have an improved therapeutic index and safety profile. It is active against all human forms of malaria. In animals tafenoquine is several times more potent than primaquine and is effective against both blood and liver stages of the malaria parasite. It has a half-life of 14 days, which makes it a good candidate for prophylaxis, with the possibility of monthly dosing.

There has been a randomized placebo-controlled study of tafenoquine as chemoprophylaxis for malaria in 426 Gabonese schoolchildren aged 12–20 years (21[C]). Children with G6PD deficiency were excluded. Radical cure of malaria was achieved with halofantrine followed by placebo or tafenoquine in the following daily doses: 250 mg, 125 mg, 62.5 mg, or 31.25 mg given for 3 days. Follow-up was for 77 days. Tafenoquine was highly effective in dosages over 62.5 mg/day.

There were 180 adverse events thought to be related to the study drug. All were mild and self-limiting and none was considered to be serious. They included *headache*, *fever*, *abdominal pain*, and *dizziness*. However, none was significantly more common with tafenoquine than placebo. On day 28, but at no other time, there was a small (0.4 g/daily) but significant *fall in hemoglobin concentration* with tafenoquine 250 mg/day.

Initial studies on tafenoquine suggest that it is promising for the prophylaxis of malaria, although further studies in non-immune travelers and more information about its safety profile are required. The safety of tafenoquine in people with G6PD deficiency is not known.

ENDOPEROXIDES

Artemisinin and its derivatives

(SED-14, 966; SEDA-22, 302; SEDA-23, 305; SEDA-24, 331)

The artemisinin derivatives derive from extracts of the sweet wormwood plant, which has been used in China for thousands of years. These compounds are useful in the treatment of uncomplicated and severe malaria. The artemisinin derivatives have short half-lives and should be used in combination with other agents.

Nervous system There has long been concern about possible *brainstem damage* caused by the artemisinin derivatives after animal studies showed brainstem damage in some species given high doses of artemether. However, a recent study of brainstem auditory evoked potentials showed no electrophysiological evidence of brainstem damage in adults treated with artemisinin derivatives (22[C]).

Artesunate plus lumefantrine

There has been a recent meta-analysis of 15 trials from Africa, Europe, and Asia of the use of varying doses of artesunate plus lumefantrine compared with several alternative antimalarials in 1869 patients conducted by the drug company Novartis into its clinical safety and tolerability in the treatment of uncomplicated malaria (23[Cr]). The most common adverse events were gastrointestinal – *nausea* (6.3%), *abdominal pain* (12%), *vomiting* (2.4%), *anorexia* (13%) – or central nervous – *headache* (21%) or *dizziness* (16%). There were 20 serious adverse events with artesunate plus lumefantrine, but only one (*hemolytic anemia*) was possibly due to artesunate plus lumefantrine. There was no QT prolongation associated with artesunate plus lumefantrine.

TETRACYCLINES (see also Chapter 25)

Doxycycline

Gastrointestinal *Esophageal ulceration* occurred in two adults taking doxycycline as malaria chemoprophylaxis (24[A]).

A 20-year-old woman returned from Africa, where she had been taking doxycycline malaria prophylaxis. Six days before admission she took a doxycycline capsule (dose not stated) before going to bed. She awoke hours later with the feeling that the capsule was stuck in her esophagus. Over the next 4 days she developed worsening dysphagia. Esophagoscopy showed an esophageal ulcer over 20% of the esophageal surface. She was treated with ranitidine and sucralfate and improved over the next 2 days.

A 27-year-old man with an 8-day history of dysphagia and retrosternal pain was taking doxycycline prophylaxis and occasional terfenadine (doses not stated). He recalled no problems with taking any of his doxycycline prophylaxis. He had an esophagoscopy, which showed a 1 cm esophageal ulcer. He improved with ranitidine.

Metabolic Although other tetracyclines have been associated with *hypoglycemia*, the first reported case of doxycycline-induced hypoglycemia has been reported (25[A]).

A 70-year-old man with type II diabetes mellitus presented with sudden confusion, which rapidly progressed to loss of consciousness. The only drug he had taken during the previous 2 months was doxycycline (100 mg/day), which he had taken for 5 days for an upper respiratory tract infection. Urine tests for sulfonylureas were negative. Routine hematological and biochemical tests and an electrocardiogram were normal. He improved with intravenous glucose and withdrawal of doxycycline and had no further episodes of hypoglycemia over the next 3 months.

Plasma insulin was not measured in this case, so the mechanism of hypoglycemia is unclear.

DRUGS USED FOR *PNEUMOCYSTIS CARINII* PNEUMONIA *(SEDA-14, 970; SEDA-22, 307; SEDA-23, 307, SEDA-24, 334)*

Co-trimoxazole (trimethoprim plus sulfamethoxazole) (see also Chapter 26)

Co-trimoxazole is the drug of choice for the treatment and prophylaxis of *Pneumocystis carinii* pneumonia. It is cheap and highly effective and there is long experience of its use in both HIV-positive and HIV-negative patients.

A high incidence of adverse events has been attributed to co-trimoxazole. The sulfamethoxazole component is the thought to be the cause of most cases of sensitivity. Adverse events to co-trimoxazole are far more common in HIV-positive patients, with a reported frequency of about 10–64%, compared with a frequency of 3% in HIV-negative cases.

A recent pharmacogenetic study has shown no differences in polymorphisms in the gene frequencies of CYP2C9, glutathione S-transferase isoforms, and slow acetylator genes between patients with co-trimoxazole hypersensitivity compared with controls without co-trimoxazole hypersensitivity (26[Cr]). This suggests that polymorphisms in these genes for drug metabolizing enzymes are not important predisposing factors to co-trimoxazole adverse events.

Cardiovascular There have been previous reports of prolongation of the *QT interval* due to co-trimoxazole, and a recent report identified a man with Marfan's syndrome with a prolonged QT interval caused by co-trimoxazole (27[Ar]). He had a single nucleotide polymorphism in the KCNE2 gene, which encodes a subunit of a potassium channel and is present in 1.6% of the general population. The investigators expressed this channel in a Chinese hamster ovary heterologous expression system and showed that potassium flux was impaired by sulfamethoxazole at therapeutic concentrations.

Nervous system There has been a further case report of *tremor* induced by co-trimoxazole (28[A]).

A 66-year-old man with diabetes mellitus, who was taking corticosteroids and home oxygen for pulmonary fibrosis, developed a lung infection with *Nocardia*. He was treated for 3 weeks with intravenous co-trimoxazole (1.92 g/day) followed by oral co-trimoxazole (3.04 g/day). He was also taking theophylline, salmeterol, budesonide, prednisolone, ranitidine, insulin, doxazosin, and simvastatin. After 3 days of he developed a severe tremor, which improved on withdrawal of co-trimoxazole. No other medication was altered and theophylline concentrations and blood O_2 and CO_2 saturation were within the expected limits.

There has been a report of *delirium* caused by co-trimoxazole in an HIV-positive man (29[A]).

A 54-year-old HIV-positive man was being treated for disseminated histoplasmosis and *Pneumo-*

cystis carinii pneumonia with amphotericin and co-trimoxazole. After 9 days he became disoriented, with visual and auditory hallucinations. An MRI scan, cerebrospinal fluid examination, and hematological tests were all normal. The co-trimoxazole was withdrawn and he was lucid again within 3 days.

Acute confusion has been associated with co-trimoxazole before, but never in a HIV-positive patient.

There have been several previous case reports of *aseptic meningitis* associated with co-trimoxazole and there have been a further three reports in HIV-negative patients with urinary or respiratory tract infections (30[Ar], 31[AR], 32[A]). It may be that aseptic meningitis is a more common adverse event with co-trimoxazole than has previously been thought.

Electrolyte balance *Hyperkalemia* associated with trimethoprim both in standard and high-dose regimens has been increasingly recognized as a problem and has been recently reviewed (33[R]). Hyperkalemia is thought to result from the amiloride-like action of trimethoprim on the distal nephron. In the presence of other risk factors, such as renal insufficiency, hypoaldosteronism, potassium-altering drugs, or older age, the hyperkalemia can be severe.

Liver A mild rise in serum transaminases or cholestatic hepatotoxicity are well reported with co-trimoxazole and usually start after a latent period of several weeks and are associated with a rash. There have been very few case reports of *fulminant hepatic failure* associated with co-trimoxazole, but recently a report of a fatal case has appeared (34[A]).

A 32-year-old woman presented with a 2-week history of a pruritic maculopapular rash and fever. She had taken a 12-day course of co-trimoxazole that had finished 5 days before and was taking no other drugs. On admission she had normal hematological indices but a raised alkaline phosphatase and aspartate aminotransferase. Serological testing for Epstein–Barr virus, hepatitis A, B, and C, cytomegalovirus, echo virus, rubella, and measles showed no evidence of recent infection. Her rash improved but her general condition worsened and steroids were started. Abdominal CT showed a large liver with a moderate amount of ascites. The aspartate aminotransferase rose to 1330 IU/l and the prothrombin time increased. She developed progressive liver failure and died while awaiting liver transplant. At autopsy the liver showed signs of massive hepatic necrosis with no other abnormalities.

There has been a further report of pancytopenia and renal and hepatic failure after a 48-year-old man had taken co-trimoxazole (35[Ar]).

Skin There has been a report of *cutaneous depigmentation* associated with co-trimoxazole (36[A]).

A 41-year-old man who was HIV-positive was given co-trimoxazole for interstitial pneumonia. Two weeks after the start of treatment he developed a fever and rash with intense desquamation. A skin biopsy was consistent with a drug eruption. The co-trimoxazole was withdrawn and he was given prednisolone. The desquamation improved but left generalized hypopigmentation. The depigmentation was so severe that he gave the impression of being albino. A further skin biopsy examined by electron microscopy showed an absence of melanocytes along the basal layer.

Depigmentation is a very rare reaction to co-trimoxazole.

There has been a single case report of *toxic epidermal necrolysis* caused by co-trimoxazole, improving with high-dose methylprednisolone (37[A]). However, previous studies of the use of steroids in toxic epidermal necrolysis have given contradictory results.

Management of adverse drug reactions There have been several recent studies that have attempted to evaluate new methods to reduce the incidence of adverse events with co-trimoxazole and methods to desensitize patients with known hypersensitivity.

In a well-designed, multicenter, randomized, double-blind study 372 HIV-positive patients were randomized to receive co-trimoxazole suspension gradually increasing to a dose of 960 mg/day over 2 weeks or co-trimoxazole tablets in a dosage of 960 mg/day (38[C]). The patients were followed up for 12 weeks. There were significantly fewer withdrawals in the gradual initiation group than in the tablet group (17% vs 33%) and fewer episodes of *rash*, *fever*, and *pruritus* in the patients who gradually started co-trimoxazole prophylaxis.

A method of oral desensitization to co-trimoxazole has been described in 17 HIV-positive patients who had previous hypersensitivity reactions to co-trimoxazole (39[C]). Desensitization was performed with a starting dose of

5 mg increasing every 12 hours up to a dose of 1 g on day 5. All but two of the patients successfully completed the course. The absence of controls makes this study hard to evaluate, but the 5-day desensitization technique was safe.

Another uncontrolled trial of a 6-day desensitization procedure in 33 cases has been reported (40[C]). The protocol started with a dose of 0.2 mg rising to 800 mg over 6 days and 32 of the subjects successfully completed the course. In addition, 12 of 14 cases were successfully rechallenged with co-trimoxazole. However, this study lacked a clear description of follow-up or the reasons for the selection of subjects for desensitization or rechallenge, and cannot be used as a basis for recommending this desensitization technique.

In a randomized study of desensitization with rechallenge in HIV-positive patients with previous adverse effects of co-trimoxazole 73 patients were given a 14-day course of trimethoprim 200 mg/day (41[C]). Fourteen had adverse reactions to trimethoprim. The remaining 59 subjects were randomized to a 2-day desensitization technique (34 subjects) or rechallenge (25 subjects). There were seven hypersensitivity reactions in both groups. Clearly there is no advantage of this 2-day desensitization technique over rechallenge with co-trimoxazole in HIV-positive individuals.

Overall it appears that desensitization to co-trimoxazole is safe in the absence of previous serious adverse events, although it is not yet certain whether desensitization is better than rechallenge or indeed what the ideal desensitization method should be.

DRUGS USED FOR TOXOPLASMOSIS

Sulfadiazine (SEDA-22, 309)

Urinary tract Sulfadiazine in combination with pyrimethamine is a highly effective treatment for cerebral toxoplasmosis. Sulfadiazine-related *nephrolithiasis* was common in the 1940s and has re-emerged with the reintroduction of sulfadiazine for HIV-related infections. There has been a further report of four cases of sulfadiazine-related nephrolithiasis presenting with oliguria, abdominal pain, and renal insufficiency (42[Ar]). All were successfully treated with rehydration and alkalinization of the urine. None required dialysis, but one required a nephrostomy tube.

DRUGS USED FOR LEISHMANIASIS

Pentavalent antimonials

(SED-14, 984; SEDA-23, 310; SEDA-24, 336)

Systemic treatment of South American leishmaniasis is recommended, because of the risk of spread of parasites to mucous membranes. There has been a further comparison of two pentavalent antimonials, meglumine antimoniate ($n = 47$) and sodium stibogluconate ($n = 64$) (43[C]). The trial was too small to examine the efficacy of the two drugs, but there were more adverse events with sodium stibogluconate, with a greater proportion with *raised transaminase and amylase activities*. There were no differences in electrocardiographic abnormalities between the two groups.

Visceral leishmaniasis has been traditionally treated with pentavalent antimonial compounds, but over the last 10 years newer drugs and combinations have become available, such as amphotericin and liposomal amphotericin, paromomycin (aminosidine), and miltefosine (a promising oral agent). The new treatment options for visceral leishmaniasis have been recently reviewed (44[R]).

There has been a open randomized comparison of sodium stibogluconate either alone ($n = 50$) or in combination with two regimens of paromomycin ($n = 52$ and $n = 48$) (45[C]). There was improved parasitological cure in both groups given combination therapy. There were no differences in adverse events or biochemical and hematological measurements between any of the treatment arms. There was one serious adverse event (*myocarditis*) in the sodium stibogluconate monotherapy group. It should be noted that there were insufficient auditory examinations performed to assess any ototoxic effects of paromomycin.

DRUGS USED FOR HUMAN AFRICAN TRYPANOSOMIASIS

Eflornithine

Melarsoprol (an arsenical compound) is still the most effective compound against stage II (CNS) disease in both East and West African trypanosomiasis. However, it is toxic and causes death in about 2–8% of subjects treated. Eflornithine, an inhibitor of polyamine synthesis, is an alternative to melarsoprol for West African trypanosomiasis (both early and late). However, eflornithine is very expensive, and its usefulness in endemic areas may therefore be limited. The standard regimen for eflornithine is 100 mg/kg intravenously 6-hourly for 14 days. There have been some anecdotal reports that a shorter 7-day course of eflornithine may be equally effective, with obvious cost-saving advantages.

There has been a recent multicenter, randomized, open comparison of treatment with eflornithine for 7 or 14 days ($n = 321$) (46[C]). The subjects were divided into new cases and relapses. The 14-day course of eflornithine was superior to the 7-day course for the new cases, but there was no difference in the relapsing cases. However, the numbers of patients who relapsed were small ($n = 47$) and this may not have allowed the detection of a small difference between the groups. The most common adverse events associated with eflornithine were *convulsions*, *altered consciousness*, *diarrhea*, *vomiting*, *nausea*, *abdominal pain*, and *secondary infections*. Diarrhea and secondary infection were more common in subjects who took the 14-day course.

OTHER COMPOUNDS

Atovaquone plus azithromycin

Human babesiosis has been traditionally treated with quinine plus clindamycin. Quinine plus clindamycin have recently been compared with atovaquone plus azithromycin in human babesiosis in a randomized, multicenter, unblinded study (47[C]). The treatments were both completely effective. There were considerably fewer adverse events with azithromycin plus atovaquone than with quinine plus clindamycin.

Metronidazole *(SED-14, 977; SEDA-21, 301; SEDA-22, 311; SEDA-23, 309)*

Metronidazole is the drug of choice for many protozoal infections, including amebiasis, giardiasis, and trichomoniasis. A *disulfiram-like reaction*, *nausea*, and a *metallic taste* are common adverse effects.

Nervous system There has been a report of *visual loss and headache* after metronidazole (48[A]).

> A 68-year-old man with a tooth abscess had a tooth extraction and received amoxicillin. A few weeks later he developed toothache again and was given amoxicillin and metronidazole 400 mg tds; he took no other drugs. Six hours after the first dose he developed a headache. He continued with metronidazole for a total of three doses and 6 hours after the last dose the headache resolved. Two days later he noticed flashing lights in both eyes. He then developed a central visual field defect and progressive visual loss. His blood pressure was 220/120 mmHg, but it settled spontaneously. Visual acuity was 6/12 in both eyes and fundoscopy showed marked disc swelling with hemorrhages, without other features of hypertensive retinopathy. Full blood count, plasma viscosity, routine biochemistry, vasculitis screen, anticardiolipin antibodies, angiotensin converting enzyme assay, chest X-ray, CT of the brain and orbits, MRI, and MRA were all normal. CSF examination showed an opening pressure of 24 cm of water and 13 white cells/μl. Over the next few months his visual symptoms slowly improved but he developed secondary optic atrophy.

In this case there was no other obvious cause for visual loss and it could have been caused by metronidazole. The exact mechanism was unclear, but it may have been related to raised intracranial pressure.

There has been a report of *convulsions* in an 87-year-old man who had taken metronidazole (49[A]) and a further report of metronidazole-associated peripheral neuropathy (50[A]), which is a relatively well recognized adverse event.

Pancreas There has been a further report of pancreatitis attributed to metronidazole in a 61-year-old woman given intravenous metronidazole 500 mg 6-hourly (51[A]). The relation between pancreatitis and metronidazole in this case was less convincing than in previously reported cases, as there was no rechallenge.

Genotoxic effects There has been concern

that metronidazole may be genotoxic, as there have been reports of mutagenicity in several bacterial species. The genotoxic effects of metronidazole (250 mg bd for 10 days) and nalixidic acid (400 mg bd for 10 days) have been assessed in women with *Trichomonas vaginalis* infection (52^C). The genotoxic potential of these drugs was evaluated using a sister chromatid exchange test in peripheral blood lymphocytes. Metronidazole had no effect but nalidixic acid caused an increase in sister chromatid exchange frequency. This result confirms that there is little evidence of genotoxicity with metronidazole.

REFERENCES

1. Molle I, Christensen KL, Hansen PS, Dragsted UB, Aarup M, Buhl MR. Use of medical chemoprophylaxis and antimosquito precautions in Danish malaria patients and their traveling companions. J Travel Med 2000; 7: 253–8.
2. Crawley J, Kokwaro G, Ouma D, Watkins W, Marsh K. Chloroquine is not a risk factor for seizures in childhood cerebral malaria. Trop Med Int Health 2000; 5: 860–4.
3. Kellner U, Kraus H, Foerster MH. Multifocal ERG in chloroquine retinopathy: regional variance of retinal dysfunction. Graefe's Arch Clin Exp Ophthalmol 2000; 238: 94–7.
4. Mitja K, Izidor K, Music E. Chloroquine-induced drug-hypersensitivity. Pneumologie 2000; 54: 395–7.
5. Reddy VG, Sinna S. Chloroquine poisoning: report of two cases. Acta Anaesthesiol Scand 2000; 44: 1017–20.
6. Boereboom FTJ, Ververs FFT, Meulenbelt J, Van DA. Hemoperfusion is ineffectual in severe chloroquine poisoning. Crit Care Med 2000; 28: 3346–50.
7. Malvy D, Receveur MC, Ozon P, Djossou F, Le Metayer P, Touze JE, Longy-Boursier M, Le Bras M. Fatal cardiac incident after use of halofantrine. J Travel Med 2000; 7: 215–16.
8. Petersen E, Ronne T, Ronn A, Bygbjerg I, Larsen SO. Reported side effects to chloroquine, chloroquine plus proguanil, and mefloquine as chemoprophylaxis against malaria in Danish travelers. J Travel Med 2000; 7: 79–84.
9. Potasman I, Beny A, Seligmann H. Neuropsychiatric problems in 2,500 long-term young travelers to the tropics. J Travel Med 2000; 7: 5–9.
10. Schwartz EI, Rotenberg M, Almog S, Sadetzki S. Serious adverse events of mefloquine in relation to blood level and gender. Am J Trop Med Hyg 2001; 65: 189–92.
11. Huzley D. Malaria chemoprophylaxis in German tourists: a prospective study on compliance and adverse effects. J Travel Med 1996; 3: 148–55.
12. Phillips M, Kass R. User acceptability patterns of mefloquine and doxycycline malaria chemoprophylaxis. J Travel Med 1996; 3: 10–15.
13. Schlagenhauf P, Steffen R, Lobel H, Johnson R, Letz R, Tschopp A, Vranjes N, Bergqvist Y, Ericsson O, Hellgren U, et al. Mefloquine tolerability during chemoprophylaxis: focus on adverse event assessments, stereo chemistry and compliance. Trop Med Int Health 1996; 1: 485–94.
14. Havaldar PV, Mogale KD. Mefloquine-induced psychosis. Pediatr Infect Dis J 2000; 19: 166–7.
15. Gotsman I, Azaz-Livshits T, Fridlender Z, Muszkat M, Ben-Chetrit E. Mefloquine-induced acute hepatitis. Pharmacotherapy 2000; 20: 1517–19.
16. Smith HR, Croft AM, Black MM. Dermatological adverse effects with the antimalarial drug mefloquine: a review of 74 published case reports. Clin Exp Dermatol 1999; 24: 249–54.
17. Kollaritsch H, Karbwang J, Wiedermann G, Mikolasek A, Na-Bangchang K, Wernsdorfer WH. Mefloquine concentration profiles during prophylactic dose regimens. Wien Klin Wochenschr 2000; 112: 441–7.
18. McGready R, Brockman A, Cho T, Cho D, Van Vugt M, Luxemburger C, Congsuphajaisiddhi T, White NJ, Nosten F. Randomized comparison of mefloquine–artesunate versus quinine in the treatment of multidrug-resistant falciparum malaria in pregnancy. Trans R Soc Trop Med 2000; 94: 689–93.
19. Lell B, Luckner D, Ndjave M, Scott T, Kremsner PG. Randomised placebo-controlled study of atovaquone plus proguanil for malaria prophylaxis in children. Lancet 1998; 351: 709–13.
20. Høgh B, Clarke PD, Camus D, Nothdurft HD, Overbosch D, Günther M, Joubert I, Kain KC, Shaw D, Roskell NS, et al. Atovaquone–proguanil versus chloroquine–proguanil for malaria prophylaxis in non-immune travellers: a randomised, double-blind study. Lancet 2000; 356: 1888–94.
21. Lell B, Faucher JF, Missinou MA, Borrmann S, Dangelmaier O, Horton J, Kremsner PG. Malaria chemoprophylaxis with tafenoquine: a randomised study. Lancet 2000; 355: 2041–5.
22. Van Vugt M, Angus BJ, Price RN, Mann C, Simpson JA, Poletto C, Htoo SE, Looareesuwan S, White NJ, Nosten F. A case-control auditory evaluation of patients treated with artemisinin derivatives for multidrug-resistant *Plasmodium falciparum* malaria. Am J Trop Med Hyg 2000; 62: 65–9.
23. Bakshi R, Hermeling-Fritz I, Gathmann I, Alteri E. An integrated assessment of the clinical safety of artemether–lumefantrine: a new oral fixed-dose combination antimalarial drug. Trans R Soc Trop Med 2000; 94: 419–24.
24. Morris TJ, Davis TP. Doxycycline-induced esophageal ulceration in the US Military Service. Mil Med 2000; 165: 316–19.

25. Odeh M, Oliven A. Doxycycline-induced hypoglycemia. J Clin Pharmacol 2000; 40: 1173–4.
26. Pirmohamed M, Alfirevic A, Vilar J, Stalford A, Wilkins EGL, Sim E, Park BK. Association analysis of drug metabolizing enzyme gene polymorphisms in HIV-positive patients with co-trimoxazole hypersensitivity. Pharmacogenetics 2000; 10: 705–13.
27. Sesti F, Abbott GW, Wei J, Murray KT, Saksena S, Schwartz PJ, Priori SG, Roden DM, George AL Jr, Goldstein SAN. A common polymorphism associated with antibiotic-induced cardiac arrhythmia. Proc Natl Acad Sci USA 2000; 97: 10613–18.
28. De Arce Borda AM, Goenaga Sanchez MA. Tremor produced by trimethoprim–sulphamethoxazole. Neurologia 2000; 15: 264–5.
29. Salkind AR. Acute delirium induced by intravenous trimethoprim-sulfamethoxazole therapy in a patient with the acquired immunodeficiency syndrome. Hum Exp Toxicol 2000; 19: 149–51.
30. Andrade A, Hilmas E, Walter C. A rare occurrence of trimethoprim/sulfamethoxazole (TMP/SMX)-induced aseptic meningitis in an older woman. J Am Geriatr Soc 2000; 48: 1537–8.
31. Capra C, Mario MG, Meazza G, Ramella G. Trimethoprim–sulfamethoxazole-induced aseptic meningitis: case report and literature review. Intensive Care Med 2000; 26: 212–14.
32. Meng MV, St Lezin M. Trimethoprim–sulfamethoxazole induced recurrent aseptic meningitis. J Urol 2000; 164: 1664–5.
33. Perazella MA. Trimethoprim-induced hyperkalaemia. Clinical data, mechanism, prevention and management. Drug Saf 2000; 22: 227–36.
34. Tse W, Singer C, Dominick D. Acute fulminant hepatic failure caused by trimethoprim–sulfamethoxazole. Infect Dis Clin Pract 2000; 9: 302–3.
35. Windecker R, Steffen J, Cascorbi I, Thurmann PA. Co-trimoxazole-induced liver and renal failure. Case report. Eur J Clin Pharmacol 2000; 56: 191–3.
36. Martinez-Ruiz E, Ortega C, Calduch L, Molina I, Montesinos E, Revert A, Cardá C, Navarro V, Jordá E. Generalized cutaneous depigmentation following sulfamide-induced drug eruption. Dermatology 2000; 201: 252–4.
37. Soylu H, Akkol N, Erduran E, Aslan Y, Gunes Z, Yildiran A. Co-trimoxazole-induced toxic epidermal necrolysis treated with high dose methylprednisolone. Ann Med Sci 2000; 9: 38–40.
38. Para MF, Finkelstein D, Becker S, Dohn M, Walawander A, Black JR, and AIDS Clinical Trials Group 268 Study Team. Reduced toxicity with gradual initiation of trimethoprim–sulfamethoxazole as primary prophylaxis for *Pneumocystis carinii* pneumonia: AIDS clinical trials group 268. J Acquired Immune Defic Syndr 2000; 24: 337–43.
39. Yoshizawa S, Yasuoka A, Kikuchi Y, Honda M, Gatanaga H, Tachikawa N, Hirabayashi Y, Oka S. A 5-day course of oral desensitization to trimethoprim/sulfamethoxazole (T/S) in patients with human immunodeficiency virus type-1 infection who were previously intolerant to T/S. Ann Allergy Asthma Immunol 2000; 85: 241–4.
40. Lopez-Serrano MC, Moreno-Ancillo A. Drug hypersensitivity reactions in HIV-infected patients. Induction of cotrimoxazole tolerance. Allergol Inmunol Clin 2000; 15: 347–51.
41. Bonfanti P, Pusterla L, Parazzini F, Libanore M, Cagni AE, Franzetti M, Faggion I, Landonio S, Quirino T. The effectiveness of desensitization versus rechallenge treatment in HIV-positive patients with previous hypersensitivity to TMP-SMX: a randomized multicentric study. Biomed Pharmacother 2000; 54: 45–9.
42. Crespo M, Quereda C, Pascual J, Rivera M, Clemente L, Cano T. Patterns of sulfadiazine acute nephrotoxicity. Clin Nephrol 2000; 54: 68–72.
43. Saldanha ACR, Romero GAS, Guerra C, Merchan-Hamann E, De Oliveira Macedo V. Comparative study between sodium stibogluconate BP 88 and meglumine antimoniate in cutaneous leishmaniasis treatment. II. Biochemical and cardiac toxicity. Rev Soc Bras Med Trop 2000; 33: 383–8.
44. Murray HW. Treatment of visceral leishmaniasis (kala-azar): a decade of progress and future approaches. Int J Infect Dis 2000; 4: 158–77.
45. Thakur CP, Kanyok TP, Pandey AK, Sinha GP, Zaniewski AE, Houlihan HH, Oliaro P. A prospective randomized, comparative, open-label trial of the safety and efficacy of paromomycin (aminosidine) plus sodium stibogluconate versus sodium stibogluconate alone for the treatment of visceral leishmaniasis. Trans R Soc Trop Med 2000; 94: 429–31.
46. Pépin J, Khonde N, Maiso F, Doua F, Jaffar S, Ngampo S, Mpia B, Mbulamberi D, Kuzoe F. Short-course eflornithine in Gambian trypanosomiasis: a multicentre randomized controlled trial. Bull WHO 2000; 78: 1284–95.
47. Krause PJ, Lepore T, Sikand VK, Gadbaw J Jr, Burke G, Telford III SR, Brassard P, Pearl D, Azlanzadeh J, Christianson D, et al. Atovaquone and azithromycin for the treament of babesiosis. New Engl J Med 2000; 343: 1454–8.
48. Allroggen H, Abbott RJ, Bibby K. Acute visual loss following administration of metronidazole: a case report. Neuro-Ophthalmology 2000; 23: 89–94.
49. Beloosesky Y, Grosman B, Marmelstein V, Grinblat J. Convulsions induced by metronidazole treatment for *Clostridium difficile*-associated disease in chronic renal failure. Am J Med Sci 2000; 319: 338–9.
50. Freedman B, Shah S, Lau A. Metronidazole-induced peripheral neuropathy. J Appl Ther Res 2000; 3: 49–54.
51. Sura ME, Heinrich KA, Suseno M. Metronidazole-associated pancreatitis. Ann Pharmacother 2000; 34: 1152–5.
52. Akyol D, Mungan T, Baltaci V. A comparative study of genotoxic effects in the treatment of *Trichomonas vaginalis* infection: metronidazole or nalidixic acid. Arch Gynecol Obstet 2000; 264: 20–3.

D.J. Jeffries

29 Antiviral drugs

DRUGS ACTIVE AGAINST *HERPES SIMPLEX* AND *VARICELLA ZOSTER* VIRUSES

Three acyclic nucleoside drugs have been licensed for the treatment of infections with α-herpesviruses (*Herpes simplex* and *Varicella zoster*). Their mode of action against a virus-specific target (herpesvirus-encoded thymidine kinase) has meant that toxicity has been generally very low.

Aciclovir *(SED-14, 990; SEDA-23, 314)*

Nervous system Neurotoxicity represents the only major adverse effect of aciclovir, and this is mainly associated with high plasma concentrations resulting from impaired renal function. Although the risk is greatest with intravenous administration, neurotoxicity has previously been noted with oral use. *Coma* has been attributed to oral aciclovir (1[A]).

A 73-year-old man with acute respiratory failure, presumed to be secondary to amiodarone toxicity, developed sepsis and acute renal insufficiency, and required intermittent hemodialysis. Following a *Herpes simplex* labial infection he was treated with oral aciclovir (400 mg tds). The next day he became sleepy, disoriented, and agitated. Over the next 48 hours his neurological condition deteriorated and he responded to pain only, had uncoordinated eye movements, tremors, facial and jaw myoclonus, increased reflexes, and hypertonia. After 7 days of aciclovir he became unresponsive and comatose. Aciclovir was withdrawn and hemodialysis carried out more frequently. His neurological status improved over a period of 4 days. Trough plasma concentrations of aciclovir were well above the upper limit of the usual target range.

This appears to be the first case of coma attributable to oral aciclovir. The fact that the patient was receiving oral rather than intravenous aciclovir and was on regular hemodialysis made neurotoxicity unlikely, and this emphasizes the need to be wary of this potentially serious complication in seriously ill elderly patients.

Immunologic *Contact sensitization* to aciclovir is rare, but frequent application to inflamed skin in relapsing *Herpes simplex* may increase the risk of allergy. Severe contact dermatitis in a teenager has been reported (2[A]).

A 16-year-old girl with an 11-year history of frequent cold sores developed an erythematous rash and severe contact dermatitis during oral and topical aciclovir therapy. Patch tests showed contact sensitization to aciclovir and to the related compound ganciclovir.

Famciclovir *(SED-14, 991; SEDA-23, 315)*

In a study of oral famciclovir versus oral aciclovir, designed to demonstrate equivalence of efficacy of the two drugs in the treatment of mucocutaneous *Herpes simplex* infection in HIV-infected individuals, there was no difference in the incidence or nature of adverse effects in the two groups (3[C]). None of the withdrawals from the trial was considered by the investigator to be related to the study medication.

DRUGS ACTIVE AGAINST CYTOMEGALOVIRUS

Cidofovir *(SED-14, 989; SEDA-23, 314; SEDA-24, 340)*

Sensory systems Iritis, uveitis, and macular edema have been recorded in previous Annu-

Side Effects of Drugs, Annual 25
J.K. Aronson, ed.

als. In a study of compassionate use of intravenous cidofovir in AIDS patients with CMV retinitis, *iritis* developed in 21 of 51 individuals (4[c]). The appearance of this inflammatory process did not fit the characteristics of the vitritis associated with immune reconstitution, or with HIV-induced vitritis. The high rate in this cohort (compared with a 5–7% incidence in randomized trials) was associated with severe CMV retinitis, and the authors suggested that breakdown of the blood–ocular barrier in these patients may promote higher intraocular concentrations of cidofovir and thus enhance local toxicity. Previous correlations of prior use of HIV protease inhibitors with iritis were not confirmed in this study, although patients with iritis had better immunological and virological status than those without the disease.

During long-term follow up of patients with AIDS treated with parenteral cidofovir for CMV retinitis, the median time to discontinuation for intolerance was 6.6 months (5[C]). Cidofovir-associated *uveitis* occurred in 10 of 58 patients and ocular hypotonia (a 50% fall in intraocular pressure from baseline to below 5 mmHg) occurred at a rate of 0.16 per person-year. There were 51 episodes of proteinuria in 30 of the 58 patients and 82% of these episodes resolved on withdrawal (median time to resolution 20 days). No nephrotoxic events required dialysis.

Fomivirsen *(SEDA-24, 341)*

The antisense phosphorothioate oligonucleotide fomivirsen has been developed for intravitreal administration in AIDS patients with CMV retinitis who are intolerant to or have a contraindication for other treatments.

Sensory systems Previously described adverse effects include uveitis and increased ocular pressure. In 309 eyes of 238 patients there were two cases of *bull's-eye maculopathy*, which resolved after withdrawal (6[A]). In another case *nyctalopia and reduced visual acuity* (20/50 od) occurred in conjunction with mid peripheral epithelial pigmentation and cotton-wool spots around the perifoveal capillary network (7[A]).

Foscarnet *(SED-14, 989; SEDA-24, 340)*

Electrolyte balance The nephrotoxic effects of foscarnet, when used to treat CMV disease in immunocompromised patients, are well-recognized. Significant *electrolyte abnormalities* have been attributed to foscarnet in a bone-marrow transplant recipient on parenteral nutrition (8[A]).

A 39-year-old man with acute myelogenous leukemia developed a fever after allogeneic bone-marrow transplantation and was given prophylactic ganciclovir and antibiotics. Parenteral nutrition was started when severe mucositis and diarrhea limited oral nutrition. On the 18th day after transplantation CMV DNA was detected in his blood and he was given foscarnet. His requirements for potassium, calcium, magnesium, and phosphorus increased dramatically, while his sodium requirements fell. Electrolyte depletion occurred within 24 hours and was accompanied by deteriorating renal function (serum creatinine 106–220, reference range 60–125 μmol/l). On withdrawal of foscarnet, the serum creatinine fell within 24 hours and the electrolyte concentrations returned to normal.

Metal metabolism Recognizing that foscarnet is a potent chelator of divalent cations, and that acute ionized *hypocalcemia* and *hypomagnesemia* are common adverse effects, a trial of intravenous magnesium sulfate has been conducted for foscarnet-induced hypocalcemia and hypomagnesemia in 12 AIDS patients with CMV infection (9[c]). Increasing doses of magnesium sulfate reduced or eliminated foscarnet-induced ionized hypomagnesemia but had no discernible effect on ionized hypocalcemia, despite significant increases in serum parathyroid hormone concentrations. On this basis, intravenous supplementation for patients with normal serum magnesium concentrations was not recommended during treatment with foscarnet.

Ganciclovir *(SED-14, 990; SEDA-24, 341)*

Hematologic The major adverse effects of *neutropenia* and *thrombocytopenia* continue to be reported in recent studies, as does the beneficial effect of granulocyte colony stimulating factor (G-CSF) in countering neutropenia. In a study of oral ganciclovir in 36 severely immunocompromised HIV-positive children with CMV disease, toxicity was minimal and manageable and similar to that in adults in controlled trials of the oral formulation (10[C]). About 20% of the children withdrew, mainly as a result of intolerance of the large volume of oral suspension or numerous capsules. As with adults, neutropenia was the main toxic effect and this was successfully treated with G-CSF.

Drug administration route Treatment options for CMV retinitis include the intravitreal insertion of ganciclovir implants. This mechanism of drug delivery has the attraction of avoiding systemic drug toxicity, but the inherent danger of introducing *bacterial infection* has been highlighted by a case report (11[A]).

A 42-year-old man with AIDS and a history of CMV retinitis developed pain in his right eye and decreased visual acuity 10 days after receiving a ganciclovir intraocular implant into that eye. A therapeutic vitrectomy was performed and a vitreal tap produced frank pus and white fluffy debris. Cultures grew oxacillin-resistant *Staphylococcus aureus* sensitive only to vancomycin, rifampicin, and co-trimoxazole. The ganciclovir implants were removed and he was given a 4-week course of vancomycin and rifampicin. The bacterial endophthalmitis left him blind in his right eye.

DRUGS ACTIVE AGAINST HEPATITIS C VIRUS

Ribavirin *(SED-14, 992; SEDA-23, 315; SEDA-24, 341)*

A rapidly increasing number of publications suggest enhanced efficacy of the combination of interferon-α with ribavirin when compared with monotherapy with interferon-α. There is also evidence that retreatment with the combination may succeed in controlling or eliminating viremia when monotherapy has failed. Although the combination may lead to some increase in the adverse effects normally associated with interferon-α (dyspnea, pharyngitis, pruritus, nausea, insomnia, and anorexia; SEDA-23, 315), there is no doubt that oral ribavirin adds to the overall toxicity of the combination by causing hemolytic anemia, which is usually mild.

The adverse effects and other safety aspects of interferon and ribavirin in the treatment of hepatitis C infection have recently been reviewed (12[R]).

Hematologic In a randomized controlled trial of high-dose interferon-α_{2b} plus oral ribavirin for 6 or 12 months in 50 patients with chronic hepatitis C, the sequential effects of treatment on hemoglobin, leukocytes, and platelets were recorded (13[C]). There was a *fall in hemoglobin*, and the lowest concentrations were recorded after 6 months of treatment in both groups. All hematological measurements returned to normal after the end of treatment.

Detailed studies of the effects of ribavirin on erythrocyte ATP content and on the hexose monophosphate shunt have been conducted in vitro. ATP concentrations were significantly reduced and the hexose monophosphate shunt increased, suggesting erythrocyte susceptibility to oxidation. In vivo, ribavirin, alone or in combination with interferon, was associated with significant *reductions in hemoglobin concentrations* and a marked *increase in absolute reticulocyte counts*. Erythrocyte Na/K pump activity was significantly reduced, whereas K/Cl co-transport and its dithiothreitol-sensitive fraction and malondialdehyde and methemoglobin concentrations increased significantly. Ribavirin-treated patients showed an increase in aggregated band 3, which was associated with significantly increased binding of autologous antibodies and complement C3 fragments, suggesting erythrophagocytic removal by the reticuloendothelial system (14[C]).

Liver As part of a multicenter, randomized, double-blind, placebo-controlled trial of ribavirin in 59 patients with hepatitis C virus infection, liver biopsies were studied for iron deposition (15[C]). *Increased total iron deposition*, preferentially in hepatocytes, occurred during a 9-month course of ribavirin. The deposition had no apparent effect on the biochemical or histological response to ribavirin therapy.

Skin *Transient acantholytic dermatosis* (Grover's disease) was first described by Grover in 1970 as a pruritic, self-limiting, papular or papulovesicular eruption, mainly distributed on the trunk of white middle-aged men. The histopathological hallmark is suprabasal acantholysis at different levels of the epidermis. Its origin is uncertain; most cases are related to sunlight, heat, or sweating. A case of Grover's disease has been attributed to ribavirin (16[A]).

A 55-year-old man with chronic hepatitis C presented with a pruritic papular eruption on the trunk lasting 2 weeks. He had multiple, erythematous, excoriated papules on the neck, trunk, upper arms, and thighs. The lesions appeared 2 weeks after combination therapy with oral ribavirin and subcutaneous interferon-α_{2b}. He had previously been treated with interferon-α alone (in the same dosage). On withdrawal of ribavirin the lesions gradually faded, but they returned 1 week after reintroduction.

DRUGS ACTIVE AGAINST HUMAN IMMUNODEFICIENCY VIRUS TYPE 1

Nucleoside analogue reverse transcriptase inhibitors (NRTI)

(SED-14, 993; SEDA-23, 319; SEDA-24, 342)

Metabolic Antiretroviral nucleoside analogues have been associated with *hepatic steatosis and lactic acidosis*. These compounds require phosphorylation to active triphosphate derivatives by cellular phosphokinases. The triphosphate nucleotide inhibits the growing proviral DNA chain, but it also inhibits host DNA polymerases, and this may result in compensatory glycolysis and lactic acidosis. Abnormal mitochondrial oxidation of free fatty acids causes the accumulation of neutral fat in liver cells, and this manifests as hepatomegaly with macrovesicular steatosis. Hepatic steatosis and lactic acidosis has been reported previously with zidovudine, didanosine, zalcitabine, Combivir (zidovudine plus lamivudine), and lamivudine. Not surprisingly, this major adverse effect continues to occur in patients who have received combination therapy including nucleoside analogues.

Three cases of steatosis–lactic acidosis syndrome associated with stavudine plus lamivudine have been reported (17[A]).

A 37-year-old HIV-infected woman receiving stavudine, lamivudine, and indinavir developed epigastric pain, anorexia, and vomiting. There was lactic acidosis (serum lactate 4.9 mmol/l), her liver enzymes were raised, and her prothrombin time was increased. She had hepatomegaly and tachypnea and required mechanical ventilation. Her progress was complicated by pancreatitis and acute respiratory distress syndrome. Antiviral medication was stopped and she was treated with co-enzyme Q, carnitine, and vitamin C. The serum lactic acid and transaminases returned to normal over 4 weeks and she was weaned off the ventilator after 4 months.

A 40-year-old HIV-infected woman receiving stavudine, lamivudine, nelfinavir, and co-trimoxazole developed dyspnea, dysphagia, and vomiting with lactic acidosis (serum lactate 9.4 mmol/l) and hepatomegaly. Despite ventilation for respiratory failure she died after 5 days. Autopsy showed massive hepatomegaly with steatosis.

A 36-year-old HIV-infected woman who had been receiving stavudine, saquinavir, ritonavir, and didanosine developed lactic acidosis (serum lactate 11.4 mmol/l) and hepatomegaly. She had acute pancreatitis and, despite ventilatory support for respiratory failure, died after 8 weeks.

There have been similar reports related to didanosine plus stavudine (18[A]) and stavudine alone (19[A]).

Drug interactions Distal sensory neuropathy is the commonest neurological complication found in HIV-infected individuals, having been documented in up to 30% of AIDS patients. Evidence has been presented from a retrospective case-notes review in 30 individuals that coadministration of stavudine and *isoniazid* increases the incidence of distal sensory neuropathy. Of 22 patients taking stavudine in combination with other drugs, all received isoniazid for tuberculosis and 12 developed distal sensory neuropathy, with a median time to onset of 5 months (20[C]). Those taking stavudine alone had an incidence of 11%.

For those who are opiate-dependent, *methadone* may facilitate adherence to highly active antiretroviral therapy (HAART) regimens. The pharmacokinetics of the tablet formulations of didanosine and stavudine have been studied in 17 individuals taking stable methadone therapy in comparison with 10 untreated controls (21[C]). Methadone reduced the $AUC_{0\rightarrow 6}$ by 63% for didanosine and by 25% for stavudine and the C_{max} by 66% and 44% respectively. These effects appeared to result primarily from reduced systemic availability. Trough concentrations of methadone were comparable to those seen in historical controls, suggesting that the nucleoside analogs did not affect methadone disposition. The authors concluded that larger doses of the tablet formulation (or another type of formulation) may be necessary to provide HAART in subjects taking methadone.

Non-nucleoside reverse transcriptase inhibitors (NNRTI)

(SED-14, 996; SEDA-22, 318; SEDA-23, 320; SEDA-24, 344)

Efavirenz

Immunologic *Hypersensitivity syndrome*, also called DRESS (drug rash with eosinophilia and systemic symptoms) syndrome, is a life-threatening reaction that typically includes a rash, fever, lymphadenopathy, hepatitis, interstitial nephritis, pneumonia, myocarditis, and hematological abnormalities, particularly eosinophilia and a mononucleosis-like atypical lymphocytosis. Hypersensitivity syndrome has been described in an HIV-infected woman treated with efavirenz (22[A]).

A 44-year-old HIV-1 infected woman from the Ivory Coast, who was taking stavudine, lamivudine, efavirenz, and pyrimethamine plus sulfadiazine for *Toxoplasma* encephalitis, developed a maculopapular rash on both arms. The sulfadiazine was withdrawn and clindamycin added. Ten days later her condition had worsened. Her temperature was 40°, pulse rate 137 beats/min, and respiratory rate 26/min. She had a generalized maculopapular rash without mucosal involvement, moderate abdominal tenderness, hepatomegaly, jaundice, and bilateral crackles. Her white cell count was 16×10^9/l with 9% eosinophils and 51% lymphocytes. Chest X-ray showed moderate bilateral interstitial pneumonitis. All drugs were withdrawn and she was given intravenous methylprednisolone. The skin rash and all systemic manifestations resolved within 1 week and HIV treatment was restarted uneventfully with lamivudine, stavudine, and nelfinavir.

Although this syndrome has been described with sulfonamides (which the patient had taken) the fact that her condition worsened after withdrawal of sulfadiazine, and the characteristic timing of the syndrome (2–6 weeks after starting a drug), suggests efavirenz as the cause.

Drug interactions Following a report of withdrawal symptoms in three patients taking *methadone* maintenance therapy, serum methadone concentrations were measured before and after starting efavirenz in one patient (23[A]). Serum methadone concentrations were as follows: (R)-methadone (the active enantiomer) 168 ng/ml and 90 ng/ml before and after efavirenz. The corresponding (S)-methadone concentrations were 100 and 28 ng/ml. The dosage of methadone was increased from 100 to 180 mg/day before the patient's withdrawal symptoms resolved. Other drugs used for the treatment of HIV (e.g. ritonavir and nelfinavir) also reduce blood concentrations of methadone.

Nevirapine

Liver The most common adverse effect of nevirapine is a hypersensitivity reaction manifesting as a rash. There have also been reports of acute hepatitis and hepatic failure. A report of significant hepatic deterioration, consistent with *cholestasis*, 5 months into a HAART regimen including nevirapine, has been reported (24[A]).

A 49-year-old man with severe factor VIII deficiency and stable chronic hepatitis C infection took stavudine, didanosine, and nevirapine. After 5 months of well-tolerated therapy, during which his viral load fell from 39 550 RNA copies/ml to under 50 ml, he developed anorexia, nausea, vomiting, fatigue, agitation, and biochemical evidence of deteriorating liver function. All drugs were withdrawn. There was no evidence of an infective cause and his hepatitis C status had not changed. Transvenous biopsy of the right hepatic lobe showed profound cholestasis and mild sinusoidal fibrosis, consistent with drug-induced cholestasis.

Skin In a review of the medical records of HIV-positive patients who had taken nevirapine, delavirdine, or both, the frequency of skin reactions was determined, as were the consequences of rechallenge with the same or the alternative agent (25[C]). The overall incidence of *rash* attributed to the use of one of the NNRTIs was 37%. While rash due to delavirdine was more common (8/20 vs 25/69), the rash due to nevirapine was more severe and necessitated more frequent hospitalization. Rash recurred in six of eight patients who were rechallenged with the same agent and in seven of 10 who were switched to the alternative agent. The conclusion was drawn that there is little value in attempting to retreat patients who have had skin reactions to NNRTIs, except possibly those with limited treatment options.

In an attempt to reduce the rate of nevirapine-associated rashes, 469 patients were randomly assigned to different schedules of induction therapy (26[C]). Using a standard procedure, 19% developed a rash compared with 11%, 8.6%, and 7.7% in subjects assigned to a slowly escalating dose, concomitant administration of prednisone, or both. The rate of drug withdrawal was also reduced by a half using the new approaches.

Immunologic The occupational risk of transmission of HIV-1 to healthcare workers by inoculation injury has been well documented. Postexposure prophylaxis guidelines, which recommend the use of combinations of nucleoside analogs with a protease inhibitor, have been published. Some have attempted to substitute a NNRTI for the protease inhibitor, but a serious warning against this has emerged from two reports of severe *hypersensitivity reactions* to nevirapine in healthcare workers exposed to HIV, one of whom required orthotopic liver transplantation to overcome the complications of acute hepatic failure and coma (27[A]).

Protease inhibitors *(SED-14, 997; SEDA-23, 316; SEDA-24, 345)*

Metabolic Remarkable improvements in the health and prognosis of HIV-infected individuals have resulted from the use of protease inhibitors in combination regimens. Unfortunately, this exciting advance has been tempered by the recognition of metabolic and morphological changes, which, although seen with nucleoside analogue therapy, have been regarded as a class effect of the protease inhibitors. The characteristic morphological changes are stigmatizing to individuals and may lead to delays in initiating therapy, to modification of existing regimens, or to temporary or permanent abandonment of therapy. Similarly, biochemical changes, including lipid abnormalities and glucose intolerance, lead to concerns over possible future morbidity, particularly vascular disease.

The main components of the lipodystrophy syndrome associated with HIV therapy include:

1. Dyslipidemia with raised total cholesterol, low HDL cholesterol, raised triglycerides, and increased lipid turnover.
2. Local accumulation of body fat, with local, visceral, and breast distribution.
3. Generalized loss of subcutaneous fat, with altered body shape.
4. Insulin resistance, with hyperglycemia.

Other metabolic changes can occur after prolonged therapy and include raised serum lactate, hypogonadism, hypertension and accelerated cardiovascular disease, reduced bone density, and avascular necrosis of the hip. These effects have been documented in previous Annuals, but two large prospective studies in 1207 patients (28[C]) and 3191 patients (29[C]) have clarified the spectrum and incidence of metabolic changes in HAART and have explored the relative importance of protease inhibitors. In addition, data on fat redistribution from a postmarketing review of HIV-infected individuals taking indinavir have been published (30[C]).

Lipemia retinalis and pancreatitis have been reported in a 39-year-old man with HIV infection associated with protease inhibitor therapy (31[A]). The ophthalmoscopic changes of lipemia retinalis include a milky-white discoloration of the retinal vessels, beginning at the periphery but progressing to involve the posterior pole as the triglyceride concentration rises. The fundus may appear salmon-colored, owing to the effect of triglycerides on the choroidal circulation. This patient developed lipemia retinalis after switching to an antiretroviral regimen including ritonavir and saquinavir (together with zalcitabine and delavirdine). He had previously been taking zidovudine, lamivudine, and indinavir. Experience from HIV-negative patients with hyperlipidemia has shown that plasma triglyceride concentrations must be at least 28 mmol/l (2500 mg/daily) for lipemia retinalis to occur (reference value below 1.52 mmol/l). This patient had a plasma triglyceride concentration of 53 mmol/l when he presented with acute pancreatitis. On withdrawal of ritonavir and saquinavir the appearance of his retinal vessels returned to normal in parallel with a fall in his plasma triglycerides.

Amprenavir

Drug interactions CYP3A4 extensively metabolizes protease inhibitors, including amprenavir, and several interactions between different protease inhibitors and between protease inhibitors and other drugs have been previously reported.

A pharmacokinetic study has shown a minor interaction of amprenavir with *clarithromycin* in healthy male volunteers (32[C]). The mean AUC, $C_{max.ss}$, and $C_{min.ss}$ of amprenavir increased by 18, 15, and 39% respectively. Amprenavir had no effect on the AUC of clarithromycin, but the median $t_{max.ss}$ increased by

2.0 hours, renal clearance increased by 34%, and the AUC for 14-(R)-hydroxyclarithromycin fell by 35%. These effects were felt not to be clinically important and dosage adjustment was not recommended.

Four HIV-infected children undergoing intense antiretroviral combination therapy were switched to regimens including amprenavir and *efavirenz* after the failure of other drugs (33^A). Pharmacokinetic studies suggested that combinations of these drugs may result in suboptimal concentrations of amprenavir. This was evident in two of the children taking amprenavir and efavirenz, in combination with two NRTIs, who had undetectable concentrations of amprenavir within 4 hours of administration. The addition of ritonavir to the combination restored the blood concentrations of amprenavir to those normally recorded (median 3500 ng/ml). The most probable reason for this effect is enhanced metabolism of amprenavir due to induction by efavirenz.

Indinavir

Hematologic Following a previous report of fatal acute hemolysis associated with indinavir, a case report of *reversible acute hemolysis*, probably caused by long-term therapy with indinavir, has been reported (34^A).

A 32-year-old Caucasian, who was taking lamivudine, stavudine, and indinavir for HIV infection, presented with pallor following a period of fatigue and headache. His hemoglobin was 8.2 g/daily and there were no clinical findings to suggest bleeding. The reticulocyte count was 3.5% and a direct Coombs' test was negative. A diagnosis of hemolytic anemia secondary to indinavir was made, the indinavir was stopped, and he was transfused with concentrated erythrocytes. The other antiretroviral drugs were continued, saquinavir was added, and a normal hemoglobin concentration was maintained.

Skin, hair, and nails Cutaneous toxicity may have a major influence on compliance with treatment and may impact adversely on the quality of life.

Of 84 patients taking indinavir plus two nucleoside reverse transcriptase inhibitors for 20 months, 48 developed *cheilitis*, 34 had *skin dryness and pruritus*, 10 developed *asteatotic dermatitis* on the trunk, arms, and thighs, and 10 complained of *scalp defluvium* (35^C). Severe alopecia was observed in one patient, while six reported that their body hair had become fairer and thinner and shed considerably. Multiple *pyogenic granulomas* were observed in the toenails of five patients and *softening of the nail plate* was noted in five. The temporal relation between starting indinavir and the onset of these effects was striking and regression occurred on withdrawal. Other cases of paronychia associated with indinavir have been reported (36^A, 37^A).

Suggested mechanisms for these adverse effects include:

1. Retinoid-like effects due to homologies of the amino acid sequences of the HIV-1 protease and cytoplasmic retinoic-acid binding protein type 1 (CRABP-1).
2. Inhibition of CYP3A by indinavir, resulting in reduced oxidation of retinoic acid and hence augmentation of its biological effects.

Drug interactions Failure of combination therapy including indinavir has been attributed to an interaction of indinavir with *carbamazepine* (38^A).

A 48-year-old HIV-positive man taking indinavir, zidovudine, and lamivudine developed *Herpes zoster*, which was treated with famciclovir. Postherpetic neuralgia was treated with carbamazepine, and his plasma indinavir concentration fell substantially. The carbamazepine was withdrawn after 2.5 months and 2 weeks later HIV-RNA was detectable in his plasma (6×10^3 copies/ml). His circulating virus was resistant to lamivudine. With a further increase in viral load, his therapy was changed to nevirapine, didanosine, and stavudine.

This treatment failure, and possibly the resistance to lamivudine, was attributed to induction of drug metabolism by carbamazepine.

Nelfinavir

Drug interactions An interaction of nelfinavir with the macrolide immunosuppressant *tacrolimus* has been reported in a patient co-infected with HIV and hepatitis C virus who had undergone orthotopic liver transplantation (39^A). The dose of tacrolimus had to be reduced to a 70th of the normal dose to avoid adverse effects. Nelfinavir serum concentrations were not affected by tacrolimus. The authors suggested that this effect had resulted from inhibition of the metabolism of tacrolimus, because both compounds are substrates of CYP3A4.

Withdrawal symptoms in a patient maintained on *methadone*, necessitating an increase in dosage, have been attributed to nelfinavir in a 40-year-old man (40[A]).

Ritonavir

Drug interactions Withdrawal symptoms and the need to increase the dose of *methadone*, in a 51-year-old man previously stable on maintenance, have been attributed to ritonavir (41[A]).

A further reminder of the potency of ritonavir as a CYP3A4 inhibitor is demonstrated by a description of an interaction with *carbamazepine* (42[A]).

A 49-year-old woman with a long history of HIV infection developed worsening ataxia leading to two falls. Four days before admission she had had her antiretroviral drugs changed from zidovudine, lamivudine, and indinavir to ritonavir, saquinavir, and efavirenz. She was also taking carbamazepine to control generalized seizures resulting from a previous right thalamic infarction. The change in antiretroviral therapy resulted in an increase in her serum carbamazepine concentration from 6.9 to 20 μg/ml. Therapeutic serum concentrations were eventually achieved by a sixth of the dose of carbamazepine that had been required before starting ritonavir.

As saquinavir is only a mild inhibitor of CYP3A4 and efavirenz is an inducer, this effect was attributed to the potent inhibitor ritonavir.

In 12 patients taking ritonavir and saquinavir for HIV infection, *ketoconazole* significantly increased the AUC, the plasma concentration at 12 hours, and the half-life of ritonavir by 29%, 62%, and 31% respectively (43[C]). Similar increases of 37%, 94%, and 38% were recorded for saquinavir. CSF concentrations of ritonavir were raised by 178% by ketaconazole, but there was no significant change in CSF concentrations of saquinavir.

DRUGS ACTIVE AGAINST INFLUENZA VIRUSES

(SED-14, 999; SEDA-23, 321; SEDA-24, 348)

Oseltamivir

Gastrointestinal Upper gastrointestinal effects (*nausea* or *nausea with vomiting*) have been reported more frequently in those taking oseltamivir in placebo-controlled studies (44[C], 45[C]). Despite this mild gastrointestinal intolerance, withdrawal rates have been low.

Zanamivir

Respiratory Zanamivir is administered by inhalation of a powder in a lactose vehicle. There is still a need for further safety data on its use in patients with asthma and chronic obstructive pulmonary disease, and this has been highlighted by a report of *bronchospasm* (46[A]).

A 63-year-old man with oxygen-dependent chronic obstructive pulmonary disease was given zanamivir because of an exacerbation attributed to influenza. Shortly after each inhalation of the drug he reported increasing respiratory difficulty and wheezing. After 3 days he developed respiratory distress, hypoxia, and wheezing, and was treated with bronchodilators, corticosteroids, and antibiotics.

Patients taking zanamivir are advised to stop using it if bronchospasm occurs, and those with underlying lung disease are advised to have a fast-acting bronchodilator to hand.

REFERENCES

1. Rajan GRC, Cobb JP, Reiss CK. Acyclovir induced coma in the intensive care unit. Anaesth Intensive Care 2000; 28: 305–7.
2. Wollenberg A, Baldauf C, Rueff F, Przybilla B. Allergic contact dermatitis and exanthematous drug eruption following aciclovir – cross reaction with ganciclovir. Allergol J 2000; 9: 96–9.
3. Romanowski B, Aoki FY, Martel AY, Lavender EA, Parsons JE, Saltzman RL. Efficacy and safety of famciclovir for treating mucocutaneous herpes simplex in HIV-infected individuals. AIDS 2000; 14: 1211–17.
4. Berenguer J, Mallolas J, Padilla B, Colmenero M, Santos I. Intravenous cidofovir for compassionate use in AIDS patients with cytomegalovirus retinitis. Clin Infect Dis 2000; 30: 182–4.
5. Jabs DA, Freeman WR, Jacobson M, Murphy R, Van Natta ML, Meinert CL. Long-term follow-up of patients with AIDS treated with parenteral cidofovir for cytomegalovirus retinitis: the HPMPC Peripheral Cytomegalovirus Trial. The Studies of Ocular Complications of AIDS Research Group in collaboration with the AIDS Clinical Trials Group. AIDS 2000; 14: 1571–81.

6. Stone TW, Jaffe GJ. Reversible bull's-eye maculopathy associated with intravitreal fomivirsen therapy for cytomegalovirus retinitis. Am J Ophthalmol 2000; 130: 242–3.
7. Amin HI, Ai E, McDonald HR, Johnson RN. Retinal toxic effects associated with intravitreal fomivirsen. Arch Ophthalmol 2000; 118: 426–7.
8. Matarese LE, Speerhas R, Seidner DL, Steiger E. Foscarnet-induced electrolyte abnormalities in a bone marrow transplant patient receiving parenteral nutrition. J Parenter Enter Nutr 2000; 24: 170–3.
9. Huycke MM, Naguib MT, Stroemmel MM, Blick K, Monti K, Martin-Munley S, Kaufman C. A double blind placebo-controlled crossover trial of intravenous magnesium sulfate for foscarnet-induced ionized hypocalcemia and hypomagnesemia in patients with AIDS and cytomegalovirus infection. Antimicrob Agents Chemother 2000; 44: 2143–8.
10. Frenkel LM, Capparelli EV, Dankner WM, Xu J, Smith IL, Ballow A, Culnane M, Read JS, Thompson M, Mohan KM, Shaver A, Robinson CA, Stempien MJ, Burchett SK, Melvin AJ, Borkowsky W, Petri A, Kovacs A, Yogev R, Goldsmith J, McFarland EJ, Spector SA. Oral ganciclovir in children: pharmacokinetics, safety, tolerance and antiviral effects. J Infect Dis 2000; 182: 1616–24.
11. Williamson JC, Virata SR, Raasch RH, Kylstra JA. Oxacillin-resistant *Staphylococcus aureus* endophthalmitis after ganciclovir intraocular implant. Am J Ophthalmol 2000; 129: 554–5.
12. Chutaputti A. Adverse effects and other safety aspects of the hepatitis C antivirals. J Gastroenterol Hepatol 2000; 15 Suppl: E156–63.
13. Di Marco V, Almasio P, Vaccaro A, Ferraro D, Parisi P, Catoldo MG, Di Stefano R, Craxi A. Combined treatment of relapse of chronic hepatitis C with high-dose $alpha_{2b}$ interferon plus ribavirin for 6 or 12 months. J Hepatol 2000; 33: 456–62.
14. De Franceschi L, Fattovich G, Turrini F, Ayi K, Brugnara C, Manzato F, Noventa F, Stanzial AM, Solero P, Corrocher R. Hemolytic anemia induced by ribavirin therapy in patients with chronic hepatitis C virus infection: role of membrane oxidative damage. Hepatology 2000; 31: 997–1004.
15. Fiel MI, Schiano TD, Guido M, Thung SN, Lindsay KL, Davis GL, Lewis JH, Seeff LB, Bodenheimer HC. Increased hepatic iron deposition resulting from treatment of chronic hepatitis C with ribavirin. Am J Clin Pathol 2000; 113: 35–9.
16. Antunes I, Azevedo F, Mesquita-Guimaraes J, Resende C, Fernandes N, Macedo G. Grover's disease secondary to ribavirin. Br J Dermatol 2000; 142: 1257–8.
17. Johri S, Alkhuja S, Siviglia G, Soni A. Steatosis–lactic acidosis syndrome associated with stavudine and lamivudine therapy. AIDS 2000; 14: 1286–7.
18. Brivet FG, Nion I, Megarbane B, Slama A, Brivet M, Rustin P, Munnich A. Fatal lactic acidosis and liver steatosis associated with didanosine and stavudine treatment: a respiratory chain dysfunction. J Hepatol 2000; 32: 364–5.
19. Mokrzycki MH, Harris C, May H, Laut J, Palmisano J. Lactic acidosis associated with stavudine administration: a report of five cases. Clin Infect Dis 2000; 30: 198–200.
20. Breen RAM, Lipman MCI, Johnson MA. Increased incidence of peripheral neuropathy with co-administration of stavudine and isoniazid in HIV-infected individuals. AIDS 2000; 14: 615.
21. Rainey PM, Friedland G, McCance-Katz EF, Andrews L, Mitchell SM, Charles C, Jatlow P. Interaction of methadone with didanosine and stavudine. J Acquir Immune Defic Syndr 2000; 24: 241–8.
22. Bossi P, Colin D, Bricaire F, Caumes E. Hypersensitivity syndrome associated with efavirenz therapy. Clin Infect Dis 2000; 30: 227–8.
23. Marzolini C, Troillet N, Telenti A, Baumann P, Decosterd LA, Eap CB. Efavirenz decreases methadone blood concentrations. AIDS 2000; 14: 1291-2.
24. Clarke S, Harrington P, Condon C, Kelleher D, Smith OP, Mulcahy F. Late onset hepatitis and prolonged deterioration in hepatic function associated with nevirapine therapy. Int J STD AIDS 2000; 11: 336–7.
25. Gangar M, Arias G, O'Brien JG, Kemper CA. Frequency of cutaneous reactions on rechallenge with nevirapine and delavirdine. Ann Pharmacother 2000; 34: 839–42.
26. Barreiro P, Soriano V, Casas E, Estrada V, Tellez MJ, Hoetelmans R, Gonzalez de Requena D, Jimenez-Nacher I, Gonzalez-Lahoz J. Prevention of nevirapine-associated exanthema using slow dose escalation and/or corticosteroids. AIDS 2000; 14: 2153–7.
27. Johnson S, Baraboutis JG, Sha BE, Proia LA, Kessler HA. Adverse effects associated with use of nevirapine in HIV post exposure prophylaxis for 2 health care workers. J Am Med Assoc 2000; 284: 2722–3.
28. Bonfanti P, Valsecchi L, Parazzini F, Carradori S, Pusterla L, Fortuna P, Timillero L, Alessi F, Ghiselli G, Gabbuti A, Di Cintio E, Martinelli C, Faggion I, Landonio S, Quirino T. Incidence of adverse reactions in HIV patients treated with protease inhibitors: a cohort study. J Acquir Immune Defic Syndr 2000; 23: 236–45.
29. Thiebaut R, Dabis F, Malvy D, Jacqmin-Gadda H, Mercie P, Daucourt Valentine V. Serum triglycerides, HIV infection and highly active antiretroviral therapy. Aquitaine Cohort, France 1996 to 1998. J Acquir Immune Defic Syndr 2000; 23: 261–5.
30. Benson JO, McGhee K, Coplan P, Grunfeld C, Robertson M, Brodovicz KG, Slater E. Fat redistribution in indinavir-treated patients with HIV infection: a review of postmarketing cases. J Acquir Immune Defic Syndr 2000; 25: 130–9.
31. Eng KT, Liu ES, Silverman MS, Berger AR. Lipemia retinalis in acquired immunodeficiency

syndrome treated with protease inhibitors. Arch Ophthalmol 2000; 118: 425–6.
32. Brophy DF, Israel DS, Pastor A, Gillotin C, Chittick GE, Symonds WT, Lou Y, Sadler BM, Polk RE. Pharmacokinetic interaction between amprenavir and clarithromycin in healthy male volunteers. Antimicrob Agents Chemother 2000; 44: 78–84.
33. Wintergerst U, Engelhorn C, Kurowski M, Hoffmann F, Notheis G, Belohradsky BH. Pharmacokinetic interaction of amprenavir in combination with efavirenz or delavirdine in HIV-infected children. AIDS 2000; 14: 1866–7.
34. Watson A. Reversible acute haemolysis associated with indinavir. AIDS 2000; 14: 465–6.
35. Calisti D, Boschini A. Cutaneous side effects of indinavir. Eur J Dermatol 2000; 10: 292–6.
36. Dauden E, Pascual-Lopez M, Martinez-Garcia C, Garcia-Diez A. Paronychia and excess granulation tissue of the toes and finger in a patient treated with indinavir. Br J Dermatol 2000; 142: 1063–4.
37. Sass JO, Jakob-Solder B, Heitger A, Tzimas G, Sarcletti M. Paronychia with pyogenic granuloma in a child treated with indinavir: the retinoid-mediated side effect theory revisited. Dermatology 2000; 200: 40–2.
38. Hugen PWH, Burger DM, Brinkman K, ter Hofstede HJM, Schuurman R, Koopmans PP, Hekster YA. Carbamazepine–indinavir interaction causes antiretroviral therapy failure. Ann Pharmacother 2000; 34: 465–70.
39. Schvarcz R, Rudbeck G, Soderdahl G, Stahle L. Interaction between nelfinavir and tacrolimus after orthotopic liver transplantation in a patient coinfected with HIV and hepatitis C virus (HCV). Transplantation 2000; 69: 2194–5.
40. McCance-Katz EF, Farber S, Selwyn PA, O'Connor A. Decrease in methadone levels with nelfinavir mesylate. Am J Psychiatry 2000; 157: 481.
41. Geletko SM, Erickson AD. Decreased methadone effect after ritonavir initiation. Pharmacotherapy 2000; 20: 93–4.
42. Burman W, Orr L. Carbamazepine toxicity after starting combination antiretroviral therapy including ritonavir and efavirenz. AIDS 2000; 14: 2793-4.
43. Khaliq Y, Gallicano K, Venance S, Kravcik S, Cameron DW. Effect of ketaconazole on ritonavir and saquinavir concentrations in plasma and cerebrospinal fluid from patients infected with human immunodeficiency virus. Clin Pharmacol Ther 2000; 68: 637–46.
44. Treanor JJ, Hayden FG, Vrooman PS, Barbarash R, Bettis R, Riff D, Singh S, Kinnersley N, Ward P, Mills RG. Efficacy and safety of the oral neuraminidase inhibitor oseltamivir in treating acute influenza. A randomised controlled trial. J Am Med Assoc 2000; 283: 1016–24.
45. Nicholson KG, Aoki FY, Osterhaus ADME, Trottier S, Carewicz O, Mercier CH, Rode A, Kinnersley N, Ward P. Efficacy and safety of oseltamivir in treatment of acute influenza: a randomised controlled trial. Lancet 2000; 355: 1845–50.
46. Williamson JC, Pegram PS. Respiratory distress associated with zanamivir. New Engl J Med 2000; 342: 661–2.

J.N. Pande

30 Drugs used in tuberculosis and leprosy

DRUGS USED IN TUBERCULOSIS

Liver damage due to antituberculous drugs

Hepatotoxicity is the most important adverse effect of antituberculous drug therapy. Isoniazid, rifampicin, and pyrazinamide are the main culprits. There is wide variability in the risk of hepatotoxic reactions reported from different parts of the world (SEDA-24, 353). Several risk factors for hepatotoxic reactions have been postulated, such as old age, pre-existing hepatic dysfunction, alcoholism, co-infection with hepatitis virus, undernutrition, and slow acetylator status (1[c]*), but there have been inconsistent findings with regard to some of these risk factors in different studies.*

The issue of hepatic dysfunction and acetylator status during treatment with isoniazid plus rifampicin has been re-examined in 77 Japanese patients with pulmonary tuberculosis (2[c]*). There was a marked increase in the risk of hepatotoxicity amongst slow acetylator NAT2* genotypes (a combination of mutant alleles) compared with the rapid acetylator genotype (homozygous NAT2*4). Using Taylor's series analysis (Epi-info Statcal) I have calculated that the relative risk was 28 (95% CI = 4.1, 192). Despite a small sample size (seven slow acetylator genotypes, 42 intermediate, and 28 rapid) the relative risk was highly significant, which is not surprising if all seven of the slow acetylators and only one of the 28 rapid acetylators developed hepatotoxicity.*

*A unique feature of this study was the determination of acetylator status by genotyping rather than phenotyping. There is generally good concordance between the two methods, but in the presence of hepatic dysfunction the phenotype assessment may not reflect the genotype. Furthermore, 42 of the 77 patients were assigned to the intermediate acetylator genotype, based on heterozygosity for NAT2*4 and a mutant allele. However, phenotyping by estimation of concentrations of metabolites of the commonly used probes does not consistently result in identification of intermediate acetylators. The Japanese are mostly fast acetylators (~90%) compared with Caucasians or Indians (40–50%). It is unlikely, however, that the observed association between slow acetylator genotype and the high risk of hepatic dysfunction was affected by any of these considerations. The dose of isoniazid was rather large (~8 mg/kg/day) and this may have increased the risk of hepatotoxicity. Furthermore, hepatotoxicity was defined as an increase in AsT or AlT to 1.5 times the top of the reference range. This degree of hepatic dysfunction is not uncommon in patients taking antituberculous drugs, and is no indication for withdrawal or modification of treatment. It is not possible to assess the risk of severe hepatotoxicity during treatment, owing to lack of detailed information in the published report.*

Old age and the presence of hepatic dysfunction on baseline evaluation are the most consistent predictors of hepatotoxicity during antituberculous therapy. The association between hepatotoxicity and hepatitis C virus and HIV seropositivity was reviewed in SEDA-23 (p. 324). A recent report from Hong Kong has suggested that the risk is much greater in hepatitis B virus carriers taking antituberculous drugs (3[c]*). Even after excluding patients who had raised baseline AlT activity or with*

Side Effects of Drugs, Annual 25
J.K. Aronson, ed.

HbeAg seroconversion during the phase of hepatic dysfunction, the risk of hepatotoxicity was still significantly higher in hepatitis B carriers taking antituberculous drugs compared with non-carriers (26% vs 8.8%). These observations are of considerable importance in regions of the world in which the prevalence of hepatitis B infection as well as tuberculosis is high, such as South-East Asia and sub-Saharan Africa.

The management of tuberculosis in patients with chronic liver disease poses a therapeutic challenge. Enhanced hepatotoxicity of conventional antituberculosis regimens has been reported in recipients of orthotopic liver transplants, which is not unexpected, because of bouts of organ rejection (4[c]). The authors recommended ofloxacin for these patients on the basis of favorable outcome in six cases. A conventional antituberculous induction regimen was used initially until hepatoxoxicity developed in all six patients. Thereafter they were treated with a combination of ofloxacin and ethambutol, with apparent cure in all. It should be noted that most of the patients took isoniazid + rifampicin for almost 2 months, which is the usual period when hepatotoxic reactions occur. Perhaps one should evaluate substitution of rifampicin with ofloxacin from the very beginning in order to minimize hepatotoxicity, as well as interference with ciclosporin leading to graft rejection noted in an earlier study (5[C]).

Isoniazid *(SED-14, 1009; SEDA-23, 324; SEDA-24, 352)*

Drug interactions A 5-fold increase in the risk of distal sensory neuropathy has been reported in patients taking *stavudine* plus isoniazid (55% vs 11%) compared with patients taking stavudine without isoniazid (6[c]). In nine of 12 patients the neuropathy resolved on changing antiretroviral drugs. Peripheral neuropathy is a distressing complication during treatment with stavudine and the risk is considerably increased with coadministration of isoniazid. This combination of drugs should be avoided, if possible, in patients with tuberculosis and AIDS.

Rifamycins *(SED-14, 1014; SEDA-22, 322; SEDA-23, 324; SEDA-24, 353)*

Drug interactions Drug interactions of rifampicin with newly introduced drugs continue to be recognized. Some of them were reviewed in SEDA-21 (p. 313) and SEDA-24 (p. 354).

Antiretroviral drugs The importance of drug interactions of rifampicin with antiretroviral drugs, particularly the protease inhibitors and non-nucleoside reverse transcriptase inhibitors (NNRTI), is well recognized. The current recommendations of the Center for Disease Control and Prevention in Atlanata regarding the use of antituberculous drugs in combination with antiretroviral drugs have recently been published (7[S]). In general, the use of rifampicin in patients taking protease inhibitors is contraindicated, except in the following circumstances:

- patients taking the NNRTI efavirenz and two NRTIs;
- patients taking the protease inhibitor ritonavir and one or more NRTIs;
- patients taking a combination of the two protease inhibitors ritonavir and saquinavir.

The use of rifampicin with the protease inhibitors indinavir, nelfinavir, and amprenavir is contraindicated. However, these agents can be used with rifabutin after appropriate dosage reduction. Failure to reduce the dosage of rifabutin may result in toxic manifestations, such arthralgia and uveitis. Rifamycins can be used with the NNRTIs nevirapine or efavirenz, but not with delavirdine.

Data on drug pharmacokinetics and drug interactions in patients taking treatment for HIV infection and tuberculosis are scanty, and the current recommendations are almost certain to be modified in the near future. Furthermore, it may be prudent to monitor rifampicin concentrations in the event of intolerance or adverse drug reactions.

Clarithromycin and fluconazole Rifabutin, which induces CYP3A4, has important interactions with other commonly used antimicrobial agents, including clarithromycin and fluconazole, which inhibit CYP3A4. The potential of these drugs to increase rifabutin concentrations has been reported before, and it has now been reported that both fluconazole and clarithromycin increased the AUC of rifabutin by 76% (8[C]).

Glimepiride The addition of rifampicin to

glimepiride (metabolized by CYP2C9) produced only a modest reduction in AUC and no significant effect on blood glucose (9[c]).

Repaglinide Coadministration of rifampicin with repaglinide considerably lowers the concentration of repaglinide and alters its therapeutic effect in diabetes mellitus (10[c]). In nine healthy volunteers, the maximum reduction in blood glucose after a single 0.5 mg dose of repaglinide fell from 1.6 to 1.0 mmol/l after pretreatment with rifampicin for 5 days. This presumably occurred by induction of CYP3A4.

Simvastatin In healthy subjects taking rifampicin the C_{max} and AUC of simvastatin were greatly reduced (11[c]), presumably by enzyme induction. It is likely that other HMG-CoA reductase inhibitors, including lovastatin and atorvastatin, may also have clinically significant interactions with rifampicin.

Tacrolimus An interaction between rifampicin and tacrolimus has been documented (12[A], 13[A]).

A 61-year-old Chinese renal transplant recipient, who had taken tacrolimus for 1 year after an episode of rejection had failed to respond to ciclosporin, took rifampicin and 12 days later had an episode of biopsy-proven graft rejection, associated with very low serum tacrolimus concentrations.

A 50-year-old woman, a renal transplant recipient, developed a brain abscess due to *Nocardia otitidiscaviarum* after craniotomy and was given meropenem and rifampicin. The dose of tacrolimus had to be increased 3-fold to maintain adequate trough concentrations.

Rifampicin has a similar interaction with ciclosporin (SEDA-21, 314). Tuberculosis is fairly common in patients taking immunosuppressive therapy after organ transplantation in developing countries. Almost half of the people in these countries are infected with tuberculosis and there is ample opportunity for contracting new exogenous infection as well. As more transplants are undertaken in developing countries the problem of tuberculosis in recipients is expected to increase. Facilities for monitoring plasma drug concentrations are limited and expensive. Furthermore, increasing the dose of ciclosporin or tacrolimus will increase the cost of treatment even more. There is therefore a need for immunosuppressive therapy that does not activate latent tuberculosis and has few drug interactions with agents used for tuberculosis.

Theophylline The clearance of theophylline in patients taking antituberculous drugs, including rifampicin, isoniazid, and ethambutol, is significantly reduced (14[c]).

DRUGS USED IN LEPROSY

Clofazimine *(SED-14, 1023)*

Gastrointestinal An *enteropathy* has been associated with clofazimine in a 32-year-old Thai patient (15[AR]). Recognized for the first time in 1967, only 14 cases of this complication, reviewed in this report, have so far appeared in the English-language literature. Acute or chronic abdominal pain was the main symptom. In most patients the diagnosis was made after exploratory laparotomy. Barium meal follow-through or CT scanning of the abdomen showed mucosal thickening in the small intestine. Mesenteric lymph node enlargement was present in the index case. Characteristic eosinophilic clofazimine crystals were demonstrated in histiocytes in all patients except three. The authors proposed the term "clofazimine-induced crystal storing histiocytosis" to emphasize causes other than B cell neoplasms for crystal-storage histiocytosis. Awareness of this complication of clofazimine may avoid unnecessary surgical exploration.

Dapsone *(SED-14, 1021; SEDA-22, 321; SEDA-23, 326)*

Drug overdose Several reports of accidental poisoning with dapsone in children have appeared since the early 1980s. Two recent reports (16[R], 17[c]) have emphasized the persistence of the problem, although the number of childhood cases has fallen over the years. Poisoning with dapsone results in cyanosis due to *methemoglobinemia*, *vomiting*, *mental confusion*, *tachycardia*, and *dyspnea*. It has been suggested (17[c]) that treatment with multiple doses of activated charcoal may be sufficient for less severely poisoned children (methemoglobin concentration below 30%) and that a single dose of methylene blue should be given to those with higher concentrations.

REFERENCES

1. Pande JN, Singh SPN, Khilnani GC, Khilnani S, Tandon RK. Risk factors for hepatotoxicity from antituberculosis drugs: a case control study. Thorax 1996; 51: 132–6.
2. Ohno M, Yamagchi I, Yamamoto I, Fukuda T, Yokota S, Maekura R, Ito M, Yamamoto Y, Ogura T, Maeda K, Komuta K, Igarashi T, Azuma J. Slow N-acetyltransferase 2 genotype affects the incidence of isoniazid and rifampicin-induced hepatotoxicity. Int J Tuberc Lung Dis 2000; 4: 256–61.
3. Wong W-M, Wu P-C, Yuen M-F, Cheng C-C, Yew W-W, Wong, P-C, Tam C-M, Leung C-C, Lai C-L. Antituberculosis drug related liver dysfunction in chronic hepatitis B infection. Hepatology 2000; 31: 201–6.
4. Meyers BR, Papanicolaou GA, Sheiner P, Emre S, Miller C. Tuberculosis in orthotopic liver transplant patients: increased toxicity of recommended agents; cure of disseminated infection with nonconventional regimens. Transplantation 2000; 69: 64–9.
5. Aguado JM, Herrero JA, Gavalda J, Torre-Cisneros J, Blanes, M, Rufi G, Moreno A, Gurgui M, Hayek M, Lumbreras C, Cantarell C. Clinical presentation and outcome of tuberculosis in kidney, liver and heart transplant recipients in Spain. Transplantation 1997; 63: 1278–86.
6. Breen RAM, Lipman MCI, Johnson MA. Increased incidence of peripheral neuropathy with co-administration of stavudine with isoniazid in HIV-infected individuals. AIDS 2000; 14: 615.
7. Updated guidelines for the use of rifabutin or rifampin for the treatment and prevention of tuberculosis among HIV-infected patients taking protease inhibitors or non-nucleoside reverse transcriptase inhibitors. MMWR Morb Mortal Wkly Rep 2000; 49: 185–9.
8. Jordan MK, Polis MA, Kelly G, Narang PK, Masur H, Piscitelli SC. Effects of fluconazole and clarithromycin on rifabutin and 25-O-deacetyl rifabutin pharmacokinetics. Antimicrob Agents Chemother 2000; 44: 2170–2.
9. Niemi M, Kivisto KT, Backman JT, Neuvonen PJ. Effect of rifampicin on the pharmacokinetics and pharmacodynamics of glimepiride. Br J Clin Pharmacol 2000; 50: 591–5.
10. Niemi M, Backman JT, Neuvonen M, Neuvonen PJ, Kivisto KT. Rifampin decreases the plasma concentrations and the effects of repaglinide. Clin Pharmacol Ther 2000; 68: 495–500.
11. Kyrklund C, Backman JT, Kivisto KT, Neuvonen M, Laitila J, Neuvonen PJ. Rifampin greatly reduces plasma simvastatin and simvastatin acid concentrations. Clin Pharmacol Ther 2000; 68: 592–7.
12. Chenhsu RY, Loong CC, Chou MH, Lin MF, Yang WC. Renal allograft dysfunction associated with rifampin–tacrolimus interaction. Ann Pharmacother 2000; 34: 27–31.
13. Hartmann A, Halvorsen CE, Jenssen T, Bjorneklett A, Brekke IB, Bakke SJ, Hirschberg H, Tonjum T, Gaustad P. Intracerebral abscess caused by *Nocardia otitidiscaviarum* in a renal transplant patient-cured by evacuation plus antibiotic therapy. Nephron 2000; 86: 79–83.
14. Ahn HC, Yang JH, Lee HB, Rhee, YK, Lee YC. Effect of combined therapy of anti-tubercular agents on theophylline. Int J Tuberc Lung Dis 2000; 4: 784–7.
15. Sukpanichnant S, Hargrove NS, Kachintorn U, Sathaporn M, Chanchairujira T, Siritanaratkul N, Akaraviputh T, Thanerngpol K. Clofazimine-induced crystal-storing histiocytosis producing chronic abdominal pain in a leprosy patient. Am J Surg Pathol 2000; 24: 129–35.
16. Carrazza MZN, Carrazza FR, Oga S. Clinical and laboratory parameters in dapsone acute intoxication. Rev Saude Publica 2000; 34: 396–401.
17. Bucaretchi F, Miglioli L, Baracat ECE, Madureira PR. Acute dapsone exposure and methemoglobinemia in children: treatment with multiple doses of activated charcoal with or without the administration of methylene blue. J Pediatr 2000; 76: 290–4.

P.J.J. van Genderen

31 Antihelminthic drugs

BENZIMIDAZOLES *(SED-14, 1030; SEDA-22, 324; SEDA-23, 327; SEDA-24, 356)*

Albendazole is a benzimidazole derivative used in the treatment of strongyloides, cutaneous larva migrans, neurocysticercosis, and in high doses in echinococcosis. Mebendazole has been successfully used to treat enterobiasis, ascariasis, trichuriasis, and hookworm infections. The antihelminthic activity of the benzimidazoles is thought to result from selective blockade of glucose uptake by adult worms lodged in the intestine and their tissue-dwelling larvae, resulting in endogenous depletion of glycogen stores and reduced formation of adenosine triphosphate, which appears to be essential for parasite reproduction and survival. However, recent developments suggest that benzimidazole antihelminthics may also have antiparasitic activity by binding to free β-tubulin, thereby inhibiting the polymerization of tubulin and microtubule-dependent glucose uptake (1[R]).

Benzimidazoles and human echinococcosis Since their introduction in 1982, the benzimidazoles have clearly contributed to improved survival in patients with alveolar echinococcosis. The epidemiology, clinical presentation, and treatment of alveolar echinococcosis of the liver have been described in French patients, diagnosed and followed between 1972 and 1993 (2[C]). From 1982 benzimidazoles were used. Of 117 patients, 72 took either albendazole or mebendazole for 4–134 months. The most common adverse effects were an *increase in alanine aminotransferase* activity to more than five times the top of the reference range (in six patients taking albendazole and in three taking mebendazole). *Neutropenia* (leukocyte count below 1.0×10^9/l) occurred in two patients taking albendazole. *Alopecia* occurred in four patients taking mebendazole. Minor adverse effects of albendazole included *malaise*, *anorexia*, and *digestive intolerance* in one patient each. In 13 patients treatment had to be withdrawn because of adverse effects (n = 10) or non-compliance (n = 3).

Albendazole is licensed only for the cyclic treatment of human alveolar echinococcosis. One treatment cycle consists of 28 days followed by a wash-out phase of 14 days without treatment, intended to reduce toxicity. Whether albendazole can also be used on a continuous basis has recently been studied in an open observational study in 35 patients with alveolar echinococcosis (in seven of 35 patients a curative operation was performed) (3[C]). The outcome (lack of progression) was compared with the results obtained with continuous treatment with mebendazole or cyclic albendazole. Albendazole 10–15 mg/kg/day and mebendazole 40–50 mg/kg/day were equally effective. Seven patients were treated with continuous albendazole for an average of 28 (range 13–50) months. All patients taking continuous albendazole had stable or even regressive disease. The continuous dosing regimen was well tolerated without increased toxicity or higher rates of adverse reactions. Therefore, continuous dosing of albendazole is a promising alternative in cases of inoperable or progressive alveolar echinococcosis.

In several reports the efficacy of albendazole in preventing hydatid disease recurrences and cyst fluid spillage complications after surgery has been studied. In one Turkish study 22 of 36 patients with echinococcosis were treated with albendazole after surgical intervention (4[C]). There was no significant benefit of perioperative albendazole over operation alone, although the recurrence rate of hepatic echinococcosis was lower than in historical controls. In contrast, in another study in 22 patients with hepatic echinococcosis there was a clear

Side Effects of Drugs, Annual 24
J.K. Aronson, ed.

benefit of peri- and postoperative cyclic albendazole (12–15 mg/kg/day in four divided doses) (5[C]). There were no cases of secondary hydatid disease or recurrence after a mean follow-up of 20 months. In two cases there were *liver function abnormalities*, which normalized after withdrawal.

Prolonged cyclic albendazole treatment (for more than 9 years) was safe and effective in a patient with isolated cervical spine echinococcosis in whom surgery was performed without preoperative antihelminthic therapy because of a delay in diagnosis (6[A]).

Benzimidazoles and human neurocysticercosis In two excellent reviews controversies in the management of neurocysticercosis have been described (7[R]–8[R]). Cysticercosis is caused by the larval stage of the pork tapeworm *Tenia solium*. Neurocysticercosis is the most severe and common clinical manifestation in humans and probably the most frequent parasitic infection of the central nervous system. *Tenia solium* is endemic in Latin America, Asia, and sub-Saharan Africa. However, with the advent of computerized neuroradiology and improved serological tests, neurocysticercosis is increasingly being diagnosed throughout the world. The management of the neurological complications of cysticercosis and in particular the role of antiparasitic drugs remain issues of debate. It is commonly believed that the use of antiparasitic drugs and steroids should be individualized, based on the presence of active or inactive disease, the location of the cysts, and the presence or absence of complications such as hydrocephalus.

Some imidazoles have been used to treat parenchymal brain cysticerci. Initially, flubendazole (40 mg/kg for 10 days) was given to 13 patients with neurocysticercosis, with promising results. However, owing to its poor intestinal absorption, the use of flubendazole is limited. Albendazole is usually well absorbed and well tolerated, and albendazole serum concentrations are not significantly affected by corticosteroids or anticonvulsants. Albendazole was given in daily doses of 15 mg/kg for 30 days. Further studies, however, showed that a treatment course could be shortened from 30 to 8 days without affecting efficacy. Direct comparative trials have shown that albendazole usually destroys 75–90% of parenchymal brain cysts, whereas praziquantel destroys 60–70%. The advantage of albendazole over praziquantel is not limited to its better efficacy, but also to better penetration of the subarachnoid space, allowing destruction of meningeal cysticerci. It also costs less than praziquantel.

Skin *Stevens–Johnson syndrome* has occasionally been described as a complication of albendazole. An outbreak of Stevens–Johnson syndrome has recently been reported in 52 Filipino overseas contract workers (aged 20–30 years, 50 women) working in China and using mebendazole for helminthic prophylaxis (9[C]). All took mebendazole at least once after the appearance of rashes and fever. Three women eventually died, mainly due to septicemia.

Hair Severe *alopecia* has been described in an almost 3-year-old child who took albendazole 400 mg/day for 3 days; 2 months later alopecia developed and resolved within 1 month (10[A]).

Diethylcarbamazine *(SED-14, 1034; SEDA-24, 357)*

Diethylcarbamazine is a microfilaricidal drug. Although ivermectin is now the preferred drug of treatment in many cases, diethylcarbamazine is still widely used, in particular for *Loa Loa* infections and lymphatic filariasis. However, diethylcarbamazine can cause significant systemic adverse effects, such as fever, headache, and myalgia, which may compromise patient compliance. These systemic inflammatory-like adverse effects resemble those seen during acute systemic inflammatory responses caused by bacterial infections and during treatment with anti-CD3 antibodies in prophylaxis of acute graft rejection. It is commonly thought that adverse reactions to diethylcarbamazine result from proinflammatory responses to antigens released from killed microfilariae rather than by direct drug or metabolite toxicity.

The involvement of inflammatory mediators in the development of adverse events has recently been studied in 29 patients with *Brugia malayi* microfilaremia treated with diethylcarbamazine (11[C]). Before and at serial time points after the start of treatment, plasma concentrations of the inflammatory mediators interleukin-6, interleukin-8, interleukin-10, tumor necrosis factor-α, and lipopolysaccharide-binding protein were measured in relation to diethylcarbamazine concentrations and adverse events. The adverse effects of diethylcarbamazine correlated well with pretreatment microfilariae counts, consistent with previous experience with diethylcarbamazine in lymphatic filariasis and onchocerciasis. Concurrent measurements of diethylcarbamazine concentrations failed to establish a clear relation between diethylcarbamazine concentrations and adverse events. Detailed kinetic studies showed the strongest association of the severity of symptoms with interleukin-6 and lipopolysaccharide-binding protein. Concentrations of interleukin-6 started to rise as early as 2–4 hours and reached a maximum after about 8 hours. Fever also occurred at 4–8 hours, consistent with the pyrogenic activity of interleukin-6. In addition, interleukin-6 plays a central role in the induction of the acute phase proteins involved in inflammatory reactions. Indeed, concentrations of the acute phase protein, lipopolysaccharide-binding protein, started to rise at 8 hours (i.e. after interleukin-6), and also peaked later than interleukin-6, at 24–48 hours after diethylcarbamazine. These observations suggest that the adverse effects of diethylcarbamazine result from an exaggerated host inflammatory response stimulated by a high load of antigen released from killed or degenerating microfilariae.

Diethylcarbamazine and lymphatic filariasis Although over 120 million individuals have lymphatic filariasis, it may be eradicable. Newer strategies for the elimination of lymphatic filariasis aim at transmission control through the use of annual doses of combinations of ivermectin, diethylcarbamazine, or albendazole, and disease control through individual patient management. Mass chemotherapy appears to be essential in the control of lymphatic filariasis. However, drug availability and the co-endemicity of onchocerciasis and loiasis play crucial roles. Although a single annual dose of diethylcarbamazine may be an effective approach towards long-term suppression of brugian and bancroftian microfilaremia, repeated multidrug chemotherapy is the preferred approach for control of lymphatic filariasis, as in other chronic infections, such as tuberculosis and leprosy. In addition, combining diethylcarbamazine with albendazole has the advantage of controlling intestinal parasites.

In order to assess the effects of retreatment in *Brugia malayi* infections, 35 asymptomatic microfilaremic patients were retreated at the end of the first year with an additional single dose of the combination they had previously received (12[C]). Eleven patients received ivermectin 200 μg/kg plus diethylcarbamazine 6 mg/kg, nine patients received ivermectin 200 μg/kg plus albendazole 400 mg, and 15 patients received diethylcarbamazine 6 mg/kg plus albendazole 400 mg. The best suppression of brugian microfilaremia 1 year after retreatment was obtained with combinations that included diethylcarbamazine. Whatever the drug regimen, both the frequency and intensity of adverse reactions after retreatment were less than after initial treatment. The greatest difference was in patients who received ivermectin plus diethylcarbamazine, who also had the lowest mean microfilarial counts immediately before retreatment. None of the adverse reactions after retreatment was severe. Most of them, including *fever*, *headache*, and *myalgia*, were easily controlled with paracetamol. *Postural hypotension* and the “string sign” (*dilated painful and inflamed lymphatic channels*) did not occur with retreatment.

In another study the cost-effectiveness of a revised mass annual single-dose regimen of diethylcarbamazine 6 mg/kg was estimated for large-scale control of lymphatic filariasis in a pilot program launched in Tamil Nadu (13[C]). This regimen gave good coverage (90% of the population studied) and high compliance of 82%. Adverse effects occurred in 22% of patients and most were non-specific (*giddiness* in 54%, *vomiting* in 11%, *nausea* in 1%, *fever* in 14%, and *headache* in 20%).

Diethylcarbamazine and onchocerciasis Mass treatment with diethylcarbamazine is a key measure for control of the transmission of bancroftian filariasis. However, severe adverse reactions can occur in patients with onchocerciasis treated with high doses of diethylcarbamazine, which may limit the prospects for the use of common salt medicated with diethylcarbamazine in many parts of Africa. However, the daily dose of diethylcarbamazine-medicated salt is considerably lower than that of conventional tablets (25–50 mg od for the first 1 or 2 days followed by 100 mg bd for 5–7 days).

The adverse effects of diethylcarbamazine-medicated salt in patients with *Onchocerca volvulus* has been assessed in a double-blind placebo-controlled trial in four groups of 10 men (14[C]). Groups I and II had *Onchocerca volvulus* microfilariae only, group III had both *Onchocerca volvulus* and *Wuchereria bancrofti* microfilariae, and group IV had *Wuchereria bancrofti* microfilariae only. Groups I, III, and IV received diethylcarbamazine-medicated salt. Group II served as a control group and received cooking salt. The medicated salt (0.33% w/w) originated from a batch previously produced for control trials. Each individual was given a total daily dose of 5.8 g of salt for 10 days, corresponding to the average daily salt intake for individuals aged over 15 years in the area. The salt supplement was spaced over three daily meals: 0.5, 2.5, and 2.8 g at breakfast, lunch, and dinner respectively. Hence, the daily dose of diethylcarbamazine was 19.1 mg.

Diethylcarbamazine-medicated salt had no significant effect on *Onchocerca volvulus* microfilarial counts, but *Wuchereria bancrofti* microfilarial counts were significantly reduced in groups III and IV. The most pronounced adverse reactions occurred in groups I and III and were mild to moderate *itching* and *rash*. They were observed on days 3–4 and lasted for the remaining medication period, but did not interfere with normal daily activities. At day 30, all the reactions had abated. There were no severe adverse events, perhaps because of low pre-existing microfilarial counts and the short duration of therapy. There was no evidence that patients with *Onchocerca volvulus* and *Wuchereria bancrofti* double infection had a different adverse reactions pattern than individuals with *Onchocerca volvulus* infection only. Thus, diethylcarbamazine-medicated salt may be an important drug for the control of bancroftian filariasis in Africa. Salt with an even lower concentration of diethylcarbamazine may still have microfilaricidal properties in Bancroftian filariasis without inducing microfilarial killing and adverse reactions in onchocerciasis, which may further improve treatment compliance and ease of use.

Ivermectin *(SED-14, 1035; SEDA-22, 326; SEDA-23, 328; SEDA-24, 357)*

Ivermectin is used to treat strongyloides, scabies, and all types of filariasis, except for *Dipalonema perstans*. Its mode of action, recently reviewed (15[R]), has tentatively been identified as agonism at GABA receptors, with inhibition of ion channels that control specific nerve cell connections. The functioning of chloride channels should thus be altered in most organisms, leading to paralysis and death of parasites. Several sites of action have been proposed:

- a postsynaptic agonist site either on the receptor or in its immediate neighborhood;
- a presynaptic site of activation of GABA release;
- potentiation of GABA binding to its receptor.

Another mechanism of action involves the binding of ivermectin to P-glycoprotein.

Ivermectin and loiasis Conjunctival hemorrhages have been recorded in patients living in areas in which loiasis is endemic. Although ivermectin is usually well tolerated, these patients had serious adverse reactions after taking ivermectin, including an encephalopathy similar to that seen after treatment with diethylcarbamazine. In retrospect, these cases all had high *Loa Loa* microfilaremia and *Loa Loa* microfilariae in the cerebrospinal fluid. The authors suggested that ivermectin might have provoked the passage of *Loa Loa* microfilariae into the cerebrospinal fluid. In a subsequent study of 1682 patients with loiasis treated with ivermectin 150 μg/kg, *conjunctival hemorrhages* were found in 41, nine of whom had previously received a microfilaricidal drug (16[C]). The initial mean *Loa Loa* microfilaremia was 14 900 microfilariae/ml (range 0–182 400; median 37 500), compared with 14.5 microfilariae/ml (range 0–97 600; median 0) in those without conjunctival hemorrhage. In addition, male sex and *Mansonella perstans* microfilaremia were associated with conjunctival hemorrhages. There was a close relation between conjunctival hemorrhages and retinal lesions. Based on observations in three patients who all developed coma after ivermectin the authors suggested that retinal lesions may reflect what occurs in the cerebral circulation in patients with high *Loa Loa* microfilaremia and neurological problems after ivermectin.

Ivermectin and lymphatic filariasis In a double-blind placebo-controlled study in Ghana single doses of ivermectin 150–200 μg/kg and albendazole 400 mg, either separately or in combination, were given to 1425 individuals for *Wuchereria bancrofti* infection (17[C]). Of these, 340 were microfilariae-positive before treatment. Ivermectin and ivermectin plus albendazole both produced statistically significant reductions in mean microfilaria counts at follow-up; the effect of ivermectin was longer lasting. Albendazole produced a non-significant reduction. Adverse reactions were few and mostly mild, and there were no severe reactions.

Ivermectin and onchocerciasis Although adverse reactions after ivermectin in onchocerciasis are usually less severe than after diethylcarbamazine, they still affect a significant number of patients with onchocerciasis after the first dose. With subsequent treatments, these reactions become less frequent and severe. The so-called *Mazzotti reaction*, a range of events that include a papular or urticarial rash, lymphedema, and fever, is ascribed to an inflammatory host response to microfilarial killing and tends to be more severe in those who have greater numbers of parasites.

The roles of chemoattractants, such as eotaxin, RANTES, and MCP-3, in the recruitment of eosinophils to the site of parasite killing has been studied in 13 patients with onchocerciasis and two control subjects before and after ivermectin (18[c]). There were adverse reactions in eight patients, but none was severe. The reactions were *fever* (54%), *pruritus* (62%), *rash* (46%), and *lymphedema* (46%). There was no significant postural hypotension. There was endothelial expression of both RANTES and eotaxin after ivermectin, suggesting that these chemoattractants have an important role in eosinophil recruitment into the skin during killing or degeneration of parasites after ivermectin.

There has been an epidemiological survey of the endemicity of human onchocerciasis and the effects of subsequent mass distribution of ivermectin in villages of the Nzerem-Ikpem community in Nigeria (19[C]). Of 1126 people studied, 527 were positive for skin microfilariae, 329 had a leopard skin (characterized by focal skin depigmentation), 385 had nodules, and 167 had onchodermatitis. There were adverse effects in 362 patients (19%) – *pruritus* in 13%, *limb swelling* in 8.5%, *facial swelling* in 2%, *weakness* in 4.8%, *nausea and vomiting* in 3.4%, *headache* in 5.8%, *diarrhea* in 3.4%, and *rheumatism* in 3.5%. There were no severe reactions.

The effects of age, sex, dosing round, time of day, and distance from the nurse monitor on adverse event reporting during mass ivermectin administration in Achi in South-East Nigeria have been examined (20[C]). There was a significant increase in adverse reporting with age, but not sex. Fewer adverse effects were reported after starting at night than after starting by day. There was no significant effect of distances up to 1 km on adverse events reporting. Both compliance and adverse reporting were less after the second dosing round than after the first. These variables should be included in the standardization of adverse events reporting.

Ivermectin and scabies Outbreaks of scabies in elderly people require special management for disease control. Owing to the frequent failure of repeated non-synchronized therapeutic efforts with conventional external antiscabies treatments, special eradication programs are required. Recently, the management of outbreaks of scabies with allethrin, permethrin, and ivermectin has been evaluated (21[C]). Healthy infested people (n = 240) were treated once simultaneously with an external scabicide, such as allethrin or permethrin; this was effective in 99%. Those with crusted scabies (n = 12) were hospitalized and treated with systemic ivermectin or ivermectin plus permethrin; seven patients received ivermectin twice after an interval of 8 days and one received permethrin three times. Unfortunately, no details of adverse effects were given.

Ivermectin and strongyloides *Strongyloides* infection is usually treated with thiabendazole, albendazole, or ivermectin. In the late stages of *Strongyloides* hyperinfection *ileus* can develop and hamper the absorption of oral medication (22[A]).

A 39-year-old Afro-Caribbean man with stage IVB T cell lymphoma due to HTLV-1 infection had invasive *Strongyloides* hyperinfection that did not respond to oral ivermectin plus albendazole because of concurrent ileus. He was treated with two 6 mg doses of a veterinary formulation of ivermectin subcutaneously. There were no adverse effects, apart from pain at the injection site.

Levamisole *(SED-14, 1037; SEDA-22, 328; SEDA-23, 330; SEDA-24, 358)*

Levamisole and colorectal cancer Levamisole was originally developed as an antihelminthic drug, but is nowadays mainly used as an immunomodulating drug in the adjuvant therapy of colorectal cancer, usually in combination with fluorouracil. However, the combination of fluorouracil plus levamisole was slightly inferior to fluorouracil plus leucovorin (23[C]). The combination of fluorouracil, levamisole, and leucovorin did not improve the disease-free or overall survival rate, but there were more adverse effects.

Fluorouracil (370 mg/m^2) plus high-dose (175 mg) or low-dose (25 mg) folinic acid and either active or placebo levamisole has been evaluated in 4927 patients with colorectal cancer (24[A]). Levamisole (50 mg) or placebo was given three times a day for 3 days, repeated every 2 weeks for 12 courses. Survival was worse with levamisole than with placebo and there were more recurrences with levamisole. Levamisole produced a significant excess of adverse *dermatological events*. Serious unexpected adverse events were rare. The authors concluded that the inclusion of levamisole in chemotherapy regimens for colorectal cancer does not delay recurrence or improve survival.

Levamisole and nephrotic syndrome The adverse effects that occur after monotherapy with levamisole in children with nephrotic syndrome include *taste disturbance (dysgeusia)*, *arthralgia*, *myalgia*, *anxiety*, *sleep disturbances*, *depression*, *neutropenia*, *diarrhea*, *nausea*, and *vomiting*. *Leukocytoclastic vasculitis* has been attributed to levamisole in a 7-year-old boy with steroid-dependent nephrotic syndrome (25[A]). The authors estimated that about 0.5% of patients treated with levamisole develop cutaneous vasculitis with circulating autoantibodies.

Levamisole and recurrent aphthous stomatitis Recurrent aphthous stomatitis is a common disorder that affects up to two-thirds of adults. Patients may present with minor recurrent aphthous stomatitis on non-keratinized mobile surfaces, such as labial and buccal mucosa, which heals without scarring, or with major recurrent aphthous stomatitis with a predilection for the lips, soft palate, and fauces, which heals with scarring. Finally, patients may suffer from herpetiform ulcers, which may be distributed throughout the oral cavity. The cause is obscure. Levamisole has been used in the treatment of recurrent aphthous stomatitis (26[C]). However, it rarely results in objective clinical improvement, whereas the associated adverse effects, such as *nausea*, *dysgeusia*, and *agranulocytosis*, discourage its use.

Praziquantel *(SED-14, 1041; SEDA-22, 329; SEDA-24, 360)*

Praziquantel and neurocysticercosis The first cysticidal drug used in humans was metrifonate, but severe cholinergic adverse effects limited its use. Praziquantel is effective in human cysticercosis in doses of 10–100 mg/kg for 3–21 days. Praziquantel is well absorbed and penetrates cyst walls, but it undergoes first-pass metabolism, especially when given together with corticosteroids and anticonvulsants. Cimetidine (20 mg/kg/day in three doses) significantly increases praziquantel serum concentrations by inhibiting its first-pass metabolism. The most common adverse effects of praziquantel result from the host inflammatory response to dying cysticerci. *Fever*, *headache*, *meningism*, and *exacerbation of neurological symptoms* have all been noted.

An important aspect of drug treatment in neurocysticercosis is the simultaneous use of corticosteroids with cysticidal drugs (7[R], 8[R]). This combination has been recommended to avoid the secondary effects of treatment due to destruction of parasites within the brain parenchyma. However, these reactions are usually mild and transient and may be ameliorated with analgesics or antiemetics, questioning the need for corticosteroids in every case. Corticosteroids are currently indicated for patients who develop *intracranial hypertension* during treatment with cysticidal drugs. This may be anticipated in patients with multiple lesions.

However, some forms of neurocysticercosis should not be treated with cysticidal drugs (7[R], 8[R]). Both albendazole and praziquantel can exacerbate the syndrome of intracranial hypertension observed in patients with cysticercotic encephalitis, and are contraindicated during the acute phase of the disease. In patients with mixed forms of neurocysticercosis, including hydrocephalus and parenchymal brain cysts, cysticidal drugs can only be used after prior ventricular shunt placement to avoid a further increase in intracranial pressure after treatment. Fatal raised intracranial pressure has been attributed to praziquantel (27[A]).

A 66-year-old man with neurocysticercosis treated with corticosteroids and praziquantel developed headache and confusion. A contrast-enhanced CT scan showed multiple focal enhancing lesions with mild edema. An MRI scan of the head was reported as being most consistent with neurocysticercosis. He was given dexamethasone 2 mg bd and praziquantel 50 mg/kg/day. A few days later his headache worsened, with nausea and drowsiness. After 2 weeks he became stuporose and had to be ventilated. A CT scan showed multiple areas of deep subcortical focal edema near the areas of previously enhancing cysts, a striatocapsular stroke, and obstructive hydrocephalus. Two weeks after the last dose of praziquantel and despite a ventriculostomy tube he died.

The authors reported that deaths related to praziquantel in neurocysticercosis are rare. However, this case had characteristics suggestive of a high risk of post-treatment complications. Death was attributed to a sudden increase in intracranial pressure, with multiple foci of edema, meningeal inflammation, and stroke, and occurred despite the concomitant use of corticosteroids.

Suramin *(SED-14, 1042; SEDA-22, 330; SEDA-23, 332; SEDA-24, 361)*

Suramin and metastatic prostate cancer Because of serious toxicity suramin is rarely used nowadays as a macrofilaricidal drug for the treatment of onchocerciasis. Its adverse effects include *neutropenia and thrombocytopenia*, *muscle weakness*, *paralysis*, *polyneuropathy*, *vortex keratopathy*, and *endocrine and skin abnormalities*. However, its potential antitumor effects have resulted in renewed interest in suramin, in particular for the treatment of prostate cancer. Metastatic disease is initially treated with androgen deprivation, which results in stabilization or regression of the disease in about 80% of patients. Despite secondary hormonal manipulations, all patients ultimately develop hormone-refractory prostate cancer, which is associated with a median survival of less than 1 year. To date, no agent has been shown to prolong survival in these patients.

The antitumor effect of suramin has been evaluated in a prospective randomized trial in 458 patients with hormone-refractory prostate cancer and significant opioid analgesic-dependent pain (28[C]). Reduction of pain and opioid requirements served as surrogates for tumor responsiveness. The patients were given either suramin (aiming at sustained plasma concentrations of 100–300 μg/ml) plus hydrocortisone (40 mg/day) or placebo plus hydrocortisone. Patients treated with suramin plus hydrocortisone had greater reductions in combined pain and opioid analgesic intake. Suramin did not reduce the quality of life or performance status. However, overall survival was similar. Most of the adverse events were mild or moderate and were easily managed medically. Frequent adverse effects of suramin were *rash*, *chills*, *fever*, and *taste disturbance*. In contrast to the results of earlier studies, in which different suramin dosage regimens were used, *neurological*, *renal*, *hepatic*, and *coagulation abnormalities* were rare.

The use of suramin plus hydrocortisone and androgen deprivation and the use of multiple courses of suramin have been assessed in 59 patients with newly diagnosed metastatic prostate cancer (29[C]). Suramin (doses aimed at plasma concentrations between a trough of 150 μg/ml and a peak of 250 μg/ml) was given in a 78-day fixed dosage schedule (one cycle) and suramin treatment cycles were repeated every 6 months to a total of four cycles. There was significant broad-spectrum toxicity throughout the study, leading to discontinuation of treatment in 33 patients. Cardiovascular events (*dysrhythmias*, *hypotension*, and *congestive heart failure*), *neurotoxic effects*, and *respiratory effects* were more frequent than expected. In consequence, repeated courses of suramin could be given in a minority of cases only. The authors felt that in the light of the relatively non-toxic palliation achieved with standard hormonal therapy, suramin in this dosage schedule has only limited use in patients with newly diagnosed metastatic prostate cancer.

OTHER ANTIHELMINTHIC DRUGS

Owing to inadequate sterilization, parenteral antischistosomal therapy, particularly during large schistosomiasis control programs, was a major factor in the spread of *hepatitis C* throughout Egypt (30[CR]). Before the development of effective oral medications against *Schistosoma*, such as metrifonate, niridazole, and praziquantel, antimony salt tartar emetic (potassium antimony tartrate) was widely used, in particular in Egypt. The lower prevalence rates of hepatitis C in children and young adults (born after parenteral antischistosomal programs) coincided with the gradual and final replacement of parenteral antischistosomal therapy by oral antischistosomal drugs like praziquantel.

REFERENCES

1. Georgiev VS. Necatoriasis: treatment and developmental therapeutics. Expert Opin Invest Drugs 2000; 9: 1065-78.
2. Bresson-Hadni S, Vuitton DA, Bartholomot B, Heyd B, Godart D, Meyer JP, Hrusovsky S, Becker MC, Mantion G, Lenys D, Miguet JP. A twenty-year history of alveolar echinicoccosis: analysis of a series of 117 patients from eastern France. Eur J Gastroenterol Hepatol 2000; 12: 327–36.
3. Reuter S, Jensen B, Buttenschoen K, Kratzer W, Kern P. Benzimidazoles in the treatment of alveolar echinococcosis: a comparative study and review of the literature. J Antimicrob Chemother 2000; 46: 451–6.
4. Mentes A, Yalaz S, Killi R, Altintas N. Radical treatment for hepatic echinococcosis. HPB 2000; 2: 49–54.
5. Erzurumlu K, Hokelek M, Gonlusen L, Tas K, Amanvermez R. The effect of albendazole on the prevention of secondary hydatidosis. Hepato-Gastroenterology 2000; 47: 247–50.
6. Garcia-Vicuna R, Carvajal I, Ortiz-Garcia A, Lopez-Robledillo JC, Laffon A, Sabando P. Primary solitary echinococcosis in cervical spine. Spine 2000; 25: 520–3.
7. Di Pentima MC, White AC. Neurocysticercosis: controversies in management. Semin Pediatr Infect Dis 2000; 11: 261–8.
8. Del Brutto OH. Medical therapy for cysticercosis: indications, risks, and benefits. Rev Ecuat Neurol 2000; 9: 13–15.
9. Ajonuma LC, Chuku Chika L. Outbreak of Stevens-Johnson syndrome among Filipino overseas contract workers using mebendazole for helminthiasis prophylaxis. Trop Doct 2000; 30: 57.
10. Herdy R. Alopecia associated to albendazole: a case report. An Bras Dermatol 2000; 75: 715–19.
11. Haarbrink M, Abadi GK, Buurman WA, Dentener MA, Terhell AJ, Yazdanbakhsh M. Strong association of interleukin-6 and lipopolysaccharide-binding protein with severity of adverse reactions after diethylcarbamazine treatment of microfilaremic patients. J Infect Dis 2000; 182: 564–9.
12. Shenoy RK, John A, Babu BS, Suma TK, Kumaraswami V. Ann Trop Med Parasitol 2000; 94: 607–14.
13. Krishnamoorthy K, Ramu K, Srividya A, Appavoo NC, Saxena NBL, Lal S, Das PK. Cost of mass annual single dose diethylcarbamazine distribution for the large scale control of lymphatic filariasis. Indian J Med Res 2000; 111: 81–9.
14. Meyrowitsch DW, Simonsen PE, Magnussen P. Tolerance to diethylcarbamazine-medicated salt in individuals infected with *Onchocerca volvulus*. Trans R Soc Trop Med Hyg 2000; 94: 444–8.
15. Bounias M. Pragmatic efficacy against conceptual precaution in parasite control: the case of avermectins. J Environ Biol 2000; 21: 275–85.
16. Fobi G, Gardon J, Santiago M, Ngangue D, Gardon-Wendel N, Boussinesq M. Ocular findings after ivermectin treatment of patients with high *Loa loa* microfilaremia. Ophthalmic Epidemiol 2000; 7: 27–39.
17. Dunyo SK, Nkrumah FK, Simonsen PE. A randomized double-blind placebo-controlled field trial of ivermectin and albendazole alone and in combination for the treatment of lymphatic filariasis in Ghana. Trans R Soc Trop Med Hyg 2000; 94: 205–11.
18. Cooper PJ, Beck LA, Espinel I, Deyampert NM, Hartnell A, Jose PJ, Paredes W, Guderian RH, Nutman TB. Eotaxin and RANTES expression by the dermal endothelium is associated with eosinophil infiltration after ivermectin treatment of onchocerciasis. Clin Immunol 2000; 95: 51–61.
19. Abanobi OC, Anosike JC. Control of onchocerciasis in Nzerem-Ikpem, Nigeria: baseline prevalence and mass distribution of ivermectin. Public Health 2000; 114: 402–6.
20. Chijioke CP. Factors affecting adverse event reporting during mass ivermectin treatment of onchocerciasis. Acta Trop 2000; 76: 169–73.
21. Paasch U, Haustein UF. Management of endemic outbreaks of scabies with allethrin, permethrin and ivermectin. Int J Dermatol 2000; 39: 463–70.
22. Chiodini PL, Reid AJC, Wiselka MJ,

Firmin R, Foweraker J. Parenteral ivermectin in *Strongyloides* hyperinfection. Lancet 2000; 355: 43–4.
23. Lavery IC, Lopez-Kostner F, Pelley RJ, Fine RM. Treatment of colon and rectal cancer. Surg Clin North Am 2000; 80: 535–69.
24. QUASAR Collaborative Group. Comparison of fluorouracil with additional levamisole, higher-dose folinic acid, or both, as adjuvant chemotherapy for colorectal cancer: a randomised trial. Lancet 2000; 355: 1588–96.
25. Bagga A, Hari P. Levamisole-induced vasculitis. Pediatr Nephrol 2000; 14: 1057–8.
26. Porter SR, Hegarty A, Kaliakatsou F, Hodgson T, Scully C. Recurrent aphthous stomatitis. Clin Dermatol 2000; 18: 569–78.
27. Chang GY, Ko DY. Isolated *Echinococcus granulosus* hydatid cyst in the CNS with severe reaction to treatment. Neurology 2000; 54: 778–9.
28. Small EJ, Meyer M, Marshall ME, Reyno LM, Meyers FJ, Natale RB, Lenehan PF, Cehn L, Slichenmyer WJ, Eisenberger M. Suramin therapy for patients with symptomatic hormone-refractory prostate cancer: results of a randomized phase III trial comparing suramin plus hydrocortisone to placebo plus hydrocortisone. J Clin Oncol 2000; 18: 1440–50.
29. Hussain M, Fisher EI, Petrylak DP, O'Connor J, Wood DP, Small EJ, Eisenberger MA, Crawford ED. Adrogen deprivation and four courses of fixed-schedule suramin treatment in patients with newly diagnosed metastatic prostate cancer: a Southwest Oncology Group study. J Clin Oncol 2000; 18: 1043–9.
30. Frank C, Mohamed MK, Strickland GT, Lavanchy D, Arthur RR, Magder LS, El Khoby T, Abdel-Wahab Y, Ohn ESA, Anwar W, Sallam I. The role of parenteral antischistosomal therapy in the spread of hepatitis C virus in Egypt. Lancet 2000; 355: 887–91.

S. Dittmann

32 Vaccines

Editor's note: Abbreviations used in this chapter include:

- *BCG: Bacillus Calmette–Guérin*
- *DT: Diphtheria + tetanus toxoids*
- *DTaP: Diphtheria + tetanus toxoids + acellular pertussis*
- *DTaP-IPV-Hib: Diphtheria + tetanus toxoids + acellular pertussis + IPV + Hib*
- *DTaP-IPV-Hib-HB: Diphtheria + tetanus toxoids + acellular pertussis + IPV + Hib + hepatitis B*
- *DTP: Diphtheria + tetanus toxoids + pertussis*
- *DTwP: Diphtheria + tetanus toxoids + whole cell pertussis*
- *HB: Hepatitis B*
- *Hib: Hemophilus influenzae type b*
- *IPV: inactivated poliomyelitis vaccine*
- *MMR: measles + mumps + rubella*
- *OPV: oral poliovirus vaccine*
- *Td: Diphtheria + tetanus toxoids (adult formulation)*
- *TdaP: Diphtheria + tetanus toxoids + acellular pertussis (adult formulation)*

R Surveillance of adverse events following immunization

Definitions *An international voluntary collaboration has been established to develop globally accepted standardized case definitions of adverse events following immunization (AEFI). The so-called Brighton Collaboration (initiated in 1999 during a vaccine meeting in Brighton, UK) took into consideration that there is a general lack of widely accepted and implemented case definitions, because only a limited set of case definitions elaborated by WHO has been available internationally. Working groups on fever, local reactions, intussusception, persistent crying, convulsions, and hypotonic–hyporesponsive episodes were already established. The website of the Brighton Collaboration contains information about the process and progress of the collaboration, the work statement for the working groups, a template format for draft definitions, and much more (1[S]).*

On behalf of the Brighton Collaboration, an electronic discussion on the wisdom of using the term "adverse event following immunization" (AEFI) has been undertaken during the year 2001. Concern has sometimes been expressed that the word "following" could imply causality. At least 10 alternative terms have been proposed and discussed. Finally, the term "adverse event possibly related to immunization" (AEPRI) received the majority of votes. However, there were many participants in the discussion who believed that the term AEFI should be kept because it is used in many countries as well as in guidelines issued by the WHO (World Health Organization) and UNICEF (United Nations International Children's Emergency Fund) and because a change will create new confusion. It therefore seems that the term AEFI will not be replaced (2[S]).

National AEFI reporting systems *Worldwide, under 10% of countries have implemented postlicensure surveillance systems. The withdrawal of rotavirus vaccine (Rotashield, Wyeth Laboratories) based on postmarketing surveillance data that showed an excess risk of intussusception after the use of the vaccine convincingly showed that such systems are essential components of vaccine program implementation. However, the event also showed the power of active surveillance systems. Active systems in Minnesota and the Northern California Kaiser Permanente Health Mainten-*

Side Effects of Drugs, Annual 25
J.K. Aronson, ed.

ance Organization have provided preliminary data that suggest an increased risk of intussusception after the administration of Rotashield. Further analysis of the data collected both from the passive US national AEFI reporting system (Vaccine Adverse Event Reporting System, VAERS) and from various active postmarketing surveillance systems led to a decision to withdraw the vaccine from the market (3[C]).

In Spain, reports on adverse events after immunization are collected through the Spanish Pharmacovigilance System by means of a yellow card. In children, the most commonly involved pharmaceutical groups were antibiotics, respiratory drugs, and vaccines. A review of reports received over 10 years (1982–91) has been provided (4[R]). In the framework of the Global Training Network, a WHO initiative to improve the quality of vaccines and their use, a model for a simple national system for dealing with vaccine safety and emergencies as they arise has been elaborated. The authors have described the model and have outlined a training program designed to help develop such a system (5[S]).

Causality assessment of adverse events following immunization (AEFI) *AEFIs can be causally related to the inherent properties of the vaccine, linked to errors in administration, quality, storage, and transport of the vaccine (programmatic errors), but also occurring coincidentally after immunization. It is therefore necessary to investigate and evaluate AEFI, particularly those that are serious or unknown.*

The most reliable way of determining the causality of an AEFI is by randomized comparisons of events in an immunized group with events in a non-immunized group. However, such trials can never be large enough to detect very rare events; postmarketing surveillance is required to identify rare events. A Global Advisory Committee on Vaccine Safety, constituted by the WHO in 1999, has developed criteria for AEFI causality assessment. Criteria to be considered are consistency (the findings should be replicable), strengths of association (in an epidemiological sense), specificity, temporal relation, and biological plausibility (according to what is known about the natural history and biology of the disease). Not all these criteria need to be present to establish causality (6[S]).

In Canada, an advisory committee on causality assessment (ACCA) has been established to evaluate serious individual adverse event reports collected through active surveillance of pediatric hospitals or a passive voluntary reporting system. The ACCA is composed of specialists in epidemiology, immunology, infectious diseases, microbiology, neurology, pathology, and pediatrics. A causality assessment form has been developed (including criteria similar to the WHO criteria described above). For final classification of the evaluated adverse events the causality assessment criteria of the WHO (see Table 1) are used. The great majority of reports collected through the surveillance system describe minor or well-known

Table 1. *WHO causality assessment criteria for adverse reactions to vaccines*

Probability	Criteria
Very likely/certain	Clinical event with a plausible time relationship to vaccine administration, and which cannot be explained by concurrent disease or other drugs or chemicals
Probable	Clinical event with a reasonable time relationship to vaccine administration, and is unlikely to be attributed to concurrent disease or other drugs or chemicals
Possible	Clinical event with a reasonable time relationship to vaccine administration, but which could also be explained by concurrent disease or other drugs or chemicals
Unlikely	Clinical event whose time relationship to vaccine administration makes a causal connection improbable, but which could plausibly explained by underlying disease or other drugs or chemicals
Unrelated	Clinical event with an incompatible time relationship to vaccine administration, and which could be explained by underlying disease or other drugs or chemicals
Unclassifiable	Clinical event with insufficient information to permit assessment and identification of the cause

reactions (over 95%); only the most serious and unusual adverse events after immunization requiring detailed review are submitted to ACCA. At each twice-yearly meeting of the ACCA 60–110 reports of severe and unusual reports are evaluated (7[C]).

Clinical Immunization Safety Assessment Centers *The National Immunization Program of the Centers for Disease Control and Prevention (CDC), Atlanta, GA, USA, is trying to set up a network of Clinical Immunization Safety Assessment Centers (CISA). Based on standardized clinical evaluation protocols the centers will assist healthcare providers in evaluating patients who may have had an adverse reaction after immunization. Furthermore, the centers will evaluate newly hypothesized syndromes or events identified through the routine Vaccine Adverse Event Reporting System (8[S]).*

Guaranteeing vaccine quality – a problem of increasing complexity *During the last 20–30 years, great progress has been achieved in both vaccine production technologies and testing technologies. In addition to sophisticated tests, vaccine regulation entails a number of procedures that ensure safety, including the characterization of starting material, cell banking, seed lot systems, principles of good manufacturing practices, independent release of vaccines on a lot-by-lot basis by national regulatory authorities, and enhanced premarketing and postmarketing surveillance for possible rare adverse events after immunization (9[R]).*

Bioterrorism and prevention through immunization

Anthrax *Human anthrax is endemic in agricultural regions of the world where animal anthrax is common; sporadic cases occur in industrialized countries.*

Cutaneous, intestinal, and pulmonary anthrax can be distinguished clinically. Untreated cutaneous anthrax has a case fatality rate of 5–10%; death occurs only rarely in properly treated patients. Intestinal and pulmonary anthrax have much higher case fatality rates, even in properly treated patients. Transmission from person to person is very rare. Recently, anthrax has been considered a leading potential agent in bioterrorism. As was first demonstrated in 1979 at Sverdlovsk, USSR (in an environmental accident in a biological weapon manufacturing facility), inhalational anthrax accounts for most of the cases and for all deaths following the use of anthrax as an aerosolized biological weapon (10[R]).

In 2001, the first bioterrorist anthrax attack occurred in the USA. From 3 October 2001 to 21 November 2001, the Centers for Disease Control and Prevention (CDC) had received reports of 23 human cases of anthrax, 18 confirmed and five suspected. There were five deaths from pulmonary anthrax (11[C]).

Three human vaccines against anthrax are currently available commercially (produced in the UK, the USA, and Russia). Two are inactivated cell-free products, whereas the Russian product contains a live attenuated vaccine. Current vaccine supplies are limited; however, even if enough vaccine were available, mass immunization would not be recommended. Immunization could be considered for essential service personnel and, following a terroristic attack, would be combined with an antibiotic to protect against residual retained spores. Limited data on efficacy and reactogenicity were provided in SEDA-23, 336.

In 1997 manufacturers in South Korea started to develop a new anthrax vaccine. However, it would take a few years more to put the vaccine to practical use (11[C]). Current US recommendations for treatment and postexposure prophylaxis of anthrax focus on the administration of antibiotics (10[R]).

Botulism *Worldwide, sporadic cases and limited outbreaks of botulism can occur when food and food products are prepared or preserved by improper methods that do not destroy the spores of Clostridium botulinum and permit the formation of botulinum toxin. In industrially developed countries, the case fatality rate of food-borne botulism is 5–10%. Person to person transmission of botulism is not known. Botulinum toxin is the most poisonous substance known and poses a major bioweapon threat. In addition to the clinical forms of natural botulism (food-borne, wound, and intestinal), there is a fourth, man-made form of inhalational botulism that results from aerosolized botulinum toxin.*

A pentavalent botulinum toxoid (botulinum toxin in different antigenic types) has been used *for more than 30 years in some countries to prevent the disease in laboratory workers and to protect troops against attack. Pre-exposure immunization for the general population is neither feasible nor desirable; the vaccine is ineffective for postexposure prophylaxis. Treatment of botulism consists of passive immunization and supportive care. Most licensed antitoxins contain antibodies against the most common toxin types A, B, and E. About 9% of recipients of equine antitoxin developed urticaria, serum sickness, or other hypersensitivity reactions. In 2% of recipients anaphylaxis occurred within 10 minutes of antitoxin administration. Before administering antitoxin the patient should be screened for hypersensitivity (12^R).*

Plague *The large plague pandemics (6th century, 14th–15th centuries, 19th century) killed millions of people worldwide and were feared as the black death. Progress in hygiene, public health, and antibiotic therapy made future pandemics improbable.*

Wild rodent plague still exists in many parts of the world, including areas of Africa, Latin America, Asia, South-Eastern Europe, and the Western half of the USA. Domestic pets, e.g. house cats and dogs, can bring infected wild rodent fleas into homes, and the bite of infected fleas can result in human disease. Bubonic, pulmonary, and septicemic plague are life-threatening diseases with very high case fatality rates in untreated patients and in patients in whom treatment is delayed. Pneumonic plague is highly communicable, particularly in overcrowded facilities.

The potential use of Yersinia pestis, the causative agent of plague, as a biological weapon is of great concern. A killed whole bacillus plague vaccine (limited data on reactogenicity – see SED-14, 1086) is no longer available in the USA. This killed vaccine was efficacious in preventing or ameliorating bubonic plague but was ineffective against primary pneumonic plague. A live plague vaccine is manufactured in Russia, but no data on its efficacy and safety are available. Recommendations for antibiotic therapy of plague are available (13^R).

Smallpox *The last natural case of smallpox occurred in 1977 in Somalia. Because of the success of worldwide coordinated efforts, particularly the use of smallpox vaccine, natural smallpox has been eradicated. In 1980, the World Health Organization declared the global eradication of this dangerous and often deadly disease (the case fatality rate in non-immunized patients was 20–40%). During natural smallpox outbreaks the secondary attack rate in non-immunized contacts was about 50%.*

The smallpox virus belongs to the limited number of organisms that could be used as a biological weapon, causing one of the most serious diseases. There is no causal treatment of smallpox available. Immunization is the most effective measure for pre-exposure prevention and postexposure infection control. However, there were severe complications associated with the use of the old vaccines: encephalitis (mainly in primary vaccinees; sometimes fatal or causing permanent neurological sequelae), progressive vaccinia (in both primary and secondary vaccinees), eczema vaccinatum (in vaccinees with either active or healed eczema), and generalized vaccinia resulting from viremia. For a full account of the complications of smallpox immunization see previous editions (SED-8, 709; SED-11, 685; SEDA-1, 247; SEDA-3, 262; SEDA-4, 227; SEDA-6, 289; SEDA-13, 289; SEDA-15, 357).

With the global eradication of smallpox, smallpox immunization was stopped in all countries of the world, and complications of smallpox vaccination became largely of historical interest. However, recently, the threat of bioterrorism has made it necessary again to consider immunization strategies and the potential hazards of immunization. The old vaccine used for prevention of smallpox contained vaccinia virus strains grown on scarified calves. Some countries and manufacturers have retained limited stocks of vaccine, and the WHO has 500 000 doses. However, there is no reserve large enough to meet more than very limited potential emergency needs (14^R). Strategies for smallpox immunization in emergencies have been elaborated, focusing on priority immunization of individuals at greatest risk and immunization to contain outbreaks (15^S). However, the old smallpox vaccine hardly meets modern safety requirements. Therefore, the development and licensure of a modern tissue cell culture vaccine and the establishment of new vaccine production facilities is necessary. Various manufacturers have initiated such developments. A British biotechnology company has already announced its intention to begin *clinical trials on immunogenicity and reactogenicity of a newly developed tissue culture smallpox vaccine in early 2002, aiming at delivery of the first doses of vaccine in 2003 or earlier (16[S]).*

Tularemia *Tularemia is a zoonotic bacterial disease that occurs in North America, China, Japan, parts of Europe, and parts of the former USSR. Various wild animals are the reservoir of the causative agent, Francisella tularensis, which is transmitted through the bite of arthropods, including ticks and mosquitoes, by eating insufficiently cooked meat, by drinking contaminated water, or by inhalation of dust from a contaminated environment. Clinically, an ulceroglandular type can be distinguished from an oropharyngeal type; inhalation of infectious material can be followed by pneumonia or septicemia, with a 30–60% case fatality rate in untreated patients. Person to person transmission of tularemia is not known.*

Francisella tularensis is considered to be a dangerous potential biological weapon. Live tularemia vaccines have been developed and used in the USSR (to protect millions of persons in endemic areas) and the USA (as an investigational vaccine to protect laboratory workers). After the administration of the US vaccine, symptoms of ulceroglandular disease were considered milder; however, the vaccine did not protect all recipients against aerosol challenge with Francisella tularensis. The live vaccine is currently under review by the US Food and Drug Administration (FDA), and its future availability is undetermined. Taking into account the short incubation period of tularemia and incomplete protection through immunization with the current live vaccine, postexposure immunization is not recommended. Treatment with antibiotics is recommended (17[R]).

BACTERIAL VACCINES

Bacille Calmette-Guérin (BCG) vaccine *(SED-14, 1056; SEDA-22, 336; SEDA-23, 337)*

Special senses Responding to the question of whether accidental inoculation of one drop of BCG vaccine into the eye of a healthcare worker could be a risk, Pless (personal communication) has reported the case of a urologist who developed a *corneal ulcer* after a similar accident.

Drug administration route Following a 6-week course of intravesical BCG a 65-year-old man with carcinoma of the bladder developed a BCG-derived *inflammatory infiltrate of the penis*. The induration and lesions resolved after treatment with isoniazid and ethambutol (18[C]).

Lyme disease vaccine *(SEDA-23, 338; SEDA-24, 366)*

In December 1998, based on many prelicensure clinical trials, the first Lyme disease vaccine (LYMErix®, manufactured by the then SmithKline Beecham) was licensed by the Food and Drug Administration for individuals aged 15–70 years and it subsequently became commercially available in the USA. In a previous Annual (SEDA-24, 366) the safety profile of the vaccine, particularly with regard to the hypothesis that it could cause a treatment-resistant form of *autoimmune arthritis*, was analysed in detail. No convincing evidence was found that the vaccine caused serious problems, but discussion about its safety continued and the demand for the vaccine did not reach a sustainable level. Therefore, in February 2002 the vaccine was withdrawn by the manufacturers.

Meanwhile, in 2000, further results of clinical trials were published. In a randomized study in 956 volunteers aged 17–72 years a shortened immunization schedule of injections at 0, 1, and 2 months were compared with a schedule of injections at 0, 1, and 12 months (19[C]). Adverse events were transient and mild to moderate. *Soreness* was the most frequently reported local symptom (82%), whereas *fatigue* (20–22%) was the most frequently reported general symptom. Two volunteers had more serious adverse events: *severe chills and shaking* in one and an episode of *syncope* (lasting a few minutes with complete recovery) on the day of the first dose in another. The authors concluded that doses at 0, 1, and 2 months would provide protection during a typical tick-transmission season.

In two overviews the results of various clinical and efficacy trials have been summarized (20[R], 21[R]) and the safety, immunogenicity, and efficacy of the vaccine were underlined. The authors considered that the intravector mode of action of the vaccine was unique and opened the door to a new method of preventing insect-borne illnesses in humans.

Hemophilus influenzae type b (Hib) vaccine *(SED-14, 1065; SEDA-22, 337; SEDA-23, 337; SEDA-24, 365)*

In 57 volunteers, 32 of whom had recently undergone splenectomy, who received Hib conjugate vaccine, antibodies to Hib were measured at 2, 6, 12, 24, and 36 months after immunization (22[C]). All tolerated the vaccine well and reached protective antibody titers. The authors concluded that the vaccine is safe and protective in patients with thalassemia.

Meningococcal vaccine *(SED-14, 1080; SEDA-22, 338; SEDA-23, 339; SEDA-24, 368)*

The first overview of the safety and immunogenicity of the different conjugated serogroup C vaccines was provided in a previous Annual (SEDA-24, 368). Polysaccharide meningococcal vaccines in various combinations against meningococcal disease caused by meningococci of groups A, C, W_{135}, and Y have been commercially available for many years. They are poorly immunogenic in children under 2 years of age. Conjugated meningococcal vaccines of serogroup C (licensure of conjugated vaccines of other serogroups is expected within the coming years), made by various manufacturers, were first licensed in 1999 in the UK and then (at the end of 2000) in many other countries, including the other member states of the European Union. They are also immunogenic in infants and young children.

The results of a further randomized, double-blind trial of safety, immunogenicity, and induction of immunological memory in 182 healthy infants has been published (23[C]). The infants received either conjugate meningococcal vaccine (conjugated to CRM_{197}, a non-toxic mutant of diphtheria toxin) of lot 1 (60 infants) or lot 2 (60 infants) or hepatitis B vaccine as a control vaccine. Diphtheria and tetanus toxoids and whole cell pertussis (DTP) vaccine reconstituted with Hib–tetanus conjugate was coadministered in the other leg. Polio vaccine was given orally. According to the UK immunization schedule, these vaccines were given at 2, 3, and 4 months of age. At 12 months the children received either meningococcal A and C polysaccharide vaccine or conjugated meningococcal serogroup C vaccine. The conjugated meningococcal vaccines were generally well tolerated and resulted in less *tenderness* and *induration* than the routine vaccines (DTP–Hib and hepatitis B) administered in the opposite leg. There was also no significant difference in systemic reactions between any of the vaccine groups. Parents of the children who received meningococcal polysaccharide vaccine as a booster dose reported significantly more *local tenderness*, *general irritability*, and *change in eating habits* than those whose children received conjugate meningococcal vaccine. There was also an *increased use of antipyretic drugs* in children who received the polysaccharide vaccine. There were no differences in *rash*, *sleepiness*, *unusual crying*, *vomiting*, or *diarrhea*. The immunological results suggested that the conjugated vaccines were highly immunogenic and able to induce both a primary response in infants and immunological memory.

Musculoskeletal A *polyarthropathy* has been reported after the administration of meningococcal serogroup C vaccine (24[C]).

A 17-year-old boy developed a widespread rash on his back and the left side of his chest and painful swelling of his left elbow, right knee, and left ankle 4 days after receiving meningococcal serogroup C vaccine. The detection of meningococcal DNA in fluid from his knee made it probable that the disease was due to natural meningococcal infection, as the meningococcal vaccine does not contain nucleic acid. As the serogroup C vaccine protects only against group C infections, natural meningococcal infection of other serogroups, particularly the commonest serogroup B, can still occur.

Pertussis vaccine (including diphtheria–tetanus–pertussis vaccine [DTP]) *(SED-14, 1083; SEDA-22, 338; SEDA-23, 340, SEDA-24, 369)*

An overview of clinical trials with a special diphtheria and tetanus toxoids and acellular pertussis (DTaP) vaccine has been published (25[R]). The vaccine contains as pertussis components purified filamentous hemagglutinin, pertactin, and genetically engineered pertussis toxin. The vaccine induces high and long-lasting immunity and is at least as efficacious as most whole-cell pertussis vaccines and similar in efficacy to the most efficacious acellular pertussis vaccines that contain three pertussis antigens. The vaccine is better tolerated than whole cell vaccines and has a similar reactogenicity profile to other acellular vaccines.

A vaccine containing diphtheria and tetanus toxoids and acellular pertussis with reduced antigen content for diphtheria and pertussis (TdaP) has been compared with a licensed reduced adult-type diphtheria–tetanus (Td) vaccine and with an experimental candidate monovalent acellular pertussis vaccine with reduced antigen content (ap) (26[C]). A total of 299 healthy adults (mean age 30 years) were randomized into three groups to receive one dose of the study vaccines. The antibody responses (antidiphtheria, antitetanus, antipertussis toxin, antipertactin, antifilamentous hemagglutinin) were similar in all groups. The most frequently reported local symptom was *pain at the injection site* (62–94%), but there were no reports of severe pain; *redness and swelling* with a diameter of 5 cm or more occurred in up to 13%. The incidence of local symptoms was similar after TdaP and Td immunization. The most frequently reported general symptoms were *headache* and *fatigue* (20–50%). The incidence of general symptoms was similar in the TdaP and Td groups. There were no reports of fever over 39° C. No serious adverse events were reported.

Data from the Third National Health and Nutrition Survey (1988–94) have been used to analyse the possible effects of DTP or tetanus immunization on allergies and allergy-related symptoms among 13 944 infants, children, and adolescents aged 2 months to 16 years in the USA (27[C]). The authors concluded that DTP or tetanus immunization increases the risk of allergies and related respiratory symptoms in children and adolescents. However, the small number of non-immunized individuals and the study design limited their ability to make firm causal inferences about the true magnitude of effect.

Combination vaccines: DTaP or DTwP vaccine combined with other antigens, such as *Hemophilus influenzae* type b (Hib), inactivated poliovirus (IPV), and hepatitis B vaccine, or simultaneous administration of these vaccines *(SED-14, 1086; SEDA-22, 342; SEDA-23, 341; SEDA-24, 371)*

The Hexavalent Study Group has compared the immunogenicity and safety of a new liquid hexavalent vaccine against diphtheria, tetanus, pertussis, poliomyelitis, hepatitis B and *Hemophilus influenzae* type b (DTP–IPV–HB–Hib vaccine, manufactured by Aventis Pasteur MSD, Lyon, France) with two reference vaccines, the pentavalent DTP–IPV–Hib vaccine and the monovalent hepatitis B vaccine, administrated separately at the same visit (28[C]). Infants were randomized to receive either the hexavalent vaccine (n = 423) or (administered at different local sites) the pentavalent and the HB vaccine (n = 425) at 2, 4, and 6 months of age. The hexavalent vaccine was well tolerated (for details see Table 2). At least one local reaction was reported in 20% of injections with hexavalent vaccine compared with 16% after the receipt of pentavalent vaccine or 3.8% after the receipt of hepatitis B vaccine. These reactions were generally mild and transient. At least one systemic reaction was reported in 46% of injections with hexavalent vaccine, whereas the respective rate for the recipients of pentavalent and HB vaccine was 42%. No vaccine-related serious adverse event occurred during the study. The hexavalent vaccine provided immune responses adequate for protection against the six diseases.

Hematologic An African-American 4-month-old girl had severe *hemolytic anemia* temporally related (4 days after receipt of the vaccines) to immunization with DTP, hepatitis B, and oral polio vaccine (29[A]). She developed severe hemolysis and died 6 weeks after admission. The authors suggested a causal relation between immunization and autoimmune hemolytic anemia. However, the report of the Institute of Medicine (cited at length in SED-12, 817 and 825) concluded that there is insufficient evidence of either the presence or

Table 2. *Percentage rates of (a) local and (b) systemic adverse events occurring within 72 hours of immunization in infants given a liquid hexavalent vaccine (Hexavac) or separate injections of the reference vaccines (DTaP-IPV reconstituting PRP-T and hepatitis B vaccine) at 2, 4, and 6 months of age (primary immunization)*

	Hexavac				Pentavac				Hepatitis B Vax II			
	1st dose	2nd dose	3rd dose	All*	1st dose	2nd dose	3rd dose	All*	1st dose	2nd dose	3rd dose	All*
Number of injections	423	420	418	1261	424	418	417	1259	424	418	417	1259
Any local reaction	22.7[1]	18.3	19.9	20.3	13.7[1]	15.6	18.2	15.8	3.3	2.6	5.5	3.8
Skin redness (≥2 cm)	10.4	11.7	14.1	12.1	3.5	7.9	9.1	6.8	0.7	1.0	2.9	1.5
Skin redness (≥5 cm)	2.8	1.2	1.0	1.6	0.5	0.7	1.0	0.7	0	0	0	0
Skin induration (≥2 cm)	15.4	14.3	13.9	14.5	11.1	14.4	16.1	13.8	2.6	2.4	4.8	3.3
Skin induration (≥5 cm)	2.6	1.5	0.7	1.6	0.3	1.0	0.7	0.6	0	0	0.3	0.1
Other local reactions[2]	2.8	0.5	1.2	1.5	0.9	0.2	0.7	0.6	0.5	0	0.2	0.2

	Hexavac				Pentavac and Hepatitis B Vax II			
	1st dose	2nd dose	3rd dose	All*	1st dose	2nd dose	3rd dose	All*
Any systemic AEs (%)	51.5[3]	47.1	38.3	45.7	44.6[3]	42.3	39.6	42.2
Fever >38.0° C	6.9	19.3	17.9	14.7	4.7	17.2	21.8	14.5
Fever 38.0–38.9° C	6.4	17.9	14.4	12.8	4.2	17.0	18.0	18.0
Fever 39.0–39.9° C	0.5	1.4	3.6	1.8	0.2	0.24	3.4	1.3
Fever ≥40.0° C	0	0	0	0	0.2	0	0.5	0.2
Drowsiness	16.8	9.5	7.7	11.3	14.4	9.3	6.0	9.9
Irritability/unusual crying	33.1	26.9	20.6	26.9	28.8	22.7	19.7	23.7
Inconsolable crying >3 hours	0.2	0.2	0.2	0.24	0	0	0	0
Vomiting/diarrhea	7.3	5.7	5.0	6.0	6.8	4.3	6.5	5.9
Insomnia	6.1	5.2	3.1	4.8	4.5	4.1	5.0	4.5
Loss of appetite	13.0	8.3	6.5	9.3	9.2	9.1	7.4	8.6
Other systemic adverse events[4]	4.3	5.0	7.7	5.6	3.8	4.1	6.2	4.7

* At least one reaction to any of the three primary doses.
[1] Statistically significant between the groups.
[2] Other local reactions: hematoma, injection site pain, local maculopapular rash, local heat.
[3] Statistically significant between the groups.
[4] Other systemic adverse events: minor childhood illnesses (e.g. respiratory or gastrointestinal disorders).

absence of a connection between this vaccine and hemolytic anemia.

Skin In temporal relation (3 weeks later) to the simultaneous administration of DTP vaccine, Hib vaccine, and oral polio vaccine, a 6-month-old boy developed *Gianotti–Crosti syndrome* (a monomorphic, non-pruritic eruption most commonly involving the face, neck, buttocks, and extremities) (30[A]). Because recent infections with most common viruses were excluded, the authors concluded that the immunization had caused the syndrome. They mentioned a report of two children with the syndrome after immunization.

Pneumococcal vaccine *(SED-14, 1086; SEDA-22, 344; SEDA-23, 343; SEDA-24, 371)*

Pneumococcal polysaccharide vaccines are not immunogenic in infants, but improved immunogenicity of polysaccharide–protein conjugates has been demonstrated. In 2000, the first heptavalent *conjugate pneumococcal vaccine*, Prevnar (containing polysaccharides of pneumococcal serotypes 4, 6B, 9V, 14, 19F, and 23F, and oligosaccharide of serotype 18C, conjugated to the protein carrier CRM 197 [non-toxic variant of diphtheria toxin]), has been licensed in the USA (covering 90% of pneumococcal serotypes found in young children in the USA), and in all EU member states, as well as in selected other countries in 2001. A comprehensive technical overview on the epidemiology and prevention of pneumococcal disease, including the use of polysaccharide and conjugate vaccines has been provided (31[R]).

Conjugated pneumococcal vaccine Further results of field trials on the efficacy, safety, and immunogenicity of heptavalent conjugated pneumococcal vaccine have been provided. Between October 1995 and August 1998, 37 868 infants were included in a double-blind trial (32[C]). At 2, 4, 6, and 12–15 months of age they were randomly assigned to receive either the pneumococcal conjugate vaccine or meningococcal conjugate vaccine. More than 95% of pneumococcal vaccine recipients developed $\geq$0.15 μg/ml antibodies against all serotypes included in the vaccine. As of April 1999, a vaccine efficacy of 97% (prevention of invasive pneumococcal disease caused by vaccine serotypes) was calculated; in addition, there was a significant impact on otitis media. Data on reactogenicity of the conjugate pneumococcal and meningococcal vaccines are provided in Tables 3 and 4. Local reactions were analysed separately for children who had received DTaP and DTwP vaccine simultaneously. Local and systemic reactions were generally relatively mild with either vaccine, and more severe local and systemic reactions were uncommon and self-limiting. There were significant differences in out-patient clinic visits for *seizures* (11 pneumococcal vaccine recipients versus 23 controls), but none of the subcategories of seizure (febrile seizures, epilepsy, afebrile seizures) was significantly different. There were four cases of *sudden infant death syndrome* (SIDS) (0.2/1000) in the pneumococcal vaccine group and eight in the controls (0.4/1000). This rate is similar to the rate of 0.5/1000 children observed in the general infant population of California.

Recent advances in conjugated pneumococcal vaccines selected from current literature have been reviewed, including studies with experimental tetravalent and pentavalent conjugated vaccines and vaccines conjugated to various proteins (33[R]).

23-valent pneumococcal polysaccharide vaccine The efficacy of polysaccharide vaccine in preventing invasive pneumococcal disease, pneumonia, and death has been assessed in a double-blind, randomized, placebo-controlled trial in 1392 HIV_1-infected adults in Uganda (34[C]). The vaccine was well tolerated. However, it was ineffective and is not recommended for use in HIV_1-infected individuals. Reassessment of recommendations for polysaccharide vaccine immunization may be necessary in some countries. The authors suggested that the vaccine causes destruction of polysaccharide-responsive B cell clones.

In another clinical trial the immunogenicity and safety of polysaccharide vaccine have been assessed in 21 renal transplant recipients (35[C]). Protective antibody titers were reached at 6 and 12 weeks after immunization in all recipients, bar one. No local or systemic adverse effects were observed.

Immunologic An *allergic reaction* has been described (36[A]).

Table 3. *Local reactions comparing pneumococcal (PNCRM7) and meningococcal (MnCC) conjugate vaccine as well as each of these with DTaP*

Reaction	PNCRM7 (%)	DTaP (%)	P value	MnCC (%)	DTaP (%)	P value	PNCRM7 vs MnCC
Redness							
Dose 1	10.0	6.7	<0.001	6.5	5.6	0.345	0.124
Dose 2	11.6	10.5	0.512	7.6	10.8	0.011	0.003
Dose 3	13.8	11.4	0.143	9.3	8.2	0.557	0.011
Dose 4	10.9	3.6	0.004	4.5	4.0	>0.999	0.226
Redness >3 cm							
Dose 1	0.3	0	0.500	0.1	0.3	>0.999	>0.999
Dose 2	0.0	0.2	>0.999	0.2	0.4	>0.999	0.481
Dose 3	0.2	0.2		1.3	0.8	0.625	0.105
Dose 4	0.6	0.6	>0.999	0.0	0.0		0.255
Swelling							
Dose 1	9.8	6.6	0.002	4.2	4.3	>0.999	0.013
Dose 2	12.0	10.5	0.312	5.1	7.4	0.080	0.001
Dose 3	10.4	10.4	>0.999	6.9	8.3	0.473	0.001
Dose 4	12.1	5.5	0.013	4.5	3.4	0.688	0.247
Swelling >3 cm							
Dose 1	0.1	0.1		0.0	0.0		>0.999
Dose 2	0.4	0.6	>0.999	0.2	0.0	>0.999	>0.999
Dose 3	0.5	1.0	0.500	0.3	0.5	>0.999	>0.999
Dose 4	0.6	0.6	>0.999	0.0	0.0		0.224
Tenderness							
Dose 1	17.9	16.0	0.053	17.9	18.9	0.265	0.970
Dose 2	19.4	17.3	0.080	15.0	15.6	0.677	0.069
Dose 3	14.7	13.1	0.265	12.3	12.0	>0.999	0.280
Dose 4	23.3	18.4	0.096	15.4	14.9	>0.999	0.052

MnCC, meningococcal conjugate.

Table 4. *Fever within 48 hours of vaccination among infants receiving PNCRM7 or MnCC vaccine**

Reaction	PNCRM7		MnCC		P value
	%	N	%	N	
Fever ≥38° C					
Dose 1	15.1	709	9.4	710	0.001
Dose 2	23.9	556	10.9	507	0.001
Dose 3	19.1	461	11.8	414	0.003
Dose 4	21.0	224	17.0	230	0.274
Fever >39° C					
Dose 1	0.9	709	0.3	710	0.178
Dose 2	2.5	556	0.8	507	0.029
Dose 3	1.7	461	0.7	414	0.180
Dose 4	1.3	224	1.7	230	>0.999

* Concomitantly with DTaP and other recommended vaccines; MnCC, meningococcal conjugate.

A 2-year-old child developed bronchospasm and cutaneous and laryngeal edema immediately after the injection of a 23-valent polysaccharide pneumococcal vaccine. The symptoms resolved within 1 hour of treatment with antihistamines, corticosteroids, and aerosols. Skin tests and specific IgE tests showed that the pneumococcal antigens were responsible for the anaphylaxis.

Typhoid fever vaccine *(SED-14, 1096; SEDA-23, 343)*

Musculoskeletal Two cases of *arthritis* temporally connected with the administration of oral typhoid vaccine have been reported (37[A]). In one case arthritis of the knees, ankles, and hands occurred 8 weeks after immunization in a 27-year-old women, and in a second case bilateral sacroiliitis was observed in a 66-year-old woman 1 day after she had completed the four-capsule series. A rheumatologist evaluated both patients and felt that the diagnosis was reactive arthritis, in his opinion most probably vaccine-related. These two cases are the first reports of reactive arthritis following oral typhoid immunization. However, the time-courses (1 day, 8 weeks) make a causal relation doubtful.

VIRAL VACCINES

Hepatitis B vaccine *(SED-14, 1067; SEDA-22, 346; SEDA-23, 345; SEDA-24, 374)*

Nervous system *Hepatitis B vaccine and multiple sclerosis* The hypothesis that hepatitis B vaccine can cause multiple sclerosis has been extensively reviewed (SED-14, 1069; SEDA-22, 346; SEDA-23, 345). Further studies have confirmed that there is no scientific evidence of a causal link (38[C]–41[C]). A European-wide study should be particularly mentioned. In 643 patients in various European countries during 1993–7, 15% of whom received various immunizations within 1 year before relapse, there was no increase in the risk in immunized patients compared with patients who did not receive any vaccine (42[C]).

The results of a hospital-based case-control study in 121 patients with a first episode of central nervous demyelination occurring within 180 days after either hepatitis B vaccine or other vaccines have been reported (43[C]). The results were compared with age- and sex-matched controls seen during the same period. No conclusion regarding a causal relation between hepatitis B vaccine and a first MS episode could be drawn, but the authors were not able to exclude such an association with certainty.

There have been reports of individual cases of *thrombocytopenia purpura* (44[A]), *pancytopenia* (45[A]), *erythema multiforme* (46[A]), *polyarteritis nodosa* and *pityriasis rosea* (47[A]), *minimal-change nephrotic syndrome* (48[A]), *Sjögren's syndrome* (49[A]), and *Guillain–Barré syndrome* (50[A]), occurring in temporal relation with hepatitis B vaccination.

Influenza vaccine *(SED-14, 1072; SEDA-22, 349; SEDA-23, 347; SEDA-24, 375)*

Various new influenza vaccines are currently under development and undergoing clinical trials, have been licensed, or are expecting licensure soon. The results of studies of the safety and immunogenicity of adjuvanted subunit influenza vaccine have been already provided (SEDA-24, 375).

The current status of adjuvanted influenza vaccines has been reviewed (51[R]). The authors concluded that the vaccine produces a higher titer of antibodies than non-adjuvanted or virosomal vaccines. *Local reactions* occur more often, but are mild and transient. The results of a trial of two doses of an intranasally administered inactivated virosome-formulated influenza vaccine containing *Escherichia coli* heat-labile toxin as a mucosal adjuvant in 106 volunteers aged 33–63 years have been reported (52[C]). About 50% of vaccinees had local adverse reactions (44% after the first dose and 54% after the second dose) or systemic adverse reactions (48% and 46%) after administration of the vaccine. *Rhinorrhea*, *sneezing*, and *headache* were the most common reactions; they were mild and transient and resolved within 24–48 hours. No febrile reactions were associated with immunization. Between 77% and 92% of vaccinees developed protective hemagglutination inhibition antibody titers against the two influenzae A strains of the vaccine, whereas protective antibody titers against the B strain of the vaccine were achieved in only 49–58%.

Drug administration route The intranasal administration of influenza vaccines has been reviewed (53[R]). Trivalent cold-adapted intranasal influenza vaccine was used to immunize 1602 healthy children aged 15–71 months in a randomized, double-blind, placebo-controlled trial (54[C]). One year later 1358 were reimmunized. The vaccine provided efficacy of 92% during 2 years against virologically-confirmed influenza. Transient, minor symptoms of respiratory illness (*rhinorrhea, nasal congestion, low-grade fever*) were reported more often in vaccinees than in controls; no significant differences were noted after dose 1 and dose 2.

There have been reports of individual cases of *giant cell arteritis* (55[A]), *pericarditis* (56[A], 57[A]), *polymyalgia rheumatica* (58[A], 59[A]), *minimal-change nephrotic syndrome* (60[A]), *pemphigus* (61[A]), and *rhabdomyolysis* (62[A]), in temporal relation to influenza vaccine.

Measles–mumps–rubella (MMR) vaccine *(SED-14, 1078; SEDA-23, 351; SEDA-24, 377)*

MMR and autism and Crohn's disease

The hypothesis that MMR vaccine can cause autism and Crohn's disease, suggested by Wakefield, has previously been discussed at length (SED-14, 1079; SEDA-23, 350; SEDA-24, 377). In a further publication Wakefield and Montgomery have raised doubts about the adequacy of the evidence that secured the licence for MMR vaccine (63[R]). Particularly in view of the immunosuppressive properties of the measles virus, they suggested that there is a potential for adverse interactions between the component live viruses. They therefore proposed that spaced monovalent measles, mumps, and rubella immunization should replace the use of the combined MMR vaccine. The continuing publications of Wakefield have led to reduced MMR coverage in some parts of the UK and to well publicized concerns about the potential for measles outbreaks among primary school entrants. In an editorial in the British Medical Journal, Elliman and Bedford replied to Wakefield's recent paper (64[R]). They considered that the current concerns were idiosyncratic and presented reviews confirming the vaccine's safety. The Medicines Control Agency and the Department of Health in the UK have rejected any suggestion by Wakefield and colleagues that combined MMR vaccines were licensed prematurely. A review of the licensing of MMR vaccines has led to the assurance that the licensing procedure was normal and was based on robust studies (65[R]). This position has been shared by the Committee on Safety of Medicines and the Joint Committee on Vaccination and Immunisation. At the end of November 2001, Wakefield left his post at the Royal Free and University College Medical School in London. The college said: "Dr Wakefield's research was no longer in line with the Department of Medicine's research strategy and he left the university by mutual agreement" (66[S]). The WHO has strongly endorsed the use of MMR vaccine. The combination vaccine is recommended rather than monovalent presentations. There is no evidence to suggest impaired safety of MMR (67[R]).

In April 2001, the Institute of Medicine's Immunization Safety Review Committee released its report "MMR vaccine and autism". Although scientists generally agree that most cases of autism result from events that occur in the prenatal period or shortly after birth, there is concern because the symptoms of autism typically do not emerge until the child's second year, and this is the same time at which MMR vaccine is first administered in most developed countries. The committee took also into consideration the papers published by Wakefield and other groups and scientists suggesting evidence of a link between MMR vaccine and Crohn's disease and autism. Following review of the numerous research efforts on the MMR–autism hypothesis the committee concluded in its report "that the evidence favors rejection of a causal relationship at the population level between MMR vaccine and autistic spectrum disorders". Epidemiological evidence showed no association between MMR vaccine and autism, and the committee did not find a proven biological mechanism that would explain such a relation. Therefore, the committee did not recommend a policy review at this time of the licensure of MMR vaccine or of the current schedules and recommendations for MMR administration (68[S]).

A conference of the American Academy of Pediatrics on "new challenges in childhood immunizations" was convened in Oak Brook, IL, on 12–13 June 2000 and reviewed data on what is known about the pathogenesis, epidemiology, and genetics of autism and the available data on hypothesized associations with Crohn's disease, measles, and MMR vaccine. The participants concluded that the available evidence does not support the hypothesis that MMR vaccine causes either Crohn's disease or autism or associated disorders. They recommended continued scientific efforts directed to the identification of the causes of autism (69[C]).

Long-term adverse events after MMR immunization When the MMR immunization program was launched in Finland in 1982, a countrywide surveillance system, including all hospitals and health centers, was established to monitor serious adverse events after immunization. From 1982 to 1996 almost 3 million doses of MMR vaccine were distributed to 1.8 million individuals, mostly children. Most of the repor-

Table 5. *Assessment of causality between MMR vaccination and 173 serious events*

Event	Number of reports	Number not causally associated with MMR	Possibly causally associated with MMR		
			Number	%	Incidence per 100 000 doses
Death (n = 1)	1	1	0	0	0
Probable allergic disorders (n = 73)					
Anaphylaxis	30	16	14	47	0.5
Asthma	10	5	5	50	0.2
Henoch-Schönlein purpura	2	1	1	50	0.03
Urticaria	30	5	25	83	0.8
Stevens-Johnson syndrome	1	0	1	100	0.03
Neurological disorders (n = 77)					
Febrile seizures	52	24	28	54	0.9
Epilepsy	3	2	1	33	0.03
Undefined seizure	4	2	2	50	0.07
Encephalitis	4	1	3	75	0.1
Meningitis	4	4	0	0	0
Guillain-Barré syndrome	2	0	2	100	0.07
Transient gait disturbance	5	0	5	100	0.2
Confusion during fever	3	1	2	67	0.07
Miscellaneous (n = 22)					
Pneumonia	12	7	5	42	0.2
Orchitis	7	6	1	14	0.03
Diabetes	3	3	0	0	0
Idiopathic thrombocytopenic purpura*					3.3

* According to a previous study.

ted adverse events were minor or self-limiting events among 437 vaccinees, e.g. *fever*, *rash*, *headache*, *fatigue*, *nausea*, *vomiting*, *transient arthralgia*, and *swelling of the parotid glands*. In all, 173 potentially serious adverse events were evaluated in detail. The assessment of causality is shown in Table 5.

One 13-month-old boy died 8 days after immunization. Autopsy showed that the cause of death was aspiration of vomit. The most commonly reported neurological adverse events were *febrile seizures*. Epilepsy was diagnosed in three children; symptoms manifested for the first time 1, 10, and 21 days after immunization. One child was later diagnosed as having severe Lennox–Gastaut syndrome; medical records subsequent to the acute phase were not available for the other two.

In the four cases of *encephalitis*, a causal relation with MMR vaccine could not be excluded, because no other specific cause was detected. One child with acute lymphoblastic leukemia (diagnosed after immunization but with symptoms leading to the diagnosis already present at the time of immunization) developed, during immunosuppressive treatment, measles encephalopathy 54 days after immunization and interstitial pneumonia a few days later; 14 years later the leukemia had not relapsed, but she had developed severe epilepsy. The fourth child had *Herpes simplex* encephalitis, with a temporal association between MMR immunization and encephalitis (70[C]).

Idiopathic thrombocytopenic purpura was excluded from the analysis, because it has been analysed before (71[C]).

Nervous system *Gait disturbance after MMR immunization* An analysis of 41 reports of "gait disturbance" in 15-month-old children in temporal relation with the first MMR immunization, collected in the framework of the

Danish surveillance system for adverse events after immunization, has been reported (72[C]). About 533 000 doses of MMR vaccine were administered to 15-month-old children in Denmark during the 10 years from 1987 to 1996. The number of reported cases of "gait disturbance" corresponded to a frequency of eight per 100 000 doses of MMR vaccine. The authors considered that the symptoms were characteristic of cerebellar ataxia. The high frequency and mainly mild course of gait disturbances might indicate a mumps-related reaction. The symptoms mainly occurred at 7–14 days after immunization, and the duration was on average 1–2 weeks (range 1 day to over 4 months). Most cases were mild and short-lasting and a longer duration of symptoms seems to be predictive of late sequelae. In the same period about the same number of doses were used for the second MMR immunization without similar reactions. Disturbance of gait has rarely been reported, and the authors listed in their paper two reports from Sweden and Germany in which symptoms were so mild that no invasive investigations were carried out.

Skin A 13-year-old girl developed toxic epidermal necrolysis 7 days after being vaccinated with live attenuated measles–mumps–rubella vaccine (73[A]).

Immunologic In a brief review of allergy and MMR vaccine the authors concluded that *anaphylactic reactions* are very rare but potentially life-threatening (74[C]). Immunization personnel must therefore be aware of this possibility and trained in its management. Most severe reactions occur within a few minutes after injection and it is extremely unlikely that a child who appears completely well after immunization will subsequently develop a severe reaction.

Mumps vaccine *(SED-14, 1080; SEDA-22, 352)*

Nervous system The risk of *aseptic meningitis* is increased after the administration of the Urabe mumps vaccine strain in mumps vaccine or MMR vaccine (SED-13, 938; SED-14, 1080). Since 1992, most vaccine manufacturers have decided to suspend the distribution of vaccines containing the Urabe strain, provided that alternative vaccines were available to maintain the immunization programs established in the various countries. In 1997, a mass immunization campaign with a Urabe vaccine strain-containing MMR vaccine was carried out in the city of Salvador, in North-East Brazil (75[C]). There was an increased risk of aseptic meningitis 3 weeks after mass immunization. The estimated risk of aseptic meningitis was 1 in 14 000 doses of MMR vaccine.

Pancreas *Acute pancreatitis* after mumps immunization is very rare and has been reported only sporadically in adolescents. A new case has been reported (76[A]).

A 13-month-old boy presented with an acute abdomen and surgery was performed for a suspected perforated appendicitis. The appendix was normal but the pancreas was enlarged, edematous, and covered with fibrin, with areas of superficial necrosis. The serum amylase activity was 528 IU (normal under 200 IU).

Unfortunately the authors reported no data on the vaccine used or the interval between immunization and disease onset.

Poliomyelitis vaccine *(SED-14, 1087; SEDA-22, 352; SEDA-23, 352; SEDA-24, 378)*

Global eradication of poliomyelitis and immunization When the final goal of global eradication (certification envisaged by 2005) is achieved, a decision on "when and how to stop polio immunization" will be necessary. Such a decision has not yet been prepared. Different scenarios are under discussion: continuation of universal immunization programs, sequential removal of one or two of the Sabin strains of OPV, change to an all-IPV program, and discontinuation of OPV immunization simultaneously worldwide or selectively country by country (77[R]). The Technical Consultative Group for the World Health Organization on the Global Eradication of Poliomyelitis has the task of elaborating a proposal for final approval by the World Health Assembly (78[S]).

Nervous system *Vaccine-associated paralytic poliomyelitis* There has been a retrospective cohort study of cases of acute flaccid paralysis reported to the Ministry of Health in Brazil between 1989 and 1995 (79[C], 80[C]). For the first dose of OPV the estimated risk was one case of vaccine-associated paralytic poliomyelitis per 2.39 million doses; for total doses of OVP the risk was one case in 13.03 million doses. Most of the cases of vaccine-associated paralytic poliomyelitis were in children with a mean age of 1 year. Paralysis of the lower limbs caused by poliovirus type 2 was dominant.

Poliomyelitis caused by vaccine-derived polioviruses Between 12 July and 18 November 2000, a total of 19 people (aged between 9 months and 21 years) with acute flaccid paralysis were identified in the Dominican Republic; one case occurred in Haiti (August 2000) (81[C]). The case in Haiti and three of the cases in the Dominican Republic were laboratory-confirmed with poliovirus type 1 isolates. All cases were either unimmunized or incompletely immunized. The outbreak was unusual, because the virus is derived from oral polio vaccine virus, with 97% genetic similarity to the parental OPV strain. Normally, vaccine-derived isolates are more than 99.5% similar to the parent strain. In contrast, wild polioviruses normally have less than 82% genetic similarity to OPV. The differences in nucleotide sequences suggest that the virus causing the outbreak has been circulating for about 2 years in the area in which immunization coverage is very low, and that the virus had accumulated genetic changes that restored the essential properties of wild poliovirus. A mass immunization with OPV brought the outbreak under control.

A similar outbreak occurred in Egypt during 1988–93, when 32 cases of polio associated with vaccine-derived poliovirus type 2 were found (82[C]). Nucleotide sequence analysis performed during 1999 showed that all isolates were related (93–96% similarity) to the OPV 2 vaccine strain. The isolates were not related (less than 81% similarity) to the wild poliovirus type 2 that had been indigenous in Egypt. OPV was probably low in the affected communities.

Between 15 March and 26 July 2001, three cases of acute flaccid paralysis associated with vaccine-derived polioviruses type 1 were reported in the Philippines (83[C]). There was a 3% genetic sequence difference between OPV type 1 virus and the vaccine-derived isolates.

What lesson is to be learned from the outbreaks caused by vaccine-derived polioviruses? That it is crucial to maintain high OPV coverage to protect against imported wild polioviruses and to prevent person-to-person transmission of OPV-derived viruses.

The first case of *acute disseminated encephalomyelitis* associated with polio vaccine has been reported (84[A]).

A 6-year-old girl developed acute disseminated encephalomyelitis, and polio vaccine virus type 2 was isolated from her cerebrospinal fluid and pharynx. The virus was sequenced throughout the 5′ non-coding region of the genome by polymerase chain reaction and was determined to have undergone various mutations at nucleotides 481, 500, 795, and 1195. The clinical signs of disease had completely disappeared 2 months later.

Gastrointestinal *Polio vaccine and intussusception* Intussusception probably causally related to rotavirus vaccine (SEDA-23, 354) prompted studies to answer the question of whether polio vaccine could also cause intussusception. A workshop held in Atlanta on 15–16 June 2000, brought together experts from various fields with the primary investigators of the studies. The participants concluded that the available evidence favored rejection of a causal relation between OPV and intussusception (85[S]).

Rotavirus vaccine *(SED-14, 1091; SEDA-23, 354; SEDA-24, 379)*

The epidemiology of hospitalizations and deaths associated with *intussusception* among US infants has been described (86[C]). Such data could be useful for further clinical trials with newly developed rotavirus vaccines.

Rubella vaccine *(SED-14, 1092; SEDA-22, 353; SEDA-24, 379)*

Acute disseminated encephalomyelitis occurred in a 14-years-old boy 22 days after rubella immunization (87[A]). The authors suggest that live rubella vaccine can occasionally trigger immunologically mediated demyelination within the CNS.

Yellow fever vaccine *(SED-14, 1097; SEDA-22, 354)*

Yellow fever vaccine containing the 17D virus vaccine strain is regarded as one of the most effective and safest vaccines. The most serious complications reported were about 20 cases of *encephalitis* collected over 40 years, mainly in infants and young children (SEDA-14, 1097).

Multiorgan failure There have been reports of seven cases of serious adverse events (including six deaths) after yellow fever immunization (88^A–92^A). The cases occurred from 1996 to 2001 in Australia (one case), Brazil (two cases), and the USA (four cases). The two people in Brazil were immunized with vaccine containing the live attenuated 17DD yellow fever strain and the others received vaccine containing the live attenuated 17D-204 strain; both strains are derived from the original 17D vaccine strain. All seven became ill within 2–5 days after immunization and required intensive care. Illness was characterized by fever, lymphocytopenia, thrombocytopenia, raised hepatocellular enzymes, hypotension, and respiratory failure. Most also had headache, vomiting, myalgia, hyperbilirubinemia, and renal insufficiency requiring hemodialysis. In some aspects the disease was similar to natural yellow fever. The causal association between multiorgan failure and the receipt of yellow fever vaccine is supported in most cases by isolation of the vaccine virus and histopathological changes; in cases with lack of specimens the temporal association and the similarity of the clinical presentations makes a causal association likely.

MISCELLANEOUS

Thimerosal-containing vaccines and neurodevelopmental disorders In 2001 the Immunization Safety Review Committee of the Institute of Medicine issued a report on thimerosal-containing vaccines and *neurodevelopmental disorders* (93^S). "The committee concluded that although the hypothesis that exposure to thimerosal-containing vaccines could be associated with neurodevelopmental disorders is not established and rests on indirect and incomplete information, primarily from analogies with methylmercury and levels of maximum mercury exposure from vaccines given in children, the hypothesis is biologically plausible. ... [However,] the evidence is inadequate to accept or reject a causal relationship between thimerosal exposure from childhood vaccines and the neurodevelopmental disorders of autism, attention deficit/hyperactivity disorder, and speech or language delay".

Routine vaccination and child survival Startling results from a prospective cohort study in Guinea–Bissau, which was performed in remarkably difficult circumstances, have been reported (94^C). Both BCG and measles vaccines halved child mortality. However, the combination of diphtheria, tetanus, and pertussis (DTP) and polio vaccines increased mortality. The paper provoked heated discussions, which can be summarized as follows: the results of the study are preliminary; this is a study from one country and conclusions regarding a change in immunization strategies would be not justified; currently there are only a few studies on the impact of immunization on mortality (positive impact of BCG and measles vaccine, negative impact of so-called high-titer measles vaccine based on the Edmonston–Zagreb strain); more studies and analyses in other countries are necessary (the WHO has established a Task Force and is ready to support research studies); future vaccine trials in countries with high mortality should not only measure the specific impact on the target disease but also the impact on general infant/childhood mortality; the study has no relevance for industrially developed countries with low general infant/childhood mortality.

Opposition to immunization Friedlander has evaluated selected websites that oppose childhood immunization, and concluded that sites containing citations to scientific papers misrepresent their contents (95^R).

REFERENCES

1. The Brighton Collaboration <http://brightoncollaboration.org/> (accessed Dec 27, 2001).
2. The term AEFI – a debate. <VACSAF-L@LIST.NIH.GOV> (accessed July 2001).
3. Delage G. Rotavirus vaccine withdrawal in the United States: the role of post-marketing surveillance. Can J Infect Dis 2000; 11: 10–12.
4. Morales-Olivas FJ, Martinez-Mir I, Ferrer JM, Rubio E, Palop V. Adverse drug reactions in children reported by means of the yellow card in Spain. J Clin Epidemiol 2000; 53: 1076–80.
5. Mehta U, Milstien JB, Duclos P, Folb PI.

Developing a national system for dealing with adverse events following immunization. Bull WHO 2000; 78: 170–7.
6. Anonymous. Causality assessment of adverse events following immunization. Wkly Epidemiol Rec 2001; 76: 85–92.
7. Collet JP, MacDonald N, Cashman N, Pless R, Halperin S, Landry M, Palkonyay L, Duclos P, Mootrey G, Ward B, LeSaux N, Caserta V. Monitoring signals for vaccine safety: the assessment of individual adverse event reports by an expert advisory committee. Bull WHO 2000; 78: 178–85.
8. Announcing funding for clinical immunization safety assessment centers. <www.cdc.gov/od/pgo/funding/01112.htm.> (accessed 27 June 2001).
9. Dellepiane N, Griffiths E, Milstien JB. New challenges in assuring vaccine quality. Bull WHO 2000; 78: 155–162.
10. Inglesby V, Henderson DA, Bartlett JG, Ascher MS, Eitzen MD, Friedlander AM, Hauer J, NcDade J, Osterholm, MT, O'Toole T, Parker G, Perl TM, Russell PK, Tonat K (for the working group on civilian biodefense). Anthrax as a biological weapon. Medical and public health management. J Am Med Assoc 1999; 281: 1735–45.
11. Anonymous. South Korea: development of anthrax vaccine close to completion. The Korea Herald, January 14, 2000.
12. Arnon SS, Schechter R, Inglesby V, Henderson DA, Bartlett JG, Ascher MS, Eitzen MD, Fine AD, Hauer J, Layton M, Lillibridge S, Osterholm, MT, O'Toole T, Parker G, Perl TM, Russell PK, Swerdlow DL, Tonat K (for the working group on civilian biodefense). Botulinum toxin as a biological weapon. Medical and public health management. J Am Med Assoc 2001; 285: 1059–70.
13. Inglesby V, Dennis DT, Henderson DA, Bartlett JG, Ascher MS, Eitzen MD, Fine AD, Friedlander AM, Hauer J, Koerner JF, McDade J, Osterholm, MT, O'Toole T, Parker G, Perl TM, Russell PK, Schoch-Spana M, Tonat K (for the working group on civilian biodefense). Plague as a biological weapon. Medical and public health management. J Am Med Assoc 2000; 283: 2281–90.
14. Henderson DA, Inglesby V,, Bartlett JG, Ascher MS, Eitzen MD, Jahrling PB, Hauer J, Layton M, McDade J, Osterholm, MT, O'Toole T, Parker G, Perl TM, Russell PK, Tonat K (for the working group on civilian biodefense). Smallpox as a biological weapon. Medical and public health management. J Am Med Assoc 1999; 281: 2127–37.
15. Centers for Disease Control and Prevention (CDC). Interim smallpox response plan and guidelines (draft 2.0 – 21 November 2001). <http://www.bt.cdc.gov/DocumentsApp/Smallpox/RPG/plan>
16. Reuters Medical News. New smallpox vaccine nears clinical trial. <http://primarycare.medscape.com/reuters/prof/2001/09/09.21/20010920drgd002.html>
17. Dennis DT, Inglesby V, Henderson DA, Bartlett JG, Ascher MS, Eitzen MD, Fine AD, Friedlander AM, Hauer J, Layton M, Lillibridge S, McDade J, Osterholm, MT, O'Toole T, Parker G, Perl TM, Russell PK, Tonat K (for the working group on civilian biodefense). Tularemia as a biological weapon. Medical and public health management. J Am Med Assoc 2001; 285: 2763–73.
18. Latini JM, Wang DS, Forgacs P, Bihrle W. Tuberculosis of the penis after intravesical BCG treatment. J Urol 2000; 163: 1870.
19. Schoen RT, Sikand VK, Caldwell MC, Van Hoecke C, Gillet M, Buscarino C, Parenti DL. Safety and immunogenicity profile of a recombinant outer-surface protein A Lyme disease vaccine: trial of a 3-dose schedule at 0, 1, and 2 months. Clin Ther 2000; 22: 315–24.
20. Thanassi WT, Schoen RT. The Lyme disease vaccine: conception, development, and implementation. Ann Intern Med 2000; 132: 661–8.
21. Onrust SV, Goa KL. Adjuvanted Lyme disease vaccine: a review of ist use in the management of Lyme disease. Drugs 2000; 59: 281–99.
22. Cimaz R, Mensi C, D'Angelo E. Safety and immunogenicity of a conjugate vaccine against *Haemophilus influenzae* type b in splenectomized and non-splenectomized patients with Cooley anemia. J Infect Dis Online 2001; 183: 1819.
23. MacLennan JM, Shackley F, Heath PT, Deeks JJ, Flamank C, Herbert M, Griffiths H, Hatzmann E, Goilav C, Moxon ER. Safety, immunogenicity, and induction of immunologic memory by a serogroup C meningococcal conjugate vaccine in infants: a randomized controlled trial. J Am Med Assoc 2000; 283: 2795–801.
24. Suresh E, Cox R, Morris I. A teenager with rash and joint swelling after meningococcal C conjugate vaccine. Lancet 2000; 356: 1486.
25. Matheson AJ, Goa KL. Diphtheria–tetanus–acellular pertussis vaccine adsorbed (Triacelluvax™ DTaP3-CB): A review of its use in the prevention of *Bordetella pertussis* infection. Paediatr Drugs 2000; 2: 139–59.
26. Van der Wielen M, Van Damme P. Tetanus–diphtheria booster in non-responding tetanus–diphtheria vaccinees. Vaccine 2000; 19: 1005–6.
27. Hurwitz EL, Morgenstern H. Effects of diphtheria–tetanus–pertussis or tetanus vaccination on allergies and allergy-related respiratory symptoms among children and adolescents in the United States. J Manip Physiol Ther 2000; 23: 81–90.
28. Mallet E, Fabre P, Pines E, Salomon H, Staub T, Schodel F, Mendelman P, Hessel L, Chryssomalis G, Vidor E, Hoffenbach A, Abeille A, Amar R, Arsene JP, Aurand JM, Azoulay L, Badescou E, Barrois S, Baudino N, Beal M, Beaude-Chervet V, Berlier P, Billard E, Billet L, Blanc B, Blanc JP, Bohu D, Bonardo C, Bossu C and the hexavalent vaccine trial study group. Immunogenicity and safety of a new liquid hexavalent combined vaccine compared with separate administration of reference licensed vaccines in infants. Pediatr Infect Dis J 2000; 19: 1119–27.
29. Downes KA, Domen RE, McCarron KF. Acute

autoimmune hemolytic anemia following DTP vaccination: report of a fatal case and review of the literature. Clin Pediatr 2001; 40: 355.
30. Murphy LA, Buckley C. Gianotti–Crosti syndrome in an infant following immunization. Pediatr Dermatol 2000; 17: 225–6.
31. Overturf GD, Peter G, Pickering LK, MacDonald NE, Chilton L, Jacobs RF, Delage G, Dowell SF, Orenstein WA, Patriarca PA, Myers MG, Ledbetter EO, Kim J. Technical report: Prevention of pneumococcal infections, including the use of pneumococcal conjugate and polysaccharide vaccines and antibiotic prophylaxis. Pediatrics 2000; 106: 367–76.
32. Black S, Shinefield H, Fireman B, Lewis E, Ray P, Hansen JR, Elvin L, Ensor KM, Hackell J, Siber G, Malinoski F, Madore D, Chang I, Kohberger R, Watson W, Austrian R, Edwards K, Aguilar J, Bartlett M, Bergen R, Burman M, Dorfman S, Easter W, Finkel A, Froehlich H, Glauber J, Herz A, Honeychurch D, Kleinrock R, and the Northern California Kaiser Permanente Vaccine Study Center group. Efficacy, safety and immunogenicity of heptavalent pneumococcal conjugate vaccine in children. Pediatr Infect Dis J 2000; 19: 187–195.
33. Dabelstein D, Cromer B. Recent advances in conjugated pneumococcal vaccination. Fam Pract 2000; 17: 435–41.
34. French N, Nakiyingi J, Carpenter LM, Lugada E, Watera C, Moi, Moore M, Antvelink D, Mulder D, Janoff EN, Whitworth J, Gilks CF. 23-valent pneumococcal polysaccharide vaccine in HIV-1-infected Ugandan adults: double-blind, randomised and placebo controlled trial. Lancet 2000; 355: 2106–111.
35. Kazancioglu R, Sever MS, Yuksel-Onel D, Eraksoy H, Yildiz A, Celik AV, Kayacan SM, Badur S. Immunization of renal transplant recipients with pneumococcal polysaccharide vaccine Clin Transplant 2000; 14: 61–5.
36. Ponvert C, Ardelean-Jaby D, Colin-Gorski AM, Soufflet B, Hamberger C, De Blic J, Scheinmann P. Anaphylaxis to the 23-valent pneumococcal vaccine in a child: a case-control study based on immediate responses to skin tests and specific IgE determination. Vaccine 2001; 19: 4588–91.
37. Adachi JA, D'Alessio FR, Ericsson CD. Reactive arthritis associated with typhoid vaccination in travelers: report of two cases with negative HLA-B27. J Travel Med 2000; 7: 35–6.
38. Hostetler L. Vaccinations and multiple sclerosis. New Engl J Med 2001; 344: 1795.
39. Gellin BG, Schaffner W. The risk of vaccination – the importance of "negative" studies. New Engl J Med 2001; 344: 372–3.
40. Asherio A, Zhang SM, Hernan MA, Olek MJ, Coplan PM, Brodovicz K, Walker AM. Hepatitis B vaccination and the risk of multiple sclerosis. New Engl J Med 2001; 344: 327–32.
41. Soubeyrand B, Boisnard F, Bruel M, Debois H, Delattre D, Gauthier A, Soum S, Thébault C. Pathologies démyélinisantes du système nerveux central rapportées après vaccination hépatite B par GenHevac B (1989–1998). Presse Méd 2000; 29: 775–80.
42. Confavreux C, Suissa S, Saddier P, Bourdes V, Vucusic S. Vaccinations and the risk of relapse in multiple sclerosis. Vaccines in multiple sclerosis study group. New Engl J Med 2001; 319–26.
43. Touzé E, Gout O, Verdier-Taillefer, Lyon-Caen O, Alpérovitch A. Premier épisode de démyelinisation du système nerveux central et vaccination contre l'hépatite B. Rev Neurol (Paris) 2000; 156: 242–6.
44. Maezono R, Escobar A. Thrombocytopenic purpura after hepatitis B vaccine. J Pediatr 2000; 76: 395–8.
45. Viallard JF, Boiron JM, Parrens M, Moreau JF, Ranchin V, Reiffers J, Leng B, Pellegrin JL. Severe pancytopenia triggered by recombinant hepatitis B vaccine. Br J Haematol 2000; 110: 230–3.
46. Loche F, Schwarze HP, Thedenat B, Carriere M, Bazex J. Erythema multiforme associated with hepatitis B immunization. Clin Exp Dermatol 2000; 25: 167–8.
47. De Keyser F, Naeyaert JM, Hindryckx P, Elewaut D, Verplancke P, Peene I, Praet M, Veys E. Immune-mediated pathology following hepatitis B vaccination. Two cases of polyarteritis nodosa and one case of pityriasis rosea-like drug eruption. Clin Exp Rheumatol 2000; 18: 81–5.
48. Islek I, Cengiz K, Cakir M Kucukoduk S. Nephrotic syndrome following hepatitis B vaccination. Pediatr Nephrol 2000; 14: 89–90.
49. Toussirot E, Lohse A, Wendling D, Mougin C. Sjögren's syndrome occurring after hepatitis B vaccination. Arthritis Rheum 2000; 43: 2139–40.
50. Sinsawaiwong S, Thampanitchawong P. Guillain-Barré syndrome following recombinant hepatitis B vaccine and literature review. J Med Assoc Thailand 2000; 83: 1124–6.
51. Dooley M, Goa KL. Adjuvanted influenza vaccine. Biodrugs 2000; 14: 61–9.
52. Gluck R, Mischler R, Durrer P, Furer E, Lang AB, Herzog C, Cryz SJ Jr. Safety and immunogenicity of intranasally administered inactivated trivalent virosome-formulated influenza vaccine containing *Escherichia coli* heat-labile toxin as a mucosal adjuvant. J Infect Dis 2000; 181: 1129–32.
53. Eyles JE, Williamson E.D, Alpar HO. Intranasal administration of influenza vaccines: current status. Biodrugs 2000; 13: 35–59.
54. Belshe RB, Gruber WC. Prevention of otitis media in children with live attenuated influenza vaccine given intranasally. Pediatr Infect Dis J 2000; 19 Suppl: S66–71.
55. Perez C, Loza E, Tinture T. Giant cell arteritis after influenza vaccination. Arch Intern Med 2000; 160: 2677.
56. Pautas E, Dulou L, Laurent M. Acute non specific pericarditis criter influenza vaccination: an infrequent effect to recognize. Rev Geriatr 2000; 25: 413–14.
57. De Meester A, Luwaert R, Chaudron JM. Symptomatic pericarditis after influenza vaccination: report of two cases. Chest 2000; 117: 1803–5.

58. Liozon E, Ittig R, Vogt N, Michel JP, Gold G. Polymyalgia rheumatica following influenza vaccination. J Am Geriatr Soc 2000; 48: 1533–4.
59. Perez C, Maravi E. Polymyalgia rheumatica following influenza vaccination. Muscle Nerve 2000; 23: 824–5.
60. Kielstein JT, Termuhlen L, Sohn J, Kliem V. Minimal change nephrotic syndrome in a 65-year-old patient following influenza vaccination. Clin Nephrol 2000; 54: 246–8.
61. Mignogna MD, Muzio LL, Ruocco E. Pemphigus induction by influenza vaccination. Int J Dermatol 2000; 39: 800.
62. Plotkin E, Bernheim J, Ben-Chetrit S, Mor A, Korzets Z. Influenza vaccine – a possible trigger of rhabdomyolysis induced acute renal failure due to the combined use of cerivastatin and bezafibrate. Nephrol Dial Transplant 2000; 15: 740–1.
63. Wakefield AJ, Montgomery SM. Measles, mumps, rubella vaccine: through a glass, darkly. Adv Drug React Toxicol Rev 2000; 19: 265–83.
64. Elliman D, Bedford H. MMR vaccine: the continuing saga. Br Med J 2001; 322: 183–4.
65. Letter from the Chief Medical Officer, the Chief Nursing Officer, and the Chief Pharmaceutical Officer, Department of Health, London: Current vaccine and immunisation issues. 1. MMR vaccine. <http://www.doh.gov.uk/cmo/cmoh.htm>
66. MMR research doctor resigns. BBC News. <http://news.bbc.co.uk/hi/english/uk/england/newsid_167000/1687967.stm>
67. WHO statement on MMR vaccine. 25 January 2001.
68. Stratton K, Gable A, Shetty P, McCormick M (editors), Immunization Safety Review Committee. Immunization safety review: measles–mumps–rubella vaccine and autism. Institute of Medicine. National Academy of Sciences, 2001.
69. Halsey NA, Hyman SL, and the conference writing panel. Electronic article: measles–mumps–rubella vaccine and autistic spectrum disorder: report from the new challenges in childhood immunizations conference convened in Oak Brook, Illinois, June 12–13, 2000. Pediatrics 2001; 107: e84.
70. Patja A, Davidkin I, Kurki T, Kallio MJT, Valle M, Peltola H. Serious adverse events after measles–mumps–rubella vaccination during a fourteen-year prospective follow-up. Pediatr Infect Dis J 2000; 19: 1127–34.
71. Nieminen U, Peltola H, Syrjälä MT, Mäkipernaa A, Kekomäki R. Acute thrombocytopenic purpura following MMR vaccination: a report on 23 patients. Acta Pediatr 1993; 82: 267–70.
72. Plesner AM, Hansen FJ, Taudorf K, Nielsen LH, Larsen C, Pedersen E. Gait disturbance interpreted as cerebellar ataxia after MMR vaccination at 15 months of age: a follow-up study. Acta Paediatr Int J Paediatr 2000; 89: 58–63.
73. Dobrosavljevic D, Milinkovic MV, Nikolic MM. Toxic epidermal necrolysis following morbilli–parotis–rubella vaccination. J Eur Acad Dermatol Venereol 1999; 13: 59–61.
74. Lakshman R, Finn A. MMR vaccine and allergy. Arch Dis Child 2000; 82: 93–5.
75. Dourado I, Cunha S, Da Gloria M, Farrington TCP, Melo A, Lucena R, Barreto ML. Outbreak of aseptic meningitis associated with mass vaccination with a Urabe-containing measles–mumps–rubella vaccine: implications for immunization programs. Am J Epidemiol 2000; 151: 524–3.
76. Feldman G, Zer M. Infantile acute pancreatitis after mumps vaccination simulating an acute abdomen. Pediatr Surg Int 2000; 16: 488–9.
77. Wood DJ, Sutter RW, Dowdle WR. Stopping poliovirus vaccination after eradication: issues and challenges. Bull WHO 2000; 78: 347–57.
78. Technical Consultative Group to the World Health Organization on the Global Eradication of Poliomyelitis: "endgame" issues for the global polio eradication initiative. Clin Infect Dis 2002; 34: 72–7.
79. De Oliveira LH, Struchiner CJ. Vaccine-associated paralytic poliomyelitis in Brazil, 1989–1995. Rev Panam Salud Publica Pan Am J Public Health 2000; 7: 219–24.
80. De Oliveira LH, Struchiner CJ. Vaccine-associated paralytic poliomyelitis: A retrospective cohort study of acute flaccid paralyses in Brazil. Int J Epidemiol 2000; 29: 757–63.
81. Anonymous. Poliomyelitis, Dominican Republic and Haiti. Wkly Epidemiol Rec 2000; 75: 397–399.
82. Anonymous. Acute flaccid paralysis associated with circulating vaccine-derived poliovirus, Philippines 2001. Wkly Epidemiol Rec 2001; 76: 319–20.
83. Anonymous. Circulation of a type 2 vaccine-derived poliovirus – Egypt 1982–1993. MMWR Morb Mortal Wkly Rep 2001; 50: 41–2, 51.
84. Ozawa H, Noma S, Yoshida Y, Sekine H, Hashimoto T. Acute disseminated encephalomyelitis associated with poliomyelitis vaccine. Pediatr Neurol 2000; 23: 177–9.
85. Anonymous. Oral poliovirus vaccine (OPV) and intussusception. Wkly Epidemiol Rec 2000; 75: 345–52.
86. Parashar UD, Holman RC, Cummings KC, Staggs NW, Curns AT, Zimmerman CM., Kaufman SF, Lewis JE, Vugia DJ, Powell KE, Glass RI. Trends in intussusception-associated hospitalizations and deaths among US infants. Pediatrics 2000; 106: 1413–21.
87. Tsuru T, Mizuguchi M, Ohkubo Y, Itonaga N, Momoi MY. Acute disseminated encephalomyelitis after live rubella vaccination. Brain Dev 2000; 22: 259–61.
88. Anonymous. Fever, jaundice, and multiple organ system failure associated with 17D-derived yellow fever vaccination, 1996–2001. MMWR Morb Mortal Wkly Rep 2001; 50: 643–5.
89. Anonymous. Adverse events following yellow fever vaccination. Wkly Epidemiol Rec 2001; 76: 217–18.
90. Vasconcelos PFC, Luna EJ, Galler R, Silva LJ, and the Brazilian Yellow Fever Vaccine Evaluation

Group. Serious adverse events associated with yellow fever 17DD vaccine in Brazil: a report of two cases. Lancet 2001; 358: 91–7.
91. Chan RC, Penney DJ, Little D, Carter IW, Roberts JA, Rawlinson WD. Hepatitis and death following vaccination with 17D-204 yellow fever vaccine. Lancet 2001; 359: 121–2.
92. Martin M, Tsai TF, Cropp B, Gwong-Jen Chang J, Holmes DA, Tseng J, Wun-Ju Shieh, Zaki SR, Al-Sanouri I, Cutrona AF, Ray G, Weld LH, Cetron MS. Fever and multisystem organ failure associated with 17D–204 yellow fever vaccination: a report of four cases. Lancet 2001; 358: 98–104.
93. Immunization Safety Review. Thimerosal-Containing Vaccines and Neurodevelopmental Disorders. Washington DC: National Academy Press, 2001.
94. Kristensen I, Aaby P, Jensen H. Routine vaccinations and child survival in Guinea–Bissau, West Africa. Br Med J 2000; 321: 1435–9.
95. Friedlander ER. Opposition to immunization: a pattern of deception. Sci Rev Alt Med 2001; 5: 18–23.

H.W. Eijkhout and W.G. van Aken

33 Blood, blood components, plasma, and plasma products

ALBUMIN *(SED-14, 1123; SEDA-23, 359; SEDA-24, 383)*

Cardiovascular In a child with chronic renal insufficiency perioperative *hypotension* occurred after plasma volume expansion using 4% albumin (1^A). The fall in blood pressure was attributed to the combination of a low concentration of prekallikrein-activating factor in albumin and the use of an angiotensin converting enzyme (ACE) inhibitor. When ACE is inhibited, the half-life of bradykinin is significantly prolonged and the concomitant administration of prekallikrein activator is likely to cause significant prolonged hypotension. To prevent this the authors suggested withdrawing ACE inhibitors 24 hours before surgery or alternatively avoiding albumin in patients taking ACE inhibitors.

Hematologic Acute normovolemic hemodilution to a hematocrit of 22% was performed in a prospective randomized study in 20 patients undergoing gynecological surgery (2^C). In one group 35% of the blood volume was replaced by 5% albumin while the other group received 6% hydroxyethyl starch solutions containing chloride concentrations of 150 and 15 mmol/l. Neither solution contained bicarbonate or citrate. After acute normovolemic hemodilution the blood volume remained constant in both groups. The plasma albumin concentration fell after hemodilution with hydroxyethyl starch and increased after hemodilution with albumin. There was a slight *metabolic acidosis* with hyperchloremia and a concomitant fall in anion gap in both groups. The acidosis, which was attributed to hyperchloremia and dilution of bicarbonate in the extracellular volume, was considered to be of no clinical relevance. The authors proposed that acidosis during acute normovolemic hemodilution can be avoided when the composition of electrolytes in colloid solutions is more physiological, as in lactate-buffered solutions.

BLOOD SUBSTITUTES *(SED-14, 1703; SEDA-23, 359; SEDA-24, 383)*

Hematologic Research continues on the evaluation of perfluorocarbon emulsions as an alternative oxygen carrier to blood transfusions in surgery. In a recent randomized, double-blind, placebo-controlled study in healthy volunteers postdosing coagulation responses (using bleeding time) and hemostasis were examined (3^C). The subjects received either saline or perfluorocarbon emulsion (1.2 or 1.8 g/kg) and were evaluated for 14 days. There were no postinfusion changes in bleeding time or differences in in vivo agonist-induced platelet aggregation. There was a *fall in platelet count*, but this recovered to baseline within 7 days. The intravascular half-life of perfluorocarbon for the first 24 hours was dose-dependent (9.4 hours and 6.1 hours with 1.8 and 1.2 g/kg respectively). The authors concluded that perfluorocarbon does not effect coagulation, at least in healthy volunteers.

BLOOD TRANSFUSION *(SED-14, 1112)*

Autologous blood transfusion

In some countries there has been a marked increase in the use of autologous blood transfusion, since it is known that blood-borne viruses,

Side Effects of Drugs, Annual 25
J.K. Aronson, ed.

such as HIV, can be transmitted by allogeneic blood transfusion (4[C]).

In 1997, 66 185 units of autologous blood (200 ml) were collected in Japan, 81% using preoperative collection and storage and 19% by perioperative hemodilution or blood salvage (4[C]). The total volume of autologous blood collected accounted for 1.1% of the total number of units of whole blood donated in the same year. Of the autologous blood donated before surgery, 78% was used, while more than 70% of the blood that was collected by hemodilution, intraoperative salvage, and postoperative salvage was used. During whole blood donations adverse reactions were reported in 1.6% of cases, and ranged from mild reactions (e.g. *dizziness*) to severe reactions, such as *angina* and *asthma*. With respect to storage and transfusion, 288 errors or problems were reported, with a frequency of 1 per 455 units during production/storage, 1 per 213 transfusion problems/errors, 1 per 23 hemodilution procedures, and 1 per 54 salvage procedures. In 3.7% of the patients hypotension occurred during hemodilution. *Clotting in blood units* (0.9%) and *bacterial contamination* (0.4%) were the most frequent problems associated with blood salvage.

Cord blood

Umbilical cord blood has recently emerged as an alternative source of hemopoietic stem cells, especially for patients who lack an HLA-matched donor (5[A]). Umbilical cord blood contains significantly more early and committed progenitor cells and is being used in patients with malignant and non-malignant hematological diseases. One of the advantages of cord blood is that it can be collected and stored in large scale in liquid nitrogen below –190° C. As the number of hemopoietic cells in umbilical cord blood is limited, current experience with this type of transplantation is predominantly restricted to children, although adults have been successfully treated with umbilical cord blood transplantation (5[A]).

In almost all patients who receive a hemopoietic stem cell transplant, *fever* and *neutropenia* will develop (6[C]). The median duration of fever in those given cord blood is substantially longer (27 days) than in those given allogeneic bone marrow (15 days), allogeneic peripheral blood stem cells (10 days), or autologous peripheral blood stem cells (6 days). In patients with a long period of fever, the time to engraftment and the period of neutropenia are longer. Therefore aggressive prevention of infection will be necessary in these patients.

Immunologic Compared with stem cells purified from bone marrow, there is no risk to donors, the risk of *graft-vs-host disease* is lower, and the ability to reconstitute hemopoiesis and immunity after transplant is improved (5[A], 7[A]). It has been suggested that the increased degree of tolerance of cord blood stem cells will yield a lower graft-vs-tumor effect (5[A]), which might be associated with an increased risk of relapse of the malignancy (7[A]). Unlike sibling marrow transplants, in which additional infusions of donor lymphocytes may be successful in inciting a graft-vs-tumor effect and salvaging relapses, there are no additional cellular therapy options for patients receiving unrelated cord units (8[A]). However, interleukin-2 has antitumor activity and can augment cytotoxic effects after cord blood transplantation (7[A], 8[A]).

In a 23-year-old man with severe aplastic anemia, graft-vs-host disease, characterized by localized erythematous plaques and papules, developed 10 months after transplantation of unrelated cord blood stem cells, but required no therapy (5[A]). Microsatellite DNA fingerprinting indicated a stable and persistent donor-recipient mixed chimerism, whilst the circulating erythrocytes remained of host origin.

Leukodepleted blood products

As in several other countries, the Health Council of the Netherlands has prepared recommendations on the need for routine leukodepletion by filtration of blood. The presence of leukocytes in blood products has no beneficial effect for the recipient, except in special cases, such as patients undergoing organ transplantation (9[R]). Leukocytes present in blood components can cause adverse effects, such as HLA immunization, non-hemolytic febrile transfusion reactions, postoperative infections, and virus transmission. It has been postulated that the theoretical risk of transmission of new variant Creutzfeldt–Jakob disease can also be prevented by using leukodepleted blood products.

The disadvantages of leukodepletion are *hypotension*, *acute respiratory distress syndrome*, and *red eye syndrome*, which is characterized by conjunctivitis, headache, and muscle aches, which resolve spontaneously ([9R]). This syndrome was caused by a specific filter, which is not being used any more.

INTRAVENOUS IMMUNOGLOBULIN *(SED-14, 1123; SEDA-22, 363; SEDA-23, 360; SEDA-24, 385)*

The efficacy and safety of intravenous immunoglobulin have been reported in patients with primary and secondary immunodeficiencies, and in some immune disorders, such as idiopathic thrombocytopenic purpura, Kawasaki disease, and Guillain–Barré syndrome ([10c]). Intravenous immunoglobulin is also used empirically in a variety of several autoimmune diseases ([11c]). Recently, the efficacy of intravenous immunoglobulin has been reported in patients with membranous and membranoproliferative lupus nephritis ([11c]).

Several mechanisms of action of intravenous immunoglobulin in autoimmune diseases have been suggested, such as enhanced suppressor activity, Fc receptor blockade, and regulation of complement, T cells, and the idiotypic network ([11c]).

Adverse effects of intravenous immunoglobulin are generally mild and self-limiting. In about 10% of cases they occur 30–60 minutes after the start of the infusion. These reactions include *flushing*, *myalgia*, *headache*, *fever*, *chills*, *low backache*, *nausea and vomiting*, *chest tightness*, *wheezing*, *changes in blood pressure*, and *tachycardia* ([12AR]). Such adverse effects can be managed by slowing or stopping the infusion, or by prior administration of hydrocortisone and/or an antihistamine.

Nervous system Cerebral vasospasm, cerebral vasculitis, and serum hyperviscosity have been implicated in the pathogenesis of cerebral infarction after intravenous immunoglobulin ([13A]).

Aseptic meningitis occurs in about 11% of the patients and is characterized by headache, meningism, photophobia, and fever. The diagnosis is confirmed by pleocytosis, eosinophilia, and raised IgG in the cerebrospinal fluid ([14C]). Patients with a history of migraine are at risk of aseptic meningitis. It has been suggested that aseptic meningitis is caused by aggregated immunoglobulin, antibody–antigen complex formation with subsequent complement activation, or stabilizing carbohydrates used during manufacture ([12c], [14C]).

Hematologic *Leukopenia* has been reported after intravenous infusion of immunoglobulin ([15c]). It has been suggested that transient neutropenia can be induced by the presence of antineutrophil antibodies present in intravenous immunoglobulin. However, the possibility that immunoglobulin-mediated neutrophil agglutination causes pseudoleukopenia has also been raised ([15c]). Increased leukocyte aggregation in the circulating pool of peripheral blood, induced by intravenous immunoglobulin, is especially observed in people with hyperfibrinogenemia ([15c]). It has been suggested that leukopenia detected by electronic counting is not necessarily associated with a real reduction in the absolute number of white blood cells in the peripheral blood, but is artefactual ([15c]).

Hemolytic anemia, which has been described after high dosages of intravenous immunoglobulin, is thought to be induced by anti-A and/or anti-B antibodies in the plasma product ([16A]).

Several cases of intravenous immunoglobulin-related *thrombosis* have been reported ([17AR], [18A]). It has been suggested that thrombosis can be caused by platelet activation and increased plasma viscosity ([17AR]). In patients with vascular risk factors, such as old age, hypertension, and a history of stroke or coronary artery disease, complications, such as myocardial infarction, pulmonary embolism, stroke, and acute spinal cord events, have been described ([18A]). Intravenous immunoglobulin enhances platelet aggregation and the release of adenosine triphosphate in human platelets in vitro. In addition, there is a dose-dependent increase in plasma viscosity with increasing plasma immunoglobulin concentration ([17AR], [18A]).

Liver Fatal *hepatic veno-occlusive disease*, characterized by hyperbilirubinemia, hepatomegaly, ascites, and weight gain, has been associated with intravenous immunoglobulin administered prophylactically to prevent transplant-related infections ([17AR]). To avoid such thrombotic complications, intravenous immunoglobulin should be infused at a slower rate in patients at risk, and high dosages (400–1000 mg/kg) should not be infused.

Urinary tract *Renal insufficiency* after high dosages of intravenous immunoglobulin has been observed, mostly in patients with preexisting renal disease (SEDA-24, 386) (19[A]). Acute renal insufficiency occurred within 7 days after the administration of intravenous immunoglobulin, with a peak at 5 days. About 40% of patients needed dialysis and 15% died despite treatment (all with severe underlying diseases); the mean time to recovery in survivors was about 10 days (20[C]). Renal histology showed extensive vacuolization of proximal tubules consistent with osmotic injury (20[C]). Cytological findings in the urine included the presence of macrophage-like tubular epithelial cells with multivacuolated cytoplasm (21[A]). Renal insufficiency has been attributed to the large quantity of sucrose that is added to the product as a stabilizer; it has been suggested that proximal tubular damage may be caused by pinocytosis of sucrose into proximal tubular cells or to an osmotic effect (20[C]). Formulations of intravenous immunoglobulin with sucrose as a stabilizer should not be used in patients with renal disease (19[A]).

In a retrospective study of a heterogeneous group of 119 patients receiving intravenous immunoglobulin, two developed irreversible renal insufficiency and six had a rise in serum creatinine. These patients had received high dosages of two different formulations of intravenous immunoglobulin, one containing sucrose 1.76 g per g of intravenous immunoglobulin; the other 0.5 g per g. There was no relation between the amount of sucrose in the intravenous immunoglobulin and the development of renal insufficiency (20[C]).

Skin Skin reactions to intravenous immunoglobulin, such as *rash*, *urticaria*, *pruritus*, and *petechiae*, have been described, but are rare (22[C]). *Pompholyx* has also been described (23[C]).

Immunologic *Anaphylaxis* occurs rarely, but mostly in patients with IgA deficiency and IgA antibodies (12[c]).

Multiorgan failure *Multiorgan failure* has recently been described after intravenous infusion of immunoglobulin (24[A]).

A 3-year-old mentally retarded girl was given intravenous sulfonated immunoglobulin for prophylaxis of measles. After infusion of about 100 mg, she became cyanotic, confused, and tachycardic. Despite hydrocortisone she developed hypotensive shock. Multiorgan failure developed, with symptoms of disseminated intravascular coagulation, acute renal insufficiency, hepatic dysfunction, respiratory distress syndrome, and rhabdomyolysis. After plasma exchange and continuous hemofiltration she recovered without sequelae. The drug-induced lymphocyte stimulation test using γ-globulin was negative. In addition, serum concentrations of IgA and IgG were normal. However concentrations of cytokines, such as interleukin-6, TNF-α, and soluble interleukin-2 receptor, were very high. Complement C3, C4, and CH_{50} were reduced but C3a was raised.

The authors suggested that an unknown mechanism associated with intravenous immunoglobulin infusion caused non-specific activation of complement systems accompanied by fulminant hypercytokinemia.

Drug contamination Recently activated *factor XIa* has been demonstrated in samples of reconstituted intravenous immunoglobulin from eight different manufacturers (10[c]). The degree of factor XIa contamination in intravenous immunoglobulin correlated with the manufacturer, suggesting that the purification process can affect residual factor XI concentration. Factor XIa can activate factor IX to factor IXa, and it can be hypothesized that there is a direct correlation between the presence of factor XIa in intravenous immunoglobulin products and an increased risk of thrombotic complications.

CLOTTING FACTORS *(SED-14, 1125; SEDA-22, 365; SEDA-23, 362; SEDA-24, 386)*

Coagulation factor concentrates became available in the 1970s, a significant step in the prevention and management of bleeding. Two major classes of complications have emerged (25[R]). First, *transfusion-related infections* with various blood-borne viruses, such as hepatitis B and C and human immunodeficiency virus (HIV). Second, *alloimmune antibodies* (inhibitors) against the deficient coagulation factor.

Fresh frozen plasma and prothrombin complex concentrate are used to reverse the effects of oral anticoagulants (e.g. during surgery or bleeding episodes) (26[c]). Prothrombin complex achieves more rapid and effective reversal of the acquired coagulation defect than fresh frozen plasma. Other disadvantages of fresh frozen plasma are the larger volume that needs to be given, the risk of viral transmission, and the variable quantities of clotting factors. Prothrombin complex products contain constant amounts of clotting factors and have been subjected to several viral inactivation processes. However, a potential disadvantage of prothrombin complex products is the risk of *thromboembolism*. Animal studies and case reports have suggested that recombinant factor VIIa will reduce the INR in patients taking oral anticoagulants and also has a clinical hemostatic effect (27[c]). It has been suggested that placebo-controlled studies with recombinant factor VIIa and comparisons with prothrombin complex products will be necessary to show whether recombinant factor VIIa is effective in reversing oral anticoagulation (27[c]).

Four cases in which there was *bleeding* at sites other than the primary site (oozing at a central line insertion site, hemarthrosis, and epistaxis), have been reported during treatment with recombinant factor VIIa (28[AR]). The authors suggested that local fibrinolysis may have contributed to or actually caused bleeding from central line insertion sites. In three cases they found raised fibrin degradation products and in two cases a 15–35% fall in plasminogen activity.

Hematologic Several serious adverse events have been reported in patients with hemophilia with antibodies to clotting factors who were treated with recombinant factor VIIa during surgery, including one fatal case of *disseminated intravascular coagulation* and one of *venous thrombosis* (25[R]).

Urinary tract In two patients with hemophilia with antibodies to both human and porcine factor VIII, continuous recombinant factor VIIa resulted in *hematuria* (29[A]). In neither case was a cause of the hematuria found. The author suggested that mucosal bleeds, such as hematuria, are characterized by high fibrinolytic activity locally and may require higher peak concentrations of factor VII to generate sufficient thrombin to achieve and sustain hemostasis. The need for a full thrombin burst could relate to the role of thrombin in the activation of thrombin-activatable fibrinolysis inhibitor.

In patients with hemophilia B with antibodies who undergo immune tolerance induction there is a risk of *nephrotic syndrome* (28[R]).

Immunologic One of the most important adverse effects of substitution therapy with clotting factors, which has important implications for further treatment, is the development of antibodies to factor VIII or factor IX. Antibodies to factor VIII occur in about 10–16% of patients, whereas 3–5% of patients with hemophilia B will develop an antibody to factor IX (SEDA-24, 387) (29[c]). If the inhibitor activity is under 10 Bethesda units/ml, patients can be treated with increased doses of factor VIII or IX concentrates (25[R]). In addition, patients with hemophilia A with low or intermediate antibody titers can also be treated with porcine factor VIII (25[R]). However, hemorrhagic episodes in patients with antibody activity over 10 Bethesda units/ml, may result in life-threatening hemorrhage that cannot be treated by conventional therapy (25[R], 29[c]). Prevention or treatment of clinically significant bleeding episodes in these patients can be achieved by using so-called bypassing therapies, such as recombinant factor VIIa and activated prothrombin complex (25[R], 29[c]).

The development of antibodies against recombinant factor VIIa or hypersensitivity reactions to recombinant factor VIIa have not so far been reported (28[R]).

In about 5% of patients with hemophilia A with antibodies treated with an activated prothrombin complex product (Autoplex®), there was a significant increase in antibody titer (30[C]).

Antibody formation in patients with mild and moderate hemophilia most likely results from the presence of structurally abnormal circulating factor VIII, so that administration of exogenous factor VIII leads to the development of antibodies by exposing the immune system to epitopes on factor VIII molecules not previously encountered (31[c]). Recent data from the UK Haemophilia Centre Directors Organization has shown that 25% of patients who developed antibodies had mild or moderate hemophilia (31[c]). It has been suggested that this high figure can be explained by improved data collection and by changes in clinical practice, namely the switch from lower purity to higher purity or recombinant products and the use of continuous infusion instead of repeated injections (31[c]).

Following the introduction of recombinant factor products, the incidence of antibody formation seemed to be higher than in patients using plasma products (32[C]). However, after considering factors such as the number of exposure days, the severity of the disease, and the frequency of prospective monitoring, the prevalence and the incidence of antibody formation for both products were similar.

Patients with hemophilia B with complete gene deletions or derangement of the factor IX gene are particularly at risk of developing antibodies after the administration of factor IX concentrate (28[R]). In patients with hemophilia B with antibodies, treatment with factor IX concentrate can result in an anaphylactic response.

Drug contamination In the past plasma factor VIII products have exposed most patients with hemophilia to foreign proteins as well as blood-borne viruses, such as *hepatitis B and C and HIV*. Before the introduction of heat-treated concentrates in 1985, about 20% of the hemophiliacs in the UK became infected with HIV (33[C]).

Virtually all patients with hemophilia who were exposed to large-pool coagulation factor concentrates before the introduction of viral inactivation procedures developed non-A, non-B hepatitis (34[R]), which is caused by hepatitis C virus. Studies using a second-generation enzyme-linked immunosorbent assay showed 89% anti-HCV positivity in a heterogeneous group of patients in the USA and in 98% of Dutch patients with hemophilia who had been exposed to large-pool, non-virally inactivated coagulation factor concentrates (34[R]). In the UK and the Netherlands increased mortality due to liver disease in patients with hemophilia has been reported (34[R]). In patients co-infected with HIV, liver disease was more severe, probably because of higher amounts of hepatitis C viral RNA (33[C]). In addition, patients infected with hepatitis C virus genotype 1 had a more rapid course of disease due to HIV (34[R]).

Dry heating at 60° C is insufficient to eliminate all hepatitis C virus, which requires dry heating at 80° C, pasteurization, or treatment with mixtures of solvents and detergents (34[R]).

Plasma-derived factor VIII concentrates have been implicated in the transmission of the non-enveloped *hepatitis A and Parvo B19 viruses* (32[R]).

Although transmission of classic *Creutzfeldt–Jakob disease* has never been observed, manufacturers have recently withdrawn plasma-derived products prepared from plasma obtained from donors who were subsequently found to have classic Creutzfeldt–Jakob disease (30[R]).

Recombinant factor VIII, used for treatment and prophylaxis in patients with hemophilia, is stabilized with human serum albumin during purification and in the final product. Although albumin has an excellent safety record and no recombinant antihemophilic factors have been associated with virus transmission, there is still concern about the safety of products that contain human- or animal-derived components (35[C]). Recently a second-generation recombinant factor VIII product has been developed with a modified manufacturing process and a formulation in which the recombinant factor VIII is stabilized by sucrose instead of albumin (35[C]).

Drug administration route The half-life of recombinant factor VIIa in patients with hemophilia is very short (2.7 hours) and the clearance is 0.5 ml/min/kg. The clearance of recombinant factor VIIa is even faster in patients aged under 15 years. In one child the half-life was no more than 1 hour (28[R]). Currently *continuous infusion* appears to offer advantages over bolus dosing, with a reduction in the total dose of recombinant factor VIIa by 50–75% (28[R], 36[c]). Studies of continuous infusion of factor VIII or IX have shown that this mode of administration is safe and cost-effective (SEDA-24, 386).

Gene therapy

Three patients with hemophilia B have been treated in a phase I trial with a recombinant adenovirus-associated vector expressing human blood-coagulation factor IX (37[c]). There was no evidence of formation of inhibitory antibodies against factor IX.

In a phase I trial with a recombinant adenovirus-associated vector expressing human blood-coagulation factor IX, there was no evidence of germ-line transmission of vector sequences (37[c]).

EPOETIN (ERYTHROPOIETIN)

(SED-14, 1128; SEDA-22, 366; SEDA-23, 364; SEDA-24, 388)

Recombinant human erythropoietin (epoetin) has been used since the latter half of the 1980s for correcting anemia in patients undergoing dialysis. Epoetin increases cognitive function and the quality of life in these patients (38[c]).

Anemia due to prematurity can also be treated with epoetin. However, there are still questions to be answered about its efficacy, dosage regimen, and route of administration (subcutaneously or intravenously) (39[C], 40[R]). A comparison of the efficacy of daily versus less frequent dosing schedules in preterm infants showed that dosage regimens that achieve lower peak serum concentrations over a more prolonged period of time may be more efficacious (40[R]).

Patients with cancer often develop anemia, and several studies have shown that recombinant human epoetin is a useful alternative to blood transfusion in such patients (41[R]). Response rates of up to about 80% have been reported in patients with cancer-related anemia, especially in patients treated with platinum-based chemotherapy (41[R]).

Whether epoetin will improve tumor control after radiotherapy is currently being investigated (42[R]). It has already been shown that epoetin corrects low hemoglobin concentrations, resulting in a better quality of life and probably improving cure rates in cancer patients undergoing radiotherapy (42[R]).

The combination of autologous predonation and epoetin treatment reduces blood requirements during and after orthopedic and cardiac surgery (43[C]). In elective open-heart surgery, 26 of 30 patients who received only iron preoperatively needed blood transfusions compared with one of 30 patients who received iron plus epoetin (43[C]).

The response to epoetin therapy in diseases such as iron deficiency, latent infection, inflammation, aluminium intoxication, and hyperparathyroidism is enhanced once these disorders are treated (44[R]).

The most common adverse effects after intravenous injection of epoetin are *bone and muscle pains* and *chills and fever*, which can be avoided by injecting epoetin subcutaneously rather than intravenously (SEDA-24, 388). Other mild adverse effects include *headache*, *conjunctivitis*, *nausea*, *vomiting*, and *diarrhea*.

Cardiovascular As the incidence of *hypertension* due to epoetin is 5–10%, it is important to monitor the blood pressure during treatment (41[R]). However, the hypertensive effect of epoetin has only been observed in patients with renal diseases (45[R]). One of the presumed mechanisms is an increase in endothelin-1, a potent vasoactive peptide produced by endothelial cells (39[C]), increased concentrations of which have been observed in adults with an increase in mean blood pressure of more than 10 mmHg. In contrast, in preterm infants receiving epoetin there were no acute effects of epoetin on endothelin-1 concentrations or mean blood pressure (39[C]).

Epoetin has vascular effects that can cause an imbalance between vasoconstrictor–pro-proliferative–proatherogenic factors (angiotensin, endothelin, thromboxane) and vasodilator–antiproliferative–antiatherogenic factors (nitric oxide, prostacyclin). These changes may be related to the occurrence or aggravation of pre-existing hypertension in humans and can cause vascular hypertrophy and potentially accelerate the development of atherosclerosis (45[R]).

Adrenomedullin, an endocrine peptide with vasodilatory and natriuretic actions, is increased in patients with hypertension and chronic renal insufficiency. In 54 patients with renal anemia, treated with epoetin 6000 IU once a week, there was a correlation between the progression of renal disease and circulating adrenomedullin; however, there was no relation between adrenomedullin and epoetin-induced hypertension (46[C]).

There have been contradictory results on the effect of epoetin on blood coagulation and fibrinolysis. There is currently no definitive evidence that epoetin further enhances hypercoagulability in uremic patients (45[R]).

Thrombotic events related to epoetin include vascular access thrombosis, renal and temporal vein thrombosis, transient ischemic attacks, and myocardial infarction (45[R]). Vascular access thrombosis has been reported in 7.5% of hemodialysis patients treated with epoetin (45[R]). It has been suggested that the increased risk of extracorporeal circuit clotting and the higher heparin requirements during hemodialysis may not be due to a hypercoagulable state, but rather to an increase in erythrocyte mass and consequently in whole blood viscosity (45[R]).

Dural sinus thrombosis has been observed in a patient with end-stage renal disease treated with epoetin-α (38[A]). It was postulated that it was caused by polycythemia, because the hematocrit more than doubled in under 2 months, reaching 0.55 (38[c]).

Strawberry hemangiomas developed in a premature infant after 1 week of treatment with epoetin (47[A]). Strawberry hemangiomas are congenital vascular lesions characterized by endothelial hyperplasia during the proliferative phase. The development and proliferation of capillary endothelium requires the presence of angiogenic factors, such as vascular endothelial growth factor. Epoetin has a proliferative effect on endothelial cells and can induce angiogenesis (37[C], 47[c]).

Nervous system Several neurological complications of epoetin, such as *seizures*, *visual hallucinations*, *headache*, *transient myalgia*, and *hypertensive leukoencephalopathy*, have been described (38[c]).

Hematologic In preterm infants treated with epoetin, increased numbers of hypochromic erythrocytes and soluble transferrin receptors were observed, despite parenteral iron; this implies that active erythropoiesis in preterm infants causes *increased iron requirements* (40[R]).

In older studies transient *neutropenia* was reported as an adverse effect of epoetin, but this has not been noted in recent studies (40[R]). Neutropenia appeared to involve reduced production of neutrophils from granulocyte progenitors and resolved after withdrawal of epoetin.

Skin A rare case of *generalized exfoliative* dermatitis secondary to epoetin has been described (48[A]). Epoetin was withdrawn and the lesions disappeared spontaneously after 20 days.

Drug administration route Epoetin can be administered in three ways: *intravenously*, *subcutaneously*, and *intraperitoneally* (44[R]). The subcutaneous route is preferred in patients undergoing dialysis, because subcutaneous epoetin provides better long-term utilization and maintains the same hematocrit with 20% lower dosages than intravenous administration. After intraperitoneal administration the absorption time is prolonged and only 5–10% of the dose is utilized (44[R]). Local reactions occur at the site of injection when epoetin is given subcutaneously (49[C]) and local pain has been reported after the administration of citrate- or phosphate-buffered epoetin (49[C], 50[C]).

REFERENCES

1. Fong SY, Hansen TG. Perioperative hypotension following plasma volume expansion with albumin in an angiotensin converting enzyme inhibited infant. Br J Anaesth 2000; 84: 537–58.
2. Rehm M, Orth V, Scheingraber S, Kreimeier U, Brechtelsbauer H, Finsterer U. Acid-base changes caused by 5% albumin versus 6% hydroxyethyl starch solution in patients undergoing acute normovolemic hemodilution. A randomized prospective study. Anesthesiology 2000; 93: 1174–83.
3. Leese PT, Noveck R , Shorr JS, Woods CM, Flaim KE, Keipert PE. Randomised safety studies of intravenous perflubron emulsion. 1. Effects on coagulation function in healthy volunteers. Anesth Analg 2000; 91: 804–11.
4. Ohto H, Fuji T, Wakimoto N, Anan M, Maeda H. A survey of autologous blood collection and transfusion in Japan in 1997. Transfus Sci 2000; 22: 13–18.
5. Mao P, Liao C, Zhu Z, Wang S, Xu X, Mo W, Ying Y, Li Q, Liu B. Umbilical cord blood transplantation from unrelated HLA-matched donor in an adult with severe aplastic anemia. Bone Marrow Transplant 2000; 26: 1121–3.
6. Mullen CA, Nair J, Sandesh S, Chan KW. Fever and neutropenia in pediatric haematopoietic stem cell transplant patients. Bone Marrow Transplant 2000; 25: 56–65.
7. Laws HJ, Nürnberger W, Körholz D, Kögler G, Fischer J, Niehues T, Wernet P, Göbel U. Successful treatment of relapsed CML after cord blood transplantation with donor leukocyte IL-2 and INFa. Bone Marrow Transplant 2000; 25: 219–22.
8. Goldberg SL, Pecora AL, Rosenbluth RJ, Jennis AA, Preti RA. Treatment of leukemic relapse following unrelated umbilical cord blood transplantation with interleukin-2: potential for augmenting

graft-versus-leukemia and graft-versus-host effects with cytokines. Bone Marrow Transplant 2000; 26: 353–5.
9. Van Aken WG, Brand A, Van der Poel CL. Leukodepletie van bloedproducten: een maatregel ten behoeve van kwaliteit en veiligheid. Ned Tijdschr Geneeskd 2000; 144; 1033–6.
10. Wolberg AS, Kon RH, Monroe DM, Hoffman M. Coagulation factor XI is a contaminant in intravenous immunoglobulin preparations. Am J Hematol 2000; 65: 30–4.
11. Levy Y, Sherer Y, George J, Rovensky J, Lukac J, Rauova L, Poprac P, Langevitz P, Fabbrizzi F, Shoenfeld Y. Intravenous immunoglobulin treatment of lupus nephritis. Semin Arthritis Rheum 2000; 29: 321–7.
12. Jolles S, Hughes J, Rustin M. The treatment of atopic dermatitis with adjuvant high-dose intravenous immunoglobulin; a report of three patients and review of the literature. Br J Dermatol 2000; 142: 551–4.
13. Turner B, Wills AJ. Cerebral infarction complicating intravenous immunoglobulin therapy in a patient with Miller Fisher syndrome. J Neurol Neurosurg Psychiatry 2000; 68: 790–1.
14. Wittstock M, Benecke R, Zettl UK. Therapie mit intravenös applizierten Immunglobulinen (IVIg). Indikationen und Nebenwirkungen. Neurol Rehabil 2000; 6: 121–4.
15. Zeltser D, Fusman R, Chapman J, Rotstein R, Shapira I, Elkayam O, Eldor A, Arber N, Berliner S. Increased leukocyte aggregation induced by γ-globulin: a clue to the presence of pseudoleukopenia. Am J Med Sci 2000; 320: 177–82.
16. Nakagawa M, Watanabe N, Okuno M, Kondo M, Okagawa M, Taga T. Severe hemolytic anemia following high-dose intravenous immunoglobulin administration in a patient with Kawasaki disease. Am J Hematol 2000; 63: 160–1.
17. Go RS, Call TG. Deep venous thrombosis of the arm after intravenous immunoglobulin infusion: case report and literature review of intravenous immunoglobulin-related thrombotic complications. Mayo Clin Proc 2000; 75: 83–5.
18. Elkayam O, Paran D, Milo R, Davidovitz Y, Almoznino-Sarafian D, Zeltser D, Yaron M, Caspi D. Acute myocardial infarction associated with high dose intravenous immunoglobulin infusion for autoimmune disorders. A study of four cases. Ann Rheum Dis 2000; 59: 77–80.
19. Dilhuydy MS, Delclaux C, De Precigout V, Haramburu F, Roger I, Deminiére C, Mercié P, Pellegrin JL, Aparicio M. Insufficance rénale aiguë aprés cure d'immunoglobulines polyvalentes. Presse Med 2000; 29: 942–3.
20. Levy JB, Pusey CD. Nephrotoxicity of intravenous immunoglobulin. Q J Med 2000; 93: 751–5.
21. Khalil M, Shin HJC, Tan A, DuBose TD, Ordóñez N, Katz RL. Macrophage-like vacuolated renal tubular cells in the urine of a male with osmotic nephrosis associated with intravenous immunoglobulin therapy. Acta Cytol 2000; 44: 86–90.
22. Noseworthy JH, O'Brien PC, Weinshenker BG, Weis JA, Petterson TM, Erickson BJ, Windebank AJ, Whisnant JP, Stolp-Smith KA, Harper CM, Low PA, Romme LJ, Johnson M, An KN, Rodriguez M. IV immunoglobulin does not reverse established weakness in MS: a double-blind, placebo-controlled trial. Neurology 2000; 55: 1135–43.
23. Peker S, Kuwert C, Paus R, Moll I. Palmar lokalisierte vesikuläre läsionen nach der intravenösen applikation van immunglobulinen. H G Z Hautkr 2000; 75: 7–8.
24. Ikeda M, Hamasaki Y, Hataya H, Honda M, Sugai K. Multiorgan failure induced by intravenous immunoglobulin. Acta Paediatr 2000; 89: 1393–5.
25. Ingerslev J. Efficacy and safety of recombinant factor VIIa in the prophylaxis of bleeding in various surgical procedures in hemophilic patients with factor VIII and factor IX inhibitors. Semin Thromb Hemost 2000; 26: 425–32.
26. Cartmill M, Dolan G, Byrne JL, Byrne PO. Prothrombin complex concentrate for oral anticoagulant reversal in neurosurgical emergencies. Br J Neurosurg 2000; 14: 458–61.
27. Berntorp E. Recombinant FVIIa in the treatment of warfarin bleeding. Semin Thromb Hemost 2000; 26: 433–5.
28. Shapiro AD. Recombinant factor VIIa in the treatment of bleeding in hemophilic children with inhibitors. Semin Thromb Hemost 2000; 26: 413–19.
29. Al-Trabolsi HA. Hematuria associated with continuous infusion of recombinant factor VIIa. Ann Saudi Med 2000; 20: 147–9.
30. White II GC. Seventeen years' experience with Autoplex®/Autoplex® T: evaluation of inpatients with severe haemophilia A and factor VIII inhibitors at a major haemophilia centre. Haemophilia 2000; 6: 508–12.
31. White B, Cotter M, Byrne M, O'Shea E, Smith OP. High responding factor VIII inhibitors in mild haemophilia – is there a link with recent changes in clinical practice? Haemophilia 2000; 6: 113–15.
32. Abshire TC, Brackmann H-H, Scharrer I, Hoots K, Gazengel C, Powell JS, Gorina E, Kellermann E, Vosburgh E. Sucrose formulated recombinant human antihemophilic factor VIII is safe and efficacious for treatment of hemophilia A in home therapy. Thromb Haemost 2000; 83: 811–16.
33. Sabin CA, Thynn Yee T, Devereux H, Griffioen A, Loveday C, Phillips AN, Lee CA. Two decades of HIV infection in a cohort of haemophilic individuals; clinical outcomes and response to highly active antiretroviral therapy. AIDS 2000; 14: 1001–7.
34. Meijer K, Smid WM, Van Der Meer J. Treatment of chronic hepatitis C in haemophilia patients. Haemophilia 2000; 6: 605-13.
35. Scharrer I, Brackmann H-H, Sultan U, Abshire T, Gazengel C, Ragni M, Gorina E, Vosburgh E, Kellerman E. Efficacy of a sucrose-formulated recombinant factor VIII used for 22 surgical procedures in patients with severe haemophilia A.

Haemophilia 2000; 6: 614–18.
36. Chuansumrit A, Isarangkura P, Angchaisuksiri P, Sriudomporn N, Tanpowpong K, Hathirat P, Jorgensen LN. Controlling acute bleeding episodes with recombinant factor VIIa in haemophiliacs with inhibitor: continuous infusion and bolus injection. Haemophilia 2000; 6: 61–5.
37. Fabb SA, Dickson JG. Technology evaluation: AAV factor IX gene therapy, Avigen Inc. Curr Opin Mol Ther 2000; 2: 601–6.
38. Finelli PF, Carley MD. Cerebral venous thrombosis associated with epoetin alfa therapy. Arch Neurol 2000; 57: 260–2.
39. Cogar AA, Hartenberger CH, Ohls RK. Endothelin concentrations in preterm infants treated with human recombinant erythropoietin. Biol Neonate 2000; 77: 105–8.
40. Ohls RK. The use of erythropoietin in neonates. Clin Perinatol 2000; 27: 681–96.
41. Engert A. Recombinant human erythropoietin as an alternative to blood transfusion in cancer-related anaemia. Dis Manage Heath Outcomes 2000; 8: 259–72.
42. Henke M, Guttenberger R. Erythropoietin in radiation oncology – a review. Oncology 2000; 58: 175–82.
43. Podesta A, Carmagnini E, Parodi E, Dottori V, Crivellari R, Barberis L, Audo A, Lijoi A, Passerone G. Elective coronary and valve surgery without blood transfusion in patients treated with recombinant human erythropoietin (epoetin-α). Minerva Cardioangiol 2000; 48: 341–7.
44. Morris AT, Ronco C. Erythropoietin therapy in peritoneal dialysis patients. Peritoneal Dial Int 2000; 20 Suppl 2; S178–82.
45. Cases A. Recombinant human erythropoietin treatment in chronic renal failure; effects on hemostasis and vasculature. Drugs Today 2000; 36: 541–56.
46. Kuriyama S, Kobayashi H, Tomonari H, Tokudome G, Hayashi F, Kaguchi Y, Horiguchi M, Ishikawa M, Hosoya T. Circulating adrenomedullin in erythropoietin-induced hypertension. Hypertens Res 2000; 23: 427–32.
47. Leung SP. Multiple strawberry haemangiomas – side effect of rHuEPO? Acta Paediatr Int J Paedriatr 2000; 89: 890.
48. Cuxart M, Just M, Sans R, Matas YM. Dermatitis exfoliativa generalizada por eritropoyetina. Med Clin 2000; 115: 158.
49. Raftery MJ, Auinger M, Hertlovà M. Safety and tolerability of a multidose formulation of epoetin beta in dialysis patients. Clin Nephrol 2000; 54: 240–5.
50. Ruiz PG, Balcke P, Martinez JM, Harris K. Tolerability of the epoetin-beta multidose formulation (Reco-Pen®) in patients with renal anaemia. Clin Drug Invest 2000; 20: 151–8.

M.C. Allwood

34 Intravenous infusions: solutions and emulsions

PLASMA SUBSTITUTES

(SED-14, 1145; SEDA-22, 371; SEDA-23, 368; SEDA-24, 393)

Dextrans

Urinary tract *Renal insufficiency* has recently been attributed to dextran (1[A]).

An 18-year-old Chinese man sustained an injury to the right ear, and the entire superior part of the helix was avulsed. The detached helix was re-attached under general anesthesia and to increase the chances of its survival 500 ml of 10% dextran 40 was infused over 2 hours at 12-hourly intervals. On day 3 he developed nausea and abdominal pain. The dextran infusion was stopped. His serum creatinine was 1092 μmol/l. Total anuria followed within 24 hours and he developed acute pulmonary edema. Renal biopsy was compatible with osmotic nephrosis caused by dextran.

Dextran is widely used in plastic surgery, but acute renal insufficiency is rare; according to one source only 60 cases have been reported (2[R]). These patients were usually either critically ill or had pre-existing renal impairment. The authors presumed that acute renal insufficiency had occurred as a result of increased plasma oncotic pressure, decreasing filtration pressure in the glomerulus; alternatively, some dextran 40 polymers may have been filtered into the tubules, causing obstruction. The amount of dextran required before acute renal insufficiency develops varies from 50 to 1000 g. This patient received 300 g over 3 days, although renal function deterioration was not recognized until uremia developed. The authors suggested that care be taken when using dextran 40, especially in patients with pre-existing renal impairment or vascular disease. Regular monitoring of urine output, electrolytes, and renal function in all dextran recipients is recommended. Administering replacement fluids before checking renal function could lead to life-threatening fluid overload. Withdrawal of dextran should be considered if there is persistent oliguria or a rise in creatinine or urea concentrations. Treatment of dextran-induced acute renal insufficiency should comprise temporary hemodialysis alternating with plasmapheresis, to remove dextran molecules from the blood.

Hydroxyethyl starch

Acid-base balance Two prospective randomized studies of acid-base changes induced by hydroxyethyl starch have recently been reported. In the first study (3[C]), healthy volunteers were given 15 ml/kg of hetastarch 6% or albumin 5% intravenously over 30 minutes. Four weeks later they were given the other colloid. Arterial blood gases and electrolyte parameters were measured at baseline and at 30-minute intervals for 5 hours. There were statistically significant changes in bicarbonate, chloride ion, and albumin concentrations, base excess, and arterial carbon dioxide tension 30 minutes after infusion of hetastarch, but only the albumin concentration changed significantly in the albumin-treated group.

In the second study (4[C]) there were acid-base changes caused by the same two colloids in patients undergoing acute normovolemic hemodilution during gynecological surgery. Two groups of 10 patients were randomly assigned to receive either albumin 5% or hydroxyethyl starch 6%, containing chloride ion concentrations of 150 and 154 mmol/l respectively. The blood volume was well maintained in both groups. Acute normovolemic hemodi-

Side Effects of Drugs, Annual 25
J.K. Aronson, ed.

lution caused slight metabolic acidosis with hyperchloremia. Plasma albumin concentrations fell after hemofiltration with hydroxyethyl starch but increased after albumin. The authors concluded that acute normovolemic hemodilution with albumin or hydroxyethyl starch led to some degree of metabolic acidosis, but not of clinical relevance.

Skin The problem of *pruritus* due to hydroxyethyl starch continues to be investigated. In a recent study, skin biopsies from 120 patients who had received plasma substitutes (including 93 who had received hydroxyethyl starch) showed lysosomal deposits in the histiocytes, some of them also in the cutaneous epithelium and endothelium (5[C]). The extent of lysosomal storage correlated with the amount of hydroxyethyl starch infused. Consecutive biopsies in some cases showed a slow reduction (over years) of hydroxyethyl starch deposits in vacuoles. The authors suggested that pruritus after high cumulative doses of hydroxyethyl starch was closely related to deposition of hydroxyethyl starch in cutaneous nerves.

Icodextrin

Skin The manufacturers have reported from pharmacovigilance data that the incidence rate of all skin reactions with icodextrin is of the order of 2.5%; in most cases the symptoms are mild, often not requiring withdrawal (6[r]).

The adverse effects associated with icodextrin in patients with renal insufficiency over 12 months have been reviewed (7[r]). There were three cases of exfoliative skin reactions in 102 patients. Each was acute and started within 3 days of icodextrin exposure. All resolved promptly on withdrawal. There were two acute *blistering reactions on sun-exposed areas*, occurring within 3–6 months after icodextrin. Both responded slowly to withdrawal, taking 6–8 weeks to resolve completely. Nine further patients reported some form of minor skin problem (*itching*, *dryness*, *rash*, and *blistering*).

PARENTERAL NUTRITION

(SED-14, 1150; SEDA-22, 373; SEDA-23, 369; SEDA-24, 395)

Nervous system Cases of *Wernicke's encephalopathy* caused by thiamine deficiency during parenteral nutrition continue to be reported (8[A]).

> A 13-year-old girl with acute myeloid leukemia received parenteral nutrition and chemotherapy. After a second cycle of chemotherapy she developed persistent nausea and vomiting, nystagmus, ophthalmoplegia, and brisk deep tendon reflexes on the left. Her level of consciousness deteriorated progressively. A CT scan was normal but MRI showed caudate nucleus lesions, cortical involvement, and typical diencephalic and mesencephalic abnomalities. She was given mannitol and dexamethasone, but without improvement. However, after intravenous thiamine her symptoms gradually improved; she recovered within 1 month and the MRI abnormalities disappeared.

The authors suggested that this case showed how MRI can play a role in the diagnosis of Wernicke's encephalopathy, but that there was unusual involvement of the frontal and parietal cortex and the caudate nuclei.

Metabolism *Hyperglycemia* has been associated with an increased risk of postoperative infection. Preoperative parenteral nutrition can be a major cause of hyperglycemia. The frequency of hyperglycemia and infectious complications has been studied in a prospective, randomized, controlled, non-blind trial in 40 patients who required parenteral nutrition for at least 5 days (9[C]). They were given either a hypocaloric regimen (1 liter containing nitrogen 70 g and dextrose 1000 kcal) or a standard weight-based regimen begun with similar amounts initially but with gradual increases in calorie and nitrogen contents to 25 kcal and 1.5 g nitrogen/kg, up to one-third of the calories being given as fat. There were no significant differences between the two groups with regard to hyperglycemia or infections. The higher calorie regimen provided significant nutritional benefit in terms of nitrogen balance compared with the hypocaloric regimen.

Mineral balance *Calcium* Calcium is normally considered to be safe in parenteral nutrition, and relatively high quantities are often included in neonatal and pediatric formulations. However, there is a risk of hypercalciuria; although the cause is unknown, it has been postulated as being due to excessive calcium or vitamin D intake or aluminium overload. *Hypercaliuric hypercalemia* has recently been reported (10[A]).

A 6-year-old girl with Hirschsprung's disease had jejunostomy at 1 month followed by parenteral nutrition. Her calcium intake was 1–1.5 mmol/kg/day. Her urinary calcium rose from 3 months of age; her serum calcium concentrations remained within the reference range but started to rise when she was 3–4 years old. At 5–6 years of age she showed growth retardation and deteriorating renal tubular function with bilateral nephrocalcinosis. The calcium content of the parenteral nutrition was reduced, her serum and urinary calcium concentrations stayed within the reference ranges, and her renal function and growth rate improved.

Metal metabolism *Copper* Micronutrient deficiencies in recipients of parenteral nutrition continue to be reported. Patients who develop cholestatic jaundice during chronic parenteral nutrition can develop significant hematological complications due to *hypocupremia* (11[A]).

A 36-year-old woman with short bowel syndrome developed progressive liver dysfunction 6 months after the start of parenteral nutrition. Trace elements had been omitted because of cholestasis and persistent hyperbilirubinemia. After 15 months she became dependent on erythrocyte transfusions and her neutrophil and platelet counts fell steadily. After 19 months her serum copper concentration was 4 (reference range 11–24) μg/l. Provision of trace elements for 2 months was associated with increased serum copper concentration and neutrophil and platelet counts, independent of erythrocyte transfusions. When the serum copper concentration reached 30 μmol/l copper was discontinued. Over the next 3 months, the copper concentration fell to 1.6 μmol/l and neutrophil and platelet counts fell precipitously. Once again, the copper concentration and neutrophil and platelet counts recovered with copper supplementation.

Copper deficiency during parenteral nutrition is associated with hematological complications (anemia and neutropenia) in adults, as well as skeletal and neurological complications, more particularly in children. However, because copper is excreted primarily in the bile, some experts advocate reducing or curtailing copper supplementation in patients with chronic hyperbilirubinemia. The earliest signs of copper deficiency are peripheral blood cytopenias (typically anemia and neutropenia) and occasionally thrombocytopenia, caused by reduced bone-marrow production. The authors recommended that serum copper should be monitored quarterly and that copper should be included in the parenteral nutrition mixture three times a week, adjusting the frequency in response to serum copper concentrations.

Manganese The dangers of *hypermanganesemia* as a result of parenteral nutrition are now well documented. These are mainly associated with neurological toxicity. The causes of hypermanganesemia are poorly understood, but cholestasis is suspected as a key factor. There has been an attempt to identify the main factors associated with increased plasma manganese in a prospective study in 21 subjects (12[C]). Hypermanganesemia was not only related to increased quantities infused, but also to persistent inflammation (which may alter manganese metabolism) and cholestasis (causing reduced manganese biliary excretion). Neurological complications appeared to be marginal, despite the fact that manganese brain deposition is frequent. The authors suggested that manganese status must be regularly monitored during long-term parenteral nutrition.

Acid-base balance *Lactic acidosis* can occur through thiamine deficiency during parenteral nutrition (13[c]).

A 13-year-old boy underwent bone-marrow transplantation and received parenteral nutrition without vitamins. After 15 days he had acute life-threatening lactic acidosis refractory to bicarbonate and Tris. Intravenous thiamine 100 mg produced satisfactory clinical and biochemical responses.

The authors suggested that in any patient receiving parenteral nutrition without added vitamins who develops lactic acidosis, thiamine deficiency should be suspected.

Liver Liver dysfunction, one of the most common problems in patients on long-term parenteral nutrition, has recently been reviewed (14[R]). In particular, cholestasis can be life-threatening.

A recent prevalence study of liver disease in patients receiving parenteral nutrition has been completed (15[C]). This prospective study included 90 patients with permanent intestinal failure who were enrolled between 1985 and

1996. They were assessed regularly clinically, biochemically, endoscopically, and ultrasonically. Liver biopsy was performed in 57 patients. Chronic cholestasis developed in 58 patients after a median of 6 (range 3–132) months, and 37 developed complicated liver disease after a median of 17 (range 2–155) months. Chronic cholestasis was significantly associated with a risk of liver disease independent of parenteral nutrition, a bowel remnant shorter than 50 cm, and a lipid intake of 1 g/kg/day or more; liver disease related to parenteral nutrition was significantly associated with chronic cholestasis and a parenteral lipid intake of 1 g/kg/day or more. The authors concluded that the prevalence of liver disease increased with the duration of parenteral nutrition and was one of the main causes of death in patients with permanent intestinal failure. Parenteral intake of long-chain lipid emulsion should be restricted to less than 1 g/kg/day.

The possible link between cholestasis and intravenous fat emulsions has been investigated in five patients (aged 2 months to 15 years) receiving parenteral nutrition, all of whom had signs of liver disease (16[c]). In particular, the possible role of phytosterols, natural contaminants of fat emulsions, in causing liver disease was evaluated. Three developed steatosis with non-icteric hepatic dysfunction. High plant phytosterol concentrations in patients receiving parenteral nutrition were related to liver dysfunction and depended on the degree of cholestasis and the dosage of fat emulsion. However, this evidence does not prove that plant phytosterols contribute to the development of liver disease in susceptible individuals, and the authors concluded that in patients with steatosis associated with parenteral nutrition, lipid emulsions should not be withdrawn.

The role of lipid emulsions in cholestasis associated with long-term parenteral nutrition has been investigated retrospectively in 10 children with a total of 23 episodes of cholestasis, associated with thrombocytopenia in 13 cases (17[c]). Changes in lipid delivery, associated with increased daily amounts, preceded complications in more than half the cases, while temporary reduction in lipid administration led to normalization of bilirubin in 17 episodes. The authors concluded that lipid supply is one of the risk factors for cholestasis associated with parenteral nutrition. They recommended that when cholestasis occurs, lipid should be temporarily withdrawn, especially if there is associated thrombocytopenia.

One cause of *deteriorating liver function* resulting from long-term parenteral nutrition is attributable to excessive or persistent calorie intake. Cyclic parenteral nutrition is a procedure of intermittent delivery (either during the day or at night over 10–12 hours). During the non-infusion period the central venous catheter is heparin-locked.

In a prospective study the effect of early use of cyclic parenteral nutrition on deterioration of liver function has been studied in 65 patients with impaired liver function (18[C]). The patients were divided into three groups based on bilirubin concentrations (over 85, 170, and 340 μmol/l). Each of the subgroups was divided into control (continuous parenteral nutrition) or test (cyclic parenteral nutrition). Patients on non-cyclic parenteral nutrition had significantly increased bilirubin and alkaline phosphatase, but the differences between the control and test groups were not significant in those patients with the most severe liver failure before the study. The authors were therefore unable to confirm the possible value of cyclic parenteral nutrition in reducing deterioration in liver function, although the results suggested that, at least in mild or moderate liver failure, there may be some benefit in reducing hepatocellular damage and progressive jaundice.

ENTERAL NUTRITION

Gastrointestinal There is a risk of *gastroesophageal reflux* during nasogastric feeding, especially in mechanically ventilated and sedated patients (19[A]).

A 77-year-old man had a ruptured abdominal aortic aneurysm repaired and developed acute renal, respiratory, and heart failure. Six days postoperatively, enteral feeding was started with a standard formulation. This was well tolerated and the volume was increased to 2000 ml/day continuously. After 9 days, the nasogastric tube was accidentally dislodged. Reinsertion was attempted but failed owing to apparent obstruction at 25 cm. Until this, the patient had been nursed supine. Esophagoscopy showed impacted enteral feed obstructing the esophagus almost completely.

Gastroesophageal reflux during enteral nutrition is caused by a number of factors, including the presence of the nasogastric tube, the supine position, leakage from the tube at the teeth, and the administration of sucralfate. While the cause in this case was not entirely clear, it does show that mechanical obstruction of the esophagus due to reflux can occur without any obvious symptoms.

REFERENCES

1. Tsang RKY, Mok JSW, Poon YS, Van Hasselt, A. Acute renal failure in a healthy young adult after dextran 40 infusion for external ear reattachment surgery. Br J Plast Surg 2000; 83: 701–3.
2. Turkoz A, Gulcan O, But AK, Hazar A, Ersoy O. Dekstran 40 sonrasi kalp durmasi. Turk Anesteziyol Reanim 2000; 28: 105–6.
3. Waters JH, Bernstein CA. Dilutional acidosis following hetastarch or albumin in healthy volunteers. Anaesthesiology 2000; 93: 1184–7.
4. Rehm M, Orth V, Scheingraber S, Kreimeier U, Brechtelsbauer H. Acid-base changes caused by 5% albumin versus 6% hydroxyethyl starch solution in patients undergoing acute normovolemic hemodilution: a randomised prosepctive study. Anaesthesiology 2000; 93: 1174–83.
5. Reimann S, Szepfalusi Z, Kraft D, Luger T, Metze D. Hydroxyethylstarke-speicherung in der haut unter besonder Berucksichtigung des Hydroxyethylstarke-assoziierten Juckreizes. Dtsch Med Wochenschr 2000; 125: 280–5.
6. Divino Filho JC. Allergic reactions to icodextrin in patients with renal failure. Lancet 2000; 355: 1364–5.
7. Goldsmith D, Jayawardene S, Sabbharwal N, Cooney K. Allergic reactions to the polymeric glucose-based peritoneal dialysis fluid icodextrin in patients with renal failure. Lancet 2000; 355: 897.
8. D'Aprile P, Tarantino A, Santoro N, Carella A. Wernicke's encephalopathy induced by total parenteral nutrition in patients with acute leukemia: unusual involvement of caudate nuclei and cerebral cortex on MRI. Neuroradiology 2000; 42: 781–3.
9. McCowen KC, Freil C, Sternberg J, Chan S, Forse RA, Forse R, Burke PA, Bistrian BR. Hypocaloric total parenteral nutrition: effectiveness in prevention of hyperglycemia and infectious complications – a randomised clinical trial. Crit Care Med 2000; 28: 3606–11.
10. Ikema S, Horikawa R, Nakano M, Yokouchi K, Yamazaki H, Tanae Y. Growth and metabolic disturbances in a patient with total parenteral nutrition: a case of hypercalciuric hypercalemia. Endocr J 2000; 47: S137–40.
11. Fuhrnan MP, Herrmann V, Masidonski P, Eby C. Pancytopenia after removal of copper from total parenteral nutrition. J Parenter Enter Nutr 2000; 24: 361–6.
12. Reimund J-M, Dietemann J-L, Warter J-M, Baumann R, Duclos B. Factors associated to hypermanganesemia in patients receiving home parenteral nutrition. Clin Nutr 2000; 19: 343–8.
13. Vossbeck S, Lindner M, Schulz A, Lindner W. Lebensbedrohliche, durch thiaminmangel bedingte, laktatazidose unter total parenteraler ernahrung ohne vitaminzufuhr. Monatsschr Kinderheilkd 2000; 148: 841–4.
14. Burstyne M, Jensen GL. Abnormal liver functions as a result of total parenteral nutrition in a patient with short-bowel syndrome. Nutrition 2000; 16: 11–12.
15. Cavicchi M, Beau P, Crenn P, Degott C, Messing B. Prevalence of liver disease and contributing factors in patients receiving home parenteral nutrition for permanent intestinal failure. Ann Intern Med 2000; 132: 525–32.
16. Bindl L, Lutjohann D, Buderus S, Lentze MJ, Bergmann KV. High plasma levels of phytosterols in patients on parenteral nutrition: a marker of liver dysfunction. J Pediatr Gastroenterol Nutr 2000; 31: 313–16.
17. Colomb V, Jobert-Giraud A, Lacaille F, Guolet O, Fournet J-C, Ricour C. Role of lipid emulsions in cholestasis associated with long-term parenteral nutrition in children. J Parenter Enter Nutr 2000; 24: 345–50.
18. Hwang T-L, Lue M-C, Chen L-L. Early use of cyclic TPN prevents further deterioration of liver functions for the TPN patients with impaired liver function. Hepato-Gastroenterology 2000; 47: 1347–50.
19. Paling A, Girbes ARJ. Esophageal obstruction: an unusual complication of enteral nutrition. Care Crit Ill 2000; 16: 224–5.

K. Peerlinck and J. Vermylen

35 Drugs affecting blood coagulation, fibrinolysis, and hemostasis

COUMARIN CONGENERS

(SED-14, 1184; SEDA-22, 386; SEDA-23, 377; SEDA-24, 398)

Drug interactions *Ciprofloxacin and other quinolones* A series of cases of coagulopathy due to interaction of warfarin with ciprofloxacin has been extracted from the FDA's Spontaneous Reporting System database, including all cases reported from 1987 to 1997, combined with two of the author's own cases (1[AM]). Soon after the introduction of ciprofloxacin in 1987, hemorrhagic events from hypoprothrombinemia were reported in patients taking warfarin. However several prospective trials of combining ciprofloxacin and other fluoroquinolones with warfarin failed to show a significant change in INR (listed in Table 1). Although it is impossible to estimate the frequency of the ciprofloxacin/warfarin interaction from these or other descriptive data, it can be concluded that potentiation of anticoagulant effect by ciprofloxacin occurs most often in older patients and those taking multiple medications.

Methylprednisolone Potentiation of the effects of vitamin K antagonists by high-dose intravenous methylprednisolone has been prospectively studied in 10 consecutive patients and five controls after the observation of a sharp increase in the International Normalized Ratio (INR) in a patient taking oral anticoagulation after concomitant administration of methylprednisolone (1g/day for 3 days) (9[c]). The mean INR was 2.8 (range 2.0–3.8) at baseline and increased to 8.0 (5.3–20). The maximum increase in INR occurred after a mean of 93 (29–156) hours. The coumarins taken by these patients were fluindione in eight and acenocoumarol in two. The prothrombin time in the controls remained stable. A similar rise in INR was previously described in two patients with multiple sclerosis taking warfarin (10[A]). The mechanism of the interaction of methylprednisolone with oral anticoagulants has not been elucidated, but it might be due to inhibition of anticoagulant catabolism. In the three patients in whom the authors assayed fluindione concentrations, these increased in parallel with the INR. The administration of high-dose methylprednisolone to patients taking oral anticoagulants is not rare; daily monitoring of INR or even reducing the anticoagulant dose before administering methylprednisolone is advised.

Methylsalicylate A rise in INR from 2.8 to 12 resulted from the application of a topical pain-relieving gel containing methylsalicylate to the knees in a 22-year-old white woman taking stable warfarin anticoagulation (11[Ar]).

NSAIDs The COX-2 selective non-steroidal anti-inflammatory drug celecoxib did not alter the pharmacokinetics or the hypoprothrombinemic effect of warfarin in 24 healthy subjects (12[c]). However, there have been at least two reports of increased INR in patients on stable warfarin therapy taking celecoxib (13[A], 14[A]). Another COX-2 selective non-steroidal anti-inflammatory drug, rofecoxib, increased plasma concentrations of the biologically less active isomer, R(+) warfarin, which accounted for an approximately 8% increase in INR at steady state in healthy volunteers (15[c]). Stand-

Side Effects of Drugs, Annual 25
J.K. Aronson, ed.

Table 1. *Prospective fluoroquinolone-warfarin interaction studies (from 1[AM])*

Study design	Number of subjects	Subjects	Drug	Coagulation effect	Reference
Single arm	9	Warfarin clinic	Ciprofloxacin	None	(2[C])
Placebo-controlled[1]	16	Warfarin clinic	Ciprofloxacin	None	(3[C])
Placebo-controlled[2]	36	Warfarin clinic	Ciprofloxacin	R-warfarin	(4[C])
Randomized crossover[3]	6	Healthy volunteers	Enoxacin	R-warfarin	(5[C])
Randomized crossover	10	Healthy volunteers	Norfloxacin	None	(6[C])
Single arm	7	Healthy volunteers	Ofloxacin	None	(7[C])
Single arm	10	Healthy volunteers	Temafloxacin	None	(8[C])

[1]Randomized, double-blind, placebo-controlled study.
[2]Randomized, double-blind, placebo-controlled, multicenter study.
[3]Randomized, two-way, crossover study.

ard monitoring of INR in patients taking warfarin should be performed when therapy with celecoxib or rofecoxib is begun or changed.

DRUGS THAT ALTER PLATELET FUNCTION

Dipyridamole *(SED-14, 1698; SEDA-22, 387; SEDA-24, 398)*

Cardiovascular Dipyridamole ^{201}thallium imaging is widely used as an alternative to exercise testing to identify patients with coronary artery disease and to stratify the risks. Although it is usually safe, it has been reported to cause *ventricular dysrhythmias* (16[A]).

A 41-year-old man with hypertension was investigated for chest tightness by dipyridamole thallium single-photon emission computed tomography. A standard dose of dipyridamole (0.56 mg/kg) was infused intravenously over 4 minutes, during which his heart rate increased from 68 to 88 beats/min and his blood pressure fell slightly (from 160/80 to 140/76 mmHg). He had no subjective symptoms, such as palpitation, dizziness, or chest tightness, but had ventricular extra beats 40 seconds after completion of the dipyridamole infusion, followed 1 minute later by a sustained ventricular tachycardia. His blood pressure fell to 80/50 mmHg and he complained of dizziness. Intravenous aminophylline 125 mg was given immediately. About 30 s later the ventricular tachycardia terminated and his hemodynamics stabilized. The ventricular extra beats persisted for another 30 s.

Respiratory Dipyridamole is also widely used as a vasodilator in the detection of coronary artery disease in conjunction with radionuclide imaging and echocardiography. The practicability of dipyridamole ^{13}N-ammonia myocardial positron emission tomography for perioperative risk assessment of coronary artery disease in patients with severe chronic obstructive pulmonary disease undergoing lung volume reduction surgery has been studied in 13 men and seven women (mean age 57 years) without symptoms of coronary artery disease (17[C]). Nine patients had intolerable dyspnea due to *bronchoconstriction* and required intravenous aminophylline. Dipyridamole cannot be recommended as a pharmacological stress in this setting.

Nervous system Dipyridamole in combination with aspirin is more effective in preventing secondary stroke than low-dose aspirin or dipyridamole alone, although only in one of several studies (18[c]). Furthermore, there is some evidence that dipyridamole can sometimes cause *transient ischemic attacks* (19[A]),

A 74-year-old woman had a 3-year history of mild dysarthria, dizziness, and gait ataxia, accompanied by two transient ischemic attacks with involuntary ballistic movements of her left arm lasting several seconds each, and another transient ischemic attack with a right homonymous hemianopia lasting 30 minutes. About 45 minutes after her first-ever oral administration of dipyridamole plus aspirin she developed a transient cerebellar deficit that reproduced features of previous vertebrobasilar ischemic events, as well as severe headache, flushing, and diarrhea.

The acute onset, the pattern of the cerebellar deficit, and the absence of features of epilepsy suggested that the episode was a transient ischemic attack. Aspirin is not known to cause transient ischemic attacks, and only rarely causes headache, flushing, and diarrhea. Since headache, flushing, and diarrhea, which can be caused by dipyridamole, occurred at the same time as the transient ischemic attacks and did not recur after withdrawal, dipyridamole may have caused the transient ischemic attacks. However, it was not clear whether the attacks occurred despite treatment rather than because of it.

Ticlopidine *(SED-14, 1193; SEDA-22, 387; SEDA-23, 378; SEDA-24, 399)*

Sensory systems Two patients developed *retinal vasculitis* 3 and 4 weeks after starting ticlopidine therapy. The symptoms and signs of retinitis resolved within 4–6 weeks after withdrawal of ticlopidine, with no reactivation within the 2 or 3 ensuing years (20[A]).

Hematologic Cases of *thrombotic thrombocytopenic purpura* have been repeatedly reported with ticlopidine, but the pathogenesis was unknown. It has recently been shown that deficiency of, or auto-antibodies to von Willebrand-cleaving metalloproteinase are pathogenic in idiopathic thrombotic thrombocytopenic purpura (21[c]). Seven consecutive patients who developed thrombotic thrombocytopenic purpura 2–7 weeks after starting to take ticlopidine, had markedly reduced concentrations of von Willebrand factor metalloproteinase. In six cases initial samples were available and were positive for immunoglobulin G inhibitors to von Willebrand factor metalloproteinase.

Skin In a 1-year prospective study of 136 patients taking ticlopidine to prevent thrombosis after coronary stenting, 16 patients had adverse skin reactions (22[C]). The most common were *urticaria*, *pruritus*, and *maculopapular eruptions*. Three patients had previously unreported reactions: *a fixed drug eruption*, *an erythromelalgia-like eruption*, and *an erythema multiforme-like eruption*.

ANTIFIBRINOLYTIC DRUGS

(SED-14, 1192; SEDA-22, 387; SEDA-23, 378; SEDA-24, 309)

Aminocaproic acid

Skin A 70-year-old man taking aminocaproic acid developed *dermatitis* with *eosinophilia* and positive patch tests on days 2 and 4 (23[A]).

Tranexamic acid

Drug interactions One case of fatal thromboembolism in acute promyelocytic leukemia during *all-trans retinoic acid* therapy combined with antifibrinolytic therapy has previously been reported (24[A]). Of 31 patients with acute promyelocytic leukemia, treated with different combinations of all-trans retinoic acid and chemotherapy, 21 were given tranexamic acid (25[A]). Of the 28 patients who received all-trans retinoic acid, seven died during the study, but of these seven, only four were early deaths (within 42 days). All four early deaths were in those who received all-trans retinoic acid plus tranexamic acid, and three of the four had sudden and rapid deterioration in their condition; post-mortem findings implicated thrombosis in the microvasculature as the predominant cause of death. Tranexamic acid has been used without thrombotic complications for the attempted prophylaxis of hemorrhage in patients with acute promyelocytic leukemia treated with combination chemotherapy, in whom hemorrhage is a significant problem. Since several studies have shown that all-trans retinoic acid can produce complete remission, it has become part of standard treatment. However, the authors suggested that in patients taking all-trans retinoic acid, tranexamic acid should be used cautiously; supportive therapy with platelets and fresh frozen plasma alone can be used.

THROMBOLYTIC AGENTS

(SED-14, 1187; SEDA-22, 387; SEDA-23, 378; SEDA-24, 399)

There have been three reports of *anaphylactoid reactions*, mostly orolingual angio-edema, following therapy of acute ischemic stroke with alteplase. In one case marked edema of the lip occurred about 45 minutes after a bolus dose of alteplase was given, and subsided within 2 hours without any intervention (26[A]). In another series two of 105 consecutive patients treated with alteplase for acute ischemic stroke developed anaphylactoid reactions (27[C]). The first had a rash and extensive bilateral swelling of the tongue, epiglottis, and uvula, requiring intubation. The second developed unilateral swelling of the tongue and lips without a rash or hypotension. In a third series, two cases of orolingual angio-edema were observed in 230 patients treated with alteplase for acute ischemic stroke (28[C]). Both presented with localized symptoms only, symmetrical in one and asymmetrical in the other. All the authors suggested that direct activation of the complement system by plasminogen activators was involved. The correlation between infarct localization and contralateral angio-edema may be the result of localized insular damage affecting sympathetic and parasympathetic innervation.

REFERENCES

1. Ellis RJ, Mayo MS, Bodensteiner DM. Ciprofloxacin–warfarin coagulopathy: a case series. Am J Hematol 2000; 63: 28–31.
2. Rindone JP, Keuy CL, Jones WN, Garewal HS. Hypoprothrombinemic effect of warfarin not influenced by ciprofloxacin. Clin Pharm 1991; 10: 136–8.
3. Bianco TM, Bussey HI, Farnett LE, Linn WD, Rousch MK, Wong YW. Potential warfarin–ciprofloxacin interaction in patients receiving long-term anticoagulation. Pharmacotherapy 1992; 12: 435–9.
4. Israel DS, Stotka J, Rock W, Sintek CD, Kamada AK, Klein C, et al. Effect of ciporofloxacin on the pharmacokineteics and pharmacodynamics of warfarin. Clin Infect Dis 1996; 22: 251–256.
5. Toon S, Hopkins KJ, Garstang FM, Aarons L, Sedman A, Rowland M. Enoxacin–warfarin interaction: pharmacokinetic and sterochemical aspects. Clin Pharmacol Ther 1987; 42: 3341.
6. Rocci ML, Vlasses PH, Distlerath LM, Gregg MH, Wheeler SC, Zing W, Bjornsson TD. Norfloxacin does not alter warfarin's disposition or anticoagulant effect. J Clin Pharmacol 1990; 30: 728–32.
7. Verho M, Malerczyk V, Rosenkranz B, Grotsch H. Absence of interaction between ofloxacin and phenprocoumon. Curr Med Res Opin 1987; 10: 474–9.
8. Wyld P, Nimmo W, Millar, Coles S, Abbott. The lack of potentiation of the anticoagulant effect of warfarin when administered concurrently with temafloxacin. 17th International Congress of Chemotherapy, Berlin; June 23–28, 1991: Abstract 413a.
9. Costedoat-Chalumeau N, Amoura Z, Aymard G, Sevin O, Wechsler B, Cacoub P, Du LTH, Diquet B, Ankri A, Piette J-C. Potentiation of vitamin K antagonists by high-dose intravenous methylprednisolone. Ann Intern Med 2000; 132: 631–5.
10. Kaufman M. Treatment of multiple sclerosis with high-dose corticosteroids may prolong the prothrombin time to dangerous levels in patients taking warfarin. Mult Scler 1997; 3: 248–9.
11. Joss JD, LeBlond RF. Potentiation of warfarin anticoagulation associated with topical methyl salicylate. Ann Pharmacother 2000; 34: 729–33.
12. Karim A, Tolbert D, Piergies A, Hubbard RC, Harper K, Wallemark CB, Slater M, Geis GS. Celecoxib does not significantly alter the pharmacokinetics or hypoprothrombinemic effects of warfarin in healthy subjects. J Clin Pharmacol 2000; 40: 655–63.
13. Haase KK, Rojas-Fernandez CH, Lane L, Frank D. Potential interaction between celecoxib and warfarin. Ann Pharmacother 2000; 34: 666–7.
14. Mersfelder TL, Stewart L. Warfarin and celecoxib interaction. Ann Pharmacother 2000; 34: 325–7.
15. Schwartz JI, Bugianesi KJ, Ebel DL, de Smet M, Haesen R, Larson PJ, Ko A, Verbesselt R, Hunt TL, Lins R, Lens S, Porras AG, Dieck J, Keymeulen B, Gertz BJ. The effect of rofecoxib on the pharmacodynamics and pharmacokinetics of warfarin. Clin Pharmacol Ther 2000; 68: 626–36.
16. Change WT, Lin LC, Huang PJ. Persistent myocardial ischemia after termination of dipyridamole induced ventricular tachycardia by intravenous aminophyline: scintigraphic demonstration. J Formos Med Assoc 2000; 99: 264–6.
17. Thurnheer R, Laube I, Kaufmaun PA, Stumpe KDM, Strammberger UZ, Bloch KE, Weder W, Russi E.W. Practicability and safety of dipyridamole cardiac imaging in patients with severe chronic obstructive pulmonary disease. Eur J Nucl Med 1999; 26: 812–17.
18. Diener HC, Cunha L, Forbes C. European Stroke Prevention Study 2. Dipyridamole and acetylsalicylic acid in the secondary prevention of stroke. J Neurol Sci 1996; 143: 1–13.
19. Siegel AM, Sandor P, Kollias SS, Baumgartner RW. Transient ischemic attacks after dipyridamole – aspirin therapy. J Neurol 2000; 247: 807–8.
20. Barak A, Morse LS, Schwab IR. Atypical retinal vasculitis associated with ticlopidine hydrochloridine use. Am J Ophthalmol 2000; 129: 684–5.
21. Tsai H-M, Rice L, Sarode R, Chow TW,

Moake JL. Antibody inhibitors to von Willebrand factor metalloproteinase and increased binding of von Willebrand factor to platelets in ticlopidine-associated thrombotic thrombocytopenic purpura. Ann Intern Med 2000; 132: 794–9.
22. Yosipovitch G, Rechavia E, Feinmesser M, David M. Adverse cutaneous reactions to ticlopidine in patients with coronary stents. J Am Acad Dermatol 1999; 41: 473–6.
23. Villarreal O. Systemic dermatitis with eosinophilia due to epsilon-aminocaproic acid. Contact Dermatitis 1999; 40: 114.
24. Hashimoto S, Koike T, Tatewaki W, Seki Y, Sato N, Azegami T, Tsukada N, Takahashi H, Kimura H, Ueno M, Arakawa M, Shibata A. Fatal thromboembolism in acute promyelocytic leukemia during all-trans retinoic acid therapy combined with antifibrinolytic therapy for prophylaxis of hemorrhage. Leukemia 1994; 8: 1113–15.
25. Brown JE, Olujohungbe A, Chang J, Ryder WDJ, Morganstern GR, Chopra R, Scarffe JH. All-trans retinoic acid (ATRA) and tranexamic acid: a potentially fatal combination in acute promyelocytic leukemia. Br J Haematol 2000; 110: 1012–14.
26. Papamitsakis NIH, Kuyl J, Lutsep HL, Clark WM. Benign angioedema after thrombolysis for acute stroke. J Stroke Cerebrovasc Dis 2000; 9: 79–81.
27. Hill MD, Barber PA, Takahashi J, Demchuk AM, Feasby TE, Buchan AM. Anaphylactoid reactions and angioedema during alteplase treatment of acute ischemic stroke. Can Med Assoc J 2000; 162: 1281–4.
28. Rudolf J, Grond M, Schmulling S, Neveling M, Heiss W-D. Orolingual angioneurotic oedema following therapy of acute ischemic stroke with alteplase. Neurology 2000; 55: 599-600.

H.J. De Silva

36 Gastrointestinal drugs

ANTIEMETICS

The efficacy and adverse effects of levosulpiride and cisapride on gastric emptying and symptoms in patients with functional dyspepsia and gastroparesis have been compared in a double-blind, crossover trial in 30 patients (1[c]). Levosulpiride 25 mg tds and cisapride 10 mg tds, for 4 weeks, were equally effective in reducing gastric emptying times, with no adverse effects. Levosulpiride had a greater impact on patients' everyday activities and produced more improvement in some symptoms such as nausea, vomiting, and early satiety.

Cisapride *(SED-14, 1223; SEDA-22, 389; SEDA-23, 380; SEDA-24, 401)*

Cardiovascular Cisapride has recently been withdrawn from the market because of the risk of *cardiac dysrhythmias*, particularly in relation to drug interactions with drugs that inhibit the metabolism of cisapride by CYP3A4 (e.g. clarithromycin, erythromycin, and troleandomycin; nefazodone; fluconazole, itraconazole, and ketoconazole; indinavir and ritonavir; and grapefruit juice). In the UK the Medicines Control Agency received 60 reports of serious cardiac adverse events between 1988 and 2000; five were fatal (2[S]). The corresponding worldwide figures were 386 serious ventricular dysrhythmias with 125 deaths and 50 unexplained deaths.

An 81-year-old woman, who had a permanent pacemaker for complete heart block with symptomatic bradycardia-dependent torsade de pointes, had breakthrough *torsade de pointes* during therapy with cisapride 10 mg tds for 22 days and paroxetine for 9 days (3[A]). She made a good recovery on withdrawal of the drugs.

In the UK cisapride is specifically contraindicated in premature babies for up to 3 months after birth, because of the risk of QT prolongation (2[S]). Between 1988 and 2000 the Medicines Control Agency received 64 reports of suspected adverse effects of cisapride in children under 13 years, of which two were cases of QT prolongation and two were sudden unexplained deaths. Another 106 cardiovascular events were reported from other countries, including 30 cases of QT prolongation, six cases of ventricular fibrillation or tachycardia, and four sudden unexplained deaths.

Electrocardiographic changes and predisposition to cardiac dysrhythmias have been investigated in 63 children (mean age 29 months) with gastro-esophageal reflux who had taken cisapride 0.2 mg/kg tds for at least 15 days and 57 control children (mean age 27 months) who were hospitalized for other reasons and were not given cisapride or other oral treatment (4[C]). All the children had an electrocardiogram performed at inclusion, and 24-hour Holter recording was performed in all children with prolonged QT intervals. When a prolonged QT interval was detected cisapride was withdrawn and a new electrocardiogram was recorded. Five children in the treatment group and six controls had *prolonged QT intervals*, which normalized in three of the five children after cisapride was withdrawn. Holter recording was normal in all children.

Nervous system *Tardive dyskinesia* with involuntary movement of muscles of mastication and the tongue has been reported in a 76-year-old man who took cisapride 10 mg tds, with complete resolution on withdrawal (5[A]).

Risk factors The cardiovascular risks of cisapride in children are discussed above.

A systematic review of randomized controlled trials of cisapride for gastro-esophageal reflux in children has been reported (6[M]). Seven

Side Effects of Drugs, Annual 25
J.K. Aronson, ed.

comparisons of cisapride with placebo (286 children in all) were included. The reflux index was significantly reduced by cisapride. However, there was no clear evidence that cisapride reduced symptoms of gastro-esophageal reflux. Adverse events (mainly *diarrhea*) were not significantly more common with cisapride.

The effects of cisapride 0.2 mg/kg tds on acid gastro-esophageal reflux in 32 formerly preterm infants receiving respiratory stimulation with caffeine have been studied using 24-hour esophageal pH monitoring (7[C]). Cisapride significantly reduced the reflux index and the frequency of reflux without impairing the systemic availability or therapeutic effects of caffeine.

The effects of cisapride 0.2–0.3 mg/kg tds on chronic constipation have been studied in a double-blind, placebo-controlled trial in 36 children (8[C]). Cisapride was effective in the treatment of chronic constipation without major adverse effects.

The effects of low-dose cisapride (0.1 mg/kg tds) on gastric emptying and the QT interval have been studied in a double-blind, placebo-controlled, crossover trial in 20 infants of low birthweights (9[C]). Low-dose cisapride significantly improved gastric emptying without prolonging the QT interval.

Domperidone *(SED-14, 1224; SEDA-22, 389; SEDA-23, 381; SEDA-24, 401)*

Few cases of extrapyramidal adverse effects due to domperidone have previously been reported. A 9-year-old child developed *dysphagia* and *involuntary movements of the facial muscles* after being treated with domperidone 0.25 mg/kg/day (10[A]). There was complete recovery after withdrawal.

Levosulpiride

The pharmacology, efficacy, and tolerability of levosulpiride for dyspepsia and emesis have been reviewed (11[M]). Levosulpiride has been evaluated in 15 double-blind, randomized trials in patients with dyspepsia (1818 patients in all, of whom 676 were treated with levosulpiride) and in 11 trials in patients with emesis (718 patients in all, of whom 383 were treated with levosulpiride). Levosulpiride was effective in the treatment of dyspepsia and emesis. The incidence of adverse effects was 11% in 840 patients with dyspepsia. Most of them were mild and resulted in treatment withdrawal in only 0.9% of cases. The common adverse effects were *drowsiness*, *breast tenderness*, and *hoarseness*.

Metoclopramide *(SED-13, 1069; SEDA-20, 316; SEDA-22, 390)*

Cardiovascular *Complete heart block* has been reported in a 65-year-old woman with type 2 diabetes, hypertension, and ischemic heart disease, who was given intravenous metoclopramide 20 mg (12[A]).

Ziprasidone

Drug interactions In 11 healthy volunteers the pharmacokinetics of ziprasidone were not affected by concurrent *cimetidine* and *co-magaldrox* (aluminium hydroxide plus magnesium hydroxide; Maalox) (13[C]). This suggests that other non-specific inhibitors of cytochrome P450 and antacids are unlikely to alter the pharmacokinetics of this drug.

5-HT_3 RECEPTOR ANTAGONISTS *(SED-14, 1225; SEDA-22, 390; SEDA-23, 381; SEDA- 24, 401)*

The efficacy and safety of oral granisetron (2 mg od) and oral ondansetron (8 mg tds for 3 days and bd on day 4) in the prophylaxis of nausea and vomiting have been studied in 34 patients receiving hyperfractionated total body irradiation in a randomized, double-blind trial (14[C]). A historical group of 90 patients who received a similar irradiation regimen but no 5HT_3 receptor antagonists acted as a control group. Both drugs were safe and effective in preventing nausea and vomiting resulting from irradiation. The most frequent adverse effects were *headache* and *diarrhea*.

Oral granisetron (1 mg bd) plus intravenous dexamethasone (10 mg) have been compared with intravenous ondansetron (8 mg tds) plus dexamethasone (10 mg) for the control of nausea and vomiting in a randomized, open trial in 51 patients receiving emetogenic chemotherapy (15[C]). The two combinations were equally effective, and the frequencies of adverse events (none serious) in the two groups were comparable. The most frequent were *diarrhea* with granisetron and constipation with ondansetron.

Alosetron

There have been several reviews of the pharmacology of alosetron and clinical experience with it (16[R]–19[R]) .

Gastrointestinal Alosetron has been evaluated in the management of irritable bowel syndrome. It increases the compliance of the colon to distension and delays colonic transit. In women with irritable bowel syndrome alosetron 1 mg bd was more effective than placebo and mebeverine in relieving abdominal pain, discomfort, and diarrhea. The most frequent adverse effect was *constipation* (16[R]–19[R]).

Alosetron (1 mg bd) was well tolerated and effective in alleviating abdominal pain, urgency, and stool frequency in a randomized, double-blind, placebo-controlled trial in 647 women with irritable bowel syndrome (20[C]). Constipation occurred in 30% of patients taking alosetron and 3% of those taking placebo. Laboratory values, including liver function tests, were unchanged by alosetron.

The efficacy of alosetron in the treatment of irritable bowel syndrome has been evaluated in a double-blind, placebo-controlled, dose-ranging study in 462 patients (21[C]). In women but not in men alosetron 2 mg bd significantly increased the proportion of pain-free days and reduced the visual analogue scale score for diarrhea. Alosetron 0.5–2 mg bd led to significant hardening of stools and reduced stool frequency in the total population. The overall incidence of adverse effects was similar with alosetron and placebo. However, the incidence of constipation was significantly higher during treatment with alosetron 0.5 mg bd and 2 mg bd. There were no changes in laboratory values associated with alosetron.

In a randomized, double-blind, placebo-controlled, crossover trial, alosetron (2 mg bd) delayed left colonic transit in both patients with irritable bowel syndrome (n = 13) and healthy volunteers (n = 12) (22[c]). In another double-blind, placebo-controlled trial in 25 non-constipated patients with irritable bowel syndrome, alosetron (1 mg and 4 mg bd) had no significant effect on gastrointestinal transit or rectal sensory and motor mechanisms (23[c]).

Granisetron

The efficacy of intravenous granisetron 40 μg/kg, droperidol 20 μg/kg, and metoclopramide 0.2 mg/kg have been compared in the treatment of nausea and vomiting after laparoscopic cholecystectomy in a double-blind trial in 120 patients (24[C]). The patients were observed for 24 hours after administration. Granisetron was significantly more effective than the other two drugs. All three drugs were equally well tolerated. The common adverse effects were *headache* and *dizziness*.

In a randomized, double-blind study, oral granisetron (1 mg) was more effective than intravenous granisetron (1 mg) in preventing emesis caused by high-dose chemotherapy in 51 patients who underwent peripheral blood progenitor cell or bone-marrow transplantation (25[c]). There was no significant difference in adverse events. The more frequent were *headache*, *diarrhea*, *extrapyramidal symptoms*, and *sedation*.

The combination of intravenous granisetron (40 μg/kg) and dexamethasone (8 mg) was more effective than granisetron alone for prophylaxis of postoperative nausea and vomiting after laparoscopic cholecystectomy in a randomized, double-blind trial in 120 patients (26[C]). There was no difference in the incidence of adverse effects between the two groups. The most frequent were *nausea*, *retching*, and *vomiting*.

In another open trial the combination of intravenous granisetron (1 mg) plus dexamethasone (10 mg) was effective and well tolerated for antiemetic control in 100 bone-marrow transplant patients receiving highly emetogenic chemotherapy with or without irradiation (27[C]). Adverse effects were mild; *headache*, *diarrhea*, and *constipation* were the most frequent.

Tropisetron

The safety and efficacy of tropisetron in the prevention of chemotherapy-induced nausea and vomiting has been reviewed (28[R]). Tropisetron monotherapy is effective for the control of acute, and to some extent delayed, nausea and vomiting in patients receiving emetogenic chemotherapy. Combining it with dexamethasone increases its efficacy. Tropisetron is as effective as ondansetron and granisetron, and more effective than metoclopramide. It is usually well tolerated by adults and children. Adverse effects are usually mild, the most common being *headache*, *constipation*, and *fatigue*. Tropisetron does not seem to potentiate the adverse effects of chemotherapeutic agents, and laboratory data and the electrocardiogram are generally unaffected.

HISTAMINE H_2 RECEPTOR ANTAGONISTS *(SED-14, 1225; SEDA-22, 391; SEDA 23, 382; SEDA 24, 402)*

The use, efficacy, and adverse effects of non-prescription H_2 receptor antagonists and alginate-containing formulations obtained from community pharmacies have been evaluated in 767 customers with dyspepsia (29[C]). Most obtained some or complete symptom relief (75%) and were completely satisfied with the product (78%). H_2 receptor antagonists were more likely to produce complete relief of symptoms than alginate-containing formulations. Only 3% reported adverse effects: *diarrhea*, *constipation*, *bloating*, and *flatulence* from alginate formulations, and *dry mouth*, *altered bowel habit*, *diarrhea*, and *constipation* from H_2 receptor antagonists.

Changes in healthcare utilization resulting from a formulary switch from nizatidine to cimetidine have been studied in 704 patients (30[C]). There was no evidence of increased healthcare utilization during the 6 months after the formulary switch, which led to considerable pharmaceutical savings. During this period only four (0.004%) adverse drug reactions associated with cimetidine were reported; *urticaria*, *nausea and vomiting*, *leg cramps*, and *impotence*.

In a retrospective case-control assessment of medical records of 56 patients who died of cardio-esophageal adenocarcinoma and 56 age- and sex-matched controls who died of myocardial infarction, subjects who died of *esophageal adenocarcinoma* were more likely to have consumed H_2 receptor antagonists (RR = 7.5; 95% CI = 1.3, 42) (31[C]). The suggested mechanism is that H_2 receptor antagonists allow asymptomatic achlorhydric reflux to continue, leading to esophageal damage.

Pancreas The risk of acute *pancreatitis* associated with the use of acid-suppressing drugs has been assessed in a retrospective cohort study with a nested case-control design within the General Practice Research Database in the UK (32[C]). The study included 180 178 people aged 20–74 years who had received at least one prescription of cimetidine, famotidine, nizatidine, ranitidine, lansoprazole, or omeprazole from January 1992 to September 1997, and who did not have major risk factors for pancreatic diseases. There were no cases of pancreatitis among users of famotidine, lansoprazole, or nizatidine. The relative risk compared with non-use, corrected for age, sex, calendar year, and use of medication known to be associated with pancreatitis was 1.3 (95% CI = 0.4, 4.1) for ranitidine, 2.1 (0.6, 7.2) for cimetidine, and 1.1 (0.3, 4.6) for omeprazole. The results do not support an association between acute pancreatitis and acid-suppressing drugs, although an increase in risk cannot be excluded.

Famotidine

Liver Famotidine-induced *cholestatic hepatitis* has been reported in a previously healthy 13-year-old boy who had taken famotidine 40 mg/day for 30 days for epigastric pain (33[A]). Other possible causes were excluded. He had a gradual and complete recovery 2 months after drug withdrawal.

Ranitidine

Effervescent ranitidine 150 mg bd has been compared with as-needed calcium carbonate antacids 750 mg in a randomized study in 115 subjects who frequently self-treated heartburn (34[C]). Effervescent ranitidine was significantly more effective than antacids in reducing heartburn, healing erosive esophagitis, alleviating pain, and improving quality of life. The overall incidences of adverse events were not significantly different in the two groups; 12% in the antacid group and 3% in the ranitidine group had adverse events related to the gastrointestinal system: *nausea*, *vomiting*, *diarrhea*, *constipation*, *gas*, *fecal incontinence*; and 1% in the antacid group and 4% in the ranitidine group had adverse events related to the central nervous system: *headache*, *dizziness*, *insomnia*, *malaise*, *fatigue*, *weakness*, *nervousness*.

Liver *Hepatitis* associated with ranitidine is rare. A case of drug hypersensitivity hepatitis with progression to fulminant hepatic failure and death has been reported in a previously healthy 66-year-old woman who had taken ranitidine for 14 days before the onset of jaundice and for 5 days after hepatitis was diagnosed (35[A]). This is the second reported case of fatal hepatitis associated with ranitidine. Another case has been reported of a 45-year-old woman with multiple sclerosis who developed severe liver injury after taking ranitidine 300 mg/day (36[A]).

PROTON PUMP INHIBITORS

(SED-14, 1230; SEDA-22, 391; SEDA-23, 383; SEDA-24, 402)

The common adverse events during treatment with proton pump inhibitors used in general practice in England have been reviewed in a prescription event monitoring study in 16 205 patients taking omeprazole, 17 329 taking lansoprazole, and 11 541 taking pantoprazole (37[C]). The commonest adverse events in all three groups were *diarrhea, nausea/vomiting, abdominal pain*, and *headache*. There was little difference in the adverse event rates between the three groups. However, *diarrhea* was more commonly associated with lansoprazole compared with omeprazole, particularly in elderly people.

To assess acid control, esomeprazole 20 mg or 40 mg/day has been compared with omeprazole 20 mg/day for 5 days in a double-blind, crossover study in 38 patients with symptoms of gastro-esophageal reflux disease (38[C]). Pharmacokinetic variables and 24-hour intragastric pH were measured on day 5 of each dosing period. Esomeprazole provided more effective acid control than omeprazole. Both dosages of esomeprazole were well tolerated, and the profile and incidence of adverse events were similar to that observed with omeprazole. The most common were *abdominal pain, nausea, diarrhea, respiratory infection*, and *headache*.

Esomeprazole 20 mg or 40 mg/day and omeprazole 20 mg/day for 8 weeks have been compared in the treatment of gastro-esophageal reflux disease in a multicenter, randomized, double-blind trial in 1960 patients (39[C]). Symptom control and healing rates were significantly better with either dose of esomeprazole than with omeprazole. There was no significant difference in reported adverse events between the treatment groups. The most commonly reported were *headache, abdominal pain*, and *diarrhea*.

The results of a therapeutic interchange program, in which 78 patients with acid peptic disease requiring proton pump inhibitor therapy (both newly diagnosed patients and those previously stabilized on omeprazole) were treated with lansoprazole, have been retrospectively analysed (40[c]). Although the switch was associated with considerable pharmaceutical savings, there was an overall lansoprazole-associated failure rate of 28%. Reported lack of efficacy required withdrawal of lansoprazole in 15%, while adverse effects required withdrawal of lansoprazole in 13% of patients (versus none with omeprazole). The main adverse effect was *diarrhea*.

The clinical and fiscal impact of replacing omeprazole with lansoprazole as the only proton pump inhibitor has been assessed by reviewing the medical records of 3833 patients requiring long-term proton pump inhibitor therapy (2224 were started on lansoprazole and 1479 were converted from omeprazole to lansoprazole) (41[C]). There were considerable pharmaceutical savings. The true lansoprazole failure rate (requiring conversion to omeprazole) was 5.3%. Withdrawal of lansoprazole was due to poor symptom control (in 69%) and/or adverse effects (in 22%). The most common adverse effects were *diarrhea* (10%), *abdominal pain* (5%), and *urticaria* (1%).

Lansoprazole 30 mg/day, lansoprazole 15 mg/day, and ranitidine 150 mg bd for 8 weeks have been compared in a randomized, double-blind, multicenter trial in the healing of NSAID-associated gastric ulceration in 353 patients (42[C]). Both doses of lansoprazole were superior to ranitidine in healing gastric ulcers. Healing rates were similar between *Helicobacter pylori* infected and non-infected patients, again with significantly better healing rates with lansoprazole than ranitidine. There were no differences in adverse effects profiles in the three groups. The most commonly reported adverse effect was *diarrhea*.

Lansoprazole 15 or 30 mg/day and ranitidine 150 mg bd for 8 weeks have been compared in the treatment of non-erosive gastro-esophageal reflux disease in two double-blind, multicenter trials in 901 patients (43[C]). Overall symptom control was significantly better with either dose of lansoprazole than with ranitidine or placebo. There was no significant difference in reported adverse events between the treatment groups. The more commonly reported were *abdominal pain* and *diarrhea*.

Pantoprazole 20 mg/day (low dose) and ranitidine 300 mg/day (standard dose) have been compared in the treatment of mild gastro-esophageal reflux disease in a double-blind, multicenter trial in 201 patients (44[C]). Overall symptom control and healing rates were significantly better with pantoprazole. There was no significant difference in reported adverse events between the treatment groups. The more commonly reported were *diarrhea*, *headache*, and *abdominal pain*.

Omeprazole 40 mg/day for 6 weeks and lansoprazole 30 mg bd have been compared for symptom control in a randomized study in 96 patients with gastro-esophageal reflux disease who had earlier failed to respond to lansoprazole 30 mg/day (45[C]). The two drugs were equally effective in symptom control. There were no significant differences in adverse events between the two groups. The most frequent adverse events reported were *diarrhea*, *abdominal pain/discomfort*, *bloating/gas*, *vomiting*, and *headache*.

Rabeprazole 10 or 20 mg bd and omeprazole 20 mg/day have been compared in the healing of erosive gastro-esophageal reflux disease in a double-blind, multicenter study in 310 patients (46[C]). Overall healing rates for rabeprazole (both dosage regimens) and omeprazole at 4 and 8 weeks of treatment were equivalent. The drugs were equally well tolerated, and there was no significant difference in reported adverse events. The more frequent were *abdominal pain*, *pharyngitis*, *bronchitis*, *headache*, and *diarrhea*.

Drug interactions The effects of proton pump inhibitors on *roxithromycin* concentrations in plasma and gastric tissue have been investigated in two crossover studies in 12 healthy volunteers who took omeprazole 20 mg bd or lansoprazole 30 mg bd with or without roxithromycin 300 mg bd over 6 days (47[c]). The medications were well tolerated, with only mild adverse events. The more frequent adverse events were *nausea*, *bloating*, and *diarrhea*. Proton pump inhibitors and roxithromycin did not alter the systemic availability of each other. However, proton pump inhibitors increased the local concentration of the antibiotic in the stomach.

Omeprazole

To test whether omeprazole accelerates healing of standardized gastroduodenal lesions in the presence of diclofenac, 12 healthy volunteers took consecutive 2-week courses of omeprazole 40 mg/day or placebo, with diclofenac given in the second week of each course, in a double-blind, crossover study (48[c]). Omeprazole did not accelerate the healing of pre-existing mucosal lesions or prevent the development of small diclofenac-induced mucosal lesions. Omeprazole *increased serum gastrin* in all subjects.

Psychiatric *Delirious psychosis* has been attributed to intravenous omeprazole 40 mg bd in a 77-year-old woman with Guillain–Barré syndrome, who also had *Helicobacter pylori* associated gastritis (49[A]). Delirium developed 2 days after omeprazole was begun and resolved completely after drug withdrawal.

Electrolyte balance Two cases of *hyponatremia* caused by omeprazole have been reported, one in a 78-year-old woman who was taking omeprazole 20 mg/day for esophagitis, and the other in a 74-year-old man (50[A]). Both recovered completely after drug withdrawal.

Gastrointestinal To evaluate the long-term safety of omeprazole, 33 patients with severe reflux esophagitis were prospectively followed up for 5–8 years (51[c]). Six were positive for *Helicobacter pylori*. There was no evidence of significant enterochromaffin-like cell hyperplasia, gastric atrophy, intestinal metaplasia, dysplasia, or neoplastic changes during 185 patient follow-up years during which 137 gastric biopsies were taken.

Urinary tract Hypercalcemia and *interstitial nephritis* has been reported in a 31-year-old pregnant woman (35 weeks gestation), possibly associated with omeprazole 20 mg/day for over 8 weeks (52[A]). Investigations excluded other causes of hypercalcemia. The patient recovered after drug withdrawal and treatment with corticosteroids. Another case of renal insufficiency due to acute interstitial nephritis has been reported in a 73-year-old man who had taken omeprazole 40 mg/day for 4 months for severe reflux esophagitis (53[A]). He too recovered completely after withdrawal of omeprazole.

Rabeprazole

The benefits and risk profile of rabeprazole have been reviewed (54[R]). Rabeprazole 10 and 20 mg/day in the morning was effective in erosive or ulcerative gastro-esophageal reflux disease, gastric and duodenal ulcers, and long-term maintenance of gastro-esophageal reflux disease healing. Healing rates were equivalent to those with omeprazole and superior (gastro-esophageal reflux disease healing and duodenal ulcer healing) or equal (gastric ulcer healing) to ranitidine. The drug has been well tolerated in both short-term and long-term studies. The overall rate of drug withdrawal because of adverse effects was 3%. Common adverse effects included *diarrhea*, *headache*, and *rash*.

In an open study in 189 patients rabeprazole 20 mg/day for 4 weeks was effective in functional dyspepsia (55[c]). The incidence of adverse events was 8%, and included *dysgeusia*, *diarrhea*, *constipation*, and *headache*.

In a double-blind, placebo-controlled trial in 288 patients with previously treated erosive or ulcerative gastro-esophageal reflux disease rabeprazole 10 or 20 mg/day was significantly more effective than placebo in preventing relapse of erosive or ulcerative gastro-esophageal reflux disease and was well tolerated (56[C]). Commonly reported adverse events were *abdominal pain*, *nausea*, *diarrhea*, *rhinitis*, *pharyngitis*, *a flu-like syndrome*, and *back pain*. Rabeprazole had no clinically significant effects on laboratory values, thyroid function tests, the electrocardiogram, vital signs, or bodyweight.

In a crossover study in 24 healthy volunteers, rabeprazole 10, 20, and 40 mg produced significant dose-related reductions in intragastric acidity associated with a significant *rise in serum gastrin concentration* (57[c]). There were no serious adverse effects. After taking into account increases in serum gastrin concentrations and interindividual variation in the antisecretory response, 20 mg appears to be the preferred dose for routine clinical use. Similar potent dose-related gastric acid inhibition and rises in serum gastrin were found with rabeprazole 5–40 mg/day in the morning for 7 days in 38 subjects infected with *Helicobacter pylori* (58[c]). There was less than 50% recovery of acid by 48 hours after the seventh dose. In this study the optimal acid inhibitory dose appeared to be 20 mg/day, and there were no serious adverse effects.

HELICOBACTER PYLORI ERADICATION REGIMENS

(SEDA-22, 392; SEDA-23, 384; SEDA-24, 404)

The number of trials investigating *Helicobacter pylori* eradication therapies continues to increase. Drugs and regimens for *Helicobacter pylori* eradication have been reviewed (59[R]). The major factor in choosing an antibiotic regimen is the pattern of antibiotic resistance in the community. Triple therapy with a proton pump inhibitor or ranitidine bismuth citrate plus two antimicrobials is the recommended first-choice regimen. In regions where metronidazole and clarithromycin resistance in common initial quadruple therapy with bismuth, metronidazole, tetracycline, and a proton pump inhibitor is recommended. In general, higher doses and longer duration of therapy are associated with better outcomes. Although therapy for 1 week has become accepted in first-line regimens, therapy for 2 weeks is better when treating nitroimidazole-resistant or clarithromycin-susceptible strains. Adverse effects are related to the individual drugs used. New triple therapies have less frequent adverse effects than classical triple therapy (which included bismuth compounds) or triple therapy including ranitidine bismuth citrate. *Diarrhea* is the most common adverse effect with all regimens. *Taste disturbance* is frequent in clarithromycin-containing therapies. Intolerable adverse effects are uncommon with any regimen.

Sucralfate 1 g tds in combination with amoxicillin 500 mg tds and clarithromycin 400 mg bd for 2 weeks was as effective as a combination of lansoprazole (30 mg bd) plus amoxicillin 500 mg tds and clarithromycin 400 mg bd for 2 weeks for *Helicobacter pylori* eradication in a randomized multicenter trail in 150 patients (60[C]). There was no significant difference in adverse effects between the two groups. *Diarrhea*, *abdominal pain*, *glossitis*, and *taste disturbance* were the adverse effects commonly reported.

In a randomized, controlled trial in 120 patients supplementation with inactivated *Lactobacillus acidophilus* tds significantly improved the efficacy of a standard 7-day regimen with rabeprazole 20 mg bd, clarithromycin 250 mg tds, and amoxicillin 500 mg tds (61[C]). There was no significant difference in adverse effects between the two groups. Those reported were *abdominal pain*, *nausea*, and *diarrhea*.

ANTIDIARRHEAL AGENTS
(SED-14, 1233)

Loperamide

The effectiveness of loperamide 4 mg, 8 mg, and 12 mg in reducing symptoms of lactose intolerance has been investigated in an open study in 19 subjects (62[c]). Loperamide 8 mg significantly improved symptom scores to a similar extent as lactase tablets. Four subjects complained of adverse effects related to loperamide: *delayed constipation* and *abdominal cramps*.

Teratogenicity To determine whether loperamide in pregnancy is associated with an increased risk of birth malformations, birth outcomes in 105 women who had taken loperamide during pregnancy (89 during the first trimester) were compared with the outcomes in women matched for age, smoking, alcohol, and other exposures (63[C]). There were no differences in the frequencies of birth malformations between the two groups. However, 21 of the cases had babies who were 200 g smaller than babies in the control group.

LAXATIVES *(SED-14, 1235; SEDA-22, 393; SEDA-23, 384; SEDA-24, 406)*

Oral sodium phosphate and oral sodium picosulfate have been compared for bowel preparation before elective colorectal surgery and colonoscopy in randomized studies in 256 patients (64[C]). Oral sodium phosphate was superior to sodium picosulfate on surgical assessment of bowel preparation, fecal residue in the resected specimen, and endoscopic score. However, there was no significant difference with regard to abdominal pain, nausea, vomiting, embarrassment, fear, and fatigue between the two groups.

Oral sodium picosulfate plus magnesium citrate (Picolax) has been compared with a self-administered phosphate enema for bowel preparation before flexible sigmoidoscopy in a randomized single-blind trial in 1142 subjects (65[C]). A single self-administered phosphate enema about 1 hour before leaving home was a more acceptable and effective method of preparing the distal bowel than oral Picolax. Although more patients felt unwell after taking the enema (15%) than after taking Picolax (7%), over 80% in both groups felt normal. More of the itemized adverse effects were rated as moderate or severe in the Picolax group, including *wind*, *incontinence*, and *sleep disturbance*. *Anal soreness* was reported more frequently in the enema group. The other reported adverse effects were *abdominal pain/cramps*, *nausea/vomiting*, and *faintness/dizziness*.

Electrolyte balance A 46-year-old woman, with hepatic encephalopathy complicating cirrhosis due to hepatitis B and C infection, developed fatal *hypernatremia*, *hyperphosphatemia*, and *hypocalcemia* following the erroneous administration of a total of six sodium phosphate enemas (133 ml each) over 36 hours (66[A]).

Gastrointestinal Four cases that suggested an association between oral sodium phosphate and *microscopic focal cryptitis* have been reported (67[A]). The three men and one woman, aged 31–56 years, all had symptoms suggestive of irritable bowel syndrome and had not taken any antibiotics, NSAIDs, or immunosuppressive drugs before the onset symptoms. Colonoscopy was normal. There was no microbiological evidence of an infective cause, and routine biochemistry and hematology laboratory tests were normal. Histology was distinct from infective, ischemic, or inflammatory bowel disease. However, an interval rebiopsy after withdrawal of the drug was not performed in any patient.

AMINOSALICYLATES
(SED-14, 1237; SEDA-22, 393; SEDA-23, 386; SEDA-24, 406)

The pharmacological properties of aminosalicylates and their potential value in the treatment of inflammatory bowel disease have been discussed in another review (68[R]). Aminosalicylates are the drugs of first choice in the acute treatment of ulcerative colitis and in maintaining remission. Their value in Crohn's disease is more modest. The variability in clinical results is at least partly caused by the different formulations and dosages of the drug used, as well as the high variation in drug disposition and topical availability of the active drug. The popular use of aminosalicylates is most likely due to the low incidence of adverse effects and good overall safety record of mesalazine. Crossover studies have clearly shown that mesalazine has about a 10-fold lower potential than sulfasalazine for inducing allergic reactions or causing intolerance. Adverse effects with all aminosalicylates include (generally more frequent with sulfasalazine) *headache*, *nausea*, *abdominal pain*, *dyspepsia*, *fatigue*, *rash*, *fever*, and rarely *exacerbation of the disease*, *pancreatitis*, *pericarditis*, *pneumonitis*, *liver disease*, *nephritis*, and *bone-marrow depression*. Watery *diarrhea* is an adverse effect unique to olsalazine, while *anorexia*, *folate malabsorption*, *hemolysis*, *neutropenia*, *agranulocytosis*, *male infertility*, and *neuropathy* are unique to sulfasalazine.

Mesalazine (mesalamine)

The therapeutic potential of prolonged-release mesalazine in the treatment of ulcerative colitis and Crohn's disease has been reviewed (69[R]). The formulation consists of ethylcellulose-coated microgranules from which mesalazine is released in the small and large intestines in a diffusion-dependent manner. Dose-dependent improvements in clinical and endoscopic parameters have been reported with prolonged-release mesalazine 2–4 g/day in trials in patients with mild to moderately active ulcerative colitis. Mesalazine also reduced the rate of relapse in ulcerative colitis; a 12 month remission rate of 64% has been reported in patients taking 4 g/day.

Prolonged-release mesalazine also reduced disease activity in patients with mild to moderately active Crohn's disease. In Crohn's disease, mesalazine was more effective in preventing relapse in patients with isolated small bowel disease than in those with colonic involvement. Prolonged-release mesalazine appears to be as well tolerated as placebo, and the incidence of adverse effects does not appear to be dose related. *Nausea/vomiting*, *diarrhea*, *abdominal pain*, and *dyspepsia* are the most commonly reported. Reports of *nephrotoxicity* with this formulation are rare.

In an 18-month double-blind, randomized, placebo-controlled trial in 318 patients, mesalazine 4 g/day did not significantly affect the postoperative course of Crohn's disease compared with placebo (70[C]). There was some relapse-preventing effect in patients with isolated small bowel disease. The overall incidence of adverse effects was similar with mesalazine and placebo. Of the serious adverse effects reported, only one case of *alopecia* was considered to be possibly or probably related to mesalazine.

In a double-blind, placebo-controlled, multicenter trial in 65 patients with ulcerative proctitis in clinical and endoscopic remission, mesalazine in suppositories (500 mg od) as sole treatment was effective, well tolerated, and safe for maintenance of remission over 24 months (71[C]). The incidence of adverse effects was similar with mesalazine and placebo. The most frequent adverse effects with mesalazine were *rectal disorders*, *abdominal pain*, and *headache*.

Mesalazine caused apoptosis and reduced cell proliferation in the colorectal mucosa in 17 patients with sporadic polyps of the large bowel (72[c]). This may be clinically relevant in lowering the rate of polyp recurrence after polypectomy, thereby contributing to chemoprevention of sporadic colonic carcinoma.

Cardiovascular Cardiac effects of mesalazine are uncommon. A case of *chest pain* has been reported (73[A]).

A 37-year-old man with ulcerative colitis developed severe retrosternal chest pain with nonspecific ST–T wave changes in the inferolateral leads of the electrocardiogram after taking mesalazine 800 mg qds for 1 week. Cardiac enzymes, coronary angiography, left ventricular function, and pulmonary angiography were normal. Mesalazine was omitted and steroids were tapered. He recovered completely and his electrocardiogram normalized. Two weeks later he was given mesalazine again 800 mg qds, and again developed retrosternal chest pain with T wave inversion in the lateral leads. Mesalazine was withdrawn and his symptoms resolved within 24 hours. His chest pain did not recur over an 18 month follow-up period while not taking mesalazine.

Respiratory *Eosinophilic pleural effusion*

has been reported for the first time in a 35-year-old male non-smoker who had been taking mesalazine 2.4 g/day orally for 2 weeks for a diarrheal illness (74[A]). He recovered after mesalazine was withdrawn.

Gastrointestinal Five cases of severe persistent *diarrhea* following the use of mesalazine in doses of 2.4–4.8 g/day have been reported (75[A]). The diarrhea was made worse by increasing doses of the drug. Symptoms resolved on withdrawal of the drug or reducing the dose.

Pancreas Three cases of mesalazine-induced acute *pancreatitis* have been reported (76[A]–78[A]).

A 10-year-old boy with ulcerative colitis developed acute pancreatitis 1 day after the dose of mesalazine was increased from 400 mg bd (which he had taken for 5 months without any adverse effect) to 800 mg bd for a mild relapse. He became asymptomatic 3 days after drug withdrawal.

A 34-year-old woman with colitis developed pancreatitis 1 week after starting mesalazine 1g tds; she recovered after drug withdrawal. She was admitted 15 months later with a relapse of colitis and was given oral prednisolone 50 mg/day and mesalazine enemas (2 g bd). Although the colitis regressed, 10 days later treatment she again developed acute pancreatitis. She recovered 3 days after prednisolone and mesalazine enemas were withdrawn. Symptoms of pancreatitis did not recur when prednisolone was restarted.

Another patient developed pancreatitis after taking mesalazine 2 g bd; the symptoms resolved when the drug was withdrawn, but recurred when azathioprine was given.

Urinary tract A 23-year-old student with ulcerative colitis who took mesalazine 1.5 g/day for 15 days developed asymptomatic *renal insufficiency* (79[A]). Renal function rapidly normalized after drug withdrawal. Two other cases of interstitial nephritis have been reported in children with Crohn's disease who were treated with mesalazine (80[A]).

Sulfasalazine

Sulfasalazine consists of sulfapyridine linked to mesalazine by an azo bond. Common adverse effects related to sulfapyridine intolerance include *headache*, *nausea*, *anorexia*, and *malaise*. Other allergic or toxic adverse effects include *fever*, *rash*, *hemolytic anemia*, *hepatitis*, *pancreatitis*, *paradoxical worsening of colitis*, and *reversible sperm abnormalities* (81[R]). Sulfasalazine appears to cause frequent severe adverse effects in adult-onset Still's disease and systemic-onset juvenile rheumatoid arthritis, as suggested by a long-term follow-up study of 41 patients with adult-onset Still's disease and 109 consecutive patients with rheumatoid arthritis (82[C]). Adverse effects included *abdominal pain*, *nausea and vomiting*, *urticaria*, *facial flushing*, *high fever*, *hypotension*, *severe myelosuppression*, and *fulminant hepatitis*, which resulted in death in one patient.

Respiratory *Peripheral lung infiltrates with blood eosinophilia* are rare effects with sulfasalazine. Sulfasalazine-induced hypersensitivity lung disease with simultaneous *Legionella pneumophila* infection has been reported for the first time (83[A]).

A 32-year-old woman with ulcerative colitis developed bilateral pulmonary infiltrates with peripheral eosinophilia 2 weeks after starting to take sulfasalazine and mesalazine enemas, and both drugs were withdrawn. Based on a high antibody titer, legionnaires' disease was diagnosed and empirical therapy with a macrolide antibiotic was started; she improved within a few days. Three months later sulfasalazine was reinstituted, followed 3 days later by acute pulmonary symptoms (bilateral confluent opacities) and blood eosinophilia. The abnormalities resolved completely after drug withdrawal and prophylactic antibiotic therapy.

Hematologic *Agranulocytosis* is a rare but serious adverse reaction to sulfasalazine, in whose metabolism *N*-acetyltransferase 2 (NAT2) plays an important role. However, in a recent study, the risk of agranulocytosis did not appear to be increased in slow acetylators (84[C]).

Sulfasalazine causes *Heinz body anemia* in patients with abnormal hemoglobin and hemolysis in patients with glucose-6-phosphate dehydrogenase deficiency (85[A]) .

A 79-year-old woman who had been taking sulfasalazine for ulcerative colitis for 5 years presented with a positive Coombs' test and a hemoglobin of 8.2 g/dl. Agglutination occurred when a mixture of sulfasalazine and the patient's serum was added to normal erythrocytes treated with the endopeptidase ficin, but there was no reactivity when control serum was used or when sulfasalazine was omitted. Preincubation of sulfasalazine with normal erythrocytes gave negative results on addition of the patient's serum, excluding the possibility of a penicillin-like reaction. The patient had normal glucose-6-

phosphate dehydrogenase activity and there were no Heinz bodies in a blood smear.

It should be remembered that about 1.7% of patients with ulcerative colitis develop immune hemolytic anemia, even in the absence of sulfasalazine.

Urinary tract In a long-term study (mean treatment time 10.1 years) in 36 patients taking sulfasalazine for ulcerative colitis, there was no nephrotoxicity (86[C]).

Skin Sulfasalazine has many adverse effects on the skin, including *maculopapular rash, pruritus, urticaria, angio-edema, eczematous dermatitis, photosensitivity, skin discoloration*, and *oral ulceration. Acute generalized exanthematous pustulosis*, which occurred in a 28-year-old man with ulcerative colitis can be added to the list (87[A]). A patch test was negative, but the lymphocyte stimulation assay for sulfasalazine showed a stimulation index of 541% (controls were not mentioned).

Immunologic Treatment with sulfasalazine was associated with *lupus-like symptoms* and systemic lupus erythematosus-related autoantibody production in 10% of patients with early rheumatoid arthritis; risk factors included a systemic lupus erythematosus-related HLA haplotype, increased serum interleukin-10 concentrations, and a speckled pattern of antinuclear antibodies (88[C]).

Sulfasalazine rarely causes *angio-immunoblastic lymphadenopathy*; a new case has been reported in a patient with juvenile chronic arthritis (89[A]).

ANTISPASMODIC AGENTS

(SED-13, 1084; SEDA-22, 394)

Mebeverine

The effectiveness and safety of two formulations of mebeverine hydrochloride (200 mg capsules bd and 135 mg tablets tds) in 213 patients with irritable bowel syndrome have been studied in a randomized, double-blind general practice study lasting 8 weeks (90[C]). The two formulations were equally effective in relieving abdominal pain. The frequencies of reported adverse events were similar in the two groups and were considered unlikely to be related to medication.

SECRETORY STIMULANTS

(SED–14, 1240)

Secretin

The pharmacology of synthetic porcine secretin and biologically derived porcine secretin has been compared in a double-blind, randomized, crossover study in 12 volunteers (91[c]). The two formulations had identical effects and were safe and well tolerated. One subject reported transient mild *flushing* with both formulations of secretin. Otherwise, physical examination, clinical laboratory assessments, and electrocardiograms were normal.

CHOLELITHOLYTIC AGENTS

Bile acids *(SED-14, 1240; SEDA-22, 395; SEDA-23, 387; SEDA-24, 408)*

The combinations of oral ursodeoxycholic acid 13–15 mg/kg/day plus interferon (3 MU thrice a week) and interferon plus placebo for 6 months have been compared in a randomized, placebo-controlled study in 91 patients with chronic hepatitis C resistant to interferon (92[C]). Combined interferon plus ursodeoxycholic acid was more effective than interferon alone in terms of normalizing AlT at 6 months (but not at 12 months), but not in terms of the virological response. The frequency of adverse effects was similar in the two groups. *Diarrhea*, which was reported by a few patients, was the only adverse effect attributable to ursodeoxycholic acid.

The long-term effects of ursodeoxycholic acid 14–16 mg/kg/day has been investigated in a double-blind, placebo-controlled, multicenter trial in 192 patients with primary biliary cirrhosis (93[C]). Ursodeoxycholic acid was associated with significant improvement in liver function tests and liver histology, but it did not affect the time to death or liver transplantation. Adverse effects were mild: *abdominal pain, flatulence*, and *diarrhea* were reported in nine patients taking ursodeoxycholic acid and six taking placebo.

The clinical and biological effects and safety of ursodeoxycholic acid in intrahepatic cholestasis of pregnancy have been reported in 19 patients, 14 of whom had clinical improvement, with reduction or disappearance of pruritus, and 11 of whom had an improvement in biochemical liver function tests (94[c]). The only birth defect reported was pyloric stenosis in a boy whose mother had taken ursodeoxycholic acid for 10 days at 34 weeks gestation.

Acknowledgement

I thank Dr Anupama De Silva for help with the manuscript.

REFERENCES

1. Mansi C, Borro P, Giacomini M, Biagini R, Mele MR, Pandolfo N, Savarino V. Comparative effects of levosulpiride and cisapride on gastric emptying and symptoms in patients with functional dyspepsia and gastroparesis. Aliment Pharmacol Ther 2000; 14: 561–9.
2. Committee on Safety of Medicines and Medicines Control Agency. Cisapride (Prepulsid) withdrawn. Curr Probl Pharmacovig 2000; 26: 9–10.
3. Ng K-S, Tham L-S, Tan H-H, Chia B-L. Cisapride and torsades de pointes in a pacemaker patient. Pace Pacing Clin Electrophysiol 2000; 23: 130–2.
4. Ramirez-Mayans J, Garrido-Garcia LM, Huerta-Tecanhuey A, Gutierrez-Castrellon P, Cervantes-Bustamante R, Mata-Rivera N, Zarate-Mondragon F. Cisapride and QT_c interval in children. Pediatrics 2000; 106: 1028–30.
5. Gomez Rodriguez MT, Mugarza Hernandez MD, Marin Perez O. Cisapride and tardive dyskinesia. Revision of one case. Medifam Rev Med Fam Comunitaria 2000; 10: 119–22.
6. Gilbert RE, Augood C, MacLennan S, Logan S. Cisapride treatment for gastro-oesophageal reflux in children: a systematic review of randomized controlled trials. J Paediatr Child Health 2000; 36: 524–9.
7. Kentrup H, Baisch H-J, Kusenbach G, Heimann G, Skopnik H. Effect of cisapride on acid gastro-oesophageal reflux during treatment with caffeine. Biol Neonate 2000; 77: 92–5.
8. Nurko S, Garcia-Aranda JA, Worona LB, Zlochisty O. Cisapride for the treatment of constipation children: a double-blind study. J Pediatr 2000; 136: 35–40.
9. Costalos C, Gounaris A, Varhalama E, Kokori F, Alexiou N, Katsarakis I. Effect of low-dose cisapride on gastric emptying and QT_c interval in preterm infants. Acta Paediatr Int J Paediatr 2000; 89: 1446–8.
10. Perez Blanco JL, Garcia Angleu F, Caceres Espejo J, Panadero Ruz Ma D. Extrapyramidal effects as a possible adverse reaction to domperidone. Rev Esp Pediatr 2000; 56: 189–92.
11. Corazza GR, Tonini M. Levosulpiride for dyspepsia and emesis. A review of its pharmacology, efficacy and tolerability. Clin Drug Invest 2000; 19: 151–62.
12. Huerta Blanco R, Hernandez Cabrera M, Quinones Morales I, Cardenes Santana MA. Total heart block after intravenous metoclopramide. An Med Interna 2000; 17: 222–3.
13. Wilner KD, Hansen RA, Folger CJ, Geoffroy P. The pharmacokinetics of ziprasidone in healthy volunteers treated with cimetidine or antacid. Br J Clin Pharmacol 2000; 49 Suppl 1: 57S–60S.
14. Spitzer TR, Friedman CJ, Bushnell W, Frankel SR, Raschko J. Double-blind, randomized, parallel-group study on the efficacy and safety of oral granisetron and oral ondansetron in the prophylaxis of nausea and vomiting in patients receiving hyperfractionated total body irradiation. Bone Marrow Transplant 2000; 26: 203–10.
15. Chiou T-J, Tzeng W-F, Wang W-S, Yen C-C, Fan FS, Liu J-H, Chen P-M. Comparison of the efficacy and safety of oral granisetron plus dexamethasone with intravenous ondansetron plus dexamethasone to control nausea and vomiting induced by moderate/severe emetogenic chemotherapy. Chin Med J Taipei 2000; 63: 729–36.
16. Barman Balfour JA, Goa KL, Perry CM. Alosetron. Drugs 2000; 59: 511–18.
17. Mucke H, Cole P, Rabasseda X. Alosetron. Drugs Today 2000; 36: 595–607.
18. Reddy P. Alosetron: A 5-HT_3 receptor antagonist for treatment of irritable bowel syndrome. Formulary 2000; 35: 404–11.
19. Camilleri M. Pharmacology and clinical experience with alosetron. Expert Opin Invest Drugs 2000; 9: 147–59.
20. Camilleri M, Northcutt AR, Kong S, Dukes GE, McSorley D, Mangel AW. Efficacy and safety of alosetron in women with irritable bowel syndrome: a randomised, placebo-controlled trial. Lancet 2000; 355: 1035–40.
21. Bardhan KD, Bodemar G, Geldof H, Schutz E, Heath A, Mills JG, Jacques LA. A double-blind, randomized, placebo-controlled dose-ranging study to evaluate the efficacy of alosetron in the treatment of irritable bowel syndrome. Aliment Pharmacol Ther 2000; 14: 23–34.
22. Houghton LA, Foster JM, Whorwell PJ. Alosetron, a 5-HT_3 receptor antagonist, delays colonic transit in patients with irritable bowel syndrome and healthy volunteers. Aliment Pharmacol Ther

2000; 14: 775–82.

23. Thumshirn M, Coulie B, Camilleri M, Zinsmeister AR, Burton DD, Van Dyke C. Effects of alosetron on gastrointestinal transit time and rectal sensation in patients with irritable bowel syndrome. Aliment Pharmacol Ther 2000; 14: 869–78.
24. Fuj II Y, Tanaka H, Kawasaki T. Randomized clinical trial of granisetron, droperidol and metoclopramide for the treatment of nausea and vomiting after laparoscopic cholecystectomy. Br J Surg 2000; 87: 285–8.
25. Abang AM, Takemoto MH, Pham T, Mandanas RA, Roy V, Selby GB, Carter TH. Efficacy and safety of oral granisetron versus i.v. granisetron in patients undergoing peripheral blood progenitor cell and bone marrow transplantation. Anti-Cancer Drugs 2000; 11: 137–42.
26. Fujii Y, Saitoh Y, Tanaka H, Toyooka H. Granisetron/dexamethasone combination for the prevention of postoperative nausea and vomiting after laparoscopic cholecystectomy. Eur J Anaesthesiol 2000; 17: 64–8.
27. Abbott B, Ippoliti C, Hecth D, Bruton J, Whaley B, Champlin R. Granisetron (Kytril) plus dexamethasone for antiemetic control in bone marrow transplant patients receiving highly emetogenic chemotherapy with or without total body irradiation. Bone Marrow Transplant 2000; 25: 1279–83.
28. Simpson K, Spencer CM, McClellan KJ. Tropisetron: an update of its use in the prevention of chemotherapy-induced nausea and vomiting. Drugs 2000; 59: 1297–315.
29. Krska J, John DN, Hansford D, Kennedy EJ. Drug utilization evaluation of nonprescription H_2-receptor antagonists and alginate-containing preparations for dyspepsia. Br J Clin Pharmacol 2000; 49: 363–8.
30. Good CB, Fultz SL, Trilli L, Etchason J. Therapeutic substitution of cimetidine for nizatidine was not associated with an increase in healthcare utilization. Am J Managed Care 2000; 6: 1141–6.
31. Suleiman UL, Harrison M, Britton A, McPherson K, Bates T. H_2-receptor antagonists may increase the risk of cardio-oesophageal adenocarcinoma: a case-control study. Eur J Cancer Prev 2000; 9: 185–91.
32. Eland IA, Huert Alvarez C, Stricker BHCh, Garcia Rodriguez LA. The risk of acute pancreatitis associated with acid-suppressing drugs. Br J Clin Pharmacol 2000; 49: 473–8.
33. Jimenez-Saenz M, Arguelles-Arias F, Herrerias-Gutierrez JM, Duran-Quintana JA. Acute cholestatic hepatitis in a child treated with famotidine. Am J Gastroenterol 2000; 95: 3665–6.
34. Earnest D, Robinson M, Rodriguez-Stanley S, Ciociola AA, Jaffe P, Silver MT, Kleoudis CS, Murdock RH. Managing heartburn at the 'base' of the GERD 'iceberg': effervescent ranitidine 150 mg b.d. provides faster and better heartburn relief than antacids. Aliment Pharmacol Ther 2000; 14: 911–18.
35. Ribeiro JM, Lucas M, Baptista A, Victorino RMM. Fatal hepatitis associated with ranitidine. Am J Gastroenterol 2000; 95: 559–60.
36. Luparini RL, Rotundo A, Mattace R, Marigliano V. Possible ranitidine-associated autoimmune hepatitis. Ann Ital Med Interna 2000; 15: 214–17.
37. Martin RM, Dunn NR, Freemantle S, Shakir S. The rates of common adverse events reported during treatment with proton pump inhibitors used in general practice in England: cohort studies. Br J Clin Pharmacol 2000; 50: 366–72.
38. Lind T, Rydberg L, Kyleback A, Jonsson A, Andersson T, Hasselgren G, Holmberg J, Rohss K. Esomeprazole provides improved acid control vs. omeprazole in patients with symptoms of gastro-oesophageal reflux disease. Aliment Pharmacol Ther 2000; 14: 861–7.
39. Kahrilas PJ, Falk GW, Johnson DA, Schmitt C, Collins DW, Whipple J, D'Amico D, Hamelin B, Joelsson B. Esomeprazole improves healing and symptom resolution as compared with omeprazole in reflux oesophagitis patients: a randomized controlled trial. Aliment Pharmacol Ther 2000; 14: 1249–58.
40. Amidon PR, Jankovich R, Stoukides CA, Kaul AF. Proton pump inhibitor therapy: preliminary results of a therapeutic interchange program. Am J Managed Care 2000; 6: 593–601.
41. Gerson LB, Hatton BN, Ryono R, Jones W, Pulliam G, Sampliner RE, Triadafilopoulos G, Fass R. Clinical and fiscal impact of lansoprazole intolerance in veterans with gastro-oesophageal reflux disease. Aliment Pharmacol Ther 2000; 14: 397–406.
42. Agrawal NM, Campbell DR, Safdi MA, Lukasik NL, Huang B, Haber MM. Superiority of lansoprazole vs ranitidine in healing nonsteroidal anti-inflammatory drug-associated gastric ulcers: results of a double-blind, randomized, multicenter study. Arch Intern Med 2000; 160: 1455–61.
43. Richter JE, Campbell DR, Kahrilas PJ, Huang B, Fludas C. Lansoprazole compared with ranitidine for the treatment of nonerosive gastroesophageal reflux disease. Arch Intern Med 2000; 160: 1803–9.
44. Van Zyl JH, Grundling HdeK, Van Rensburg CJ, Retief FJ, O'Keefe SJD, Theron I, Fischer R, Bethke T. Efficacy and tolerability of 20 mg pantoprazole versus 300 mg ranitidine in patients with mild reflux-oesophagitis: a randomized, double-blind, parallel, and multicentre study. Eur J Gastroenterol Hepatol 2000; 12: 197–202.
45. Fass R, Murthy U, Hayden CW, Malagon IB, Pulliam G, Wendel C, Kovacs TOG. Omeprazole 40 mg once a day is equally effective as lansoprazole 30 mg twice a day in symptom control of patients with gastro-oesophageal reflux disease (GERD) who are resistant to conventional-dose lansoprazole therapy – a prospective, randomized, multi-centre study. Aliment Pharmacol Ther 2000; 14: 1595–603.
46. Delchier J-C, Cohen G, Humphries TJ. Rabeprazole, 20 mg once daily or 10 mg twice daily, is equivalent to omeprazole, 20 mg once

daily, in the healing of erosive gastro-oesophageal reflux disease. Scand J Gastroenterol 2000; 35: 1245–50.

47. Kees F, Holstege A, Ittner KP, Zimmermann M, Lock G, Scholmerich J, Grobecker H. Pharmacokinetic interaction between proton pump inhibitors and roxithromycin in volunteers. Aliment Pharmacol Ther 2000; 14: 407–12.
48. Dorta G, Nicolet M, Vouillamoz D, Margalith D, Saraga E, Bouzourene H, Hacki WH, Stolte M, Blum AL, Armstrong D. The effects of omeprazole on healing and appearance of small gastric and duodenal lesions during dosing with diclofenac in healthy subjects. Aliment Pharmacol Ther 2000;14: 535–41.
49. Heckmann JG, Birklein F, Neundorfer B. Omeprazole-induced delirium. J Neurol 2000; 247: 56–7.
50. Bechade D, Algayres J-P, Henrionnet A, Texier F, Bili H, Coutant G, Helie C, Daly J-P. Hyponatremia caused by omeprazole administration. Gastroenterol Clin Biol 2000; 24: 684–5.
51. Singh P, Indaram A, Greenberg R, Visvalingam V, Bank S. Long term omeprazole therapy for reflux esophagitis: follow-up in serum gastrin levels, EC cell hyperplasia and neoplasia. World J Gastroenterol 2000; 6: 789–92.
52. Wall CAM, Gaffney EF, Mellotte GJ. Hypercalcaemia and acute interstitial nephritis associated with omeprazole therapy. Nephrol Dial Transplant 2000; 15: 1450–2.
53. Post AT, Voorhorst G, Zanen AL. Reversible renal failure after treatment with omeprazole. Neth J Med 2000; 57: 58–61.
54. Johnson D, Perdomo C, Barth J, Jokubaitis L. The benefit/risk profile of rabeprazole, a new proton-pump inhibitor. Eur J Gastroenterol Hepatol 2000; 12: 799–806.
55. Mundo-Gallardo F, De Mezerville-Cantillo L, Burgos-Quiroz H, Izquierdo E, Chang-Mayorga J, Azteguieta L, Passarrelli-Sandhoff LF. Latin American open-label study with rabeprazole in patients with functional dyspepsia. Adv Ther 2000; 17: 190–4.
56. Birbara C, Breiter J, Perdomo C, Hahne W. Rabeprazole for the prevention of recurrent erosive or ulcerative gastro-oesophageal reflux disease. Eur J Gastroenterol Hepatol 2000; 12: 889–97.
57. Williams MP, Blanshard C, Millson C, Sercombe J, Pounder RE. A placebo-controlled study to assess the effects of 7-day dosing with 10, 20 and 40 mg rabeprazole on 24-h intragastric acidity and plasma gastrin in healthy male subjects. Aliment Pharmacol Ther 2000; 14: 691–9.
58. Ohning GV, Barbuti RC, Kovacs TOG, Sytnik B, Humphries TJ, Walsh JH. Rabeprazole produces rapid, potent, and long-acting inhibition of gastric acid secretion in subjects with *Helicobacter pylori* infection. Aliment Pharmacol Ther 2000; 14: 701–8.
59. Nakajima S, Graham DY, Hattori T, Bamba T. Strategy for treatment of *Helicobacter pylori* infection in adults II. Practical policy in 2000. Curr Pharm Des 2000; 6: 1515–29.
60. Adachi K, Ishihara S, Hashimoto T, Hirakawa K, Niigaki M, Takashima T, Kaji T, Kawamura A, Sato H, Okuyama T, Watanabe M, Kinoshita Y. Efficacy of sucralfate for *Helicobacter pylori* eradication triple therapy in comparison with a lansoprazole-based regimen. Aliment Pharmacol Ther 2000; 14: 919–22.
61. Canducci F, Armuzzi A, Cremonini F, Cammarota G, Bartolozzi F, Pola P, Gasbarrini G, Gasbarrini A. A lyophilized and inactivated culture of *Lactobacillus acidophilus* increases *Helicobacter pylori* eradication rates. Aliment Pharmacol Ther 2000; 14: 1625–9.
62. Szilagyi A, Torchinsky A, Calacone A. Possible therapeutic use of loperamide for symptoms of lactose intolerance. Can J Gastroenterol 2000; 14: 581–7.
63. Einarson A, Mastroiacovo P, Arnon J, Ornoy A, Addis A, Malm H, Koren G. Prospective, controlled, multicentre study of loperamide in pregnancy. Can J Gastroenterol 2000; 14: 185–7.
64. Yoshioka K, Connolly AB, Ogunbiyi OA, Hasegawa H, Morton DG, Keighley MRB. Randomized trial of oral sodium phosphate compared with oral sodium picosulphate (Picolax) for elective colorectal surgery and colonoscopy. Dig Surg 2000; 17: 66–70.
65. Atkin WS, Hart A, Edwards R, Cook CF, Wardle J, McIntyre P, Aubrey R, Baron C, Sutton S, Cuzick J, Senapati A, Northover JMA, Wulff HR, Taylor M. Single blind, randomised trial of efficacy and acceptability of oral Picolax versus self administered phosphate enema in bowel preparation for flexible sigmoidoscopy screening. Br Med J 2000; 320: 1504–9.
66. Egesel T, Sivri B, Asik M, Altun B, Bayraktar Y. A fatal complication of sodium-phosphate enema. Turk J Gastroenterol 2000; 11: 338–40.
67. Wong NAC, Penman ID, Campbell S, Lessells AM. Microscopic focal cryptitis associated with oral sodium phosphate bowel preparation. Histopathology 2000; 36: 476–8.
68. Klotz U. The role of aminosalicylates at the beginning of the new millennium in the treatment of chronic inflammatory bowel disease. Eur J Clin Pharmacol 2000; 56: 353–62.
69. Clemett D, Markham A. Prolonged-release mesalazine: a review of its therapeutic potential in ulcerative colitis and Crohn's disease. Drugs 2000; 59: 929–56.
70. Lochs H, Mayer M, Fleig WE, Mortensen PB, Bauer P, Gienser D, Petritsch W, Rathel M, Hoffmann R, Gross V, Plauth M, Staun M, Niesje LB, Hinterleitner T, Holtz J, Plein K, Otto P, Thilo A, Raedler A, Jenss H, Kaskas B, Koop I, Frank M, Loeschke K, Dotzel W, Scheurien C, Gross V, Caesar I, Reissmann A. Prophylaxis of postoperative relapse in Crohn's disease with mesalamine: European Cooperative Crohn's Disease Study VI. Gastroenterology 2000; 118: 264–73.
71. Hanauer S, Good LI, Goodman MW, Pizinger RJ, Strum WB, Lyss C, Haber G, Williams

CN, Robinson M. Long-term use of mesalamine (Rowasa) suppositories in remission maintenance of ulcerative proctitis. Am J Gastroenterol 2000; 95: 1749–54.
72. Reinacher-Schick A, Seidensticker F, Petrasch S, Reiser M, Philippou S, Theegarten D, Freitag G, Schmiegel W. Mesalazine changes apoptosis and proliferation in normal mucosa of patients with sporadic polyps of the large bowel. Endoscopy 2000: 32: 245–54.
73. Amin HE, Della Siega AJ, Whittaker JS, Munt B. Mesalamine-induced chest pain: a case report. Can J Cardiol 2000; 16: 667–9.
74. Trisolini R, Dore R, Biagi F, Luinetti O, Pochetti P, Carrabino N, Luisetti M. Eosinophilic pleural effusion due to mesalamine. Report of a rare occurrence. Sarcoidosis Vasc Diffuse Lung Dis 2000; 17: 288–91.
75. Goldstein F, DiMarino AJ Jr. Diarrhea as a side effect of mesalamine treatment for inflammatory bowel disease. J Clin Gastroenterol 2000; 31: 60–2.
76. Paul AC, Oommen SP, Angami S, Moses PD. Acute pancreatitis in a child with idiopathic ulcerative colitis on long-term 5-aminosalicylic acid therapy. Indian J Gastroenterol 2000; 19: 195–6.
77. Schworer H, Ramadori G. Acute pancreatitis caused by 5-aminosalicylic acid (mesalazine) administered orally or by enema. Dtsch Med Wochenschr 2000; 125: 1328–30.
78. Glintborg B. Pancreatitis in a patient with Crohn's disease treated with mesalazine and azathioprine. Ugeskr Laeg 2000; 162: 4553–4.
79. Musil D. Early renal failure caused by mesalazine. Vnitr Lek 2000; 46: 728–731.
80. Benador N, Grimm P, Lemire J, Griswold W, Billman G, Reznik V, Narchi H, Chellapa C. Interstitial nephritis in children with Crohn's disease. Clin Pediatr 2000; 39: 253–4.
81. Stein RB, Hanauer SB. Comparative tolerability of treatments for inflammatory bowel disease. Drug Saf 2000; 23: 429–48.
82. Jung JH, Jun JB, Yoo DH, Kim TH, Jung SS, Lee IH, Bae SC, Kim SY. High toxicity of sulfasalazine in adult-onset Still's disease. Clin Exp Rheumatol 2000; 18: 245–8.
83. Gunnarsson I, Nordmark B, Hassan Bakri A, Grondal G, Larsson P, Forslid J, Bielecki JW, Avar S, Joss R. Sulfasalazine-induced pulmonary infiltrates and *Legionella pneumonia*. Schweiz Med Wochenschr 2000; 130: 1078–83.
84. Wadelius M, Stjernberg E, Wiholm BE, Rane A. Polymorphisms of NAT2 in relation to sulfasalazine-induced agranulocytosis. Pharmacogenetics 2000; 10: 35–41.
85. Teplitsky V, Virag I, Halabe A. Immune complex haemolytic anaemia associated with sulfasalazine. Br Med J 2000; 320: 1113.
86. Birkevedt GS, Berg KJ, Fausa O, Florholmen J. Glomerular and tubular renal functions after long-term medication of sulfasalazine, olsalazine, and mesalazine in patients with ulcerative colitis. Inflamm Bowel Dis 2000; 6: 275–9.
87. Kawaguchi M, Mitsuhashi Y, Kondo S. Acute generalized exanthematous pustulosis induced by salazosulfapyridine in a patient with ulcerative colitis. J Dermatol 1999; 26: 359–62.
88. Gunnarsson I, Nordmark B, Hassan Bakri A, Grondal G, Larsson P, Forslid J, Klareskog L, Ringertz B. Development of lupus-related side-effects in patients with early RA during sulfasalazine treatment – the role of IL-10 and HLA. Rheumatology 2000; 39: 886–93.
89. Pay S, Dinc A, Simsek I, Can C, Erdem H. Sulfasalazine-induced angioimmunoblastic lymphadenopathy developing in a patient with juvenile chronic arthritis. Rheumatol Int 2000; 20: 25–7.
90. Gilbody JS, Fletcher CP, Hughes IW, Kidman SP. Comparison of two different formulations of mebeverine hydrochloride in irritable bowel syndrome. Int J Clin Pract 2000; 54: 461–4.
91. Jowell PS, Robuck-Mangum G, Mergener K, Branch MS, Purich ED, Fein SH. A double-blind, randomized, dose response study testing the pharmacological efficacy of synthetic porcine secretin. Aliment Pharmacol Ther 2000; 14: 1679–84.
92. Poupon RE, Bonnand A-M, Queneau P-E, Trepo C, Zarski J-P, Vetter D, Raabe J-J, Thieffin G, Larrey D, Grange J-D, Capron J-P, Serfaty L, Chretien Y, St Marc Girardin M-F, Mathiex-Fortunet H, Zafrani ES, Guechot J, Beuers U, Paumgartner G, Poupon R. Randomized trial of interferon-alpha plus ursodeoxycholic acid versus interferon plus placebo in patients with chronic hepatitis C resistant to interferon. Scand J Gastroenterol 2000; 35: 642–9.
93. Pares A, Caballeria L, Rodes J, Bruguera M, Rodrigo L, Garcia-Plaza A, Berenguer J, Rodriguez-Martinez D, Mercader J, Velicia R, Gines A, Linares-Rodriguez A, Cano-Ruiz A, Martin-Scapa A, Berenguer M, Fernandez-Rodriguez C, Obrador A, Vaquer P, Clemente G, Arenas-Mirave JI, Castiella A, Vargas V, Martin-Vivaldi R, Vidan JM, Zozaya JM, Planas R, Viver JM, De la Mata M, Pons F, Diaz F. Long-term effects of ursodeoxycholic acid in primary biliary cirrhosis: results of a double-blind controlled multicentric trial. J Hepatol 2000; 32: 561–6.
94. Berkane N, Cocheton J-J, Brehier D, Merviel P, Wolf C, Lefevre G, Uzan S. Ursodeoxycholic acid in intrahepatic cholestasis of pregnancy: a retrospective study of 19 cases. Acta Obstet Gynaecol Scand 2000; 79: 941–6.

Thierry Vial and Jacques Descotes

37 Drugs acting on the immune system

INTERFERONS *(SED-14, 1246; SEDA-22, 399; SEDA-23, 391; SEDA-24, 411)*

Interferon-α

A wide range of persistent symptoms has been reported during interferon-α treatment for chronic hepatitis C. An analysis of 222 patients from the USA and France enrolled in a multicenter trial suggested that pretreatment symptoms were an important predictor of moderate or severe (defined as debilitating) adverse effects during interferon-α treatment (1^C). Compared with baseline, the incidences of moderate and severe *fatigue*, *myalgia*, *arthralgia*, *headache*, *dry eyes*, and *dry mouth* increased significantly after 6 months of treatment. In each case the development of these debilitating adverse effects was associated with the presence of that symptom at baseline. They were more often reported in patients who received interferon-α daily than three times weekly, and in US than French patients, suggesting possible differences in cultural attitudes toward illness. There was also increased usage of antidepressants during the 6-month survey.

Pegylated interferon-α_{2a} is a modified form of interferon-α; it produces higher serum concentrations and has greater efficacy. Two studies have shown that peginterferon-α_{2a} once weekly is more effective than unmodified interferon-α_{2a} three times weekly in patients with chronic hepatitis C (2^C, 3^C). The frequency and severity of adverse effects with the two treatments were very similar and were consistent with the known adverse effects of interferon-α. In one study a neutrophil count below 0.5×10^9/l was more frequent with peginterferon-α than unmodified interferon-α (12/265 vs 4/261), but none of these patients required treatment withdrawal or had serious infections in relation to *neutropenia* (3^C). In the other study, the proportion of patients who required dosage modification because of *thrombocytopenia* was also higher with peginterferon-α (18% vs 6%), but no patients had clinically significant bleeding disorders (2^C). Taken together, these studies suggest that pegylated interferon-α may produce more frequent or more severe hemotoxic effects than unmodified interferon-α.

Respiratory The first case of pleural effusion with interferon-α has been reported (4^A).

A 54-year-old man received daily interferon-α_{2a} (9 MIU) for chronic hepatitis C. He developed an asymptomatic right pleural effusion after 14 days. Although his serum titer of antinuclear antibodies was slightly increased, a more complete screening for autoimmune disease was negative. An infectious origin was also ruled out. The pleural effusion spontaneously disappeared after interferon-α withdrawal and did not recur.

Although the mechanism of this adverse effect is purely speculative, it was suggested that interferon-α might have induced a reaction similar to the immunopathological mechanism involved in serositis associated with systemic lupus erythematosus.

Nervous system Various forms of interferon-α-induced neuropathy have been reported (SED-14, 1249), but *chronic inflammatory demyelinating polyneuropathy* has seldom been described (5^A, 6^A).

In two patients with chronic hepatitis C or malignant melanoma, paresthesia and tiredness occurred after 6 weeks and 9 months of treatment respectively. Despite interferon-α withdrawal, the neurolo-

Side Effects of Drugs, Annual 25
J.K. Aronson, ed.

gical symptoms worsened initially and a diagnosis of chronic inflammatory demyelinating polyneuropathy was finally confirmed several weeks later. One patient improved after an extended course of plasma exchange and the other required immunoglobulins and prednisolone. Mild to moderate neurological abnormalities persisted at follow-up in both patients.

Interferon-α-induced immune dysregulation in an immunologically predisposed patient was suggested to account for this complication.

There have been previous reports of interferon-α-induced cranial nerve palsies (SED-14, 1249), but Bell's palsy has not been previously reported. Two patients, one of whom also received ribavirin, had facial nerve palsy after 5 and 8 months of interferon-α therapy (7[A]). Complete resolution of the palsy was obtained in one patient by withdrawing interferon-α and giving prednisolone; however, in the other case the palsy resolved without drug withdrawal, suggesting coincidence.

Sensory systems A case of *anosmia* has previously been reported (SEDA-22, 403), and interferon-α has now been deemed to be the cause in another patient (8[A]).

A 37-year-old man received interferon-α for chronic hepatitis C. After 2 weeks he complained of smelling difficulties and subsequently developed complete anosmia. There were no other neurological symptoms and complete neurological examination was normal. Anosmia still persisted 13 months after drug withdrawal.

In both patients, the persistence of anosmia late after interferon-α was resumed indicates that a causal relation to treatment is purely speculative.

Psychiatric Neuropsychiatric disorders during interferon-α treatment continue to occur. The clinical features, management, and prognosis of psychiatric symptoms in patients with chronic hepatitis C have been reviewed using data from 943 patients treated with interferon-α (85%) or interferon-β (15%) for 24 weeks (9[C]). Interferon-induced psychiatric symptoms were identified in 40 patients (4.2%) of those referred for psychiatric examination. They were classified in three groups according to the clinical profile: 13 cases of *generalized anxiety disorder* (group A), 21 cases of *mood disorders with depressive features* (group B), and six cases of other psychiatric disorders, including *psychotic disorders with delusions/hallucinations* (four patients), *mood disorders with manic features* (one patient), and *delirium* (one patient) (group C). The time to onset of the symptoms differed significantly between the three groups: 2 weeks in group A, 5 weeks in group B, and 11 weeks in group C. Women were more often affected than men. There was no difference in the incidence or nature of the disorder according to the type of interferon used. Whereas most patients who required psychotropic drugs were able to complete treatment, 10 had to discontinue interferon treatment because of severe psychiatric symptoms, five from group B and five from group C. Twelve patients still required psychiatric treatment for more than 6 months after interferon withdrawal. In addition, residual symptoms (anxiety, insomnia, and mild hypothymia) were still present at the end of the survey in seven patients. Delayed recovery was mostly observed in patients in group C and in patients treated with interferon-β. Although several patients with a previous history of psychiatric disorders are sometimes successfully treated with interferon-α, severe decompensation with persistent psychosis should be regarded as a major possible complication (10[A]).

The risk of *manic symptoms* during or after interferon-α treatment is still not fully recognized. The clinical features of this complication have been described in four patients with malignant melanoma, with a detailed review of nine other published cases (11[AR]). Although seven suffered from depression during treatment, the onset of mania or hypomania was often associated with interferon-α dosage fluctuation (withdrawal or dose reduction) or introduction of an antidepressant for interferon-α-induced depression. In these patients, the risk of mood fluctuations persisted for several months after interferon-α withdrawal, and low-dose gabapentin was considered useful in treating manic disorders and in preventing mood fluctuations.

Several recent studies have prospectively assessed mood disorders in patients treated with interferon-α and have focused on risk factors or tools to identify patients at risk of depression during treatment. Of 91 patients treated with interferon-α_{2b} and low-dose cytarabine for chronic myelogenous leukemia, 22 developed severe neuropsychiatric toxicity (12[C]). Their symptoms consisted mostly of *severe depression or psychotic behavior*, which resolved on withdrawal in all patients. The time to toxicity ranged from as early as 2 weeks to as long as 184 weeks after the start of treatment. Five of six patients had recurrent or worse symptoms after readministration of both drugs. Several baseline factors were analysed, but only a pretreatment history of neurological or psychiatric disorders was considered to be a reliable risk factor. Severe neuropsychiatric toxicity developed during treatment in 63% of patients with previous neuropsychiatric disorders compared with 10% in patients without. It is unlikely that the combination of interferon-α_{2b} with low-dose cytarabine potentiated the neuropsychiatric adverse effects of interferon-α in this study. Indeed, previous experience with this combination, but after exclusion of patients with a psychiatric history, was not associated with such a high incidence of neuropsychiatric toxicity or any significant difference in toxicity between interferon-α alone and interferon-α plus low-dose cytarabine.

In another study of 67 patients with chronic viral hepatitis, the self-administered Minnesota Multiphasic Personality Inventory (MMPI), which determines the patient's psychological profile, significantly correlated with the clinical evaluation and was a sensitive and reliable tool for identifying patients at risk of depressive symptoms before the start of interferon-α therapy (13[C]). It was also successfully used to monitor patients during treatment.

The first controlled trial of an antidepressant in interferon-α-induced depression has now been fully reported (14[C]). Forty patients with high-risk malignant melanoma were randomized to receive paroxetine (mean maximal dose of 31 mg) or placebo, starting 2 weeks before adjuvant high-dose interferon-α. Paroxetine significantly reduced the incidence of major depression (45% in the placebo group and 11% in the paroxetine group) and the rate of interferon-α withdrawal (35% vs 5%). Although the number of patients was small and the duration of the survey short (12 weeks), this suggests that paroxetine effectively prevents the risk of depressive disorders in patients eligible for high-dose interferon-α. However, these results are limited, because patients with melanoma who receive adjuvant high-dose interferon-α are particularly likely to developing depression. The safety of prophylaxis with paroxetine also requires additional data, because three patients taking paroxetine developed retinal hemorrhages, including one with irreversible loss of vision.

In contrast to this study, a 31-year-old woman with major depressive disorder, which responded to paroxetine and trazodone, had progressive recurrence of mood disorders after the introduction of interferon-α for essential thrombocythemia (15[A]). This suggests that interferon-α can also reverse the antidepressant response.

Endocrine *Worsening of insulin-dependent diabetes mellitus* has sometimes been reported (SED-14, 1250), and interferon-α may produce more severe changes than interferon-β (16[A]).

A 39-year-old diabetic man, stabilized with insulin 22 U/day for 13 years, received interferon-β (6 MU/day) for chronic hepatitis C. His diabetes progressively worsened, necessitating insulin 50 U/day. After 4 weeks, interferon-β was replaced by interferon-α (10 MU/day). Shortly afterwards he developed severe diabetic ketoacidosis and shock, which reversed after hemodynamic support and continuous hemodiafiltration.

Hematologic The kinetics of the hemotoxic effects of interferon-α have been studied in 76 patients with chronic hepatitis C (17[c]). There were significant *falls in white blood cell count and platelet count* within 12 hours after the first injection, and a second fall in platelet count after 2 weeks, but not further thereafter. This rapid time-course suggests that liver or spleen sequestration of blood cells, rather than direct bone-marrow suppression or immune-mediated hematological toxicity, is the most likely explanation for this acute hemotoxic effect, which does not preclude continuation of treatment.

Isolated *anemia* is not a common feature of the hemotoxic effects of interferon-α, and pure red cell aplasia has been reported in two patients with chronic leukemia for several months (18[A], 19[A]). Both patients improved progressively after replacement of interferon-α by hydroxyurea. However, one required erythrocyte transfusions for 14 months.

The development of an *acquired factor VIII inhibitor* is rare outside patients with hemophilia, and a possible role of interferon-α has previously been discussed (SED-14, 1252). A further case associated with significant bleeding disorders and hematomas has been reported in a 58-year-old man who took interferon-α for 1 year for chronic myelogenous leukemia (20[A]). The factor VIII inhibitor, which was markedly raised, disappeared within 6 weeks of interferon-α withdrawal and prednisone treatment.

Gastrointestinal Since the first two cases of celiac disease attributed to interferon-α (SEDA-24, 413), three additional cases have been reported after 1–5 months of treatment for chronic hepatitis C (21[A], 22[A]). The diagnosis was confirmed in all three patients, based on the presence of total villous atrophy on distal duodenal biopsy, positivity of antiendomysial antibodies, and recovery with a gluten-free diet. Pretreatment antiendomysial antibodies were positive in the two patients tested. As suggested in one patient, interferon-α can be safely continued providing that a gluten-free diet is strictly respected.

Several forms of *colitis* (microscopic, ulcerative, or ischemic) have already been described, and eosinophilic enteritis has now also been reported (23[A]).

A 23-year-old man with no previous history of digestive disorders took interferon-α for chronic hepatitis C. After 2 weeks of treatment, he had severe abdominal pain and diarrhea. The absolute eosinophil count was 7.5×10^9/l, with 40% eosinophils on bone-marrow aspiration and a markedly high IgE concentration. Radiological examination showed diffuse jejunal and ileal wall thickening and gross ascites with numerous eosinophils. Complete resolution was obtained after interferon-α withdrawal and prednisolone treatment. There was no recurrence after prednisolone was withdrawn.

Pancreas Although interferon-α-induced acute *pancreatitis* has been seldom reported, two recent cases in patients treated for chronic hepatitis C were particularly convincing, because other causes were carefully ruled out and clinical symptoms or biological abnormalities recurred after rechallenge in both patients (24[A]). Although one patient also took ribavirin, recurrence was observed after interferon-α readministration alone. Lipid disorders were not found in these patients, confirming that interferon-α-induced pancreatitis is not due to hypertriglyceridemia.

Skin Severe *injection site reactions* sometimes occur after subcutaneous administration. This has been extensively detailed in six patients who had local cutaneous necrosis or indurated erythema after 1–10 months of treatment with low-dose interferon-α (25[A]). Four patients had concomitant risk factors known to reduce microcirculation, i.e. β-blockers, dihydroergotamine, and cigarette smoking. The lesions healed after medical treatment in five patients, but one required surgical excision. The ulcers healed slowly and full recovery occurred only after a mean of 16 weeks after drug withdrawal. The lesions did not recur after interferon-α readministration at the other injection sites. Cutaneous ulcers have also been reported in one patient treated with peginterferon-α_{2b} (26[A]).

Cutaneous polyarteritis nodosa has been attributed to interferon-α for the first time (27[A]).

A 50-year-old woman was given interferon-α for chronic hepatitis C and primary biliary cirrhosis, and within 2 months became febrile and developed a diffuse nodular erythematous rash. The skin biopsy showed typical features of necrotizing angiitis and cutaneous periarteritis nodosa was diagnosed. Full recovery was obtained after interferon-α withdrawal and prednisolone treatment.

According to the authors, it is not known whether this complication was directly due to interferon-α, represented the triggering of latent periarteritis nodosa in a patient with primary biliary cirrhosis, or was a coincidental adverse event.

Bullous lesions with specific infiltrates of *mycosis fungoides* have been reported in a 67-year-old woman who took interferon-α for 2 months for mycosis fungoides (28[A]). Although the syndrome could not be definitely attributed to interferon-α, the authors noted that bullous mycosis fungoides is an extremely rare variant of this disease and withdrawal of interferon-α led to healing of the blisters without further recurrence.

Musculoskeletal A 26-year-old man with malignant melanoma had two episodes of acute severe *rhabdomyolysis* after each exposure to a chemotherapy regimen containing interferon-α and dacarbazine (29[A]). As a few cases of rhabdomyolysis have been previously reported after interferon-α alone (SEDA-19, 336; SEDA-20, 330; SEDA-22, 403), interferon-α was suggested as the most likely cause.

There have been two reports of *polymyositis* in association with interferon-α treatment for hematological malignancies (30[A], 31[A]). In both cases, clinical and/or electrophysiological recovery occurred after drug withdrawal, spontaneously or after a short course of corticosteroids. Another case suggested that interferon-α can also cause *dermatomyositis* (32[A]).

A 57-year-old woman received adjuvant high-dose interferon-α 16 months after removal of a malignant melanoma. About 6 weeks later, she developed hand swelling, fatigue, myalgia, arthralgia, and weakness. Interferon-α was withdrawn. She had multiple joint involvement, and radiological imaging showed bilateral interstitial pulmonary infiltrates. Anti-Jo antibodies were positive but other autoantibodies were negative. She also had violet eyelid discoloration with edema, tenderness in various muscle groups, and reduced strength in the shoulders. The muscle biopsy showed scattered necrotic fibers and basophilic regenerative fibers. She gradually recovered with methotrexate and corticosteroids, and the titer of anti-Jo antibodies fell dramatically.

These cases of polymyositis and dermatomyositis add further to the clinical diversity of interferon-α-associated autoimmune diseases.

Three patients developed unilateral or bilateral *avascular necrosis of the femoral head* after 3–54 months of treatment with interferon-α for chronic myelogenous leukemia (33[AR]). One required bilateral hip replacement and two significantly improved after interferon-α withdrawal. One patient received further interferon-α without exacerbation. Although there were risk factors for avascular necrosis in two of the patients (a short course of methylprednisolone and moderate alcohol consumption), the authors did not consider them to be significant. The authors identified seven other reported cases of avascular necrosis in patients with chronic myeloid leukemia, including two patients who were taking interferon-α at the time of the complication. One patient with pre-existing avascular necrosis had an acute exacerbation within 1 month of interferon-α and required hip replacement. Although any causal relation with treatment remains purely speculative, the authors argued that the known antiangiogenic effects of interferon-α could have predisposed patients to avascular necrosis.

Infection risk Possible *exacerbation of latent parasitic infection* by interferon-α has previously been reported (SEDA-22, 403). Two patients receiving interferon-α plus ribavirin for chronic hepatitis C developed symptomatic strongyloidiasis within 2–3 weeks of treatment (34[A]). Because both drugs have immunomodulatory effects, it was not determined which one was the more likely cause.

Miscellaneous Cutaneous or systemic *sarcoidosis* is sometimes associated with interferon-α, alone or in association with ribavirin. This has been exemplified in further reports (35[A], 36[A]), including one patient whose sarcoidosis resolved with prednisone and despite interferon-α continuation (37[A]).

Interferon-β

Respiratory The first case of *bronchiolitis obliterans organizing pneumonia* in a patient taking interferon-β has been very briefly reported (38[A]).

A 49-year-old man had a progressive unproductive cough and right hemithoracic pain after 3 months of interferon-β_{1a} 30 μg/week for multiple sclerosis. A CT scan showed a right basal pulmonary infiltrate and transbronchial biopsies showed features consistent with bronchiolitis obliterans organizing pneumonia. The lesions resolved fully on interferon-β_{1a} withdrawal and prednisone treatment.

Nervous system Moderate *exacerbation of multiple sclerosis* sometimes occurs in the first 3 months of interferon-β treatment. A 21-year-old man had an acute and very severe clinical relapse, with multiple disseminated demyelinating lesions and axonal injury on MRI and cerebral biopsy, after the third injection of interferon-β_{1a} (39[A]). Whether this case was due to interferon-β or resulted from spontaneous exacerbation was open to question.

Endocrine Interferon-β is sometimes associated with autoimmune *hypothyroidism*. Two patients took thyroxine replacement and continued to receive interferon-β_{1b} (40[A]). As suggested in a more comprehensive long-term follow-up study, interferon-β-induced thyroid dysfunction is often transient or has limited clinical consequences (41[C]). Of 31 patients with multiple sclerosis regularly assessed for 30–42 months for thyroid function, 13 developed thyroid disorders during treatment with interferon-β_{1b}. None withdrew because of thyroid disorders. Of the eight patients with no previous thyroid disorders, one had a persistent but isolated increase in antithyroglobulin titer, six developed transient signs of hypothyroidism or hyperthyroidism during the first year of therapy, and only one had overt hypothyroidism after 12 months of treatment and required thyroxine replacement. Of the five patients with baseline signs of Hashimoto's thyroiditis, one had a transiently positive antithyroglobulin titer, one developed transient hyperthyroidism, and the three patients who had previously had or who newly developed subclinical hypothyroidism remained stable throughout the study. Overall, thyroid disorders occurred only during the first 12 months of treatment and no additional cases were detected after the first year of therapy. In the authors' opinion, pre-existing or new thyroiditis is not a contraindication to continuing interferon-β_{1b} treatment.

Metabolic Severe *hypertriglyceridemia*, a well known adverse effect of interferon-α, has been reported and fully investigated in a 39-year-old man receiving interferon-β for chronic hepatitis C (42[A]).

Liver A case of *fulminant liver failure* has been attributed to interferon-β_{1a} (43[A]).

A 59-year-old woman with no history of liver disease and no particular risk factors started to use interferon-β_{1a} for multiple sclerosis. Anorexia and nausea occurred after 4 weeks of treatment, jaundice 1 week later, and encephalopathy and hepatorenal syndrome 2 weeks later, by when she had received a cumulative dose of 215 μg. Virological tests for cytomegalovirus and hepatitis A, B, and C were negative. Antimicrosomal antibodies were positive. Emergency liver transplantation was performed. Liver histology showed submassive hepatic necrosis.

Cases of liver failure with interferon-α have mostly occurred in patients with chronic viral hepatitis, and no cases of interferon-β-induced fulminant liver failure have previously been reported.

Urinary tract Interferon-β has previously been implicated in *glomerulopathies* in patients with chronic hepatitis C (SEDA-24, 416). Nephrotic syndrome with segmental glomerulosclerosis has been reported in a 32-year-old woman with multiple sclerosis (44[A]).

Immunologic One debatable case of an *anaphylactoid reaction* to interferon-β_{1a} has previously been reported (SEDA-23, 397). Urticaria developed after 9 months of treatment with interferon-β_{1b} in a 32-year-old woman with a previous history of penicillin allergy (45[A]). She also had an exacerbation of asthma shortly after starting treatment. A positive intradermal test to interferon-β_{1b}, but not to interferon-β_{1a} or the diluents, suggested a specific IgE allergic reaction.

INTERLEUKINS *(SED-14, 1260; SEDA-22, 406; SEDA-23, 398; SEDA-24, 416)*

Interleukin-2 (IL-2)

Denileukin diftitox, a fusion protein formed by human IL-2 binding to diphtheria toxin, has been approved for treatment of cutaneous T cell lymphoma. Its more severe adverse effects consisted of *acute hypersensitivity* reactions during or within 24 hours of infusion in 69% of patients, and a vascular leak syndrome in 27% of patients, which was severe in 6%. In contrast to acute hypersensitivity reactions, the vascular leak syndrome was typically delayed and occurred within the first 2 weeks of infusion (46[Ar]). Whether this was due to a direct action of denileukin diftitox or to tumor lysis syndrome is unknown.

Cardiovascular IL-2-induced *cardiac eosinophilic infiltration* has not previously been reported (47[A]).

After 25 days of treatment with continuous IL-2 infusion (up to 150 000 IU/kg/day) for stage IV Hodgkin's disease a 26-year-old woman had increased fatigue, tachycardia, hypotension, and hypothermia. Echocardiography showed bilateral intraventricular masses. Her maximal absolute eosinophil count was 11.4×10^9/l and the platelet count was 17×10^9/l. Despite IL-2 withdrawal, her condition deteriorated and she died. Post-mortem examination showed biventricular thrombi and prominent eosinophilic infiltration of the endomyocardium.

Of 10 subsequent patients who received prolonged infusions of IL-2 and were monitored by echocardiography, one developed asymptomatic changes in cardiac function, with features suggestive of early thrombus formation and a reduced ejection fraction during weeks 6–8. The maximal absolute eosinophil count was 5×10^9/l. These abnormalities resolved on IL-2 withdrawal.

Nervous system Neurotoxicity of IL-2 has

repeatedly been reported, but few reports have focused on the short-term occurrence of *depressive symptoms*. This has been investigated by using the Montgomery and Asberg Depression Rating Scale (MADRS) before and after 3 and 5 days of treatment in 48 patients without a previous psychiatric history and treated for renal cell carcinoma or melanoma with IL-2 alone (20 patients), IL-2 plus interferon-α_{2b} (6 patients), or interferon-α_{2b} alone (22 patients) (48[C]). On day 5, patients in the IL-2 groups had significantly higher MADRS scores, whereas there were no significant changes in the patients who received interferon-α_{2b} alone. At this time, eight of 26 patients in the IL-2 groups and only three of 22 given interferon-α_{2b} alone had severe depressive symptoms. Depressive symptoms occurred as early as the second day of IL-2 treatment and were more severe in the patients who received both cytokines. Early detection of mood changes can be useful in pinpointing patients at risk of subsequent severe neuropsychiatric complications.

Immunologic Because IL-2 stimulates T cells, it has been suggested to have favored the development of successive episodes of multifocal *fixed drug eruption* in response to chemically unrelated drugs (paracetamol, ondansetron, and tropisetron) in a 43-year-old patient (49[A]). Similarly, IL-2 was deemed to be the triggering factor in the occurrence of sarcoidosis in a 36-year-old AIDS patient stabilized for a long time by highly active antiretroviral therapy (50[A]).

Interleukin-10 (IL-10)

Hematologic The mechanisms of mild *thrombocytopenia* after multiple doses of IL-10 have been extensively explored in 12 healthy volunteers, of whom four received placebo and eight received subcutaneous IL-10 (8 μg/kg/day for 10 days) (51[c]). Compared with placebo, there was a 40% fall in platelet count during IL-10 treatment and prompt normalization after IL-10 withdrawal. There were also moderate changes in hemoglobin concentration. Bone-marrow function, platelet production, and serum thrombopoietin concentrations suggested that a reduction in bone-marrow platelet production was the primary cause.

Interleukin-12 (IL-12, edodekin-α)

Hematologic One case of complete agranulocytosis and one case of *Coombs' negative hemolytic anemia* have been attributed to twice-weekly IL-12 in 28 patients with renal cell cancer or melanoma (52[A]). The patients responded only to cyclophosphamide and/or steroids, and the causative role of IL-12 was therefore inconclusive.

Immunologic IL-12 has been involved in the pathogenesis of several autoimmune disorders, and this may explain *exacerbation of severe rheumatoid arthritis* after each course of IL-12 for cervical carcinoma in a 53-year-old woman with previously mild and stable rheumatoid disease (53[A]).

COLONY-STIMULATING FACTORS *(SED-14, 1270; SEDA-22, 407; SEDA-23, 399; SEDA-24, 417)*

Few studies have directly compared the safety of the various available colony-stimulating factors. The frequency and severity of adverse effects associated with the prophylactic use of filgrastim (a bacterial cell-derived G-CSF) or sargramostim (a yeast cell-derived GM-CSF) have been assessed in a retrospective review of the medical records of 490 cancer patients from 10 centers (54[C]). Sargramostim-treated patients had significantly more frequent non-infectious *fever*, *fatigue*, *diarrhea*, *injection site reactions*, *edema*, and *dermatological adverse effects*, whereas *skeletal pain* was more frequent with filgrastim. In addition, switching to the alternative treatment was more frequent in the sargramostim group (18% of patients) than in the filgrastim group (none of the patients). The authors tried to minimize selection bias, but the strength of the results was limited by the retrospective nature of the study.

Granulocyte colony-stimulating factor (G-CSF)

G-CSF is being increasingly used in healthy donors to mobilize granulocytes or peripheral blood stem cells, and most short-term adverse effects have been rated as mild or moderate (SEDA-24, 417). Less is known about long-term safety and possible late adverse effects. In one study, 101 healthy donors who had received filgrastim for a median of 6 days were questioned after a median of 43 (range 34–74) months to assess their current health; 70 donors also had a complete blood count (55[c]). No unusual disease was detected and the blood counts were within the reference range.

Cardiovascular Arterial thrombotic events due to growth factors are rare. *Microthrombotic necrotizing panniculitis* has recently been reported (56[A]).

A 49-year-old woman received subcutaneous filgrastim 300 μg/day into the upper thighs for neutropenia prophylaxis after treatment of relapsing Hodgkin's disease with mitoguazone, etoposide, vinorelbine, and ifosfamide. After 3 days she suddenly developed fever, painful livedo, deeply infiltrated edema on the legs and thighs, and inflamed livedoid erythema on both soles. Deep biopsy specimens showed small vessel thrombosis with subcutaneous necrosis and hemorrhage. She recovered over the next 4 weeks after filgrastim withdrawal and prednisone treatment.

Although a causal relation was difficult to ascertain in the context of malignancy and cytotoxic chemotherapy, the short time to occurrence after G-CSF favored a causative role.

Respiratory Fatal non-cardiac *pulmonary edema* has been reported in a 59-year-old man with renal amyloidosis who received G-CSF for 3 days for stem cell mobilization (57[AR]). The authors also extensively reviewed the available experimental and clinical data on the pulmonary toxicity of growth factors.

Hematologic The possibility of adverse effects after transfusion performed with G-CSF-mobilized granulocytes has been recently suggested in a 53-year-old man with aplastic anemia, who had clinically asymptomatic and reversible *hypercoagulability* after the transfusion of granulocytes obtained from G-CSF-stimulated donors (58[A]). The authors stressed the recurrence of the disorder after each of the three granulocyte transfusions that the patient received.

Carcinogenicity There is still concern about whether G-CSF favors the development of *myelodysplasia* or leukemia in patients who receive long-term treatment for severe chronic neutropenia or aplastic anemia. The results of two recent studies have offered contrasting conclusions. In the first study in severe aplastic anemia the frequencies of cytogenetic abnormalities and myelodysplasia or leukemia were similar in 87 patients treated with G-CSF in addition to immunosuppressive treatment compared with 57 patients who did not receive G-CSF (59[C]). Although the authors stated that a leukemogenic effect of G-CSF was unlikely, they mentioned that the median interval of appearance of cytogenetic abnormalities was shorter in the G-CSF group. In the other study the data from an international register of patients with severe chronic neutropenia were analysed (60[C]). Of 352 patients treated with G-CSF for congenital neutropenia and followed for a mean of 6 years (maximum 11 years), 31 developed myelodysplasia or leukemia, whereas there were no cases in 344 patients with idiopathic or cyclic neutropenia. Associated cytogenetic clonal changes consisted of partial or complete loss of chromosome 7 in 18 patients and abnormalities in chromosome 21 in nine. Isolated cytogenic abnormalities were also found in nine other patients. None of the patients had abnormal marrow cytogenetic changes before G-CSF therapy. A more complete analysis failed to identify any correlation between G-CSF dose and treatment duration in patients who developed myelodysplasia or leukemia compared with those who were not affected. Although this argues against a role of G-CSF in the conversion of congenital neutropenia to myelodysplasia or leukemia, the authors recognized that a direct leukemogenic role of G-CSF could not be completely ruled out.

MONOCLONAL ANTIBODIES

(SED-14, 1308; SEDA-22, 409; SEDA-23, 401; SEDA-24, 419)

According to a recent review, the mechanisms of adverse effects of monoclonal antibodies include sensitization due to the xenogenetic nature of the product, specific suppression of physiological functions, and secondary activation of inflammatory cells or mediators, which might be characterized by the cytokine release syndrome, as observed with muromonab-CD3 or rituximab (61[r]). Although sensitization may be frequent, its clinical relevance is still limited, with only rare cases of *hypersensitivity reactions*. Although this has been strongly debated with muromonab-CD3 (orthoclone; SED-14, 1309), the available information on the risk of infections or cancers with other monoclonal antibodies is still limited, but does not suggest an increased risk.

Basiliximab

Drug interactions Basiliximab, an interleukin-2 receptor antibody used in the prophylaxis of acute renal rejection, has been reported to inhibit *ciclosporin* metabolism transiently in children with renal transplants (62[c]). Despite the use of lower daily doses, the ciclosporin trough concentrations were significantly higher during the first 10 days after transplantation in 24 children who received basiliximab at days 0 and 4 after transplantation compared with 15 children who did not receive basiliximab. Ciclosporin dosage requirements again increased by 20% to achieve the target blood concentration at days 28–50 after transplantation. It is noteworthy that all seven acute episodes of rejection in the basiliximab group occurred during this period of time. However, these results have been debated and there were no changes in ciclosporin dosage requirements in 54 liver transplant children (63[c]).

Edrecolomab

Edrecolomab (17-1A antibody) is being developed for the adjuvant treatment of colorectal cancer. One case of severe *exacerbation of Wegener's granulomatosis* with multiorgan involvement has been reported after the first infusion (500 mg over 2 hours) in a 64-year-old man (64[A]).

Infliximab

There were severe infusion reactions, defined by any significant change in vital signs or the development of *chest pain*, *wheeze*, *dyspnea*, *vomiting*, *abdominal pain*, or *rash*, in 16 of 100 patients with refractory Crohn's disease (65[C]). Half of them occurred during the first infusion, and the rate of infusion reactions was similar in patients taking concurrent immunosuppressants or corticosteroids compared with those who were not. One patient had *anaphylactic shock*, five had significant *hypotension*, six had acute *pulmonary symptoms*, two had *pruritus*, *flushing*, or *rash*, and one had *vomiting*. The final patient, who had a previous history of chronic pancreatitis, had acute *pancreatitis* within 1 hour of treatment.

Liver The first case of *acute hepatitis* with infliximab has been described (66[A]).

A 44-year-old woman, who had used oral contraceptives for many years and had taken mesalazine, mercaptopurine, and prednisone for Crohn's disease for 7 years, developed clinical and biological signs of acute mixed hepatitis 19 days after a single dose of infliximab 5 mg/kg. There were no symptoms suggestive of hypersensitivity and liver histology showed cholestasis without inflammation or eosinophilia. Other causes, such as a recent viral infections (hepatitis A, B, C, cytomegalovirus, *Herpes simplex*) or gallstones, were ruled out. Among various autoantibodies, only antinuclear antibody titers were slightly raised. Complete normalization was observed 2 months later.

Although the patient took other potentially hepatotoxic drugs, the time-course suggested that infliximab was the cause.

Skin In three patients with severe Crohn's disease who required digestive surgery, infliximab before or immediately after surgery was discussed as a additional possible cause of postoperative *poor wound healing* with serious complications (67[A]).

Infection risk An important warning was issued in December 2000 regarding the risk of *tuberculosis and other opportunistic infections* that may occur during infliximab treatment. An analysis of 70 cases of tuberculosis reported to the FDA has recently been published (68[c]). Two-thirds of the cases were noted after three or fewer infusions and 57% of the patients had extrapulmonary disease. There were 64 cases from countries with a low incidence of tuberculosis. From these reports and the number of patients treated with infliximab, the estimated rate of tuberculosis in patients with rheumatoid arthritis treated with infliximab was four times higher than the background rate.

Muromonab-CD3 (orthoclone, OKT3)

Sensory systems *Ototoxicity* from muromonab has previously been described, but the incidence is unknown (SEDA-21, 380). Audiograms performed before and 48–72 hours after administration of muromonab showed sensorineural hearing loss of at least 15 db in five of seven renal transplant patients (69[A]). A third audiogram 2 weeks after muromonab treatment showed amelioration or complete recovery in all four of the patients who were tested.

Rituximab

Cardiovascular *Cardiac dysrhythmias* have been reported in 8% of patients treated with the anti-CD20 monoclonal antibody rituximab in patients with lymphomas (70[C]).

Sensory systems A variety of ocular adverse effects, including conjunctivitis, transient ocular edema, and visual changes occurred in 7% of patients receiving rituximab (70[C]).

Infection risk Rituximab produces prolonged depletion of B lymphocytes. This effect was suggested as a likely explanation for the occurrence of chronic *parvovirus B19 infection* complicated by pure red cell aplasia in a 45-year-old patient (71[A]).

Etanercept

Although etanercept is not an antibody, it is included here for convenience. In a study of weekly oral methotrexate in two different doses (10 or 25 mg) or a twice-weekly etanercept regimen in 632 patients, etanercept produced fewer systemic adverse effects than methotrexate, but a higher incidence of *injection site reactions* (72[C]). Despite theoretical concerns about the development of autoimmune reactions in patients taking etanercept, no evidence of clinical autoimmune disease emerged from this large trial.

Endocrine *Type 1 diabetes mellitus* occurred after 5 months treatment with etanercept for juvenile rheumatoid arthritis in a 7-year-old girl (73[A]). Antiglutamic acid decarboxylase antibodies were positive both before and during treatment, suggesting that etanercept may have prematurely triggered an underlying disease.

Skin *Injection site reactions* are very common during the first month of treatment. Histological findings in one patient showed a mild transient inflammatory response that did not suggest sensitization (74[A]).

Other types of skin reactions have been described: *urticaria-like eruptions with prurigo* in two infants with juvenile arthritis (75[A]) and purpuric lesions with histological features of *leukocytoclastic vasculitis* in a 58-year-old man (76[A]). It is not known whether the latter resulted from the deposition of specific immune complexes.

Urinary tract *Glomerulonephritis* has been discussed as a possible consequence of etanercept treatment in two patients, with biopsy-proven mesangial deposits of IgA in one (77[A]).

Interference with laboratory assays *Non-neutralizing antibodies* to etanercept have been identified in clinical trials. Although there was no correlation between these antibodies and the development of adverse effects (72[C]), their presence was suggested as a likely explanation of *false-positive rises in troponin* concentrations in an assay that used mouse antihuman troponin (78[A]).

IMMUNOSUPPRESSIVE DRUGS

Azathioprine and mercaptopurine

(SED-14, 1280; SEDA-22, 409; SEDA-23, 401; SEDA-24, 422)

Respiratory Although azathioprine-associated pulmonary toxicity mostly occurs as part of the azathioprine hypersensitivity reaction, isolated *interstitial pneumonitis* has been reported in a 13-year-old girl with autoimmune chronic active hepatitis (79[A]).

Acute *upper airway edema* has been observed after a single dose of azathioprine (80[A]).

A 57-year-old woman with a history of several drug allergies underwent renal transplantation for end-stage polycystic kidney disease and 1 hour later was given intravenous azathioprine 400 mg. She developed profound hypotension and bradycardia within 30 minutes, reversed by sympathomimetics. Shortly after extubation, she had severe breathing difficulties with loss of consciousness. Laryngoscopy showed massive swelling of the tongue and upper airways. Later, while still taking corticosteroids, she was rechallenged with azathioprine and had milder hypotension and airways edema.

Even if no clear mechanism can account for this adverse effect, positive rechallenge strongly suggested that azathioprine was the culprit.

Hematologic In 30 heart transplant patients treated with azathioprine the myelosuppressive effects of azathioprine/mercaptopurine were predicted by systematic genotypic screening of thiopurine methyltransferase deficiency (81[C]). However, myelosuppression can also be observed in patients without the thiopurine methyltransferase mutation. Of 41 patients with *leukopenia* or *thrombocytopenia* taking azathioprine/mercaptopurine for Crohn's disease, four were classified as low methylators, seven as intermediate methylators, and 30 as high methylators by genotypic analysis (82[C]). Thus, only 27% of the patients had the typical mutations associated with enzyme deficiency and a risk of myelosuppression. The delay in bone-marrow toxicity was shorter in the four homozygous patients (median 1 month) than in the others (median 3–4 months). Many other causes, including viral infections, associated drugs, or another azathioprine/mercaptopurine metabolic pathway, were suggested to account for most of the cases of late hemotoxicity. This confirmed that continuous hematological monitoring is required, even in patients with no thiopurine methyltransferase mutations.

Liver A 50-year-old woman with nodular sclerosis developed azathioprine-induced *hepatotoxicity* within the first weeks of treatment (83[A]), the usual time-course. Positive rechallenge confirmed the role of azathioprine. Delayed occurrence of hepatitis is also possible, and canalicular cholestasis with portal fibrosis and ductal proliferation has been reported after 24 years of azathioprine in a 57-year-old woman with myasthenia gravis (84[A]).

Pancreas *Pancreatitis* has been reported after a progressive increase in dose of 6-thioguanine in a 10-year-old infant (85[A]). She had had two previous episodes of pancreatitis after mercaptopurine. The chemical structure of 6-thioguanine, which results from the metabolism of azathioprine/mercaptopurine, is very similar to that of mercaptopurine. Therefore, a history of previous adverse effects with mercatopurine should be noted in patients considered for 6-thioguanine treatment.

Ciclosporin *(SED-14, 1286; SEDA-22, 411; SEDA-23, 402; SEDA-24, 424)*

Nervous system Ciclosporin neurotoxicity is frequent, and very severe or fatal outcomes have been reported in isolated patients only. Based on post-mortem findings in a 32-year-old woman who died from acute encephalopathy (86[A]) and another report of two patients investigated with transcranial Doppler ultrasound and MRI for symptoms of ciclosporin neurotoxicity (87[A]), vascular changes with vasospasm and dissection of the vascular intima strongly suggest that vasculopathy is a possible mechanism of ciclosporin-induced *encephalopathy*.

Sensory systems In two large randomized controlled trials in 977 patients, the adverse effects associated with ciclosporin ophthalmic emulsion for the treatment of dry eye disease were minimal and consisted mostly of mild *ocular burning and stinging* (88[C]). However, topical application of ciclosporin eye-drops was the suspected cause of severe visual loss with bilateral white corneal deposits in a 45-year-old patient with dry eye syndrome caused by graft-vs-host disease (89[A]). Infrared spectroscopy and X-ray analysis suggested that the deposits contained ciclosporin. A reduction in tear clearance and compromised epithelial barrier function caused by the concomitant use of oxybuprocaine may have precipitated this adverse effect.

Liver Ciclosporin has been associated with *intrahepatic cholestasis* in transplant patients, and is now being used in the treatment of inflammatory bowel disease. Since many patients with inflammatory bowel disease also rely on parenteral nutrition, ciclosporin may enhance the associated loss of liver function. In a retrospective study (90[C]), this possible association was examined in a series of 50 consecutive patients who received both parenteral nutrition and corticosteroids, with or without the addition of ciclosporin, at some stage in their management. There was no evidence that ciclosporin caused more liver dysfunction than that associated with parenteral nutrition.

Urinary tract Nephrotoxicity is a major adverse effect of ciclosporin, but there is as yet no predictor of renal dysfunction. From a prospective study in 36 heart transplant patients with stable renal function for at least 6 months after transplantation, it was suggested that high urinary retinol-binding protein concentrations may indicate *tubulointerstitial damage* and therefore detect patients who are at risk of ciclosporin nephrotoxicity (91[C]). At the start of the study, 13 patients had high urinary retinol-binding protein concentrations and 23 had normal concentrations. After 5 years of follow-up, five of the 13 patients developed end-stage renal insufficiency requiring dialysis, whereas none of the 23 other patients had terminal renal insufficiency. Although these data await confirmation, the authors suggested that ciclosporin dosage reduction should be considered in patients with high urinary retinol-binding protein concentrations, in order to limit renal damage.

Skin Mild *flushing* often occurs during ciclosporin treatment, but more severe extensive erythema is infrequent. Recurrent episodes of diffuse flushing of the arms, the face, and the trunk reportedly occurred about 2 hours after each dose of ciclosporin in a 24-year-old man who had received a renal transplant 6 years before (92[A]). These episodes were noted from the beginning of treatment, worsened after he changed to Neoral®, the microemulsion form of ciclosporin, and completely resolved after ciclosporin was replaced by tacrolimus.

Ciclosporin sometimes causes *chronic inflammatory dermatitis*, and there have been two recent reports of four male transplant recipients who developed clinical and histopathological features of keloid acne of the posterior scalp or neck (93[A], 94[A]). *Staphylococcus aureus* infection was identified in three patients. Ciclosporin-induced hypertrichosis was suggested as a possible cause, with local bacterial infection and immunosuppression as trigger factors. Multiple large epidermoid cysts have also been described in a 23-year-old man (95[A]).

Second-generation effects There are few data on the long-term consequences of prolonged in utero exposure to ciclosporin. Renal function in 14 children born to women with transplants treated throughout pregnancy with a ciclosporin-based regimen has been extensively investigated at a mean of 2.6 years after delivery (96[C]). No renal function abnormalities were found. In particular, glomerular filtration rate was within the reference range.

Drug overdose It is generally agreed that ciclosporin overdose in adults has only limited consequences, with moderate symptoms and a low risk of acute renal insufficiency. However, two reports, including one fatal case, have shown that accidental intoxication sometimes produces severe complications (97[A], 98[A]).

A 29-year-old man received a double lung transplantation for end-stage cystic fibrosis. After uneventful surgery, he was accidentally given 10 times the intended dose of ciclosporin (30 instead of 3 mg/kg) and 18 hours later became anuric. His blood ciclosporin concentration was 4100 ng/ml. Hemodialysis was required for 6 weeks. A renal biopsy 7 weeks later showed typical features of acute tubular necrosis and lesions that resembled chronic nephrotoxicity. Renal function was still abnormal when he died from another cause 14 weeks after the accidental overdose.

A 51-year-old man underwent double lung transplantation for pulmonary fibrosis, accidentally received an infusion of ciclosporin 30 mg/hour instead of 3 mg/hour, and 3 hours later had bilateral reactive mydriasis and absence of tendon reflexes. A CT brain scan showed diffuse cerebral edema, and massive intracranial hypertension rapidly developed. He died 5 hours later from brainstem compression, and pathological examination showed diffuse cerebral edema with neuronal necrosis.

The first case suggested that acute renal dysfunction secondary to acute overdose can lead to renal sequelae. In the second patient, an isolated neurotoxic effect of ciclosporin was suggested because no predisposing factor except overdose was identified.

Drug interactions Many drugs are known to interact with ciclosporin (SED-14, 1294), and there is potential for numerous other drug interactions. From an analysis of changes in ciclosporin clearance and systemic availability obtained from the medical records of 100 transplant patients, 22 drugs were confirmed to affect ciclosporin pharmacokinetics, and 12 previously unknown or unconfirmed drug interactions were detected (99[C]). The following drugs were suggested to reduce the clearance of ciclosporin: *aciclovir*, *alendronic acid*, *atorvastatin*, *fluvastatin*, *pravastatin*, *simvastatin*, *losartan*, *valsartan*, *sertraline*. The following drugs were suggested to alter its systemic availability: *digoxin* and *quinidine* (increase), *oxycodone* (decrease). Obviously, more data are required to confirm these findings.

Other reports on ciclosporin drug interactions have mostly focused on drugs that reduce ciclosporin trough concentrations either by reduced absorption or enhanced metabolism.

At least three additional case reports have clearly confirmed that *Hypericum perforatum* (St John's wort) is dangerous in transplant patients, because it produced a rapid and dramatic reduction in blood ciclosporin concentration, and resulted in acute organ rejection in two patients (100[A]–102[A]). Induction of CYP3A4 and/or P-glycoprotein was the most likely mechanism.

Orlistat, which inhibits intestinal lipases and reduces fat absorption, can cause reduced absorption of ciclosporin, which is highly lipophilic (103[A], 104[A]).

In 120 heart transplant patients, *sulfinpyrazone* (200 mg/day) for ciclosporin-associated hyperuricemia was associated with lowered blood ciclosporin concentrations despite an increase in the daily dose (105[C]). The authors cited evidence (106[E]) that sulfinpyrazone induces ciclosporin metabolism.

Cyclophosphamide *(SED-14, 1283; SEDA-22, 410; SEDA-23, 405; SEDA-24, 427)*

Cyclophosphamide has been investigated in a wide range of diseases, but recent experiences in aplastic anemia and idiopathic pulmonary fibrosis have been disappointing. In a low dose (2 mg/kg/day), it produced minimal efficacy in 19 patients with idiopathic pulmonary fibrosis who had failed to respond to a corticosteroid or who had had adverse effects (107[C]). Moreover, 13 patients had cyclophosphamide-induced adverse effects, which required drug withdrawal in nine. The most frequent were severe *gastrointestinal effects*, *leukopenia*, and *skin rashes*. In another study, high-dose cyclophosphamide plus ciclosporin (50 mg/kg/day for 4 days) was compared with antithymocyte globulin plus ciclosporin in patients with severe aplastic anemia, but the trial was prematurely stopped after only 31 patients had been enrolled because of three early deaths in patients taking cyclophosphamide (108[C]). Subsequent analysis showed excess morbidity and mortality in patients taking cyclophosphamide, with six proven or suspected cases of systemic fungal infection (including the three deaths) compared with no cases in the other group, but no significant difference in the hematological response rates between the groups. In addition, the durations of hospital stay, neutropenia, and antibacterial treatment were longer with cyclophosphamide. Based on these results, the authors concluded that cyclophosphamide should not be used in aplastic anemia.

In 155 patients with Wegener's granulomatosis, of whom 142 took daily oral cyclophosphamide, the most frequent long-term cyclophosphamide-related adverse effects were *cystitis* despite mesna therapy (12%) and *myelodysplasia* (8%) (109[C]). Patients who took a cumulative dose of cyclophosphamide over 100 g had a 2-fold greater risk of developing cystitis and/or myelodysplasia than patients who took under 100 g. The authors emphasized that cyclophosphamide therapy should be as short as possible, with mesna and close surveillance in order to reduce treatment-associated morbidity.

Liver Late *hepatotoxicity* has been reported with low-dose cyclophosphamide (110[A]).

A 67-year-old man with Sjögren's syndrome took cyclophosphamide for 2 years, a cumulative dose of 40.5 g. He then developed severe progressive jaundice due to acute hepatocellular injury. Gallstones and acute viral hepatitis were excluded, and only antismooth muscle antibodies were weakly positive. Liver histology showed marked ballooning of the hepatocytes and cell loss, cytoplasmic and canalicular cholestasis, and infiltration of the portal tract with inflammatory cells. Complete resolution occurred 6 weeks after cyclophosphamide withdrawal.

The authors emphasized this was the first case suggesting a cumulative hepatotoxic effect of low-dose cyclophosphamide. Previous rare cases of low-dose cyclophosphamide-induced acute hepatitis have usually occurred within the first 2 months.

Carcinogenicity It has been suggested that cyclophosphamide can contribute to the risk of *cervical dysplasia*. In a retrospective study of 110 patients with systemic lupus erythematosus, cervical dysplasia was significantly more frequent in patients who had received intravenous cyclophosphamide (10 of 61) than in a control group who did not receive cyclophosphamide (two of 49) (111[C]). In addition, cervical pathology worsened during cyclophosphamide therapy in all four patients with pre-existing cervical dysplasia, and one patient developed in situ cervical carcinoma.

A 54-year-old man with polyarteritis nodosa developed *hepatic angiosarcoma* after taking cyclophosphamide for 13 years (112[A]). Although this may have been coincidental, the authors found two other published reports of this very rare tumor in patients taking long-term cyclophosphamide.

Methotrexate *(SED-14, 1297; SEDA-22, 416; SEDA-23, 406; SEDA-24, 427)*

Folic acid supplementation is now commonly given to reduce the adverse effects of methotrexate, in particular *mucosal and gastrointestinal toxic effects* (SED-14, 1297; SEDA-23, 406), but less is known about how long this should be continued in patients taking long-term treatment. This issue has been examined in 75 patients with rheumatoid arthritis taking methotrexate (up to 20 mg/week) and folic acid (5 mg/day) (113[C]). After folic acid withdrawal, the patients were randomized to restart folic acid (n = 38) or to take placebo (n = 37) double-blind, and were regularly assessed for 1 year. There were more withdrawals with placebo (46%) than with folic acid (21%), and more nausea. There were no obvious differences in efficacy. This suggests that folic acid supplementation is still helpful in the long term.

Cardiovascular It has been suggested that methotrexate increases mortality in patients with rheumatoid arthritis with cardiovascular co-morbidity (114[C]). This assumption was based on a retrospective analysis of 632 patients with rheumatoid arthritis, of whom 73 died. The simultaneous presence of methotrexate and evidence of cardiovascular disease was an independent predictor of mortality. There was no such association with other disease-modifying antirheumatic drugs. The authors suggested that this effect may result from a methotrexate-induced increase in serum homocysteine, encouraging atherosclerosis.

Hematologic Impaired renal function is an important risk factor for hematological toxicity due to methotrexate. A report of severe complications, mostly *bone-marrow suppression* and related complications, in three patients on regular hemodialysis for end-stage renal disease, has confirmed that methotrexate should not be used in this setting (115[A]).

Skin In the context of a case of severe reactivation of recent sunburn after a single injection of methotrexate for ectopic pregnancy in a 40-year-old woman, the authors reviewed the literature on methotrexate *photosensitivity* (116[AR]). Photodermatitis reactivation is the only well-documented type of photosensitivity associated with methotrexate. It can occur if methotrexate is given at 2–5 days after excessive exposure to ultraviolet or X-radiation.

A previously unreported skin reaction mimicking *Stevens–Johnson syndrome* has been reported (117[A]).

A 61-year-old woman inadvertently took a high dose of methotrexate (10 mg/day) for psoriasis, and developed mucosal ulcers after 3 months. One month later, methotrexate (20 mg/week) was restarted, but she developed painful oral ulceration and burning skin lesions 3 days later. She had an erythema multiform-like rash and several buccal ulcers. There was a moderate pancytopenia. Histological examination of the skin showed features consistent with an acute graft-vs-host reaction. All medications except aspirin were withdrawn, and she recovered fully after treatment with calcium folinate and prednisolone.

The authors speculated that concomitant aspirin may have contributed to this severe reaction.

Musculoskeletal There has been a controversy about whether long-term low-dose methotrexate caused *reduced bone mass* in patients with rheumatoid arthritis (118[R]). A new study has provided evidence that it is disease activity rather than methotrexate that accounts for changes in bone mass (119[C]). This 2-year longitudinal study involved 22 patients taking methotrexate and 18 patients taking other disease-modifying antirheumatic drugs; it was strictly controlled for the use of corticosteroids. There were significant and equal reductions in trabecular bone mineral density in both groups. Bone loss was most marked in patients with active disease.

Immunologic *Vasculitis* has been infrequently reported in patients taking low-dose methotrexate (SEDA-21, 388; SEDA-22, 417). Although most cases have been observed in patients with rheumatoid arthritis, suggesting that the underlying disease plays a part, vasculitis has also been described in a patient with ankylosing spondylitis (120[A]). Methotrexate was also reported to have exacerbated pre-existing urticarial vasculitis in a 32-year-old woman; the lesions recurred after rechallenge (121[A]).

Mycophenolate mofetil

(SED-14, 1303; SEDA-22, 418; SEDA-23, 406; SEDA-24, 429)

Mycophenolate mofetil has been used not only to prevent allograft rejection, but also to replace ciclosporin in patients with ciclosporin-associated adverse effects. When mycophenolate replaced ciclosporin in 17 renal transplant patients with ciclosporin nephropathy serum creatinine concentrations fell by a mean of 26% (122[C]). There were no cases of acute allograft rejection. Adverse effects of mycophenolate were not mentioned.

Similar beneficial effects on blood pressure, lipid profile, and glomerular hemodynamics by switching from ciclosporin to mycophenolate were also found in open an study in 17 renal transplant patients with stable renal function. who took ciclosporin and prednisone in two steps (123[C]). In step I mycophenolate was added and the dose of ciclosporin was progressively reduced to produce one-third of the original trough concentration; this took about 20 weeks. In step II ciclosporin was gradually withdrawn over 6 weeks. During step I, two patients dropped out, one with severe *diarrhea* which reversed after mycophenolate withdrawal and one with biopsy-proven *acute rejection*, with recovery after mycophenolate withdrawal and an increase in the dose of ciclosporin. During step II there was no acute rejection. At 1 year after the end of the study, two patients had stopped taking mycophenolate, one because of *recurrent upper airway infections* (probably not related to mycophenolate) and one because of *Kaposi's sarcoma of the leg*. In the last case a possible role of mycophenolate could not be ruled out (SEDA-24, 429).

Hematologic Although leukopenia is common, *abnormalities of neutrophil morphology* have not previously been reported with mycophenolate. In two transplant patients, changes in circulating neutrophils (nuclear hypolobulation and abnormal clumping of nuclear chromatin) were identified after 4–5 months of treatment with mycophenolate (124[A]). A bone-marrow aspirate in one patient showed hypocellularity, abnormal clumping of chromatin beyond the promyelocyte stage, and almost no segmented neutrophils. These morphological abnormalities preceded the appearance of peripheral neutropenia in both patients and normalized after mycophenolate withdrawal. The authors suggested that neutrophil dysplasia had resulted from inhibition of guanosine nucleoside synthesis.

Liver In two renal transplant patients serum *bilirubin concentrations increased* to 46 and 63 μmol/l within 3–7 days of mycophenolate treatment, and further increased to 98 μmol/l in one patient after the dose was increased (125[A]). The bilirubin concentration returned to normal or pretreatment values after withdrawal or dosage reduction. Although both patients also received ciclosporin, which has been associated with hyperbilirubinemia, the temporal relation and a possible dose-dependent effect favored a causative role of mycophenolate.

Gastrointestinal *Ischemic colitis* has been attributed to mycophenolate (126[A]).

A 49-year-old woman taking ciclosporin, prednisolone, and mycophenolate developed acute refractory rejection 4 days after renal transplantation. After an unsuccessful steroid pulse, her immunosuppressive regimen was successively changed to OKT3 and tacrolimus with mycophenolate maintenance. Twelve days after transplantation she had abdominal pain and watery/bloody diarrhea. Colonoscopy showed multiple ulcers with mucosal injection and colon edema. A biopsy suggested ischemic colitis and cytomegalovirus infection was ruled out. Her symptoms persisted until mycophenolate was withdrawn and further colonoscopy showed complete resolution.

Skin and nails *Onycholysis with blisters and loose toenails* has been observed in a 45-year-old man who took tacrolimus, prednisone, and mycophenolate for 3 weeks after renal transplantation (127[A]). The lesions improved after withdrawal and recurred after two subsequent re-exposures.

Infection risk *Staphylococcal septicemia* complicated by endocarditis has been reported in a 50-year-old woman after 5 months of treatment with mycophenolate for atopic dermatitis (128[A]). As the skin of most patients with atopic dermatitis may be colonized with

Staphylococcus aureus, the authors suggested caution in using mycophenolate, which can also cause leukopenia. This patient had previously taken ciclosporin and azathioprine, which were ineffective, but without apparent infectious complications. A specific role of mycophenolate is therefore debatable and the occurrence of bacterial septicemia may have been purely coincidental.

The role of mycophenolate in the rate and severity of *cytomegalovirus infection* in transplant patients has been debated (SEDA-23, 407) and is difficult to evaluate in otherwise immunosuppressed patients. Severe cytomegalovirus pancolitis has been reported in a 59-year-old man taking only mycophenolate and prednisone for Wegener's granulomatosis (129[A]). In a retrospective study of 84 cytomegalovirus seronegative renal transplant patients who received a kidney from a cytomegalovirus seropositive donor without cytomegalovirus prophylaxis, the incidence of primary cytomegalovirus infection was similar in the 24 patients who took mycophenolate plus ciclosporin and prednisone, compared with the 60 patients who took ciclosporin and prednisone alone (130[C]). However, the incidence of cytomegalovirus disease was nearly twice as high in the mycophenolate group (67% vs 30%), but with no difference in the severity of the disease. The authors speculated that the more frequent incidence of symptomatic cytomegalovirus disease might have been due to some specific effects of mycophenolate on the primary immune response to cytomegalovirus.

Body temperature Isolated and intermittent drug fever with a spiking pattern has been attributed to mycophenolate in a 41-year-old man with a renal transplant (131[A]). The relation to treatment was confirmed by the exclusion of numerous infectious causes, the persistence of fever despite ciclosporin withdrawal, the subsidence of fever after mycophenolate withdrawal, and the absence of further episodes of fever during follow-up.

Sirolimus (rapamycin)

(SED-14, 1304; SEDA-24, 430)

Respiratory Since sirolimus became available, several cases of *interstitial pneumonitis* have been reported (SEDA-24, 432); the FDA is now aware of at least 34 cases (132[r]). Although the reports were insufficient to conclude that sirolimus was responsible in most cases, eight patients recovered after sirolimus withdrawal.

Bronchiolitis obliterans organizing pneumonia has been attributed to sirolimus in two renal transplant patients (133[A]). Both improved rapidly after sirolimus withdrawal or dosage reduction.

Hematologic In 119 patients taking sirolimus, *thrombocytopenia* (defined as a platelet count below 150×10^9/l) and *leukopenia* (white blood cell count below 5.0×10^9/l) occurred in 78% and 63% respectively (134[C]). The incidence, but not the severity, of these effects correlated with sirolimus whole-blood trough concentrations. Most cases occurred within the first 4 weeks of treatment and the severity was usually limited. There was spontaneous resolution in 89% of the patients and sirolimus dosage reduction or temporary withdrawal was necessary in only 7% and 4% of the patients respectively. None of the patients required permanent withdrawal.

Tacrolimus *(SED-14, 1304; SEDA-24, 431)*

The clinical pharmacology, clinical use, and adverse effects profile of tacrolimus in organ transplantation have been extensively reviewed (135[R]).

Cardiovascular Cardiac symptoms manifesting as *myocardial ischemia* are uncommon, but may occur through tacrolimus toxicity (136[A]).

A 20-year-old woman with chest pain, dyspnea, and protracted electrocardiographic ST depression had very high blood tacrolimus concentrations (45 ng/ml). Subsequent coronary angiography ruled out any significant organic lesions, but showed vasospastic coronary arteries. She had no other cardiac symptoms when tacrolimus was restarted with careful surveillance of serum concentrations.

Nervous system Tacrolimus-induced *neurotoxicity* has been well described, and several recent reports have shown that complete resolution is not always obtained after tacrolimus withdrawal or dosage reduction (137[A]).

A 48-year-old man developed acute loss of speech and swallowing apraxia shortly after liver transplantation. Tacrolimus serum concentrations were very high. Although there was progressive improvement after tacrolimus withdrawal, residual speech deficits were still present 3 weeks later. A PET scan showed a marked reduction in metabolic rate in the temporal lobes and the adjacent parieto-occipital region bilaterally.

Other cases of severe neurotoxicity have been seen during tacrolimus treatment for graft-vs-host disease after allogeneic bone-marrow transplantation. A 16-year-old girl had hypertension and generalized convulsions, which recurred after tacrolimus readministration; she subsequently died from cerebral hemorrhage and respiratory failure (138[AR]). Based on this report and a review of previously published cases, concomitant hypertension and the use of high-dose methylprednisolone were discussed as precipitating factors of tacrolimus neurotoxicity. In two other patients aged 4 and 15 years who had prolonged leukoencephalopathy, the underlying chronic graft-vs-host disease was thought to be a risk factor (139[A]).

Sensory systems *Optic neuropathy*, not previously described, has been reported in a 58-year-old liver transplant patient who had taken tacrolimus for 2 months (140[A]). Further deterioration of vision occurred despite withdrawal.

Endocrine The incidence, mechanism, and risk factors of tacrolimus-associated *diabetes mellitus* are still debated. In 58 patients investigated 1–3 years after liver transplantation there was a significantly higher incidence of diabetes mellitus with tacrolimus ($n = 32$) compared with ciclosporin ($n = 26$) (141[C]). Newly diagnosed diabetes was found in nine of 28 tacrolimus-treated patients, of whom six required insulin, and in none of 25 ciclosporin-treated patients. Five patients taking tacrolimus also had islet cell-specific autoantibodies that correlated significantly with HLA risk haplotypes.

A 32-year-old woman with previous autoimmune disorders and a susceptible HLA haplotype developed diabetes with newly positive glutamic acid decarboxylase antibody after taking tacrolimus for 5 months (142[A]).

Together, these reports suggest that tacrolimus did not suppress the production of autoantibodies in patients genetically prone to develop autoimmune diabetes, with induction of an autoimmune phenomenon. This also suggests that tacrolimus treatment should be undertaken cautiously in predisposed patients.

Pancreas Acute *pancreatitis* has rarely been reported in clinical trials, but no detailed cases were available before the following report (143[A]).

A 28-year-old woman was switched from ciclosporin to tacrolimus for prophylaxis of graft-vs-host disease after allogeneic stem cell transplantation for chronic myelogenous leukemia. She also took methylprednisolone and inhaled pentamidine. After 2 weeks she developed acute abdominal pain, tachypnea, hypoxia, and oliguria. Amylase and lipase peaked at about four and five times the upper limits of the reference ranges, and urinary analysis was consistent with acute tubular necrosis. An abdominal CT scan showed an enlarged edematous pancreas with a peripancreatic inflammatory exudate. There was no biliary obstruction or dyslipidemia. Shortly after tacrolimus withdrawal, she became anuric and had an episode of acute respiratory distress, but then improved over the next days.

Although treatment with methylprednisolone, pentamidine, and total parenteral nutrition could have contributed in this patient, they were either continued or readministered without ill effect.

Skin The long-term safety of topical tacrolimus ointment 0.1% for 6–12 months has been assessed in 316 patients with atopic dermatitis (144[C]). The most common adverse effects clearly attributed to tacrolimus were a *local burning sensation* (47%), *pruritus* (24%), and *erythema* (12%); the incidences fell with time. The observed incidence of infections did not exceed the expected incidence in patients with atopic dermatitis, and there were no effects on circulating cell-mediated immunity.

Immunologic A *diffuse, follicular, erythematous eruption* has been reported in a 45-year-old patient with a previous history of allergies to multiple medications, including clarithromycin (145[A]). It resolved after tacrolimus withdrawal. The authors speculated on possible cross-sensitivity between tacrolimus and clarithromycin, which are both macrolides, but confirmatory skin testing was not performed. In addition, the patient had taken many other drugs that might have been responsible.

Drug interactions Significant interactions between tacrolimus and *protease inhibitors*, substrates of CYP3A4, are expected. An acute drug interaction with nelfinavir has been described in a 49-year-old liver transplant man with HIV and hepatitis C infections (146[A]). The patient had three consecutive episodes of increased blood tacrolimus concentrations during nelfinavir administration. Both drugs were finally continued, but the dose of tacrolimus was only one-seventieth of the usual dose.

An increase in tacrolimus trough blood concentrations has been attributed to concomitant *theophylline* therapy in a 33-year-old man with a renal transplant (147[A]). A subsequent pharmacokinetic study showed that theophylline increased the AUC of oral tacrolimus 6-fold.

Carcinogenicity It has generally been considered that the incidence and pathological features of tacrolimus-induced cancers after transplantation are similar to those observed with other immunosuppressive agents, in particular ciclosporin (148[R]). However, in a recent retrospective study in 392 children, who survived for more than 6 months after liver transplantation and were followed for a mean of 4.3 years, there was a 5-fold higher rate of *lymphoproliferative disease* after transplantation in children who took tacrolimus (n = 141) than in those who took ciclosporin (n = 251) (149[C]). As a result, the incidence density rate of lymphoproliferative disease was 4.8 per 100 person-years in tacrolimus-treated patients, with no difference among age groups. In addition, the mean time to lymphoproliferative disease (12.6 months) was 5-fold shorter with tacrolimus than with ciclosporin. Most of the patients with lymphoproliferative disease had a primary Epstein–Barr virus infection after transplantation. The authors suggested that the 10-fold higher in vivo immunosuppressive effect of tacrolimus might have accounted for these findings.

IMMUNOENHANCING DRUGS

(SED-14, 1311; SEDA-22, 421; SEDA-23, 410; SEDA-24, 433)

Levamisole

See Chapter 31.

REFERENCES

1. Cotler SJ, Wartelle CF, Larson AM, Gretch DR, Jensen DM, Carithers RL Jr. Pretreatment symptoms and dosing regimen predict side-effects of interferon therapy for hepatitis C. J Viral Hepat 2000; 7: 211–17.
2. Heathcote EJ, Shiffman ML, Cooksley GE, Dusheiko GM, Lee SS, Balart L, Reindollar R, Wright TL, Lin A, Hoffman J, De Pampjilis J. Peginterferon alfa-2a in patients with chronic hepatitis C and cirrhosis. New Engl J Med 2000; 343: 1673–80.
3. Zeuzem S, Feinman SV, Rasenack J, Heathcote EJ, Lai MY, Gane E, O'Grady J, Reichen J, Diago M, Lin A, Hoffman J, Brunda MJ. Peginterferon alfa-2a in patients with chronic hepatitis C. New Engl J Med 2000; 343: 1666–72.
4. Takeda A, Ikegame K, Kimura Y, Ogawa H, Kanazawa S, Nakamura H. Pleural effusion during interferon treatment for chronic hepatitis C. Hepato-Gastroenterology 2000; 47: 1431–5.
5. Anthoney DA, Bone I, Evans TRJ. Inflammatory demyelinating polyneuropathy: a complication of immunotherapy in malignant melanoma. Ann Oncol 2000; 11: 1197–200.
6. Meriggioli MN, Rowin J. Chronic inflammatory demyelinating polyneuropathy after treatment with interferon-alpha. Muscle Nerve 2000; 23: 433–5.
7. Ogundipe O, Smith M. Bell's palsy during interferon therapy for chronic hepatitis C infection in patients with haemorrhagic disorders. Haemophilia 2000; 6: 110–12.
8. Kraus I, Vitezic D. Anosmia induced with alpha interferon in a patient with chronic hepatitis C. Int J Clin Pharmacol Ther 2000; 38: 360–1.
9. Hosoda S, Takimura H, Shibayama M, Kanamura H, Ikeda K, Kumada H. Psychiatric symptoms related to interferon therapy for chronic hepatitis C: clinical features and prognosis. Psychiatry Clin Neurosci 2000; 54: 565–72.
10. Schäfer M, Boetsch T, Laakmann G. Psychosis in a methadone-substituted patient during interferon-alpha treatment of hepatitis C. Addiction 2000; 95: 1101–4.
11. Greenberg DB, Jonasch E, Gadd MA, Ryan BF, Everett JR, Sober AJ, Mihm MA, Tanabe KK, Ott M, Haluska FG. Adjuvant therapy of melanoma with interferon-alpha-2b is associated with mania and bipolar syndromes. Gabapentin may serve as a mood stabilizer. Cancer 2000; 89: 356–62.
12. Hensley ML, Peterson B, Silver RT, Larson RA, Schiffer CA, Szatrowski TP. Risk factors for severe neuropsychiatric toxicity in patients receiving interferon alfa-2b and low-dose cytarabine for chronic myelogenous leukemia: analysis of cancer

and leukemia group B 9013. J Clin Oncol 2000; 18: 1301–8.
13. Scalori A, Apale P, Panizutti F, Mascoli N, Pioltelli P, Pozzi M, Redaelli A, Roffi L, Mancia G. Depression during interferon therapy for chronic viral hepatitis: early identification of patients at risk by means of a computerized test. Eur J Gastroenterol Hepatol 2000; 12: 505–9.
14. Musselman DL, Lawson DH, Gumnick JF, Manatunga AK, Penna S, Goodkin RS, Greiner K, Nemeroff CB, Miller AH. Paroxetine for the prevention of depression induced by high-dose interferon alfa. New Engl J Med 2001; 344: 961–6.
15. McAllister-Williams RH, Young AAH, Menkes DB. Antidepressant response reversed by interferon. Br J Psychiatty 2000; 176: 93.
16. Hayakawa M, Gando S, Morimoto Y, Kemmotsu O. Development of severe diabetic ketoacidosis with shock after changing interferon-beta into interferon-alpha for chronic hepatitis C. Intensive Care Med 2000; 26: 1008.
17. Dormann H, Krebs S, Muth-Selbach U, Brune K, Schuppan D, Hahn EG, Schneider T. Rapid onset of hematotoxic effects after interferon alpha in hepatitis C. J Hepatol 2000; 32: 1041–2.
18. Hirri HM, Green PJ. Pure red cell aplasia in a patient with chronic granulocytic leukaemia treated with interferon-alpha. Clin Lab Haematol 2000; 22: 53–4.
19. Tomita N, Motomura S, Ishigatsubo Y. Interferon-alpha induced red cell aplasia following chronic myelogenous leukemia. Anti-Cancer Drugs 2001; 12: 7–8.
20. English KE, Brien WF, Howson-Jan K, Kovacs MJ. Acquired factor VII inhibitor in a patient with chronic myelogenous leukemia receiving interferon-alpha therapy. Ann Pharmacother 2000; 34: 737–9.
21. Cammarota G, Cuoco L, Cianci R, Pandolfi F, Gasbarrini G. Onset of coeliac disease during treatment with interferon for chronic hepatitis C. Lancet 2000; 356: 1494–5.
22. Bourlière M, Oulès V, Perrier H, Mengotti C. Onset of coeliac disease and interferon treatment. Lancet 2001; 357: 803–4.
23. Kakumitsu S, Shijo H, Akiyoshi N, Seo M, Okada M. Eosinophilic enteritis observed during alpha-interferon therapy for chronic hepatitis C. J Gastroenterol 2000; 35: 548–51.
24. Eland IA, Rasch MC, Sturkenboom MJCM, Bekkering FC, Brouwer JT, Delwaide J, Belaiche J, Houbiers G, Stricker BHC. Acute pancreatitis attributed to the use of interferon alfa-2b. Gastroenterology 2000; 119: 230–3.
25. Sparsa A, Loustaud-Ratti V, Liozon E, Denes E, Soria P, Bouyssou-Gauthier ML, Le Brun V, Boulinguez S, Bédane C, Scribe-Outtas M, Outtas O, Labrousse F, Bonnetblanc JM, Bordessoule D, Vidal E. Réactions cutanées ou nécrose à l'interféron alpha: peut-on reprendre l'interféron? A propos de six cas. Rev Med Interne 2000; 21: 756–63.
26. Heinzerling L, Dummer R, Wildberger H, Burg G. Cutaneous ulceration after injection of polyethylene-glycol-modified interferon alpha associated with visual disturbances in a melanoma patient. Dermatology 2000; 201: 154–7.
27. Dohmen K, Miyamoto Y, Irie K, Takeshita T, Ishibashi H. Manifestation of cutaneous polyarteritis nodosa during interferon therapy for chronic hepatitis C associated with primary biliary cirrhosis. J Gastroenterol 2000; 35: 789–93.
28. Pföhler C, Ugurel S, Seiter S, Wagner A, Tilgen W, Reinhold U. Interferon-alpha-associated development of bullous lesions in mycosis fungoides. Dermatology 2000; 200: 51–3.
29. Hauschild A, Möller M, Lischner S, Christophers E. Repeatable acute rhabdomyolysis with multiple organ dysfunction because of interferon alpha and dacarbazine treatment in metastatic melanoma. Br J Dermatol 2001; 144: 215–16.
30. Hengstman GJD, Vogels OJM, ter Laak HJ, de Witte T, van Engelen BGM. Myositis during long-term interferon-alpha treatment. Neurology 2000; 54: 2186–7.
31. Schleinitz N, Veit V, Labarelle A, Figarella-Branger D, Harlé JR. La polymyosite: une complication rare du traitement par interféron-alpha. Rev Med Interne 2000; 21: 113–14.
32. Dietrich LL, Bridges AJ, Albertini MR. Dermatomyositis after interferon alpha treatment. Med Oncol 2000; 17: 64–9.
33. Kozuch P, Talpaz M, Faderl S, O'Brien S, Freireich EJ, Kantarjian H. Avascular necrosis of the femoral head in chronic myeloid leukemia patients treated with interferon-alpha. A synergistic correlation? Cancer 2000; 89: 1482–9.
34. Parana R, Portugal M, Vitvitski L, Cotrim H, Lyra L, Trepo C. Severe strongyloidiasis during interferon plus ribavirin therapy for chronic HCV infection. Eur J Gastroenterol Hepatol 2000; 12: 245–6.
35. Savoye G, Goria O, Herve S, Riachi G, Noblesse I, Bastien L, Courville P, Lerebours E. Probable sarcoïdose cutaneé après bi-thérapie associant ribavirine et interferon-alpha pour une hépatite chronique virale C. Gastroenterol Clin Biol 2000; 24: 679–80.
36. Vanders Els NJ, Gerdes H. Sarcoidosis and IFN-alpha treatment. Chest 2000; 117: 294.
37. Fiorani C, Sacchi S, Bonacorsi G, Cosenza M. Systemic sarcoidosis associated with interferon-alpha treatment for chronic myelogenous leukemia. Haematologica 2000; 85: 1006–7.
38. Ferriby D, Stojkovic T. Clinical picture: bronchiolitis obliterans with organising pneumonia during interferon beta-1a treatment. Lancet 2001; 357: 751.
39. Von Raison F, Abboud H, Saint Val C, Brugières P, Césaro P. Acute demyelinating disease after interferon beta-1a treatment for multiple sclerosis. Neurology 2000; 55: 1416–17.
40. McDonald ND, Pender MP. Autoimmune hypothyroidism associated with interferon beta-1b treatment in two patients. Aust NZ J Med 2000; 30:278–9.

41. Monzani F, Caraccio N, Casolaro A, Lombardo F, Moscato G, Murri L, Ferrannini E, Meucci G. Long-term interferon beta-1b therapy for MS. Is routine thyroid assessment always useful? Neurology 2000; 55: 549–52.
42. Homma Y, Kawazoe K, Ito T, Ide H, Takahashi H, Ueno F, Matsuzaki S. Chronic hepatitis C beta-interferon-induced severe hypertriglyceridaemia with apolipoprotein E phenotype E3/2. Int J Clin Pract 2000; 54: 212–16.
43. Yoshida EM, Rasmussen Sl, Steinbrecher UP, Erb SR, Scudamore CH, Chung SW, Oger JJ, Hashimoto SA. Fulminant liver failure during interferon beta treatment of multiple sclerosis. Neurology 2001; 56: 1416.
44. Gotsman I, Elhallel-Darnitski M, Friedlander Z, Haviv YS. Beta interferon-induced nephrotic syndrome in a patient with multiple sclerosis. Clin Nephrol 2000; 54: 425–6.
45. Brown DL, Login IS, Borish L, Powers PL. An urticarial Ig-E-mediated reaction to interferon beta-1b. Neurology 2001; 56: 1416–17.
46. Railan D, Fivenson DP, Wittenberg G. Capillary leak syndrome in a patient treated with interleukin 2 fusion toxin for cutaneous T-cell lymphoma. J Am Acad Dermatol 2000; 43: 323–4.
47. Junghans RP, Manning W, Safar M, Quist W. Biventricular cardiac thrombosis during interleukin–2 infusion. New Engl J Med 2001; 344: 859–60.
48. Capuron L, Ravaud A, Dantzer R. Early depressive symptoms in cancer patients receiving interleukin 2 and/or interferon alfa-2b therapy. J Clin Oncol 2000; 18: 2143–51.
49. Bernand S, Scheidegger EP, Dummer R, Burg G. Multifocal fixed drug eruption to paracetamol, tropisetron and ondansetron induced by interleukin–2. Dermatology 2000; 201: 148–50.
50. Blanche P, Gombert B, Rollot F, Salmon D, Sicard D. Sarcoidosis in a patient with acquired immunodeficiency syndrome treated with interleukin–2. Clin Infect Dis 2000; 31: 1493–4.
51. Sosman JA, Verma A, Moss S, Sorokin P, Blend M, Bradlow B, Chachlani N, Cutler D, Sabo R, Nelson M, Bruno E, Gustin D, Viana M, Hoffman R. Interleukin 10-induced thrombocytopenia in normal healthy adult volunteers: evidence for decreased platelet production. Br J Haematol 2000; 111: 104–11.
52. Gollob JA, Veenstra JW, Mier JW, Atkins MB. Agranulocytosis and hemolytic anemia in patients with renal cell cancer treated with interleukin–12. J Immunother 2001; 24: 91–8.
53. Peeva E, Fishman AD, Goddard G, Wadler S, Barland P. Rheumatoid arthritis exacerbations caused by exogenous interleukin-12. Arthritis Rheum 2000; 43: 461–3.
54. Milkovich G, Moleski J, Reitan JF, Dunning DM, Gibson GA, Paivanas TA, Wyant S, Jacobs RJ. Comparative safety of filgrastim versus sargramostim in patients receiving myelosuppressive chemotherapy. Pharmacotherapy 2000; 20: 1432–40.
55. Cavallaro AM, Lilleby K, Majolino I, Storb R, Appelbaum FR, Rowley SD, Bensinger WI. Three to six year follow-up of normal donors who received recombinant human granulocyte colony-stimulating factor. Bone Marrow Transplant 2000; 25: 85–9.
56. Dereure O, Bessis D, Lavabre-Bertrand T, Exbrayat C, Fegueux N, Biron C, Guilhou JJ. Thrombotic and necrotizing panniculitis associated with recombinant human granulocyte colony-stimulating factor treatment. Br J Dermatol 2000; 142: 834–6.
57. Gertz MA, Lacy MQ, Bjornsson J, Litzow MR. Fatal pulmonary toxicity related to the administration of granulocyte colony-stimulating factor in amyloidosis: a report and review of growth factor-induced pulmonary toxicity. J Hematother Stem Cell Res 2000; 9: 635–43.
58. Mizuno SI, Okamura T, Iwasaki H, Ohno Y, Akashi K, Inaba S, Niho Y. Hypercoagulable state following transfusions of granulocytes obtained from granulocyte colony-stimulating factor-stimulated donors. Int J Dermatol 2000; 72: 115–17.
59. Locasciulli A, Arcese W, Locatelli F, Di Bona E, Bacigalupo A, for the Italian Aplastic Anemia Study Group. Treatment of aplastic anaemia with granulocyte-colony stimulating factor and risk of malignancy. Lancet 2001; 357: 43–4.
60. Freedman MH, Bonilla MA, Fier C, Bolyard AA, Scarlata D, Boxer LA, Brown S, Cham B, Kannourakis G, Kinsey SE, Mori PG, Cottle T, Welte K, Dale DC. Myelodysplasia syndrome and acute myeloid leukemia in patients with congenital neutropenia receiving G-CSF therapy. Blood 2000; 96: 429–36.
61. Breedveld F. Therapeutic monoclonal antibodies. Lancet 2000; 355: 735–40.
62. Strehlau J, Pape L, Offner G, Nashan B, Ehrich JHH. Interleukin-2 receptor antibody-induced alterations of ciclosporin dose requirements in paediatric transplant recipients. Lancet 2000; 356: 1327–28.
63. Ganschow R, Grabhorn E, Burdelski M. Basiliximab in paediatric liver-transplant patients. Lancet 2001; 357: 388.
64. Franz A, Bewersdorf H, Hartung G, Dencausse Y, Queiber W. Exacerbation of Wegener's granulomatosis following single administration of monoclonal antibody 17-1A (Panorex Rm) during adjuvant immunotherapy of colon cancer. Onkologie 2000; 23: 472–4.
65. Farrell RJ, Shah SA, Lodhavia PJ, Alsahlki M, Falchuk KR, Michetti P, Peppercorn MA. Clinical experience with infliximab therapy in 100 patients with Cronh's disease. Am J Gastroenterol 2000; 95: 3490–7.
66. Menghini VV, Arora AS. Infliximab-associated reversible cholestatic liver disease. Mayo Clin Proc 2001; 76: 84–6.
67. Griffin SP, Selby WS. Poor wound healing following surgery in three patients who received infliximab for Crohn's disease. J Gastroenterol

Hepatol 2000; 15 Suppl: 78.
68. Keane J, Gershon S, Wise RP, Mirabile-Levens E, Kasznica J, Schwieterman WD, Siegel JN, Braun MM. Tuberculosis associated with infliximab, a tumor necrosis factor a-neutralizing agent. New Engl J Med 2001; 345: 1098–104.
69. Smith RV, Greenstein S, Tellis V, Ruben RJ. Reversible sensorineural hearing loss following administration of muromonab-CD3 (OKT3) for cadaveric renal transplant immunosuppression. Ann Otol Rhinol Laryngol 2000; 109: 45–7.
70. Foran JM, Rohatiner AZS, Cunimgham D, Popescu RA, Solal-Celigny P, Ghielmini M, Coiffier B, Johnson PWM, Gisselbrecht C, Reyes F, Radford JA, Bessell EM, Souleau B, Benzohra A, Lister TA. European Phase II study of rituximab (chimeric anti CD20 monoclonal antibody) for patients with newly diagnosed mantle-cell lymphoma and previously treated mantle-cell lymphoma, immunocytoma, and small B-cell lymphocytic lymphoma. J Clin Oncol 2000; 18: 317–24.
71. Sharma VR, Fleming DR, Slone SP. Pure red cell aplasia due to parvovirus B19 in a patient treated with rituximab. Blood 2000; 96: 1184–6.
72. Bathon JM, Martin RW, Fleischmann RM, Tesser JR, Schiff MH, Keystone EC, Genovese MC, Wasko MC, Moreland LW, Weaver AL, Markenson J, Finck BF. A comparison of etanercept and methotrexate in patients with early rheumatoid arthritis. New Eng J Med 2000; 343: 1586–93.
73. Bloom BJ. Development of diabetes mellitus during etanercept therapy in a child with systemic-onset juvenile rheumatoid arthritis. Arthritis Rheum 2000; 43: 2606–8.
74. Murphy FT, Enzenauer RJ, Battafarano DF, David-Bajar K. Etanercept-associated injection-site reactions. Arch Dermatol 2000; 136: 556–7.
75. Skyttä E, Pohjankoski H, Savolainen A. Etanercept and urticaria in patients with juvenile idiopathic arthritis. Clin Exp Rheumatol 2000; 18: 533–4.
76. Galaria NA, Werth VP, Schumacher HR. Leukocytoclastic vasculitis due to etanercept. J Rheumatol 2000; 27: 2041–4.
77. Kemp E, Nielsen H, Petersen LJ, Gam AN, Dahlager J, Horn T, Larsen S, Olsen S. Newer immunomodulating drugs in rheumatoid arthritis may precipitate glomerulonephritis. Clin Nephrol 2001; 55: 87–8.
78. Russell E, Zeihen M, Wergin S, Litton T. Patients receiving etanercept may develop antibodies that interfere with monoclonal antibody laboratory assays. Arthritis Rheum 2000; 43: 944.
79. Perreaux F, Zenaty D, Capron F, Trioche P, Odièvre M, Labrune P. Azathioprine-induced lung toxicity and efficacy of cyclosporin A in a young girl with type 2 autoimmune hepatitis. J Pediatr Gastroenterol Nutr 2000; 31: 190–2.
80. Jungling AS, Shangraw RE. Massive airway edema after azathioprine. Anesthesiology 2000; 92: 888–90.
81. Sebbag L, Boucher P, Davelu P, Boissonnat P, Champsaur G, Ninet J, Dureau G, Obadia JF, Vallon JJ, Delaye J. Thiopurine s-methyltransferase gene polymorphism is predictive of azathioprine-induced myelosuppression in heart transplant recipients. Transplantation 2000; 69: 1524–7.
82. Colombel JF, Ferrari N, Debuysere H, Marteau P, Gendre JP, Bonaz B, Soulé JC, Modigliani R, Touze Y, Catala P, Libersa C, Broly F. Genotypic analysis of thiopurine s-methyltransferase in patients with Crohn's disease and severe myelosuppression during azathioprine therapy. Gastroenterology 2000; 118: 1025–30.
83. Eaton VS, Casanova JM, Kupa A. Azathioprine hepatotoxicity confirmed by rechallenge. Aust J Hosp Pharm 2000; 30: 58–9.
84. Muszkat M, Pappo O, Caraco Y, Haviv YS. Hepatocanalicular cholestasis after 24 years of azathioprine administration for myasthenia gravis. Clin Drug Invest 2000; 19: 75–8.
85. Bisschop D, Germain ML, Munzer M, Trenque T. Thioguanine, pancréatotoxicité? Thérapie 2001; 56: 67–9.
86. Koide T, Yamada M, Takahashi S, Igarashi S, Masuko M, Furukawa T, Kuroha T, Koike T, Sato M, Tanaka R, Tsuji S, Takahashi H. Cyclosporine A-associated fatal central nervous system angiopathy in a bone marrow transplant recipient: an autopsy case. Acta Neuropathol 2000; 99: 680–4.
87. Shbarou RM, Chao NJ, Morgenlander JC. Cyclosporin A-related cerebral vasculopathy. Bone Marrow Transplant 2000; 26: 801–4.
88. Sall K, Stevenson OD, Mundorf TK, Reis BL, and the CsA Phase 3 Study Group. Two multicenter, randomized studies of the efficacy and safety of cyclosporine ophthalmic emulsion in moderate to severe dry eye disease. Ophtalmology 2000; 107: 631–9.
89. Kachi S, Hirano K, Takesue Y, Miura M. Unusual corneal deposit after the topical use of cyclosporine as eyedrops. Am J Ophtalmol 2000; 130: 667–9.
90. Chicharro ML, Guarner L, Vilaseca J, Planas M, Malagelada J-R. Does cyclosporin A worsen liver function in patients with inflammatory bowel disease and total parenteral nutrition? Rev Esp Enferm Dig 2000; 92: 68–77.
91. Câmara NOS, Matos ACC, Rodrigues DA, Pereira AB, Pacheco-Silva A. Early detection of heart transplant patients with increased risk of ciclosporin nephrotoxicity. Lancet 2001; 357: 856–7.
92. Ramsay HM, Harden PN. Cyclosporin-induced flushing in a renal transplant recipient resolving after substitution with tacrolimus. Br J Dermatol 2000; 142: 832–3.
93. Azurdia RM, Graham RM, Weismann K, Geurin DM, Parslew R. Acne keloidalis in caucasian patients on cyclosporin following organ transplantation. Br J Dermatol 2000; 143: 465–6.
94. Carnero L, Silvestre JF, Guijarro J, Albares MP, Botella R. Nuchal acne keloidalis associated with cyclosporin. Br J Dermatol 2001; 144: 429–30.

95. Gupta S, Radotra BD, Kumar B, Pandhi R, Rai R. Multiple, large, polypoid infundibular (epidermoid) cysts in a cyclosporin-treated renal transplant recipient. Dermatology 2000; 201: 78.
96. Lo Giudice P, Dubourg L, Hadj-Aïssa A, Saïd MH, Claris O, Audra P, Martin X, Cochat P. Renal function of children exposed to cyclosporin in utero. Nephrol Dial Transplant 2000; 15: 1575–9.
97. Dussol B, Reynaud-Gaubert M, Saingra Y, Daniel L, Berland Y. Acute tubular necrosis induced by high level of cyclosporine A in a lung transplant. Transplantation 2000; 70: 1234–6.
98. De Perrot M, Spiliopoulos A, Cottini S, Nicod L, Ricou B. Massive cerebral edema after i.v. cyclosporin overdose. Transplantation 2000; 70: 1259–60.
99. Lill J, Bauer LA, Horn JR, Hansten PD. Cyclosporine-drug interactions and the influence of patient age. Am J Health-Syst Pharm 2000; 57: 1579–84.
100. Barone GW, Gurley BJ, Ketel BL, Lightfoot ML, Abul-Ezz SR. Drug interaction between St. John's wort and cyclosporine. Ann Pharmacother 2000; 34: 1013–16.
101. Karliova M, Treichel U, Malago M, Frilling A, Gerken G, Broelsch CE. Interaction of *Hypericum perforatum* (St. John's wort) with cyclosporin A metabolism in a patient after liver transplantation. J Hepatol 2000; 33: 853–5.
102. Mai I, Krüger H, Budde K, Johne A, Brockmöller J, Neumayer HH, Roots I. Hazardous pharmacokinetic interaction of Saint John's wort (*Hypericum perforatum*) with the immunosuppressant cyclosporin. Int J Clin Pharmacol Ther 2000; 38: 500–2.
103. Le Beller C, Bezie Y, Chabatte C, Guillemain R, Amrein C, Billaud EM. Co-administration of orlistat and cyclosporine in a heart transplant recipient. Transplantation 2000; 70: 1541–2.
104. Schnetzler B, Kondo-Oestreicher M, Vala D, Khatchatourian G, Faidutti B. Orlistat decreases the plasma level of cyclosporine and may be responsible for the development of acute rejection episodes. Transplantation 2000; 70: 1540–1.
105. Caforio ALP, Gambino A, Tona F, Feltrin G, Marchini F, Pompei E, Testolin L, Angelini A, Dalla Volta S, Casarotto D. Sulfinpyrazone reduces cyclosporine levels: a new drug interaction in heart transplant recipients. J Heart Lung Transplant 2000; 19: 1205–8.
106. Pichard L, Fabre I, Fabre G, Domergue J, Saint-Aubert B, Mourad G, Maurel P. Cyclosporin A drug interactions. Screening for inducers and inhibitors of cytochrome P-450 (cyclosporin A oxidase) in primary cultures of human hepatocytes and in liver microsomes. Drug Metab Dispos 1990; 18: 595–606.
107. Zisman DA, Lynch JP, Toews GB, Kazerooni EA, Flint A, Martinez FJ. Cyclophosphamide in the treatment of idiopathic pulmonary fibrosis. A prospective study in patients who failed to respond to corticosteroids. Chest 2000; 117: 1619–26.
108. Tisdale JF, Dunn DE, Geller N, Plante M, Nunez O, Dunbar CE, Barrett AJ, Walsh TJ, Rosenfeld SJ, Young NS. High-dose cyclophosphamide in severe aplastic anaemia: a randomised trial. Lancet 2000; 356: 1554–9.
109. Reinhold-Keller E, Beuge N, Latza U, de Groot K, Rudert H, Nölle B, Heller M, Gross WL. An interdisciplinary approach to the care of patients with Wegener's granulomatosis. Long-term outcome in 155 patients. Arthritis Rheum 2000; 43: 1021–32.
110. Mok CC, Wong WM, Shek TWH, Ho CTK, Lau CS, Lai CL. Cumulative hepatotoxicity induced by continuous low-dose cyclophosphamide therapy. Am J Gastroenterol 2000; 95: 845–6.
111. Bateman H, YaziciY, Leff L, Peterson M, Paget SA. Increased cervical dysplasia in intravenous cyclophosphamide-treated patients with SLE: a preliminary study. Lupus 2000; 9: 542–4.
112. Rosenthal AK, Klausmeier M, Cronin ME, McLaughlin JK. Hepatic angiosarcoma occurring after cyclophosphamide therapy. Case report and review of the literature. Am J Clin Oncol 2000; 23: 581–3.
113. Griffith SM, Fisher J, Clarke S, Montgomery B, Jones PW, Saklatvala J, Dawes PT, Shadforth MF, Hothersall TE, Hassell AB, Hay EM. Do patients with rheumatoid arthritis established on methotrexate and folic acid 5 mg daily need to continue folic acid supplements long term? Rheumatology 2000; 39: 1102–9.
114. Landewé RBM, Van den Borne BEEM, Breedveld FC, Dijkmans BAC. Methotrexate effects in patients with rheumatoid arthritis with cardiovascular comorbidity. Lancet 2000; 355: 1616–17.
115. Chatham WW, Morgan SL, Alarcon GS. Renal failure: a risk factor for methotrexate toxicity. Arthritis Rheum 2000; 43: 1185–6.
116. Khan AJ, Brook S, Marghoob AA, Prestia AE, Spector IJ. Methotrexate and photodermatitis reactivation reaction: a case report and review of the literature. Cutis 2000; 66: 379–82.
117. Hani N, Casper C, Groth W, Krieg T, Hunzelmann N. Stevens-Johnson syndrome-like exanthema secondary to methotrexate histologically simulating acute graft-versus-host disease. Eur J Dermatol 2000; 10: 548–50.
118. Mazzantini M, Di Munno O. Methotrexate and bone mass. Clin Exp Rheumatol 2000; 18 Suppl 1: S87–92.
119. Mazzantini M, Di Munno O, Incerti-Vecchi L, Pasero G. Vertebral bone mineral density in female rheumatoid arthritis patients treated with low-dose methotrexate. Clin Exp Rheumatol 2000; 18: 327–31.
120. Borman P, Bodur H, Güleç AT, Uçan H, Seçkin U, Mocan G. Atypical methotrexate dermatitis and vasculitis in a patient with ankylosing spondylitis. Rheumatol Int 2000; 19: 191–3.
121. Borcea A, Greaves MW. Methotrexate-induced exacerbation of urticarial vasculitis: an

unusual adverse reaction. Br J Dermatol 2000; 143: 203–4.
122. Houde I, Isenring P, Boucher D, Noel R, Lachanche JG. Mycophenolate mofetil, an alternative to cyclosporin for long-term immunosuppression in kidney transplantation. Transplantation 2000; 70: 1251–3.
123. Schrama YC, Joles JA, Van Tol A, Boer P, Koomans HA, Hené RJ. Conversion to mycophenolate mofetil in conjunction with stepwise withdrawal of cyclosporine in stable renal transplant recipients. Transplantation 2000; 69: 373–83.
124. Banerjee R, Halil O, Bain BJ, Cummins D, Banner NR. Neutrophil dysplasia caused by mycophenolate mofetil. Transplantation 2000; 70: 1608–10.
125. Chueh SC, Huang CY, Lai MK. Mycophenolate mofetil-induced hyperbilirubinemia in renal transplant recipients. Transplant Proc 2000; 32: 1901–2.
126. Kim HC, Park SB. Mycophenolate mofetil-induced ischemic colitis. Transplant Proc 2000; 32: 1896–7.
127. Rault R. Mycophenolate-associated onycholysis. Ann Intern Med 2000; 133: 921–2.
128. Satchell AC, Barnetson RSC. Staphylococcal septicaemia complicating treatment of atopic dermatitis with mycophenolate. Br J Dermatol 2000; 143: 202–3.
129. Woywodt A, Choi M, Schneider W, Kettritz R, Gobel U. Cytomegalovirus colitis during mycophenolate mofetil therapy for Wegener's granulomatosis. Am J Nephrol 2000; 20: 468–72.
130. Ter Meulen CG, Wetzels JFM, Hilbrands LB. The influence of mycophenolate mofetil on the incidence and severity of primary cyctomegalovirus infections and disease after renal transplantation. Nephrol Dial Transplant 2000; 15: 711–14.
131. Chueh SC, Hong JC, Huang CY, Lai MK. Drug fever caused by mycophenolate mofetil in a renal transplant recipient. A case report. Transplant Proc 2000; 32: 1925–6.
132. Singer SJ, Tiernan R, Sullivan EJ. Interstitial pneumonitis associated with sirolimus therapy in renal-transplant recipients. New Engl J Med 2000; 343: 1815–16.
133. Mahalati K, Murphy DM, West ML. Bronchiolitis obliterans and organizing pneumonia in renal transplant recipients. Transplantation 2000; 69: 1531–2.
134. Hong JC, Kahan BD. Sirolimus-induced thrombocytopenia and leukopenia in renal transplant recipients: risk factors, incidence, progression, and management. Transplantation 2000; 69: 2085–90.
135. Plosker GL, Foster RH. Tacrolimus. A further update of its pharmacology and therapeutic use in the management of organ transplantation. Drugs 2000; 59: 323–89.
136. Uchida N, Taniguchi S, Harada N, Shibuya T. Myocardial ischemia following allogeneic bone marrow transplantation: possible implication of tacrolimus overdose. Blood 2000; 96: 370–2.
137. Bronster DJ, Gurkan A, Buchsbaum MS, Emre S. Tacrolimus-associated mutism after orthotopic liver transplantation. Transplantation 2000; 70: 979–82.
138. Mori A, Tanaka J, Kobayashi S, Hashino S, Yamamoto Y, Ota S, Asaka M, Imamura M. Fatal cerebral hemorrhage associated with cyclosporin-A/FK506-related encephlalopathy after allogeneic bone marrow transplantation. Ann Hematol 2000; 79: 588–92.
139. Misawa A, Takeuchi Y, Hibi S, Todo S, Imashuku S, Sawada T. FK506-induced intractable leukoencephalopathy following allogeneic bone marrow transplantation. Bone Marrow Transplantation 2000; 25: 331–4.
140. Brazis PW, Spivey JR, Bolling JP, Steers JL. A case of bilateral optic neuropathy in a patient on tacrolimus (FK506) therapy after liver transplantation. Am J Ophtalmol 2000: 129: 536–8.
141. Lohmann T, List C, Lamesch P, Kohlhaw K, Wenzke M, Schwarz C, Richter O, Hauss J, Seissler J. Diabetes mellitus and islet cell specific autoimmunity as adverse effects of immunsuppressive therapy by FK506/tacrolimus. Exp Clin Endocrinol Diabetes 2000; 108: 347–52.
142. Kawai T, Shimada A, Kasuga A. FK506-induced autoimmune diabetes. Ann Intern Med 2000; 132: 511.
143. Nieto Y, Russ P, Everson G, Bearman SI, Cagnoni PJ, Jones RB, Shpall EJ. Acute pancreatitis during immunosuppression with tacrolimus following an allogeneic umbilical cord blood transplantation. Bone Marrow Transplant 2000; 26: 109–11.
144. Reitamo S, Wollenberg A, Schöpf E, Perrot JL, Marks R, Ruzicka T, Christophers E, Kapp A, Lahfa M, Rubins A, Jablonska S, Rustin M. Safety and efficacy of 1 year of tacrolimus ointment monotherapy in adults with atopic dermatitis. Arch Dermatol 2000; 136: 999–1006.
145. Riley L, Mudd L, Baize T, Herzig R. Cross-sensitivity reaction between tacrolimus and macrolide antibiotics. Bone Marrow Transplant 2000; 25: 907–8.
146. Schvarcz R, Rudbeck G, Söderdahl G, Stahle L. Interaction between nelfinavir and tacrolimus after orthoptic liver transplantation in a patient coinfected with HIV and hepatitis C virus (HCV). Transplantation 2000; 69: 2194–5.
147. Boubenider S, Vincent I, Lambotte O, Roy S, Hiesse C, Taburet AM, Charpentier B. Interaction between theophylline and tacrolimus in a renal transplant patient. Nephrol Dial Transplant 2000; 15: 1066–8.
148. Penn I. Post-transplant malignancy. The role of immunosuppression. Drug Saf 2000; 23: 101–13.
149. Younes BS, McDiarmid SV, Martin MG, Vargas JH, Goss JA, Busuttil RW, Ament ME. The effect of immunosuppression on posttransplant lymphoproliferative disease in pediatric liver transplant patients. Transplantation 2000; 70: 94–9.

H.D. Reuter

38 Vitamins

VITAMIN A (RETINOL)

(SED-14, 1340; SEDA-21, 405; SEDA-22, 433; SEDA-23, 418; SEDA-24, 443)

R

Are β-carotene and carotenoids carcinogenic in smokers?

Negative outcomes in several supplementation trials of β-carotene, especially the results of the Finnish α-Tocopherol β-Carotene (ATBC) Cancer Prevention Study (1[C]) (SEDA-20, 363) has again revived discussion about the carcinogenic potential of β-carotene. The ATBC trial showed that there was a statistically significant increase in the incidence of lung cancer in heavy smokers who took β-carotene. Problems concerning the interactions of cigarette smoking, cancer, and carotenoids have been reviewed (2[R]).

Over several decades, evidence has accumulated that a diet rich in fruit and vegetables is associated with a lower risk of cardiovascular disease and various forms of cancer, principally cancer of the lung and stomach, but also esphageal, oral, breast, and prostate cancer (3[R], 4[E]).

β-carotene and other micronutrients have been claimed to counteract oxidative processes that participate in various stages of carcinogenesis, and increased consumption of fruit and vegetables rich in carotenoids lowered urinary indices of oxidized lipids and DNA in healthy subjects (5[C]). Although β-carotene and other carotenoids are excellent in vitro quenchers of singlet oxygen and β-carotene, and may also protect lipids from radical-initiated peroxidation under certain conditions, evidence for antioxidant properties of β-carotene in vivo is much less compelling (6[E]). Assessment of the antioxidant benefit of β-carotene is especially complicated by the fact that carcinogenesis is a very complex multistage process, in which oxidative pathways play variable and incompletely understood roles. While a few early supplementation trials suggested a beneficial role of β-carotene (4[E]), many other studies did not show such an effect. The proposed beneficial properties of carotenoids appear to be consistent with findings that cigarette smokers generally have subnormal serum concentrations of various carotenoids and other micronutrients, such as vitamin C, supposed to be caused by the increased oxidative stress associated with smoking and its attendant activation of the inflammatory and immune systems. On the other hand, the low concentrations in smokers could also result from lower intake of these micronutrients. Lower concentrations of carotenoids and other micronutrients are also observed in passive smokers (7[R], 8[C]).

The constituents of cigarette smoke can degrade β-carotene (9[E], 10[E]), but the conclusion that smoking causes increased carotenoid metabolism demands the demonstration of raised carotenoid oxidation products. Moreover, the consistent oservation of subnormal carotenoid concentrations but unchanged α-tocopherol concentrations (8[C]) suggests that factors other than oxidative stress contribute to the relative carotenoid deficiency.

The assumption that remedying the carotenoid deficit would minimize the risks of cancer and heart disease associated with passive smoking has not been supported by several large randomized supplemention trials. In two major trials there was an increased incidence of cancer with β-carotene supplementation in both smokers and asbestos workers. Of course, both high-risk groups might already have been in the early stages of cancer development at the start of the studies (1[C], 2[R]).

These surprising findings have raised an interesting apparent paradox: how can sup-

Side Effects of Drugs, Annual 25
J.K. Aronson, ed.

plementation with β-carotene, a presumed antioxidant and possible chemoprotective agent, enhance cancer formation, even though this is thought to involve oxidative processes? In some experimental systems carotenoids have pro-oxidant properties at high concentrations, but these are not reached in vivo (7[R], 8[C]). Another mechanism is an increase or alteration in carotenoid metabolism in high-risk groups, resulting in the formation of metabolites or oxidation products that could be procarcinogenic (for instance by interfering with retinoid signaling pathways, by promoting DNA damage, or by inducing cytochrome P450 enzymes that might promote carcinogen activation) (4[E], 11[R]). Such induction of cytochrome P450 enzymes might also enhance the catabolism of retinoic acid, which plays an important role in lung epithelial proliferation and differentiation. Downregulation of the retinoic acid receptor, RARβ, by β-carotene supplementation has been shown in recent studies in ferrets (11[R]). RARβ may act as a tumor suppressor gene. Moreover, lung expression of the proto-oncogenes c-jun and c-fos was increased in animals exposed to cigarette smoke and also receiving β-carotene supplements (11[R]).

In general, the negative outcomes of several supplementation trials and the lack of proof that carotenoids form the primary beneficial component of fruit and vegetables should serve as a warning against unregulated supplementation with these individual micronutrients, especially in view of the potential carcinogenic effect of carotenoids.

The carcinogenic effect of β-carotene has recently been found to be reduced by vitamin E (12[E]), suggesting that, rather than individual micronutrient supplementation, combinations of various such substances might be more advantageous.

All-*trans* retinoic acid

A *dry scaling skin rash* and *cheilitis* were the most common adverse effects in 14 patients with prostate cancer treated with all-*trans* retinoic acid and 20 patients treated with a combination of *cis*-retinoic acid and interferon-α_{2a} (13[C]). There was anorexia and significant weight loss in under 10% of the patients, but one patient discontinued treatment because of persistent *fatigue* and *anorexia*. Hematological toxic effects included *leukopenia*, *neutropenia*, *anemia*, and *thrombocytopenia*. Two patients with mild urinary hesitancy had *acute urinary outlet obstruction* within 1 week of starting *cis*-retinoic acid plus interferon. There were mild *rises in hepatic transaminases* and *serum triglycerides* in over half of the patients. Most triglyceride concentrations were below 2.3 (reference range 0.6-1.9) mmol/l, but one patient had an extreme rise of triglycerides to 3280 mg/daily. *Sensory and mood changes* were mild and occurred mostly in those given *cis*-retinoic acid plus interferon. *Headaches* were the most common neurological abnormality with all-*trans* retinoic acid. Pulmonary adverse effects were *dyspnea* and a non-fatal *pulmonary embolism* in one patient treated with all-*trans* retinoic acid. Other adverse effects included *constipation, fever, nausea, vomiting, diarrhea, fatigue*, and *stomatitis*.

In 21 patients with squamous cell carcinomas of the head and neck randomized to all-*trans* retinoic acid 45, 50, or 150 mg/m^2 either once daily or as divided doses every 8 hours for 1 year, severe adverse effects included *headache* in five patients, *hypertriglyceridemia* in six, *mucositis* in two, and *hyperbilirubinemia, raised alkaline phosphatase, colitis, raised lipase, xerostomia, eczema*, and *arthritis* in one patient each (14[C]). The dose had to be reduced in seven of eight patients with severe toxicity at 90 mg/m^2/day. Three of nine patients taking 45 mg/m^2/day required dose reductions. The plasma AUC of all-*trans* retinoic acid did not correlate with the severity or frequency of adverse effects. From these results it can be concluded that 15 mg/m^2/day every 8 hours is a tolerable dose for 1 year in patients with squamous cell carcinomas of the head and neck.

Retinoic acid syndrome The *retinoic acid syndrome*, its incidence and clinical course, has been investigated in 167 patients taking all-*trans* retinoic acid as induction and maintenance therapy for acute promyelocytic leukemia (15[C]). The syndrome did not occur during maintenance therapy. During induction it occurred in 44 patients (26%) at a median of 11 (range 2–47) days. The major manifestations included *respiratory distress* (84%), *fever* (81%), *pulmonary edema* (54%), *pulmonary infiltrates* (52%), *pleural or pericardial effusions* (36%), *hypotension* (18%), *bone* *pain* (14%), *headache* (14%), *congestive heart failure* (11%), and *acute renal insufficiency* (11%). The median white blood cell count was 1.45×10^9/l at diagnosis and 31×10^9/l (range $6.8–72 \times 10^9$/l) at the time the syndrome developed. All-*trans* retinoic acid was continued in eight of the 44 patients, with subsequent resolution in seven. It was withdrawn in 36 patients and then reintroduced in 19, after which the syndrome recurred in three, with one death attributable to reintroduction of the drug. Ten of these 36 patients received chemotherapy without further all-*trans* retinoic acid, and eight achieved complete remission. Of seven patients in whom all-*trans* retinoic acid was not reintroduced and who were not given chemotherapy, five achieved complete remission and two died. Two deaths were definitely attributable to the syndrome.

In 63 patients with acute promyelocytic leukemia taking all-*trans* retinoic acid (60 mg/day) the rates of leukocytosis, intracranial hypertension, and retinoic acid syndrome were 57%, 9.5%, and 3.2% respectively; the death rate was 11% (16[C]). The authors suggested that progressive leukocytosis during all-*trans* retinoic acid therapy should be an indication for chemotherapy (for example, with homoharringtonine); if the white cell count exceeds 10×10^9/l before treatment, the patient should be given homoharringtonine only; if it is below 5.0×10^9/l homoharringtonine plus all-*trans* retinoic acid should be used.

A syndrome similar to that of the retinoic acid syndrome occurred after 10 days of all-*trans* retinoic acid therapy in a patient with a relapse of acute myeloblastic leukemia (17[A]).

A 75-year-old woman whose acute myeloblastic leukemia relapsed was treated with one dose of intravenous idarubicin (10 mg/m^2), cytarabine 20 mg subcutaneously for 10 days, and oral all-*trans* retinoic acid 45 mg/m^2/day. Ten days later she developed a persistent fever. A chest X-ray and a CT scan showed bilateral pleural efflusions and interstitial infiltrates, but no pulmonary embolus. All-*trans* retinoic acid was withdrawn and she was given intravenous dexamethasone 10 mg every 12 hours. Her fever disappeared within 24 hours and her respiratory distress gradually improved during the next 24–48 hours. A chest X-ray 7 days later showed total resolution.

Respiratory *Adult respiratory distress syndrome* has been attributed to all-*trans* retinoic acid (18[A]).

A 24-year-old woman with acute promyelocytic leukemia took all-*trans* retinoic acid, and 2 days later developed dyspnea and general aching. Her total leukocyte count was 5.04×10^9/l, her PaO_2 42.5 was mmHg, and a chest X-ray showed bilateral parenchymal infiltration consistent with respiratory distress syndrome. She recovered within 3 days of treatment with low-dose cytarabine and corticosteroids, without withdrawal of the retinoic acid.

Although the retinoic acid syndrome involves the lungs, *pulmonary hemorrhage* has only rarely been reported. Two patients with acute promyelocytic leukemia developed severe lung hemorrhage during the first 3 weeks of treatment with all-*trans* retinoic acid, shortly after the administration of chemotherapy (19[A]).

A 36-year-old man with acute promyelocytic leukemia was given all-*trans* retinoic acid 45 mg/m^2/day, daunorubicin, and cytarabine. A week later his platelet count fell to 10×10^9/l, and the next day he developed dyspnea, hemoptysis and fever. A chest X-ray showed diffuse bilateral patchy pulmonary infiltrates. All-*trans* retinoic acid was withdrawn, but despite high doses of corticosteroids and blood products, hemoptysis and respiratory failure continued for 6 weeks, when he improved.

A 59-year-old man with acute promyelocytic leukemia was given all-*trans* retinoic acid 45 mg/m^2/day and chemotherapy. On day 6, his fibrinogen concentration fell to 940 mg/l and he developed a fever (39° C), dyspnea, and hypotension. A chest X-ray showed a right pleural effusion. All-*trans* retinoic acid was withdrawn and he was given dexamethasone. However he deteriorated and developed hemoptysis. Despite corticosteroids and blood products his pulmonary bleeding continued unabated. On day 29 he developed Gram-negative sepsis and died.

Nervous system *Pseudotumor cerebri* has been attributed to all-*trans* retinoic acid in a child with acute promyelocytic leukemia (20[A]).

An 8-year-old girl with acute promyelocytic leukemia was given cytarabine, etoposide, idarubicin, and all-*trans* retinoic acid 25 mg/m^2/day. Five days later she developed fever, pleural effusions, and ascites, but the symptoms resolved spontaneously. On day 65 (cumulative dose of all-*trans* retinoic acid 1.6 g/m^2) she had nausea and vomiting, severe headache, and diplopia. There was paralysis of the left trochlear nerve bilateral papilledema. A cranial MRI scan was normal. The intracranial pressure was not meaured. All-*trans* retinoic acid was withdrawn and she was given corticosteroids, mannitol, acetazolamide. and pethidine. Her symptoms resolved within 2 days.

Hematologic All-*trans* retinoic acid often causes a persistent *procoagulant tendency*, which may explain why it is associated with an increase in thrombotic events.

Of 31 patients with acute promyelocytic leukemia (15 men and 16 women, median age 43 years) four received all-*trans* retinoic acid 45 mg/m^2/day and intravenous tranexamic acid 1-2 g for 6 days, nine received all-*trans* retinoic acid, daunorubicin, and cytarabine followed by thioguanine, 15 received chemotherapy, all-*trans* retinoic acid, and tranexamic acid, two received chemotherapy and tranexamic acid, and one received chemotherapy only (21[C]). Three of the four patients who received all-*trans* retinoic acid plus tranexamic acid had sudden and rapid detoriation in their condition, leading to early death. At post mortem there were widespread microvascular thromboses in unusual sites (e.g. the brain and kidney). The rapid progression to multiorgan failure and the widespread nature of the microthrombi suggests the need for caution in the simultaneous use of all-*trans* retinoic acid and tranexamic acid.

Another case of thrombosis during induction treatment with all-*trans* retinoic acid, aprotinin, and chemotherapy has been described (22[A]).

Liver *Acute liver damage* has been attributed to all-*trans* retinoic acid (23[A]).

A 40-year-old man with acute promyelocytic leukemia was given all-*trans* retinoic acid 45 mg/m^2/day and intravenous daunorubicin. After 3 weeks his alkaline phosphatase rose to 370 (reference range 82–198) U/L, the γ-glutamyltranspeptidase to 198 (reference range 7–43) U/l, and the direct bilirubin to 39 (reference range below 10) μmol/l. He had painful hepatomegaly without splenomegaly. Abdominal Doppler ultrasound ruled out biliary tract injury. Percutaneous liver biopsy showed intracellular cholestasis with preservation of hepatic architecture. He was given dexamethasone and all-*trans* retinoic acid was withdrawn. After 3 days the symptoms and hepatomegaly abated.

Skin Three cases of *scrotal ulceration* during all-*trans* retinoic acid therapy for a microgranular variant of acute promyelocytic leukemia (24[A], 25[A]), together with eight other reported cases (26[A]–28[A]), suggest that this adverse effect is specific for all-*trans* retinoic acid. The incidence has been estimated at 12% (24[A]). The pathogenesis is unknown, but it has been suggested to be a manifestation of the retinoic acid syndrome (24[A]). Improvement after the withdrawal of all-*trans* retinoic acid and the administration of corticosteroids supports this assumption. However, activation of neutrophils by superoxide production may also be involved.

In patients with acute promyelocytic leukemia all-*trans* retinoic acid can cause *Sweet's syndrome* (29[A]).

A 39-year-old man with acute promyelocytic leukemia was given all-*trans* retinoic acid 45 mg/m^2. His leukocyte count rose to 34.3×10^9/l on day 11. On day 18 he developed rigors, mild dyspnea, and a fever (39° C). He had exquisite pain in the right posterior tibial muscle and had several 2-mm erythematous papular and pustular lesions on his limbs and trunk. He was given a cephalosporin and developed painful bilateral nodules in the quadriceps, posterior tibial, and right biceps muscles. An MRI scan showed focal areas of increased T2 signals in the quadriceps muscles bilaterally, in most of the left sartorius and soleus muscles, and in all the compartments of the right leg. There was thickening of the adjacent fascia with subcutaneous edema. All-*trans* retinoic acid was withdrawn and he was given dexamethasone 16 mg/day. The cutaneous lesions improved dramatically and all-*trans* retinoic acid 45 mg/m^2 was restarted. The symptoms did not recur.

A 35-year-old woman with acute promyelocytic leukemia was given all-*trans* retinoic acid 45 mg/m^2/day. On day 9 she became febrile (39.5° C), and had a sore throat with pharyngeal erythema and tender lymphadenopathy. The fever persisted despite cephalosporins, vancomycin, and antibiotics for anerobic cover. On day 20 she developed severe bilateral anterior leg pain and both anterior tibial muscles were tender. Creatine kinase activity was 348 (reference range 38–176) U/L. All-*trans* retinoic acid was withdrawn and she was given intravenous dexamethasone 10 mg/day. Her fever resolved, her pain abated, and her muscles legs felt softer and less tender. All-*trans* retinoic acid was reintroduced and her symptoms returned.

Isotretinoin (*cis*-retinoic acid)

(see also p. 179)

Sensory systems Xerophthalmia, carrying a high risk of blindness, requires the immediate administration of massive doses of vitamin A. An infant who received intramuscular vitamin A for xerophthalmia secondary to cystic fibrosis developed an acute *sixth nerve palsy* (30[A]).

A 5-month-old boy with cystic fibrosis and xerophthalmia was given intramuscular vitamin A 50 000 IU (water-miscible retinyl palmitate). After the first dose prominent bulging of the fontanelle developed, but the infant remained alert and was feeding well. Two days later another dose of 50 000 IU was given in two divided doses over 2 days. These doses were well tolerated, with gradual improvement of the bulging fontanelle over 1 week. Five days later, a complete abduction deficit of the left eye developed, in keeping with an acute sixth nerve palsy. There were no other signs of raised intracranial pressure. The sixth nerve palsy resolved fully over the next 2 months. There were no other neurological sequelae. After discharge the infant continued to take oral vitamin A supplements.

Teratogenicity *Multiple congenital anomalies* occurred after exposure to isotretinoin in the first trimester (31[A]).

A neonate whose mother had taken isotretinoin 40 mg/day during the first 2 months of pregnancy had absent auricles, tachypnea, and feeding difficulties. There were signs of heart failure, and echocardiography showed a large subpulmonary ventricular septal defect (Taussig-Bing malformation) and a secundum atrial septal defect. Both great arteries originated from the anterior right ventricle, and there was tricuspid insufficiency. A cranial CT scan showed atresia of the external ear canal, tympanic membrane, middle ear, and antrum. Other ear structures were normal. The child died at home.

Previously published information on outcomes after maternal exposure to topical tretionin has been limited to three case reports (32[A]–34[A]). A fourth case has now been reported (35[A]).

A boy, born at 41 weeks weighing 4090 g, had no right auricle or external auditory canal. Before conception and during the first months of pregnancy his mother had used topical tretinoin (Retin A 0.025%) on her face and a large area of her back. She had also used vitamins during pregnancy. His father had used oral isotretinoin before conception. At 16 months the baby was babbling. Optokinetic response was diminished and there was no oculovestibular response. At 20 months he was non-verbal and had poor receptive language, compatible with cognitive impairment. A cranial CT scan showed calcification of the right posterior hemisphere and MRI showed reduction in the volume of the right cerebral hemisphere, an infarct in the deep basal ganglia, focal atrophy, and encephalomalacia of the right parieto-occipital lobe. MRA showed marked attenuation of the posterior cerebral artery with poor declination of the more distal cortical, temporal, and occipital branches. A PET scan showed severe hypometabolism of the right posterior parietal, occipital, and temporal lobes, right basal ganglia, and thalamus, and mild hypometabolism of the left cerebellum.

Risk factors The concentration of vitamin A is raised in *chronic renal insufficiency*, because reduced filtration of low molecular proteins results in increased concentrations of retinol binding protein. A retrospective evaluation of 18 liver biopsies in 71 patients on hemodialysis taking therapeutic doses of vitamin A showed hyperplasia of stellate cells in seven, but no evidence of fibrosis (36[C]).

In a patient with renal insufficiency *stellate cell hyperplasia* was accompanied by fibrosis (37[A]).

A 51-year-old man, with a 9-year history of renal insufficiency and an alcohol intake of 4 units/week, underwent transplant nephrectomy. At surgery, ascites and liver cirrhosis were noted. A needle biopsy of the liver 1 month later showed nodular regenerative hyperplasia but no cirrhosis. There were subendothelial vacuolated cells, suggestive of modified stellate cells, and there was adjacent focal perisinusoidal fibrosis. His medications included one multivitamin/mineral supplement per day containing vitamin A 4000 IU. His vitamin A concentration was 1045 (reference range 490–720) μg/l. Viral and antibody studies were negative.

VITAMINS OF THE B GROUP

(SED-14, 1344; SEDA-22, 436; SEDA-23, 419; SEDA-24, 446)

Nicotinic acid (niacin), nicotinamide

The safety and efficacy of escalating doses of modified-release tablets of niacin (Niaspan) have been evaluated in a multicenter, placebo-controlled study in 131 patients with primary hyperlipidemia (38[C]). The dose of niacin was initially 375 mg/day, then 500 mg/day, and then increasing in 500-mg increments at 4-week intervals to a maximum of 3000 mg/day. Changes in biochemical measurements in patients taking niacin were significant only for uric acid and phosphorus. Fasting blood glucose, bilirubin, AsT, AlT, alkaline phosphatase, lactate dehydrogenase, and amylase were not altered. Of the 131 patients 80 completed the study. Of the patients who withdrew, 31 did so for medical reasons (3% taking niacin and 11% placebo). Eight of the 26 patients who stopped taking niacin withdrew because of *flushing* (all before the 2000 mg/day dose) and five because of a *rash*. These reasons accounted for half of the dropouts with niacin. The number of patients who had episodes of flushing fell with each dose increment of niacin, suggesting tolerance.

Of other adverse events, only *nausea* (18% and 9%), *vomiting* (10% and 2%), *pruritus* (11% and 0%), and *rash* (10% and 0%) were more common with niacin.

Gastrointestinal In patients with squamous cell carcinomas of the head and neck accelerated radiotherapy with carbogen and nicotinamide 6 g/day (ARCON) was carried out to determine the feasibility and the adverse effects of this therapeutic approach (39[C]). Accelerated fractionation was combined with carbogen (n = 11), daily nicotinamide (n = 10), or both (n = 17). There were no significant differences in local adverse effects in the three groups. Systemic adverse effects took the form of *nausea* or *vomiting*. The authors concluded that in future ARCON trials a lower dose of nicotinamide will be needed to reduce severe upper gastrointestinal toxicity.

Of 61 patients with ischemic heart diease and dyslipidemia treated with niacin 1.5 and 3.0 g/day, 32 patients were withdrawn, 18 because of adverse effects and 14 for reasons not related to niacin (40[C]). Of the 29 patients who finished the study, adverse effects include *dryness of the skin* (14%), *acanthosis nigricans* (10%), *fatigue* (6.9%), *nausea* (6.9%), *abdominal pain* (3.4%), *diarrhea* (3.4%), and *anorexia* (3.4%); the figures in parentheses were the incidences at 33 weeks. Flushing occurred more often at 18 weeks than at 33 weeks (24% vs 6.9%), as did pruritus (35% vs 28%), suggesting tolerance to these effects.

Immunologic A *pseudoallergic reaction* has been reported in a patient who took several niacin-containing formulations (41[A]).

A previously healthy 40-year-old woman developed a generalized macular erythematous rash associated with palpitation and light-headness, recurring every few days. The rash started behind the neck and arms, with a sensation of tingling, progressing to a general feeling of heat. She felt ill and had to lie down until the episode subsided after 45–90 minutes, with residual fatigue for several hours. Laboratory findings were all in the reference ranges. She was taking two multivitamin tablets a day, each containing niacin 20 mg, one B-complex tablet containing niacin 50 mg, and 1–3 tablets of an antiemetic containing niacin 50 mg. Thus, she had unknowingly taken niacin up to 240 mg/day. Graded oral challenge with niacin 20–200 mg reproduced her symptoms.

Vitamin B_6 (pyridoxine)

Pyridoxine-induced *photosensitivity* has been reported in a patient with hypophosphatasia (42[A]).

A 30-year-old woman, a heterozygote for hypophosphatasia, who had been taking two tablets of a multivitamin formulation (pyridoxine hydrochloride 100 mg, riboflavin butyrate 30 mg, nicotinic amide 40 mg biotin, 0.05 mg, ascorbic acid 100 mg) once daily for 6 years, had severe skin eruptions and pruritus on exposure to the sun. The minimum erythema doses for UVB (20 mJ/cm^2) and UVA (4 J/cm^2) were lower than normal only for UVB (reference ranges 60–100 mJ/cm^2 UVB and below 10 J/cm^2 UVA). Patch and photopatch tests with the constituents of the tablets produced reactions to pyridoxine and pyridoxalphosphate only.

The authors suggested that photosensitivity in this patient may have been caused by abnormal metabolism of vitamin B_6 because of hypophosphatasia.

Vitamin B_1 (thiamine)

Immunologic Despite its enormous safety profile, it cannot be assumed that thiamine is completely innocuous. Thiamine hydrochloride is routinely given to patients with Wernicke's encephalopathy or malnourished states (such as malabsorption, beri-beri, cancer, aquired immunodeficiency syndrome, and chronic alcohol abuse). Systemic reactions to thiamine hydrochloride are rare but deaths can occur. *Anaphylactic shock* is a major adverse effect that can be life-threatening. It usually occurs after multiple parenteral dosages (43[r]–47[r]), and is IgE-mediated (47[r]). Most cases of anaphylaxis to thiamine were seen when the vitamin was first introduced for routine use 60 years ago. Another case has been reported (48[A]).

A 51-year-old woman with diabetes mellitus, chronic alcoholism, and anxiety disorder became acutely confused and was given 50% dextrose 25 g and thiamine hydrochloride 100 mg intravenously; 20 min later she became deeply cyanosed with shallow labored breathing at 28 breaths/minute, hypertensive, and tachycardic, with respiratory and metabolic acidosis and a blood alcohol concentration of 124 mg/daily (27 mmol/l). The next morning she was communicative and oriented and her vital signs and blood gases were normal. She was given thiamine hydrochloride intravenously and within moments developed shortness of breath, warmth, and tightness of the throat. She had a tachycardia, hypotension, hypoxia, and central cyanosis. She recovered within 24 hours.

VITAMIN C (ASCORBIC ACID)

(SED 13, 1175; SEDA-22, 438; SEDA-23, 423)

The adverse effects of high-dose vitamin C have been reviewed in the context of its pharmacokinetics (49[r]).

Urinary tract Oxalate-induced *renal damage* has been related to excessive doses of vitamin C (50[A]).

A 31-year-old man developed a headache, nausea, and vomiting. He had taken vitamin C, 2–2.5 g/day and before the onset of symptoms up to 5 g/day. He had a raised serum creatinine (1000 μmol/l). Renal ultrasound showed increased cortical echogenicity, and a renal biopsy showed acute tubular necrosis and massive oxalate deposition. He was given pyridoxine and two sessions of hemodialysis.

Immunologic Ascorbic acid and citric acid are used as food additives, ascorbic acid (E300) as an acidifier, antioxidant, and an additive in wheat, and citric acid as an acidifying complex-binding agent. Because additives are widely used in foods, beverages, and drugs, people with hypersensitivity or intolerance have to be carefully instructed. Caution must also be taken when scratch tests are performed with these substances (51[A]).

A 62-year-old man had frequent angio-edema, and a scratch test was performed with several food additives. Scratching with 1% ascorbic acid and 1% citric acid in vaseline resulted in a +3 reaction, and 20 minutes later he developed angio-edema with swelling of the glottis, reddening of the face and hands, itching, vertigo, tachycardia, and hypotension. He was given a corticosteroid and an antihistamine and recovered within half an hour.

VITAMIN D (CALCIFEROL) AND ANALOGS *(SED-14, 1351; SEDA-22, 438; SEDA-23, 423; -SEDA-24, 446)*

Calcitriol (1α,25-dihydroxycholecalciferol)

Mineral metabolism Calcitriol + calcium carbonate has been compared with calcium carbonate alone over 12 months in a prospective, randomized trial in 15 patients with secondary hyperparathyroidism (52[C]). Calcitriol 2 μg was given after each dialysis; the dose of calcium carbonate was adjusted as needed to maintain calcium and phosphate concentrations at 2.4–2.6 and 1.0–1.5 mmol/l respectively. During the first 6 months, one patient taking calcitriol had an asymptomatic episode of *hypercalcemia* (2.8 mmol/l), which resolved by reducing the dose of calcitriol to 1 μg. In the control group two patients had asymptomatic episodes of hypercalcemia (each 2.9 mmol/l) during the first 6 months. There were two episodes of asymptomatic hypercalcemia (3.2 and 2.9 mmol/l) in two patients taking calcitriol during the last 6 months of the study, requiring a reduction in dose to 0.5 μg in one patient. There was one epidose of hypercalcemia (2.8 mmol/l) in the control group during the last 6 months of the study.

Metal metabolism Primary infantile hypomagnesemia is an uncommon cause of neonatal hypocalcemic seizures, but it is an important condition to recognize, because magnesium supplementation corrects the magnesium deficit, reverses the hypocalcemia due to hypoparathyroidism, and prevents further seizures (53[C]). There is evidence of genetic heterogeneity, but the number of gene loci is not known and phenotypic classification is still evolving. Several reports have described primary infantile hypomagnesemia in children of unaffected Arab parents (54[R], 55[R]). One of the first reported patients, now an affected adult, used calcitriol as an alternative to the parenteral magnesium injections that had been part of his life for more than 20 years and developed *hypomagnesemia* (56[A]).

A 22-year-old man, first reported at 4 months of age and currently free of neurological deficits, had had intermittent and chronic diarrhea due to large oral doses of magnesium for hypomagnesemic tetany. Hypothesizing that modest hypercalcemia might prevent the tetany, he was given calcitriol 5 μg/day for 5 days. Despite the resultant increase in serum calcium concentration, he developed tetany and a fall in serum magnesium concentration from 0.63 to 0.39 mmol/l (reference range over 0.65 mmol/l). The calcitriol was withdrawn, and 33% of his usual oral magnesium supplement was given by continuous nasogastric infusion; the serum magnesium concentration rose to 0.60 mmol/l.

Skin The efficacy, safety, and tolerability of twice-daily calcitriol ointment 3 μg/g ($n = 60$) has been investigated and compared with 0.25–2% dithranol cream (once daily for 30 min; $n = 54$) in an 8-week prospective, randomized, open, parallel-group trial in 114 patients with plaque psoriasis (57[C]). *Skin irritation* was reported by three patients who used calcitriol and by 39% of those who used dithranol. Three patients who used calcitriol and four who used dithranol reported adverse effects on the skin (pruritus, erythema, rash, dry skin, eczema). One patient with 75% skin involvement, used 3.38 mg of calcitriol over 56 days (about 140 g of ointment per week without any effect on serum calcium.

Vitamin D_3 has been reported to cause *hyper-reactivity of skin* with pseudoxanthoma elasticum (58[A]).

A 68-year-old woman with pseudoxanthoma elasticum was given oral vitamin D_3, 0.25 μg/day. After 2 weeks she developed new yellow papules on the pre-existing plaques on the neck and abdomen without itching or pain. Biopsy showed a thicker epidermis and more abundant calcium deposition than in a biopsy before treatment. Electon microscopy showed electron-dense deposits between the degenerated elastic fibers, which had been surrounded by normal collagen fibers before treatment. After treatment with vitamin D_3 there were lucent areas that suggested unusual mineralization in association with electron-dense deposits. Serum concentrations of calcium were within the reference range throughout.

VITAMIN K (PHYTOMENADIONE) *(SED-14, 1356; SEDA-22, 439; SEDA-23, 423; SEDA-24, 448)*

Skin reactions to vitamin K_1

Presentation *The English-language literature on adverse skin reactions associated with intramuscular or subcutaneous vitamin K_1 has been reviewed (59[AR]). Vitamin K is generally well tolerated subcutaneously or intramuscularly. However, erythematous eczematous plaques have been well documented. Of 39 skin reactions due to vitamin K_1, 32 were eczematous and 91% of the patients were women, average age 39 (range 9–64) years; in four cases there were small vesicles within the plaques (60[A]–63[A]).*

A case of localized eczema at the site of subcutaneous injection has been reported (59[AR]).

A 50-year-old woman taking warfarin had an INR of 8 and was given vitamin K_1 10 mg subcutaneously (Sabex, containing propylene glycol 2% and polyethylene glycol 10%) and 12 hours later another 5 mg. One week later she developed two red, pruritic, warm, indurated areas, measuring 2×4 and 8×10 cm, at the two separate injection sites. A skin biopsy showed minimal spongiosis of the epidermis and an edematous dermis with a dense perivascular lymphocytic infiltrate and numerous eosinophils.

Timing *The median number of days between the administration of vitamin K_1 and the appearance of the eruption was 13 days, but eruptions have appeared as early as 30 minutes and as late as 4 weeks after injection. In 13 of 32 cases it took more than 2 months for the reaction to resolve.*

Relation to dose *In some early reports it was postulated that a minimum dose was necessary to cause eruptions, but there have been later reports of adverse skin reactions after small doses (range 10–440 mg).*

Histopathology *Histopathological examination typically shows epidermal changes, including spongiosis with or without intraepidermal vesicles. In the dermis there is a perivascular mononuclear cell infiltrate, which may also be interstitial, often containing eosinophils.*

Mechanism *Various formulations of vitamin K_1 contain different inactive ingredients, including polysorbate 80, propylene glycol, sodium acetate, glacial acetic acid, polyethoxylated castor oil (Cremophor EL), dextrose, and benzyl alcohol. Based on negative results with these ingredients, it appears that vitamin K_1 itself is the antigen that leads to adverse skin reactions. Of ten patients with liver disease* *and prior exposure to vitamin K_1 (Konakion) four had positive results to patch testing with vitamin K (64[C]). Intracutaneous tests have supported the generally accepted hypothesis that the phenomenon is due to type IV hypersensitivity.*

Treatment *No particular therapy is effective. It is not known whether the minute quantities of vitamin K_1 that are present in some foods, such as parsley, kale, Brussels sprouts, spinach, cucumber, soy bean oil, and green and black tea leaves, preclude effective dietary therapy. Since the mechanism of this reaction is thought to delayed hypersensitivity, another potential therapeutic approach is topical application of tacrolimus (FK-506), a potent inhibitor of interleukin-2 and T-cell activation. Tacrolimus up to now has only been shown to suppress allergic contact dermatitis to dinitrophenol.*

REFERENCES

1. The Alpha-Tocopherol, β-Carotene and Cancer Prevention Study Group. The effect of vitamin E and β-carotene on the incidence of lung cancer and other cancers in male smokers. New Engl J Med 1994; 330: 1029–35.
2. Van der Vliet A. Cigarettes, cancer, and carotenoids: a continuing, unresolved antioxidant paradox. Am J Clin Nutr 2000; 72: 1421–3.
3. Block G, Patterson B, Subar A. Fruit, vegetables and cancer prevention. A review of the epidemiological studies. Nutr Cancer 1992; 18: 1–29.
4. Pryor WA, Stahl W, Rock CL. Beta carotene: from biochemistry to clinical trials. Nutr Rev 2000; 58: 39–53.
5. Thompson HJ, Helmendinger J, Haegele A, Sedlacek SM, Gillette C, O'Neill C, Wolfe P, Conry C. Effect of increased vegetable and fruit consumption on markers of oxidative cellular damage. Carcinogenesis 1999; 20: 2261-6.
6. Krinsky NI. The antioxidant and biological properties of the caretenoids. Ann NY Acad Sci 1998; 854: 443–7.
7. Cross CE, Traber M, Eiserich J, Van der Vliet A. Micronutrient antioxidants and smoking. Br Med Bull 1999; 55: 691–704.
8. Alberg AJ, Chen JC, Zhao H, Hoffman SC, Comstock GW, Helzlsouer KJ. Household exposure to passive cigarette smoking and serum micronutrient concentrations. Am J Clin Nutr 2000; 72: 1576–82.
9. Handelman GJ, Packer L, Cross CE. Destruction of tocopherols, carotenoids, and retinol in human plasma by cigarettte smoke. Am J Clin Nutr 1996; 63: 559–65.
10. Baker DL, Krol ES, Jacobsen N, Liebler DC. Reactions of β-carotene with cigarette smoke oxidants. Identification of carotenoid oxidation products and evaluation of the prooxidant/antioxidant effect. Clin Res Toxicol 1999; 12: 535–43.
11. Wang X-D, Russell RM. Procarcinogenic and anticarcinogenic effects of β-carotene. Nutr Rev 1999; 57: 263–72.
12. Perocco P, Mazzullo M, Broccoli M, Rocchi P, Ferreri AM, Paolini M. Inhibitory activity of vitamin E and α-naphthoflavone on β-carotene-enhanced transformation of BALB/c 3T3 cells by benzo(a)pyrene and cigarette-smoke condensate. Mutat Res Genet Toxicol Environ Mutagen 2000; 465: 151–8.
13. Kelly WK, Osman I, Reuter VE, Curley T, Heston WDW, Nanus DM, Scher HI. The development of biologic end points in patients treated with differentiation agents. An experience of retinoids in prostate cancer. Clin Canc Res 2000; 6: 838–46.
14. So Hyang Park, Gray WC, Hernandez I, Jacobs M, Ord RA, Sutharalingam M, Smith RG, Van Echo DA, Wu S, Conley BA. Phase I trial of all-trans retinoic acid in patients with treated head and neck squamous carcinoma. Clin Canc Res 2000; 6: 847–54.
15. Tallman MS, Andersen JW, Schiffer CA, Appelbaum FR, Feusner JH, Ogden A, Shepherd L, Rowe JM, Francois C, Larson RS, Wiernik PH. Clinical description of 44 patients with acute promyelocytic leukemia who developed the retinoic acid syndrome. Blood 2000; 95: 90–5.
16. Han Z-P, Lu H-B, Shen Z-S. Severe side effects of the treatment of acute promyelocytic leukemia with all-trans retinoic acid. Bull Hunan Med Univ 2000; 25: 283–4.
17. Lehmann S, Paul C. The retinoic acid syndrome in non-M3 acute myeloid leukaemia: a case report. Br J Haematol 2000; 108: 198–9.
18. Kim C, Ki Ko W, Hyun Kwon S, Myung Kang S, Nyun Kim C, Gyoo Yang D, Kyu Kim S, Chang J, Kyu Kim S, Young Lee W, Ik Yang W. A case of acute respiratory distress syndrome induced by all-*trans* retinoic acid. Tuberc Respir Dis 2000; 49: 93–8.
19. Raanani P, Segal E, Levi I, Bercowicz M, Berkenstat H, Avigdor A, Perel A, Ben-Bassat I. Diffuse alveolar hemorrhage in acute promyelocytic leukemia patients treated with ATRA – a manifestation of the basic disease or the treatment. Leuk Lymphoma 2000; 37: 605–10.

20. Schroeter T, Lanvers C, Herding H, Suttorp M. Pseudotumor cerebri induced by all-*trans* retinoic acid in a child treated for acute promyelocytic leukemia. Med Pediatr Oncol 2000; 34: 284–6.
21. Brown JE, Olujohungbe A, Chang J, Ryder WDJ, Morganstern GR, Chopra R, Scarffe JH. All-trans retinoic acid (ATRA) and tranexamic acid: a potentially fatal combination in acute promyelocytic leukaemia. Br J Haematol 2000; 110: 1010–12.
22. Kocak U, Gursel T, Ozturk G, Kantarci S. Thrombosis during all-*trans* retinoic acid therapy in a child with acute promyelocytic leukemia and factor VQ 506 mutation. Pediatr Hematol Oncol 2000; 17: 177–80.
23. Perea G, Salar A, Altes A, Brunet S, Sierra J. Acute hepatomegaly with severe liver toxicity due to all-*trans* retinoic acid. Haematologica 2000; 85: 551–2.
24. Charles KS, Kanaa M, Winfield DA, Reilly JT. Scrotal ulceration during all-*trans* retinoic (ATRA) therapy for acute promyelocytic leukaemia. Clin Lab Haematol 2000; 22: 171–4.
25. Esser AC, Nossa R, Shoji T, Sapadin AN. All-*trans* retinoic acid-induced scrotal ulcerations in a patient with acute promyelocytic leukemia. J Am Acad Dermatol 2000; 43: 316–17.
26. Sun GL. Treatment of acute promyelocytic leukemia (APL) with all-*trans* retinoic acid (ATRA): a report of five year experience. Zhonghua Zhong Liu Za Zhi 1993; 15: 125–9.
27. Tajima K, Sagae M, Yahagi A, Akiba J, Suzuki K, Hayashi T, Satoh S. Scrotum exfoliative dermatitis with ulcers associated with treatment of acute promyelocytic leukemia with all-*trans* retinoic acid. Rinsho Ketsueki 1998; 39: 48–52.
28. Mori A, Tamura T, Nishimura Y, Ito T, Saheki K, Takatsuka H, Wada H, Fujimori Y, Okamoto T, Takemoto Y, Kakishita E. Scrotal ulcer occurring in patients with acute promyelocytic leukemia during treatment with all-*trans* retinoic acid. Oncol Rep 1999; 6: 55–8.
29. Van der Vliet HJJ, Roberson AE, Hogan MC, Morales CE, Crader SC, Letendre L, Pruthi RK. All-*trans* retinoic acid-induced myositis: a description of two patients. Am J Hematol 2000; 63: 94–8.
30. Ng EWM, Congdon NG, Sommer A. Acute sixth nerve palsy in vitamin A treatment of xerophthalmia. Br J Ophthalmol 2000; 84: 931–2.
31. Ceviz N, Ozkan B, Eren S, Ors R, Olgunturk R. A case of isotretinoin embryopathy with bilateral anotia and Taussig-Bing malformation. Turk J Pediatr 2000; 42: 239–41.
32. Camera G, Pregliasco P. Ear malformation in baby born to mother using tretinoin cream. Lancet 1992; 339: 687.
33. Lipson AH, Collins F, Webster WS. Multiple congenital defects associated with maternal use of topical tretinoin. Lancet 1993; 341: 1352–3.
34. Navarre-Belhassen C, Blanchet P, Hillaire-Buys D, Sarda P, Blayac JP. Multiple congenital maldeformations associated with topical tretionin. Ann Pharmacother 1998; 32: 505–6.
35. Selcen D, Seidman S, Nigro MA. Otocerebral anomalies associated with topical tretinoin use. Brain Dev 2000; 22: 218–20.
36. Vannucchi MT, Vannuchi H, Humphreys M. Serum levels of vitamin A and retinol binding protein in chronic renal patients treated by continuous ambulatorial peritoneal dialysis. Int J Vitam Nutr Res 1992; 62: 107–12.
37. Doyle S, Conlon P, Royston D. Vitamin A induced stellate cell hyperplasia and fibrosis in renal failure. Histopathology 2000; 36: 90–1.
38. Goldberg A, Alagona DP Jr, Capuzzi DM, Guyton J, Morgan JM, Rodgers J, Sachson R, Samuel P. Multiple-dose efficacy and safety of an extended-release form of niacin in the management of hyperlipidemia. Am J Cardiol 2000; 85: 1100–5.
39. Bernier J, Denekamp J, Rojas A, Minatel E, Horiot J-C, Hamers H, Antognoni P, Dahl O, Richaud P, Van Glabbeke M, Pierart M. ARCON: Accelerated Radiotherapy with Carbogen and Nicotinamide in head and neck squamous cell carcinomas. The experience of the Co-operative Group of Radiotherapy of the European Organization for Research and Treatment of Cancer (EORTC). Radiother Oncol 2000; 55: 111–19.
40. Morato Hernandez MDL, Del Sagrario Ichazo Cerro M, Alvarado Vega AG, Zamora Gonzalez J, Cardoso Saldana GC, Posadas Romero C. Immediate release niacin in the treatment of ischemic heart disease. Arch Inst Cardiol Mex 2000; 70: 367–76.
41. Grouhi M, Sussman G. Pseudoallergic toxic reaction. Ann Allergy Asthma Immunol 2000; 85: 269–71.
42. Kawada A, Kashima A, Shiraishi H, Gomi H, Matsuo I, Yasuda K, Sasaki G, Sato S, Orimo H. Pyridoxine-induced photosensitivity and hypophosphatasia. Dermatology 2000; 201: 356–60.
43. Stephen JM, Grant R, Yeh CS. Anaphylaxis from administration of intravenous thiamine. Am J Med 1992; 10: 61–3.
44. Leung R, Puy R, Czarny D. Thiamine anaphylaxis. Med J Aust 1993; 159: 355.
45. Van Haecke P, Ramaekers D, Vanderwegen L. Thiamine induced anaphylactic shock. Am J Med 1995; 13: 371–2.
46. Wrenn KD, Slovis CM. Is intravenous thiamine safe? Am J Emerg Med 1992; 10: 165.
47. Fernandez M, Barcelo M, Munoz C. Anaphylaxis to thiamine (vitamin B1). Allergy 1997; 52: 958–9.
48. Johri S, Shetty S, Soni A, Kumar S. Anaphylaxis from intravenous thiamine-long forgotten? Am J Emerg Med 2000; 18: 642–3.
49. Aronson JK. Forbidden fruit. Nature Med 2001; 7: 7–8.
50. Mashour S, Turner JF Jr, Merrell R. Acute renal failure, oxalosis, and vitamin C supplementation: a case report and review of the literature. Chest 2000; 118: 561–3.
51. Thumm EJ, Jung EG, Bayerl C. Anaphylaktische Reaktion nach Scratchtestung mit Ascorbin-

säure (E 300) und Zitronensäure (E 330). Allergologie 2000; 23: 354–9.
52. Delmez JA, Kelber J, Norwood KY, Giles KS, Slatopolsky E. A controlled trial of the early treatment of secondary hyperparathyroidism with calcitriol in hemodialysis patients. Clin Nephrol 2000; 54: 301–8.
53. Cole DEC, Carpenter TO, Goltzman D. Calcium homeostasis and disorders of bone and mineral metabolism. In: Collu R, Ducharme JR, Guyda HJ (editors). Pediatric Endocrinology. Raven Press: New York, 1989: 509–80.
54. Abdulrazzaq YM, Smigura FC, Wettrel G. Primary infantile hypomagneseamia: report of two cases and review of literature. Eur J Pediatr 1989; 148: 459–61.
55. Dudin KI, Teebi AS. Primary hypomagnesaemia. A case report and literature review. Eur J Pediatr 1987; 146: 303–5.
56. Cole DEC, Kooh SW, Vieth R, Primary infantile hypomagnesaemia: outcome after 21 years and treatment with continuous nocturnal nasogastric magnesium infusion. Eur J Pediatr 2000; 159: 38–43.
57. Hutchinson PE, Marks R, White J. The efficacy, safety and tolerance of calcitriol 3 μg/g ointment in the treatment of plaque psoriasis: a comparison with short-contact dithranol. Dermatology 2000; 201:139–45.
58. Hamamoto Y, Nagai K, Yasui H, Muto M. Hyperreactivity of pseudoxanthoma elasticum-affected dermis to vitamin D3. J Am Acad Dermatol 2000; 42: 685–7.
59. Wilkins K, DeKoven J, Assaad D. Cutaneous reactions associated with vitamin K_1. J Cutaneous Med Surg 2000; 4: 163–7.
60. Bruynzeel I, Hebeda CI, Folkers E, Bruynzeel DP. Cutaneous hypersensitivity reactions to vitamin K: 2 case reports and a review of the literature. Contact Dermatitis 1995; 32: 78–82.
61. Pigatto PD, Bigardi A, Fumagalli M, Altomare GF, Riboldi A. Allergic dermatitis from parenteral vitamin K. Contact Dermatitis. 1990; 22: 307–8.
62. Joyce JP, Hood AF, Wiess MM. Persistent cutaneous reaction to intramuscular vitamin K injection. Arch Dermatol 1988; 124: 27–8.
63. Keough GC, English JC, Meffert JJ. Eczematous hypersensitivity from aqueous vitamin K injection. Cutis 1998; 61: 81–3.
64. Bullen AW, Miller JP, Cuncliffe WJ, Losowsky MS. Skin reactions caused by vitamin K in patients with liver disease. Br J Dermatol 1978; 98: 561–5.

J. Costa and M. Farré

39 Corticotrophins, corticosteroids, and prostaglandins

Editor's note: *In this chapter adverse effects arising from the oral or intravenous administration of corticosteroids are covered in the section on systemic glucocorticosteroids. Other routes of administration are dealt with in the section after that, apart from inhalation and nasal administration, which are dealt with in Chapter 16, and topical administration, which is covered in Chapter 14.*

CORTICOTROPHINS *(SED-14, 1365; SEDA-24, 450)*

Cardiovascular Corticotrophin has been reported to cause *enlargement of cardiac tumors* in tuberous sclerosis (1^A).

A female infant with tuberous sclerosis had multiple large cardiac tumors in the left and right ventricles. Corticotrophin was given (dose not stated; once a day for 2 weeks, tapering over 3 months) at 4 months for infantile spasms. At 6 months a heart murmur was detected. Echocardiography showed pronounced enlargement of the tumors in both ventricles and a small tumor extending from the upper portion of the interventricular septum into the left ventricular outflow tract. An electrocardiogram showed 2–3 mm ST segment depression in leads I, aVL, and V4-6. Gated single photon emission CT showed low perfusion at the lateral and inferior regions of the left ventricle, indicating myocardial ischemia. Corticotrophin was withdrawn and 3 months later the patient was asymptomatic. An echocardiogram showed that the tumors had reduced in size, and there was concomitant improvement in the electrocardiogram.

Nervous system *Cerebral shrinkage* and *subdural hematoma* occurred after the administration of high doses of ACTH for West syndrome (total dose 4.5–6.75 mg) and subdural hematoma occurred in two children (aged 2 and 5 months) during the administration of low doses of synthetic ACTH (0.01 mg/kg/day; total dose 0.24–0.26 mg) (2^A).

SYSTEMIC GLUCOCORTICOSTEROIDS *(SED-14, 1369; SEDA-23, 427; SEDA-24, 450))*

In 539 patients with systemic lupus erythematosus organ damage was associated with corticosteroid therapy compared with controls (3^C). Oral prednisone 10 mg/day for 10 years (cumulative dose 36.6 g) was significantly associated with *osteoporotic fractures* (RR = 2.5; 95%CI = 1.7, 3.7), symptomatic *coronary artery disease* (RR = 1.7; CI = 1.1, 2.5), and *cataracts* (RR = 1.7; CI = 1.4, 2.5). *Avascular necrosis* was associated with high-dose prednisone (at least 60 mg/day for at least 2 months; RR = 1.2; CI = 1.1, 1.4). Intravenous pulses of methylprednisolone (1000 mg for 1–3 days) were associated with a small increase in the risk of osteoporotic fractures (RR 1.3; CI = 1.0, 1.8).

Nervous system Dexamethasone is widely used for the prevention and treatment of chronic lung disease in premature infants, in whom follow-up studies have raised the possibility of an association with *alterations in neuromotor*

Side Effects of Drugs, Annual 25
J.K. Aronson, ed.

function and somatic growth. In 159 survivors (mean age 53 months) of a previous placebo-controlled study the children who had received dexamethasone had a significantly higher incidence of *cerebral palsy* (39/80 vs 12/79; OR = 4.62, 95%CI = 2.38, 8.98) (4[C]). The most common form of cerebral palsy was spastic diplegia. Developmental delay was more frequent in the dexamethasone group (44/80 vs 23/79; OR = 2.9, CI = 1.5, 5.4).

Prednisone, 10 mg/day for 1 year, has been evaluated in 136 patients with probable Alzheimer's disease in a double-blind, randomized, placebo-controlled trial (5[C]). There were no differences in the primary measures of efficacy (cognitive subscale of the Alzheimer Disease Assessment Scale), but those treated with prednisone had significantly greater *memory impairment* (Clinical Dementia sum of boxes), and *agitation* and *hostility/suspicion* (Brief Psychiatric Rating Scale). Other adverse effects in those who took prednisone were *reduced bone density* and a small *rise in intraocular pressure.*

A rare case of osteoporotic spine fracture associated with epidural lipomatosis causing paraplegia has been described after long-term cortisone therapy (6[A])

A 40-year-old woman with ulcerative colitis took cortisone 20 mg/day and developed progressive paraplegia. There was kyphosis of the thoracic spine from T7 to T9, with pathological fractures. An MRI scan showed massive epidural fat extending from T1 to T9. She recovered 3 months after surgical removal of the epidural fat.

Psychiatric Glucocorticoids can cause *impaired memory* (SEDA-23, 428) and some have found correlations between impairment of some elements of memory performance and cortisol concentrations associated with physical and psychological stress (SEDA-24, 453). A recent study in healthy individuals undergoing acute stress cortisone has shown specifically impaired retrieval of declarative long-term memory for a word list, suggesting that cortisol-induced impairment of retrieval may add significantly to the memory deficits caused by prolonged treatment (7[c]).

Endocrine One unanswered question is whether the *growth suppression* that occurs in children during glucocorticoid treatment persists after treatment is withdrawn and affects final adult height. In an attempt to answer this question, growth 6–7 years after withdrawal of alternate-day treatment with prednisone has been evaluated in children (aged 6–14 years) with cystic fibrosis who had participated in a multicenter trial from 1986 to 1991 (8[C]). Of 224 children, 161 had been randomized to prednisone (1 or 2 mg/kg) and 73 to placebo. At the time of the study 68% were aged 18 years or more. Height fell during prednisone therapy, but catch-up growth began 2 years after withdrawal. However, the heights of the boys treated with prednisone remained significantly lower by 4 cm than those who took placebo. In contrast, in the girls there were no differences in height at 2–3 years after prednisone withdrawal.

Many protocols for treating children with early B cell acute lymphoblastic leukemia involve 28 consecutive days of high-dose glucocorticoids during induction. The effect of this therapy on adrenal function has been prospectively evaluated (9[A]) in 10 children by co-syntropin (corticotrophin 1–24) stimulation before the start of dexamethasone therapy and every 4 weeks thereafter until adrenal function returned to normal. All had normal adrenal function before dexamethasone treatment and impaired adrenal responses 24 hours after completing therapy. Each child felt ill for 2–4 weeks after completing therapy. Seven patients recovered normal adrenal function after 4 weeks, but three did not have normal adrenal function until 8 weeks after withdrawal. Thus, high-dose dexamethasone therapy can cause adrenal insufficiency lasting more than 4 weeks after the end of treatment. This problem might be avoided by tapering doses of glucocorticoids and providing supplementary glucocorticoids during periods of increased stress.

An *acute adrenal crisis* occurred in a woman who received an intra-articular corticosteroid for pseudogout of the knee (10[A]).

An 87-year-old woman received intra-articular betamethasone (Diprophos®) 7 mg on three occasions for painful knee joints over 6 months. Six weeks after the last injection she developed diffuse pain and contractures in the legs, fatigue, nausea, abdominal pain, and weight loss of 6 kg. Both knee joints were tender but there was no effusion. Her serum sodium concentration was 123 mmol/l, serum osmolality 254 mOsm/kg, urine sodium 136 mmol/l, and urinary osmolality 373 mOsm/kg. The syndrome of inappropriate antidiuretic hormone secretion was diagnosed, but despite treatment she remained drowsy and hyponatremic. About a week later, she developed hypotension and symptoms of an acute abdomen.

Further investigations showed that her basal cortisol concentration was low (36 nmol/l) but it increased to 481 nmol/l after a short Synacthen test, consistent with acute adrenal crisis. She recovered rapidly after treatment with oral hydrocortisone, but still required corticosteroid substitution several months later.

Liver Fatal *liver failure* after high-dose methylprednisolone pulse therapy for thyroid eye disease has been reported (11[A]).

A 71-year-old white woman with a compressive optic neuropathy was given five cycles of intravenous methylprednisolone 1 g/day for 3 days followed by tapering oral cortisone for 10–14 days. The intervals between cycles were 14 days to 6 weeks. She was otherwise healthy and had no history of liver disease. Her liver function tests were normal or only slightly raised during the first five cycles. She then developed raised liver enzymes, a prolonged prothrombin time, and fatal liver failure. Post-mortem examination showed necrosis of the liver parenchyma. Hepatitis serology (A, B, and C) was negative as was in situ hybridization for immunohistochemical proof of hepatitis Bs and Bc or delta virus antibodies in the liver.

Skin A delayed hypersensitivity reaction, characterized by a *skin rash*, due to dexamethasone has been reported (12[A]). These kinds of reactions to systemic corticosteroids are rarely reported.

A 59-year-old woman, who had not used corticosteroids before, developed an exfoliative rash on her face, upper chest, and skin folds after 3 days treatment with oral dexamethasone (dosage not stated) for an acute episode of encephalomyelitis disseminata. Dexamethasone was immediately withdrawn and her skin lesions resolved over several days. Patch tests were positive to dexamethasone, betamethasone, and clobetasol, but negative to other corticosteroids, including prednisolone, hydrocortisone butyrate, methylprednisolone, and triamcinolone. Prick tests with all of these corticosteroids were negative. She tolerated oral methylprednisolone without adverse effects.

Musculoskeletal The risk of *vertebral deformity* is increased by the combination of an oral corticosteroid and advanced age, according to the findings in 229 patients (69% women) taking long-term oral corticosteroids (prednisone equivalents of 5 mg/day or more) and 286 untreated controls (13[C]). The duration of treatment was 0.5–37 (median 4.8) years. More than 60% of the treatment group were aged over 60 years, and most (62%) had been treated for rheumatoid arthritis. Bone mineral density data were analyzed in 194 patients. The researchers identified at least one vertebral deformity (defined as a more than 20% reduction in anterior, middle, or posterior vertebral height) in 65 (28%) of the patients in the treatment group, and two or more fractures were identified in 25 (11%). In the treatment group, vertebral deformities were significantly more common in men than in women, and the prevalence of deformities increased with age. Compared with patients aged under 60 years, corticosteroid-treated patients aged 70–79 years had a 5-fold increased risk of vertebral deformity (OR = 5.1; 95%CI = 2.0, 13). The prevalence of vertebral deformities increased significantly with age in the corticosteroid group. While the mean spine and femoral bone mineral density scores were lower in the corticosteroid group, logistic regression analysis showed that bone mineral density was only a modest predictor of deformity. Age is an important independent risk factor, with very high prevalence rates in those over 70 years. Increasing duration of corticosteroid use may increase the risk of fracture.

Osteonecrosis (*aseptic necrosis* or *avascular necrosis*) is a well-recognized adverse effect of high-dose corticosteroid therapy, and the risk has been assessed in a nested case-control study using computer records (14[C]). There were 31 cases during 720 000 person-years. Avascular necrosis was strongly associated with corticosteroid exposure (RR = 16). When total prednisone exposure over 35 months was stratified into three levels (under 440 mg, 440–1290 mg, and over 1290 mg), there was no excess risk for cumulative doses of up to 440 mg (RR = 0, 95% CI = 0, 5). The relative risk was increased at doses between 440–1290 mg (RR = 6, CI = 1, 43) and indeterminately increased at doses over 1290 mg (CI = 26, infinity).

Glucocorticoid therapy is associated with *bone loss*, *osteoporosis*, and an *increased risk of fracture*. The clinical implications of recent clinical trials in the management of corticosteroid-induced osteoporosis have been reviewed (15[R]). Although corticosteroids can cause changes in trabecular microarchitecture, loss of bone (reduced bone density) seems to be the major determinant of osteoporosis (16[C]). The risk of vertebral fractures is not different in patients taking or not taking corticosteroids, in whom bone mineral density is similar (17[C]). Reduced bone mineral density induced by corticosteroids is related to the route of administration, the dose, the duration of treatment, and the cumulative dose.

A reduction in bone mineral density has been described in 23 patients (19 men) with chronic fatigue syndrome taking low-dose glucocorticoids in a double-blind, randomized, placebo-controlled study (18[C]). The patients took hydrocortisone 25–35 mg/day or matched placebo for 3 months. Mean bone mineral density in the spine fell by 2% with hydrocortisone and increased by 1% with placebo.

Bone loss caused by steroids can be prevented in non-osteoporotic patients with calcium and vitamin D, bisphosphonates, and calcitonin. Other agents are effective in special populations. Vitamin K prevented bone loss in 20 patients with chronic glomerulonephritis treated with prednisolone (19[c]) and ciclosporin 4.8 mg/kg/day prevented steroid-induced osteopenia in 52 patients taking prednisone 10 mg/day after kidney transplantation (20[c]).

Risedronate, a bisphosphonate, has similar efficacy to other bisphosphonates in the treatment of corticosteroid-induced osteoporosis. The effects of risedronate on bone density and vertebral fracture have been studied in 518 patients (mean age 59 years, 40% with rheumatoid arthritis, 56% men, 64% of the women postmenopausal) taking moderate to high doses of oral corticosteroids (equivalent to prednisone 7.5 mg/day or more) (21[C]). The patients were randomized double-blind to placebo, or risedronate 2.5 or 5 mg/day for 1 year. All took elemental calcium 1000 mg/day and vitamin D 400 IU/day. The mean density of the lumbar spine fell by 1% in the placebo group and increased by 1.3% and 1.9% with risedronate 2.5 and 5 mg respectively. There was a significant reduction of 70% in the risk of vertebral fracture with risedronate 5 mg compared with placebo. There were similar incidences of adverse effects in all the groups.

Similar results have been reported in a clinical trial in 290 patients (38% men, 55% of the women postmenopausal) taking high-dose corticosteroid therapy (prednisone over 7.5 mg/day or equivalent) (22[C]). The subjects were randomized to receive placebo or risedronate 2.5 or 5 mg/day for 1 year. All took elemental calcium 1000 mg/day and vitamin D 400 IU/day. Risedronate 5 mg increased bone mineral density at 1 year by a mean of 2.9% in the lumbar spine, 1.8% in the femoral neck, and 2.4% in the trochanter. The values for placebo were 0.4%, −0.3%, and 1.0% respectively. The results for risedronate 2.5 mg were positive but not significant compared with placebo. The incidence of spinal fractures was reduced by 70% in the combined risedronate treatment groups compared with placebo. Risedronate and placebo caused similar adverse effects.

Immunologic *Exacerbation of giant cell arteritis*, with clinical signs of an evolving vertebrobasilar stroke, has been attributed to prednisolone (23[A]).

A 64-year-old man with giant cell arteritis was given prednisolone 60 mg/day. Within 5 days he developed double vision and agitation and became drowsy and confused. A cranial MRI scan showed recent cerebral lesions and a Doppler scan showed high-resistant blood flow in both vertebral arteries. He had an episode of complete loss of vision and was given dexamethasone and intravenous heparin followed by warfarin. He gradually improved over the next few weeks but was left with cognitive and memory deficits.

Budesonide has recently been marketed in oral form for intestinal inflammatory disease. An *anaphylactic-like reaction* has been associated with oral budesonide (24[A]).

A 32-year-old woman with Crohn's disease, who had taken prednisone 20 mg/day and azathioprine 150 mg/day, switched to budesonide 9 mg/day because of weight gain, and 5 minutes after the first capsule her tongue and throat swelled, accompanied by wheeziness and diarrhea. She was given clemastine and recovered after 4 days. Intracutaneous tests with diluted budesonide suggested a non-IgE mediated reaction. She had a previous history of a similar reaction to mesalazine. One year later her tongue and throat swelled after intravenous dexamethasone.

Erythema multiforme has been attributed to deflazacort (25[A]).

A 27-year-old woman, a pharmacist, had dermatitis on three separate occasions a few hours after she started to take oral deflazacort 6 mg for vesicular hand eczema. On each occasion, her symptoms included a widespread macular rash mainly on the inner aspects of her arms and legs and buttocks. She also had severe scaling, fever, nausea, vomiting, malaise, and hypotension. A skin biopsy was consistent with erythema multiforme, and direct immunofluorescence showed granular deposits at the dermoepidermal junction. Patch tests to the commercial formulation of deflazacort 6 mg (1% aq) and to pure deflazacort (1% aq) were positive, but there were no cross-reactions to other corticosteroids.

The author commented that the patient probably developed hypersensitivity to deflazacort as a result of occupational exposure.

A case of *fever* and *leukopenia* with methylprednisolone and prednisolone has been reported in a 29-year-old woman with systemic lupus erythematosus (26[A]). The authors commented that fever associated with corticosteroids occurs frequently, whereas leukopenia is rare. Fever and leukopenia are important signs of an exacerbation of systemic lupus erythematosus, and it would be difficult to distinguish between an exacerbation of the disease and an adverse effect of corticosteroids.

Infection risk Patients taking corticosteroids have an increased risk of infections, including those produced by rare pathogens. Singleton pregnancies delivered at 24–34 weeks after antenatal betamethasone exposure have been prospectively analysed, in order to study the incidence of perinatal infection (27[C]). There were 453 patients, 267 of whom took a single course of betamethasone (two doses of 12 mg in 24 hours), and 186 of whom took a multiple course (more than two doses in the 24 hours after the initial course). Multiple courses were significantly associated with early-onset *neonatal sepsis* (OR = 5.0, 95%CI = 1.0, 23), *neonatal death* (OR = 2.9, CI = 1.3, 6.9), *chorioamnionitis* (OR = 10, CI = 2.1, 65), and *endometritis* (OR = 3.6, CI = 1.7, 8.1). Respiratory distress and intraventricular hemorrhage were similar in the two groups. Although the study was nonrandomized the results suggest an increased risk of neonatal infection and death after multiple courses of dexamethasone during pregnancy.

Of 31 patients who received 1 ml (40 mg) of methylprednisolone epidurally at the end of microdiscectomy, three developed *epidural abscesses* (28[A]). These results were compared with a historical series of 400 patients not taking steroids, who had no deep infection. Although the data were limited, epidural steroids after discectomy should not be recommended.

Fatal pulmonary infection with *Aspergillus fumigatus* and *Nocardia asteroides* has been described in a patient who took prednisone 1 mg/kg/day for 1 month for bronchiolitis obliterans (29[A]).

Cutaneous alternariosis (infection with *Alternaria alternata*) has been described in a 78-year-old farmer with idiopathic pulmonary fibrosis taking oral prednisone 20 mg/day (30[A]).

Carcinogenicity *Kaposi's sarcoma* has been associated with prednisolone therapy in two elderly women (31[A]).

An 84-year-old woman with polymyalgia rheumatica and a 79-year-old woman with undifferentiated connective tissue disease and leukocytoclastic vasculitis were given prednisolone 20 mg/day with subsequent dosage reductions. The first patient developed a raised purpuric rash and lymphedema of the left leg within 5 months and the second developed large purple nodules on the soles of her feet and the backs of her hands accompanied by periorbital and peripheral oedema. Skin biopsies showed Kaposi's sarcoma, and both patients had raised IgG antibody titers to human herpesvirus-8.

Prior infection with herpesvirus-8 is a requisite for the development of Kaposi's sarcoma. The question arises as to how steroid treatment alone can lead to the emergence of this malignancy. In vitro evidence supports the hypothesis that glucocorticoids have a direct role in stimulating tumor development and the activation of herpesvirus-8.

SECOND-GENERATION EFFECTS

Teratogenicity The teratogenic effects of prednisone have been evaluated in a placebo-controlled study in 372 women and a meta-analysis (32[CM]). There was no statistical difference in the rate of major anomalies between the corticoid-exposed women and the controls. The meta-analysis included 10 studies (six cohort and four case-control) with data from 535 exposed and 50 845 non-exposed women. The odds ratios for major malformations were 1.5 (95%CI = 0.8, 2.6) for the cohort studies and 3.4 (CI = 2.0, 5.7) for the case-control studies. The results suggest that although prednisone does not represent a major teratogenic risk in humans in therapeutic doses, it does increase the risk of oral cleft defects by an order of 3.4-fold.

Pregnancy Treatment of pregnant women with a single course of antenatal corticosteroids to enhance fetal lung maturation significantly reduces neonatal mortality and morbidity. However, the safety and efficacy of repeated courses of antenatal corticosteroids have not been adequately studied. The risks of early-onset neonatal sepsis and neonatal death were significantly increased in neonates exposed in utero to multiple antenatal courses of β-methasone (27[C]) (see above under Infection risk).

In a retrospective study in 609 mothers and their 713 infants who were treated with 1–12 courses of antenatal corticosteroids, data from 369 singleton preterm infants born at 34 weeks or later, 210 multiple gestations, and 134 infants delivered at 35 weeks or later were analysed (33[c]). The incidence of respiratory distress syndrome was 45% for single courses and 35% for multiple courses of corticosteroids (OR = 0.44; 95%CI = 0.25, 0.79). The multiple-course group also had significantly less cases of patent ductus arteriosus (20% vs 13%). The incidences of death before discharge and other neonatal morbidities were similar. The multiple-course group had a significant reduction of 0.46 cm in head circumference at birth when adjusted for gestational age and pre-eclampsia. The two groups had similar birth weights. Infants born at more than 35 weeks, multiple-gestation infants, and infants who were born more than 7 days after the last dose of corticosteroid had similar outcomes, regardless of the number of courses they had received. Mothers treated with multiple courses compared with a single course had a significantly higher incidence of post-partum endometritis, even though they had a lower incidence of prolonged rupture of membranes (24% vs 33%) and similar cesarean delivery rates. In conclusion, antenatal exposure to multiple courses of corticosteroids compared with a single course resulted in a significant reduction in the incidence of respiratory distress syndrome in singleton preterm infants delivered within a week of the last corticosteroid dose. This was associated with a reduction in head circumference at birth and an increased incidence of maternal endometritis. Whether the potential benefits of repeated therapy outweigh the risks will ultimately be determined in randomized controlled trials.

A study in 10 women has been conducted to determine whether betamethasone administered at risk of preterm delivery causes adrenal suppression (34[c]). After adrenal stimulation with ACTH 1 μg at 24–25 weeks each woman received two intramuscular doses of betamethasone 12 mg 24 hours apart; 1 week later another ACTH test was followed by another two doses of betamethasone; a third ACTH stimulation test was carried out 1 week later. All the women had normal baseline and stimulated cortisol concentrations during the first ACTH stimulation test. Mean baseline serum cortisol concentrations fell with each ACTH stimulation test, from 25.4 μg/dl (700 nmol/l) before betamethasone to 4.3 μg/dl (120 nmol/l) 1 week after the second course of betamethasone). The mean stimulated cortisol concentrations also fell significantly, from 33.0 μg/dl (910 nmol/l) to 11.8 μg/dl (326 nmol/l). There was evidence of adrenal suppression in four patients after the first course of betamethasone and in seven patients after the second course. There was no evidence of Addisonian crisis antepartum or intrapartum.

Drug interactions Most glucocorticosteroids are metabolized in part by CYP3A4, which can be induced and inhibited in pharmacokinetic interactions. The following interactions can be attributed to this mechanism.

- In one study *ketoconazole* was given orally as 200 mg od for 4 days, followed a single oral dose of budesonide 3 mg either at the same as ketoconazole or 12 hours before (35[c]). Ketoconazole increased budesonide concentrations (C_{max} and AUC) 6.8- to 7.6-fold when the two drugs were coadministered; with a 12 hour separation, budesonide concentrations increased only 1.7- to 2.1-fold. Another imidazole, *itraconazole*, given orally increased oral prednisolone concentrations by only 24% (36[c]) but increased intravenous dexamethasone concentrations 3.3-fold and oral dexamethasone 3.7-fold (37[c]).
- *Oral contraceptives* increased budesonide concentrations by only 22%, but prednisolone concentrations increased by 131%, suggesting a clinically relevant interaction (38[c]).
- Methylprednisolone concentrations increased with the coadministration of *diltiazem* (2.6-fold), *mibefradil* (3.8-fold), and *grapefruit juice* (1.75-fold) (39[c], 40[c]).
- Budesonide for collagenous colitis caused Cushing's syndrome in a patient with

chronic renal insufficiency taking *amiodarone* for paroxysmal atrial fibrillation (41[A]).

An 81-year-old man with persistent diarrhea was given oral budesonide 9 mg/day, following unsuccessful treatment with mesalazine and prednisone. He was also taking amiodarone 100 mg/day. His diarrhea resolved within 6 weeks, and attempts to reduce the dosage of budesonide resulted in recurrent diarrhea. After 11 months he developed Cushing's syndrome, which persisted despite a reduction in dosage to 3 mg/day. His mild diarrhea recurred and the dosage of budesonide was increased to 6 mg/day with worsening of Cushing's syndrome; the dosage was reduced to 3 mg/day. Four weeks later amiodarone was withdrawn. The symptoms of Cushing's syndrome resolved within 4 weeks.

The authors suggested that the development of Cushing's syndrome and its persistence at a low dosage of budesonide was caused by inhibition of the metabolism of budesonide by amiodarone.

Patients taking budesonide with drugs that are metabolized by CYP3A should be carefully monitored.

Conversely, intravenous methylprednisolone (1 g/day for 3 days) has been reported to inhibit the metabolism of *oral anticoagulants* (acenocoumarol and fluindinone) in 10 patients, increasing the INR by 8 (range 5–20) (42[c]).

In a probable pharmacodynamic interaction, severe peripheral edema followed treatment with *montelukast* and prednisone for asthma (43[A]).

A 23-year-old man, with a history of asthma, house dust mite allergy, and rhinoconjunctivitis, presented with acute respiratory symptoms. He was given oral cetirizine, inhaled salmeterol and fluticasone propionate, and oral prednisone 40 mg/day for 1 week and 20 mg/day for 1 week. His asthma recurred when prednisone was withdrawn and he took oral prednisone 60 mg/day for 1 week and 40 mg/day for 1 week. He also took montelukast 10 mg/day. He then developed severe peripheral edema with a gain in weight of 13 kg. Prednisone was withdrawn and his edema resolved. Montelukast was continued.

The author commented that the patient had tolerated prednisone without montelukast and montelukast without prednisone. However, he had severe edema when both drugs were used together. Montelukast may have potentiated corticosteroid-induced renal tubular sodium and fluid retention. Both have previously been associated with edema.

SPECIAL ROUTES OF ADMINISTRATION OF CORTICOSTEROIDS *(SED-14, 1387; SEDA-23, 431; SEDA-24, 459)*

Epidural and intrathecal administration Cervical epidural steroid injection is often used for the treatment of cervical radiculopathy. Subjective patient satisfaction has been reported, but controlled trials have not yet delineated the effectiveness of this procedure. Three cases of severe *pain* consistent with nerve injury have been reported immediately after cervical epidural steroid injection, bringing into question the benefit-harm ratio of this technique (44[A]).

Intra-articular administration *Anaphylaxis* occurred in two women after intra-articular administration of paramethasone plus mepivacaine 2% (45[A]).

A 44-year-old woman developed generalized pruritus 10 minutes after intra-articular paramethasone and mepivacaine and 30 minutes later developed generalized urticaria, tachycardia, and dyspnea. She received emergency treatment and her condition initially improved. However, her symptoms recurred after 6 hours and she was treated again and then discharged taking oral dexchlorpheniramine. She had a history of allergic contact dermatitis due to nickel sulfate sensitization, and 7 years before had had generalized urticaria and dyspnea after intra-articular administration of a corticosteroid.

A 31-year-old woman developed generalized pruritus and urticaria, facial edema, and dyspnea 2 hours after the intra-articular administration of paramethasone and mepivacaine. She was treated with an intramuscular corticosteroid and antihistamines, with worsening of her symptoms. She received intravenous fluids and dexchlorpheniramine, but her symptoms recurred after 1 hour, when she was given subcutaneous adrenaline, intravenous fluids and dexchlorpheniramine. She was later discharged taking oral diphenhydramine. She had a history of a systemic reaction after the administration of a corticosteroid and a local anesthetic.

Skin prick tests were positive for isolated paramethasone in both patients, but negative for mepivacaine. There has only been one previous report of anaphylaxis in association with paramethasone.

Osteomyelitis after three steroid injections for tennis elbow has been reported; the second injection was given 3 months after the first and the third 2 days later (46[A]). This case illustrates the need for vigilance, even after common procedures, and that exacerbation of symptoms after local steroid injections should prompt the doctor to review the diagnosis and consider the need for further investigation.

PROSTAGLANDINS *(SED-14, 1396; SEDA-23, 432; SEDA-24, 459)*

Alprostadil (prostaglandin E_1)

Cardiovascular Moderate or severe *phlebitis* can occur at the site of venipuncture in some patients who receive prostaglandin E_1 (PGE_1) infusion therapy. It is sometimes severe enough to necessitate withdrawal of therapy. The frequency and severity of phlebitis has been investigated in 18 men, mean age 63 (range 47–78) years, with peripheral vascular disease who received a 2-hour infusion twice daily (47[c]). Although 60 μg of PGE_1 is usually dissolved in 500 ml of fluid to avoid phlebitis, in this study 200 ml was used to prevent volume overload. The solution was neutralized to pH 7.4 with 4 ml of 7% sodium bicarbonate. Two patients had grade 0, four grade 1, 11 grade 2, and one grade 3 phlebitis (by Dinley's criteria (48[R])). Age correlated negatively with the severity of phlebitis. Usually PGE_1 infusion therapy is stopped when phlebitis reaches grade 4 or more, but there were no such cases in this study.

Skin A neonate with transposition of the great vessels developed *urticaria* during treatment with alprostadil (49[A]). While flushing and peripheral edema are well recognized, urticaria has not been described before.

Musculoskeletal Alprostadil infusion can produce *bone cortical hyperostosis*. Periosteal changes have been described in 15 neonates after the administration of alprostadil for more than 1 week (50[c]). Serum alkaline phosphatase activity was significantly raised. The long bones and clavicles were most commonly involved and symmetrically affected. The scapula was involved in two cases and the ribs in seven. The involvement of clavicles has not been previously reported.

Gemeprost

Cardiovascular Two women developed *myocardial ischemia* during treatment with gemeprost for termination of pregnancy (51[A]).

A 29-year-old woman, a smoker with a history of renal insufficiency, obesity, hypertension, hypercholesterolemia, and cardiac dysrhythmias, underwent termination of pregnancy at 10 weeks with a pessary of gemeprost 1 mg and 5 hours later dilatation and evacuation, followed by tubal ligation. After surgery, her blood pressure became unmeasurable, her heart rate dropped to 40 beats/min, and she developed ventricular fibrillation. She was given streptokinase and intravenous heparin for suspected pulmonary embolism; her blood pressure rose and was maintained with adrenaline and noradrenaline. Angiography showed an 80% stenosis of her right coronary artery and complete occlusion of the anterior interventricular branch. Blood flow was re-established by coronary angioplasty.

A 32-year-old woman, a smoker, had an evacuation after the death of her fetus at 18 weeks. Two pessaries of gemeprost 1 mg were inserted 7.25 hours apart, and about 90 minutes later she became unconscious, apneic, and cyanotic, and had dilated pupils and no detectable blood pressure or pulse. She was given 100% oxygen, intravenous adrenaline and dobutamine, and a crystalloid infusion. Her systolic pressure rose to 100 mmHg. Coronary angiography showed left and circumflex coronary artery spasm.

The author commented that the myocardial ischemia experienced by both of these patients was thought to be due to prostaglandin-induced coronary spasm. It would be prudent to monitor every woman treated with gemeprost during the course of an abortion.

Latanoprost

Sensory systems Latanoprost can produce *darkening of the iris* in 10–25% of patients treated for 0.5–2 years. In a 50-year-old man with peripheral iris darkening after latanoprost treatment, the darkening did not change appreciably for several years after withdrawal (52[A]).

Cystoid macular edema has been associated with latanoprost, but a review of the published literature (28 eyes in 25 patients) has shown that in all cases there were other associated risk factors, so that a definitive conclusion about a causal relation cannot be reached (53[R]). Nevertheless, latanoprost should be used with caution in patients with risk factors for cystoid macular edema and special surveillance must be done.

Skin *Hyperpigmentation of the eyelids* can occur during latanoprost therapy (54[A]).

A 62-year old Korean woman treated with latanoprost for 4 months developed eyelid pigmentation in both upper and lower eyelids of both eyes. There was no increase in iris pigmentation. The eyelid pigmentation gradually diminished after withdrawal, but minimal brownish coloration remained along the lower eyelid folds in both eyes at 4 months.

Hair, nails, and sweat glands Latanoprost has been reported to have caused *regrowth of eyelash hair* (55[A]).

A 53-year-old woman, with glaucoma and loss of the eyelashes secondary to alopecia following an allergic response to ibuprofen was given latanoprost. After 3 weeks her eyelashes were noticeable and 2 months later full growth had occurred.

Misoprostol

The manufacturers GD Searle have distributed a "Dear Health Care Provider" letter in the USA, emphasizing the fact that misoprostol, by any route of administration, is not intended for the induction of labor or as a cervical ripening agent before termination of pregnancy (56[S]). Searle has become aware of instances in which misoprostol was used for such purposes, in spite of its being specifically contraindicated for use during pregnancy. The following serious adverse events have been reported after such off-label use: *maternal or fetal death*; *uterine hyperstimulation*; *uterine rupture or perforation* requiring surgical repair, hysterectomy, or salpingo-oophorectomy; *amniotic fluid embolism*; severe *vaginal bleeding*; *retained placenta*; *shock*; *fetal bradycardia*; and *pelvic pain*. Searle does not intend to study or support the use of misoprostol for pregnancy termination or labor induction. The company is therefore unable to provide complete risk information for misoprostol when it is used for such purposes. Furthermore, the effects of misoprostol on the later growth, development, and functional maturation of children who are exposed to it during induction of labor have not been established.

Reproductive system A single intravaginal dose of misoprostol 800 μg can obtain an abortion. The success rate has been assessed in 102 pregnant patients with amenorrhea for less than 42 weeks (57[C]). After 1 day and 3 days of administration the abortion rates were 72% and 87% respectively. A second dose 7 days later increased the cumulative rate to 92%. The main complaints were *pain* (85%), *nausea* (21%), and *headache* (18%). Similar results were obtained in 2295 pregnant women (up to 56 days of gestation), who took a single oral dose of mifepristone (200 mg) and were randomized to self-administer misoprostol 800 μg/day at home for 1, 2, or 3 days (58[C]). Complete abortion rates were 98%, 98%, and 96% among those who took misoprostol for 1, 2, and 3 days respectively. There were similar frequencies of adverse effects in all groups (*cramping*, *nausea*, *fever/chills*, *dizziness*, *vomiting*, *headache*, and *diarrhea*).

New cases of *uterine rupture* have been described after misoprostol vaginal administration during labor in patients with prior cesarean section (59[A], 60[A]), but also in a patient without previous cesarean section (two normal deliveries and a curettage after abortion) (61[A]). *Uterine dehiscence* occurred in one and *uterine rupture* in three of 48 women with prior cesarean sections treated with intravaginal misoprostol 50 μg for cervical ripening (62[A]). In comparison, uterine rupture occurred in one of 89 women who had an oxytocin infusion and none of 24 patients who received intravaginal prostaglandin E_1.

Teratogenicity Mothers who used misoprostol during pregnancy as an abortifacient had an increased risk of having a baby with *congenital anomalies* (OR = 2.4; 95% CI = 1.0, 6.2), as reported in a case-control study in Fortaleza, Brazil (63[C]).

In another case-control study in Brazil, 93 cases of prenatal exposure to misoprostol and 279 controls were recruited (64[C]). *Vascular disruption defects* (transverse terminal limb reductions, Moebius and/or Poland sequences, hypoglossia–hypodactyly sequence, arthrogryposis, intestinal atresia, hemifacial microsomia, microtia, and porencephalic cyst) were identified in 32 exposed infants compared with only 12 controls.

In another case-control study in Brazil, congenital anomalies were compared in 34 misoprostol-exposed children and 4639 unexposed controls (65[C]). Misoprostol exposure significantly increased the risk of arthrogryposis (OR = 8.5, 95% CI = 2, 37), hydrocephalus (OR = 4.2, CI = 1.5, 12), terminal transverse limb reduction (OR = 12, CI = 3.5, 41), and limb constriction ring or skin scars (OR = 40, CI = 11,

153). There were 13 different defects not previously described in the misoprostol-exposed cases, but only holoprosencephaly and bladder exstrophy significantly exceeded the expected number.

Misoprostol-induced arthrogryposis has been reported in 15 Brazilian patients (66[c]).

Sulprostone

Reproductive system Sulprostone can cause *rupture of the uterine cervix* (67[A]).

A 43 year-old woman, who had previously had a first trimester miscarriage that required evacuation of the uterus and a normal vaginal delivery at term 4 years before, was admitted for an abortion at 16 weeks. Ripening of the cervix was started with a pessary of gemeprost 1 mg. After 3 hours, when the cervix was 1 cm dilated, an intramuscular injection of sulprostone 500 μg was given. After 30 minutes she developed persistent abdominal pain, which became a continuous cramping and then a shooting pain; a male fetus of 170 g was aborted. There was a 3 cm longitudinal cervical rupture located posteriorly that reached the posterior fornix.

PROSTACYCLIN ANALOGS

(SEDA-23, 436; SEDA-24, 463)

Beraprost

A stable orally active prostacyclin analogue, cicaprost, was withdrawn at an early stage of clinical development in the 1980s because of too narrow a margin between efficacy and tolerance. Beraprost, another stable orally active prostacyclin analogue, has recently been tested in patients with intermittent claudication in a randomized placebo-controlled trial (68[C]). Beraprost improved walking distance more often than placebo. It also reduced the incidence of critical cardiovascular events, but the trial was not powered for statistical validation of this effect. As with iloprost, *headache* and *flushing* were the most common adverse effects.

Epoprostenol

Epoprostenol has become the preferred long-term treatment for patients with primary pulmonary hypertension who continue to have symptoms despite conventional therapy. *Pulmonary edema* has been described during such treatment (69[A]).

A 66-year-old woman with scleroderma and severe pulmonary hypertension was given continuous intravenous epoprostenol 2 and then 4 ng/kg/min (total duration 48 hours). Two weeks later her dyspnea had improved, but her leg was swollen and her oxygen saturation had fallen. Her dosage of epoprostenol was increased to 5 ng/kg/min. One month later she developed increasing dyspnea, a non-productive cough, severe edema of her legs, and severe hypoxemia. She had gained 5 kg in weight and there were new bibasal lung crackles. A chest X-ray showed bilateral air-space opacities and bilateral effusions. Her PaO2 was 5.7 kPa, PaCO2 3.9 kPa, and the arterial pH 7.51. Pulmonary veno-occlusive disease was diagnosed and the infusion of epoprostenol was gradually tapered over the next 48 hours. She died 6 days later with right-sided heart failure. At autopsy, histological examination showed thickening of the alveolar septa by proliferation of dilated capillaries on both sides of the alveolar walls, consistent with pulmonary capillary hemangiomatosis.

Iloprost

The stable prostacyclin analogue iloprost is mainly used in patients with chronic critical leg ischemia due to atherosclerosis or to Buerger's disease. Episodic digital ischemia in patients with systemic sclerosis or related disorders is another use. The most frequently observed adverse effects, *facial flushing* and *headache*, are caused by profound vasodilatation.

Four women with CREST syndrome or systemic sclerosis had *pain and eventually contracture of the masseter muscles* during infusion of iloprost for severe attacks of Raynaud's phenomenon (70[A]). The adverse effect was quickly reversed by reducing the infusion rate. There were no electrocardiographic or cardiac enzyme changes. The mechanism of this effect is obscure.

Inhalation of aerosolized iloprost is being tested in patients with severe primary or secondary pulmonary hypertension refractory to conventional therapy. The aim is to produce predominantly pulmonary vasodilatation without significant systemic effects. In an uncontrolled series of 19 patients, the most common adverse effects of inhaled iloprost were *coughing*, *nausea*, *edema*, and *thoracic pain* (71[c]). In most patients these effects were transient and rarely required a change in therapy.

REFERENCES

1. Hiraishi S, Iwanami N, Ogawa N. Enlargement of cardiac rhabdomyoma and myocardial ischaemia during corticotropin treatment for infantile spasm. Heart 2000; 84: 170.
2. Ito M, Miyajima T, Fujii T, Okuno T. Subdural hematoma during low-dose ACTH therapy in patients with West syndrome. Neurology 2000; 54: 2346–7.
3. Zonana-Nacach A, Barr SG, Magder LS, Petri M. Damage in systemic lupus erythematosus and its association with corticosteroids. Arthritis Rheum 2000; 43: 1801–8.
4. Shinwell ES, Karplus M, Reich D, Weintraub Z, Blazer S, Bader D, Yurman S, Dolfin T, Kogan A, Dollberg S, Arbel E, Goldberg M, Gur I, Naor N, Sirota L, Mogilner S, Zaritsky A, Barak M, Gottfried E. Early postnatal dexamethasone treatment and increased incidence of cerebral palsy. Arch Dis Child Fetal Neonatal Ed 2000; 83: F177–81.
5. Aisen PS, Davis KL, Berg JD, Schafer K, Campbell K, Thomas RG, Weiner MF, Farlow MR, Sano M, Grundman M, Thal LJ, for the Alzheimer's Disease Cooperative Study. A randomized controlled trial of prednisone in Alzheimer's disease. Neurology 2000; 54: 588–93.
6. Andress HJ, Schürmann M, Heuck A, Schmand J, Lob G. A rare case of osteoporotic spine fracture associated with epidural lipomatosis causing paraplegia following long-term cortisone therapy. Arch Orthop Trauma Surg 2000; 120: 484–6.
7. De Quervein D-JF, Roozendaal B, Nitsch RM, McGaugh JL, Hock C. Acute cortisone administration impairs retrieval of long-term declarative memory in humans. Nat Neurosci 2000; 3: 313–14.
8. Lai H-C, FitzSimmons SC, Allen DB, Kosorok MR, Rosenstein BJ, Campbell PW, Farrell PM. Risk of persistent growth impairment after alternate-day prednisone treatment in children with cystic fibrosis. New Engl J Med 2000; 342: 851–9.
9. Felner EI, Thompson MT, Ratliff AF, White PC, Dickson BA. Time course of recovery of adrenal function in children treated for leukemia. J Pediatr 2000; 137: 21–4.
10. Wicki J, Droz M, Cirafici L, Vallotton MB. Acute adrenal crisis in a patient treated with intraarticular steroid therapy. J Rheumatol 2000; 27: 510–11.
11. Weissel M, Hauff W. Fatal liver failure after high-dose glucocorticoid pulse therapy in a patient with severe thyroid eye disease. Thyroid 2000; 10: 521.
12. Reinhold K, Schneider L, Hunzelmann N, Krieg T, Scharffetter-Kochanek K. Delayed-type allergy to systemic corticosteroids. Allergy 2000; 55: 1095–6.
13. Naganathan V, Jones G, Nash P, Nicholson G, Eisman J, Sambrook PN. Vertebral fracture risk with long-term corticosteroid therapy: prevalence and relation to age, bone density, and corticosteroid use. Arch Intern Med 2000; 160: 2917–22.
14. Bauer M, Thabault P, Estok D, Chrinstiansen C, Platt R. Low-dose corticosteroids and avascular necrosis of the hip and knee. Pharmacoepidemiol Drug Saf 2000; 9: 187–91.
15. Sambrook PN. Corticosteroid osteoporosis: practical implications of recent trials. J Bone Miner Res 2000; 15: 1645–9.
16. Lespessailles E, Siroux V, Poupon S, Andriambelosoa N, Pothuaud L, Harba R, Benhamou CL. Long-term corticosteroid therapy induces mild changes in trabecular bone texture. J Bone Miner Res 2000; 15: 747–53.
17. Selby PL, Halsey JP, Adams KRH, Klimiuk P, Knight SM, Pal B, Stewart IM, Swinson DR. Corticosteroids do not alter the threshold for vertebral fracture. J Bone Miner Res 2000; 15: 952–6.
18. Mckenzie R, Reynolds JC, O'Fallon A, Dale J, Deloria M, Blackwelder W, Straus SE. Decreased bone mineral density during low dose glucocorticoid administration in a randomized, placebo controlled trial. J Rheumatol 2000; 27: 2222–6.
19. Yonemura K, Kimura M, Miyaji T, Hishida A. Short-term effect of vitamin K administration on prednisolone-induced loss of bone mineral density in patients with chronic glomerulonephritis. Calcif Tissue Int 2000; 66: 123–8.
20. Westeel FP, Mazouz H, Ezaitouni F, Hottelart C, Ivan C, Fardellone P, Brazier M, EL Esper I, Petit J, Achard JM, Pruna A, Fournier A. Cyclosporine bone remodeling effect prevents steroid osteopenia after kidney transplantation. Kidney Int 2000; 58: 1788–96.
21. Wallach S, Cohen S, Reid DM, Hughes RA, Hosking DJ, Laan RF, Doherty SM, Maricic M, Rosen C, Brown J, Barton I, Chines AA. Effects of risedronate treatment on bone density and vertebral fracture in patients on corticosteroid therapy. Calcif Tissue Int 2000; 67: 277–85.
22. Reid DM, Hughes RA, Laan RFJM, Sacco-Gibson NA, Wenderoth DH, Adami S, Eusebio RA, Devogelaer JP. Efficacy and safety of daily risedronate in the treatment of corticosteroid-induced osteoporosis in men and women: a randomized trial. J Bone Miner Res 2000; 15: 1006–13.
23. Staunton H, Stafford F, Leader M, O'Riordain D. Deterioration of giant cell arteritis with corticosteroid therapy. Arch Neurol 2000; 57: 581–4.
24. Heeringa M, Zweers P, de Man RA, de Groot H. Anaphylactic-like reaction associated with oral budesonide. Br Med J 2000; 321: 927.
25. Garcia-Bravo B, Repiso JB, Camacho F. Systemic contact dermatitis due to deflazacort. Contact Dermatitis 2000; 43: 359–60.
26. Maeshima E, Yamada Y, Yukawa S. Fever and leucopenia with steroids. Lancet 2000; 355: 198.
27. Vermillion ST, Soper DE, Newman RB. Neonatal sepsis and death after multiple courses of antenatal betamethasone therapy. Am J Obstet Gynecol 2000; 183: 810–14.
28. Lowell TD, Errico TJ, Eskenazi MS. Use of epidural steroids after discectomy may predispose to

infection. Spine 2000; 25: 516–19.
29. Fernández JM, Sánchez E, Polo FJ, Sáez L. Infección pulmonar por *Aspergillus fumigatus* y *Nocardia* asteroides como complicación del tratamiento con glucocorticoides. Med Clin (Barc) 2000; 114: 358.
30. Ioannidou DJ, Stefanidou MP, Maraki SG, Panayiotides JG, Tosca AD. Cutaneous alternariosis in a patient with idiopathic pulmonary fibrosis. Int J Dermatol 2000; 39: 293–5.
31. Vincent T, Moss K, Colaco B, Venables PJW. Kaposi's sarcoma in two patients following low-dose corticosteroid treatment for rheumatological disease. Rheumatology 2000; 39: 1294–6.
32. Park-Wyllie L, Mazzotta P, Pastuszak A, Moretti ME, Beique L, Hunnisett L, Friesen MH, Jacobson S, Kasapinovic S, Chang D, Diav-Citrin O, Chitayat D, Nulman I, Einarson TR, Koren G. Birth defects after maternal exposure to corticosteroids: prospective cohort study and meta-analysis of epidemiological studies. Teratology 2000; 62: 385–92.
33. Abbasi S, Hirsch D, Davis J, Tolosa J, Stouffer N, Debbs R, Gerdes JS. Effect of single versus multiple courses of antenatal corticosteroids on maternal and neonatal outcome. Am J Obstet Gynecol 2000; 182: 1243–9.
34. Helal KJ, Gordon MC, Lightner CR, Barth WH. Adrenal suppression induced by betamethasone in women at risk for premature delivery. Obstet Gynecol 2000; 96: 287–90.
35. Seidegård J. Reduction of the inhibitory effect of ketoconazole on budesonide pharmacokinetics by separation of their time of administration. Clin Pharmacol Ther 2000; 67: 13–17.
36. Varis T, Kivistö KT, Neuvonen PJ. The effect of itraconazole on the pharmacokinetics and pharmacodynamics of oral prednisolone. Eur J Clin Pharmacol 2000; 56: 57–60.
37. Varis T, Kivistö KT, Backman JT, Neuvonen PJ. The cytochrome P450 3A4 inhibitor itraconazole markedly increases the plasma concentrations of dexamethasone and enhances its adrenal-suppressant effect. Clin Pharmacol Ther 2000; 68: 487–94.
38. Seidegård J, Simonsson M, Edsbäcker S. Effect of an oral contraceptive on the plasma levels of budesonide and prednisolone and the influence on plasma cortisol. Clin Pharmacol Ther 2000; 67: 373–81.
39. Varis T, Backman JT, Kivistö KT. Neuvonen PJ. Diltiazem and mibefradil increase the plasma concentrations and greatly enhance the adrenal-suppressant effect of oral methylprednisolone. Clin Pharmacol Ther 2000; 67: 215–21.
40. Varis T, Kivistö KT, Neuvonen PJ. Grapefruit juice can increase the plasma concentrations of oral methylprednisolone. Eur J Clin Pharmacol 2000; 56: 489–93.
41. Ahle GB, Blum AL, Martinek J, Oneta CM, Dorta G. Cushing's syndrome in an 81-year-old patient treated with budesonide and amiodarone. Eur J Gastroenterol Hepatol 2000; 12: 1041–2.
42. Costedoat-Chalumeau N, Amoura Z, Aymard G, Sevin O, Wechsler B, Cacoub P, Du LTH, Diquet B, Ankri A, Piette JC. Potentiation of vitamin K antagonist by high-dose intravenous methylprednisolone. Ann Intern Med 2000; 132: 631–5.
43. Geller M. Marked peripheral edema associated with montelukast and prednisone. Ann Intern Med 2000; 132: 924.
44. Field J, Rathmell JP, Stephenson JH, Katz NP. Neuropathic pain following cervical epidural steroid injection. Anesthesiology 2000; 93: 885–8.
45. Montoro J, Valero A, Serra-Baldrich E, Amat P, Lluch M, Malet A. Anaphylaxis to paramethasone with tolerance to other corticosteroids. Allergy 2000; 55: 197–8.
46. Jawed S, Allard SA. Osteomyelitis of the humerus following steroid injections for tennis elbow. Rheumatology 2000; 39: 923–4.
47. Fujita M, Hatori N, Shimizu M, Yoshizu H, Segawa D, Kimura T, Iizuka Y, Tanaka S. Neutralization of prostaglandin E_1 intravenous solution reduces infusion phlebitis. Angiology 2000; 51: 719–23.
48. Lewis GBH, Hecker JF. Infusion thrombophlebitis. Br J Anaesth 1985; 57: 220–33.
49. Carter EL, Garzon MC. Neonatal urticaria due to prostaglandin E_1. Pediatr Dermatol 2000; 17: 58–61.
50. Nadroo AM, Shringari S, Garg M, Al-Sowailem AM. Prostaglandin induced cortical hyperostosis in neonates with cyanotic heart disease. J Perinat Med 2000; 28: 447–52.
51. Schulte-Sasse U. Life threatening myocardial ischaemia associated with the use of prostaglandin E_1 to induce abortion. Br J Obstet Gynaecol 2000; 107: 700–2.
52. Camras CB, Neely DG, Weiss EL. Latanoprost-induced iris color darkening: a case report with long-term follow-up. J Glaucoma 2000; 9: 95–8.
53. Schumer RA, Camras CB, Mandahl AK. Latanoprost and cystoid macular edema: is there a causal relation? Curr Opin Ophthalmol 2000; 11: 94–100.
54. Kook MS, Lee K. Increased eyelid pigmentation associated with use of latanoprost. Am J Ophthalmol 2000; 129: 804–6.
55. Mansberguer SL, Cioffi GA. Eyelash formation secondary to latanoprost treatment in a patient with alopecia. Arch Oftalmol 2000; 118: 718–19.
56. GD Searle. Important drug warning concerning unapproved use of intravaginal or oral misoprostol in pregnant women for induction of labor or abortion. Media Release, 23 August 2000.
57. Bugalho A, Mocumbi S, Faúndes A, David E. Termination of pregnancies of < 6 weeks gestation with a single dose of 800 μg of vaginal misoprostol. Contraception 2000; 61: 47–50.
58. Schaff EA, Fielding SL, Westhoff C, Ellertson C, Eisinger SH, Stadalius LS, Fuller L. Vaginal misoprostol administered 1, 2, or 3 days after mifepristone for early medical abortion. A randomized trial. J Am Med Assoc 2000; 284; 1948–53.
59. Gherman RB, McBrayer S, Browning J. Ute-

rine rupture associated with vaginal birth after cesarean section: a complication of intravaginal misoprostol? Gynecol Obstet Invest 2000; 50: 212–13.
60. Jwarah E, Greenhalf JO. Rupture of the uterus after 800 micrograms misoprostol given vaginally for termination of pregnancy. Br J Obstet Gynaecol 2000; 107: 807.
61. Mathews JE, Mathai M, George A. Uterine rupture in a mutiparous woman during labor induction with oral misoprostol. Int J Gynecol Obstet 2000; 68: 43–4.
62. Hill DA, Chez RA, Quinlan J, Fuentes A, LaCombe J. Uterine rupture and dehiscence associated with intravaginal misoprostol cervical ripening. J Reprod Med 2000; 45: 823–6.
63. Brasil R, Coelho HL, D'Avanzo B, La Vecchia C. Misoprostol and congenital anomalies. Pharmacoepidemiol Drug Saf 2000; 9: 401–3.
64. Vargas FR Schuler-Faccini L, Brunoni D, Kim C, Meloni VFA, Sugayama SMM, Albano L, Llerena JC, Almeida JCC, Duarte A, Cavalcanti DP, Goloni-Bertollo E, Conte A, Koren G, Addis A. Prenatal exposure to misoprostol and vascular disruption defects: a case-control study. Am J Med Genet 2000, 95: 302–6.
65. Orioli IM, Castilla EE. Epidemiological assessment of misoprostol teratogenicity. Br J Obstet Gynaecol 2000; 107: 519–23.
66. Coelho K-EFA, Sarmento MvF, Veiga CM, Speck-Martins CE, Safatle HPN, Castro CV, Niikawa N. Misoprostol embryotoxicity: clinical evaluation of fifteen patients with arthrogryposis. Am J Med Genet 2000; 95: 297–301.
67. Corrado F, D'Anna R, Cannata ML. Rupture of the cervix in a sulprostone induced abortion in the second trimester. Arch Gynecol Obstet 2000; 264: 162–3.
68. Lievre M, Morand S, Besse B, Fiessinger JN, Boissel JP. Oral beraprost sodium, a prostaglandin I(2) analogue, for intermittent claudication: a double-blind, randomized, multicenter controlled trial. Beraprost et Claudication Intermittente (BERCI) Research Group. Circulation 2000; 102: 426–31.
69. Gugnani MK, Pierson C, Vanderheide R, Girgis RE. Pulmonary edema complicating prostacyclin therapy in pulmonary hypertension associated with scleroderma: a case of pulmonary capillary hemangiomatosis. Arthritis Rheum 2000; 43: 699–703.
70. Boubakri C, Bouchou K, Guy C, Roy M, Cathebras P. Douleurs masseterines: un effet indesirable meconnu de l'iloprost. Presse Med 2000; 29: 1935–6.
71. Olschewski H, Ghofrani HA, Schmehl T, Winkler J, Wilkens H, Hoper MM, Behr J, Kleber FX, Seeger W. Inhaled iloprost to treat severe pulmonary hypertension. An uncontrolled trial. German PPH Study Group. Ann Intern Med 2000; 132: 435–43.

M.N.G. Dukes

40 Sex hormones and related compounds, including hormonal contraceptives

GONADOTROPHINS AND OVULATION-INDUCING DRUGS

(SED-14, 1464; SEDA-22, 465; SEDA-23, 444; SEDA-24, 473)

Hematological A further case of *activated protein C resistance and deep calf vein thrombosis* has been reported during controlled ovarian stimulation for in vitro fertilization (1[AR]). The thrombosis occurred on the eighth day of human menopausal gonadotrophin use and before human chorionic gonadotrophin was given.

Reproductive system The efficacy and safety of recombinant human follicle stimulating hormone (r-hFSH) has been compared with that of highly purified urinary FSH (u-hFSH-HP) in women undergoing ovarian stimulation for in vitro fertilization, including intracytoplasmic sperm injection, in a prospective randomized study in 278 patients, who were treated with gonadotrophin-releasing hormone and then received one of the two formulations in doses of 150 IU/day subcutaneously for the first 6 days; on day 7 the dose was adjusted, if necessary, according to the ovarian response (2[C]). Human chorionic gonadotrophin (HCG, 10 000 IU subcutaneously) was administered once there was more than one follicle 18 mm in diameter and two others of 16 mm or larger. R-hFSH was more effective than u-hFSH-HP in inducing multiple follicular development. There were seven cases (5.0%) of *ovarian hyperstimulation syndrome* in those given r-hFSH and three (2.2%) in those given u-hFSH-HP; this difference was not significant.

Immunologic Even the most highly purified gonadotropins of natural origin can on occasion elicit *hypersensitivity reactions*. A case of general hypersensitivity-like allergic reactions to intramuscular injections of highly purified urinary follicle stimulating hormone (uFSH-HP) has been described (3[A]). The problem was successfully managed by changing the treatment to intramuscular recombinant FSH (rFSH). A generalized allergic reaction to human menopausal gonadotrophin (Pergonal) has been described during controlled ovarian hyperstimulation (4[Ar]). In this case a desensitization protocol allowed the patient to complete her treatment cycle without further problems. Subsequently recombinant follicle stimulating hormone was used successfully and uneventfully.

ESTROGENS *(SED-14, 1448; SEDA-22, 458; SEDA-23, 440; SEDA-24, 467)*

Diethylstilbestrol

Although it is more than 25 years since the full extent became clear of the injury to offspring by the ill-advised use of diethylstilbestrol (DES) during pregnancy (SEDA-24, xxiii), details of that injury are still being filled in as the individuals concerned grow older. The total picture will continue to be filled in as long as this generation of individuals lives, and it is even possible that findings in the third generation will throw light on the persisting injury to the family. Psychological research among "DES daughters"

Side Effects of Drugs, Annual 25
J.K. Aronson, ed.

has shown how traumatic it can be for a woman to learn of her prenatal exposure to diethylstilbestrol, and the extent to which this creates persistent uncertainty as to her health status; the failure of a physician to provide reliable information and continuing support may severely undermine her faith in healthcare (5[C]).

Long-term studies of the pregnancy experiences of women exposed to diethylstilbestrol in utero, compared with unexposed women, now include one in the US National Collaborative Diethylstilbestrol Adenosis cohort and one in the Chicago cohort and their respective non-exposed comparison groups. A review of questionnaire replies from 3373 exposed daughters and from controls has confirmed that diethylstilbestrol-exposed women were less likely than unexposed women to have had full-term live births and more likely to have had premature births, spontaneous pregnancy losses, or ectopic pregnancies (6[Cr]). The data are shown in Table 1. Second-trimester spontaneous pregnancy losses were much more common in diethylstilbestrol-exposed women.

Table 1. *Outcomes of first pregnancies in women exposed or not exposed to diethylstilbestrol in utero*

Outcome	Not exposed (%)	Exposed (%)
Full-term delivery	85	64
Spontaneous absorption	10	19
Pre-term delivery	4.1	12
Ectopic pregnancy	0.77	4.2

Long-term data are also accumulating on the actual incidence of *genital cancer* in women exposed to diethylstilbestrol in utero (7[R]). In the Netherlands, a country in which diethylstilbestrol was used intensively in pregnancy, there is now evidence that the risk of cervical cancer in these women is trebled, rather than doubled as was previously supposed (8[Cr]).

Hormone replacement therapy (HRT)

The multiplicity of HRT regimens in use (involving one or two drugs, continuous or intermittent treatment, and various forms of administration) makes it difficult to express any general conclusion about the benefit:harm ratio of hormonal replacement therapy, and there has been a thoughtful review of the obstacles to assessing these matters objectively and scientifically, including questions of both ethics and trial design (9[R]). Even the ultimate effect of HRT on the incidence of *ischemic heart disease* remains subject to dispute (10[R]), and incidental reports of cardiac complications, sometimes in women with entirely healthy coronary vessels, continue to cause concern (11[Ar]). For such reasons, much work has now been devoted to determining the lowest effective dose of estrogen needed to achieve particular results.

For the acute treatment of climacteric vasomotor symptoms it now seems clear that micronized 17-β-estradiol in a dose as low as 0.25 mg can be sufficient; however, a starting dose of 1 mg is advisable, with subsequent adjustments as necessary. At a dose of 2 mg the proportion of women withdrawing from treatment with the active product because of adverse effects was twice that seen with placebo (12[Cr]). To provide longer-term protection against early postmenopausal bone loss, treatment with estradiol in a dose of 1 mg/day, balanced by a progestogen, is adequate (13[CR]). Most workers believe that the estrogen is best counterbalanced by a progestogen when used in the long term, but here there is still some disagreement about the doses needed.

The minimum dose of continuously administered norethindrone acetate needed to reduce significantly the incidence of *endometrial hyperplasia* associated with the use of β-estradiol 1 mg/day has been investigated in a large controlled comparative study in 1146 women over 12 months (14[C]). The results suggested that continuous norethindrone acetate at doses as low as 0.1 mg/day is fully effective, at least during the first year of treatment.

In assessing the overall risks of HRT it may also be productive to examine various types of known risks and to determine to what extent they vary with the form of treatment used. Large comparative studies have suggested that a series of alternative regimens for HRT should be available, so that for each individual woman the most appropriate form of treatment can be chosen; no one regimen is ideal for all, and finding the best approach for a given patient may be a matter of trial and error (15[C]).

In a randomized multicenter study in Denmark 376 perimenopausal women with climacteric symptoms were randomly allocated to oral sequential combined treatment with regimens based on estrogen plus either desogestrel or medroxyprogesterone acetate (16[Cr]). Both treatments effectively alleviated menopausal complaints within 6 months and gave good cycle control. Bleeding pattern and mood disturbances were more favorably affected by desogestrel, but overall the differences in adverse effects (*irregular bleeding* and a slight tendency to *hypotension*) were not large. It should be noted, however, that with cyclic combined HRT treatment, the bleeding pattern alone does not seem to be a reliable means of distinguishing cases in which the endometrium is atrophic or inactive from those in which it is proliferative or hyperplastic (17[C]).

A Japanese study of the use of estriol 2 mg/day for 12 months in 68 postmenopausal women with climacteric symptoms showed a significant effect in relieving hot flushes, night sweats, and insomnia (18[C], 19[C]). There were significant *falls in serum follicle stimulating hormone (FSH) and luteinizing hormone (LH) concentrations*, but no effect on lipids, bone demineralization, or blood pressure. There was slight *vaginal bleeding* in 14% of women treated during a natural menopause, but histological and ultrasound evaluation showed no changes in the endometrium or breasts. It is evident, however, that higher doses might be needed when treating women of other races with a higher bodyweight. Other workers have found that when given with a progestogen over long periods, estriol 2.0 mg/day seems much less likely to cause undesirable lipid changes than are equine conjugated estrogens, which can cause *increased HDL cholesterol and triglyceride concentrations* (20[C]).

Cardiovascular Despite biologically plausible mechanisms whereby estrogens might be expected to confer cardioprotection in postmenopausal women, as well as observational data suggesting cardiovascular benefit, the literature continues to provide contradictory outcomes on this. Electrocardiographic work suggests that not only the estrogen but also the progestogen component of HRT may have some impact on the electrophysiological properties of the heart (21[C]), the clinical significance of which, if any, is not understood. The picture is further confused by evidence that a particular regimen may initially increase the risk, yet confer long-term benefit, as in the Heart and Estrogen/progestin Replacement Study (HERS), while in other well-planned work, such as the recent Estrogen Replacement and Atherosclerosis trial (ERA), no benefit has been seen (22[R]).

There has been a randomized trial in 270 postmenopausal women to evaluate the effects on cardiovascular risk markers of two continuous combined estrogen–progestogen replacement products (17-β-estradiol 1 mg with or without norethindrone acetate 0.25 or 0.5 mg) compared with unopposed estrogen or placebo (23[CR]). LDL cholesterol was reduced to a similar extent in all those who took the active treatment (10–14% from baseline). Compared with unopposed 17-β-estradiol, 17-β-estradiol plus norethindrone acetate 0.5 mg enhanced the reductions in total cholesterol and apolipoprotein B concentrations. The combination of 17-β-estradiol plus norethindrone blunted or reversed the increases in concentrations of high-density lipoprotein cholesterol, apolipoprotein A-I, and triglycerides produced by 17-β-estradiol alone. The effects of 17-β-estradiol plus norethindrone on hemostatic variables were similar to those of 17-β-estradiol alone, except for factor VII activity, which was significantly reduced by 17-β-estradiol plus norethindrone acetate 0.25 and 0.5 mg. The combination of 17-β-estradiol plus norethindrone blunted reductions in C peptide and insulin concentrations produced by unopposed 17-β-estradiol, but did not affect them compared with placebo. The authors concluded that 17-β-estradiol plus norethindrone produced favorable changes in most cardiovascular risk markers and had a profile distinct from that of unopposed estrogen, but the long-term significance of these differences demands further study

Sensory systems *Visual hallucinations* have been associated with estrogen in a patient with Charles Bonnet syndrome (24[Ar]).

An 84-year-old woman with poor visual acuity secondary to bilateral, non-exudative, age-related macular degeneration had non-threatening visual hallucinations 2 weeks after starting oral estrogen for osteoporosis. The estrogen was withdrawn and the hallucinations subsided. She was given estrogen twice more and each time the hallucinations recurred.

In this patient estrogen may have promoted release phenomena and triggered the hallucinatory episodes.

Hematologic There has been a randomized, placebo-controlled study in 25 postmenopausal women to investigate the mechanisms that could underlie the induction of *thrombosis* by unopposed estrogens (25[Cr]). Fasting and fat-load-stimulated plasma concentrations of clotting factor VII were measured after 8 weeks of oral 17-β-estradiol (2 mg/day). The estrogen increased the mean fasting and postprandial plasma concentrations of total factor VII by 17% and 21% respectively, but did not affect the fasting and/or postprandial plasma concentrations of active factor VII. These findings argue against the idea that raised concentrations of total factor VII underlie the increased risk of arterial thromboembolism in these women.

The thrombotic complications of combined HRT in a potentially high-risk group have been further assessed in a randomized, multicenter study in the USA in 2763 women, average age 67 years (26[C]). All had some degree of pre-existing coronary heart disease but no previous venous thromboembolism, and none had undergone hysterectomy. They took either conjugated equine estrogens 0.625 mg plus medroxyprogesterone acetate 2.5 mg or a placebo. During an average 4.1 years of follow-up, 34 women in the hormone therapy group and 13 in the placebo group had venous thromboembolism (relative risk = 2.7, excess risk = 3.9 per 1000 woman-years). The mean risk for venous thromboembolism was increased among women who had leg fractures (relative risk = 18) or cancer (relative risk = 4) and it was also raised several-fold for 3 months after in-patient surgery or non-surgical hospitalization. The risk was approximately halved by the use of aspirin or statins.

Immunologic Two healthy young women took estrogen supplements for some 3 years and then developed classic *Sjögren's syndrome* (27[Ar]). The syndrome was most severe in the woman who had taken the higher dose. These cases seem to have confirmed earlier reports that estrogens can play a role in the pathogenesis of Sjögren's syndrome in susceptible patients.

Gene toxicity A finding that needs further study is that when estrogens are used for the treatment of osteoporosis they may have some genotoxic potential, as evidenced by their ability to cause an *increased frequency of sister chromatid exchange* (28[C]).

Carcinogenicity *Endometrial cancer* Because sequential combined hormone replacement therapy with estrogen and progestogen for 10–24 days per month may increase the risk of endometrial cancer in the long run, attention has been devoted to the possibility of giving the two types of hormone continuously. In one retrospective case-control study in the USA it was concluded that the risk of endometrial cancer among users of continuous combined treatment, relative to women who had never used hormone replacement therapy, was 0.6 (95% CI = 0.3, 1.3); the risk relative to women who used intermittent combined therapy was 0.4 (CI = 0.2, 1.1) (29[CR]). The authors' conclusions were cautious, since most continuous combined hormonal therapy had been fairly short-term (under 72 months), but the figures suggested that women taking continuous combined hormone replacement therapy for several years did not appear to be at an increased risk of endometrial cancer relative to women who had never taken hormone replacement therapy and might in fact be at reduced risk of endometrial cancer.

In the meantime others have concluded that the risk of endometrial cancer is present, but is less with combined therapy than with unopposed estrogen. However, the picture is not simple; the contradictions could be explained by the fact that risks appear to vary both by usage patterns and by patient characteristics, such as bodyweight and history of diabetes (30[C]).

Breast cancer The complexity of the relation between hormonal replacement therapy and breast cancer has been stressed in previous volumes (SED-14, 1454; SEDA-22, 465), and much depends on the type of replacement therapy given and the class of tumor studied. This latter point has been underscored by a recent US study that has provided evidence that the use of combined hormonal replacement therapy increases the risk of lobular, but not ductal, breast carcinoma in middle-aged women (31[C]).

An American cohort study designed to determine whether increases in risk associated with the estrogen–progestogen regimen are greater than those associated with estrogen alone has been carried out based on follow-up data for 1980–95 from the National Breast Cancer Detection Demonstration Project (32[CR]). From 46 355 postmenopausal women, mean age at the start of follow-up 58 years, 2082 cases of breast cancer were identified. Increases in risk with estrogen only and estrogen plus progestogen were restricted to use within the previous 4 years, the relative risks being 1.2 and 1.4 respectively. The relative risk increased by 0.01 with each year of estrogen use and by 0.08 with each year of estrogen plus progestogen use. Among women with a BMI of 24.4 kg/m^2 or less, the mean increases in relative risk were 0.03 and 0.12 with each year of estrogen use and estrogen plus progestogen use respectively. These associations were evident for the majority of invasive tumors with ductal histology and regardless of the extent of invasive disease. The risk in heavier women did not increase with the use of estrogen only or estrogen plus progestogen. These data suggest that estrogen plus progestogen increases the risk of breast cancer beyond that associated with estrogen alone.

Risk factors In women with pre-existing morbidity, such as *diabetes mellitus* or *hypertension*, an appropriate form of HRT can apparently be found. When 16 diabetic and hypertensive postmenopausal women aged 47–57 years were treated cyclically with estradiol plus norgestrel, existing proteinuria and even creatinine clearance often improved (33[C]). The effects were unrelated to conventional risk factors for vascular complications, such as raised blood pressure, plasma glucose, or serum cholesterol.

Estrogen replacement therapy may also have untoward effects in patients with *renal disease*, including an increased risk of thrombosis of dialysis access and potentially worsening of coronary artery disease, probably because the excretion of estrogens is impaired (34[R]).

Young women When a young woman undergoes a surgical menopause it is clear that estrogen replacement treatment, if given at all, is likely to be needed for many years, and in the present state of knowledge this is probably justifiable, provided that the effects are monitored. The dilemma that the physician faces in such cases has been discussed in the light of a patient in whom gross obesity compounded the possible risk of thrombosis; the patient was nevertheless treated with an implant and has remained well for 4 years (35[Ar]).

Men Following castration for cancer of the prostate, a high proportion of men have hot flushes, and estrogens can provide relief. In a study in 12 such men, estrogen in a low dose (0.05 mg) or high dose (0.10 mg) given as patches twice weekly for 4 weeks provided considerable improvement (36[c]). In this dosage, mild painless breast swelling or nipple tenderness was noted in two and five of the 12 men treated with the low- and high-dose patches respectively. Estradiol concentrations increased from 12 pg/ml to 16 and 27 pg/ml with the low- and high-dose patches respectively. There were no significant changes in serum testosterone or luteinizing hormone concentrations. This was a small study, and data on the tolerability of this topical treatment in a larger series would be welcome.

Various centers have expressed interest in the longer-term use of estrogen in men. There is evidence for a role of estrogen in male bone metabolism, notably from studies in a man with a genetic defect in estrogen receptors and in men with aromatase deficiencies. Estrogen is likely to affect bone turnover in men throughout life, and it has been suggested that older men could have reduced bone resorption in response to estrogen therapy. In a study of this possibility, in 14 men with osteopenia of the femoral neck using micronized estradiol 1 mg/day for 9 weeks, i.e. a dose that is effective in postmenopausal women, estradiol and estrone concentrations increased significantly by more than 6-fold and 15-fold respectively (37[cr]). Concentrations of serum hormone binding globulin increased significantly by 17%, but testosterone and free testosterone concentrations fell significantly by 27% and 34% respectively. Markers of bone resorption showed wide variations both at baseline and during treatment; they were too inconsistent to justify conclusions as to the potential usefulness of the treatment. However, the adverse effects of treatment were minimal, including (as might be expected) breast tenderness and reduced libido, which reversed after treatment.

Drug administration route *Vaginal administration* Because weak estrogens, such as estriol and estrone (the main component of conjugated estrogens), are claimed to act primarily on the lower part of the genital tract, they have long been used topically for atrophic conditions of the vagina and vulva, and are reputed to have useful effects in doses that do not cause marked endometrial or systemic changes. However, everything may in fact be a question of dosage; it could well be that even a low dose of a potent estrogen would have a similarly selective effect. In 159 menopausal women with atrophic vaginitis who used either a conjugated equine estrogen vaginal cream (2 g/day containing conjugated estrogens 1.25 mg) or 17-β-estradiol 25 μg pessaries (one daily for 2 weeks), the two treatments provided equivalent relief of the symptoms of atrophic vaginitis, but at weeks 2, 12, and 24 there were increases in serum estradiol concentrations and suppression of follicle-stimulating hormone in significantly more patients who used the conjugated estrogen cream than in those who used the estradiol pessaries; the patients themselves rated the estradiol treatment more highly (38[C]).

Another effective alternative to the use of weak estrogens is the administration of estradiol from an estradiol-releasing vaginal ring, which has been studied as a means of alleviating lower urinary tract symptoms after the menopause. It appears to be well tolerated and enjoys better patient acceptance than the use of local estriol (39[Cr]).

Transdermal administration New topical formulations of estrogens continue to be studied and marketed, although most studies have shown little difference between the various formulations available (40[CR]). In a randomized, placebo-controlled, cross-over study for 12 weeks, the estrogen matrix patch Estraderm MX, which unlike some other patches contains no alcohol, significantly relieved climacteric symptoms in both lower and higher strengths (50 and 100 μg of estradiol) (41[c]). Local tolerability was good, but there was a slight increase in estrogen-related adverse effects (*breast tenderness, leukorrhea*) with the higher dose; there was a 4.8% overall incidence of *endometrial hyperplasia* in patients with an intact uterus. In women who have local reactions to alcohol a patch of this type may be helpful.

Other work has confirmed the similar value of two patch formulations, Menorest and Climara; the latter has been reported to cause a much higher incidence of local reactions, but they are mild (42[C]). The Fem 7 patch, which delivers estradiol 50 μg/day, was also well tolerated (43[C]). Another effective and well accepted variant on the patch theme is Demestril, which releases estradiol 25 or 37.5 μg/day depending on the formulation used (44[C]). Differences in effect and tolerability between all these various estradiol patches are primarily a question of dosage and release rate, but it also seems that acceptance may be better when the drug is incorporated into the adhesive rather than being stored in a separate reservoir. The former type of patch shows better adhesion and is cosmetically more acceptable (45[C]).

When low-dose patch therapy results in *breakthrough bleeding* it is supposedly more likely to occur in women with large, thin-walled, superficial endometrial vessels (46[A]). If this finding is correct it might also apply to breakthrough bleeding with other forms of hormonal therapy.

Intranasal administration Intranasal estradiol gives results comparable to transdermal estradiol, but substantially higher doses are needed. In 300 postmenopausal women 17-β-estradiol 300 μg/day was as effective as two patches per week delivering 50 μg/day (47[C]). Adverse events rates were similar but moderate, and severe *mastalgia* was significantly less frequent with intranasal estradiol (7.2%) than with the patch (15.5%); 66% of the patients chose to continue the intranasal therapy and 34% the transdermal therapy.

Drug interactions Preclinical studies (as well as anecdotal clinical reports in the course of the years) seem to show that estrogens, through their effects on the central nervous system, may influence behavioral responses to psychoactive drugs. In an unusual cross-over study, the subjective and physiological effects of oral *d-amphetamine* 10 mg have been assessed after pretreatment with estradiol (48[Cr]). One group of healthy young women used estradiol patches (Estraderm TTS, total dose 0.8 mg), which raised plasma estradiol concentrations to about 750 pg/ml, and a control group used placebo patches. Most of the subjective and physiological effects of amphetamine were not affected by acute estradiol treatment, but the estrogen did increase the magnitude of the effect of amphetamine on subjective ratings of "pleasant stimulation"and reduced ratings of "want more". Estradiol also produced some subjective effects when used alone, raising ratings of "feel drug", "energy and intellectual efficiency", and "pleasant stimulation".

HORMONAL CONTRACEPTIVES

(SED-14, 1405; SEDA-22, 462; SEDA-23, 442; SEDA-24, 471)

℞ *Third-generation oral contraceptives: tracking a risk*

As a rule the study of adverse reactions must relate to current and emergent issues. However, now and again it can be instructive to look back into recent history. When a drug problem has been fairly clearly defined, and particularly when it has for a time been the subject of debate and even frank controversy, one can learn something from the processes involved. How did the facts become known? Why did the controversy emerge? And could the risk have been detected and eliminated earlier?

Since their appearance in the late 1950s, oral contraceptives have gone through several stages of development. What are now in retrospect referred to as first-generation oral contraceptives were high-dose combinations of progestogens (more particularly norethynodrel, norethisterone, and lynestrenol in doses of 2.5 mg or more) and the estrogen mestranol 75 μg. A decade later a second generation came to the fore, with substantially lower doses, commonly half of those used earlier; some new progestogens, notably the more potent levonorgestrel, also came into use. Finally, in the early 1980s some manufacturers introduced so-called third-generation products, a particular characteristic of which was the use of entirely new, very potent progestogens, among them desogestrel and gestodene. Clinical studies of gestodene- and desogestrel-based contraceptives have suggested that they are very similar to one another, although differences in dosage and potency could account for reports that gestodene-containing products provide better cycle control (49[Cr]).

Almost from the earlier years, the risk of thromboembolic complications among users of "the pill" was recognized, and by the mid-1960s it was well documented (50[R], 51[C]). Progressive reductions in dosage, in particular that of the estrogenic component, during the period that first- and second-generation products held sway were widely regarded as having reduced this risk to manageable proportions, although it was not eliminated. The relative risk with first-generation products was highly variable (2–11), but the best work in the UK and the USA fairly consistently reached an estimate of 4–6 (52[C]–54[C]). With the second-generation products the relative risk of thromboembolic complications was again variously estimated, but a large cohort study published in 1991 set it at 1.5 with products containing the lowest doses of estrogen, and 1.7 with products containing intermediate doses of estrogen (55[C]).

The fact that both prescribers and users of medicines are likely to anticipate that a new generation of drugs will be in some way better than that which has gone before means that both groups are in principle receptive to claims and suggestions in this regard. By the time the third-generation oral contraceptives were marketed, this type of contraception had been around for a quarter of a century; the risk of thromboembolism, the most widely publicized problem in the field, seemed by that time to have receded with progressive reductions in dosage. There was every reason to hope that it would recede further with the newest generation of products. That expectation was further nurtured by the even lower doses now attainable. It also seems to have been fostered by some of the suggestive promotion that appeared, although that in fact related as a rule merely to an improved lipid spectrum, which in turn raised the theoretical possibility, also discussed but not documented by some clinical investigators (56[CR]), that arterial and cardiac risks might be less.

What in fact happened was that by 1989 alarm bells began to ring in Germany, where the regulatory authorities were alerted to the submission of an unusually high number of spontaneous reports of thromboembolic complications thought to be associated with the new products. Cases continued to accumulate, long-term studies already begun were completed, and in 1995 Britain's Committee on Safety of Medicines made a public statement to the effect that the risk of thromboembolic complications among hitherto healthy users of third-generation products was approximately twice that seen with second-generation products (SEDA-19, xix). The studies in question, including work by the World Health Organization and others (SED-14, 1410), were subsequently published and confirmed that conclusion, as did later work (57[C]). It was further reinforced by others (58[Ec]), who worked on a smaller scale but provided well-documented evidence that while a factor V Leiden mutation or a biased family history could increase the risk in individual cases, they did not explain the higher thrombosis risk seen with a product based on desogestrel than with contraceptives that incorporated levonorgestrel, norethisterone, or lynestrenol.

Currently one must ask why the particular risk of the third-generation contraceptives was identified so late. These third-generation products had been in development since the late 1970s and the first had been marketed in 1981–2, some 14 years before the Committee on Safety of Medicines issued its statement. Could society not have done better and thereby reduced the risks to which women were exposed? There are two principal answers, both of them at least partly in the affirmative.

The first is that products of this type could well have been entered at an earlier date into large studies of oral contraception and their effects. A series of university centers around the world, as well as bodies such as Britain's Royal College of Physicians and Royal College of General Practitioners, have throughout the oral contraceptive era either sponsored or participated in prolonged cohort and case-control studies of these products. Experience with data on thromboembolism suggests that significant data are likely to be obtainable in a cohort study of manageable size within some 5–7 years. The use of third-generation products may have been small in the early years, but they were aggressively promoted in major oral contraceptive markets to ensure rapid growth, in all probability sufficient to provide adequate recruitment. One would hesitate to argue that such studies should be a universal condition of the marketing of drugs, but when the products concerned have immense social significance and considerable potential for good and harm, as the oral contraceptives do, and when the compounds involved are entirely new, there is at least a sound medical reason for such work in every case. That work was performed with successive forms of the earlier oral contraceptive products, in which dosages were progressively reduced, and there was particular reason to set it in motion on the introduction of products that contained new chemical components with some significant structural and pharmacological differences from the older progestogens. A little statistical effort will show that an early cohort study involving some 30 000–50 000 women taking a third-generation product could within 2 years have shown the degree of increase in the thrombotic risk, which was actually not elicited until much later.

The second answer with respect to the earlier acquisition of risk data must come from the laboratory. Not from animal studies, which in this field are of very restricted value, but from biochemical and particularly hematological work. When during the 1990s various groups began to examine in detail the effects of the third-generation contraceptives on processes related to the clotting system, they identified a series of properties that could very well explain an increased incidence of thrombosis.

The first of these was an increase in circulating concentrations of factor VII produced by the desogestrel plus estrogen combination, which was some 20–30% higher than that seen with a second-generation product based on levonorgestrel (59[E]). The methods used to carry out this work were available before 1988 (60[E]), and it is not at all clear from the published material whether there was a failure to compare the two generations in this respect at an early date, or whether such work was performed and either overlooked or misinterpreted.

A second finding related to the effects of activated protein C on thrombin generation in low-platelet plasma via the intrinsic or extrinsic clotting pathways. Using a method developed on the basis of work first published in 1997 (61[E]), a Dutch group in Maastricht found that all types of combined oral contraceptives induced acquired resistance to activated protein C. With the third-generation contraceptives, however, the effect was significantly more marked than with those of the second generation: in other words, these drugs significantly reduced the ability of activated protein C to downregulate the formation of thrombin (62[C]). However, this work only became feasible in the late 1990s.

A third underlying mechanism seems to involve a reduction in concentrations of free protein S, again more pronounced with products of the third generation. When protein S falls, the antifibrinolytic effect of the so-called thrombin-activated fibrinolysis inhibitor is increased; in other words, fibrinolysis is impeded, with an increased risk of clotting problems (63[E]). Again, however, these are recent methods, which were not available when the third-generation products were launched.

The laboratory findings therefore suggest that a greater thrombosis-inducing effect of the third-generation oral contraceptives can be explained and even anticipated on the basis of known mechanisms. Not all the relevant methods were available in the early years, but that relating to factor VII most certainly was. It is unfortunate, to say the least, that such work was either not performed or not properly interpreted.

All in all, had a combination of hematological methods and field studies been initiated sufficiently soon, the increased risk of thromboembolism with the third-generation oral contraceptives could have been detected some years earlier, sufficient for society to take decisions on the benefit:harm ratio of these drugs before so much needless injury was incurred.

Hematological One possible risk factor for *thrombosis*, about which too little has been known, is the presence of inherited clotting defects. Data from the Leiden Thrombophilia Study have been used to construct a case-control study, based on contraceptive users who had experienced a first episode of objectively proven deep vein thrombosis (64[CR]). Patients and controls were considered thrombophilic when they had protein C deficiency, protein S deficiency, antithrombin deficiency, factor V Leiden mutation, or a prothrombin 20210 A mutation. Among healthy women the risk of developing deep vein thrombosis was trebled in the first 6 months and doubled in the first year of contraceptive use. Among women with thrombophilia, the risk of deep vein thrombosis was increased 19-fold during the first 6 months and 11-fold (95%CI = 2.1, 57) in the first year of use. Venous thrombosis during the first period of oral contraceptive use might actually point to the presence of an inherited clotting defect.

Mild hematological effects can occur with any form of hormonal contraception, including progestogen implants. During 1 year of observation of 23 healthy fertile African women, beginning at the time that a Norplant device was inserted, the mean packed cell volume rose slightly but significantly from 40.5 to 42.2, but the mean total leukocyte, neutrophil, and lymphocyte counts all fell significantly, as did the mean platelet count (65[Cr]). In four patients the platelet counts were only $50–80 \times 10^9$/l. The rise in packed cell volume might, according to the authors, help to counter anemia in people in developing countries. However, the fall in the platelet count is hard to explain.

Metabolic Adolescents with polycystic ovary syndrome are regarded as candidates for long-term treatment combined hormonal treatment using a product of the oral contraceptive type, and there has been some concern about possible unfavorable late metabolic effects, notably on lipids. The risks with two combined products, one based on cyproterone acetate 2 mg and the other on desogestrel 0.15 mg, both with estrogen, have been estimated in 24 women (66c[r]). After 12 months the hirsutism score was improved, but while *triglycerides and HDL cholesterol were significantly increased* by cyproterone the only relevant effect of the desogestrel combination was a *raised apolipoprotein A1 concentration*. The authors concluded that the desogestrel combination was therefore to be preferred in such patients

Biliary tract The precise nature of the changes in the liver that can occur during treatment with various types of hormonal contraceptives continues to be elucidated. Formation of *biliary sludge* is one phenomenon that may have been largely overlooked (67[Ar]).

A 21-year-old woman developed increasing jaundice, with severe pruritus and weight loss, after a bout of dyspepsia. She had been taking contraceptives for 4 years (cyproterone acetate 2 mg, ethinylestradiol 0.035 mg). Laboratory tests at first suggested cholestatic hepatitis, but ultrasonography showed biliary sludge in the gall bladder and dilatation of the common bile duct and the smaller biliary passages. There was a space-occupying lesion near the papilla: it was not fixed and had no vascular supply. At endoscopic retrograde cholangiopancreatography the lesion was removed. It consisted of jelly-like viscous streaky bile without calculi. Within a few days the jaundice disappeared, the pruritus ceased, and liver function returned to normal.

Reproductive system One problem with the hormonal implant Norplant is the relatively high incidence of *irregular uterine bleeding*, which in some countries has reduced the acceptability of the treatment (68[R]). It is not clear why some women are more susceptible to this complication than others. In a Thai study in a large number of Norplant users with irregular bleeding were characterized by low estradiol concentrations, absence of luteal activity, and a thin hyperechoic pattern in the endometrium (69[C]). The possible role of cellular apoptosis in the endometrial response to Norplant has been investigated using immunohistochemistry, but with negative results (70[E]). However, among Norplant users the superficial endometrial blood vessels are more fragile than in controls and even more fragile than in untreated women with dysfunctional uterine bleeding (71[cE]).

An unusual approach to dealing with this irregular bleeding has been to give an antiprogestogen simultaneously. In 50 Chinese women with implants, the effect of mifepristone 50 mg once every 4 weeks has been compared with placebo (72[c]). In all the women, regardless of treatment, the frequency of bleeding fell significantly over 1 year of observation, as it commonly does. However, women who took mifepristone had significantly shorter episodes of bleeding during treatment than during the 90 days before treatment started; the duration of bleeding episodes fell more gradually in the controls. Women who used mifepristone were more likely to find the treatment acceptable than the women who used placebo. Despite concerns that antiprogestogenic effects may jeopardize contraception, there were no pregnancies. In the view of the investigators, this approach may offer a useful strategy to relieve unwanted adverse effects of implants until bleeding patterns improve spontaneously with time.

A second unusual approach to the bleeding problem has been to give vitamin E. There is evidence that there is a poor angiogenic response in the endometrium of Norplant users, and it has been hypothesized that this might be caused by an imbalance of pro-oxidant and antioxidant processes. A placebo-controlled study has suggested that vitamin E (200 mg/day for 10 days monthly) significantly reduces the number of monthly bleeding days (73[cr]). However, there was also some reduction in bleeding days with placebo, and this approach would need further study before the results could be accepted as clinically useful.

The appearance of *enlarged ovarian follicles* is a recognized complication of Norplant, but the reported incidence varies, probably because different methods are used to recognize them. Serial ultrasonography produces much higher figures than clinical methods and has led to exaggerated concern; the enlarged follicles are transient and do not require intervention (74[c]).

Immunologic Estrogens have some adverse immunological effects (SED-14, 1463), and it has even been suggested that they could predispose to infections, although one would hardly expect this to be significant with the "physiological" doses used in estrogen treatment or hormonal contraception. However, this needs to be followed up.

The immunological effects of two contraceptive combinations, namely Valette (dienogest 2.0 mg plus ethinylestradiol 0.03 mg) and Lovelle (desogestrel 0.15 mg plus ethinylestradiol 0.02 mg), have been examined during one treatment cycle (75[c]). The latter significantly increased the numbers of lymphocytes, monocytes, and granulocytes. Valette reduced the CD4 lymphocyte count after 10 days and Lovelle did the opposite. Lovelle increased CD19 and CD23 cell counts after 21 days. Phagocytic activity was unaffected by either treatment. After 10 days both contraceptives reduced serum IgA, IgG, and IgM, which remained low at day 21 with Lovelle but returned to baseline with Valette. Secretory IgA was unaffected by either contraceptive. Neither treatment affected concentrations of interleukins, except for a significant difference between the treatment groups in interleukin-6 after 10 days, which resolved after 21 days. Concentrations of non-immunoglobulin serum components fluctuated; macroglobulin was increased by Valette. However, total protein and albumin concentrations were reduced more by Lovelle than Valette. Complement factors also fluctuated. There was no evidence of sustained immunosuppression with either Valette or Lovelle.

Drug administration routes *Implantable formulations* have been reviewed (76[R]).

Intrauterine devices have been reviewed (68[R], 77[R]). One of the newer variants on this theme contains levonorgestrel; the formulation, which has been approved for 5-year use, releases 20 μg/day from a polymer cylinder covered with a membrane that controls the rate of release. *Extrauterine pregnancies* occur in 1 per 5000 users per year. Both the volume of menstrual blood loss and the number of bleeding days are reduced, and during the first year of use 20% of women develop *amenorrhea*. There is an initial increase in the mean number of bleeding and spotting days, but in 3–6 months the number of bleeding and spotting days is the same as observed in users of copper IUCDs. The variation between individuals is wide and unpredictable, but the method is claimed to be well accepted by users, with typical annual continuation rates above 80% in various studies (78[Cr]). However, premature removal of the system because of unwanted effects is now well documented; in a nationwide study in Finland, the continuation rates at 1, 2, 3, 4, and 5 years were 93, 87, 81, 75, and 65% respectively (79[CR]). The symptoms most strongly associated with premature removal were *excessive bleeding and spotting*, *infections*, and *pain*. The risk of premature removal was markedly lower among women who had occasional or total absence of menstruation. Premature removal was less likely in the oldest age group. British experience shows a clear need to counsel women in advance about the possibility of early disruption of the bleeding pattern, including the chance of oligomenorrhea or amenorrhea, if they are not to become discouraged and abandon the treatment entirely (80[CR]).

The authors of a balanced review of this and other hormone-releasing intrauterine systems concluded that while with large-size devices that release high doses (e.g. 20 μg/day) pregnancy rates and the incidence of ectopic pregnancy are extremely low, users are more likely to have *amenorrhea* and *device expulsion* (81[R]). Compared with users of a subdermal hormonal implant (Norplant-2), women who used LNG-20 were more likely to have oligomenorrhea but less likely to have prolonged bleeding and spotting.

The FibroPlant is another levonorgestrel-releasing device derived from the earlier Gyne-Fix principle and has been well tolerated in studies in postmenopausal women. Experience with two forms of this frameless "fibrous delivery system", which releases smaller doses (10 or 14 μg/day) suggests that it is as effective and well tolerated as other types of device (82[c]). However, it has been pointed out by others that the *irregular bleeding* that can occur with devices of this type can complicate and delay the recognition of endometrial cancer (83c[r]).

Progesterone-only vaginal rings Vaginal administration of steroid-containing polymer rings has been studied for at least 20 years as a means of contraception, without gaining wide acceptance. In a large multicenter WHO trial with a levonorgestrel ring, releasing 20 μg/day, the 1-year pregnancy rate was 4.5% (84[cR]). The main reason for discontinuation was *menstrual disturbances* (17%), followed by frequent *expulsion of the ring* and *vaginal symptoms*.

The finding of erythematous lesions in the vagina in some women has led to the development of a more flexible device. The Population Council is also developing a vaginal ring containing Nestorone progestin (16-methylene-17-acetoxy-19-norpregn-4-ene-3,20-dione) for 6 months of continuous use (85[S]). Ovulation inhibition was achieved in over 97% of the segments studied, with rings releasing either 50, 75, or 100 μg/day. No pregnancies occurred in women who used the low-dose ring, while one pregnancy each occurred with the intermediate- and high-dose rings, for 6-month cumulative pregnancy rates of 0.0, 1.9, and 2.1% respectively; it is not clear why the reported pregnancy rates were higher with the higher doses. However, *bleeding irregularities* were common, and this form of contraception still demands further development work.

Drug interactions In standard reference works, oral contraceptives are commonly listed as increasing the circulating concentrations of *corticosteroids* (84[S]), but it has not been clear whether this is of clinical importance. A study in 40 healthy women has shown that in fact oral contraceptives have a greater effect on prednisolone than budesonide (86[c]). In oral contraceptive users, the average plasma concentration of simultaneously administered prednisolone was 131% higher than in a control group, whereas the average plasma concentration of budesonide was only 22% higher. Mean plasma cortisol concentrations were suppressed by 90% and 82% with prednisolone and by 22% and 28% with budesonide in oral contraceptive users and controls respectively. Ethinylestradiol plasma concentrations were not affected by either glucocorticoid. The authors concluded that the oral contraceptive made no difference to the plasma concentrations of budesonide or cortisol suppression after the administration of budesonide capsules. These findings suggest that oral budesonide can be used in the usual doses without problems in women using oral contraceptives.

The newer *anticonvulsants* have not been studied as intensively as older drugs as regards the possibility of interference with the effects of oral contraceptives. The available data suggest that women taking oral contraceptives can also take *gabapentin*, *lamotrigine*, *tiagabine*, and *vigabatrin* without significant pharmacokinetic interactions, but that the use of higher-dose contraceptives (or of backup contraceptive measures) is advisable during treatment with *felbamate*, *oxcarbazepine*, and *topiramate*, as these agents have enzyme-inducing activity, leading to reduced plasma steroid concentrations; the effect of *zonisamide* is uncertain (87[R]).

A kinetic study in which *ziprasidone* (40 mg/day) or placebo were coadministered with a second-generation oral contraceptive has provided evidence that ziprasidone is unlikely to interfere with oral contraception (88[c]).

In a small study the degree of erythrocyte aggregation during oral contraception was, at least in the short term, partially reversed by treatment with *acetylsalicylic acid* 100 mg/day, as one would probably have anticipated (89[c]).

"Morning after" contraception

The "morning after" method of suppressing pregnancy is usually less well tolerated than normal hormonal contraception, and variants on the dosage schedule continue to be studied in an attempt to improve tolerability without undermining the reliability of the method. An impartial and well documented review from France has examined large-scale work comparing the use of two doses of levonorgestrel (750 μg per dose) and two doses of a combination of ethinylestradiol (100 μg) plus levonorgestrel (500 μg) (90[M]). Levonorgestrel alone was more reliable, with only one-third of the pregnancy rate of the combined treatment. However, *nausea and vomiting*, *dizzy spells*, and *fatigue* were only half as frequent in the women who used levonorgestrel alone. In both groups nearly one-third of the women had abnormal periods after treatment. In the light of this work there is every reason to use levonorgestrel alone.

Hormonal contraception in men

The notion that an oral contraceptive closely similar to that used in women might be developed for men has been discussed for nearly 40 years, but the concept has not yet found wide acceptance. Of the many possible formulations tested all have proved to have unacceptable facets, generally including a very slow onset of azoospermia, uncertain reliability, and undesirable effects on biochemistry, bodyweight, or sexual function. However, some progress is now being made. A combination of oral desogestrel 150 or 300 μg plus intramuscular testosterone 50 or 100 mg has been tested in 24 young men and compared with historical data from studies on a combination of oral levonorgestrel plus intramuscular testosterone (91[C]). All the doses tested achieved azoospermia. All the groups tended to *gain weight* compared with their baseline, but the weight gain was greatest (and statistically significant) in men who received the higher dose of testosterone. Adverse effects were acceptably low; *acne* occurred in occasional cases, but no-one developed gynecomastia.

In a similar study limited to 8 weeks the various formulations rapidly suppressed LH and FSH to a similar extent irrespective of dosage, while testosterone concentrations fell slightly during treatment, with evidence of a linear dose-response relation (92[C]). There were minor changes in plasma concentrations of inhibin B, but in seminal fluid it was suppressed, becoming undetectable in all the men who took desogestrel 300 μg/day. There were no significant changes in lipoproteins, fibrinogen, or sexual behavior during treatment, and only minor falls in hematocrit and hemoglobin concentration.

ANTIESTROGENS *(SED-14, 1466; SEDA-23, 223; SEDA-24, 475)*

Tamoxifen

Tamoxifen is used as a form of HRT to reduce bone loss and the incidence of fractures in high-risk cases (93[cR]), but its main use is in oncology, and it sometimes appears capable of replacing more toxic drugs. In particular, it appears increasingly likely that in the treatment of breast cancer a combination of tamoxifen with ovarian suppression is as effective as the use of cytostatic drugs, and it has been claimed to be better tolerated (94[CR], 95[R], 96[R]). However, the balance between wanted and unwanted effects when using tamoxifen to prevent breast cancer in cases considered to be at risk is a delicate one. The matter has nowhere been more extensively studied than in the Breast Cancer Prevention Trial (P-1), initiated by the National Surgical Adjuvant Breast and Bowel Project (NSABP) in 1992 (97[CR]). In all, more than 13 000 eligible women were randomized to tamoxifen 20 mg/day or placebo for 5 years. During 69 months of follow-up tamoxifen reduced the risk of both invasive and non-invasive cancer and reduced fractures of the hip, radius, and spine; however, the rate of *endometrial cancer* increased (RR = 2.53; 95% CI = 1.35, 4.97), as did the frequency of *vascular events*.

On the other hand, when tamoxifen 20 mg/day was compared with equieffective doses of anastrozole in 668 patients with advanced breast tumors that were hormone receptor-positive or of unknown receptor status, tamoxifen produced too high a rate of *thromboembolism and vaginal bleeding* to be considered the treatment of choice (98[Cr], 99[Cr]).

The effect of high-dose tamoxifen as an adjunct to postoperative brain irradiation has been studied for 40 weeks in 12 patients with glioblastoma multiforme, but without controls (100[c]). Two weeks after surgery, the patients were given high-dose oral tamoxifen (120 mg/m^2 bd for 3 months) and 2 weeks later external beam radiotherapy (59.4 Gy, 3 qd fractions every 6.5 weeks). In one patient tamoxifen was associated with severe *vomiting*, necessitating dosage reduction and subsequent withdrawal; another patient had bilateral *deep venous thrombosis* after 51 weeks, but a causal relation was not firmly established. The authors concluded that adjuvant high-dose tamoxifen is relatively well tolerated, although in this series it did not appear to improve the prognosis.

Nervous system A short supplementary report on the US National Surgical Adjuvant Breast and Bowel Project, originally published in 1999, has now corrected the original data on adverse effects: among the women who had used tamoxifen for an average of 29 months to complement irradiation after lumpectomy for intraductal carcinoma there were five cases of *stroke*, compared with only one of the women who had not used tamoxifen (101[c]). In a parallel trial on breast cancer prevention there was also a slight but non-significant increase in the incidence of stroke in those taking tamoxifen. The investigators have more recently excluded from tamoxifen studies all women with a history of stroke, transient ischemic attacks, uncontrolled hypertension, diabetes mellitus, or atrial fibrillation. It may be wise to regard these conditions as relative contraindications to tamoxifen.

Liver Occasional reports of *hepatic damage* attributable to tamoxifen continue to appear, but the prognosis may be favorable. In one case multifocal steatohepatitis was found in an elderly woman with a history of breast cancer, but after tamoxifen was withdrawn the CT features improved dramatically, and the hepatic transaminases normalized (102[A]).

Skin Tamoxifen has several adverse effects on the skin, including *edema*, *flushing*, *rashes*, *hyperhidrosis*, *urticaria*, *alopecia*, and *hypertrichosis*. *Radiation recall dermatitis*, a severe painful inflammatory skin reaction in sites that have previously been exposed to ionized radiation, was reported for the first time in 1992 (103[A]), and a further case has been reported in a patient taking tamoxifen (104[Ar]). The tamoxifen was withdrawn and the skin healed spontaneously in 7 weeks. The patient was restarted on toremifene, a tamoxifen analogue, which was well tolerated: during 18 months of continuous treatment no signs of radiation recall developed.

Reproductive system *Uterus Intermenstrual bleeding* is a practical problem during tamoxifen therapy, particularly since it obliges the physician to undertake repeated endometrial investigations to exclude malignancy. Monitoring of the uterine cavity in women taking tamoxifen is mandatory, especially when there is postmenopausal bleeding (105[CR]).

Some preliminary but well-designed work has suggested that by inserting a levonorgestrel-releasing intrauterine system it may be possible to limit considerably the problems posed by unscheduled uterine bleeding (106[C]).

Benign thickening of the endometrium is also common during tamoxifen treatment, but appears to be fully reversible within a few months of withdrawal (107[Ar], 108[Cr]). Polyps are not uncommon (109[C]). As to more serious consequences, it would seem that certain women have a genetic predisposition to develop endometrial malignancy during tamoxifen treatment. There were significant amounts of tamoxifen-DNA adducts in the endometrium in eight of 16 women who took the drug but none at all in others, suggesting that a genotoxic mechanism may be responsible for tamoxifen-induced endometrial cancer (110[Cr]). There is, however, some biochemical and histological evidence that tamoxifen-associated endometrial carcinoma is likely to be similar to type I and will therefore have a relatively favorable prognosis (111[E]).

Although the *endometrial cancers* associated with tamoxifen are usually pure adenocarcinomas, other types of rare tumors have also been reported. There is one recent report of a mesodermal mixed tumor of the endometrium occurring 5 years after 5 years of tamoxifen therapy (112[AR]). The tumor responded only to combined treatment with doxorubicin, cyclophosphamide, 5-fluorouracil, and carboplatin. It is possible that this type of tumor arises later than adenocarcinomas and should be looked for during long-term use of tamoxifen.

Two well-documented cases of *uterine carcinosarcoma* have been reported in elderly women after 6 and 7 years of tamoxifen treatment (113[A]). At laparotomy, a heterologous malignant mixed Mullerian tumor with peritoneal spread was found in each case and rapidly proved fatal; large uterine polyps with special histological features may represent an intermediate step in the formation of such tumors (114[AR]). Ten similar cases have been described before.

The pathology of tamoxifen-associated cases of *myometrial adenomyosis* has been compared with that in five cases of postmenopausal adenomyosis not associated with tamoxifen. The tumors were not identical: morphological features more often present in the tamoxifen-associated cases were cystic dilatation of glands (which sometimes resulted in grossly visible intramural cystic lesions), fibrosis of the stroma, and various forms of epithelial metaplasia. The proliferative activity in the adenomyosis, as determined by MIB1 staining, was higher in the tamoxifen group (115[C]), and this could be another mechanism of postmenopausal bleeding among tamoxifen users.

When assessing the risk of endometrial malignancy in women with breast cancer taking tamoxifen, it is worth taking into account evidence that patients with breast cancer may at the outset have some endometrial pathology. In patients with breast cancer scheduled for tamoxifen there were endometrial polyps in 9.3%, endometrial cysts in 16%, and synechiae in 12% at the outset. Tamoxifen significantly increased the incidence of these benign endometrial lesions, usually after less than 1 year of treatment. There were no cases of endometrial carcinoma in 34 patients who had taken tamoxifen for 12–24 months, and only one in 78 patients who had taken it for 5–72 months (116[Cr]).

Ovaries Macroscopically visible *cystic endosalpingiosis* in the paraovarian region has been described in a woman who had been taking tamoxifen for breast cancer (117[Ar]). A 2.5 cm multicystic lesion was seen on the external surface of the right ovary, and histological examination showed a mass of dilated glands lined by ciliated tubal-type epithelium and set in a fibrovascular stroma. Cystic endosalpingiosis resulting in a tumor-like mass is rarely described and is probably not well recognized by histopathologists. Although unlikely to be mistaken for malignancy, the lesion may result in diagnostic confusion. The role of tamoxifen in the development of the lesion in this case is not clear, but the estrogenic effects of tamoxifen may have contributed.

Diagnosis and management of adverse drug reactions The usefulness of transvaginal ultrasound in detecting serious uterine changes in tamoxifen users is currently disputed. According to one group it is a dependable diagnostic method (118[C]), whereas another has found it disappointing, with a high proportion of false-positive findings, even when the assessment criteria were chosen so as to exclude mild endometrial thickening (119[C]). Setting these two papers beside one another it seems that one can detect marked endometrial changes but that ultrasound is not a dependable means of determining whether there is malignancy.

The *hot flushes* that are the main and recurrent problem with tamoxifen in usual doses have now been found to respond well to oral clonidine 0.1 mg/day (120[C]).

Toremifene

Toremifene is an antiestrogen that in animals was less carcinogenic than tamoxifen. An early study to determine whether this promise was fulfilled has been carried out in 20 postmenopausal women with breast cancer; they were switched from tamoxifen 20 mg/day to toremifene 60 mg/day and the effects on the uterus were evaluated prospectively by transvaginal ultrasound (121[c]). In 14 women who had *endometrial thickening or polyps* while taking tamoxifen there were no significant changes during a median of 18 months of toremifene treatment. Of six women who had entered the study because of intolerance to tamoxifen three tolerated toremifene well.

In a multicenter trial in 900 postmenopausal women toremifene 40 mg/day has been compared with tamoxifen 20 mg/day, both given orally for 3 years after breast surgery (122[C]). Subjective adverse effects were similar in the two groups. There were slightly more vascular complications (*deep vein thromboses*, *cerebrovascular events*, and *pulmonary emboli*) among tamoxifen-treated patients (5.9%) than toremifene-treated patients (3.5%), whereas *bone fractures* and *vaginal leukorrhea* were more common with toremifene. The number of subsequent second cancers was similar, as was the breast cancer recurrence rate. If such findings are confirmed in further studies they could provide a reason for using toremifene in patients who do not tolerate tamoxifen.

Raloxifene

The use and adverse effects of raloxifene have been reviewed (123[R]–125[R]). Many centers continue to examine this and other selective estrogen receptor modulators (SERMs), for example in countering menopausal bone loss (126[C]), in the hope that they can take the place of tamoxifen and provide a means of avoiding the risks of such complications as *endometrial cancer*, *cataract*, and *stroke* (127[R]–129[R]).

Cardiovascular There have been conflicting reports on the incidence and severity of symptoms such as *hot flushes* (also known as hot flashes) during long-term treatment with raloxifene for the prevention of osteoporosis. In fact the difference between raloxifene and placebo does not seem to be very great. In a review of three identical randomized trials in which raloxifene 60 mg was given for long periods to healthy postmenopausal women of various ages it was concluded that after 30 months the cumulative incidence of hot flushes was 21% for placebo and 28% for raloxifene, but the difference in frequency was confined to the first 6 months of therapy (130[M]). There was no difference between placebo and raloxifene in the maximum severity of symptoms or the rate of early discontinuation, while the period during which hot flushes continued was only a little shorter in the raloxifene group. In a US study in more than 1100 postmenopausal women who took raloxifene 30–150 mg/day the only significant adverse effect of therapy was hot flushes (25% with 60 mg/day and 18% in the placebo group) (131[CR]).

Reproductive system Several sources have suggested that raloxifene can on occasion either cause *uterine endometrial polyps* or cause preexistent polyps to enlarge considerably (132[A]).

Retinamide and derivatives

Retinamide and tamoxifen have been shown in preclinical studies to have synergistic antitumor and chemopreventive activity against mammary cancer, and they have now been tested together clinically. In 32 women at high risk of breast cancer, treated with four cycles of oral retinamide (200 mg for 25 days of each cycle) and tamoxifen (20 mg od for 23 months beginning after 1 month of retinamide alone), symptomatic reversible *nyctalopia* developed in two patients taking 4-hydroxyretinamide (fenretinide), but three-quarters of the patients had reversible *changes in dark adaptation*, which correlated with a relative fall in plasma retinol concentrations (133[C]). Most of the patients had hot flushes, but only four stopped treatment because of adverse effects. Other unwanted symptoms, all reversible, included skin and ocular dryness, fatigue, and mood changes. Serum HDL cholesterol increased and total cholesterol fell from baseline to month four. The combination appeared to have acceptable tolerability for a high-risk group of patients.

PROGESTERONE ANTAGONISTS

(SED-14, 1471; SEDA-21, 422)

Mifepristone

There has sometimes been reluctance to use higher doses of mifepristone because of a supposedly greater risk of severe adverse effects. However, a recent randomized comparison of a single oral dose of mifepristone (either 200 mg or 600 mg) followed 48 hours later by oral misoprostol 400 μg showed that the two regimens produced identical results as regards the induction of abortion and the incidence of adverse effects (134[Cr])

ANABOLIC STEROIDS, ANDROGENS, AND RELATED COMPOUNDS *(SED-14, 1471; SEDA-22, 463; SEDA-23, 444; SEDA-24, 476)*

Anabolic steroids

One possible use of anabolic agents is in the treatment of the physical wasting associated with HIV infection. Some experience has been gained, but it is still not clear whether such treatment is warranted, bearing in mind the limited benefits that can be expected and the well-documented risks of anabolic drug therapy (135[R]).

Liver The long familiar but low risk of *hepatic adenomas* with anabolic steroids has come to the fore again with the presentation of a Japanese case involving a girl aged 20 years who had been legitimately treated with oxymetholone (30 mg/day) for 6 years for aplastic anemia (136[Ar]). In this case, in contrast to some earlier reports, there was a predisposing factor in the form of familial adenomatous polyposis.

Reversible hepatotoxicity, in the form of abnormal liver function tests, also led to the withdrawal of stanozolol in a patient with lipodermatosclerosis; since some dermatologists continue to have faith in anabolic steroids in this condition, the patient was then given oxandrolone, which is reputed to be less hepatotoxic (137[Ar]). The hepatic problems did not recur, although several months later the patient developed a cardiomyopathy, which may have been coincidental.

Endocrine One residual medical use for oxandrolone in some centers is as a growth-promoting treatment for girls with Turner's syndrome, in which it is regarded by certain workers as an acceptable supplement (in a dose of 0.06 mg/kg/day) to recombinant human growth hormone. A risk of this treatment is *altered glucose metabolism*, but this effect is usually transient. In a series of 18 patients, one girl developed *non-ketotic hyperglycemia* 50 months after the end of treatment; in the other 17 girls the effect of treatment on glucose metabolism was reversible (138[c]). There was a moderate, but not significant, rise in fasting blood glucose throughout the course of the longitudinal study. Fasting insulin increased continuously during treatment but fell after the end of treatment; subsequent concentrations were slightly higher than before treatment, but this could have been an effect of age.

Drug abuse An Australian study of 41 past and present users of anabolic steroids, together with controls from a similar population ("potential users") has vividly portrayed the risks that prolonged use of these products bring (139[C]). Complications included *alterations in libido* (61%), *changes in mood* (48%), *reduced testicular volume* (46%), and *acne* (43%). The mean systolic and diastolic blood pressures were raised in 29% of current users, 37% of past users, and only 8% of controls, although these differences were not significant. *Gynecomastia* was found in 10 past users (37%), two current users (12%), and none of the controls, while mean testicular volume was significantly smaller in current users (18 ml). There were *abnormal liver function tests* in 20 past users (83%), eight present users (62%), and five potential users (71%).

Drug dependence With continuing study of the misuse of anabolic steroids, both in sport and for recreational purposes, the phenomenon of dependence on anabolic steroids is becoming better defined; among the mental changes noted, *aggression* is more prominent than has previously been realized (140[A]).

Androgens

Age-related falls in the concentrations of sex hormones in men are well established in elderly healthy men, although the changes are small compared with the changes in estrogen that occur in postmenopausal women. There have been frequent attempts to develop a male form of hormonal replacement therapy as a "fountain of youth", but the work that continues to appear is either poorly designed or based only on brief and limited studies. The safety of such therapy, even if effective, remains uncertain (141[R]). However, it continues to be in demand for the treatment of hypogonadal men (as well as on the medical fringe as a supposed aphrodisiac), and a recent development is the use of testosterone-impregnated scrotal patches, which have proved acceptable to men who complain of the adverse effects of oral testosterone (142[c], 143[c]).

As noted elsewhere, however, the long-term risks of androgen replacement have still not been properly quantified, and classical complications, such as *polycythemia vera*, continue to be reported (144[A]).

Carcinogenicity Two observations have supported the view that the risks of *prostate cancer* from using testosterone hormone replacement in men may not be as great as was at first feared (145[R]). First, prostate cancers arising in men with low serum testosterone concentrations are more malignant and frequently non-responsive to hormones. Second, breast cancers diagnosed in women taking HRT, although more frequent, are less malignant, possibly because of enhanced sensitivity to hormone therapy, and the situation may prove to be analogous with prostate cancer and testosterone replacement.

ANTIANDROGENS *(SED-14, 1475; SEDA-22, 464; SEDA-23, 445; SEDA-24, 479)*

Complete androgen blockade for the treatment of metastatic prostatic cancer is now facing increasing criticism. All the published data from 27 phase III clinical trials in which medicinal androgen deprivation was used have been reviewed (146[M]). The authors were impressed by the evidence of a higher rate of toxicity and a reduced quality of life with complete androgen blockade. They concluded that the data do not support the routine use of antiandrogens in combination with medical or surgical castration as first-line hormonal therapy in patients with metastatic prostate cancer.

Musculoskeletal Femoral neck bone mineral density has been examined in 26 men before orchidectomy or chemical castration as initial hormone therapy for prostate cancer and at intervals thereafter for up to 42 months (147[C]). The average age-corrected baseline femoral neck bone mineral density was higher in controls than in those who were treated and remained essentially unchanged for 2 years. *Bone loss* was similar after chemical castration to that after orchidectomy: average bone mineral density fell by 1.4–2.6% per year. Bone loss after castration was greater in men who took no regular exercise or were obese or younger than 75 years.

Bicalutamide

Comparative studies of bicalutamide have shown that medical and surgical castration are equally effective in terms of survival or time to progression, but there were statistically significant benefits with bicalutamide monotherapy as regards sexual interest and physical capacity (148[C]). The only common adverse events were *hot flushes* in the surgical castration group, and *breast pain and gynecomastia* in the bicalutamide group. The rates of occurrence of other adverse events were low.

Finasteride

Endocrine Reversible painful *gynecomastia* has been reported as a complication of the use of finasteride in a dose as low as 1 mg/day (149[C]). Such complications call for careful diagnosis, as shown by the case of a 53-year-old man who developed unilateral gynecomastia following finasteride therapy for alopecia (150[A]). On needle biopsy the mammary mass was diagnosed as adenocarcinoma on the basis of nuclear atypia and particularly because of cytoplasmic vacuolization, but excision biopsy showed only benign gynecomastia with no evidence of malignant change. It is possible that in other patients taking finasteride these changes will similarly be wrongly diagnosed as cancerous.

Sexual function Antiandrogens have often been used to treat sexual offenders, but when they are used therapeutically, notably in prostatic cancer, it is not clear what their effect on sexual function may be. In an open, prospective, randomized study, 310 patients with metastatic prostate cancer (median age 71 years) were treated with either flutamide or cyproterone acetate monotherapy, and effects on sexual performance were evaluated periodically using a questionnaire (151[C]). Sexual function depended on age but not on prostate cancer-related parameters. Sexual function at entry was similar in the two treatment groups, with spontaneous erections and sexual activity in 43–51% and 29–35% respectively. During treatment, sexual function in both groups fell slowly over 6–14 months; with an average observation time in excess of 2 years, loss of spontaneous erections and of sexual activity occurred in 80% vs 92% and in 78% vs 88% of men taking flutamide and cyproterone acetate respectively, but these differences were not statistically significant.

Reproductive system Of 65 hirsute women who received either finasteride 5 mg/day or the long-acting GnRH agonist leuprorelin (3.75 mg intramuscular depot monthly), none had either menstrual abnormalities or adverse effects (152[C]). However, the question arises whether adequate doses were used, since the hirsutism score improved only in some 36% of the patients in the GnRH group and in only some 14% of those who received finasteride. Serum total testosterone, free testosterone, androstenedione, and dihydroepiandrosterone fell in patients treated with the GnRH agonist, but only serum total testosterone and free testosterone concentrations fell significantly with finasteride.

Flutamide

While flutamide 250 mg 8-hourly has usually been used in prostatic cancer, comparative work now seems to show that using double this dose produces a more rapid therapeutic response without increasing the risks (153[C]).

Liver Reports on the *hepatotoxicity* of flutamide continue to appear. The authors of a Japanese study in which flutamide was compared with chlormadinone acetate in prostate cancer have again stressed the problem of liver damage with flutamide, but have not provided information on pre-existing risk factors (154[C]). Knowledge of the latter may prove crucial in avoiding this complication (SEDA-24, 480). Liver dysfunction (grade 2) has been noted in another series of Japanese patients treated with flutamide for advanced prostatic cancer (155[Cr]), and there has been a further dramatic account from a Spanish group of acute liver failure during treatment (156[Ar]).

MISCELLANEOUS COMPOUNDS

Tibolone *(SEDA-24, 480)*

Tibolone has estrogenic, progestogenic, and androgenic properties and has been used in different conditions, including hormonal replacement therapy. One positive aspect of its use could be that when equieffective doses are used there is no significant increase in uterine volume or in the number and size of myomas, which can occur when estrogen plus progestogen treatment is used in equieffective doses. Nor does tibolone increase the thickness of the endometrium (157[C]). It has even been claimed, on the basis of one single-blind study, that the use of tibolone in HRT improves sexual desire and performance and coital frequency compared with equieffective continuous treatment with conjugated estrogen 0.625 mg with added progestogen (158[C]). A similar finding has emerged from a recent study in which oral tibolone 2.5 mg/day was claimed to be superior to conventional transdermal 17-β-estradiol 50 μg/day over 12 months in women with surgical menopause. There were similar reductions in climacteric symptoms in the two groups, but there were lower concentrations of HDL and triglycerides in the women who took tibolone, who also had greater improvement in psychological problems and sexual behavior (159[C]). Adverse effects were similar in the two groups.

One of the more unusual applications proposed for tibolone is in combination with the estrogen mestranol and the corticosteroid paramethasone to counter age-related degeneration of the skin in postmenopausal women. The very limited work done so far has provided no basis for a proper assessment of the usefulness or safety of such a long-term blunderbuss approach (160[c]).

Cardiovascular Precisely because of the unusual hormonal profile of tibolone it is still unclear what the biological effects of long-term treatment will be or whether it will be suitable for women with particular diseases, such as hypertension. The effects of tibolone 2.5 mg/day for 6 months on blood pressure and lipids in 29 hypertensive women have been studied, using placebo controls and randomization (161[c]). At 6 months systolic and diastolic blood pressures had fallen slightly more with tibolone than with placebo, but the differences were not statistically significant. The biochemical effects were mixed. Triglycerides fell by a mean of 33% vs 7.6% and HDL cholesterol by a mean of 22 vs 3.8%% in the tibolone and placebo groups respectively. There were no significant differences in total cholesterol, LDL cholesterol, or lipoprotein (a). Fibrinogen concentrations fell by a mean of 14% with tibolone and rose by 19% with placebo. This study suggests that tibolone has no deleterious effect on blood pressure in women with hypertension but is inconclusive about its effects on biochemical risk factors. More work will be needed to determine the overall effect of tibolone on cardiovascular morbidity and mortality.

Hematologic Thrombosis does not seem to be a risk with tibolone. Hematological studies have clearly confirmed that tibolone, and to a lesser extent combined hormonal replacement therapy, changes hemostasis parameters toward a more fibrinolytic profile, which may well reduce the risk of venous thrombosis (162[Ec]).

Reproductive system *Metrorrhagia* is a problem with tibolone in some patients (163[C]). It seems to be related to endometrial proliferation (which can be treated with progestogens, after which tibolone can be restarted), or sometimes to endometrial polyps (which, when small, are likely to be recognized only at hysterectomy), and in certain cases to the formation of ovarian cysts or of intramural myomata.

REFERENCES

1. Ludwig M, Felberbaum RE, Diedrich K. Deep vein thrombosis during administration of HMG for ovarian stimulation. Arch Gynecol Obstet 2000; 263: 139–41.
2. Frydman R, Howles CM, Truong F. A double-blind, randomized study to compare recombinant human follicle stimulating hormone (FSH; Gonal-F) with highly purified urinary FSH (Metrodin HP) in women undergoing assisted reproductive techniques including intracytoplasmic sperm injection. Hum Reprod 2000; 15: 520–5.
3. Battaglia C, Salvatori M, Regnani G, Primavera MR, Genazzani AR, Artini PG, Volpe A. Allergic reaction to a highly purified urinary follicle stimulating hormone preparation in controlled ovarian hyperstimulation for in vitro fertilization. Gynecol Endocrinol 2000; 14: 158–61.
4. Harrison S, Wolf T, Abuzeid MI. Administration of recombinant follicle stimulating hormone in a woman with allergic reaction to menotropin: a case report. Gynecol Endocrinol 2000; 14: 149–52.
5. Duke SS, McGraw SA, Avis NE, Sherman A. A focus group study of DES daughters: implications for health care providers. Psycho-Oncology 2000; 9: 439–44.
6. Kaufman RH, Adam E, Hatch EE, Noller K, Herbst AL, Palmer JR, Hoover RN. Continued follow-up of pregnancy outcomes in diethylstilbestrol-exposed offspring. Obstet Gynecol 2000; 96: 483–9.
7. Herbst AL. Behavior of estrogen-associated female genital tract cancer and its relation to neoplasia following intrauterine exposure to diethylstilbestrol (DES). Gynecol Oncol 2000; 76: 147–56.
8. Verloop J, Rookus MA, Van Leeuwen FE. Prevalence of gynecologic cancer in women exposed to diethylstilbestrol in utero. New Engl J Med 2000; 342: 1838–9.
9. Ylikorkala O. Balancing between observational studies and randomized trials in prevention of coronary heart disease by estrogen replacement: HERS study was no revolution. Acta Obstet Gynecol Scand 2000; 79: 1029–36.
10. Lloyd G. Hormone replacement therapy and ischaemic heart disease: continuing questions but still no answers. Int J Clin Pract 2000; 54: 416–17.
11. Steiner MK, Clarkson PBM, Lip GYH. Myocardial infarction complicating hormone replacement therapy in a young woman with normal coronary arteries. Int J Clin Pract 2000; 54: 475–7.
12. Notelovitz M, Lenihan JP Jr, McDermott M, Kerber IJ, Nanavati N, Arce JC. Initial 17-beta-estradiol dose for treating vasomotor symptoms. Obstet Gynecol 2000; 95: 726–31.
13. Bjarnason NH, Byrjalsen I, Hassager C, Haarbo J, Christiansen C. Low doses of estradiol in combination with gestodene to prevent early postmenopausal bone loss. Am J Obstet Gynecol 2000; 183: 550–60.
14. Kurman RJ, Felix JC, Archer DF, Nanavati N, Arce J-C, Moyer DL. Norethindrone acetate and estradiol-induced endometrial hyperplasia. Mech Dev 2000; 96: 373–9.
15. Heikkinen JE, Vaheri RT, Ahomaki SM, Kainulainen PMT, Viitanen AT, Timonen UM. Optimizing continuous–combined hormone replacement therapy for postmenopausal women: a comparison of six different treatment regimens. Am J Obstet Gynecol 2000; 182: 560–7.

16. Saure A, Planellas J, Poulsen HK, Jaszczak P. A double-blind, randomized, comparative study evaluating clinical effects of two sequential estradiol–progestogen combinations containing either desogestrel or medroxyprogesterone acetate in climacteric women. Maturitas 2000; 34: 133–42.
17. Burch D, Biesheuvel E, Smith S, Fox H. Can endometrial protection be inferred from the bleeding pattern on combined cyclical hormone replacement therapy? Maturitas 2000; 34: 155–60.
18. Takahashi K, Manabe A, Okada M, Kurioka H, Kanasaki H, Miyazaki K. Efficacy and safety of oral estriol for managing postmenopausal symptoms. Maturitas 2000; 34: 169–77.
19. Takahashi K, Okada M, Ozaki T, Kurioka H, Manabe A, Kanasaki H, Miyazaki K. Safety and efficacy of oestriol for symptoms of natural or surgically induced menopause. Hum Reprod 2000; 15: 1028–36.
20. Itoi H, Minakami H, Iwasaki R, Sato I. Comparison of the long-term effects of oral estriol with the effects of conjugated estrogen on serum lipid profile in early menopausal women. Maturitas 2000; 36: 217–22.
21. Haseroth K, Seyffart K, Wehling M, Christ M. Effects of progestin–estrogen replacement therapy on QT-dispersion in postmenopausal women. Int J Cardiol 2000; 75: 161–5.
22. Wenger NK. Hormonal and nonhormonal therapies for the postmenopausal woman: what is the evidence for cardioprotection? Am J Geriatr Cardiol 2000; 9: 204–9.
23. Davidson MH, Maki KC, Marx P, Maki AC, Cyrowski MS, Nanavati N, Arce J-C. Effects of continuous estrogen and estrogen–progestin replacement regimens on cardiovascular risk markers in postmenopausal women. Arch Intern Med 2000; 160: 3315–25.
24. Fernandes LHS, Scassellati-Sforzolini B, Spaide RF. Estrogen and visual hallucinations in a patient with Charles Bonnet syndrome. Am J Ophthalmol 2000; 129: 407.
25. De Valk-De Roo GW, Stehouwer CDA, Emeis JJ, Nicolaas-Merkus A, Netelenbos C. Unopposed estrogen increases total plasma factor VII, but not active factor VII: a short-term placebo-controlled study of healthy postmenopausal women. Thromb Haemostasis 2000; 84: 968–72.
26. Grady D, Wenger NK, Herrington D, Khan S, Furberg C, Hunninghake D, Vittinghoff E, Hulley S. Postmenopausal hormone therapy increases risk for venous thromboembolic disease: the heart and estrogen/progestin replacement study. Ann Intern Med 2000; 132: 689–96.
27. Nagler RM, Pollack S. Sjögren's syndrome induced by estrogen therapy. Semin Arthritis Rheum 2000; 30: 209–14.
28. Sahin F, Sahin I, Ergun MA, Saracoglu OF. Effects of estrogen and alendronate on sister chromatid exchange (SCE) frequencies in postmenopausal osteoporosis patients. Int J Gynecol Obstet 2000; 71: 49–52.
29. Hill DA, Weiss NS, Beresford SAA, Voigt LF, Daling JR, Stanford JL, Self S. Continuous combined hormone replacement therapy and risk of endometrial cancer. Am J Obstet Gynecol 2000; 183: 1456–61.
30. Jain MG, Rohan TE, Howe GR. Hormone replacement therapy and endometrial cancer in Ontario, Canada. J Clin Epidemiol 2000; 53: 385–91.
31. Li CI, Weiss NS, Stanford JL, Daling JR. Hormone replacement therapy in relation to risk of lobular and ductal breast carcinoma in middle-aged women. Cancer 2000; 88: 2570–7.
32. Schairer C, Lubin J, Troisi R, Sturgeon S, Brinton L, Hoover R. Menopausal estrogen and estrogen–progestin replacement therapy and breast cancer risk. J Am Med Assoc 2000; 283: 485–91.
33. Szekacs B, Vajo Z, Varbiro S, Kakucs R, Vaslaki L, Acs N, Mucsi I, Brinton EA. Postmenopausal hormone replacement improves proteinuria and impaired creatinine clearance in type 2 diabetes mellitus and hypertension. Br J Obstet Gynaecol 2000; 107: 1017–21.
34. Matrix H, Singh AK. Estrogen replacement therapy: implications for postmenopausal women with end-stage renal disease. Curr Opin Nephrol Hypertens 2000; 9: 207–14.
35. Ewies AAA, Olah KSJ. Endometrial adenocarcinoma treated by hysterectomy and bilateral salpingo-oophorectomy at age 22 – the dilemma of long-term HRT. J Obstet Gynaecol 2000; 20: 639–40.
36. Gerber GS, Zagaja GP, Ray PS, Rukstalis DB. Transdermal estrogen in the treatment of hot flushes in men with prostate cancer. Urology 2000; 55: 97–101.
37. Taxel P, Kennedy D, Fall P, Willard A, Shoukri K, Clive J, Raisz LG. The effect of short-term treatment with micronized estradiol on bone turnover and gonadotrophins in older men. Endocr Res 2000; 26: 381–98.
38. Rioux JE, Devlin MC, Gelfand MM, Steinberg WM, Hepburn DS. 17-beta-estradiol vaginal tablet versus conjugated equine estrogen vaginal cream to relieve menopausal atrophic vaginitis. Menopause 2000; 7: 156–61.
39. Lose G, Englev E. Oestradiol-releasing vaginal ring versus oestriol vaginal pessaries in the treatment of bothersome lower urinary tract symptoms. Br J Obstet Gynaecol 2000; 107: 1029–34.
40. Rovati LC, Setnikar I, Genazzani AR. Dose-response efficacy of a new estradiol transdermal matrix patch for 7-day application: a randomized, double-blind, placebo-controlled study. Gynecol Endocrinol 2000; 14: 282–91.
41. De Vrijer B, Snijders MPM, Troostwijk AL, The S, Iding RJ, Friese S, Smit DA, Schierbeek JM, Brandts H, Van Kempen PJH, Van Buuren I, Monza G. Efficacy and tolerability of a new estradiol delivering matrix patch (Estraderm MX) in postmenopausal women. Maturitas 2000; 34: 47–55.
42. Andersson TLG, Stehle B, Davidsson B, Hoglund P. Bioavailability of estradiol from two mat-

rix transdermal delivery systems: Menorest and Climara. Maturitas 2000; 34: 57–64.
43. Von Holst T, Salbach B. Efficacy and tolerability of a new 7-day transdermal estradiol patch versus placebo in hysterectomized women with postmenopausal complaints. Maturitas 2000; 34: 143–53.
44. De Aloysio D, Rovati LC, Giacovelli G, Setnikar I, Bottiglioni F. Efficacy on climacteric symptoms and safety of low dose estradiol transdermal matrix patches – a randomized, double-blind placebo-controlled study. Arzneim-Forsch Drug Res 2000; 50: 293–300.
45. Lake Y, Pinnock S. Improved patient acceptability with a transdermal drug-in-adhesive oestradiol patch. Aust NZ J Obstet Gynaecol 2000; 40: 313–16.
46. McGavigan CJ, Metaxa-Mariatou V, Dockery P, Rodger MW, Cameron IT, Campbell S. Large, thin walled, superficial endometrial vessels: the cause of breakthrough bleeding in women with Mirena? Br J Fam Plann 2000; 26: 235–6.
47. Lopes P, Merkus HMWM, Nauman J, Bruschi F, Foidart J-M, Calaf J. Randomized comparison of intranasal and transdermal estradiol. Obstet Gynecol 2000; 96: 906–12.
48. Justice AJH, De Wit H. Acute effects of estradiol pretreatment on the response to d-amphetamine in women. Neuroendocrinology 2000; 71: 51–9.
49. Bruni V, Croxatto H, De La Cruz J, Dhont M, Durlot F, Fernandes MTMS, Andrade RP, Weisberg E, Rhoa M. A comparison of cycle control and effect on well-being of monophasic gestodene-, triphasic gestodene- and monophasic desogestrel-containing oral contraceptives. Gynecol Endocrinol 2000; 14: 90–8.
50. Marks LV. Sexual chemistry. A history of the contraceptive pill. New Haven: Yale University Press, 2001: 138–57.
51. Sartwell PE, Masi AT, Arthes FG, Greene GR, Smith HE. Thromboembolism and oral contraceptives: an epidemiologic case-control study. Am J Epidemiol 1969; 90, 365–80.
52. Royal College of General Practitioners. Oral contraception and thromboembolic disease. J R Coll Gen Pract 1967; 13: 267–9.
53. Vessey MP, Doll R. Investigation of relation between use of oral contraceptives and thromboembolic disease. Br Med J 1968; 2: 199–205.
54. Vessey MP, Doll R. Investigation of relation between use of oral contraceptives and thromboembolic disease. Br Med J 1969; 2: 651–7.
55. Gerstman BB, Piper JM, Tomita DKJ, Ferguson WJ, Stadel BV, Lundin FE. Oral contraceptive estrogen dose and the risk of deep venous thromboembolic disease. Am J Epidemiol 1991; 133: 32–7.
56. Creatsas G, Koliopoulos C, Mastorakos G. Combined oral contraceptive treatment of adolescent girls with polycystic ovary syndrome: lipid profile. Ann NY Acad Sci 2000; 900: 245–52.
57. Jick H, Kaye JA, Vasilakis-Scaramozza C, Jick SS. Risk of venous thromboembolism among users of third generation oral contraceptives compared with users of oral contraceptives with levonorgestrel before and after 1995: cohort and case-control analysis. Br Med J 2000; 321: 1190–5.
58. Bloemenkamp KW, Rosendaal FR, Helmerhorst FM, Buller HR, Vandenbroucke JP. Enhancement by factor V Leiden mutation of risk of deep-vein thrombosis associated with oral contraceptives containing a third-generation progestagen. Lancet 1995; 346: 1593–6.
59. Kemmeren JM, Algra A, Grobbee D.E. Third generation oral contraceptives and risk of venous thrombosis: meta-analysis. Br Med J 2001; 323: 131–4.
60. Bonnar J, Daly L, Carroll E. Blood coagulation with a combination pill containing gestodene and ethinyl estradiol. Int J Fertil 1987; 32 Suppl: 21–8.
61. Nicolaes GAF, Thomassen MCLGD, Tans G, Rosing J, Hemker HC. Effect of activated protein C on thrombin generation and on the thrombin potential in plasma of normal and APC-resistant individuals. Blood Coag Fibrinol 1997; 8: 28–38.
62. Rosing J, Tans G, Nicolaes GAF, Thomassen MCLGD, Van der Ploeg PM, Heijnen P, Hamulyak K, Hemker HC. Oral contraceptives and venous thrombosis: different sensitivities to activated protein C in women using second- and third-generation oral contraceptives. Br J Haematol 1997; 97: 233–8.
63. Meijers JCM, Middeldorp S, Tekelenburg W, Van den Ende AE, Tans G, Prins MH, Rosing J, Buller HR, Bouma BN. Increased fibrinolytic activity during use of oral contraceptives is countered by enhanced factor XI-independent down regulation of fibrinolysis: a randomized cross-over study of two low-dose oral contraceptives. Thromb Haemostasis 2000; 84: 9–14.
64. Bloemenkamp KWM, Rosendaal FR, Helmerhorst FM, Vandenbroucke JP. Higher risk of venous thrombosis during early use of oral contraceptives in women with inherited clotting defects. Arch Intern Med 2000; 160: 49–52.
65. Aisien AO, Sagay AS, Imade GE, Ujah IAO, Nnana OU. Changes in menstrual and haematological indices among Norplant acceptors. Contraception 2000; 61: 283–6.
66. Creatsas G, Koliopoulos C, Mastorakos G. Combined oral contraceptive treatment of adolescent girls with polycystic ovary syndrome. Lipid profile. Ann NY Acad Sci 2000; 900: 245–52.
67. Riederer J. Obstructive jaundice due to sludge in the common bile duct. Dtsch Med Wochenschr 2000; 125: 11–14.
68. Rehan N, Inayatullah A, Chaudhary I. Norplant: reasons for discontinuation and side-effects. Eur J Contracept Reprod Health Care 2000; 5: 113–18.
69. Kaewrudee S, Taneepanichskul S. Norplant users with irregular bleeding: ultrasonographic assessment and evaluation of serum concentration of estradiol and progesterone. J Reprod Med Obstet Gynecol 2000; 45: 983–6.

70. Rogers PAW, Lederman F, Plunkett D, Affandi B. Bcl-2, Fas and caspase 3 expression in endometrium from levonorgestrel implant users with and without breakthrough bleeding. Hum Reprod 2000; 15 Suppl: 152–61.
71. Hickey M, Dwarte D, Fraser IS. Superficial endometrial vascular fragility in Norplant users and in women with ovulatory dysfunctional uterine bleeding. Hum Reprod 2000; 15: 1509–14.
72. Cheng L, Zhu H, Wang A, Ren F, Chen J, Glasier A. Once a month administration of mifepristone improves bleeding patterns in women using subdermal contraceptive implants releasing levonorgestrel. Hum Reprod 2000; 15: 1969–72.
73. Subakir SB, Setiadi E, Affandi B, Pringgoutomo S, Freisleben HJ. Benefits of vitamin E supplementation to Norplant users – in vitro and in vivo studies. Toxicology 2000; 148: 173–8.
74. Alvarez-Sanchez F, Brache V, De Oca VM, Cochon L, Faundes A. Prevalence of enlarged ovarian follicles among users of levonorgestrel subdermal contraceptive implants (Norplant). Am J Obstet Gynecol 2000; 182: 535–9.
75. Klinger G, Graser T, Mellinger U, Moore C, Vogelsang H, Groh A, Latterman C, Klinger G. A comparative study of the effects of two oral contraceptives containing dienogest or desogestrel on the human immune system. Gynecol Endocrinol 2000; 14: 15–24.
76. French RS, Cowan FM, Mansour DJA, Morris S, Procter T, Hughes D, Robinson A, Guillebaud J. Implantable contraceptives (subdermal implants and hormonally impregnated intrauterine systems) versus other forms of reversible contraceptives: two systematic reviews to assess relative effectiveness, acceptability, tolerability and cost-effectiveness. Health Technol Assess 2000; 4: 1–98.
77. Riphagen FE. Intrauterine application of progestins in hormone replacement therapy: a review. Climacteric 2000; 3: 199–211.
78. Lahteenmaki P, Rauramo I, Backman T. The levonorgestrel intrauterine system in contraception. Steroids 2000; 65: 693–7.
79. Backman T, Huhtala S, Blom T, Luoto R, Rauramo I, Koskenvuo M. Length of use and symptoms associated with premature removal of the levonorgestrel intrauterine system: a nation-wide study of 17,360 users. Br J Obstet Gynaecol 2000; 107: 335–9.
80. Cox M, Blacksell S. Clinical performance of the levonorgestrel intra-uterine system in routine use by the UK Family Planning and Reproductive Health Research Network: 12-month report. Br J Fam Plann 2000; 26: 143–7.
81. French RS, Cowan FM, Mansour D, Higgins JPT, Robinson A, Procter T, Morris S, Guillebaud J. Levonorgestrel-releasing (20 mg/day) intrauterine systems (Mirena) compared with other methods of reversible contraceptives. Br J Obstet Gynaecol 2000; 107: 1218–25.
82. Wildemeersch D, Schacht E. Endometrial suppression with a new "frameles" levonorgestrel releasing intrauterine system in perimenopausal and postmenopausal women: a pilot study. Maturitas 2000; 36: 63–8.
83. Wong CY. Irregular bleeding with levonorgestrel IUS may delay cancer diagnosis Br J Fam Plann 2000; 26: 61.
84. Brache V, Alvarez-Sanchez F, Faundes A, Jackanicz T, Mishell DR Jr, Lahteenmaki P. Progestin-only contraceptive rings. Steroids 2000; 65: 687–91.
85. British National Formulary. 2001; September: 624.
86. Seidegard J, Simonsson M, Edsbacker S. Effect of an oral contraceptive on the plasma levels of budesonide and prednisolone and the influence on plasma cortisol. Clin Pharmacol Ther 2000; 67: 373–81.
87. Wilbur K, Ensom MHH. Pharmacokinetic drug interactions between oral contraceptives and second-generation anticonvulsants. Clin Pharmacokinet 2000; 38: 355–65.
88. Muirhead GJ, Harness J, Holt PR, Oliver S, Anziano AJ. Ziprasidone and the pharmacokinetics of a combined oral contraceptive. Br J Obstet Gynaecol 2000; 49 Suppl 1: 49S–56S.
89. El Bouhmadi A, Laffargue F, Raspal N, Brun JF. 100 mg acetylsalicylic acid acutely decreases red cell aggregation in women taking oral contraceptives. Clin Hemorheol Microcirc 2000; 22: 99–106.
90. Anonymous. Levonorgestrel new preparation: emergency contraceptive. Prescrire Int 2000; 9: 202–4.
91. Anawalt BD, Herbst KL, Matsumoto AM, Mulders TMT, Coelingh-Bennink HJT, Bremner WJ. Desogestrel plus testosterone effectively suppresses spermatogenesis but also causes modest weight gain and high-density lipoprotein suppression. Fertil Steril 2000; 74: 707–14.
92. Martin CW, Riley SC, Everington D, Groome NP, Riemersma RA, Baird DT, Anderson RA. Dose-finding study of oral desogestrel with testosterone pellets for suppression of the pituitary-testicular axis in normal men. Hum Reprod 2000; 15: 1515–24.
93. Rosenfeld JA. Can the prophylactic use of raloxifene, a selective estrogen-receptor modulator, prevent bone mineral loss and fractures in women with diagnosed osteoporosis or vertebral fractures? West J Med 2000; 173: 186–8.
94. Boccardo F, Rubagotti A, Amoroso D, Mesiti M, Romeo D, Sismondi P, Giai M, Genta F, Pacini P, Distante V, Bolognesi A, Aldrighetti D, Farris A Cyclophosphamide, methotrexate, and fluorouracil versus tamoxifen plus ovarian suppression as adjuvant treatment of estrogen receptor-positive pre-/perimenopausal breast cancer patients: results of the Italian Breast Cancer Adjuvant Study Group O2 randomized trial. J Clin Oncol 2000; 18; 4 2718–27.
95. Goldstein SR. Drugs for the gynecologist to prescribe in the prevention of breast cancer: cur-

rent status and future trends. Am J Obstet Gynecol 2000; 182: 1121–6.

96. Reddy P, Chow MSS. Safety and efficacy of antiestrogens for prevention of breast cancer. Am J Health-Syst Pharm 2000; 57: 1315–25.

97. Dunn BK, Ford LG. Prevention of breast cancer. Sem Breast Dis 2000; 3: 90–9.

98. Bonneterre J, Thurlimann B, Robertson JFR, Krzakowski M, Mauriac L, Koralewski P, Vergote I, Webster A, Steinberg M, Von Euler M. Anastrozole versus tamoxifen as first-line therapy for advanced breast cancer in 668 postmenopausal women: results of the Tamoxifen or Arimidex Randomized Group Efficacy and Tolerability Study. J Clin Oncol 2000; 18: 3748–57.

99. Nabholtz JM, Buzdar A, Pollak M, Harwin W, Burton G, Mangalik A, Steinberg M, Webster A, Von Euler M. Anastrozole is superior to tamoxifen as first-line therapy for advanced breast cancer in postmenopausal women: results of a North American multicenter randomized trial. J Clin Oncol 2000; 18: 3758–67.

100. Muanza T, Shenouda G, Souhami L, Leblanc R, Mohr G, Corns R, Langleben A. High dose tamoxifen and radiotherapy in patients with glioblastoma multiforme: a phase IB study. Can J Neurol Sci 2000; 27: 302–6.

101. Dignam JJ, Fisher B. Occurrence of stroke with tamoxifen in NSABP B-24. Lancet 2000; 355: 848–9.

102. Cai Q, Bensen M, Greene R, Kirchner J. Tamoxifen-induced transient multifocal hepatic fatty infiltration. Am J Gastroenterol 2000; 95: 277–9.

103. Parry BR. Radiation recall. Lancet 1992; 340: 49.

104. Bostrom A, Sjolin-Forsberg G, Wilking N, Bergh J. Radiation recall – another call with tamoxifen. Acta Oncol 1999; 38: 955–9.

105. Prevedourakis C, Makris N, Xygakis A, Dachlythras M, Michalas S. Endometrial abnormalities in breast cancer patients with tamoxifen therapy. Gynaecol Endosc 2000; 9: 23–6.

106. Gardner FJE, Konje JC, Abrams KR, Brown LJR, Khanna S, Al-Azzawi F, Bell SC, Taylor DJ. Endometrial protection from tamoxifen-stimulated changes by a levonorgestrel-releasing intrauterine system: a randomised controlled trial. Lancet 2000; 356: 1711–17.

107. Love CDB, Dixon JM. Thickened endometrium caused by tamoxifen returns to normal following tamoxifen cessation. Breast 2000; 9: 156–7.

108. Cohen I, Beyth Y, Azaria R, Flex D, Figer A, Tepper R. Ultrasonographic measurement of endometrial changes following discontinuation of tamoxifen treatment in postmenopausal breast cancer patients. Br J Obstet Gynaecol 2000; 107: 1083–7.

109. Bakour SH, Khan KS, Newton JR. Evaluation of the endometrium in abnormal uterine bleeding associated with long-term tamoxifen use. Gynaecol Endosc 2000; 9: 19–22.

110. Shibutani S, Ravindernath A, Suzuki N, Terashima I, Sugarman SM, Grollman AP, Pearl ML. Identification of tamoxifen-DNA adducts in the endometrium of women treated with tamoxifen. Carcinogenesis 2000; 21: 1461–7.

111 . Roy RN, Gerulath AH, Cecutti A, Bhavnani BR. Effect of tamoxifen treatment on the endometrial expression of human insulin-like growth factors and their receptor mRNAs. Mol Cell Endocrinol 2000; 165: 173–8.

112. Dumortier J, Freyer G, Sasco AJ, Frappart L, Zenone T, Romestaing P, Trillet-Lenoir V. Endometrial mesodermal mixed tumor occurring after tamoxifen treatment: report on a new case and review of the literature. Ann Oncol 2000; 11: 355–8.

113. Jessop FA, Roberts PF. Mullerian adenosarcoma of the uterus in association with tamoxifen therapy. Histopathology 2000; 36: 91–2.

114. Fotiou S, Hatjieleftheriou G, Kyrousis G, Kokka F, Apostolikas N. Long-term tamoxifen treatment: a possible aetiological factor in the development of uterine carcinosarcoma: two case-reports and review of the literature. Anticancer Res 2000; 20: 2015–20.

115. McCluggage WG, Desai V, Manek S. Tamoxifen-associated postmenopausal adenomyosis exhibits stromal fibrosis, glandular dilatation and epithelial metaplasias. Histopathology 2000; 37: 340–6.

116. Andia D, Lafuente P, Matorras R, Usandizaga JM. Uterine side effects of treatment with tamoxifen. Eur J Obstet Gynecol Reprod Biol 2000; 92: 235–40.

117. McCluggage WG, Weir PE. Paraovarian cystic endosalpingiosis in association with tamoxifen therapy. J Clin Pathol 2000; 53: 161–2.

118. Strauss H-G, Wolters M, Methfessel G, Buchmann J, Koelbl H. Significance of endovaginal ultrasonography in assessing tamoxifen-associated changes of the endometrium. A prospective study. Acta Obstet Gynecol Scand 2000; 79: 697–701.

119. Gerber B, Krause A, Muller H, Reimer T, Kulz T, Makovitzky J, Kundt G, Friese K. Effects of adjuvant tamoxifen on the endometrium in postmenopausal women with breast cancer: a prospective long-term study using transvaginal ultrasound. J Clin Oncol 2000; 18: 3464–70.

120. Pandya KJ, Raubertas RF, Flynn PJ, Hynes HE, Rosenbluth RJ, Kirshner JJ, Pierce HI, Dragalin V, Morrow GR. Oral clonidine in postmenopausal patients with breast cancer experiencing tamoxifen-induced hot flashes: a University of Rochester Cancer Center Community Clinical Oncology Program study. Ann Intern Med 2000; 132: 788–93.

121. Bertelli G, Queirolo P, Vecchio S, Angiolini C, Bergaglio M, Del Mastro L, Signorini A, Valenzano M, Venturini M. Toremifene as a substitute for adjuvant tamoxifen in breast cancer patients. Anticancer Res 2000; 20: 3659–62.

122. Holli K, Valavaara R, Blanco G, Kataja V, Hietanen P, Flander M, Pukkala E, Joensuu H.

Safety and efficacy results of a randomized trial comparing adjuvant toremifene and tamoxifen in postmenopausal patients with node-positive breast cancer. J Clin Oncol 2000; 18: 3487–94.
123. Snyder KR, Sparano N, Malinowski JM. Raloxifene hydrochloride. Am J Health-Syst Pharm 2000; 57: 1669–78.
124. Sismondi P, Biglia N, Roagna R, Ponzone R, Ambroggio S, Sgro L, Cozzarella M. How to manage the menopause following therapy for breast cancer. Is raloxifene a safe alternative? Eur J Cancer 2000; 36 Suppl 4: S74–6.
125. Body JJ, Sternon J. Raloxifene. Rev Med Brux 2000; 21: 35–41.
126. Brandi ML. Raloxifene reduces vertebral fracture risk in postmenopausal women with osteoporosis. Clin Exp Rheumatol 2000; 18: 309–10.
127. Smith SMR, Osborne MP. Breast cancer chemoprevention. Am J Surg 2000; 180: 249–51.
128. Dardes RC, Jordan VC. Future directions in endocrine therapy for the treatment and prevention of breast cancer. Sem Breast Dis 2000; 3: 119–30.
129. Goldstein SR, Siddhanti S, Ciaccia AV, Plouffe L Jr. A pharmacological review of selective oestrogen receptor modulators. Hum Reprod Update 2000; 6: 212–24.
130. Cohen FJ, Lu Y. Characterization of hot flashes reported by healthy postmenopausal women receiving raloxifene or placebo during osteoporosis prevention trials. Maturitas 2000; 34: 65–73.
131. Johnston CC Jr, Bjarnason NH, Cohen FJ, Shah A, Lindsay R, Mitlak BH, Huster W, Draper MW, Harper KD, Heath III H, Gennari C, Christiansen C, Arnaud CD, Delmas PD. Long-term effects of raloxifene on bone mineral density, bone turnover, and serum lipid levels in early postmenopausal women: three-year data from two double-blind, randomized, placebo-controlled trials. Arch Intern Med 2000; 160: 3444–50.
132. Maia H Jr, Maltez A, Oliveira M, Almeida M, Coutinho EM. Growth of an endometrial polyp in a postmenopausal patient using raloxifene. Gynaecol Endosc 2000; 9: 117–21.
133. Conley B, O'Shaughnessy J, Prindiville S, Lawrence J, Chow C, Jones E, Merino MJ, Kaiser-Kupfer MI, Caruso RC, Podgor M, Goldspiel B, Venzon D, Danforth D, Wu S, Noone M, Goldstein J, Cowan KH, Zujewski J. Pilot trial of the safety, tolerability, and retinoid levels of N-(4-hydroxyphenyl) retinamide in combination with tamoxifen in patients at high risk for developing invasive breast cancer. J Clin Oncol 2000; 18: 275–83.
134. Wu YM, Gomez-Alzugaray M, Haukkamaa M, Ngoc NTN, Ho PC, Pretnar-Darovec A, Healy DL, Sotnikova E, Shah RS, Pavlova NG, Chen JK, Song S, Bygdeman M, Kovacs L, Khomassuridze A, Song LJ, Hamzaoui R, Alexaniants S, Von Hertzen H. Comparison of two doses of mifepristone in combination with misoprostol for early medical abortion: a randomised trial. Br J Obstet Gynaecol 2000; 107: 524–30.
135. Taiwo BO. HIV-associated wasting: brief review and discussion of the impact of oxandrolone. AIDS Patient Care STDs 2000; 14: 421–5.
136. Nakao A, Sakagami K, Nakata Y, Komazawa K, Amimoto T, Nakashima K, Isozaki H, Takakura N, Tanaka N. Multiple hepatic adenomas caused by long-term administration of androgenic steroids for aplastic anemia in association with familial adenomatous polyposis. J Gastroenterol 2000; 35: 557–62.
137. Segal S, Cooper J, Bolognia J. Treatment of lipodermatosclerosis with oxandrolone in a patient with stanozolol-induced hepatotoxicity. J Am Acad Dermatol 2000; 43: 558–9.
138. Joss EE, Zurbrugg RP, Tonz O, Mullis PE. Effect of growth hormone and oxandrolone treatment on glucose metabolism in Turner syndrome: a longitudinal study. Horm Res 2000; 53: 1–8.
139. O'Sullivan AJ, Kennedy MC, Casey JH, Day RO, Corrigan B, Wodak AD. Anabolic–androgenic steroids: medical assessment of present, past and potential users. Med J Aust 2000; 173: 323–7.
140. Copeland J, Peters R, Dillon P. Anabolic–androgenic steroid use disorders among a sample of Australian competitive and recreational users. Drug Alcohol Depend 2000; 60: 91–6.
141. Janssens H, Vanderschueren DMOI. Endocrinological aspects of aging in men: is hormone replacement of benefit? Eur J Obstet Gynecol Reprod Biol 2000; 92: 7–12.
142. Asscheman H, Gooren LJG. Scrotal testosterone patches: a good supplement to treatment possibilities of hypogonadal men. Ned Tijdschr Geneeskd 2000; 144: 847–50.
143. Marcq P, Vanderschueren D. Experiences with scrotal testosterone patches in intolerance or contraindications to intramuscular administration of testosterone esters. Tijdschr Geneeskd 2000; 56: 447–50.
144. Viallard JF, Marit G, Mercie P, Leng B, Reiffers J, Pellegrin JL. Polycythaemia as a complication of transdermal testosterone therapy. Br J Haematol 2000; 110: 237–8.
145. Slater S, Oliver RTD. Testosterone: its role in development of prostate cancer and potential risk from use as hormone replacement therapy. Drugs Aging 2000; 17: 431–9.
146. Laufer M, Denmeade SR, Sinibaldi VJ, Carducci MA, Eisenberger MA. Complete androgen blockade for prostate cancer: what went wrong? J Urol 2000; 164: 3–9.
147. Daniell HW, Dunn SR, Ferguson DW, Lomas G, Niazi Z, Stratte PT. Progressive osteoporosis during androgen deprivation therapy for prostate cancer. J Urol 2000; 163; 181–6.
148. Iversen P, Tyrrell CJ, Kaisary AV, Anderson JB, Van Poppel H, Tammela TLJ, Chamberlain M, Carroll K, Melezinek I. Bicalutamide monotherapy compared with castration in patients with nonmetastatic locally advanced prostate cancer: 6.3 years of followup. J Urol 2000; 164: 1579–82.
149. Wade MS, Sinclair RD. Reversible painful gynaecomastia induced by low dose finasteride (1 mg/day). Australas J Dermatol 2000; 41: 55.

150. Zimmerman RL, Fogt F, Cronin D, Lynch R. Cytologic atypia in a 53-year-old man with finasteride-induced gynecomastia. Arch Pathol Lab Med 2000; 124: 625–7.
151. Schroder FH, Collette L, De Reijke TM, Whelan P, Pavone-Macaluso M, Mattelaer J, Van Velthoven RPF, Newling DWW, Studer UE, Brausi M, Akdas A, Denis L, De Pauw M. Prostate cancer treated by anti-androgens: is sexual function preserved? Br J Cancer 2000; 82: 283–90.
152. Bayhan G, Bahceci M, Demirkol T, Ertem M, Yalinkaya A, Erden AC. A comparative study of a gonadotropin-releasing hormone agonist and finasteride on idiopathic hirsutism. Clin Exp Obstet Gynecol 2000; 27: 203–6.
153. Thrasher JB, Deeths J, Bennety C, Iyer P, Dineen MK, Zhai S, Figg WD, McLeod DG, Bostwick D, Klotz L, Fourcroy J, Stone N. Comparative study of the clinical efficacy of two dosing regimens of flutamide. Mol Urol 2000; 4: 259–63, 265.
154. Ozono S, Okajima E, Yamaguchi A, Yoshikawa M, Iwai A, Moriya A, Yoshida K, Samma S, Maruyama Y, Hirao Y, Kaneko Y, Ohara S, Tabata S, Natsume O, Watanabe S, Aoyama H, Morita N, Hiramatsu T, Ikuma S, Yamada K, Shiomi T, Hayashi Y, Tokizane M. A prospective randomized multicenter study of chlormadinone acetate versus flutamide in total androgen blockade for prostate cancer. Jap J Clin Oncol 2000; 30: 389–96.
155. Tanaka M, Murakami S, Suzuki N, Hamano S, Kinsui H, Oikawa T, Shimazaki J. Endocrine therapy of stage D2 prostate cancer – comparison of drugs used for total androgen blockade. Acta Urol Jpn 2000; 46: 9–14.
156. Rodriguez Gomez SJ, Martinez Moreno J, Martin Arribas MI, Perez Villoria A, De la Serna Higuera C, Betancourt Gonzalez A. Fulminant hepatic failure associated with flutamide. Rev Esp Enferm Dig 2000; 92: 411.
157. Fedele L, Bianchi S, Raffaelli R, Zanconato G. A randomized study of the effects of tibolone and transdermal estrogen replacement therapy in postmenopausal women with uterine myomas. Eur J Obstet Gynecol Reprod Biol 2000; 88: 91–4.
158. Kokcu A, Cetinkaya MB, Yanik F, Alper T, Malatyalioglu E. The comparison of effects of tibolone and conjugated estrogen–medroxyprogesterone acetate therapy on sexual performance in postmenopausal women. Maturitas 2000; 36: 75–80.
159. Mendoza N, Suarez AM, Alamo F, Bartual E, Vergara F, Herruzo A. Lipid effects, effectiveness and acceptability of tibolone versus transdermic 17-beta-estradiol for hormonal replacement therapy in women with surgical menopause. Maturitas 2000; 37: 37–43.
160. Kalogirou D, Aroni K, Kalogirou O, Antoniou G, Botsis D, Kontoravdis A. Histological changes induced by tibolone and estrogen/glucocorticoid on aging skin. Int J Fertil Women's Med 2000; 45: 273–8.
161. Lloyd G, McGing E, Cooper A, Patel N, Lumb PJ, Wierzbicki AS, Jackson G. A randomised placebo controlled trial of the effects of tibolone on blood pressure and lipids in hypertensive women. J Hum Hypertens 2000; 14: 99–104.
162. Winkler UH, Altkemper R, Kwee B, Helmond FA, Coelingh Bennink HJT. Effects of tibolone and continuous combined hormone replacement therapy on parameters in the clotting cascade: a multicenter, double-blind, randomized study. Fertil Steril 2000; 74: 10–19.
163. Ribes C, Montero JJ, Rubira JL, Juarez MA, Ribes M, Ballesteros G, Cavero A, Ceballos C, Berrazueta JR. Metrorrhagia during treatment with tibolone. Toko-Ginecol Pract 2000; 59: 7–10.

J.A. Franklyn

41 Thyroid hormones and antithyroid drugs

THYROID HORMONES

(SED-14, 1485; SEDA-22, 469; SEDA-23, 451; SEDA-24, 484)

Drug interactions Levothyroxine is more than 80% absorbed in the small intestine, peak serum concentrations being reached after 6–12 hours. Non-compliance is by far the commonest cause of persistent hypothyroidism, despite adequate prescription. Rarely severe gastrointestinal disease can reduce absorption. Certain drugs can also affect levothyroxine absorption, including *cholestyramine*, *aluminium hydroxide*, and *ferrous sulfate* (SEDA-24, 484). Now it has been reported that *calcium carbonate* can also reduce levothyroxine absorption (1[A]).

A 49-year-old woman, taking levothyroxine 150 μg/day and calcium carbonate (3 tablets daily) for prevention of osteoporosis, developed symptoms of hypothyroidism and had a raised serum thyrotropin (TSH) concentration (22 mU/l). She was advised to continue taking the same dose of levothyroxine but to separate her medications. Repeat biochemical testing 8 months later showed a normal serum TSH (3.3 mU/l).

Because of the possibility that calcium carbonate might impair levothyroxine absorption, another group carried out a prospective study in 20 patients taking stable long-term levothyroxine for hypothyroidism, who were given elemental calcium as calcium carbonate 1200 mg/day, taken with their levothyroxine for 3 months (2[CE]). Mean serum concentrations of free thyroxine and total thyroxine were significantly reduced during the calcium treatment period and rose after withdrawal. Mean concentrations of triiodothyronine did not change, but serum TSH rose during the calcium period, and 20% of the subjects had a serum TSH concentration above the reference range. The authors also reported the results of an in vitro study of thyroxine binding to calcium, which showed that there is adsorption of thyroxine to calcium at acidic pH. These findings show that calcium can have a modest but potentially clinically significant effect on levothyroxine treatment, probably by binding it and reducing its absorption; patients should be advised to separate their medications.

ANTITHYROID DRUGS

(SED-14, 1489; SEDA-22, 468; SEDA-23, 451; SEDA-24, 484)

Hematologic The most feared complication of thionamide drugs is *bone-marrow suppression*. The reported incidence of agranulocytosis is 0.1–0.3%. In a Japanese study, using an adverse drug reactions database, 24 of 91 cases of presumed drug-induced leukopenia were associated with methimazole (3[R]). The estimated overall risk was 3 per 10 000, largely in the first 3 months (RR = 182, 95% CI = 74, 449). Although full recovery usually follows drug withdrawal, treatment of this complication remains controversial. There have been many reports of the use of granulocyte-colony stimulating factor (G-CSF) in severe cases of thionamide-induced agranulocytosis, with the objective of shortening the period of neutropenia and hence the risk of infection. In 24 patients with Graves' disease who developed agranulocytosis during antithyroid drug therapy, randomized to receive G-CSF ($n = 14$) or an antibiotic only, recovery time (defined as the number of days required for neutrophil counts to exceed 0.5×10^9/l) did not differ between the treatments in patients with

Side Effects of Drugs, Annual 25
J.K. Aronson, ed.

moderate or severe agranulocytosis, arguing against its routine use (4[C]). These conclusions have been supported by retrospective data from a further 12 patients, four of whom received G-CSF (5[c]). Again, there was no significant difference in terms of the speed of hematological recovery, the number of days of antibiotic treatment, or the duration of hospitalization.

Methimazole has also been implicated in cases of immune *thrombocytopenia* and *hemolytic anemia*. Laboratory studies have provided new insights into the immune mechanisms underlying these complications (6[E]). Sera from five patients taking methimazole who presented with immune thrombocytopenia showed antibodies to the platelet cell adhesion molecule-1. Similar antibodies were present in the serum of a patient with carbimazole-associated neutropenia and mild thrombocytopenia, together with antibodies to the neutrophil-specific FC-γ receptor IIIb (7[E]). Antibodies against the rhesus component of erythrocyte proteins have also been described in patients with carbimazole-associated anemia, leading to the conclusion that carbimazole can induce cell lineage-specific drug-dependent antibodies that cause cytopenias.

Immunologic The other important group of adverse effects of the thionamides is vasculitis. Antineutrophil cytoplasmic antibody (ANCA)-associated vasculitis is well described, particularly with propylthiouracil and to a lesser extent with carbimazole, and has been most often described in patients with Graves' disease. The size of the problem has been addressed using serum samples from 117 patients with Graves' disease treated either with propylthiouracil or methimazole, and from untreated patients (8[C]). Myeloperoxidase antineutrophil cytoplasmic antibodies (MPO-ANCA) and proteinase-3 antineutrophil cytoplasmic antibodies (PR3-ANCA) were tested by enzyme-linked immunosorbent assay. MPO-ANCA was negative in all untreated patients and patients taking methimazole, but positive in 21 of 56 patients taking propylthiouracil. In contrast, PR3-ANCA was not detected in any patient in the study. The proportion of patients who were positive for MPO-ANCA increased with the duration of propylthiouracil therapy. Of the 21 MPO-ANCA-positive patients, 12 had no symptoms, but nine complained of myalgia, arthralgia, or coryza-like symptoms after the appearance of the antibody; none had abnormal urinary findings. These findings suggest a specific association between propylthiouracil therapy and the development of MPO-ANCA in patients with Graves' disease.

Drug use has also been examined in 30 patients with ANCA-positive vasculitis, selected as having the highest ANCA titers (defined as more than 12 times the median titer in 250 patients with vasculitis and anti-MPO-ANCA antibodies) (9[C]). Three of the 30 patients had been exposed to propylthiouracil, ten to hydralazine, and five to other candidate drugs, leading to the view that drug exposures should be actively sought in patients with ANCA-positive vasculitis, particularly those with high antibody titers.

Several new reports have described cases of MPO-ANCA-positive cases of vasculitis presenting in a variety of ways in both adults and children treated with propylthiouracil (10[A]–13[A]). Other reports have described serious complications of propylthiouracil in the absence of ANCA, including interstitial nephritis and fatal Stevens–Johnson syndrome in a 90-year-old woman treated for 5 weeks (14[A]) and disseminated intravascular coagulation and vasculitis 2 weeks after the introduction of propylthiouracil in a 42-year-old woman (15[A]). The latter was treated successfully by drug withdrawal and intravenous methylprednisolone.

Teratogenicity *Aplasia cutis congenita* has been attributed to carbimazole, or its active metabolite methimazole, during early pregnancy (16[AM]). The defects can be restricted to a region of the body or can be widespread. Several causes have been documented, including chromosomal abnormalities (e.g. trisomy 13) and single gene mutations, such as Goltz syndrome. A few cases are believed to result from in utero exposure to teratogens, including thionamide drugs. To date, 16 cases of solitary skin defects associated with intrauterine exposure to methimazole have been reported. Additional cases of aplasia cutis congenita in thionamide-exposed infants associated with other congenital abnormalities, such as bilateral atresia of the nasal choana, esophageal atresia, imperforate anus, and cardiovascular defects have also been reported (16[AM]). A 3-year-old child, whose mother had been treated for Graves' hyperthyroidism with methimazole throughout pregnancy, had two scalp lesions and other abnormalities of tissues of ectodermal origin, including dystrophic nails and syndactyly. The authors suggested that a history of in utero exposure to methimazole should be sought in all children with aplasia cutis congenita, as well as other ectodermal tissue abnormalities, to allow better definition of so-called "methimazole embryopathy". However, cautious interpretation of the literature is required, given the small number of methimazole-associated cases of aplasia cutis congenita compared with the widespread prescription of this drug in pregnant women with hyperthyroidism. On the other hand, the absence of an apparent association with the use of the alternative thionamide, propylthiouracil, argues in favor of using the latter in pregnant patients.

IODINE AND THE IODIDES

(SED-14, 1492; SEDA-22, 470; SEDA-23, 452; SEDA-24, 485)

It has been estimated that in 1990 iodine deficiency affected almost one-third of the world's population and represented the greatest single cause of preventable brain damage and mental retardation. Fortification of all salt for animal and human consumption has been chosen as the preferred method for the prevention of iodine deficiency disorders, and this approach is effective in reducing the incidence of such disorders. However, iodine supplementation is not without risk, particularly iodine-induced *hyperthyroidism*, *thyroiditis*, and *thyroid cancer*. The issue of benefit versus risk has been reviewed and the view, previously expressed, that the benefits of correcting iodine deficiency far outweigh risk of iodine supplementation has been reiterated (17[R]). Complications of iodine administration are not confined to those taking dietary supplements to correct deficiency, but can also occur in those given iodine-containing contrast media and with the use of iodine-containing antiseptic solutions (see Chapter 24).

Endocrine Acute *hyperthyroidism* can follow the use of intravenous iodine-containing contrast media (18[A]).

A 54-year-old man developed Graves' hyperthyroidism and hypoadrenalism secondary to adrenocorticotropin deficiency soon after a cranial CT scan with iodine-containing contrast medium. It was presumed that the iodine load (about 30 g) had precipitated thyrotoxicosis in this patient, who had antibodies to the thyrotropin receptor, which in turn precipitated collapse due to adrenal insufficiency.

Salivary glands Acute *sialadenitis* ("iodide mumps") has been described in a 70-year-old man who underwent femoral artery angiography with an iodine-containing contrast agent; he gave a history of a similar episode 24 hours after a previous angiogram (19[A]).

REFERENCES

1. Butner LE, Fulco PP, Feldman G. Calcium carbonate-induced hypothyroidism. Ann Intern Med 2000; 132: 595.
2. Singh N, Singh PN, Hershman JM. Effect of calcium carbonate on the absorption of levothyroxine. J Am Med Assoc 2000: 283: 2822–5.
3. Ohtsu F, Yano R, Inagaki K, Sakakibara J. Estimation of adverse drug reactions by the evaluation scores of subjective symptoms and background of patients. III. Drug-induced leucopenia. Yakugaku Zasshi 2000; 120: 397–407.
4. Fukata S, Kuma K, Sugawara M. Granulocyte colony stimulating factor does not improve recovery from antithyroid drug-induced agranulocytosis: a prospective study. Thyroid 1999; 9: 29–31.
5. Andres E, Maloise F, Ruellan A. Use of colony stimulating factors for the treatment of antithyroid drug-induced agranulocytosis: a retrospective study in 12 patients. Thyroid 2000; 10: 103.
6. Kroll H, Sun Q, Santoso S. Platelet endothelial cell adhesion molecule-1 is a target glycoprotein in drug-induced thrombocytopenia. Blood 2000; 96: 1409–14.
7. Bux J, Ernst-Schlegel M, Rothe B, Panzer C. Neutropenia and anaemia due to carbimazole-dependent antibodies. Br J Haematol 2000; 109: 243–7.
8. Sera N, Ashizawa K, Ando T, Abe Y, Ide A, Usa T, Tominaga T, Ejima E, Yokoyama N, Eguchi K. Treatment with propylthiouracil is associated with appearance of antineutrophil cytoplasmic antibodies in some patients with Graves' disease. Thyroid 2000; 10: 595–9.
9. Choi HK, Merkel PA, Walker AM, Niles JL. Drug-associated antineutrophil cytoplasmic antibody-positive vasculitis. Arthritis Rheum 2000; 43: 405–13.
10. Morita S, Ueda Y, Eguchi K. Antithyroid drug-

induced ANCA-associated vasculitis: a case report and review of the literature. Endocr J 2000; 47: 467–70.

11. Sera N, Yokoyama N, Abe Y, Ide A, Usa T, Tominaga T, Ejima E, Kawakami A, Ashizawa K, Eguchi K. Antineutrophil cytoplasmic antibody-associated vasculitis complicating Graves' disease: report of two adult cases. Acta Med Nagasaki 2000; 45: 33–6.
12. Otsuka S, Kinebuchi A, Tabata H, Yamakage A, Yamazaki S. Myeloperoxidase-antineutrophil cytoplasmic antibody-associated vasculitis following propylthiouracil therapy. Br J Dermatol 2000; 142: 828–9.
13. Matsubara K, Nigami H, Harigaya H, Osaki M, Baba K. Myeloperoxidase-antineutrophil cytoplasmic antibody positive vasculitis during propylthiouracil treatment: successful management with oral corticosteroids. Pediatr Int 2000; 42: 170–3.
14. Dysseleer A, Buysschaert M, Fonck C, Van Ginder Deuren K, Jadoul M, Tennstedt D, Cosyns JP, Daumerie Ch. Acute interstitial nephritis and fatal Stevens–Johnson syndrome after propylthiouracil therapy. Thyroid 2000; 10: 713–16.
15. Khursid I, Sher J. Disseminated intravascular coagulation and vasculitis during propylthiouracil therapy. Postgrad Med J 2000; 76: 185–6.
16. Martin-Denavit T, Edery P, Plauchu H, Attia-Sobol J, Raudrant D, Aurand JM, Thomas L. Ectodermal abnormalities associated with methimazole intrauterine exposure. Am J Med Genet 2000; 94: 338–40.
17. Delange F, Lecomte P. Iodine supplementation – benefits outweigh risks. Drug Saf 2000; 22: 89–95.
18. Beckers EAM, Strack van Schijndel RJM, Weijmer MC. A contrast crisis. Lancet 2000; 356: 908.
19. Chuen J, Roberts N, Lovelock M, King B, Beiles B, Frydman G. "Iodide mumps" after angioplasty. Eur J Vasc Endovasc Surg 2000; 19: 217–18.

H.M.J. Krans

42 Insulin, glucagon, and hypoglycemic drugs

INSULIN *(SED-14, 1501; SEDA-22, 472; SEDA-23, 454; SEDA-24, 487)*

Nervous system Risk factors for cerebral edema during ketoacidosis in children have been investigated in 61 cases of cerebral edema during 6977 hospital admissions (1[C]). They were matched with two types of controls for each case – three children with ketoacidosis randomly selected and three children matched for age (within 2 years), onset of diabetes, blood pH, and serum glucose at entry. The results suggested that high initial serum urea concentrations and a low P_aCO_2 are associated with an increased probability of cerebral edema. Children with these abnormalities should be monitored for signs of neurological deterioration, and hyperosmolar therapy should be immediately available. Treatment with bicarbonate was associated with an increased risk and should be avoided. In an accompanying editorial it was stated that high doses of insulin, hypotonic fluids, and bicarbonate are often seen as culprits, but it is also possible that it is an idiosyncratic response to diabetic ketoacidosis; there is no proof of either theory (2[r]).

Metabolic The authors of a systematic review of whether there is a difference in the frequency and awareness of *hypoglycemia* induced by human or animal insulins identified 52 randomized controlled trials; 37 were double-blind (3[M]). They found no support for the supposition that human insulin per se affects the frequency, severity, or symptoms of hypoglycemia. In a few studies, mainly of less rigorous design, there was an effect when people were transferred from animal to human insulin, indicating increased frequency or reduced awareness of hypoglycemia.

Using evidence from auditory-evoked brain potentials and hypoglycemic clamps, it has been argued that antecedent hypoglycemia not only reduces awareness, but also that several aspects of cognitive function are attenuated during subsequent hypoglycemia 18–24 hours later (4[R]).

A retrospective questionnaire was sent to 195 consecutive patients addressing questions of severe hypoglycemia, coma, awareness of hypoglycemia, and fear of hypoglycemia (5[c]). The mean duration of diabetes was 20 years and 82% had received intensive therapy. Coma was reported in 19% and severe hypoglycemia in 41%. Coma was independently related to neuropathy, β-blockers, and alcohol.

In reaction to a report of *pulmonary edema* and *hypoglycemia* (SEDA-24, 488) it has been noted that in many cases one or more seizures precede pulmonary edema (acute respiratory distress syndrome), suggesting a neurogenic mechanism (6[r]).

The opinions of experts about when and how to treat asymptomatic hypoglycemia in children vary greatly (7[r]). Hypoglycemia in children is often undetected. Using a subcutaneous continuous glucose monitoring system (8[r]) or the non-invasive Glucowatch biographer (9[C]) hypoglycemic periods were more frequent and prolonged than when only fingerprick testing was available. For treating hypoglycemia in children small doses of glucagon are suggested. The contents of a 1 mg/ml ampoule can be drawn into a 1 ml U100 syringe. For children under 2 years 20 μg should be given initially; 10 μg is added for every year, up to 150 μg at age 15. When the effect is insufficient, the dose can be repeated once or twice (10[c]).

Twice-daily NPH insulin for 6 months has been compared with once-daily ultralente in-

Side Effects of Drugs, Annual 25
J.K. Aronson, ed.

sulin in 60 patients (11[C]). NPH was associated with fewer attacks of hypoglycemia, lower HbA_{1c}, lower evening glucose concentrations, and greater patient satisfaction.

Immunologic *Insulin allergy* is rare, but can occur even with new insulins, which are often used in patients with allergic reactions.

A 54-year-old woman with gestational diabetes was later found to be allergic to chromium, pollen, dust, penicillin, acarbose, and metformin (12[A]). She was treated with diet and glibenclamide, but later required insulin. With Humulin N insulin she developed a wheal of 15 mm immediately after the injection, which resolved in a few hours. However, a painful itchy induration appeared 2–3 hours after the injection and lasted a few days. She had an immediate reaction to NPH insulin, with induration, but insulin lispro was well tolerated.

A 5-year-old child with diabetes, Pierre Robin syndrome, cleft palate, allergic rhinitis, recurrent sinusitis, and obstructive sleep apnea, who had previously had skin rashes after penicillin, sulfonamides, and clindamycin, was given soluble and NPH human insulins (13[A]). Three years later she developed local reactions, 2–5 cm in area, 30–120 minutes after injection. Skin-prick tests were negative for the diluent, NPH, and soluble insulin, but intradermal testing was positive with both insulins. Cetirizine and dexamethasone added to the insulin gave temporary relief. She was then given lispro insulin by pump. After about 8 months she started to develop local reactions again, but with cetirizine and the pump her reactions were manageable.

A 6-year-old boy developed recurrent generalized urticaria 1 year after he started to use human Mixtard insulin (14[A]). The rash started 10 minutes after injections in the arms, thighs, and buttocks, at sites where earlier injections had been given, and disappeared within 12 hours. When he was changed to lispro insulin he had three urticarial reactions in the first 2 weeks and then sporadically. The reactions were treated with chlorpheniramine for 2 years.

Drug administration route *Continuous subcutaneous insulin infusion* was found to be feasible in 56 children and adolescents (aged 7–23 years) (15[C]). HbA_{1c} improved in 36 and deteriorated in six. The rate of severe attacks of hypoglycemia fell, but not significantly. Hypoglycemia and seizure frequency were less overall in the group, with better HbA_{1c} concentrations. One patient had a catheter infection and was treated with local antibiotics and a new infusion system at an other site.

Short-acting neutral buffered insulin by pump is sometimes ineffective. Treatment with non-buffered insulin may make things worse, but short-acting acidified insulin can improve HbA_{1c}. This type of insulin is well tolerated for over 3 years. The acid insulin may contain more monomers than neutral insulin, which may act less rapidly, as it contains more polymers (16[r]).

There was no macrophage activation in 10 patients with obstructed (n = 3) or non-obstructed (n = 7) catheters in implantable pumps (17[C]).

Inhaled insulin has been studied in 72 patients in an open, parallel-group, randomized trial for 12 weeks; 35 used inhaled insulin (18[C]). The inhaled insulin was given three times before meals with NPH insulin at bedtime. Controls used their regular insulin two or three times a day with a long-acting insulin at bedtime. HbA_{1c} did not differ between the groups and there was no difference in the frequency or severity of attacks of hypoglycemia. Pulmonary function tests were stable and showed no differences between the groups. There were no serious or major adverse effects.

A warning has been given that over 0.3 μl of blood (and viruses) can reflux in insulin cartridges in pen-like injectors. Reflux was measured using a rubber tube containing a dye solution. A questionnaire study in 193 patients using cartridges showed that 20 patients sometimes noted a reddish cartridge and that two patients shared their cartridges with other patients (19[C]).

An 89-year-old man wrongly read the glucose concentrations in his home glucose meter (20[A]). The meter read 561 mg/dl and 591 mg/dl but testing in the clinic 2 hours later showed concentrations of 175 mg/dl and 188 mg/dl. He had read the digital *display upside down*: 591 instead of 165 and 561 instead of 195. Patients should be instructed about the correct orientation of digital meters.

Drug overdose Suicide by insulin has been reported in a 68-year-old non-diabetic physician who had also taken metoprolol and alcohol. The blood metoprolol concentration was 0.4 μg/ml (usual target range 0.035–0.5 μg/ml) and alcohol 122 mg/dl (27 mmol/l). C-peptide could not be detected, serum insulin was 1849 μU/ml (normal fasting concentration below 16 μU/ml) (21[A]). Insulin overdose has also been reported in four other patients without diabetes (22[A]) and in a 25-year-old man with Munchausen's syndrome (23[A]).

Hypokalemia, *hypophosphatemia*, and *hypomagnesemia* can occur after insulin overdose (24[A]).

A 47-year-old man with type 2 diabetes attempted suicide by taking a bottle of wine, triazolam 2 mg, zoplicone 75 mg, and subcutaneous insulin (soluble 300 U and NPH 1800 U). His blood glucose was 1.5 mmol/l, potassium 2.4 mmol/l, phosphate 0.74 mmol/l, and magnesium 1.06 mmol/l. After 80 ml of 50% glucose and gastric lavage he needed a glucose infusion 6.6 mg/kg/min for 24 hours to keep his blood glucose at 5.5–11.1 mmol/l. There was no brain damage on neurological examination or CT scan.

NEW SYNTHETIC INSULINS

(SED-14, 1506; SEDA-22, 442; SEDA-23, 446; SEDA-24, 489)

Glargine insulin

The long-acting analogue glargine insulin has been reviewed (25[R]). It did not cause a peak in blood insulin concentration, compared with NPH and ultralente insulin. The effect lasted 24 hours, almost comparable to continuous subcutaneous infusion of a short-acting insulin (26[R]).

Metabolic Glargine plus a short-acting insulin has been compared with NPH insulin for 4 weeks in a double-blind study in 256 patients with type 1 diabetes (27[C]). The patients used glargine with zinc 30 μg/ml or 80 μg/ml plus a short-acting insulin at bedtime or once or twice daily NPH insulin. In the patients who used twice-daily NPH the dose of glargine, which was first equal to the total dose of NPH used by the patient, had to be lowered by 6–8%. The patients who used glargine had more attacks of *hypoglycemia* at the start of the study than those who used NPH, but this tended to equalize during the 4 weeks. Fasting plasma glucose was lower in the glargine group. HbA_{1c} concentrations were not reported.

In 619 patients with type 1 diabetes treated with NPH insulin and lispro randomized to once-daily glargine or to once- or twice-daily NPH insulin for 16 weeks in an open study, there was no difference in the frequency of hypoglycemic episodes, severe hypoglycemia, or HbA_{1c} (28[C]). Fasting plasma glucose concentrations were lower with glargine.

In 518 patients with type 2 diabetes using NPH with or without short-acting insulin, randomized to glargine or NPH insulin, there was less nocturnal hypoglycemia with glargine (29[C]). HbA_{1c} and mild symptomatic hypoglycemia was the same in both groups.

In 426 patients with type 2 diabetes poorly controlled with oral therapy, randomized to NPH insulin or glargine, glucose concentrations after dinner were lower with glargine and there were significantly fewer attacks of hypoglycemia (30[C]). HbA_{1c} was 8.2% and 8.1% with glargine and NPH respectively.

Immunologic Glargine insulin solved a problem in a man with type 1 diabetes after pork, beef, and human insulins had elicited allergic reactions (31[A]). Antihistamines ameliorated the reactions but did not resolve them. Glargine insulin elicited no reactions, even when regular insulin was given. This case suggests that the A chain, which is modified in glargine, is part of the allergic epitope. Tolerance to glargine insulin appeared to suppress allergy to regular insulin.

Insulin aspart

Insulin aspart has been compared with regular insulin in 1065 patients for 26 weeks (32[C]). HbA_{1c} improved significantly with aspart. The number of major attacks of *hypoglycemia* fell in the aspart group from 11% to 8%; there were no other differences.

Insulin aspart has been compared with buffered regular insulin by continuous subcutaneous infusion (33[C]). There was some crystal formation with both formulations, but less with insulin aspart. Patients who used aspart required a slightly higher basal dose of insulin but had fewer unexplained attacks of hypoglycemia.

Insulin detemir

Insulin detemir, a new long-acting insulin with a fatty-acid side-chain, has been developed for a constant blood glucose lowering profile. It has been compared with NPH insulin in 59 patients with type 1 diabetes (34[r]). All used detemir for 6 weeks and NPH insulin for 6 weeks in a randomized order. About 2.35 times higher doses of detemir were necessary than NPH. Fasting blood glucose concentrations were lower at the end of the detemir period and there were fewer attacks of hypoglycemia.

Lispro insulin

The pharmacodynamic and pharmacokinetic properties of regular soluble insulin and lispro have been investigated in 12 patients with and without nephropathy in a double-blind cross-over study with euglycemic glucose clamping (35[C]). Insulin clearance was reduced by 30–40% in patients with nephropathy, but in both groups the time to reach the maximal effect was shorter with lispro insulin. The overall metabolic effect of regular soluble insulin but not of lispro insulin was lower in nephropathy, in which a 50% higher dose of regular insulin may be necessary.

When lispro insulin and insulin aspart were compared in a single-blind randomized cross-over study in 14 patients with type 1 diabetes, lispro insulin had a faster onset of action but a shorter duration (36[C]). However, in another study the pharmacokinetic and the pharmacodynamic profiles of insulin aspart compared with human insulin were the same in 24 healthy Japanese as in non-Japanese (37[C]).

Skin *Lipoatrophy* is rare with human recombinant insulin. Two cases of lipoatrophy induced by lispro insulin during continuous subcutaneous insulin infusion have been reported (38[A]).

An 8-year-old girl was switched to continuous subcutaneous insulin infusion using lispro insulin for better regulation after 4 years of diabetes. After 12 months she developed lipoatrophy of the abdominal wall, which progressed during the next months. When she changed to neutral buffered regular human insulin no further lipoatrophy developed, but the existing atrophy did not improve either.

A 51-year-old woman started to use continuous subcutaneous insulin and after 2 years the insulin was changed to lispro. She developed lipoatrophy in the abdomen and buttocks 1 year later and there was an increase in the time before the bolus started to peak. Buffered regular human insulin stopped progression of the lipoatrophy.

Drug administration route Lispro insulin by repeated injection has been compared with lispro insulin by continuous subcutaneous infusion in 41 patients who were C peptide negative (39[c]). HbA_{1c}, mean blood glucose concentrations, and mean insulin doses were significantly lower during continuous subcutaneous infusion; the frequency of attacks of hypoglycemia was the same.

GLUCAGON-LIKE PEPTIDE-1

Glucagon-like peptide-1 is an intestinal hormone that stimulates insulin secretion and inhibits glucagon secretion. Its effects are glucose-dependent and it should not cause hypoglycemia, in contrast to the sulfonylureas. It also reduces the appetite. However, in high doses it causes hypoglycemia in healthy individuals. In eight patients with type 2 diabetes and seven matched non-diabetics subcutaneous glucagon-like peptide-1 and intravenous glucose caused reactive hypoglycemia in five controls but not in the patients (40[r]). Glucagon was suppressed.

In a randomized, cross-over study with glucagon-like peptide-1, metformin, or the combination, there were no differences between the monotherapies (41[r]). The combination had additive effects in lowering blood glucose and tended to reduce the appetite.

ORAL HYPOGLYCEMIC DRUGS

(SED-14, 1508; SEDA-22, 475; SEDA-23, 457; SEDA-24, 491)

Pregnancy Recently attention has given to the use of oral hypoglycemic drugs during pregnancy and more specifically in gestational diabetes. A sulfonylurea (68 women) or metformin (50 women) have been compared retrospectively with insulin (42 women) in pregnancy (42[C]). There were no severe attacks of hypoglycemia, no jaundice, and no differences in neonatal morbidity. However, in those who took metformin *pre-eclampsia* and *perinatal deaths* were more common. Since metformin was given to obese women, and since obesity contributes to pre-eclampsia and perinatal mortality, this may have been an effect of obesity.

In 404 pregnant women at 11–33 weeks of gestation, with a fasting blood glucose of 5.3–7.8 mmol/l, randomly assigned to insulin or glibenclamide there were no differences in perinatal outcome (43[C]). Glibenclamide was not found in cord blood. The data were analysed separately for women with mean glucose concentrations at home above and below 5.8 mmol/l. In the high blood glucose group there were large children for gestational age in 19% (insulin) and 17% (glibenclamide), compared with 10% (insulin) and 11% (glibenclamide) in the low glucose group; it is not clear whether these differences were significant. There were no other differences (e.g. macrosomia, insulin in cord blood) between the groups.

SULFONYLUREAS *(SED-14, 1508; SEDA-22, 475; SEDA-23, 457; SEDA-24, 492)*

There were no differences in episodes of hypoglycemia, concentrations of glucose, insulin, HbA_{1c}, or lipids, or bodyweight when glibenclamide was given in one daily dose instead of divided doses (44[r]).

Maturity-onset diabetes of the young (MODY) is characterized by type 2 diabetes at or before adolescence. It is a genetically heterogeneous disease, for which at least five different genes have been identified. MODY3, one of the most common forms, is characterized by a mutation in the hepatocyte nuclear factor (HNF)-1α gene. MODY3, can be very sensitive to sulfonylureas (SEDA-22, 475; 45[A], 46[c]). Three new cases have been presented, all with a mutation in the HNF-1α gene (47[A]).

The patients were aged 20–25 years. Two took glibenclamide 2.5 mg and chlorpropamide 250 mg for 11 and 3.5 years respectively. HbA_{1c} was low (5.25% and 4.8% respectively). In the first patient glibenclamide was changed to metformin after 11 years as his weight increased. His HbA_{1c} deteriorated rapidly (10%). Reintroduction of glibenclamide lowered the HbA_{1c} to 5.3%. In the second patient chlorpropamide was withdrawn because of hypoglycemia. This led to rapid deterioration (HbA_{1c} 11%). After reintroduction the HbA_{1c} fell. In the third patient tolbutamide, glibenclamide, and chlorpropamide caused recurrent hypoglycemia and he was managed with a very low dose of glibenclamide.

Hematologic *Thrombocytopenia* has been attributed to glimepiride (48[A]).

A 68-year-old man, who had taken pipotiazine and trihexyphenidyl for 12 years for chronic psychosis, took glimepiride for hyperglycemia. No platelet counts were performed before or during this. He had no symptoms of bleeding. He developed a petechial rash and hematomas on his trunk, legs, and face, hemorrhagic bullae in his mouth, and gingival bleeding. There was thrombocytopenia (1×10^9/l), with no malignant cells in a bone-marrow aspirate and no serological evidence of recent viral infection. All medications were withdrawn and he was given prednisone and human immunoglobulin. After 7 days the hemorrhagic syndrome abated, although his platelet count was still 2×10^9/l. After four weeks the platelet count was 23×10^9/l and the prednisone was gradually withdrawn. After 6 months the platelet count was normal (346×10^9/l).

Liver *Acute hepatitis* has been attributed to gliclazide (49[A]).

A 60-year-old woman with normal liver function tests developed acute hepatitis 6 weeks after starting to take gliclazide. No viruses, autoimmune factors, or metabolic factors that could have caused hepatitis could be found. A lymphocyte transformation test was not performed. A liver biopsy was compatible with drug-related acute hepatitis. When gliclazide was withdrawn she improved. She took glibenclamide and recovered fully within 6 weeks.

Risk factors Prolonged hypoglycemia in patients with *end-stage renal disease* prompted a search for predisposing factors in such patients with type 2 diabetes taking oral therapy only (50[R]). Seven patients with and 31 without prolonged attacks of hypoglycemia, all on hemodialysis, were studied. All were using glibenclamide, except for three controls who took tolbutamide. The hypoglycemic episodes lasted 28–256 hours and 83–2000 g of glucose was given for each episode. A recent fall in food intake, previous hypoglycemic episodes, longer duration of episodes, and a history of cerebrovascular disease were associated with prolonged hypoglycemia. There were no relations to age, sex, β-blockers, ACE inhibitors, or drug doses. There were no cases of liver disease or alcohol abuse. Glibenclamide is seven times more highly concentrated in the pancreatic islets than other sulfonylureas, it has a long half-life, and its degradation products have hypoglycemic activity (SED-14, 1510).

Drug formulations Gliclazide MR is a modified-release formulation that allows once-a-day dosing. In a double-blind study 800 patients were randomized to gliclazide or gliclazide MR (51[r]). There were no differences in adverse reactions or hypoglycemia.

Drug overdose Glibenclamide self-poisoning has been reported in a 48-year-old man with von

Willebrand disease, Prinzmetal angina, hepatitis C, and depression (52[A]). He had frequent hypoglycemic attacks, which were not reduced by reducing the dose of glibenclamide. Laparotomy for an insulinoma was considered until a glibenclamide concentration of 0.32 μg/ml was found, although glibenclamide was supposed to have been withdrawn.

To study the impact of Munchausen's syndrome, 129 patients with unexplained hypoglycemia in France had blood tests for sulfonylureas, which were found in 22 cases – glibenclamide in 19 patients and gliclazide in three (53[CR]). The concentrations were usually higher than the usual target concentration – in seven cases they were five times higher and the highest value was 18 times higher. In most cases an insulinoma was suggested and pancreatectomy was planned.

Drug interactions Tolbutamide is mainly metabolized by CYP2C9, which also has a role in the metabolism of sulfonamides. Of various sulfonamides, *sulfaphenazole* had the largest inhibitory effect on the metabolism of tolbutamide in vitro (54[E]). This gives a theoretical basis for being careful when tolbutamide and sulfonamides are coadministered.

Reduced efficacy of gliclazide has been attributed to induction of CYP2C9 by *rifampicin* (55[c])

A 65-year-old man who had taken gliclazide 80 mg/day for 2 years took rifampicin for an infection with *Mycobacterium gordonae*, after which the dose of gliclazide had to be increased to 120 and later to 160 mg/day. After 75 days of combined therapy gliclazide 80 mg/day gave a plasma concentration of 1.4 μg/ml; 7 months after stopping rifampicin it increased to 4.7 μg/ml. Gliclazide was than reduced to 80 mg/day.

It is important to check the blood glucose concentration if rifampicin is given in combination with oral hypoglycemic drugs.

MEGLITINIDES *(SEDA-22, 479; SEDA-23, 462; SEDA-24, 494)*

Repaglinide binds to an unique receptor on the β-cell, different from the sulfonylurea receptor. Meglitinide-stimulated insulin secretion depends on the glucose concentration; insulin secretion is not stimulated in vitro or in fasted animals.

Repaglinide

Repaglinide is a carbamoylmethyl benzoic acid derivative. It is metabolized by CYP3A4. When given preprandially it improves glucose control without increasing the risk of adverse effects (56[C]). There were no differences in action in healthy younger or older volunteers (57[c]). Repaglinide has been extensively reviewed recently, both in monotherapy or in combination with other blood glucose-lowering drugs. It is short-acting and seems to be associated with significantly fewer episodes of serious *hypoglycemia* (58[R]). In a short review of a number of clinical studies the following contraindications were reported (59[r]):

- known hypersensitivity to repaglinide or one of the constituents of Novonorm®;
- type 1 diabetes;
- renal or hepatic impairment.

In a multicenter, double-blind, randomized, fixed-dose trial of placebo and repaglinide 1 and 4 mg for 24 weeks in 361 patients there were no episodes of severe hypoglycemia (60[C]). Most patients withdrew from the placebo group because of hyperglycemia, hypoglycemia, erythematous rash, headache, diarrhea, fatigue, or abnormal vision. Adverse effects had about the same frequencies in the two groups.

Risk factors The clearance of repaglinide is reduced and the half-life prolonged (2.5-fold) in patients with *chronic liver disease* (61[r]).

Drug interactions In theory, drugs such as *ketoconazole* and *erythromycin* should inhibit repaglinide metabolism and drugs that induce CYP3A4, such as *rifampicin*, *barbiturates*, and *carbamazepine*, should increase the dose of repaglinide needed to maintain its hypoglycemic effect. Rifampicin 600 mg reduced the repaglinide AUC by 57% and shortened its half-life from 1.5 to 1.1 hours in nine healthy volunteers after 5 days (62[c]). The effect may even be greater when rifampicin is used for a longer period.

Nateglinide

Nateglinide is a phenylalanine derivative. Single doses of nateglinide 120 mg, repaglinide 0.5 and 2 mg, and placebo 10 minutes preprandially or 2 mg repaglinide 1 minute preprandially have been compared in 15 healthy volunteers (63[C]). Nateglinide stimulated early insulin secretion more than repaglinide, and insulin concentrations returned more promptly to the preprandial values. The highest but slowest rise was seen with placebo. There were no episodes of hypoglycemia.

In a prospective, randomized, double-blind, placebo-controlled study for 24 weeks 701 patients took nateglinide 120 mg before the three main meals, or metformin 500 mg tds, or the combination of the two, or placebo (64[C]). The most frequent adverse effect was *hypoglycemia*, and it was most common in the combination group. There were no differences between those who took nateglinide only or metformin only and there were no episodes of serious hypoglycemia. Diarrhea was more frequent in those taking metformin or the combination, but infection, nausea, headache, and abdominal pain were comparable in the two groups.

In a randomized, double-blind, placebo-controlled comparison of glibenclamide and nateglinide for 8 weeks in 152 patients nateglinide produced higher postprandial insulin concentrations (65[C]). Hypoglycemia and low blood glucose concentrations were more common with glibenclamide.

BIGUANIDES *(SED-14, 1512; SEDA-22, 475; SEDA-23, 459; SEDA-24, 495)*

Metformin

Metabolic *Lactic acidosis* due to metformin continues to be reported, mostly in patients with reduced renal function and taking a high dose of metformin (850 mg tds). The following are the details of several cases:

- a 62-year-old woman: pH 6.60, blood lactate 45 mmol/l, creatinine 133 μmol/l (66[A]);
- a 72-year-old woman: pH 6.84, creatinine 125 μmol/l (67[A]);
- a 75-year-old woman: pH 6.73, lactate 18 mmol/l (67[A]);
- creatinine 91 μmol/l, creatinine clearance 52 ml/min, metformin concentration 61 mg/l (target under 5 mg/l) (68[A]);
- a 52-year-old woman, a chronic alcohol user: pH 6.74, lactate over 30 mmol/l, creatinine 710 μmol/l (69[A]).

All survived but all needed hemodialysis. In all cases there were contraindications to metformin.

Gastrointestinal Three patients who had taken metformin for more than 2 years developed *diarrhea* (70[A]). After withdrawal of metformin the diarrhea resolved within a month. A fourth patient developed diarrhea after taking metformin for 4 months, which stopped after withdrawal; rechallenge with metformin 8 months later led to recurrence. Three patients had bowel disease (diverticulosis, irritable bowel syndrome, and diabetic neuropathy).

Drug overdose The regional poison centers certified by the American Association of Poison Control have reported 55 cases of metformin ingestion by children (71[C]). Unintentional ingestion of 1700 mg of metformin did not pose health risks. In 21 children tested for blood glucose, lactate, or electrolytes there was no evidence of lactic acidosis. Plasma metformin concentrations were not determined.

α-GLUCOSIDASE INHIBITORS *(SED-14, 1513; SEDA-22, 477; SEDA-23, 460; SEDA-24, 495)*

α-glucosidase inhibitors are competitive inhibitors of 1α-glucosidases, enzymes located in the brush border of epithelial cells in the small intestine. The enzymes degrade complex carbohydrates into monosaccharides, which are absorbed.

Acarbose

Acarbose increases insulin sensitivity but not insulin release in elderly patients (72[C]).

Gastrointestinal In a randomized, double-blind, placebo-controlled, cross-over study 12 healthy subjects took acarbose 100 mg or voglibose 0.3 mg tds (73[c]). Postprandial glucose, the rise in plasma immunoreactive insulin, and in immunoreactive C-peptide in the urine increased more with acarbose than voglibose. The *flatus score* was higher with acarbose than voglibose but the stool score was not different and was higher than with placebo. Voglibose before the evening meal may improve nocturnal hypoglycemia during intensive insulin therapy (74[c]).

Lymphocytic colitis activated by acarbose has been reported (75[A]).

A 52-year-old man developed watery diarrhea 6–8 times a day 2 weeks after he had started to take acarbose 100 mg. In 3 weeks he lost 3 kg. Duodenal biopsies were normal; colon biopsies showed a large increase in intraepithelial lymphocytes. The mononuclear cells expressed CD-25 and HLA-DR antigen was increased in the epithelial cells. Within 4 days of acarbose withdrawal the diarrhea had disappeared and biopsies 4 months later showed that CD-25 expression in the cells of the lamina propria was improved and HLA-DR was no longer expressed by the epithelial cells. On rechallenge the diarrhea recurred within 3 days. Biopsies showed pronounced HLA-DR in the epithelial cells and CD-25 expression in some mononuclear cells in the lamina propria.

Paralytic ileus with intestinal pneumatosis cystoides has been reported (76[A]).

An 87-year-old woman, who took acarbose, glibenclamide, and mannitol (for constipation), developed abdominal distension and loss of appetite. An X-ray showed distension of the small intestine, with pockets of small gas bubbles in submucosal space. When her drugs were withdrawn her symptoms subsided and the radiological evidence of ileus disappeared by 5 days. Although she had an atonic bladder, there were no signs of neuropathy. She was also hypothyroid, which could have contributed.

Non-digestible sugar substitutes and α-glucosidase inhibitors should probably not be used in combination.

Liver Hepatitis (SED-14, 1514; SEDA-23, 461) has been attributed to acarbose (77[A]).

A 57-year-old woman developed hepatitis 2 months after starting to take acarbose 100 mg tds. No other causes of hepatitis were found. Liver function tests normalized 3 months after withdrawal. Acarbose was reintroduced 3 years later and she again developed acute hepatitis. Liver function tests became normal 2 months after withdrawal.

Pregnancy In six women with gestational diabetes acarbose 50 mg before meals normalized fasting and postprandial glucose concentrations (78[c]). The pregnancies were uneventful and the neonates were healthy. Internal discomfort persisted during the whole pregnancy.

Drug interactions Acarbose can reduce *digoxin* concentrations, requiring increased doses of digoxin (79[A]).

An 82-year-old man with type 2 diabetes, taking digoxin and voglibose 0.9 mg/day, had digoxin serum concentrations in the target range. He was given acarbose 300 mg/day instead of voglibose and his digoxin concentrations fell from 0.8–2.0 ng/ml to 0.2–0.4 ng/ml. One month after restarting voglibose the digoxin concentrations were again in the target range.

Miglitol

A recent review of miglitol included data on adverse effects in 3585 patients in well-designed clinical trials (80[M]). Only the adverse effects in the gastrointestinal tract occurred with a significantly greater incidence with miglitol 50 mg or 100 mg tds. The adverse effects were the same as with other drugs in this class: *flatulence*, *diarrhea*, *dyspepsia*, and *abdominal pain*. There were no differences with monotherapy or combination therapy or in relation to age or ethnicity. There were more episodes of *hypoglycemia* when miglitol was combined with insulin but not with oral agents. The incidence of cardiovascular events was the same as with placebo.

Drug interactions In a placebo-controlled study of 154 patients taking glibenclamide or metformin, miglitol (starting at 25 mg tds and increasing to 50 or 100 mg tds for 24 weeks) caused more *meteorism*, *flatulence*, and *diarrhea* (81[C]). When miglitol was added to metformin, HbA_{1c} improved and there was weight loss. In another study in 318 patients, more of the patients taking miglitol only or miglitol plus metformin withdrew because of flatulence and diarrhea than in the other groups (82[C]).

THIAZOLIDINEDIONES

(SED-14, 1514; SEDA-22, 478; SEDA-23, 461; SEDA-24, 496)

The thiazolidinediones (glitazones) reduce insulin resistance, specifically in adipose tissue, by binding to the peroxisome proliferator-activated receptor γ (PPARγ). They are sometimes called insulin sensitizers. They increase the number of glucose transporters and reduce concentrations of triglycerides and dense LDL and increase HDL. Troglitazone has been withdrawn because of hepatotoxicity. Rosiglitazone and pioglitazone are being registered in an increasing number of countries. They have been recently reviewed (83[r]).

In a multicenter, double-blind, placebo-controlled study 408 patients took pioglitazone 7.5, 15, 30, or 45 mg/day (84[C]). There was no hepatotoxicity and the overall adverse events profiles did not differ, except for *edema* in 12 of 329 patients who took pioglitazone. There was a significant fall in triglycerides and a small fall in LDL. However, in another study in 150 patients postprandial triglycerides were not reduced by pioglitazone (85[r]).

In a placebo-controlled study 959 patients took placebo, rosiglitazone 4 mg od, 2 mg bd, 8 mg od, or 4 mg bd for 26 weeks (86[C]). In the placebo group 38% withdrew and in the rosiglitazone groups 20%. Two patients (one in the placebo and one in the 4 mg bd group) had changes in AlT of more than three times the upper limit of the reference range. Other adverse events related to edema were seen in 1.6% of the placebo group and in 4.1% of those taking 2 mg bd and 6.6% in those taking 4 mg bd. There were small dose-dependent *falls in hemoglobin and hematocrit*.

In a multicenter, randomized, double-blind study 116 patients were treated for 26 weeks with metformin plus placebo, 119 with metformin plus rosiglitazone 4 mg/day, and 113 with metformin plus rosiglitazone 8 mg/day (87[C]). In both rosiglitazone groups there were small but statistically significant falls in hemoglobin and hematocrit. Edema was rare but more common in the rosiglitazone groups (2.5% with 4 mg/day and 3.5% with 8 mg/day). Bodyweight fell by 1.2 kg from baseline with placebo but increased by 0.7 kg with rosiglitazone 4 mg/day and by 1.9 kg with 8 mg/day. No one taking rosiglitazone had an increase in AlT greater than three times the upper limit of the reference range.

Cardiovascular Reduction in VLDL, cholesterol, LDL-cholesterol, and chylomicrons may contribute to a reduction in cardiac complications. Pioglitazone reduced both lipoprotein(a) and the remnant particles (cholesterol-rich particles after the release of triglycerides from the chylomicrons), whereas troglitazone caused *increases in lipoprotein(a)* (88[r]).

Metabolism The thiazolidinediones *increase bodyweight*. With troglitazone the increase in bodyweight is accompanied by changed fat distribution, but central fat, in part responsible for the cardiovascular changes seen in diabetes, remains the same; weight gain is accompanied by increased subcutaneous fat (89[c]). In a study of pioglitazone in 23 patients for 16 weeks, fasting and mean glucose concentrations and mean free fatty acid concentrations fell; weight gain of 3.6 kg was associated with an increase in peripheral fat without edema (90[c]).

Fluid balance One of the complications of pioglitazone is *fluid retention*, possibly because of increased production of vascular endothelial growth factor (91[r]).

Liver The *hepatotoxicity* of the thiazolidinediones has recently been discussed (92[R]). For troglitazone there were two patterns: “rapid risers”, in whom liver failure took only a few days to develop, and “slower risers”. There were no differences in outcome. The estimated death rate was 1 in 100 000, but the estimate of the FDA advisory committee was 1 in 15 154 at 8 months of treatment. It is unclear whether hepatotoxicity is a class effect of thiazolidinediones or whether the lipophilic α-tocopherol moiety of troglitazone is responsible for this effect. The basic quinone structure of α-tocopherol is common to other drugs that can form hepatotoxic free radicals by CYP2E1-mediated oxidation. No hepatotoxicity has hitherto been reported with pioglitazone. The frequency with rosiglitazone is much lower than for troglitazone and the reported cases seem to have been less serious. No deaths have been reported.

A 61-year-old man developed hepatotoxicity 8 days after starting to take rosiglitazone 4 mg/day, which was withdrawn (93[A]). The AlT was 28 μkat/l,

AsT 23 μkat/l, alkaline phosphatase 8.7 μkat/l, total bilirubin 14 μmol/l, and direct bilirubin 13 μmol/l. All the tests were normal 5 months later. He had taken troglitazone for 1 week 8 months before this incident but had stopped because of nausea and an upset stomach.

A 69-year-old man taking rosiglitazone 4 mg/day and metformin 500 mg/day developed hepatic failure within a week and both drugs were withdrawn (94[A]). His AlT was 32 μkat/l, AsT 47 μkat/l, total bilirubin 65 μmol/l, and direct bilirubin 41 μmol/l. He became comatose and the AsT rose to 185 μkat/l. The enzyme activities were normal 7 weeks after withdrawal.

A 58-year-old woman started to feel ill 2 weeks after starting to take rosiglitazone 4 mg/day (95[A]). One week later her peak AsT was 5.2 μkat/l, AlT 4.2 μkat/l, and bilirubin 41 μmol/l. Four weeks later all the values had returned to normal.

In a 47-year-old woman, who took rosiglitazone 4 mg/day for a short, unspecified time, the alkaline phosphatase increased (11 μkat/l) and returned to normal 2 weeks after withdrawal (96[A]).

There has been a report of hepatic injury with troglitazone but not with rosiglitazone (97[A]).

A 38-year-old woman was given insulin when glibenclamide and acarbose failed. Troglitazone 400 mg/day was added and increased to 800 mg/day 1 month later. After 2 months her liver function tests were normal, but she developed jaundice after 4 months. Total and direct bilirubin were 127 and 101 μmol/L and AlT was 34 μkat/l. After withdrawal of troglitazone her symptoms disappeared and her liver function tests normalized within several months. Metformin 1000 mg bd reduced her insulin requirement. Rosiglitazone 4 mg bd was added and her liver function tests remained normal for 10 months.

Drug interactions In 16 healthy men taking metformin 500 mg bd and/or rosiglitazone 2 mg bd for 4 days there were no significant effects on the steady-state pharmacokinetics of either drug (98[r]).

REFERENCES

1. Glaser N, Barnett P, McCaslin I, Nelson D, Trainor J, Louie J, Kaufman F, Quayle K, Roback M, Malley R, Kuppermann N. Risk factors for cerebral edema in children with diabetic ketoacidosis. New Engl J Med 2001; 344: 264–9.
2. Dunger DB, Edge JA. Predicting cerebral edema during diabetic acidosis. New Engl J Med 2001; 344: 302–3.
3. Airey CM, Williams DRR, Martin PG, Bennett CMT, Spoor PA. Hypoglycaemia induced by exogenous insulin – human and animal insulin compared. Diabetic Med 2000; 17: 416–32.
4. Freuhwald-Schultes B, Born J, Kern W, Peters A, Fehm HL. Adaptation of cognitive function in healthy men. Diabetes Care 2000; 23: 1059–66.
5. ter Braak EWMT, Appelman AMMF, van de Laak ME, Stolk RP, van Haeften TW, Erkelens DW. Clinical characteristics of type 1 diabetic patients with and without severe hypoglycemia. Diabetes Care 2000; 23: 1467–71.
6. Matz R. Hypoglycemia, seizures, and pulmonary edema. Diabetes Care 2000; 23: 1715.
7. Tupola S, Sipilä I, Huttunen NP, Salo S, Nuuja A, Åkerblom HK. Management of asymptomatic hypoglycaemia in children and adolescents with type 1 diabetes mellitus. Diabetic Med 2000; 17: 752–3.
8. Deiss D, Kordonouri O, Meyer K, Danne T. Long hypoglycaemic periods detected by subcutaneous continuous glucose monitoring in toddlers and pre-school children with diabetes mellitus. Diabetic Med 2001; 38: 337–8.
9. Pitzer KR, Desai S, Dunn T, Edelman S, Jayalakshmi Y, Kennedy J, Tamada JA, Potts RO. Detection of hypoglycemia with the GlucoWatch biographer. Diabetes Care 2001; 24: 881–5.
10. Haymond MW, Schreiner B. Mini-dose glucagon rescue for hypoglycemia in children with type 1 diabetes. Diabetes Care 2001; 24: 643–5.
11. Taylor R, Davies R, Fox C, Sampson M, Weaver JU, Wood L. Appropriate insulin regimens for type 2 diabetes. Diabetes Care 2000; 23: 1612–18.
12. Pánczél P, Hosszúfalusi N, Horváth MM, Horváth A. Advantages of insulin lispro in suspected insulin allergy. Allergy Eur J Allergy Clin Immunol 2000; 55: 409–10.
13. Eapen SS, Connor EL, Gern JE. Insulin desensitization with insulin lispro and an insulin pump in a 5-year-old child. Ann Allergy Asthma Immunol 2000; 85: 395–7.
14. Sackey AH. Recurrent generalized urticaria at insulin injection sites. Br Med J 2000; 321: 7274.
15. Maniatis K, Klingensmith GJ, Slover RH, Mowry CJ, Chase HP. Continuous subcutaneous infusion therapy for children and adolescents: an option for routine diabetes care. Pediatrics 2001; 107: 351–6.
16. Kamoi K, Sasaki H, Kobayashi T. Effect on glycemic control of short-acting acidified insulin administered for three years in patients treated by continuous subcutaneous insulin infusion. J Jpn Diabetes Soc 2000; 43: 847–52.
17. Kessler L, Tritschler S, Bohbot A, Sigrist S, Karsen V, Boivin S, Dufour P, Belcourt A, Pinget M. Macrophage activation in type 1 diabetic patients with catheter obstruction during peritoneal delivery with an implantable pump. Diabetes Care 2001; 24: 302–7.

18. Sonoki K, Yoshinari M, Iwase M, Tashiro K, Iino K, Wakisaka M, Fujishima M. Regurgitation of blood into insulin cartridges in the pen-like injectors. Diabetes Care 2001; 24: 603–4.
19. Skyler JS, Cefalu WT, Kourides IA, Landschulz WH, Balagtas CC, Cheng S-L, Gelfand RA. Efficacy of human insulin in type 1 diabetes mellitus: a randomised proof-of-concept study. Lancet 2001; 357: 331–5.
20. Steward DE, Khardori R. An avoidable cause of false home glucose measurements. Diabetes Care 2000; 24: 794.
21. Junge M, Tsokos M, Püschel K. Suicide by insulin injection in combination with beta-blocker application. Forensic Sci Int 2000; 113: 457–60.
22. Winston DC. Suicide via insulin overdose in nondiabetics. Am J Forensic Med Pathol 2000; 21: 237–40.
23. Bretz SW, Richards JR. Munchausen syndrome presenting acutely in the emergency department. J Emerg Med 2000; 18: 417–20.
24. Matsumura M, Nakashima A, Tofuku Y. Electrolyte disorders following massive insulin overdose in a patient with type 2 diabetes. Intern Med 2000; 39: 55–7.
25. Bolli GB, Owens DR. Insulin glargine. Lancet 2000; 356: 443–5.
26. Lepore M, Pampanelli S, Fanelli C, Porcellati F, Bartocci L, Di Vincenzo A, Cordoni C, La Costa E, Brunetti P, Bolli GB. Pharmacokinetics and pharmacodynamics of subcutaneous injection of long-acting human insulin analog glargine, NPH insulin, and ultralente human insulin and continuous subcutaneous infusion of insulin lispro. Diabetes 2000; 49: 2142–8.
27. Rosenstock J, Park G, Zimmerman J. Basal insulin glargine (HOE 901) versus NPH Insulin in patients with type 1 diabetes on multiple daily insulin regimens. Diabetes Care 2000; 23: 1137–42.
28. Raskin P, Klaff L, Bergenstal R, Hallé J-P, Donley D, Mecca T. A 16-week comparison of the novel insulin analog insulin glargine (HOE 901) and NPH human insulin used with insulin lispro in patients with type 1 diabetes. Diabetes Care 2000; 23: 1666–71.
29. Rosenstock J, Schwartz SL, Clark Jr CM, Park GD, Donley DW, Edwards MB. Basal insulin therapy in type 2 diabetes. 28-week comparison of insulin glargine (HOE 901) and NPH insulin. Diabetes Care 2001; 24: 631–6.
30. Yki-Järvinen H, Dressler A, Ziemen M. Less nocturnal hypoglycemia and better post-dinner glucose control with bedtime insulin glargine compared with bedtime NPH insulin during insulin combination therapy in type 2 diabetes. Diabetes Care 2000; 23: 1130–6.
31. Moriyama H, Nagata M, Fujihira K, Yamada K, Chowdhuri SA, Chakrabarty S, Jin Z, Yasuda H, Ueda H, Yokono K. Treatment with human analog (GlyA21, ArgB31, ArgB32) insulin glargine (HOE 901) resolves a generalized allergy to human insulin in type 1 diabetes. Diabetes Care 2001; 24: 411–12.
32. Home PD, Lindholm A, Riist A. Insulin aspart vs human insulin in the management of long-term blood glucose control in Type 1 diabetes mellitus: a randomized controlled trial. Diabetic Med 2000; 17: 762–70.
33. Bode WB, Strange P. Efficacy, safety, and pump compatibility of insulin aspart used in continuous subcutaneous insulin infusion therapy in patients with type 1 diabetes. Diabetes Care 2001; 24: 69–72.
34. Hermansen K, Madsbad S, Perrild H, Kristensen A, Axelsen M. Comparison of the soluble basal analog insulin detemir with NPH insulin. Diabetes Care 2001; 24: 296–301.
35. Rave K, Heise T, Pfützner A, Heinemann L, Sawicki PT. Impact of diabetic nephropathy on pharmacodynamic and pharmacokinetic properties of insulin in type 1 diabetic patients. Diabetes Care 2001; 24: 886–90.
36. Hedman CA, Lindstrom T, Arnquist HJ. Direct comparison of insulin lispro and aspart show small differences in plasma insulin profiles after subcutaneous injection in type 1 diabetes. Diabetes Care 2001; 24: 1120–1.
37. Kaku K, Matsuda M, Urae K, Irie S. Pharmacokinetics and pharmacodynamics of insulin aspart, a rapid-acting analog of human insulin, in healthy Japanese volunteers. Diabetes Res Clin Pract 2000; 49: 119–26.
38. Griffin ME, Feder A, Tamborlane WV. Lipoatrophy associated with lispro in insulin pump therapy. Diabetes Care 2001; 24: 174.
39. Hanaire-Broutin H, Melki V, Bessieres-Lacombe S, Tauber J-P. Comparison of continuous subcutaneous insulin infusion and multiple daily injection regimens using insulin lispro in type 1 diabetic patients on intensified treatment. Diabetes Care 2000; 23: 1232–5.
40. Vilsbøll K, Krarup T, Madsbad S, Holst JJ. No reactive hypoglycaemia in type 2 patients after subcutaneous administration of GLP-1 and intravenous glucose. Diabetic Med 2001; 18: 144–9.
41. Zander M, Taskiran M, Toft-Nielsen M-B, Madsbad S, Holst JJ. Additive glucose-lowering effects of glucagon-like peptide-1 and metformin in type 2 diabetes. Diabetes Care 2001; 24: 720–5.
42. Hellmuth E, Damm P, Mølsted-Pedersen L. Oral hypoglycaemic agents in 118 diabetic pregnancies. Diabetic Med 2000; 17: 507–11.
43. Langer O, Conway DL, Berkus MD, Xenakis EM-J, Gonzales O. A comparison of glyburide and insulin in women with gestational diabetes mellitus. New Engl J Med 2000; 343: 1134–8.
44. Mohamad WBW, Fizi AT, Ismail RB, Mafauzy M. Efficacy and safety of single versus multiple daily doses of glibenclamide in type 2 diabetes mellitus. Diabetes Res Clin Pract 2000; 49: 93–9.
45. Hathout EH, Cockburn BN, Mace JW, Sharkey J, Chen-Daniel J, Bell GI. A case of hepatic nuclear factor-1 alpha diabetes/MODY3 masquerading as type 1 diabetes in a Mexican–American adolescent and responsive to a low dose of sulfonylurea.

Diabetes Care 1999; 22: 867–8.

46. Hansen T, Eiberg H, Rouard M, Vaxillaire M, Møller AM, Rasmussen SK. Novel MODY3 mutations in the nuclear factor-1 alpha gene. Evidence for a hyperexcitability of pancreatic beta-cells to intravenous secretagogues in a glucose-tolerant carrier of a P447L mutation. Diabetes 1997; 46: 726–30.
47. Pearson ER, Liddell WG, Shepherd M, Corrall RJ, Hattersley AT. Sensitivity to sulfonureas in patients with hepatocyte nuclear factor-1 alpha gene mutations: evidence for pharmocogenetics in diabetes. Diabetic Med 2000; 17: 534–5.
48. Cartron G, Jonville-Bera A-P, Autret-Leca E, Colombat P. Glimepiride-induced thrombocytopenic purpura. Ann Pharmacother 2000; 34: 120.
49. Dourakis SP, Tzemanakis E, Sinani C, Kafiri G, Hadziyannis SJ. Gliclazide induced acute hepatitis. Eur J Gastroenterol Hepatol 2000; 12: 119–21.
50. Krepisky J, Ingram AJ, Clase CM. Prolonged sulfonylurea-induced hypoglycemia in diabetic patients with end-stage renal disease. Am J Kidney Dis 2000; 35: 500–5.
51. Drouin P. Diamicron-MR once daily is effective and well tolerated in type 2 diabetes. A double-blind, randomized, multinational study. J Diabetes Complications 2000; 14: 185–91.
52. Torelló AL, Canonge RS, Pascual CH, Manteca JM. Occult ingestion of sulfonylureas: a diagnostic challenge. Endocrinol Nutr 2000; 47: 174–5.
53. Trenque T, Hoizey G, Lamiable D. Serious hypoglycemia: Munchausen's syndrome? Diabetes Care 2001; 24: 792–3.
54. Komatsu K, Kiyomi I, Nakajima Y, Kanamitsu S-I, Imaoka S, Funae Y, Green CE, Tyson CA, Shimada S, Sugiyama Y. Prediction of in vivo drug-interactions between tolbutamide and various sulfonamides in humans based on in vitro experiments. Drug Metab Dispos 2000; 28: 475–81.
55. Kihara Y, Otsuki M. Interaction of gliclazide and rifampicin. Diabetes Care 2000; 23: 1204–5.
56. Moses RG, Gomis R, Frandson KB, Schlienger J-L, Dedov I. Flexible meal-related dosing with repaglinide facilitates glycemic control in therapy-naive type 2 diabetes. Diabetes Care 2001; 24: 11–15.
57. Hatorp V, Huang WC, Strange P. Pharmacokinetic profiles of repaglinide in elderly subjects with type 2 diabetes. J Clin Endocrinol Metab 1999; 84: 1475–8.
58. Massi-Benedetti M, Damsbo P. Pharmacology and clinical experience with repaglinide. Exp Opin Invest Drugs 2000; 9: 885–98.
59. Bouhanick B, Barbosa SS. Repaglinide: Novonorm®, une alternative chez le diabétique de type 2. Presse Méd 2000; 29: 1059–61.
60. Jovanovic L, Dailey III G, Huang WC, Strange P, Goldstein BJ. Repaglinide in type 2 diabetes: a 24-week, fixed-dose efficacy and safety study. J Clin Pharmacol 2000; 40: 49–57.
61. Anonymous. Clinical news. Interactions and pharmacokinetics of repaglinide. Pharm J 2000; 264: 503.
62. Niemi M. Backman JT, Nuevonen M, Nuevonen PJ, Kivistö KT. Rifampicin decreases the plasma concentrations and effects of repaglinide. Clin Pharmacol Ther 2000; 68: 495–500.
63. Kalbag JB, Walter YH, Nedelman JR, McLeod JF. Mealtime glucose regulation with nateglinide in healthy volunteers. Diabetes Care 2001; 24: 73–7.
64. Horton ES, Clinkingbeard C, Gatlin M, Foley J, Mallows S, Sharon S. Nateglidine alone and in combination with metformin improves glycemic control by reducing mealtime glucose levels in type 2 diabetes. Diabetes Care 2000; 23: 1660–5.
65. Hollander PA, Schwartz SL, Gatlin MR, Haas SJ, Zheng H, Foley JE, Dunning BE. Importance of early insulin secretion: comparison of nateglinide and glyburide in previously diet-treated patients with type 2 diabetes. Diabetes Care 2001; 24: 983–8.
66. Reeker W, Schneider G, Felgenhauer N, Tempel G, Kochs E. Metformin-induced lactacidosis. Dtsch Med Wochenschr 2000; 125: 249–51.
67. Løvås K, Fadnes DJ, Dale A. Metformin associated lactic acidosis. Tidsskr Nor Lægeforen 2000; 121: 1539–41.
68. Soomers AJM, Tack CJ. Severe lactic acidosis after use of metformin in a patient with contra-indications to metformin. Ned Tijdschr Geneeskd 2001: 145: 104–5.
69. Houwerzijl EJ, Snoek WJ, Van Haastert M, Holman ND. Severe lactic acidosis after use of metformin in a patient with contraindications to metformin. Ned Tijdschr Geneeskd 2000: 144: 1923–6.
70. Raju B, Resta C, Tibaldi JT. Metformin and late gastrointestinal complications. Am J Med 2000; 109: 261–2.
71. Spiller HA, Weber JA, Winter ML, Klein-Schwartz W, Hofman M, Gorman SE, Stork CM, Krenzelok EP. Multicenter case series of pediatric metformin ingestion. Ann Pharmacother 2000; 34: 1385–8.
72. Meneilly GS, Ryan EA, Radziuk J, Lau DCW, Yale J-F, Morais J, Chiasson J-L, Rabasa-Lhoret R, Maheux P, Tessier D, Wolever T, Josse RG, Elahi D. Effect of acarbose on insulin sensitivity in elderly patients with diabetes. Diabetes Care 2000; 23: 1162–7.
73. Kageyama S, Nakamichi N, Sekino H, Fujita H, Nakano S. Comparison of the effects of acarbose and voglibose on plasma glucose, endogenous insulin sparing, and gastrointestinal adverse events in obese subjects: a randomized, placebo-controlled, double-blind, three-way crossover study. Curr Ther Res Clin Exp 2000; 61: 630–45.
74. Taira M, Takasu N, Komiya I, Taira T, Tanaka H. Voglibose administration before the evening meal improves nocturnal hypoglycemia in insulin-dependent diabetic patients with insulin therapy. Metabolism 2000; 49: 440–3.
75. Piche T, Raimondi V, Schneider S, Héburterne V, Rampal P. Acarbose and lymphocytic colitis. Lancet 2000; 356: 9237.

76. Azami Y. Paralytic ileus accompanied by pneumatosis cystoides intestinalis after acarbose treatment in an elderly diabetic patient with a history of heavy intake of mannitol. Intern Med 2000; 39: 826–9.
77. De la Vega J, Crespo M, Escudero JM, Sánchez L, Rivas LL. Acarbose-induced hepatitis. A report of two events in the same patient. Gastroenterol Hepatol 2000; 23: 282–4.
78. Zárate A, Ochoa R, Hernández M, Basurto l. Efficacy of acarbose to control deterioration of glucose tolerance during gestation. Ginecol Obstet Mex 2000; 68: 42–5.
79. Nagai Y, Hayakawa T, Abe T, Nomura G. Are there different effects of acarbose and voglibose on serum levels of digoxin in a diabetic patient with congestive heart failure? Diabetes Care 2000; 23: 1703.
80. Scott LJ, Spencer CM. Miglitol: a review of its therapeutic potential in type 2 diabetes mellitus. Drugs 2000; 59: 521–49.
81. Standl E, Schernthaner G, Rybka J, Hanefeld M, Raptis SA, Naditch L. Improved glycaemic control with miglitol in inadequately-controlled type 2 diabetics. Diabetes Res Clin Pract 2001; 52: 205–13.
82. Chiasson J-L, Naditch L. The synergistic effect of miglitol plus metformin combination therapy in the treatment of type 2 diabetes. Diabetes Care 2001; 24: 989–94.
83. Docubo J, Sternon J. Les glitazones (thiazolidinediones). Rev Med Brux 2000; 21: 441–6.
84. Aronoff S, Rosenblatt S, Braithwaite S, Egan JW, Mathisen AL, Schneider RL. Pioglitazone hydrochloride monotherapy improves glycemic control in the treatment of patients with type 2 diabetes. Diabetes Care 2000; 23: 1605–11.
85. Shimono D, Kuwamura N, Nakamura Y, Koshiyama H. Lack of effect of pioglitazone on postprandial triglyceride levels in type 2 diabetes. Diabetes Care 2001; 24: 971–2.
86. Phillips LS, Grunberger G, Miller E, Patwardhan R, Rappaport EB, Salzman A. Once- and twice-daily dosing with rosiglitazone improves glycemic control in patients with type 2 diabetes. Diabetes Care 2001; 24: 308–15.
87. Fonseca V, Rosenstock J, Patwardhan R, Salzman A. Effect of metformin and rosiglitazone combination therapy in patients with type 2 diabetes mellitus. J Am Med Assoc 2000; 283: 1695–702.
88. Nagai Y, Abe T, Nomura G. Does pioglitazone like troglitazone increase serum levels of lipoproteine(a) in diabetic patients? Diabetes Care 2001; 24: 408–9.
89. Akazawa S, Sun F, Ito M, Kawasaki E, Eguchi K. Efficacy of troglitazone on body fat distribution in type 2 diabetes. Diabetes Care 2000; 23: 1067–71.
90. Miyazaki Y, Mahankali A, Matsuda M, Glass L, Mahankali S, Ferrannini E, Cusi K, Mandarino L, DeFronzo RA. Improved glycemic control and enhanced insulin sensitivity in type 2 diabetic subjects treated with pioglitazone. Diabetes Care 2001; 24: 710–19.
91. Baba T, Shimada K, Neugebauer S, Yamada D, Hashimoto S, Watanabe T. The oral insulin sensitizer, thiazolidinedione, increases plasma vascular endothelial growth factor in type 2 diabetic patients. Diabetes Care 2001; 24: 953–4.
92. Tolman KG. Thiazolidinedione hepatotoxicity: a class effect? Int J Clin Pract 2000; 54 Suppl: 29–34.
93. Al-Salman J, Arjomand H, Kemp DG, Mittal M. Hepatocellular injury in a patient receiving rosiglitazone: a case report. Ann Intern Med 2000: 132: 121–4.
94. Forman LM, Simons DA, Diamond RH. Hepatic failure in a patient taking rosiglitazone. Ann Intern Med 2000; 132: 118–21.
95. Ravinuthala RS, Nori U. Rosiglitazone toxicity. Ann Intern Med 2000; 132: 658.
96. Hachey DM, O'Neil MP, Force RW. Isolated elevation of alkaline phosphatase level associated with rosiglitazone. Ann Intern Med 2000; 133: 752.
97. Lenhard MJ, Funk WB. Failure to develop hepatic injury from rosiglitazone in a patient with a history of troglitazone-induced hepatitis. Diabetes Care 2001; 24: 168–9.
98. Di Cicco RA, Allen A, Carr A, Fowles S, Jorkasky DK, Freed MI. Rosiglitazone does not alter the pharmacokinetics of metformin. J Clin Pharmacol 2000; 40: 1280–5.

P. Coates

43 Miscellaneous hormones

Calcitonin *(SED-14, 1520; SEDA-22, 483; SEDA-23, 466; SEDA-24, 503)*

The intranasal formulation of calcitonin is associated with fewer adverse effects than the subcutaneous form, probably because of lower systemic availability.

Ear, nose, and throat In a randomized placebo-controlled trial 22% of 1255 postmenopausal women taking active treatment compared with 15% of women taking placebo had *rhinitis* (nasal congestion, discharge, or sneezing) (1[C]). Almost all cases were mild to moderate.

Immunologic *Calcitonin allergy* is very rare and only the second case has been reported (2[A]).

A 60-year-old woman tolerated daily intranasal calcitonin for 6 months of the year for 4 years. She developed *nasal watering*, *nasal and ocular pruritus*, and *sweating* immediately after the administration of nasal calcitonin when she restarted after a 6-month break. These symptoms recurred 2 years later, with *abdominal pain and hypotension*, after 10 months of intramuscular calcitonin, and were again reproduced by a lower dose intramuscularly.

Gonadotrophin-releasing hormone (GnRH, gonadorelin) and analogs

(SED-14, 1523; SEDA-22, 483; SEDA-23, 466; SEDA-24, 503)

Gonadotrophin-releasing hormone analogs cause an initial surge in FSH, LH, and gonadal steroids. Receptor downregulation and gonadotrophin suppression occurs after prolonged administration. Thus, both the clinical and adverse effects depend on the duration of administration. Biological activity and adverse effects also vary between GnRH agonists. In 67 premenopausal Japanese women randomized to 4-weekly low-dose buserelin 1.8 mg or leuprorelin 1.88 mg, women given leuprorelin had a more rapid clinical response and a higher rate of *hot flushes* (3[C]).

Nervous system *Pituitary apoplexy* (hemorrhagic infarction, presenting with sudden severe headache and often followed by pituitary hormone deficiency) has been described in isolated cases when GnRH was given to patients with pre-existing pituitary adenomas.

A 43-year-old woman with a pituitary macroadenoma, who took quinagolide 37.5 μg/day for 33 months, developed *severe headache*, *nausea and vomiting*, and *photophobia* 30 minutes after diagnostic testing with GnRH 50 μg intravenously (4[A]). Although a CT scan at the time showed no evidence of hemorrhage, an MRI scan 18 months later showed a partial empty sella.

It is unclear whether pituitary apoplexy in this case was due to GnRH or quinagolide.

There has been one previous report of seizure exacerbation during leuprorelin treatment, in a girl with pre-existing brain damage (5[A]), and now a case of de novo seizures has been reported (6[A]).

A 13-year-old girl, who had previously had surgery and radiotherapy for a medulloblastoma, developed *atypical absence seizures* for the first time after 3 months of therapy with leuprorelin. The seizures stopped 1 month after treatment was withdrawn and did not recur until 30 months later. The seizures were not related to estradiol concentrations or the menstrual cycle.

Neuromuscular Prolonged GnRH administration is commonly associated with *reduced*

Side Effects of Drugs, Annual 25
J.K. Aronson, ed.

muscle bulk and voluntary muscle function. In a prospective uncontrolled study of 62 men with prostate cancer, treatment with cyproterone acetate and goserelin caused an *increase in fatigue scores* and *increased muscle fatiguability* on objective testing within 6 weeks, in 66% of subjects (7[c]). Fatigue was unrelated to psychological complaints or to self-reported functional ability.

Endocrine Hypogonadal adverse effects, such as *hot flushes*, *mood changes*, and *reduced libido and potency*, are extremely common with gonadorelin analogs. "Draw-back" therapy, in which the dose of nafarelin was reduced after 4 weeks, had similar efficacy, but a lesser degree of bone loss and fewer vasomotor adverse effects compared with full-dose therapy, in a randomized study in 15 premenopausal women (8[c]).

There has been a single case report of *transient thyroiditis* associated with antithyroid antibodies in a 45-year-old woman taking leuprorelin (9[A]). She had other risk factors for autoimmune thyroid disease, and the association was probably coincidental, but the episode may have been precipitated by low estrogen concentrations, as is hypothesized in postpartum thyroiditis.

Musculoskeletal *Osteoporosis* is common in both sexes after gonadorelin therapy. Cross-sectional (10[C]) and longitudinal (11[C]) studies of men with prostate cancer have shown a significant relation between the duration of gonadorelin treatment and bone loss. Hormone replacement therapy has been proposed as prophylaxis against bone loss in women treated with gonadorelin agonists. In a prospective study of 49 women treated with goserelin and randomized to estradiol plus norethisterone or placebo, bone loss persisted 6 years after stopping therapy, and the hormone replacement therapy had only a minor protective effect (12[C]).

Teratogenicity Pregnancies have occurred both after low-dose GnRH agonist therapy for ovulation induction and after higher-dose therapy for endometriosis or other indications: these have been reviewed in the context of a report of a 36-year-old woman who stopped monthly goserelin injections at 16 weeks of gestation and delivered a healthy girl. *Congenital abnormalities* have been reported in a few cases, including one child with *trisomy 13*, one with *trisomy 18*, and an *intrauterine death* due to thrombosis; however, most pregnancies have had normal outcomes (13[Ar]).

Gonadotrophin-releasing hormone antagonists *(SED-14, 1523; SEDA-24, 504)*

Competitive GnRH receptor antagonists cause immediate inhibition of gonadotrophin secretion without downregulation of the GnRH receptor. Although early GnRH receptor antagonists had low potency and caused histamine-related adverse effects, ganirelix and cetrorelix are better tolerated (14[R], 15[C]). *Hot flushes* are rare, in contrast to GnRH receptor agonist therapy: in a prospective uncontrolled study of 346 women given cetrorelix, there was only one case of hot flushes (16[C]). *Ovarian hyperstimulation syndrome* is far less common with GnRH receptor antagonists than agonists in induction of ovulation (15[C], 16[C]).

Skin *Local injection reactions* are common and probably dose-related. In an open study of cetrorelix in its lowest effective dose of 0.25 mg/day, three of 346 women described local reactions (16[C]). In another study of 154 women, 115 of whom were randomized to one 3 mg dose of cetrorelix, 25% had *transitory redness or itching* at the injection site (15[C]). In a multicenter European study of 463 women randomized to ganirelix and 238 to buserelin, 17% of those given ganirelix had moderate *skin redness*, *bruising*, *pain*, or *itching* 1 hour after subcutaneous injection; this had mostly disappeared after 4 hours (17[C]).

Growth hormone (human growth hormone, hGH, somatotropin) *(SED-14, 1520; SEDA-22, 484; SEDA-23, 467; SEDA-24, 504)*

The adverse effects of human growth hormone are dose related, and also more common in men than women, owing to their greater sensitivity to growth hormone. It is common practice to start with a low dose, increase gradually, and titrate against age-specific concentrations of IGF-1, to minimize adverse events (SED-14, 1521).

Nervous system The fatal neurodegenerative condition *Creutzfeldt–Jakob disease* was associated with an earlier form of human growth hormone, manufactured from human pituitary tissue. It was discontinued in the 1980s because of this adverse effect (SED-14, 1521). The condition may take up to 30 years after treatment to develop, and new cases continue to be reported (18[A]).

Endocrine *Hyperinsulinemia* is common in recipients of human growth hormone. In a postmarketing review of 23 333 children and adolescents (52 375 treatment years), the incidence of type I diabetes was not significantly increased. However, *type II diabetes* occurred in 46 and 28 per 100 000 treatment years in children aged 10–19 and 6–14 years respectively (six times greater in both age groups than published reference values). There was no difference in incidence between boys and girls. A further 42 children developed *abnormal glucose tolerance* (19[C]). Diabetes and glucose intolerance did not resolve after growth hormone was withdrawn. Children who became diabetic were usually pubertal and had received growth hormone for a longer period. Obesity, a risk factor for type II diabetes in the general population, was uncommon in these children.

Experience in adults is more limited, and monitoring is essential (20[r]). Studies of human growth hormone in adults have consistently shown *increased plasma concentrations of glucose*, *glycated hemoglobin*, and *insulin* (21[C], 22[C]). Glucose intolerance and frank diabetes mellitus have been frequently reported in small series (21[C], 23[C]), but the overall incidence has not been compared with that in the general population.

Three adolescent boys with chronic renal insufficiency, treated with human growth hormone during the pubertal growth spurt, developed severe *hyperparathyroidism* (24[Ar]). It is unclear whether this was coincidental or whether growth hormone and sex steroid hormones had a synergistic effect.

Enhanced peripheral conversion of thyroxine to triiodothyronine is a well-described effect of human growth hormone (SED-13, 1308). One child with Prader–Willi syndrome had a *fall in serum thyroxine concentration* during growth hormone therapy and needed thyroxine replacement (25[R]).

Hematologic *Leukemia* has been reported in several patients treated with human growth hormone. However, when other risk factors are accounted for, there is no current evidence that it increases the risk significantly above population levels (SEDA-23, 468) (26[C]). Acute myelogenous leukemia was diagnosed in a 25-year-old man with hypopituitarism, 4 months after he started to use human growth hormone three times a week (27[A]). The time interval in this case was too short to implicate growth hormone as a definite cause.

Drug interactions Growth hormone increases the activity and regulates the gene expression of hepatic CYP3A4 (28[E]). Mean blood concentrations of ciclosporin were lower during human growth hormone therapy in an open study in 16 prepubertal kidney transplant recipients, despite stable weight-related doses, suggesting that the metabolism of ciclosporin was increased by growth hormone. Two patients had acute episodes of rejection during growth hormone therapy: one of these may have been related to the drop in ciclosporin concentration (29[A]).

Growth hormone release-inhibiting hormone (somatostatin) and analogs *(SED-14, 1522; SEDA-22, 486; SEDA-23, 469; SEDA-24, 505)*

Cardiovascular Somatostatin and octreotide both cause a *transient increase in mean arterial pressure*, which is rarely significant; this might be either direct or mediated by inhibition of gut vasodilatory peptides (SEDA-24, 505) (30[Ar]). *Severe hypertension with associated headache*, *nausea*, and *vomiting* was reported within 2 weeks of administration of octreotide LAR 20 mg in a 26-year-old diabetic woman with autonomic neuropathy (30[Ar]). Rechallenge with octreotide 75 μg resulted in a transient hypertensive episode lasting 3 hours. Exacerbation of pre-existing hypertension was also reported in a 22-month-old boy during octreotide infusion (31[A]).

Hematologic A 42-year-old woman treated with octreotide infusion 50 μg/hour for cirrhosis-related gastrointestinal bleeding on two occasions 9 months apart, had an immediate *fall in platelet count* on both occasions, resolving after octreotide withdrawal (32[A]). Thrombocytopenia was not severe (nadir platelet counts 62 and 55×10^9/l), comparable to two previously reported cases, and did not require specific treatment. The rapid fall in platelet count suggests an immunological mechanism, although this was not directly demonstrated.

Immunologic *Antibodies* to somatostatin analogs have previously been reported only rarely. However, octreotide antibodies were demonstrated in 63 (27%) of 231 patients treated with subcutaneous octreotide for more than 3 years, rising to 57% after 5 years and 72% after 8 years (33[C]). The antibodies did not reduce clinical efficacy.

Melatonin

Melatonin (N-acetyl-5-methoxytryptamine) is a hormone secreted by the pineal gland from the amino acid precursor L-tryptophan. Its endogenous secretion is photosensitive and has a circadian rhythm – plasma melatonin concentrations are highest at night in both diurnal and nocturnal animals, and fall with age (34[R]). The nocturnal melatonin peak coincides with a drop in body temperature and increased sleepiness in healthy humans.

Because melatonin is present in small amounts in some foods, it is licensed as a nutritional supplement in the USA. However, the reliability and consistency of commercial melatonin has been questioned (35[R]). One group analysed three commercial melatonin formulations and identified analogs of the contaminant of L-tryptophan compounds implicated in an epidemic of eosinophilia–myalgia syndrome in the 1980s (36[E]). There have been no reports of this condition associated with melatonin consumption, but food supplements are not required to comply with the same manufacturing and monitoring quality control standards as drugs.

Melatonin has been promoted as a treatment for conditions ranging from jet lag to cancer (34[R], 35[R], 37[R], 38[M]) and is sometimes used for sleep induction (34[R]). The effects of chronic treatment have not been studied, and adverse effects have not been systematically reported.

Oral melatonin has a short half-life of 30–50 minutes and extensive first-pass metabolism. Its clearance is reduced in severe liver disease (39[c]). Timing is critical for melatonin to be effective: if given at the wrong time for sleep disorders or jet lag, it can cause increased daytime sleepiness (38[M], 40[c]) and worsened mental performance (41[c]). Drowsiness and a small fall in body temperature are commonly reported effects of melatonin (42[r]), particularly after daytime administration, when endogenous concentrations are low.

Cardiovascular *There was an increase in blood pressure throughout 24 hours in a double-blind, placebo-controlled, cross-over study in 47 hypertensive patients who were also taking nifedipine (43[c]). This finding differs from other studies in which melatonin had a mild hypotensive effect (44[c]), and may indicate an interaction between melatonin and nifedipine. Tachycardia, chest pain, and cardiac dysrhythmias have also been reported, although the relation to melatonin was not clearly established (38[M]).*

Nervous system *Four of six children with preexisting severe neurological disorders had increased seizure activity within 2 weeks of starting oral melatonin 5 mg at bedtime (45[c]). Seizure frequency returned to baseline after treatment was stopped, and increased again after rechallenge with melatonin 1 mg. A convulsion during melatonin treatment, which recurred when medication was continued, has been reported to the WHO database but not published (38[M]). Headache, which recovered after melatonin was withdrawn, has also been reported in a few cases (38[M]).*

Dyskinesia and akathisia has been reported after withdrawal of long-term melatonin (46[A]).

A 22-year-old woman with cerebral palsy, severe mental retardation, and insomnia had taken melatonin 5 mg each night for 1 year with a good response. However, 1 week after melatonin was stopped because of repeated vomiting she gradually developed involuntary lip-smacking movements and tongue protrusion, with extreme restlessness, moaning, and shouting. These symptoms continued for 2 weeks, accompanied by marked worsening of insomnia with restlessness. Melatonin was reintroduced in gradually increasing doses, and 2 days after a dose of 5 mg was reached, the involuntary movements disappeared and her agitated state and insomnia improved. A month later, another episode of abdominal pain and vomiting made her discontinue melatonin again. Within 2 days she developed identical involuntary lip and tongue movements and akathisia. Melatonin 5 mg was readministered and by the next day all her symptoms had disappeared.

This case raises an important question regarding the dopamine-blocking effect of melatonin. Like dopamine receptor antagonists, melatonin should be used with care because of the risk of tardive dyskinesia, which has serious morbidity and a low remission rate. It should be used with special caution in patients with organic brain damage.

Sensory systems *Loss of visual acuity, reduced color vision, and altered light adaptation developed in a 42-year-old woman 2 weeks after starting a high protein diet and melatonin 1 mg/day. She had also been taking sertraline for the past 4 years. Her vision improved within 2 months of stopping the melatonin and the high protein diet (47[A]). Her retinal melatonin concentration may have been high because of increased serotonin (a melatonin precursor) from sertraline and a high protein intake, plus the exogenous melatonin. Retinal damage was reported as an adverse effect of melatonin in an NIH workshop (42[r]) but the report has not been formally published.*

Psychiatric *One severely depressed woman developed a mixed affective state after taking melatonin for 7 days in a clinical trial (48[A]). Confusion, hallucinations, and paranoia temporally related to melatonin have also been described (38[M]).*

Endocrine *Impaired insulin-dependent glucose utilization occurred in a double-blind study of postmenopausal women given melatonin 1 mg in the morning (49[c]). The authors also cited isolated reports of increased blood glucose in healthy individuals and in two men with Parkinson's disease taking melatonin.*

There was suppression of endogenous melatonin secretion in two of five patients with bipolar disorder after 12 weeks of treatment with high-dose melatonin (10 mg/day) (50[c]).

Gynecomastia has been attributed to melatonin (42[r], 51[A]).

A 56-year-old man complained of painful asymmetrical breast enlargement, gradually developing over 3 months (51[A]). He had had amyotrophic lateral sclerosis for 3 years and had taken riluzole 50 mg bd for 2 years and melatonin for 1.5 years (1 mg/day during the first year then gradually increasing to 2 mg/day). He had bilateral painful gynecomastia and homogeneously enlarged breasts. There was no galactorrhea. There were no signs or symptoms of other endocrine dysfunction. Withdrawal of melatonin resulted in complete regression of the gynecomastia within a few weeks.

This is a warning against the uncontrolled use of apparently innocuous substances. The absence of adverse effects in healthy people taking melatonin for various reasons does not mean safety in certain diseased populations.

Liver *Autoimmune hepatitis was diagnosed in a previously healthy 39-year-old woman 4 weeks after she started to take melatonin 3 mg at bedtime (52[A]). It is unclear whether this was a direct hepatotoxic effect of melatonin (or a contaminant), or if hepatitis was caused indirectly by an immunomodulatory mechanism.*

Skin *Vesicular plaques and erosions developed on the penis in two men after they took melatonin for jet lag: one man had two such episodes 4 months apart (53[A]). The lesions resolved within 10 days without any sequelae, and recurred within 8 hours of rechallenge.*

Reproductive system *Melatonin affects reproduction in seasonally breeding animals. In humans, findings of increased endogenous melatonin in hypogonadism and low concentrations in precocious puberty imply an interaction between melatonin and gonadotrophins; however, data on the effects of exogenous melatonin are limited (34[R]). In a randomized study in 16 women, melatonin enhanced LH and FSH responses to submaximal GnRH stimuli in the follicular but not the luteal phase of the menstrual cycle (54[c]). A very high dose of melatonin (300 mg) partially inhibited ovulation in healthy young women: norethisterone enhanced the effect (55[c]).*

Immunologic *There has been a single report of a subject in a controlled trial of melatonin who had difficulty in swallowing and breathing within 20 minutes of taking melatonin 0.5 mg. The symptoms resolved without treatment after 45 minutes and recurred to a milder degree after rechallenge (56[c]).*

Withdrawal effects *There was suppression of endogenous melatonin secretion in two of five patients with bipolar disorder after 12 weeks of treatment with high-dose melatonin (10 mg/day) (50[C]). One woman developed an unentrained sleep-wake cycle after melatonin was withdrawn (not previously a feature of her illness), which persisted for several months.*

Involuntary movements of the lip and tongue, restlessness, and insomnia developed twice when chronic melatonin therapy was abruptly withdrawn in a young woman with cerebral palsy: these symptoms resolved when melatonin was restarted, but did not recur with gradual withdrawal over 2 months (46[A]). This again suggests that endogenous melatonin secretion is suppressed after chronic use.

Drug interactions *There have been several unpublished reports of altered prothrombin time in patients taking warfarin and melatonin. In some cases bleeding or purpura was the presenting symptom, despite a reduced prothrombin time (38[M]). This potentially serious interaction has not yet been formally studied.*

Fluvoxamine increases the systemic availability of oral melatonin, probably by reducing its first-pass clearance (57[C]). In a cross-over study in seven healthy subjects serum melatonin concentration was increased by fluvoxamine but not citalopram (58[C]). In another study fluoxetine, paroxetine, citalopram, imipramine, and desipramine did not affect the biotransformation of melatonin at therapeutic concentrations in vitro (59[E]).

Drug overdose *Melatonin overdose has been reported in three patients, all of whom were also taking psychotropic drugs. Drug interactions with antidepressants may have played a part in the resulting symptoms, which were not reported in cancer trials using higher doses of melatonin (34[R]).*

A 73-year-old woman developed an acute psychosis after taking melatonin 30 mg as well as her usual fluoxetine (60[A]). A 14-year-old girl became drowsy and dizzy and complained of blurred vision after taking melatonin 24–36 mg as well as her usual trazodone and paroxetine (61[A]). A 66-year old man became lethargic, confused, and disoriented after taking melatonin 24 mg with his usual amitriptyline and chlordiazepoxide (62[A]).

All three patients recovered fully within 24 hours without specific treatment.

Parathyroid hormone and analogs *(SED-14, 1520; SEDA-20, 402)*

Parathyroid hormone has potent anabolic effects on the skeleton if given intermittently; both the intact molecule and smaller N-terminal fragments are being used in clinical trials. Initial concerns about the development of osteosarcoma in rats after prolonged high-dose treatment have not been confirmed in human trials, but surveillance continues (63[R]). In one study there was a mild increase in creatinine, which was thought not to have clinical significance (64[C]). Mild nausea (65[C]) and arthralgia (65[C], 66[C]) have also been reported.

Mineral metabolism There is a *transient increase in serum calcium* within the reference range after injection of parathyroid hormone. Transient *mild hypercalciuria* and *increased serum phosphate* are common but do not usually limit therapy. In a randomized study in premenopausal women also treated with nafarelin, four of 23 women randomized to PTH(1–34) 500 IU/day had a serum calcium concentration over 2.67 mmol/l 4 hours after the injection; the concentration normalized after the dose of parathyroid hormone was reduced and other treatment was continued (65[C]). In another study, two of 10 men who were randomized to receive subcutaneous PTH(1-34) 400 IU/day for 18 months had serum calcium concentrations over 2.6 mmol/l after 1 or 3 months; the concentrations normalized after reduction of the dose of parathyroid hormone (66[C]).

Skin Local reactions at sites of subcutaneous injection are common but are usually limited to *transitory redness* (65[C], 66[C]). *Subcutaneous nodules* at the injection site developed in two of 17 women after more than 2 years of administration in a clinical trial (67[C]).

VASOPRESSIN AND ANALOGS

(SED-14, 1522; SEDA-22, 487; SEDA-23, 469; SEDA-24, 506)

Terlipressin (triglycyl-lysine vasopressin)

Terlipressin, a long-acting vasopressin analog,

is metabolized to the active drug lysine vasopressin.

Cardiovascular Terlipressin has similar, but less pronounced, systemic hemodynamic effects to vasopressin, including *increases in mean arterial pressure* and *reduced heart rate* (68[c]). Of 105 patients who had continuous terlipressin infusions for variceal bleeding in a multicenter study, *lower limb ischemia* developed in two and *cardiac ischemia* in one (69[C]).

Electrolyte balance Four of 105 patients in the study mentioned above developed *hyponatremia*, which was severe in one case (69[C]).

Skin Mild *lymphangitis* was reported in one of 105 patients in the same multicenter study (69[C]).

Bullous necrosis developed within 48 hours of starting terlipressin infusion in a 44-year-old man (70[A]). There have been only four previous reports of skin necrosis.

REFERENCES

1. Chesnut CH III, Silverman S, Andriano K, Genant H, Gimona A, Harris S, Kiel D, LeBoff M, Maricic M, Miller P, Moniz C, Peacock M, Richardson P, Watts N, Baylink D. A randomized trial of nasal spray salmon calcitonin in postmenopausal women with established osteoporosis: The Prevent Recurrence Of Osteoporotic Fractures Study. Am J Med 2000; 109: 267–76.
2. Porcel SL, Cumplido JA, De La Hoz B, Cuevas M, Losada E. Anaphylaxis to calcitonin. Allergol Immunopathol 2000; 28: 243–5.
3. Takeuchi H, Kobori H, Kikuchi I, Sato Y, Mitsuhashi N. A prospective randomized study comparing endocrinological and clinical effects of two types of GnRH agonists in cases of uterine leiomyomas or endometriosis. J Obstet Gynaecol Res 2000; 26: 325–31.
4. Foppiani L, Piredda S, Guido R, Spaziante R, Giusti M. Gonadotropin-releasing hormone-induced partial empty sella clinically mimicking pituitary apoplexy in a woman with a suspected non-secreting macroadenoma. J Endocrinol Invest 2000; 23: 118–21.
5. Minagawa K, Sueoka H. Seizure exacerbation by the use of leuprorelin acetate for treatment of central precocious puberty in a female patient with symptomatic localized-related epilepsy. No To Hattatsu 1999; 31: 466–8.
6. Akaboshi S, Takeshita K. A case of atypical absence seizures induced by leuprolide acetate. Pediatr Neurol 2000; 23: 266–8.
7. Stone P, Hardy J, Huddart R, A'Hern R, Richards M. Fatigue in patients with prostate cancer receiving hormone therapy. Eur J Cancer 2000; 36: 1134–41.
8. Tahara M, Matsuoka T, Yokoi T, Tasaka K, Kurachi H, Murata Y. Treatment of endometriosis with a decreasing dosage of a gonadotropin-releasing hormone agonist (nafarelin); a pilot study with low-dose agonist therapy ("draw-back" therapy). Fertil Steril 2000; 73: 799–804.
9. Kasayama S, Miyake S, Samejima Y. Transient thyrotoxicosis and hypothyroidism following administration of the GnRH agonist leuprolide acetate. Endocr J 2000; 47: 783–5.
10. Wei JT, Gross M, Jaffe CA, Gravlin K, Lahaie M, Faerber GJ, Cooney KA. Androgen deprivation therapy for prostate cancer results in significant loss of bone density. Urology 1999; 54: 607–11.
11. Daniell HW, Dunn SR, Ferguson DW, Lomas G, Niazi Z, Stratte PT. Progressive osteoporosis during androgen deprivation therapy for prostate cancer. J Urol 2000; 163: 181–6.
12. Pierce SJ, Gazvani MR, Farquharson RG. Long-term use of gonadotropin-releasing hormone analogs and hormone replacement therapy in the management of endometriosis: a randomized trial with a 6-year follow-up. Fertil Steril 2000; 74: 964–8.
13. Jimenez-Gordo AM, Espinosa E, Zamora P, Feliu J, Rodriguez-Salas N, Gonzalez-Baron M. Pregnancy in a breast cancer patient treated with a LHRH analogue at ablative doses. Breast 2000; 9: 110–12.
14. Gillies PS, Faulds D, Balfour JAB, Perry CM. Ganirelix. Drugs 2000; 59: 107–11.
15. Olivennes F, Belaisch-Allart J, Emperaire J-C, Dechaud H, Alvarez S, Moreau L, Nicollet B, Zorn J-R, Bouchard P, Frydman R. Prospective, randomized, controlled study of in vitro fertilization-embryo transfer with a single dose of a lutenizing hormone-releasing hormone (LH-RH) antagonist (cetrorelix) or a depot formula of an LH-RH agonist (triptorelin). Fertil Steril 2000; 73: 314–20.
16. Felberbaum RE, Albano C, Ludwig M, Riethmuller-Winzen H, Grigat M, Devroey P, Diedrich KHR. Ovarian stimulation for assisted reproduction with HMG and concomitant midcycle administration of the GnRH antagonist cetrorelix according to the multiple dose protocol: a prospective uncontrolled phase III study. Hum Reprod 2000; 15: 1015–20.
17. Abyholm T, Barlow D, for The European Orgalutran Study Group. Treatment with the gonadotrophin-releasing hormone antagonist ganirelix in women undergoing ovarian stimulation with recombinant follicle-stimulating hormone is effective, safe and convenient: results of a controlled, randomized, multicentre trial. Hum Reprod 2000; 15: 1490–8.

18. Gibbons RV, Holman RC, Belay ED, Schonberger LB. Creutzfeldt–Jakob disease in the United States: 1979–1998. J Am Med Assoc 2000; 284: 2322–3.
19. Cutfield WS, Wilton P, Bennmarker H, Albertsson-Wikland K, Chatelain P, Ranke MB, Price DA. Incidence of diabetes mellitus and impaired glucose tolerance in children and adolescents receiving growth hormone treatment. Lancet 2000; 355: 610–13.
20. Jeffcoate W. Can growth hormone therapy cause diabetes? Lancet 2000; 355: 589–90.
21. Florakis D, Hung V, Kaltsas G, Coyte D, Jenkins PJ, Chew SL, Grossman AB, Besser M, Monson JP. Sustained reduction in circulating cholesterol in adult hypopituitary patients given low dose titrated growth hormone replacement therapy: a two year study. Clin Endocrinol 2000; 53: 453–9.
22. Rosenfalck AM, Maghsoudi S, Fisker S, Jorgensen JOL, Christiansen JS, Hilsted J, Volund AA, Madsbad S. The effect of 30 months of low-dose replacement therapy with recombinant human growth hormone (rhGH) on insulin and C-peptide kinetics, insulin secretion, insulin sensitivity, glucose effectiveness, and body composition in GH-deficient adults. J Clin Endocrinol Metab 2000; 85: 4173–81.
23. Fernholm R, Bramnert M, Hagg E, Hilding A, Baylink D, Mohan S, Thoren M. Growth hormone replacement therapy improves body composition and increases bone metabolism in elderly patients with pituitary disease. J Clin Endocrinol Metab 2000; 85: 4104–12.
24. Picca S, Cappa M, Rizzoni G. Hyperparathyroidism during growth hormone treatment: a role for puberty? Pediatr Nephrol 2000; 14: 56–8.
25. Lindgren AC. Side effects of growth hormone treatment in Prader–Willi syndrome. Endocrinologist 2000; 10 Suppl 1: 63S–64S.
26. Nishi Y, Tanaka T, Takano K, Fujieda K, Igarashi Y, Hanew K, Hirano T, Yokoya S, Tachibana K, Saito T, Watanabe S. Recent status in the occurrence of leukemia in growth-hormone treated patients in Japan. J Clin Endocrinol Metab 1999; 84: 1961–5.
27. Aktan M, Tanakol R, Nalcaci M, Dincol G. Leukemia in a patient treated with growth hormone. Endocr J 2000; 47: 471–3.
28. Liddle C, Goodwin BJ, George J, Tapner M, Farrell GC. Separate and interactive regulation of cytochrome P450 3A4 by triiodothyronine, dexamethasone, and growth hormone in cultured hepatocytes. J Clin Endocrinol Metab 1998; 83: 2411–16.
29. Sanchez CP, Salem M, Ettenger RB. Changes in cyclosporine A levels in pediatric renal allograft recipients receiving recombinant human growth hormone therapy. Transplant Proc 2000; 32: 2807–10.
30. Pop-Busui R, Chey W, Stevens MJ. Severe hypertension induced by the long-acting somatostatin analogue sandostatin LAR in a patient with diabetic autonomic neuropathy. J Clin Endocrinol Metab 2000; 85: 943–6.
31. Beckman RA, Siden R, Yanik GA, Levine JE. Continuous octreotide infusion for the treatment of secretory diarrhea caused by acute intestinal graft–versus–host disease in a child. J Pediatr Hematol Oncol 2000; 22: 344–50.
32. Demirkan K, Fleckenstein JF, Self TH. Thrombocytopenia associated with octreotide. Am J Med Sci 2000; 320: 296–7.
33. Kaal A, Orskov H, Nielsen S, Pedroncelli AM, Lancranjan I, Marbach P, Weeke J. Occurrence and effects of octreotide antibodies during nasal, subcutaneous and slow release intramuscular treatment. Eur J Endocrinol 2000; 143: 353–61.
34. Brzezinski A. Melatonin in humans. New Engl J Med 1997; 336: 186–95.
35. Caley CF. Dehydroepiandrosterone and melatonin: two neurohormones. J Pharm Pract 1999; 12: 251–65.
36. Williamson BL, Tomlinson AJ, Naylor S, Gleich GJ. Contaminants in commercial preparations of melatonin. Mayo Clin Proc 1997; 72: 1094–5.
37. Avery D, Lenz M, Landis C. Guidelines for prescribing melatonin. Ann Med 1998; 30: 122–30.
38. Herxheimer A, Petrie KJ. Melatonin for preventing and treating jet lag. (Cochrane Review). In: The Cochrane Library, 2, 2001. Oxford: Update Software.
39. Lane EA, Moss HB. Pharmacokinetics of melatonin in man: first pass hepatic metabolism. J Clin Endocrinol Metab 1985; 61: 1214–16.
40. Middleton BA, Stone BM, Arendt J. Melatonin and fragmented sleep patterns. Lancet 1996; 348: 551–2.
41. Rogers NL, Phan O, Kennaway DJ, Dawson D. Effect of daytime oral melatonin administration on neurobehavioral performance in humans. J Pineal Res 1998; 25: 47–53.
42. Lamberg L. Melatonin potentially useful but safety, efficacy remain uncertain. J Am Med Assoc 1996; 276: 1011–14.
43. Lusardi P, Piazza E, Fogari R. Cardiovascular effects of melatonin in hypertensive patients well controlled by nifedipine: a 24-hour study. Br J Clin Pharmacol 2000; 49: 423–7.
44. Arangino S, Cagnacci A, Angiolucci M, Vacca AMB, Longu G, Volpe A, Melis GB. Effects of melatonin on vascular reactivity, catecholamine levels and blood pressure in healthy men. Am J Cardiol 1999; 83: 1417–19.
45. Sheldon, SH. Pro-convulsant effects of oral melatonin in neurologically disabled children. Lancet 1998; 351: 1254.
46. Giladi N, Shabtai H. Melatonin-induced withdrawal emergent dyskinesia and akathisia. Mov Disord 1999; 14: 381–2.
47. Lehman NL, Johnson LN. Toxic optic neuropathy after concomitant use of melatonin, Zoloft, and a high-protein diet. J Neuro-Ophthalmol 1999; 19: 232–4.
48. Dalton EJ, Rotondi D, Levitan RD, Kennedy

SH, Brown GM. Use of slow-release melatonin in treatment-resistant depression. J Psychiatry Neurosci 2000; 25: 48–52.
49. Cagnacci A, Arangino S, Renzi A, Paoletti AM, Melis GB, Cagnacci P, Volpe A. Influence of melatonin administration on glucose tolerance and insulin sensitivity of postmenopausal women. Clin Endocrinol 2001; 54: 339–46.
50. Leibenluft E, Feldman-Naim S, Turner EH, Wehr TA, Rosenthal NE. Effects of exogenous melatonin administration and withdrawal in five patients with rapid-cycling bipolar disorder. J Clin Psychiatry 1997; 58: 383–8.
51. De Bleecker JL, Lamont BH, Verstraete AG, Schelfhout, VJ. Melatonin and painful gynecomastia. Neurology 1999; 53: 435–6.
52. Hong YG, Riegler JL. Is melatonin associated with the development of autoimmune hepatitis? J Clin Gastroenterol 1997; 25: 376–8.
53. Bardazzi F, Placucci F, Neri I, D'Antuono A, Patrizi A. Fixed drug eruption due to melatonin. Acta Derm-Venereol 1998; 78: 69–70.
54. Cagnacci A, Paoletti AM, Soldani R, Orru M, Maschio E, Melis GB. Melatonin enhances the luteinizing hormone and follicle-stimulating hormone responses to gonadotropin-releasing hormone in the follicular, but not in the luteal, menstrual phase. J Clin Endocrinol Metab 1995; 80: 1095–9.
55. Voordouw BC, Euser R, Verdonk RE, Alberda BT, De Jong FH, Drogendijk AC, Fauser BC, Cohen M. Melatonin and melatonin–progestin combinations alter pituitary-ovarian function in women and can inhibit ovulation. J Clin Endocrinol Metab 1992; 74: 108–17.
56. Spitzer RL, Terman M, Williams JBW, Terman JS, Malt UF, Singer F, Lewy AJ. Jet lag: clinical features, validation of a new syndrome-specific scale, and lack of response to melatonin in a randomized, double-blind trial. Am J Psychiatry 1999; 156: 1392–6.
57. Hartter S, Grozinger M, Weigmann H, Roschke J, Hiemke C. Increased bioavailability of oral melatonin after fluvoxamine coadministration. Clin Pharmacol Ther 2000; 67: 1–6.
58. Von Bahr C, Ursing C, Yasui N, Tybring G, Bertilsson L, Rojdmark S. Fluvoxamine but not citalopram increases serum melatonin in healthy subjects – an indication that cytochrome P450 CYP1A2 and CYP2C19 hydroxylate melatonin. Eur J Clin Pharmacol 2000; 56: 123–7.
59. Hartter S, Wang X, Weigmann H, Friedberg T, Arand M, Oesch F, Hiemke C. Differential effects of fluvoxamine and other antidepressants on the biotransformation of melatonin. J Clin Psychopharmacol 2001; 21: 167–74.
60. Force RW, Hansen L, Bedell M. Psychotic episode after melatonin. Ann Pharmacother 1997; 31: 1408.
61. Balentine J, Hagman J. More on melatonin. J Am Acad Child Adolesc Psychiatry 1997; 36: 1013.
62. Holliman BJ, Chyka PA. Problems in assessment of acute melatonin overdose. South Med J 1997; 90: 451–3.
63. Whitfield J, Morley P, Willick G. The parathyroid hormone, its fragments and analogues – potent bone-builders for treating osteoporosis. Expert Opin Invest Drugs 2000; 9: 1293–315.
64. Hodsman AB, Fraher LJ, Watson PH, Ostbye T, Stitt LW, Adachi JD, Taves DH, Drost D. A randomized controlled trial to compare the efficacy of cyclical parathyroid hormone versus cyclical parathyroid hormone and sequential calcitonin to improve bone mass in postmenopausal women with osteoporosis. J Clin Endocrinol Metab 1997; 82: 620–8.
65. Finkelstein JS, Klibanski A, Arnold AL, Toth TL, Hornstein MD, Neer RM. Prevention of estrogen deficiency-related bone loss with human parathyroid hormone-(1—34). J Am Med Assoc 1998; 280: 1067–73.
66. Kurland ES, Cosman F, McMahon DJ, Rosen CJ, Lindsay R, Bilezikian JP. Parathyroid hormone as a therapy for idiopathic osteoporosis in men: effects on bone mineral density and bone markers. J Clin Endocrinol Metab 2000; 85: 3069–76.
67. Lindsay R, Nieves J, Formica C, Henneman E, Woelfert L, Shen V, Dempster D, Cosman F. Randomised controlled study of effect of parathyroid hormone on vertebral-bone mass and fracture incidence among postmenopausal women on oestrogen with osteoporosis. Lancet 1997; 350: 550–5.
68. Romero G, Kravetz D, Argonz J, Bildozola M, Suarez A, Terg R. Terlipressin is more effective in decreasing variceal pressure than portal pressure in cirrhotic patients. J Hepatol 2000; 32: 419–25.
69. Escorsell A, Ruiz Del Arbol L, Planas R, Albillos A, Banares R, Cales P, Pateron D, Bernard B, Vinel J-P, Bosch J, et al. Multicenter randomized controlled trial or terlipressin versus sclerotherapy in the treatment of acute variceal bleeding: the TEST study. Hepatology 2000; 32: 471–6.
70. Tomassini E, Guiot P, Poussel JF, De Cubber J, Schnitzler B. Bullous disease following intravenous terlipressin infusion. Réanim Urgences 2000; 9: 313–14.

I. Aursnes

44 Drugs that affect lipid metabolism

FIBRATES *(SED-14, 1527; SEDA-22, 490; SEDA-23, 472; SEDA-24, 510)*

Musculoskeletal Unexpected *acute renal insufficiency* occurred in four patients after uncomplicated cardiac surgery; each was taking a fibrate (1^A). Renal insufficiency occurred rapidly within 3 days of surgery and was associated with increased concentrations of skeletal muscle-derived creatine kinase. One patient developed myoglobinuria. Presumably patients taking lipid-lowering drugs are at higher risk of acute renal insufficiency after cardiac surgery, due to rhabdomyolysis. This suggests that patients taking either statins or fibrates should discontinue them before cardiac surgery.

HMG COENZYME-A REDUCTASE INHIBITORS *(SED-14, 1530; SEDA-22, 490; SEDA-23, 472; SEDA-24, 510)*

Nervous system HMG-CoA reductase inhibitors can cause a *peripheral neuropathy* (SEDA-24, 510), and another case has been reported with atorvastatin (2^A).

A 60-year-old woman had painless horizontal diplopia, vertigo, blurry vision, and paresthesia in both arms after taking atorvastatin 10 mg/day. Neurological improvement began 2 days after drug withdrawal. Antiacetylcholine receptor antibodies were 10 times the upper limit of the reference range.

Although some features of this patient's external ophthalmoplegia were similar to myasthenia and there was a reversible rise in antiacetylcholine receptor antibody titer, a negative edrophonium test and a negative repetitive stimulation test on electromyography argued against a myasthenia-like drug reaction.

Sensory systems *Lens opacities* have been suspected in patients taking HMG-CoA reductase inhibitors, but according to a recent review there is no danger and there should be no requirement for regular ophthalmological examination (3^R).

Psychological Animal and cross-sectional studies have suggested that serum lipid concentrations can cause *altered cognitive function*, *mood*, and *behavior*. In a double-blind study, 209 healthy adults were randomized to placebo or lovastatin 20 mg/day for 6 months. Placebo-treated subjects improved between baseline and post-treatment periods on neuropsychological tests in all performance domains (neuropsychological performance, depression, hostility, and quality of life), consistent with the effects of practice on test performance, whereas those treated with lovastatin improved only on tests of memory recall. Comparisons of the changes in performance between placebo and lovastatin showed small but significant differences for tests of attention and psychomotor speed, and were consistent with greater improvement with placebo. Psychological well-being was not affected by lovastatin. The authors concluded that treatment of hypercholesterolemia with lovastatin did not cause psychological distress or substantially alter cognitive function. Treatment did result in slight impairment of performance in neuropsychological tests of attention and psychomotor speed, the clinical importance of which is uncertain (4^C). Other reports on this subject can be found in a recent review (3^R).

Side Effects of Drugs, Annual 25
J.K. Aronson, ed.

Liver HMG-CoA reductase inhibitors can cause mild *rises in aminotransferase activities*, but this effect has not been definitely correlated with severe morbidity involving altered hepatic function. There seems to be no difference between the various drugs in this respect (3[R]).

Pancreas *Pancreatitis* has been observed during treatment with various statins (SED-14, 1530). This has also now been described with atorvastatin (5[A]).

Musculoskeletal HMGCoA reductase inhibitors can cause *rhabdomyolysis* (SED-14, 1533), and more cases have been reported with simvastatin (6[A], 7[A]).

Simvastatin 5 mg/day caused rhabdomyolysis in a 61-year-old man who was not taking concomitant interacting drugs (6[A]). An elderly lady with chronic renal insufficiency developed rhabdomyolysis during simvastatin therapy (7[A]). Her symptoms of muscle pain, fatigue, myoglobulinuria, oliguria, and pulmonary edema occurred 48 hours after the first dose of simvastatin. Simvastatin was immediately withdrawn, and she was dialysed for 1 week.

Extreme care should be exercised in prescribing simvastatin in elderly patients with renal impairment.

Symptomatic rises in creatine kinase activity to over 10 times the upper end of the reference range occurred in 0%, 1%, and 0.9% of patients taking placebo, cerivastatin 0.4 mg, or cerivastatin 0.8 mg respectively (8[C]), and rhabdomyolysis has been described in patients taking cerivastatin (9[A], 10[A]). However, in a review of the pharmacological properties and therapeutic efficacy of cerivastatin in hypercholesterolemia, it was stated that cerivastatin only infrequently causes rhabdomyolysis when given alone (11[R]) (see also Drug interactions below).

℞ *Drug interactions with HMG-CoA reductase inhibitors*

Mechanisms *Many statins are metabolized by CYP3A4, and this and other mechanisms of drug interactions involving statins have been reviewed (12[R]). Other drugs metabolized by CYP3A4 can greatly increase statin concentrations in the body and precipitate rhabdomyolysis. Although the statins are similar in their ability to lower cholesterol concentrations, there are dissimilarities in their interactions with other drugs.*

Like other statins the chance of rhabdomyolysis increases when cerivastatin is taken together with certain other drugs. Although cerivastatin is degraded by two different isoforms of P450 in the liver, and therefore should be less likely to take part in drug interactions than most of the other statins, clinically important interactions do occur, and reports of drug interactions in 2001 triggered the withdrawal of cerivastatin.

Ciclosporin *The main concern about drug interactions with cerivastatin has been with ciclosporin. Cerivastatin 0.2 mg/day was well tolerated when given together with ciclosporin, although there were 3- to 5-fold increases in the plasma concentrations of cerivastatin and its metabolites when single-dose cerivastatin was given to 12 kidney transplant recipients taking ciclosporin 200 mg bd and to 12 healthy controls (13[C]). Ciclosporin may have affected both the distribution of cerivastatin and its biotransformation in the liver.*

Diltiazem *Diltiazem interacts with lovastatin but not with pravastatin (SEDA-24, 511). The results of a study in 10 healthy volunteers given lovastatin orally with a randomized two-way cross-over design with or without intravenous diltiazem have suggested that the interaction of diltiazem with lovastatin is primarily a first-pass effect, due to inhibition of CYP3A4 (14[C]). Thus, drug interactions with diltiazem may become evident when a patient is switched from intravenous to oral dosing.*

Fibrates *Combination therapy with fluvastatin and bezafibrate 400 mg/day in 71 patients with persistent hypertriglyceridemia resulted in no significant increase in creatine phosphokinase activity or in the frequency of myalgia (15[C]).*

In contrast, although in vitro studies have not shown any evidence of pharmacokinetic interactions between cerivastatin and gemfibrozil (11[R]), there was myalgia and a marked increase in creatine kinase in a 74-year-old woman with normal renal function who took gemfibrozil 1200 mg/day 3 weeks after she started to take cerivastatin 0.3 mg/day (10[A]). Since then several other cases, one in a 64-year-old woman (16[A]), one in a 63-year-old man with diabetes mellitus (17[A]), one in a 75-year-old man (18[A]), and one in a 68-year-old man (19[A]) have been described. The last patient fared well on a combination of gemfibrozil and cerivastatin until he received influenza vaccination. Rhabdomyolysis has been reported with various viruses, including influenza A and B and inactivation of the virus does not totally prevent this.

Gemfibrozil also increased plasma concentrations of simvastatin and its active form, simvastatin acid, in a randomized, double-blind, cross-over study in 10 healthy volunteers given gemfibrozil or placebo orally for 3 days before a single dose of simvastatin (20[c]). This suggests that the increased risk of myopathy in combination treatment is at least partly pharmacokinetic in origin. Because gemfibrozil does not inhibit CYP3A4 in vitro, the mechanism of the pharmacokinetic interaction is probably inhibition of non-CYP3A4-mediated metabolism of simvastatin acid.

Grapefruit juice *When 10 healthy volunteers took simvastatin 24 hours after a large amount of grapefruit juice in a non-randomized cross-over study, the effect on the AUC of simvastatin was only about 10% of the effect observed when grapefruit juice and simvastatin were taken together (21[c]). The interaction potential of even large amounts of grapefruit juice with CYP3A4 substrates dissipates within 3–7 days after ingestion of the last dose.*

Imidazoles *In a randomized, double-blind, cross-over study in 12 healthy volunteers fluconazole increased the plasma concentrations of fluvastatin and prolonged its elimination; the mechanism was probably inhibition of the CYP2C9-mediated metabolism of fluvastatin (22[c]). Care should be taken if fluconazole or other potent inhibitors of CYP2C9 are given to patients using fluvastatin.*

The effects of itraconazole, a potent inhibitor of CYP3A4, on the pharmacokinetics of atorvastatin, cerivastatin, and pravastatin have been evaluated in an open, randomized, cross-over study in 18 healthy subjects who took single doses of atorvastatin 20 mg, cerivastatin 0.8 mg, or pravastatin 40 mg, with and without itraconazole 200 mg (23[C]). Itraconazole markedly raised atorvastatin plasma concentrations (2.5-fold) and produced modest rises in the plasma concentrations of cerivastatin (1.3-fold) and pravastatin (1.5-fold). These results suggest that in patients taking itraconazole, cerivastatin, or pravastatin may be preferable to atorvastatin.

Rifampicin *Rifampicin greatly reduced the plasma concentrations of simvastatin and simvastatin acid in 10 healthy volunteers in a randomized, cross-over study (24[c]). Because the half-life of simvastatin was not affected by rifampicin, induction of CYP3A4-mediated first-pass metabolism of simvastatin in the intestine and liver probably explains this interaction. Concomitant use of potent inducers of CYP3A4 can lead to considerably reduced cholesterol-lowering efficacy of simvastatin.*

Troglitazone *In four men with diabetes using insulin and taking atorvastatin troglitazone was added (25[c]). Serum LDL cholesterol and triglycerides increased by 23% and 21% respectively. This suggests a drug interaction, but further studies of troglitazone and atorvastatin are warranted to substantiate this.*

NICOTINIC ACID DERIVATIVES

(SED-11, 923; SEDA-15, 480)

Acipimox

Acipimox (S-methylpyrazine-2-carboxylic acid 4-oxide) is structurally related to nicotinic acid. Of 32 patients with hypertriglyceridemia, excessive hypertriglyceridemia, and combined hyperlipidemia, acipimox had to be withdrawn in 10 cases, because of adverse effects or absence of clinical response (26[c]). The other 22 completed 6 months of treatment with no adverse effects. The authors claimed that acipimox is much better tolerated than nicotinic acid; it has fewer adverse effects and can therefore be used as a second-line drug.

REFERENCES

1. Sharobeem KM, Madden BP, Millner R, Rolfe LM, Seymour CA, Parker J. Acute renal failure after cardiopulmonary bypass: a possible association with drugs of the fibrate group. J Cardiovasc Pharmacol Ther 2000; 5: 33–9.
2. Negvesky GJ, Kolsky MP, Laureno R, Yau TH. Reversible atorvastatin-associated external ophthalmoplegia, anti-acetylcholine receptor antibodies, and ataxia. Arch Ophthalmol 2000; 118: 427–8.
3. Farmer JA, Torre-Amione G. Comparative tolerability of the HMG-CoA reductase inhibitors. Drug Saf 2000; 23: 197–213.
4. Muldoon MF, Barger SD, Ryan CM, Flory JD, Lehoczky JP, Matthews KA, Manuck SB. Effects of lovastatin on cognitive function and psychological well-being. Am J Med 2000; 108: 538–46.
5. Belaiche G, Ley G, Slama JL. Pancreatite aiguë associée a la prise d'atorvastatine. Gastroenterol Clin Biol 2000; 24: 471–2.
6. Pershad A, Cardello FP. Simvastatin and rhabdomyolysis – a case report and brief review. J Pharm Technol 1999; 15: 88–9.
7. Al Shohaib S. Simvastatin-induced rhabdomyolysis in a patient with chronic renal failure. Am J Nephrol 2000; 20: 212–13.
8. Insull W Jr, Isaacsohn J, Kwiterovich P, Brazg PM, Dujovne C, Shan M, Shugrue-Crowley E, Ripa S, Tota R. Efficacy and safety of cerivastatin 0.8 mg in patients with hypercholesterolaemia: the pivotal placebo-controlled clinical trial. J Int Med Res 2000; 28: 47–68.
9. Rodriguez ML, Mora C, Navarro JF. Cerivastatin-induced rhabdomyolysis. Ann Intern Med 2000; 132: 598.
10. Pogson GW, Kindred LH, Carper BG. Rhabdomyolysis and renal failure associated with cerivastatin-gemfibrozil combination therapy. Am J Cardiol 1999; 83: 1146.
11. Plosker GL, Dunn CJ, Figgitt DP. Cerivastatin: a review of its pharmacological properties and therapeutic efficacy in the management of hypercholesterolaemia. Drugs 2000; 60: 1179–206.
12. Horsmans Y. Differential metabolism of statins: importance in drug-drug interactions. Eur Heart J Suppl 1999; 1 Suppl T: T7–12.
13. Muck W, Mai I, Fritsche L, Ochmann K, Rohde G, Neymayer H-H, Kuhlmann J. Increase in cerivastatin systemic exposure after single and multiple dosing in cyclosporine-treated kidney transplant recipients. Clin Pharmacol Ther 1999; 65: 251–61.
14. Masica AL, Azie NE, Brater C, Hall SD, Jones DR. Intravenous diltiazem and CYP3A-mediated metabolism. Br J Clin Pharmacol 2000; 50: 273–6.
15. Spieker LE, Noll G, Hannak M, Lüscher TF. Efficacy and tolerability of fluvastatin and bezafibrate in patients with hyperlipidemia and persistently high triglyceride levels. J Cardiovasc Pharmacol 2000; 35: 361–5.
16. Bermingham RP, Whitsitt TB, Smart ML, Nowak DP, Scalley RD. Rhabdomyolysis in a patient receiving the combination of cerivastatin and gemfibrozil. Am J Health-Syst Pharm 2000; 57: 461–4.
17. Özdemir Ö, Boran M, Gökce V, Uzun Y, Kocak B, Korkmaz S. A case with severe rhabdomyolysis and renal failure associated with cerivastatin-gemfibrozil combination therapy: a case report. Angiology 2000; 51: 695–7.
18. Alexandridis G, Pappas GA, Elisaf MS. Rhabdomyolysis due to combination therapy with cerivastatin and gemfibrozil. Am J Med 2000; 109: 261–2.
19. Plotkin E, Bernheim J, Ben-Chetrit S, Mor A, Korzets Z. Influenza vaccine – a possible trigger of rhabdomyolysis induced acute renal failure due to the combined use of cerivastatin and bezafibrate. Nephrol Dial Transplant. 2000; 15: 740–1.
20. Backman JT, Kyrklund C, Kivistö KT, Wang J-S, Neuvonen PJ. Plasma concentrations of active simvastatin acid are increased by gemfibrozil. Clin Pharmacol Ther 2000; 68: 122–9.
21. Lilja JJ, Kivistö KT, Neuvonen PJ. Duration of effect of grapefruit juice on the pharmacokinetics of the CYP3A4 substrate simvastatin. Clin Pharmacol Ther 2000; 68: 384–90.
22. Kantola T, Backman JT, Niemi M, Kivistö KT, Neuvonen PJ. Effect of fluconazole on plasma fluvastatin and pravastatin concentrations. Eur J Clin Pharmacol 2000; 56: 225–9.
23. Mazzu AL, Lasseter KC, Shamblen EC, Agarwal V, Lettieri J, Sundaresen P. Itraconazole alters the pharmacokinetics of atorvastatin to a greater extent than either cerivastatin or pravastatin. Clin Pharmacol Ther 2000; 68: 391–40.
24. Kyrklund C, Backman JT, Kivistö KT, Neuvonen M, Laitila J, Neuvonen PJ. Rifampin greatly reduces plasma simvastatin and simvastatin acid concentrations. Clin Pharmacol Ther 2000; 68: 592–7.
25. DiTusa L, Luzier AB. Potential interaction between troglitazone and atorvastatin. J Clin Pharm Ther 2000; 25: 279–82.
26. Yeshurun D, Hamood H, Morad N, Naschitz J. Acipimox as a secondary hypolipidemia in combined hypertriglyceridemia and hyperlipidemia. Harefuah 2000; 138: 650–3.

Judith Fraser, Chris Twelves, and Andrew Stanley

45 Cytostatic drugs

Editor's note: *The wide range of cytostatic drugs, the multitude of their adverse effects, and the fact that they are generally used in combinations of several agents all make it impossible to provide as detailed a review of the adverse effects of all the drugs in this field as the Annual gives in others. This year most of this chapter is devoted to a special review of the adverse effects of the anthracycline antibiotics by Dr Fraser and Dr Twelves. The rest of the chapter is by Dr Stanley, who thanks those clinicians and researchers who have sent him copies of their original research papers.*

Anthracyclines

Anthracyclines form a broad group of antitumor drugs within the group of cytotoxic antibiotics. The lead compounds were doxorubicin and daunorubicin; analogues include epirubicin, idarubicin, and aclarubicin. Mitoxantrone is a related compound of the anthracenedione family. Liposomal forms of doxorubicin (Caelyx®, Myocet®) and daunorubicin (DaunoXome®) are in use. These drugs are licensed for the treatment of a wide range of tumors (Table 1). Much information regarding the anthracyclines has been previously published in major reviews and textbooks (1^R, 2^R). With this in mind we have outlined their major toxic effects, but have concentrated in more detail on new findings, such as the interaction with trastuzumab.

Doxorubicin, daunorubicin, epirubicin, and idarubicin

Mechanism of action *The specific mechanism of cytotoxicity of these drugs has not been fully elucidated. Doxorubicin and epirubicin are both thought to act principally as inhibitors of the enzyme topoisomerase II.*

Pharmacokinetics *The anthracyclines are given intravenously, except for idarubicin, which can be given either intravenously or orally. The parent compound is the active moiety in all cases, but the major metabolite of idarubicin, idarubicinol, is also pharmacologically active. In most cases the principal route of excretion is via the biliary tract; renal excretion is of minor importance. There is extensive tissue distribution and subsequent slow release from these sites. In the case of doxorubicin only about 33–50% of the drug or its degradation products can be accounted for in urine, bile, or feces for up to 5 days after intravenous administration; the remainder appears to be retained for long periods in the body tissues.*

Epirubicin has a mean half-life of about 40 hours, which is somewhat shorter than doxorubicin. Biliary excretion is the main route of elimination. Neither crosses the intact blood–brain barrier.

Cardiovascular *Anthracyclines can cause the late complication of a cardiomyopathy, which can be irreversible and can proceed to congestive cardiac failure, ventricular dysfunction, conduction disturbances, or dysrhythmias several months or years after the end of treatment (3^R). The development of cardiomyopathy is closely associated with the cumulative lifetime dose of the anthracycline. The recommended maximum cumulative lifetime dose of doxorubicin is 450–550 mg/m^2 (4^R) and of daunorubicin 900–1000 mg/m^2 (1^R, 2^R). About 5% of doxorubicin-treated patients develop congestive cardiac failure at this dose; however, the in-*

Side Effects of Drugs, Annual 25
J.K. Aronson, ed.

Table 1. *Licensed indications for anthracyclines*

Drug	Where licensed	Licensed for treatment of
Doxorubicin	USA and EU	Acute leukemia, lymphomas, soft tissue and osteogenic sarcomas, pediatric malignancies, and adult solid tumors (particularly lung and beast cancers)
Epirubicin	EU	Breast, ovarian, gastric, lung, and colorectal cancers, malignant lymphomas, leukemias, and multiple myeloma, superficial and in-situ bladder carcinomas
Daunorubicin	USA and EU	Acute leukemia
Idarubicin	USA and EU	Relapsed or first-line treatment refractory advanced breast cancer, acute leukemia
Liposomal doxorubicin (Caelyx®, Doxil®)	USA and EU	Kaposi's sarcoma in AIDS
Liposomal daunorubicin (DaunoXome®)	USA and EU	Kaposi's sarcoma in AIDS
Liposomal doxorubicin (Myocet®)	EU	Breast cancer

cidence approaches 50% at cumulative doses of 1000 mg/m² (4[R], 5[R], 6[C]). These figures are derived from experience with doxorubicin administered as a bolus or by infusion of very short duration (under 30 minutes). The incidence of clinical cardiotoxicity falls dramatically with other schedules of administration (i.e. weekly doses or continuous infusion for more than 24 hours). The risk of cardiotoxicity is greater in children, elderly people, and patients with pre-existing cardiac disease or concomitant or prior mediastinal or chest wall irradiation (7[C], 8[C]).

All anthracyclines have cardiotoxic potential. However, because only a few cycles of treatment are administered in most regimens, few patients reach the cardiotoxic threshold of cumulative anthracycline dose. There is therefore limited information about the comparative cardiotoxic potential of these agents. However, it appears that on a molar basis epirubicin is substantially less cardiotoxic than doxorubicin (9[R]). Indeed, data from large clinical series, and from morphological examination of endomyocardial biopsies in smaller series of patients, suggest that the incidence and severity of cumulative cardiac toxicity associated with epirubicin 900 mg/m² is similar to that associated with doxorubicin 450–550 mg/m² (10[R]). Both mitoxantrone and the oral formulation of idarubicin are also thought to be less cardiotoxic than doxorubicin (11[R], 12[R]).

The diagnosis of anthracycline cardiomyopathy is based on the clinical presentation and investigations such as radionuclide cardiac angiography, which can show a reduced ejection fraction, and echocardiography, which can show reduced or abnormal ventricular function. Dysrhythmias can be detected by electrocardiography. Radioimmunoscintigraphy can be used to highlight damaged myocytes, and changes such as myocardial fibrosis are characteristic on endomyocardial biopsy (8[C], 13[c]).

Several mechanisms contribute to anthracycline cardiotoxicity. The principal mechanism is thought to be oxidative stresses placed on cardiac myocytes by reactive oxygen species. Amelioration of this toxicity is possible using dexrazoxane, an intracellular metal-chelating agent of the dioxopiperazine class (3[R]). Dexrazoxane acts by depleting intracellular iron, thus reducing the formation of cardiotoxic anthracycline–iron complexes. In patients without heart failure, in vivo measurements of myocardial oxidative metabolism and blood flow did not change in patients with cancer receiving doxorubicin (14[c]).

Anthracycline cardiomyopathy. although reportedly difficult to treat, often responds to current methods used to manage congestive cardiac failure.

Other cardiotoxic events occur only rarely. Occasionally acute transient electrocardiographic changes (ST-T wave changes, prolongation of the QT interval) and dysrhythmias can occur. Acute conduction disturbances, acute myopericarditis, and acute cardiac failure are also rare. In a study of the effects of anthracyclines on myocardial function in 50 long-term survivors of childhood cancer there was cardiac failure in one patient and electrocardiographic abnormalities (non-specific ST segment and T wave changes) in two (8[C]). In one patient with a VVI pacemaker, who received the combination of vincristine, doxorubicin, and dexamethasone, the pacemaker had to be reset after each cycle of treatment, as the pacing threshold had increased, resulting in bradycardia (15[A]).

The combination of doxorubicin plus paclitaxel is cardiotoxic. Various authors have suggested that after a median cumulative dose of 480 mg/m^2, 50% of patients will have a reduced left ventricular ejection fraction and 20% will develop congestive heart failure. Two studies of the combination of epirubicin plus paclitaxel have shown less reduction in left ventricular ejection fraction and no clinical evidence of cardiac failure (16[c], 17[c]). Clinically significant cardiac insufficiency has also been reported in a patient who was given epirubicin (316 mg/m^2) followed by six cycles of docetaxel (100 mg/m^2/cycle) (18[A]).

Hematologic Myelosuppression, principally neutropenia, occurs in 60–80% of patients who receive conventional doses of anthracyclines (single-agent standard doses: doxorubicin 60–75 mg/m^2, epirubicin 60–90 mg/m^2 given 3-weekly) (19[R]). On an equimolar basis, in both the single-agent and combination regimens, epirubicin causes less hematological toxicity than doxorubicin (10[R]). The incidence and severity of myelosuppression is related to dose; it has been suggested that severe neutropenia occurs in all patients who are given high-dose anthracyclines (doxorubicin 100 mg/m^2 or more and epirubicin 120 mg/m^2 or more) (20[R]). Neutrophil nadirs occur at 7–10 days after treatment, and full neutrophil recovery usually occurs by day 21 (10[R]). Platelets are less affected; about 35% of patients receiving epirubicin 120 mg/m^2 have grade 3 thrombocytopenia (21[c]). Anemia occurs rarely (10[R]).

Although the extent of leukopenia is not related to cumulative anthracycline dose, patients who have received extensive prior chemotherapy develop more severe leukopenia, possibly because of diminished bone-marrow reserve (10[R]). There was a strong correlation between dose and both leukocyte nadirs and platelet nadirs in 287 patients who received single-agent epirubicin 40, 60, 90, or 135 mg/m^2 every 3 weeks (22[C]). Myelosuppression correlates with exposure to epirubicin, as reflected by the plasma AUC (23[c]).

Myelosuppression is not prevented by prolonged doxorubicin infusion (19[R]), although this may mitigate other adverse effects. Hematological toxicity associated with high-dose regimens may be partially ameliorated by giving hemopoietic growth factors, with or without autologous bone marrow or peripheral blood progenitor cell rescue (24[c], 25[c], 26[C]). Unfortunately, however, other adverse effects, mainly mucositis, then become dose limiting. It has been suggested that mitoxantrone 14 mg/m^2 is more myelosuppressive than doxorubicin 70 mg/m^2, which in turn is more myelosuppressive than epirubicin 70 mg/m^2, each given at 3-week intervals (27[c]).

Secondary acute myeloid leukemia, with or without a preleukemic phase, has been rarely reported in patients being concurrently treated with epirubicin or doxorubicin in association with DNA-damaging antineoplastic agents; such cases have a short latency period (1–3 years) (28[C], 29[r]). In one study three of 77 patients who received epirubicin plus cisplatin and two who received other epirubicin-containing combinations developed acute myelogenous leukemia 15–33 months after the start of epirubicin treatment for advanced breast cancer (28[C]). However, all had received prior treatment with alkylating agents and/or radiotherapy, which are recognized independent leukemogenic risk factors. Despite high mean lifetime epirubicin doses in this study (mean 800 mg/m^2), there was no relation between cumulative dose and the risk of acute myelogenous leukemia. In a second study, four of 351 patients with metastatic breast cancer who received fluorouracil + epirubicin + cyclophosphamide , but none of 359 who received cyclophosphamide + methotrexate + 5-fluorouracil developed leukemia (three acute myelogenous leukemia, one acute lymphoblastic leukemia) (29[r]). No secondary leukemias were documented in other large comparative studies of epirubicin-containing regimens (30[C], 31[r]). Nevertheless, a retrospective analysis of case reports, published in abstract form without references or methods, concluded that when epirubicin was combined with alkylating agents it was associated with an increased risk of *secondary acute myelogenous leukemia in women with breast cancer (32[M]).*

Gastrointestinal *The anthracyclines are classed as moderately to strongly emetogenic. Nausea and vomiting occurs in 21–55% of patients, but is substantially reduced by pretreatment with antiemetic drugs (19[R], 21[c]). In one randomized study epirubicin 70 mg/m^2, doxorubicin 70 mg/m^2, and mitoxantrone 14 mg/m^2 were compared (27[c]). The first cycles of epirubicin and mitoxantrone were given without antiemetic drugs, unless specifically requested, but thereafter antiemetic drugs were given as required; doxorubicin was given with antiemetic drugs from cycle one. Doxorubicin and epirubicin were significantly more emetogenic than mitoxantrone; there was grade 3 nausea and vomiting in 22% of those who received doxorubicin, 18% of those who received epirubicin, and none of those who received mitoxantrone. Oral idarubicin may cause more emesis, which is quoted as occurring in 25–86% of patients; however, these effects are said to be usually mild to moderate (12[R]).*

With the advent of the 5-hydroxytryptamine (5-HT$_3$) receptor antagonists (ondansetron, granisetron, tropisetron), used in conjunction with dexamethasone, nausea and vomiting can be ameliorated in most patients.

Mucositis and stomatitis are potentially severe and dose-limiting adverse effects of the anthracyclines. Both the frequency and the severity are dose dependent (22[C], 33[C]). Their onset and recovery generally parallel the hematological toxicity, but they can occur earlier (5–10 days after treatment starts). Commonest are areas of painful erosions, mainly along the side of the tongue and on the sublingual mucosa. Mucositis occurs in about 9% of patients who receive oral idarubicin in standard doses (12[R]).

Diarrhea has also been reported with the anthracyclines. In a typical study, in which epirubicin 100 mg/m^2 was given for 1–8 cycles, one of 39 patients had grade 1/2 diarrhea and two of 39 had grade 3/4 diarrhea (34[c]). Of patients who take oral idarubicin 10–38% are said to develop diarrhea, again generally mild to moderate (12[R]).

Urinary tract *All anthracyclines can cause discoloration of the urine and other body fluids (i.e. tears) (1[R], 2[R]).*

Skin *Anthracyclines can cause local irritant reactions. These range from erythema and phlebitis at the injection site to potentially severe vesicant reactions requiring skin grafting (10[R]). Care appropriate to the administration of a vesicant must be observed during infusion. Various treatments have been used immediately after extravasation in an attempt to lessen the injury, including ice, steroids, vitamin E, topical dimethylsulfoxide (35[c]), and bicarbonate. None of these has been established convincingly. Reactivation of skin damage can also occur at sites of prior radiation therapy ("radiation recall") (36[R]).*

A syndrome of palmar–plantar erythema (progressing in some patients to blistering and desquamation) has been reported in seven of eight patients with advanced breast or ovarian cancer who received high-dose doxorubicin (125–150 mg/m^2) (37[c]). By contrast, in a similar dose intensification study in which patients received epirubicin 200 mg/m^2 with cyclophosphamide and growth factor support, the palmar–plantar syndrome did not occur (38[R]).

Hair *Complete or partial alopecia occurs in the majority (60–90%) of patients who receive anthracyclines, and although it is reversible it can be distressing (10[R]). Scalp cooling during chemotherapy to minimize hair loss is now little used, because of limited efficacy, discomfort of scalp cooling techniques, and concern about the potential creation of a "sanctuary" for circulating tumor cells. Alopecia is less frequent (about 35% of patients) in those who take oral idarubicin 40–45 mg/m^2 every 3 weeks (12[R]).*

Mutagenicity *There was an increased number of chromosomally aberrant lymphocytes in nurses who handled cytostatic agents (doxorubicin, cyclophosphamide, vincristine, fluorouracil, and methotrexate) many years ago, before modern facilities for the preparation of chemotherapeutic drugs were in use (39[c]). No long-term fertility problems were identified in 205 men who were treated with doxorubicin during childhood (40[C]).*

Teratogenicity *There is no conclusive evidence about whether anthracyclines adversely affect human fertility or are teratogenic. In 26 of 28 pregnancies three or more chemotherapeutic agents were used to treat acute leukemia* *(n = 20), non-Hodgkin's lymphoma (n = 3), Ewing's sarcoma (n = 2), breast cancer (n = 2), and myoblastoma (n = 1) (41[R]). The anthracyclines were introduced at various gestational ages, ranging from time of conception to 38 weeks, but in most cases chemotherapy was started in the second trimester. The outcomes were 24 normal infants, including a set of twins. Four of the five cases of infant death occurred in those with hematological malignancies (acute leukemia and non-Hodgkin's lymphoma), one each due to maternal death and therapeutic abortion and two resulting from spontaneous abortion. Neonatal pathological examination showed no congenital anomalies or organ defects, one case of marrow hypoplasia, and one case of neonatal sepsis. These findings suggest that anthracyclines have no detectable effect on the offspring up to the age of 54 months. However, bias inherent in reporting pregnancies with a successful outcome is obvious, so extreme caution must be exercised in the use of anthracyclines in pregnancy, and they should be avoided if at all possible.*

Fetotoxicity *Cardiac failure occurred in a 3-day-old neonate whose mother had been given idarubicin 9 mg/m^2 as part of induction therapy for acute lymphoblastic leukemia at 22 weeks; the baby was delivered at 28 weeks (109[A]). In the absence of another known cause, the cardiotoxicity was attributed to idarubicin exposure 6 weeks before.*

Risk factors *Since the main route of metabolism and elimination of anthracyclines is via the bile, dosage reduction is recommended if there is hepatic impairment. This was first suggested after a report of increased toxicity in patients with liver metastases who received full-dose anthracycline, followed by a second report that suggested that the clearance of anthracyclines is reduced in patients with hepatic metastases (42[c], 43[c]). These reports led to the current recommendations for anthracycline doses, based on serum bilirubin concentration or sulphobromophthalein clearance. However, the question of whether liver dysfunction significantly affects anthracycline clearance is unclear, and the dosage modifications suggested (see Table 2) have never been validated. Indeed, there is evidence that anthracycline kinetics are altered in patients with raised serum transaminases alone, which may be a better basis for dosage modification (44[c]). In practice many clinicians make empirical dosage modifications in patients with abnormal liver biochemistry tests (23[c]).*

Drug administration route *The anthracyclines are most commonly given intravenously, either as bolus doses or, less often, as infusions over varying lengths of time. Alternative routes have been tried, such as the intraperitoneal, intrapleural, and intravesical routes (45[R], 46[c]).*

Intraperitoneal *Intraperitoneal instillation of doxorubicin has been used in the early postoperative period in patients with retroperitoneal or visceral sarcoma, in an attempt to eradicate microscopic residual disease after complete macroscopic surgical excision (47[c]). Three of 17 patients had pyrexia, one peritoneal sclerosis, one a pancreatic fistula, and two abdominal pain. There were no anastomotic disruptions or intra-abdominal hemorrhages.*

Intrapleural *Adverse effects associated with the intrapleural instillation of doxorubicin in doses of 10–40 mg consist of fever (11–15%), anorexia (24–29%), nausea (20–29%), and chest pain (28–29%) (46[c], 48[R]). Cardiomyopathy and myelosuppression were not reported (48[R]).*

Intravesical *Intravesical epirubicin has been used to treat superficial bladder cancers. At a dose of 50 mg, the overall incidence of adverse events was 16–25% (45[R]). The frequency of adverse events tended to increase with dose but not the number of instillations. Most adverse events were mild and transient; the commonest were localized to the bladder and included chemical cystitis (10–38%), urinary tract infection (2–13%), and hematuria (2–33%). Contracted bladder or hemorrhagic cystitis have been reported in 1–6% of patients (45[R]).*

Adverse events occurred in 31 of 194 patients who received epirubicin 80 mg intravesically compared with 12 of 205 who received placebo after transurethral resection (49[C]). Systemic adverse events (usually cardiac or hematological adverse events or hypersensitivity) generally occurred in under 5% of patients. In two studies of intravesical epirubicin, there were reports of myocardial infarction (9%), stroke (3%), angina pectoris (3%), or atrioventricular block (2%) (50[c], 51[C]). There were

Table 2. *Effects of liver function on doses of doxorubicin and epirubicin*

Drug	Serum bilirubin concentration	BSP retention	Recommended dose
Doxorubicin	20–50 μmol/l	9–15%	50% of normal
	>50 μmol/l	>15%	25% of normal
Epirubicin	25–50 μmol/l		50% of normal
	>50 μmol/l		25% of normal

no reports of myelosuppression in clinical trials of intravesical epirubicin, apart from thrombocytopenia in one of 37 patients in one cancer trial (50[c]) and hemoglobinemia in two of 40 patients in another (52[C]).

Biochemical abnormalities have been reported in trials of intravesical epirubicin. In one trial liver function tests were impaired in seven of 40 patients who received epirubicin and in 10 of 35 patients who received epirubicin and verapamil concomitantly (53[c]). In another study, liver function tests were impaired in one of 69 patients who received combination prophylaxis with epirubicin 50 mg and BCG 150 mg after transurethral resection (54[c]).

Hypersensitivity has been reported in 0–8% of patients in trials of intravesical epirubicin; the symptoms included generalized skin rash, vulval irritation, or urinary frequency and dysuria, or were not stated (52[C], 55[c], 56[C]). One of 34 patients developed symptoms characterized as allergic (dizziness, nausea, hypotension) 1 hour after instillation of epirubicin (57[c]). Two patients who received epirubicin developed severe allergic reactions and one died (58[A], 59[A]).

Non-specific systemic adverse events (flu-like symptoms, malaise, fever, nausea, vomiting, anorexia, rash) occurred in under 5% of patients who received intravesical epirubicin (50[c], 55[c], 60[C]). Alopecia was reported in one of 37 patients (50[c]).

Intravesical epirubicin and doxorubicin appear to have similar tolerability profiles (56[C], 61[c]–63[c], 64[C]).

Valrubicin (a novel N-trifluoroacetyl, 14-valerate derivative of doxorubicin) is currently licensed in the USA for intravesical use in prophylaxis in patients with BCG-refractory carcinoma in situ after transurethral resection. It has a similar toxicity profile to that of epirubicin and doxorubicin (65[R]).

Drug overdose *Very high single doses of anthracyclines can cause acute myocardial degeneration within 24 hours and severe myelosuppression within 10–14 days. Treatment should aim to support the patient during this period and should include such measures as blood transfusion and reverse barrier nursing. Delayed cardiac failure can occur up to 6 months after overdosage.*

Drug interactions *An interaction of doxorubicin with the anti-HER2 receptor humanized monoclonal antibody, trastuzumab (Herceptin®), has recently been reported. Most patients who received trastuzumab in early trials had been pretreated with anthracyclines. Despite this, preliminary information suggested that reduced systolic cardiac function was an adverse effect of trastuzumab (66[C]). More recently this problem has been further highlighted in a study of women with metastatic breast cancer (67[C]). Patients who had not received prior anthracycline-containing adjuvant chemotherapy were at greater risk of cardiotoxicity when they received trastuzumab in combination with doxorubicin or cyclophosphamide (27% and 75% respectively), compared with only 11% of patients who received trastuzumab in combination with paclitaxel (67[C], 68[C]). The risk of cardiac events in patients treated with doxorubicin, cyclophosphamide, and trastuzumab increased markedly after a cumulative doxorubicin dose of 360 mg/m^2. This suggests synergistic cardiotoxicity with trastuzumab and doxorubicin. Trastuzumab is therefore currently licensed only for use in conjunction with paclitaxel and not with doxorubicin.*

The mechanism of trastuzumab-induced cardiotoxicity and its synergy with doxorubicin is as yet unknown. However, the cardiac fail-

ure responds to standard medical management (69[R]).

Since trastuzumab is active as a single agent and in combination with chemotherapy in patients whose tumors overexpress HER2, the interaction with doxorubicin is clearly of concern. Although it is possible to avoid this problem by not combining trastuzumab with doxorubicin, there are compelling reasons for further exploring its use with anthracyclines. For example, follow-up results from the CALGB 8541 study have shown that patients who received high and moderate (standard) doses of cyclophosphamide plus doxorubicin plus fluorouracil survived longer than those who received low doses (70[C]). Moreover, examination of patients' HER2 status in this trial showed that those whose tumors expressed large amounts of the HER2 protein had a significantly worse survival if treated with moderate or low doses of cyclophosphamide plus doxorubicin plus fluorouracil, compared with high doses (71[C]). These results suggest that patients whose tumors express large amounts of the HER2 receptor protein may require high-dose anthracyclines, presenting the problem of how then to treat them with trastuzumab without causing cardiotoxicity.

In an attempt to avoid cardiotoxicity after the administration of trastuzumab with doxorubicin, alternative adjuvant regimens have been suggested. Trastuzumab could be combined with other anthracyclines (epirubicin or liposomal formulations), which are inherently less cardiotoxic, or given sequentially rather than concomitantly with the anthracycline. Alternatively, non-anthracycline combinations, such as cyclophosphamide plus doxorubicin plus fluorouracil or based around taxanes, cisplatin, and vinorelbine are being investigated (72[R]).

Caution should of course be exercised when giving other cytotoxic drugs, especially myelotoxic agents or agents that cause significant mucositis/stomatitis, in combination with anthracyclines.

Liposomal anthracyclines

Liposomes are microscopic particles composed of a lipid bilayer membrane enclosing active drug in a central aqueous compartment (73[R]). The aim of liposomal encapsulation of a drug is to alter its pharmacokinetics, thus improving efficacy and/or reducing toxicity (74[R]). Current formulations of liposomes can be divided into two broad classes, based on their recognition by the reticuloendothelial system. Examples are:

- pegylated liposomal doxorubicin (Caelyx/Doxil) and liposomal daunorubicin, which conceal themselves from the reticuloendothelial system;
- liposomal doxorubicin (Myocet), which uses the reticuloendothelial system.

Sterically stabilized liposomal doxorubicin (pegylated liposomal doxorubicin; Caelyx/Doxil) is coated with polyethylene glycol (75[R]). In liposomal daunorubicin the liposome consists of a lipid bilayer of distearoylphosphatidylcholine and cholesterol in a 2:1 molar ratio (76[R]). Both formulations have a hydrophilic outer layer and so lead to a coating of water around the liposomal shell. This significantly increases circulation time, by making the liposomes virtually invisible to the reticuloendothelial system. There are differences in the adverse effects associated with pegylated liposomal doxorubicin and liposomal daunorubicin.

The second liposome system (Myocet) was designed to preserve the antitumor effects of doxorubicin but with reduced cardiotoxicity. This type of liposome is readily recognized and phagocytosed by the mononuclear phagocyte system. In animals most of the injected cytotoxic agent is rapidly taken up by phagocytes, minimizing exposure of normal tissues, and thus diminishing some acute and chronic adverse effects (77[E], 78[E]). The doxorubicin is then released by the phagocytes in a controlled fashion, similar to a slow infusion.

Pharmacokinetics The differences between pegylated liposomal doxorubicin and liposomal daunorubicin are due to the differences in their liposomal packaging. Pegylated liposomal doxorubicin (Caelyx/Doxil) and liposomal daunorubicin produce lower peak plasma concentrations and longer circulation times than free drug (79[C]).

Doxorubicin in Myocet has systemic availability, metabolism, and excretion similar to that of conventional doxorubicin, but at a slower rate (80[C]). In dogs the plasma concentrations of doxorubicin from Myocet were

1000-fold greater than conventional doxorubicin at 6 hours, but the difference diminished at 24 hours (81[E]). This distinguishes Myocet from Doxil, which persists in the circulation for significantly longer.

Caelyx has linear pharmacokinetics and its disposition occurs in two phases, the first relatively short (5 hours) and the second prolonged (55 hours). Unlike free doxorubicin, most of the pegylated liposomal doxorubicin is confined to the vascular fluid volume, and its blood clearance depends on the liposomal carrier. Liposomal daunorubicin acts similarly to Caelyx, but produces a lower AUC and has a higher clearance and shorter terminal half-life (82[R]).

Pegylated liposomes (diameter about 70–100 nm) and liposomal daunorubicin (diameter 45 nm) are small enough to pass intact through defective blood vessels that supply tumors. This, rather than any particular affinity for tumor cells, is the reason for their accumulation in tumor tissue (74[R]). Caelyx provides a greater concentration of doxorubicin in Kaposi's sarcoma tumors than in normal skin.

Cardiovascular *The incidence of cardiotoxicity in anthracycline-treated patients has been related to the peak plasma drug concentration (83[c], 84[r]). One of the aims in developing pegylated liposomal doxorubicin was to reduce plasma concentrations of free doxorubicin and restrict myocardial penetration, to minimize cardiotoxicity. Preclinical data suggested that the liposomal formulation was indeed less cardiotoxic than the free drug: about 50% more pegylated liposomal doxorubicin than free doxorubicin can be given to rabbits without producing the same frequency of cardiotoxicity (85[E]).*

Cardiac adverse events that have been considered probably or possibly related to pegylated liposomal doxorubicin have been reported in 3–9% of patients (86[M], 87[C], 88[c]). These include hypotension, pericardial effusion, thrombophlebitis, heart failure, and tachycardia (86[M], 87[C]).

Left ventricular failure has been reported in a few patients, particularly those who received high cumulative lifetime doses of pegylated liposomal doxorubicin (over 550 mg/m^2) (86[M], 87[C]). However, cumulative doses of 450 mg/m^2 or more and 550 mg/m^2 have been administered without significant reduction in ejection fraction or the development of cardiac failure (89[c], 90[c]). To date, no or minimal cardiotoxicity has been observed in patients with AIDS-related Kaposi's sarcoma who received pegylated liposomal doxorubicin in high cumulative doses (91[R]).

Both peak and overall concentrations of doxorubicin in myocardial tissue are reduced by 30–40% after Myocet relative to conventional doxorubicin (81[E]). This reduced myocardial exposure resulted in a significant reduction in cardiotoxicity, assessed both functionally and histologically (77[E], 78[E]). Compared with free doxorubicin 75 mg/m^2 given 3-weekly, Myocet 75 mg/m^2 caused significantly less congestive cardiac failure (1% vs 6%) (92[c]). However, a high dose of Myocet (135 mg/m^2, median cumulative dose 405 mg/m^2) caused a significant increase in cardiac toxicity: 38% of patients had a protocol-defined cardiac event, including 13% who developed congestive heart failure (93[c]).

In one study there was a significant (over 20%) reduction in the shortening fraction with liposomal daunorubicin measured by echocardiography (94[c]). In contrast, in another study there was no significant fall in cardiac function, even after cumulative doses of liposomal daunorubicin over 1000 mg/m^2 (95[c]).

Respiratory *Acute dyspnea, low back pain, and/or pain at the site of tumor have been described beginning within 1–5 minutes of the start of infusion of pegylated liposomal doxorubicin (96[E]). Three of 35 patients were described as suffering acute dyspnea, two with back pain and two with abdominal pain. In each case the symptoms resolved within 5–15 minutes of stopping the infusion, which was restarted without adverse effects. The mechanism of these symptoms was unclear. However, because the dyspnea was reminiscent of that seen in hemodialysis neutropenia, complete blood counts were obtained from four patients about 2 minutes after the onset of symptoms. All four had relative neutropenia (neutrophil counts of 3–46% of pretreatment), which resolved by the end of the infusion. In vitro, pegylated liposomal doxorubicin, in concentrations predicted to be present in the plasma during the start of treatment, stimulates neutrophil adhesion to human umbilical vein endothelial cells (96[E]). Thus, pegylated liposomal doxorubicin may* *cause transient sequestration of neutrophils in the pulmonary circulation, resulting in reduced lung compliance and associated dyspnea.*

Hematologic *In a phase I dose-finding study of pegylated liposomal doxorubicin, myelosuppression was not a major problem with the doses tested (20–80 mg/m^2, redosing every 3–4 weeks). Median nadir white cell and platelet counts were well above 2 × 10^9/l and 100 × 10^9/l respectively. In the occasional patient in whom profound granulocytopenia developed there was quick recovery of the cell counts within less than 7 days. Neutropenic fever was documented in only one patient at the top dose of 80 mg/m^2 (89[c]). There was no significant indication of cumulative myelosuppression. Treatment-related anemia was generally mild and blood transfusions were not required. However, two patients with head and neck malignancies and extensive pretreatment were given erythropoietin to maintain hemoglobin concentrations above 9.0 g/dl (89[c]).*

Pooled data from 12 phase I or II studies, in 308 patients with solid tumors who received pegylated liposomal doxorubicin in doses of 10–80 mg/m^2, showed that there was neutropenia (neutrophil count below 1 × 10^9/l) in 50%, anemia in 19%, and thrombocytopenia in 9.2% (97[M]).

Of 71 patients with metastatic breast cancer treated with pegylated liposomal doxorubicin in doses of 45–60 mg/m^2 given 3- or 4-weekly, grade 3/4 neutropenia occurred in 10% and thrombocytopenia in 1% (97[M]).

Pegylated liposomal doxorubicin and liposomal daunorubicin are predominantly used to treat AIDS related Kaposi's sarcoma, in which other factors also affect the white cell count. In patients with HIV/AIDS, myelosuppression was the most frequent dose-limiting adverse effect of liposomal anthracyclines (94[c], 95[c]). In one study of 30 patients with Kaposi's sarcoma given liposomal daunorubicin 40 mg/m^2, 53% developed granulocytopenia (white cell count below 1 × 10^9/l); 17% had a hemoglobin concentration below 8.0 g/dl, but none had thrombocytopenia (94[c]).

In another study in 53 patients with AIDS-related Kaposi's sarcoma given pegylated liposomal doxorubicin 20 mg/m^2 every 3 weeks, 21 had leukopenia and three had thrombocytopenia (98[c]).

At doses of 20 mg/m^2 liposomal doxorubicin, combined tolerability data from 705 patients with AIDS-related Kaposi's sarcoma showed that neutropenia (below 1 × 10^9/l) and anemia were the most common adverse events, affecting 50% and 19% of patients respectively (86[M]).

In summary, myelosuppression after treatment with pegylated liposomal doxorubicin appears not to be a major problem in patients with solid tumors and relatively intact immunological systems, but is the dose-limiting adverse effect in immunocompromised patients with HIV/AIDS.

High-dose Myocet (135 mg/m^2) caused significant hematological toxicity, namely grade 4 neutropenia in 98% and thrombocytopenia in 46 of 52 patients (93[c]). However, Myocet 75 mg/m^2 3-weekly caused less hematological toxicity than conventional doxorubicin (92[c]).

Gastrointestinal *Stomatitis and pharyngitis have been confirmed, along with hand–foot syndrome, as dose-limiting adverse effects of pegylated liposomal anthracyclines (89[c]). Stomatitis was dose limiting at high single doses over 70 mg/m^2. Similarly, 12 of 35 patients who received pegylated liposomal doxorubicin 50 mg/m^2 every 3 weeks for advanced ovarian carcinoma required dose reduction (to 40 mg/m^2) or treatment delay (to 4 weeks) because of mucositis (90[c]). Stomatitis and mucositis are dose dependent (99[R]). In the treatment of Kaposi's sarcoma in patients with HIV/AIDS, mucositis and stomatitis are rarely problematic and are not dose limiting. Presumably this is because significantly lower doses of pegylated liposomal doxorubicin are used in these patients.*

Nausea and vomiting have been reported but appear to be a mild and infrequent adverse effects of pegylated liposomal anthracyclines and liposomal daunorubicin (95[c], 100[c]). In most patients pegylated liposomal doxorubicin can be given without prophylactic antiemetics. In one study there was only mild nausea and vomiting in eight of 53 patients who had not received prophylactic antiemetics (98[c]). Further reviews in patients with AIDS-related Kaposi's sarcoma have reported nausea and vomiting in 17% and 8% of patients respectively (99[R]). Pooled data from 12 phase I and II studies in patients with solid tumors showed that 3.6% of patients had had grade 3/4 nausea or vomiting (97[M]). Diarrhea has similarly been recog-

nized as a mild and infrequent adverse effect of pegylated liposomal doxorubicin (three of 53 patients) (98[c]).

The authors of a case report suggested that pegylated liposomal doxorubicin was the probable cause of hepatic failure in a patient who, 2 weeks after treatment with pegylated liposomal doxorubicin 10 mg/m^2 (cumulative dose 20 mg/m^2), developed jaundice and ascites (101[r]). Despite withdrawal of other potentially hepatotoxic drugs, the patient died of hepatorenal failure 12 weeks later. This may have been an idiosyncratic effect augmented by hepatitis B viral infection (87[C], 102[r]), as there have been no other reports of hepatorenal failure (86[M], 103[C]).

Myocet (75 mg/m^2) causes significantly less vomiting (11% vs 23%) than conventional free doxorubicin (75 mg/m^2) (92[c]). It also leads to lower peak free doxorubicin concentrations in the gastrointestinal mucosa compared with conventional doxorubicin, and less gastrointestinal toxicity (77[E]). However, high-dose Myocet (135 mg/m^2) caused grade 4 mucositis in 10 of 52 patients (93[c]).

Skin *Skin toxicity, manifesting primarily as palmar–plantar erythrodysesthesia or hand–foot syndrome, is one of the principal dose-limiting adverse effects of pegylated liposomal anthracyclines. Skin toxicity is tolerable with Caelyx either 50 mg/m^2 given every 3 weeks or 60 mg/m^2 every 4 weeks (89[c], 90[c]). In pooled tolerability data (97[M]) grade 3/4 hand–foot syndrome was reported in 17.5% of 308 patients. The median time to the development of grade 3/4 hand–foot syndrome was 51 days, corresponding to the second or third cycle of treatment (97[M]). Myocet, even when given in a high dose (135 mg/m^2), was not associated with the hand–foot syndrome characteristic of pegylated liposomal doxorubicin (92[c], 93[c]). This was presumed to be due to differences in the liposomal formulation. Pegylated liposomes circulate for prolonged periods and extravasate through leaky capillary beds, whereas with Myocet the liposome is phagocytosed by the reticuloendothelial system and the active drug is then slowly released into the circulation, similar to a slow infusion.*

Conjunctivitis and skin pigmentation have been reported but are mild (95[c], 97[M], 98[c]).

Unlike extravasation of conventional doxorubicin, which can cause severe local inflammation and tissue damage, extravasation of liposomal doxorubicin was associated with only mild transient irritation at the infusion site in the eight documented cases (104[r], 105[r]).

Four cases of extravasation of liposomal daunorubicin have been reported and were associated with only mild irritation and transient erythema and swelling, similar to pegylated liposomal doxorubicin (106[A]).

In 60 patients receiving polyethylene glycol-coated liposomal doxorubicin (Doxil) 35–70 mg/m^2 by infusion over 1–2 hours there were four patterns of skin eruption: hand–foot syndrome (40%), a diffuse follicular rash (10%), an intertrigo-like eruption (8%), and new melanotic macules (0.5%) (107[CR]).

Hair *Alopecia is generally mild and occurs in 6–9% of patients. There have been no reports of alopecia with single-agent Myocet.*

Immunologic *Acute hypersensitivity reactions have been reported with the first infusion of pegylated liposomal doxorubicin (86[M], 87[C]). The symptoms included flushing, shortness of breath, facial swelling, headache, chills, back pain, tightness in the chest and throat, and hypotension. Similar reactions have been reported after the intravenous administration of colloid imaging agents and unloaded liposomes.*

Acute reaction to infusion have been observed on first exposure to the drug in six of 56 patients treated with pegylated doxorubicin 20–60 mg/m^2 (89[c]). The reactions developed at 3–25 minutes after the start of the infusion and were characterized by flushing, sensation of choking, back pain, and in one instance hypotension. All the symptoms disappeared shortly after discontinuation of the infusion. Three patients were retreated successfully using premedication (hydrocortisone, cimetidine, and diphenhydramine) and a slower infusion rate (under 1 mg/m^2). Similarly acute onset symptoms of dyspnea, back pain, and tumor site pain have been reported in other studies (96[E]). Since this reaction generally improves on rechallenge with or without premedication, it has been termed pseudoallergic.

Carcinogenicity *Two patients with acute promyelocytic leukemia developed therapy-related myelodyspasia 2–2.5 years after complete remission and then acute myeloid* *leukemia; both had received anthracyclines (108[AR]). In both cases the cytogenetic changes that usually occur after the use of alkylating agents were observed. There has only been one previous similar report after successful therapy with anthracyclines, but these observations suggest that anthracyclines can cause acute myeloid leukemia similar to that caused by alkylating agents.*

Teratogenicity *Pegylated liposomal doxorubicin is embryotoxic in rats and embryotoxic and abortifacient in rabbits. Teratogenicity cannot therefore be ruled out, but there is no reported experience in pregnant women. Equally, it is not known if the drug is excreted into human breast milk, so breastfeeding should be discontinued before the administration of pegylated liposomal doxorubicin.*

Risk factors *Since Caelyx has activity in Kaposi's sarcoma, many studies have been performed in patients with HIV/AIDS. Thus, assessment of the tolerability of Caelyx and Doxil has been complicated by underlying immune suppression, neutropenia, and co-morbidity commonly present in patients with HIV/AIDS. This has led to a difference in the dose-limiting adverse effects in patients with solid tumors compared to those with Kaposi's sarcoma. Tolerance differs in patients with HIV/AIDS (standard dose 20 mg/m^2 Caelyx given 2–3 times a week) and those with solid tumors (standard dose 50–80 mg/m^2 given 3–4 times a week).*

Drug overdose *Acute overdose with pegylated liposomal doxorubicin worsens the toxic effects of mucositis, leukopenia, and thrombocytopenia. There have been no reports of overdose of liposomal daunorubicin, but the primary anticipated toxic effect would be myelosuppression.*

Drug administration route *Intra-arterial Pegylated liposomal doxorubicin has been given to three patients via a catheter located in the hepatic artery (110[A]). No severe adverse effects, such as nausea, vomiting, stomatitis, alopecia, or cardiotoxicity, were observed. There was mild leukopenia (2.8 × 10^9/l) in one patient; neither anemia nor thrombocytopenia were reported.*

Drug interactions *No formal drug interaction studies have been conducted with pegylated liposomal doxorubicin, liposomal daunorubicin, or Myocet. Caution should be exercised in the concomitant use of drugs known to interact with doxorubicin or daunorubicin. Equally, caution should be exercised when giving any other cytotoxic drugs, especially myelotoxic agents, at the same time.*

GENERAL

Recent reviews, which have improved our understanding of the adverse effects profiles of individual drugs and groups of drugs, have dealt with the scale and causative factors of chemotherapy-induced *anemia* (111[M]) and *nausea and vomiting* (112[M]). The relation between a drug's complete adverse effects spectrum and either its pharmacological action (113[c]) or its dosage regimen have recently been described and reviewed by several authors (114[c]–116[c]). From a pooled collection of data from four phase II studies, a raft of interconnected prognostic factors has emerged, which predict tumor response, progression-free survival, and toxicity in patients with metastatic colorectal cancer given irinotecan as second-line chemotherapy after failure of fluorouracil (117[M]). Finally, there have been two treatment reviews, one on colon and rectal cancers (118[R]) and the other on melanoma (119[R]).

Cardiovascular In an attempt to clarify further the cardiotoxicity of paclitaxel, its effect on cardiovascular autonomic regulation has been investigated in 14 women (120[c]). The authors concluded that *autonomic modulation of heart rate is impaired* by paclitaxel, but they were unable to say whether it would return to normal on withdrawal. They also investigated the effect of docetaxel on neural cardiovascular regulation in women with breast cancer, previously treated with anthracyclines (121[c]). They concluded that docetaxel did not impair vagal cardiac control. The changes that they observed in blood pressure suggest that docetaxel *changes sympathetic vascular control*, although these changes seemed to be related to altered cardiovascular homeostasis rather than peripheral sympathetic neuropathy.

Corrected QT dispersion was a predictor of acute heart failure after high dose cyclophosphamide chemotherapy (5.6 g/m^2 over 4 days) in 19 patients (122[r]).

Venous discomfort and venous chemical phlebitis have been reported with vinorelbine 30 mg/m^2, with an incidence of up to 23% (123[c], 124[c]).

Two women who survived childhood malignancies were left with *cardiovascular compromise* and *short stature* (125[A]). One had been treated with nephrectomy, adrenalectomy, radiotherapy, and chemotherapy (vincristine, cyclophosphamide, and doxorubicin) and the other with radiotherapy and chemotherapy.

An *acute cardiomyopathy* has been reported after the use of cisplatin and 5-fluorouracil (126[A]). and an occlusive thromboembolic event (127[A]).

A 52-year-old man with a squamous cell carcinoma of the soft palate finished a first course of cisplatin (30 mg/m^2/day for 3 days), 5-fluorouracil (1000 mg/m^2 daily for 4 days), and radiotherapy. An electrocardiogram showed sinus tachycardia and left ventricular hypertrophy with repolarization changes. There was cardiomegaly on the chest X-ray. An echocardiogram showed severely depressed left ventricular function, an ejection fraction of 20%, and a mobile thrombus at the apex. He was immediately given heparin. Three days later he developed severe pain in the back and both legs. There was bluish discoloration of the feet and absent femoral pulses. MRI angiography of the abdominal aorta showed embolic obstruction at the aortic bifurcation, with evidence of infarction in the kidneys. Bilateral transfemoral thrombectomy was performed, following which circulation to the lower extremities was restored.

A *thrombotic stroke* has been reported after the use of cisplatin, etoposide, and bleomycin (127[A]).

A 31-year-old man with a seminoma had an orchidectomy, followed by chemotherapy with cisplatin, etoposide, and bleomycin. A day after the end of the second course of chemotherapy he became comatose with a heart rate of 150/min and a systolic blood pressure of 80 mmHg. Cranial angiography showed a thrombosis of the basilar artery and a cranial CT scan showed cerebellar infarction but no brain metastases.

Respiratory Two cases of *respiratory failure* occurred during induction chemotherapy for acute myelomonocytic leukemia with cytarabine and all-trans-retinoic acid (128[A]). The authors attributed this to a manifestation of the retinoic acid syndrome. Both cases developed acute respiratory failure with widespread pulmonary infiltrates about 60 hours after starting chemotherapy. Both cases were managed successfully using high-dose dexamethasone and ventilation.

Methotrexate can cause *lung damage*. A recent case in a 34-year-old woman followed exposure to only 232 mg, and despite drug withdrawal lung function deteriorated for a further 2 months (reduced CO transfer factor to 66% of predicted) and improved only by the fifth month (129[A]).

Nervous system *Peripheral neuropathy* occurred in 13 of 37 patients treated with paclitaxel 175 mg/m^2 and carboplatin (130[c]). The authors concluded that clinically important neurotoxicity increases with every cycle of chemotherapy. The peripheral neuropathy mainly affected sensory fibers without involving motor nerves. The same paclitaxel/carboplatin chemotherapy in 28 women caused no signs of acute central neurotoxicity or neuropsychological deterioration; however, 11 patients had a peripheral neuropathy (131[c]).

In 12 of 52 patients treated with ifosfamide there was *neurocortical toxicity* greater than grade 2 (132[A,c]). They were successfully treated with intravenous methylene blue 50 mg 3-hourly, which was also prophylactic in three patients.

In the context of two children treated with methotrexate it was proposed that progressive hypomethylation in the CNS may be responsible for demyelinization in the *leukoencephalopathy* caused by high-dose systemic or intrathecal methotrexate (133[A]).

Sensory systems A woman developed *bilateral blindness* and *lumbosacral myelopathy* within 1 month of having received an autologous bone-marrow transplant, cisplatin 55 mg/m^2, carmustine 600 mg/m^2, and cyclophosphamide 1875 mg/m^2 (134[A]).

Fluid balance *Fluid retention* has previously been reported with docetaxel. Some believe that this effect depends on the dose and the duration of infusion (135[c], 136[c]) and that high concentrations of M4, the cyclized oxazolidinedione metabolite of docetaxel, cause more pronounced fluid retention.

Hematologic The authors of a study in 101 patients concluded that in addition to the dose of chemotherapy and the administration of hemopoietic growth factors, poor performance status and a high concentration of soluble p75-R-TNF can predict the occurrence of chemotherapy-induced *myelosuppression* in lymphoma (137[C]).

In another study in 43 patients, raised plasma concentrations of FLT3-L (an fms-like tyrosine kinase) in patients who had previously received chemotherapy predicted the stage of recovery of the bone-marrow compartment (138[c]). FLT3-L seems to identify the likelihood that the patient will have severe thrombocytopenia if additional cytotoxic therapy is given. Knowledge of bone-marrow activity should permit more aggressive therapy, by establishing the earliest possible time for dosing with any cytotoxic agent for which myelosuppression is the dose-limiting toxic effect.

In 46 chemotherapy-naive patients docetaxel had an important but reversible nonspecific *lymphopenic effect*, thought to be associated with an increased risk of non-neutropenic infections (139[C]).

Concern about the toxicity of hydroxyurea expressed in a report from the AIDS Clinical Trials Group (ACTG 5025 report) have led to a retrospective study of the antiviral activity, immunological effects, and tolerability of hydroxyurea in combination with didanosine (140[C]). Hematological adverse events were the most frequent and involved 37 of the 65 patients. *Neutropenia* was the commonest adverse event (26 patients) and was occasionally accompanied by *anemia* or *thromobocytopenia*. However, these effects normalized spontaneously, despite continued therapy.

Of 16 children receiving hydroxyurea in combination with nucleoside analogues, four developed *neutropenia* (below 1.5×10^9/l) by weeks 2 or 4 (141[C]). Hydroxyurea was temporarily withdrawal and then reintroduced without further ill effects after the neutrophil count had returned to normal.

Mouth and teeth In the study quoted above (140[C]), *mouth ulceration* was recorded in eight of the 65 patients and this led to discontinuation in one patient.

Gastrointestinal Three of 14 patients in a phase I study of docetaxel plus vinorelbine for metastatic breast cancer developed colitis (142[Ar]). A further three patients were identified in other studies of docetaxel.

Pancreas In the study quoted above (140[C]), *hyperamylasemia* occurred in 15 of the 65 patients. Although asymptomatic, it occasioned withdrawal of therapy in four patients.

Urinary tract Both cisplatin and ifosfamide are *nephrotoxic*. Cisplatin fractionated over 5 days, cisplatin combined with ifosfamide in standard doses. and high-dose carboplatin plus ifosfamide have been compared in 52 patients (143[c]). The high-dose regimen with the less nephrotoxic drug carboplatin was associated with a comparable or even higher rate of nephrotoxicity. In another study in 22 patients the degree of albuminuria (as an early marker of cisplatin-induced renal damage) was related to the urinary monoaquoplatin concentration (144[c]).

The Late Effects Group of the UK Children's Cancer Study Group, showed that higher total doses of ifosfamide correlated significantly with greater glomerular and tubular toxicity (145[c]). They concluded that restriction of the total dose of ifosfamide to below 84 g/m^2 will reduce the frequency of significant nephrotoxicity but not abolish it, while doses over 119 g/m^2 are associated with a very high risk of severe toxicity.

Skin *Calciphylaxis* is a rare, often fatal disease characterized clinically by progressive cutaneous necrosis and ulceration and histologically by vascular calcification and thrombosis. It has been described in association with end-stage renal disease and hyperparathyroidism. A case of calciphylaxis has been described in a 64-year-old woman who 3 months before had finished a course of cyclophosphamide, doxorubicin, and fluorouracil chemotherapy for breast carcinoma (146[A]). She had no renal disease and had normal renal function and parathyroid hormone concentrations. The authors speculated that the cause may have been chemotherapy-induced functional deficiency of protein C and protein S.

Four cases of fixed plaques of *erythrodysesthesia* have been attributed to intravenous docetaxel (147[A]). There had been no extravasation or previous skin injury. While this was a new presentation, the authors did not explain why the lesions were not just late presentations of small-volume extravasation injuries.

In 60 patients receiving polyethylene glycol-coated liposomal doxorubicin (Doxil) 35–70 mg/m^2 by infusion over 1–2 hours there were four patterns of skin eruption: *hand-foot syndrome* (40%), a *diffuse follicular rash* (10%), an *intertrigo-like eruption* (8%), and new *melanotic macules* (0.5%) (107[CR]).

Nails *Onycholysis* occurred in five of 21 patients who received more than six doses of paclitaxel 100 mg/m^2/week (148[CR]). The authors also provided a useful review of onycholysis caused by other chemotherapy. Onycholysis has also been reported in patients receiving docetaxel (149[A]).

Immunologic There was a 9% incidence of clinically important hypersensitivity reactions to paclitaxel in 450 women with gynecological malignancies treated with paclitaxel either alone or in combination regimens (150[C]). There was a significant association between bee sting or animal allergy and paclitaxel hypersensitivity in 57 patients with a variety of tumors (151[c])

There were no allergic reactions to pegylated asparaginase compared with 30% with non-pegylated asparaginase in 70 children with acute lymphoblastic leukemia or non-Hodgkin's lymphoma, and other toxic effects were also less common (152[c]).

Body temperature Drug-induced *fever* has been reported in a 64-year-old woman with essential thrombocythemia after 3 weeks of treatment with hydroxyurea 1000 mg/day; the fever subsided on withdrawal and reappeared on rechallenge (153[A]).

Carcinogenicity Of 1774 patients with breast cancer, nine (0.005%) developed secondary *myelodysplasia* or *acute myeloid leukemia* after mitoxantrone-based therapy (154[R]). The median time to presentation was 2.5 years. This level of occurrence is 10 times higher than that in the general population.

During long-term follow-up of patients treated with busulfan and hydroxyurea for essential thrombocythemia, seven patients (13%) taking hydroxyurea developed secondary *acute leukemia*, *myelodysplasia*, or *solid tumors*, compared with only one of the no treatment control group; none of the 20 patients who had never been treated with chemotherapy developed secondary malignancies compared with three of the 77 given hydroxyurea only and five of the 15 given busulfan plus hydroxyurea. This suggests that the combination of busulfan plus hydroxyurea causes a significantly increased risk of secondary malignancies (155[c]).

REFERENCES

1. Chabner BA, Longo DL. Cancer Chemotherapy and Biotherapy: Principles and Practice. 2nd edition. Lippincott Williams and Wilkins, 2001.
2. Souhami RL, Tannock I, Hohenberger P, Horiot JC. Oxford Textbook of Oncology. 2nd edition. Oxford: Oxford University Press, 2002.
3. Wiseman LR, Spencer CM. Dexrazoxane. A review of its use as a cardioprotective agent in patients receiving anthracycline-based chemotherapy. Drugs 1998; 56: 385–403.
4. Launchbury AP, Habboubi N. Epirubicin and doxorubicin: a comparison of their characteristics, therapeutic activity and toxicity. Cancer Treatment Rev 1993; 19: 197–228.
5. Shan K, Lincoff AM, Young JB. Anthracycline-induced cardiotoxicity. Ann Int Med 1996; 125: 47–58.
6. Von Hoff DD, Layard MW, Basa P, Davis HL, Von Hoff AL, Rozencweig M, Muggia FM. Risk factors for doxorubicin-induced congestive heart failure. Ann Int Med 1979; 91: 710–17.
7. Pihkala J, Saarinen UM, Lundstrom U, Virtanen K, Virkola K, Siimes MA, Pesonen E. Myocardial function in children and adolescents after therapy with anthracyclines and chest irradiation. Eur J Cancer 1996; 32: 97–103.
8. Hesseling PB, Kalis NN, Wessels G, Van der Merwe P-L. The effect of anthracyclines on myocardial function in 50 long-term survivors of childhood cancer. Cardiovasc J South Afr 1999; 89 Suppl 1: C25–8.
9. Coukell AJ, Faulds D. Epirubicin. An updated review of its pharmacodynamic and pharmacokinetic properties and therapeutic efficacy in the management of breast cancer. Drugs 1997; 53: 453–82.
10. Plosker GL, Faulds D. Epirubicin: a review of its pharmacodynamic and pharmacokinetic properties, and therapeutic use in cancer chemotherapy. Drugs 1993; 45: 788–856.
11. Booser DJ, Hortobagyi GN. Anthracycline antibiotics in cancer therapy: focus on drug resistance. Drugs 1994; 47: 223–58.

12. Buckley MM, Lamb HM. Oral idarubicin. A review of its pharmacological properties and clinical efficacy in the treatment of haematological malignancies and advanced breast cancer. Drugs Aging 1997; 11: 61–86.
13. Vici P, Ferraironi A, Di Lauro L, Carpano S, Conti F, Belli F, Paoletti G, Maini CL, Lopez M. Dexrazoxane cardioprotection in advanced breast cancer patients under high-dose epirubicin treatment. Clin Ter 1998; 149: 15–20.
14. Nony P, Guastalla J-P, Rebattu P, Landais P, Lievre M, Itti LBR, Beaune J, Andre-Fouet X, Janier M. In vivo measurement of myocardial oxidative metabolism and blood flow does not show changes in cancer patients undergoing doxorubicin therapy. Cancer Chemother Pharmacol 2000; 45: 375–80.
15. Wilke A, Hesse H, Gorg C, Maisch B. Elevation of the pacing threshold: a side effect in a patient with pacemaker undergoing therapy with doxorubicin and vincristine. Oncology 1999; 56: 110–11.
16. Rischin D, Smith J, Millward M, Lewis C, Boyer M, Richardson G, Toner G, Gurney H, McKendrick J. A phase II trial of paclitaxel and epirubicin in advanced breast cancer. Br J Cancer 2000; 83: 438–42.
17. Lalisang RI, Voest EE, Wils JA, Nortier JW, Erdkamp FL, Hillen HF, Wals J, Schouten HC, Blijham GH. Dose-dense epirubicin and paclitaxel with G-CSF: a study of decreasing intervals in metastatic breast cancer. Br J Cancer 2000; 82: 1914–19.
18. Salminen E, Bergman M, Huhtala S, Jekunen A, Ekholm E. Docetaxel, a promising novel chemotherapeutic agent in advanced breast cancer. Anticancer Res 2000; 20: 3663–8.
19. Abraham R, Basser RL, Green MD. A risk-benefit assessment of anthracycline antibiotics in antineoplastic therapy. Drug Saf 1996; 15: 406–29.
20. Zuckerman KS. Efficacy of intensive, high-dose anthracycline-based therapy in intermediate and high-grade non-Hodgkin's lymphomas. Semin Oncol 1994; 21 Suppl 1: 59–64.
21. Lissoni A, Cormio G, Colombo N, Gabriele A, Landoni F, Zanetta G, Mangioni C. High-dose epirubicin in patients with advanced or recurrent uterine sarcoma. Int J Gynaecol Cancer 1997; 7: 241–4.
22. Bastholt L, Dalmark M, Gjedde SB, Pfeiffer P, Pedersen D, Sandberg E, Kjaer M, Mouridsen HT, Rose C, Nielsen OS, et al. Dose-relationship of epirubicin in the treatment of postmenopausal patients with metastatic breast cancer: a randomised study of epirubicin at four different dose levels performed by the Danish Breast Cancer Cooperative Group. J Clin Oncol 1996; 14: 1146–55.
23. Dobbs NA, Twelves CJ. Anthracycline doses in patients with liver dysfunction: do UK oncologists follow current recommendations? Br J Cancer 1998; 77: 1145–8.
24. Scinto AF, Ferraresi V, Campioni N, Tonachella R, Piarulli L, Sacchi I, Giannarelli D, Cognetti F. Accelerated chemotherapy with high-dose epirubicin and cyclophosphamide plus r-met-HIG-CSF in locally advanced and metastatic breast cancer. Ann Oncol 1995; 6: 665–71.
25. Hansen F, Stenbygaard L, Skovsgaard T. Effect of granulocyte-macrophage colony-stimulating factor (GM-CSF) on hematologic toxicity induced by high-dose chemotherapy in patients with metastatic breast cancer. Acta Oncol 1995; 34: 919–24.
26. Chevallier B, Chollet P, Merrouche Y, Roche H, Fumoleau P, Kerbrat P, Genot JY, Fargeot P, Olivier JP, Fizames C, et al. Lenograstim prevents morbidity from intensive induction chemotherapy in the treatment of inflammatory breast cancer. J Clin Oncol 1995; 13: 1564–71.
27. Lawton PA, Spittle MF, Ostrowski MJ, Young T, Madden F, Folkes A, Hill BT, MacRae K. A comparison of doxorubicin, epirubicin and mitozantrone as single agents in advanced breast carcinoma. Clin Oncol 1993; 5: 80–4.
28. Pedersen-Bjergaard J, Sigsgaard TC, Nielsen D, Gjedde SB, Philip P, Hansen M, Larsen SO, Rorth M, Mouridsen H, Dombernowsky P. Acute monocytic or myelomonocytic leukaemia with balanced chromosome translocations to band 11q23 after therapy with 4-epi-doxorubicin and cisplatin or cyclophosphamide for breast cancer. J Clin Oncol 1992; 10: 1444–51.
29. Shepherd L, Ottaway J, Myles J, Levine M. Therapy-related leukaemia associated with high-dose 4-epi-doxorubicin and cyclophosphamide used as adjuvant chemotherapy for breast cancer. J Clin Oncol 1994; 12: 2514–15.
30. Coombes RC, Bliss JM, Wils J, Morvan F, Espie M, Amadore D, Gambrosier P, Richards M, Aapro M, Villar-Grimalt A, et al. Adjuvant cyclophosphamide, methotrexate, and fluorouracil versus fluorouracil, epirubicin, and cyclophosphamide chemotherapy in pre-menopausal women with axillary node-positive operable breast cancer: results of a randomised trial. J Clin Oncol 1996; 14: 35–45.
31. Marty M. International CCGSC. Epirubicin and the risk of leukemia: not substantiated? J Clin Oncol 1993; 11: 1431–2.
32. Ragaz J, Yun J, Spinelli J. Analysis of incidence of secondary acute myelogenous leukemias (2nd AML) in breast cancer patients (BCP) treated with adjuvant therapy (AT) – association with therapeutic regimens. (Abstract no. 147). Proc Am Soc Clin Oncol 1995; 14: 112.
33. Focan C, Andrien JM, Closon MT, Dicato M, Driesschaert P, Focan-Henrard D, Lemaire M, Lobelle JP, Longree L, Ries F. Dose-response relationship of epirubicin-based first-line chemotherapy for advanced breast cancer: a prospective randomised trial. J Clin Oncol 1993; 11: 1253–63.
34. Bissett D, Paul J, Wishart G, Jodrell D, Machan MA, Harnett A, Canney P, George WD, Kaye S. Epirubicin chemotherapy and advanced breast cancer after adjuvant CMF chemotherapy. Clin Oncol 1995; 7: 12–15.

35. Bertelli G, Gozza A, Forno GB, Vidili MG, Silvestro S, Venturini M, Del Mastro L, Garrone O, Rosso R, Dini D. Topical dimethylsulphoxide for the prevention of soft tissue injury after extravasation of vesicant cytotoxic drugs: a prospective clinical study. J Clin Oncol 1995; 13: 2851–5.
36. Perry MC. Complications of chemotherapy. In: Moosa AR, Schimpff SC, Robson MC, editors. Comprehensive textbook of oncology. 2nd ed. Baltimore, Maryland: Williams and Wilkins, 1991: 1706–19.
37. Bronchud MH, Howell A, Crowther D, Hopwood P, Souza L, Dexter TM. The use of granulocyte colony-stimulating factor to increase the intensity of treatment with doxorubicin in patients with advanced breast and ovarian cancer. Br J Cancer 1989; 60: 121–5.
38. Green M. Dose-intensive chemotherapy with cytokine support. Semin Oncol 1994; 1 Suppl 1: 1–6.
39. Nikula E, Kiviniitty K, Leisti J, Tskinen PJ. Chromosome aberration in lymphocytes of nurses handling cytostatic agents. Scand J Work Environ Health 1984; 10: 71–4.
40. Aubier F, Patte C, De Vathaire F, Tournade MF, Oberlin O, Sakiroglu O, Lemerle J. Male fertility after chemotherapy during childhood. Ann Endocrinol 1995; 56: 141–2.
41. Turchi JJ, Villasis C. Anthracyclines in the treatment of malignancy in pregnancy. Cancer 1988; 61: 435–40.
42. Benjamin RS, Wiernik PH, Bachur NR. Doxorubicin chemotherapy, efficacy, safety and pharmacologic basis of an intermittent single high dosage schedule. Cancer 1973; 33: 19–27.
43. Camaggi CM, Strocchi E, Tamassia V, Martoni A, Giovannini M, Lafelice G, Canova N, Marraro D, Martini A, Pannuti F. Pharmacokinetic studies of 4′-epi-doxorubicin in cancer patients with normal and impaired renal function and with hepatic metastases. Cancer Treat Res 1982; 66: 1819–24.
44. Twelves CJ, Dobbs NA, Michael Y, Summers LA, Gregory W, Harper PG, Rubens RD, Richards MA. Clinical pharmacokinetics of epirubicin: the importance of abnormal liver biochemistry tests. Br J Cancer 1992; 66: 765–9.
45. Onrust SV, Wiseman LR, Goa KL. Epirubicin: a review of its intravesical use in superficial bladder cancer. Drugs Aging 1999; 15: 307–33.
46. Masuno T, Kishimoto S, Ogura T, Honma T, Niitani H, Fukuoka M, Ogawa N. A comparative trial of LC9018 plus doxorubicin and doxorubicin alone in the treatment of malignant pleural effusion secondary to lung cancer. Cancer 1991; 68: 1495–500.
47. Sugarbaker PH, Sweatman TW, Graves T, Cunliffe W, Israel M. Early postoperative intraperitoneal adriamycin. Pharmacological studies and a preliminary report. Reg Cancer Treat 1991; 4: 127–31.
48. Walker-Renard PB, Vaughan LM, Sahn SA. Chemical pleurodesis for malignant pleural effusions. Ann Intern Med 1994; 120: 56–64.
49. Oosterlinck W, Kurth KH, Schroder F, Bultinck J, Hammond B, Sylvester R. A prospective European Organisation for Research and Treatment of Cancer Genitourinary Group randomized trial comparing transurethral resection followed by a single intravesical instillation of epirubicin or water in single stage Ta, T1 papillary carcinoma of the bladder. J Urol 1993; 149: 749–52.
50. Cumming JA, Kirk D, Newling DW, Hargreave TB, Whelan P. A multi-centre phase-2 study of intravesical epirubicin in the treatment of superficial bladder tumour. Eur Urol 1990; 17: 20–2.
51. Okamura K, Murase T, Obata K, Ohshima S, Ono Y, Sakata T, Hasegawa Y, Shimoji T, Miyake K. A randomised trial of early intravesical instillation of epirubicin in superficial bladder cancer. Cancer Chemother Pharmacol 1994; 35 Suppl: S31–5.
52. Bono AV, Hall RR, Denis L, Lovisolo JA, Sylvester R. Chemoresection in Ta-T1 bladder cancer: members of the EORTC Genito-urinary Group. Eur Urol 1996; 29: 385–90.
53. Lukkarinen O, Paul C, Hellstrom P, Kontturi M, Nurmi M, Puntala P, Ottelin J, Tammela T, Tidefelt U. Intravesical epirubicin with and without verapamil for the prophylaxis of superficial bladder tumours. Scand J Urol Nephrol 1991; 25: 25–8.
54. Bono AV, Lovisolo JA, Saredi G. Conservative treatment of primary T1G3 bladder carcinoma: results from a phase II trial. Br J Urol 1997; 80 Suppl 2: 117.
55. Melekos MD, Dauaher H, Fokaefs E, Barbalias G. Intravesical instillations of 4-epi-doxorubicin (epirubicin) in the prophylactic treatment of superficial bladder cancer: results of a controlled prospective study. J Urol 1992; 147: 371–5.
56. Ali-El-Dein B, El-Baz M, Aly ANM, Shamaa S, Ashamallah A. Intravesical epirubicin versus doxorubicin for superficial bladder tumours (stages pTa and pT1): a randomized prospective study. J Urol 1997; 158: 68–74.
57. Kurth K, Van der Vijgh WJF, Ten Kate F, Bogdanowicz JF, Carpentier PJ, Van Reyswoud I. Phase 1/2 study of intravesical epirubicin in patients with carcinoma in situ of the bladder. J Urol 1991; 146: 1508–13.
58. Hermenegildo Caudevilla M, Climente Marti M, Polo i Peris A, Poveda Andres JL, Gasso Matoses M. Fatal adverse reaction after intravesical administration of epirubicin. Farm Hosp 1996; 20: 395–6.
59. Michelena Hernandez L, Iruin Sanz A, Martinez Lopez de Castro N, Sarobe Carricas M, Oderiz Mendioroz N, Vivanco Arana M, Alfaro Basarte J. Systemic reaction due to intravesical epirubicin. Farm Hosp 1996; 20: 393–4.
60. Melekos MD, Zarakovitis IE, Fokaefs ED, Dandinis K, Chionis H, Bouropoulos C, Dauaher H. Intravesical bacillus Calmette–Guerin versus epirubicin in the prophylaxis of recurrent and/or multiple superficial bladder tumours. Oncology 1996; 53: 281–8.

61. Gohji K, Hara I, Taguchi I, Ueno K, Yamada Y, Eto H, Arakawa S, Kamidono S, Obe S, Ogawa T, et al. Long-term results of a randomised study of intravesical instillation of epirubicin and doxorubicin as a prophylaxis against superficial bladder recurrence. Nishinihon J Urol 1997; 59: 785–91.
62. Schon G, Merkle W. Epirubicin vs doxorubicin for the treatment of superficial bladder cancer: a randomised study (abstract no P1.13). Urologe A 1998; Suppl 1: S18.
63. Shuin T, Kubota Y, Noguchi S, Hosaka M, Miura T, Kondo I, Fukushima S, Ishizuka E, Furuhata A, Moriyama M, et al. A phase II study of prophylactic intravesical chemotherapy with 4-epirubicin in recurrent superficial bladder cancer: comparison of 4-epirubicin and adriamycin. Cancer Chemother Pharmacol 1994; 35 Suppl: S52–6.
64. Eto H, Oka Y, Ueno K, Nakamura I, Yoshimura K, Arakawa S, Kamidono S, Obe S, Ogawa T, Hamami G. Comparison of the prophylactic usefulness of epirubicin and doxorubicin in the treatment of superficial bladder cancer by intravesical instillation: a multicentre randomised trial. Cancer Chemother Pharmacol 1994; 35 Suppl: S46–51.
65. Onrust SV, Lamb HM. Valrubicin. Drugs Aging 1999; 15: 69–75.
66. Cobleigh MA, Vogel CL, Tripathy D, Robert NJ, Scholl S, Fehrenbacher L, Wolter JM, Paton V, Shak S, Lieberman G, Slamon DJ. Multinational study of the efficacy and safety of humanized anti-HER2 monoclonal antibody in women who have HER2-overexpressing metastatic breast cancer that has progressed after chemotherapy for metastatic disease. J Clin Oncol 1999; 17: 2639–48.
67. Slamon DJ, Leyland-Jones B, Shak S, Fuchs H, Paton V, Bajamonde A, Fleming T, Eiermann W, Wolter J, Pegram M, et al. Use of chemotherapy plus a monoclonal antibody against HER2 for metastatic breast cancer that overexpresses HER2. New Engl J Med 2001; 344: 783–92.
68. Slamon D, Leyland-Jones B, Shak S, Paton V, Bajamonde A, Flemiong T, Eirmann W, Wolter J. Baselga J, Norton L. Addition of Herceptin, (humanized anti-HER2 antibody) to first line chemotherapy for HER2 overexpressing metastatic breast cancer (HER2+/MBC) markedly increases anticancer activity: A randomised, multinational, controlled phase III trial. Proc Am Soc Clin Oncol 1998; 17: 98a (Abstract 377).
69. Gianni L. Tolerability in patients receiving trastuzumab with or without chemotherapy. Ann Oncol 2001; 12 Suppl 1: S63–8.
70. Budman DR, Berry DA, Cirrincione CT, Henderson IC, Wood WC, Weiss RB, Ferree CR, Muss HB, Green MR, Norton L, Frei E III. Dose and dose intensity as determinants of outcome in the adjuvant treatment of breast cancer. The Cancer and Leukemia Group B. J Natl Cancer Inst 1998; 90: 1205–11.
71. Thor AD, Berry DA, Budman DR, Muss HB, Kute T, Henderson IC, Barcos M, Cirrincione C, Edgerton S, Allred C, et al. erbB-2, p53 and efficacy of adjuvant therapy in lymph node positive breast cancer. J Natl Cancer Inst 1998; 90: 1346–60.
72. Smith I. Future directions in the adjuvant treatment of breast cancer: the role of trastuzumab. Ann Oncol 2001; 12 Suppl 1: S75–9.
73. Kim S. Liposomes as carriers of cancer chemotherapy: current status and future prospects. Drugs 1993; 46: 618–38.
74. Gabizon AA. Liposomal anthracyclines. Hematol Oncol Clin N Am 1994; 8: 431–50.
75. Verrill M. Anthracyclines in breast cancer: therapy and issues of toxicity. Breast 2001; Suppl 2: S8–15.
76. Forssen EA, Ross ME. DaunoXome treatment of solid tumours: preclinical and clinical investigations. J Liposome Res 1994; 4: 481–512.
77. Kanter PM, Bullard GA, Pilkiewicz FG, Mayer LD, Cullis PR, Pavelic ZP. Preclinical toxicology study of liposome encapsulated doxorubicin (TLC D-99): comparison with doxorubicin and empty liposomes in mice and dogs. In Vivo 1993; 7: 85–95.
78. Kanter PM, Bullard GA, Ginsberg RA, Pilkiewicz FG, Mayer LD, Cullis PR, Pavelic ZP. Comparison of the cardiotoxic effects of liposomal doxorubicin (TLC D-99) versus free doxorubicin in beagle dogs. In Vivo 1993; 7: 17–26.
79. Schuller J, Czejka M, Bandak S, Borow D, Pietrzak C, Marei I, Schernthaner G. Comparison of pharmacokinetics (PK) of free and liposome encapsulated doxorubicin in advanced cancer patients. Onkologie 1995; 18 Suppl 2: 184.
80. Batist G, Ramakrishnan G, Rao CS, Chandrasekharan A, Gutheil J, Guthrie T, Shah P, Khojasteh A, Nair MK, Hoelzer K, et al. Reduced cardiotoxicity and preserved antitumor efficacy of liposome-encapsulated doxorubicin and cyclophosphamide compared with conventional doxorubicin and cyclophosphamide in a randomised, multicenter trial of metastatic breast cancer. J Clin Oncol 2001; 19: 1444–54.
81. Kanter PM, Klaich G, Bullard GA, King JM, Pavelic ZP. Preclinical toxicology study of liposome encapsulated doxorubicin (TLC D–99) given intraperitoneally to dogs. In Vivo 1994; 8: 975–82.
82. Sparano JA, Winer EP. Liposomal anthracyclines for breast cancer. Semin Oncol 2001; 28: 32–40.
83. Legha SS, Benjamin RS, Mackay B, Ewer M, Wallace S, Valdivieso M, Rasmussen SL, Blumenschein GR, Freireich EJ. Reduction of doxorubicin cardiotoxicity by prolonged continuous intravenous infusion. Ann Intern Med 1982; 96: 133–9.
84. Workman P. Infusional anthracyclines. Is slower better? If so why? Ann Oncol 1992; 3: 591–4.
85. Working PK, Dayan AD. Pharmacological–toxicological expert report: Caelyx^{tm} (Stealth® liposomal doxorubicin HCl). Hum Exp Toxicol 1996; 15: 752–85.
86. Dezube BJ. Safety assessment: Doxil (doxorubicin HCl liposome injection) in refractory AIDS-

related Kaposi's sarcoma. Doxil Clinical Series Vol. 1, No. 2; SEQUUS Pharmaceuticals Inc, Menlo Park, California, 1996.
87. Goebel F-D, Goldstein D, Goos M, Jablonowski H, Stewart JS. Efficacy and safety of Stealth liposomal doxorubicin in AIDS-related Kaposi's sarcoma. Br J Cancer 1996; 73: 989–94.
88. Harrison M, Tomlinson D, Stewart S. Liposomal-entrapped doxorubicin: an active agent in AIDS-related Kaposi's sarcoma. J Clin Oncol 1995; 13: 914–20.
89. Uziely B, Jeffers S, Isacson R, Kutsch K, Wei Ysao D, Yehoshua Z, Libson E, Muggia FM, Gabizon A. Liposomal doxorubicin: antitumor activity and unique toxicities during two complimentary phase 1 studies. J Clin Oncol 1995; 13: 1777–85.
90. Muggia FM, Hainsworth J, Jeffers S, Miller P, Groshen S, Tan M, Roman L, Uziely B, Muderspach L, Garcia A, et al. Phase II study of liposomal doxorubicin in refractory ovarian cancer: antitumor activity and toxicity modification by liposomal encapsulation. J Clin Oncol 1997; 15: 987–93.
91. Gabizon A, Martin F. Polyethylene glycol-coated (pegylated) liposomal doxorubicin. Rationale for use in solid tumours. Drugs 1997; 54 Suppl 4: 15–21.
92. Harris L, Winer E, Batist G, Rovira D, Navari R, Lee L, and the TLC D–99 Study Group. Phase III study of TLC D-99 (liposome encapsulated doxorubicin) vs. free doxorubicin in patients with metastatic breast cancer. Proc Am Soc Clin Oncol 1998; 17: A474 (Abstract 26).
93. Shapiro CL, Ervin T, Welles L, Azarnia N, Keating J, Hayes DF, for the TLC D–99 Study Group. Phase II trial of high-dose liposome-encapsulated doxorubicin with granulocyte colony-stimulating factor in metastatic breast cancer. J Clin Oncol 1999; 17: 1435–41.
94. Girard PM, Bouchaud O, Goetschel A, Mukwaya G, Eestermans G, Ross M, Rozenbaum W, Saimot AG. Phase II study of liposomal encapsulated daunorubicin in the treatment of AIDS-associated mucocutaneous Kaposi's sarcoma. AIDS 1996; 10: 753–7.
95. Gill PS, Espina BM, Muggia F, Cabriales S, Tulpule A, Esplin JA, Liebman HA, Forssen E, Ross ME, Levine AM. Phase I/II clinical and pharmacokinetic evaluation of liposomal daunorubicin. J Clin Oncol 1995; 13: 996–1003.
96. Skubitz KM, Skubitz APN. Mechanism of transient dyspnoea induced by pegylated-liposomal doxorubicin (Doxil). Anti-Cancer Drugs 1998; 9: 45–50.
97. SEQUUS Pharmaceuticals Inc. Doxil safety report (07 Apr 1997). Menlo Park, California, USA.
98. Northfelt DW, Dezube BJ, Thommes JA, Levine R, Von Roenn JH, Dosik GM, Rios A, Krown SE, DuMond C, Mamelok RD. Efficacy of pegylated liposomal doxorubicin in the treatment of AIDS-related Kaposi's sarcoma after failure of standard chemotherapy. J Clin Oncol 1997; 15: 653–9.
99. Alberts DS, Garcia DJ. A safety review of pegylated liposomal doxorubicin in the treatment of various malignancies. Oncology 1997; 11 Suppl 11: 54–62.
100. Ranson MR, Carmichael J, O'Byrne K, Stewart S, Smith D, Howell A. Treatment of advanced breast cancer with sterically stabilised liposomal doxorubicin: results of a multicentre phase II trial. J Clin Oncol 1997; 15: 3185–91.
101. Hengge UR, Brockmeyer NH, Rasshofer R, Goos M. Fatal hepatic failure with liposomal doxorubicin. Lancet 1993; 341: 383–4.
102. Coker RJ, James ND, Stewart JSW. Hepatic toxicity of liposomal encapsulated doxorubicin. Lancet 1993; 341: 756.
103. Stewart S, Jablonowski H, Goebel FD, Arasteh K, Spittle M, Rios A, Aboulafia D, Galleshaw J, Dezube B. A randomised comparative trial of Doxil versus bleomycin and vincristine (BV) in the treatment of AIDS-related Kaposi's sarcoma. J Clin Oncol 1998; 16: 683–91.
104. Madhavan S, Northfelt DW. Lack of vesicant injury following extravasation of liposomal doxorubicin. J Natl Cancer Inst 1995; 87: 1556–7.
105. Madhavan S, Northfelt DW. Lack of vesicant injury following extravasation of liposomal doxorubicin. Breast Cancer Res Treat 1996; 37 Suppl: 77.
106. Cabriales S, Bresnahan J, Testa D, Espina BM, Scadden DT, Ross M, Gill PS. Extravasation of liposomal daunorubicin in patients with AIDS-associated Kaposi's sarcoma: a report of four cases. Oncol Nurs Forum 1998; 25: 67–70.
107. Lotem M, Hubert A, Lyass O, Goldenhersh MA, Ingber A, Peretz T, Gabizon A. Skin toxic effects of polyethylene glycol-coated liposomal doxorubicin. Arch Dermatol 2000; 136: 1475–80.
108. Zompi S, Legrand O, Bouscary D, Blanc CM, Picard F, Casadeevall N, Dreyfus F, Marie JP, Viguie F. Therapy-related acute myeloid leukaemia after successful therapy for acute promyelocytic leukaemia with t(15; 17): a report of two cases and a review of the literature. Br J Haematol 2000; 110: 610–13.
109. Achtari C, Hohfeld P. Cardiotoxic transplacental effect of idarubicin administered during the second trimester of pregnancy. Am J Obstet Gynecol 2000; 183: 511–12.
110. Konno H, Maruo Y, Matsuda I, Nakamura S, Baba S. Intra-arterial liposomal adriamycin for metastatic adenocarcinoma of the liver. Eur Surg Res 1995; 27: 301–6.
111. Barrett-Lee PJ, Bailey NP, O'Brien MER, Wager E. Large-scale UK audit of blood transfusion requirements and anaemia in patients receiving cytotoxic chemotherapy. Br J Cancer 2000; 82: 93–7.
112. Tsavaris N, Kosmas C, Mylonakis N, Bacoyiannis C, Kalergis G, Vadiaka M, Boulamatsis D, Iakovidis V, Kosmidis P. Parameters that influence the outcome of nausea and emesis in cisplatin based chemotherapy. Anticancer Res 2000; 20; 4777–84.

113. Lyass O, Uziely B, Ben-Yosef R, Tzemach D, Heshing NI, Lotem M, Brufman G, Gabizon A. Correlation of toxicity with pharmacokinetics of pegylated liposomal doxorubicin (Doxil) in metastatic breast carcinoma. Cancer 2000; 89: 1037–47.
114. Cure H, Chevalier V, Pezet D, bousquet J, Focan C, Levi F, Garufi C, Chipponi J, Chollet P. Phase II trial of chronomodulated infusion of 5-fluorouracil and folinic acid in metastatic colorectal cancer. Anticancer Res 2000; 20: 4649–54.
115. Hartmann JT, Kanz L, Bokemeyer C. Phase II study of continuous 120-hour-infusion of mitomycin C as salvage chemotherapy in patients with progressive or rapidly recurrent gastrointestinal adenocarcinoma. Anticancer Res 2000; 20: 1177–82.
116. Bogliolo G, Pannacciulli I, Desalvo L, Barsotti B, Lerza R, Mencoboni M, Arboscelo E. Advanced colorectal cancer: quality of life and toxicity in patients after weekly 24-hour continuous infusion of biomodulated 5-fluorouracil; Anticancer Res 2000; 20: 501–4.
117. Freyer G, Rougier P, Bugat R, Droz J-P, Marty M, Bleiberg H, Mignard D, Awad L, Culine S, Trillet-Lenoir V, and CPT–11 F205, F220, F221, and V222 Study Groups. Prognostic factors for tumour response, progression-free survival and toxicity in metastatic colorectal cancer patients given irinotecan (CPT–11) as second-line chemotherapy after 5FU failure. Br J Cancer 2000; 83: 431–7.
118. Lavery IC, Lopes-Kostner F, Pelley RJ, Fine RM. Treatment of colon and rectal cancer. Surg Clin North Am 2000; 80: 535–69.
119. Reeves ME, Coit DG. Melanoma: a multidisciplinary approach for the general surgeon. Surg Clin North Am 2000; 80: 581–601.
120. Ekholrn EMK, Salrninen EK, Huikuri HV, Jalonen J, Antila K, Salmi T, Rantanen V. Impairment of heart rate variability during paclitaxel therapy. Cancer 2000; 88: 2149–53.
121. Ekholm E, Rantanen V, Bergman M, Vesalainen R, Antila K, Salminen E. Docetaxel and autonomic cardiovascular control in anthracycline treated breast cancer patients. Anticancer Res 2000; 20: 2045–8.
122. Nakamae H, Tsumura K, Hino M, Hayashi T, Tatsumi N. QT dispersion as a predictor of acute heart failure after high-dose cyclophosphamide. Lancet 2000; 355: 805–6.
123. Feun LG, Savaraj N, Hurley J, Marini A, Lai S. A clinical trial of intravenous vinorelbine tartrate plus tamoxifen in the treatment of patients with advanced malignant melanoma. Cancer 2000; 88: 584–8.
124. Miller KD, Munshi N, Loesch D, Einhorn LH, Sledge GW Jr. A phase II trial of high dose epirubicin in patients with advanced breast cancer. Cancer 2000; 88: 375–80.
125. Gortin H, Wilson R, Robinson A, Lyons G. Survivors of childhood cancers: implications for obstetric anaesthesia. Br J Anaesth 2000; 85: 911–13.
126. Cheriparambil KM, Vasireddy H, Kuruvilla A, Gambarin B, Makan M, Saul BI. Acute reversible cardiomyopathy and thromboembolism after cisplatin and 5-fluorouracil chemotherapy – a case report. Angiology 2000; 5: 873–8.
127. Doehn C, Buttner H, Fornara P, Jocham D. Fatal basilar artery thrombosis after chemotherapy for testicular cancer. Urol Int 2000; 65: 43–5.
128. Lester WA, Hull DR, Fegan CD, Morris TCM. Respiratory failure during induction chemotherapy for acute myelomonocytic leukaemia (FAB M4Eo) with Ara-C and all-*trans* retinoic acid. Br J Haematol 2000; 109: 847–50.
129. McKenna KE, Burrows D. Pulmonary toxicity in a patient with psoriasis receiving methotrexate therapy. Clin Exp Dermatol 2000; 25: 24–7.
130. Mayerhofer K, Bodner-Aldr B, Bodner K, Leodolter S, Kainz C. Paclitaxel/carboplatin as first-line chemotherapy in advanced ovarian cancer: efficacy and adverse effects with special consideration of peripheral neurotoxicity. Anticancer Res 2000 20: 4047–50.
131. Mayerhofer K, Bodner-Aldr B, Bodner K, Saletu B, Schindl M,Kaider A, Hefler L, Leodolter S, Kainz C. A paclitaxel-containing chemotherapy does not cause central nervous adverse effects; a prospective study in patients with ovarian cancer. Anticancer Res 2000; 20: 4051–5.
132. Pelfrims J, De Vos F, Van Den Brande J, Schrijvers D, Prove A, Vermorken JB. Methylene blue in the treatment and prevention of ifosfamide-induced encephalopathy: report of 12 cases and a review of the literature. Br J Cancer 2000; 82: 2914.
133. Kishi T, Tanaka Y, Ueda K. Evidence for hypomethylation in two children with acute lymphoblastic leukaemia and leukoencephalopathy. Cancer 2000; 89: 925–31.
134. Wang MY, Arnold AC, Vinters HV, Glasgow BJ. Bilateral blindness and lumbosacral myelopathy associated with high-dose carmustine and cisplatin therapy. Am J Ophthalmol 2000; 130: 367–8.
135. Shin E, Ishhtobi M, Hiraoia M, Kazumasa F, Hideyuki M, Nishisho I, Toshiro S, Yasunori H, Tosimasa T. Phase I study of docetaxel administered by bi-weekly infusion to patients with metastatic breast cancer. Anticancer Res 2000; 26: 4721–6.
136. Rosing H, Lustig V, Van Warmedan LJC, Huizing MT, Ten Bokkel Huinink WW, Schellens JHM, Rodenhuis S, Bult A, Beijnen JH. Pharmacokinetics and metabolism of docetaxel administered as a 1-h intravenous infusion. Cancer Chemother Pharmacol 2000; 45: 213–18.
137. Voog E, Bienenu J, Warzocha K, Moullet I, Dumontet C, Thieblemont C, Monneret G, Gutowski M-C, Coiffier B, Salles G. Factors that predict chemotherapy-induced myelosuppression in lymphoma patients: role of the tumour necrosis factor Ligand-Receptor system. J Clin Oncol 2000; 18: 325–31.
138. Blumenthal RD, Lew W, Juweid M, Al-

isauskas R, Ying Z, Goldenberg DM. Plasma FLT3-L levels predict bone marrow recovery from myelosuppressive therapy. Cancer 2000; 88: 333–43.

139. Kotsakis A, Sarra E, Peraki M, Koukourakis M, Apostolaki S, Souglakos J, Mavromanomakis E, Vlachonikolis J, Georgoulias V. Docetaxel-induced lymphopenia in patients with solid tumors. Cancer 2000; 89: 1380–6.
140. Biron F, Ponceau B, Bouhour D, Boibieux A, Verrier B, Peyramond D. Long-term safety and antiretroviral activity of hydroxyurea and didanosine in HIV-infected patients. J Acquir Immune Defic Syndr 2000; 25: 329–36.
141. Kline MW, Calles NR, Simon C, Schwarzwold MD. Pilot study of hydroxyurea in human immunodeficiency virus-infected children receiving didanosine and/or stavudine. Pediatr Infect Dis J 2000; 19: 1083–6.
142. Ibrahim NK, Sahin AA, Dubrow RA, Lynch PM, Boenke-Michaud L, Valero V, Buzdar A, Hortobagyi GN. Colitis associated with docetaxel-based chemotherapy in patients with metastatic breast cancer. Lancet 2000; 355: 281–3.
143. Hartman JT, Fels LM, Franzke A, Knop S, Renn M, Maess B, Panagiotou P, Lampe H, Kanz L, Stolte H, Bokemeyer C. Comparative study of the acute nephrotoxicity from standard dose cisplatin ± ifosfamide and high dose chemotherapy with carboplatin and ifosfamide. Anticancer Res 2000; 20: 3767–73.
144. Kern W, Braess J, Kaufmann CC, Wilde S, Schleyer E, Hiddemann W. Microalbuminuria during cisplatin therapy: relation with pharmacokinetics and implications for nephroprotection. Anticancer Res 2000; 20: 3679–88.
145. Skinner R, Cotterill SJ, Stevens MCG. Risk factors for nephrotoxicity after ifosfamide treatment in children: a UKCCSG Late Effects Group study. Br J Cancer 2000; 82: 1636–45.
146. Goyal S, Huhn KM, Provost TT. Calciphylaxis in a patient without renal failure or elevated parathyroid hormone: possible aetiological role of chemotherapy. Br J Dermatol 2000; 143: 1087–90.
147. Chu C-Y, Yang C-H, Yang C-Y, Hsiao G-H, Chiu H-C. Fixed erythrodysaesthesia plaque due to intravenous injection of docetaxel. Br J Dermatol 2000; 142: 808–11.
148. Hussain S, Anderson DN, Salvatti ME, Adamson B, McManus M, Braverman A. Onycholysis as a complication of systemic chemotherapy. Cancer 2000; 88: 2367–71.
149. Correia O, Azevedo C, Pinto Ferreira E, Braga Cruz F, Polonia J. Nail changes secondary to docetaxel (Taxotere). Dermatology 1999; 198: 288–90.
150. Markman M, Kennedy A, Webster K, Kulp B, Peterson G, Belinson J. Paclitaxel-associated hypersensitivity reactions: experience of the Gynaecologic Oncology Program of the Cleveland Clinic Cancer Center. J Clin Oncol 2000; 18: 102–5.
151. Grosen E, Siitari E, Larrison E, Tiggelaar C, Roecker E. Paclitaxel hypersensitivity reactions related to bee-sting allergy. Lancet 2000; 355: 288–9.
152. Muller H-J, Loning L, Horn A, Schwabe D, Gunkel M, Schrappe M, Von Schutz V, Henze G, Casimiro Da Palma J, Ritter J, Pinheiro JPV, Winkelhorst M, Boos J. Pegylated asparaginase (Oncaspar^{tm}) in children with ALL: drug monitoring in reinduction according to the ALL/NHL-BFM 95 protocols. Br J Haematol 2000; 110: 379–84.
153. Braester A, Quitt M. Hydroxyurea as a cause of drug fever. Acta Haematol 2000; 104: 50–1.
154. Saso R, Kulkarni S, Mitchell P, Treleaven J, Swansbury GJ, Mehta J, Powles R, Ashley S, Kuan A, Powles T. Secondary myelodysplastic syndrome/acute myeloid leukaemia following mitoxantrone-based therapy for breast carcinoma. Br J Cancer 2000; 83: 91–4.
155. Finazzi G, Ruggeri M, Rodeghiero F, Barbui T. Second malignancies in patients with essential thromocythaemia treated with busulphan and hydroxyurea: long-term follow-up of a randomised clinical trial. Br J Haematol 2000; 110: 577–83.

Sameh K. Morcos and Baskaran Sundaram

46 Radiological contrast agents

TYPES OF CONTRAST MEDIA

Iodinated water-soluble contrast media are of four types:

- high-osmolar ionic monomers (e.g. diatrizoate, iothalamate, metrizoate);
- low-osmolar ionic dimers (e.g. ioxaglate);
- low-osmolar non-ionic monomers (e.g. iobitridol, iohexol, iomeprol, iopamidol, iopromide, ioversol);
- iso-osmolar non-ionic dimers (e.g. iodixanol, iotrolan).

They are mainly used intravascularly but can also be injected into body cavities, including the bile ducts and pancreatic ducts, which can be outlined during endoscopic retrograde cholangiopancreatography (ERCP).

There are also contrast agents that enhance the diagnostic information provided by ultrasound imaging and magnetic resonance imaging (MRI). The latter are mainly gadolinium based, but new non-gadolinium paramagnetic contrast agents have recently become available.

Ultrasound contrast agents are microbubbles that provide acoustic enhancement.

Liposomal contrast agents have recently been developed, mainly for hepatic CT imaging. They are not yet available for routine use and their safety is currently under evaluation.

Adverse reactions to contrast media are generally few, and serious reactions are uncommon. Ultrasound contrast agents are particularly safe.

Side Effects of Drugs, Annual 25
J.K. Aronson, ed.

WATER-SOLUBLE INTRAVASCULAR IODINATED CONTRAST AGENTS

(SED-14, 1596; SEDA-22, 498; SEDA-23, 494; SEDA-24, 519)

Adverse reactions to intravascular iodinated agents are usually classified into minor, intermediate, or severe life-threatening. All types of reactions to low-osmolar contrast media are five times less common than reactions to high-osmolar contrast agents (SEDA-22, 489; SEDA-23, 494; SEDA-24, 519). However, there are no important differences in the safety profiles of low-osmolar non-ionic monomers (1[C]).

In a study from France the incidence of adverse drug reactions following 1480 injections of low-osmolar iodinated contrast media was 0.34%; the frequency was higher in patients with a history of allergy (1.5%) (2[C]). The prevalence of adverse drug reactions amongst in-patients in a North Indian referral hospital over 3 years has been assessed in a similar study (3[C]). In all, 317 adverse reactions were reported (0.3%). *Skin reactions* (123 cases, 39%) and *gastrointestinal disturbances* (90 cases, 28%) made up a large proportion of the reported adverse reactions. Of all the adverse reactions, 15% (48 cases) were due to iodinated contrast media (details of the types of contrast media used were not provided in the report) and the common reactions were *nausea/vomiting* (24 cases, 7.5%) and *rashes* (16 cases, 5%); however, there was serious life threatening *anaphylaxis* in three cases (0.9%).

Very severe adverse reactions to contrast media are rare, with a frequency of about 0.04% with high-osmolar agents and 0.004% with low-osmolar agents. A report from Japan has documented *non-cardiogenic pulmonary edema* complicating intravenous injection of a low-osmolar non-ionic monomer, iomeprol (4[A]).

A 68-year-old man with chronic obstructive pulmonary disease underwent CT examination of the abdomen with intravenous infusion of iomeprol for suspected hepatocellular carcinoma and 2 hours later developed severe dyspnea. A chest X-ray showed bilateral diffuse shadowing of the lungs and the heart shadow was not enlarged. A diagnosis of non-cardiogenic pulmonary edema was made and he improved with corticosteroids.

Preheating contrast media before injection for intravenous urography has been suggested to be beneficial in facilitating the rate of injection and in reducing the frequency of adverse drug reactions. The incidence of adverse reactions in patients receiving the non-ionic medium iopromide with preheating (5670 patients) and without (6448 patients) for intravenous urography has been studied in Taiwan (5[C]). There was no obvious difference in the incidence of the ADRs between the two groups. The authors concluded that there is no benefit in preheating contrast media before injection.

Delayed reactions Delayed contrast reactions usually occur after 1 hour but within 7 days of contrast injection. Reported incidences vary from 1% to 15%. Occasionally prolonged immediate reactions can be confused with delayed reactions. A patient's anxiety and the molecular structure of the contrast medium can play important roles in the incidence of delayed reactions as in immediate reactions.

The incidence of delayed reactions has been assessed in 403 Italian patients who received intravenous iopamidol during CT or urographic examination (6[C]). A total of 50 patients (12%) developed delayed reactions. Allergy, previous exposure to a contrast agent, and being female were associated with a significantly higher incidence of delayed reactions. The most frequently reported delayed reactions were *nausea and vomiting*, *drowsiness*, *rash*, *itching*, and *headache*. All reported reactions were mild and resolved spontaneously.

In a questionnaire study of 11 121 Japanese patients, 216 (1.4%) developed immediate adverse reactions and 1058 (9.5%) reported having had delayed reactions after intravenous contrast administration during various CT examinations (7[C]). Delayed reactions were reported by 18 patients (13%) of the 136 patients with immediate reactions who answered the questionnaire. All the patients, with the exception of 360 who received the non-ionic dimer iotrolan, were given non-ionic monomeric contrast media. The dose was 60–200 ml. Delayed reactions were more frequent in patients with a history of allergy, past adverse reactions to contrast media or with a serum creatinine over 180 μmol/l. Delayed reactions were also more frequent in women and in patients who had not previously received contrast media. There was no significant relation between the occurrence of immediate adverse reactions and the development of delayed reactions. The commonest delayed reactions were *itching* and *skin reactions*, which developed in 5.5% and 3.0% of the patients respectively. Skin reactions were observed twice as often in patients who were given iotrolan compared with those who were given monomeric agents. In the iotrolan group 7.3% of the patients developed a skin reaction, 9.9% reported itching, and 60% of the reactions were severe or moderate. A quarter of the delayed reactions occurred within 6 hours after the examination and more than half occurred within 24 hours. Most of the reactions occurred within the first 3 days.

Cardiovascular Low-osmolar contrast media are better tolerated than high-osmolar ionic media in cardiac and coronary angiography. However, it has been suggested that ionic contrast media may be advantageous during percutaneous transluminal coronary angioplasty, as they have some anticoagulant effect, which is lacking with non-ionic media (SEDA-22, 501). The effects of the iso-osmolar non-ionic dimer iodixanol (320 mg I/ml) and the low-osmolar ionic dimer ioxaglate (320 mg I/ml) have been compared in 1411 patients, mean age 62 years, undergoing percutaneous transluminal coronary angioplasty in a multicenter, randomized, double-blind study (8[C]). The groups were comparable in relation to the prevalence of cardiac and other medical conditions, including diabetes, obesity, and smoking habits. All the patients received heparin and all but four received an antiplatelet agent (100 mg or more of aspirin and/or ticlopidine). There was no significant difference between the two groups–the incidence of major adverse cardiac events was 4.7% (192 patients) after iodixanol and 3.9% (197 patients) after ioxaglate. However, hypersensitivity reactions and adverse drug reactions were significantly less common with iodixanol (five cases) than with ioxaglate (18 cases). The reactions to iodixanol were mainly *rashes* and *urticaria-like reactions*. The reactions to ioxaglate were one case of *anaphylaxis*, 12 cases of *urticaria*, 12 of *coughing and throat tightness*, and in one patient *rigors*, *fever*, *vomiting*, and *flushing*.

In another comparison of the electrophysiological effects of iodixanol and ioxaglate during coronary angiography, 22 patients received ioxaglate for the first injection into the left coronary artery and iodixanol for the next injections, and 20 patients received the media in the reverse order (9[C]). Those who received ioxaglate first received a mean of 102 ml of contrast medium and the iodixanol group 104 ml. The first three injections into the left coronary artery were subjected to electrocardiographic analysis. Deviation from baseline was greater in those who received ioxaglate first. The most pronounced effects of ioxaglate were on the ST segment and T wave: the T wave change vector magnitude increased 11-fold from baseline after ioxaglate and 5-fold after iodixanol; the increase in ST change vector magnitude was 4-fold with ioxaglate and 3-fold with iodixanol. The authors concluded that iodixanol caused less pronounced electrocardiographic changes than ioxaglate. These findings are in accord with experimental evidence that iodixanol is well tolerated by the myocardium.

Nervous system The adverse effects of myelography with low-osmolar non-ionic contrast media include *nausea*, *vomiting*, *headache*, and *backache*. Acute encephalopathy after myelography with iohexol has previously been documented (SEDA-23, 496). A case of aseptic meningitis after iohexol myelography has now been reported (10[A]).

A 74-year-old woman underwent lumbar myelography with iohexol (12 ml, 240 mg I/ml) for low back pain, having had iohexol myelography 2 years before with no complications, and 18 hours later developed headache, pyrexia (39° C), shivering, sweating, neck stiffness, nausea, and mild confusion. She had a leukocytosis (16.4×10^9/l) and a high C-reactive protein (145 mg/l). There were leukocytes in the cerebral spinal fluid (11.5×10^9/l, 98% polymorphonuclear leukocytes), with protein 6.6 g/l and glucose 3 mmol/l, but a Gram stain was negative and no micro-organisms were grown. She recovered spontaneously.

The authors suggested that this was a meningeal reaction to iohexol, since the interval between the injection of iohexol and the onset of symptoms was short, the symptoms resolved quickly, and there was no evidence of an infection.

Sensory systems *Transient cortical blindness* is a well recognized complication of vertebral angiography (SEDA-23, 497; SEDA-24, 521) and another case has been reported (11[A]).

A 64-year-old man developed transient cortical blindness after right subclavian, aortic, and femoral arteriography for ischemic pain in his left leg. Iopromide 250 ml (300 mg I/ml) was used. The patient was hemodynamically stable throughout the procedure, at the end of which he had blurred vision and a slight headache. He could see shapes and colors but could not focus. There were no field defects. His pupillary reflexes and eye movements were normal. His vision improved 3 hours later and fully recovered after 48 hours.

Endocrine *Hyperthyroidism* and *hypothyroidism* have both been reported to be precipitated by the administration of iodinated contrast media (SEDA 21, 478; SEDA 23, 497). Blockade of iodide absorption by the thyroid gland has been assumed to be partly responsible. Infants of very low birthweights are highly susceptible, and because thyroid function during the neonatal period is critical for neurological development and metabolism, it is advisable to avoid exposure of preterm infants to iodine if possible; if an iodinated contrast medium is required the choice of contrast medium is important to minimize the risk of thyroid complications.

The effects of the iopromide on thyroid function have been investigated in 20 preterm infants with very low birthweights and 26 matched premature infants who did not receive contrast medium (12[C]). The dose of iopromide (300 mg I/ml) was 0.3–1.0 ml. Iopromide did not affect the concentrations of free thyroxine and thyroid stimulating hormone. This was attributed to the small amount of free iodide that iopromide contains (0.6 mg/l) compared with other contrast media, in which the free iodide concentration ranges from 1.8 mg/l (iohexol) to 4 mg/l (ioxaglate). Furthermore, hypothyroidism has previously been described after the injection of less than 1 ml of ioxaglate 320 in 13 premature infants of less than 34 weeks gestational age and in other children after the injection of iopamidol. The authors concluded that iopromide may be superior to other contrast media in protecting infants of very low birthweight from thyroid dysfunction. It is advisable to monitor thyroid function when contrast media are given to such infants.

Hematologic The effects of contrast media on blood coagulation and platelet aggregation have received great interest over the last decade (SEDA-21, 478; SEDA-22, 501; SEDA-23, 497). *Disseminated intravascular coagulation* has been described in a 63-year-old man who received 50 ml of the non-ionic monomer iobitridol (300 mg I/ml) for arteriography (13[A]).

Pancreas *Acute pancreatitis* is a well recognized complication of endoscopic retrograde cholangiopancreatography (ERCP), and contrast media have been incriminated in its pathogenesis. It has been suggested that the use of low-osmolar non-ionic contrast media may minimize the risk. However, this has not been proven conclusively.

The iso-osmolar non-ionic dimer iotrolan and the low-osmolar non-ionic monomer iopromide (osmolarity about twice that of the blood) have been compared in 40 patients who underwent ERCP (14[C]). They were randomized to receive either iopromide (300 mg I/ml, 770 mosmol/kg, mean dose 15 ml) or iotrolan (300 mg I/ml, 320 mosmol/kg, mean dose 12 ml). Pancreatitis after ERCP occurred in two patients given iopromide and in five given iotrolan. There were no significant differences between the groups in the time-course of *changes in serum pancreatic enzyme activities*, *changes in acute-phase proteins*, or the incidence of *abdominal pain*.

Experimental data suggest that high-osmolar ionic contrast media are more likely to cause chemical irritation of the pancreas, precipitating pancreatitis (14[C]). However, clinical trials have not shown a clear advantage in using non-ionic media in ERCP. The authors suggested that overfilling of the pancreatic duct with contrast medium could be an important factor in the pathogenesis of ERCP-induced pancreatitis and that careful technique is important to avoid this complication.

Urinary tract The causes of *acute renal insufficiency* have been surveyed in elderly patients (over 60 years) admitted to a hospital in India over 12 months (15[C]). Of 4176 patients 59 (1.4%) developed acute renal insufficiency during hospitalization. Contrast medium injection was the culprit in 10 patients.

There have been several studies of potential methods of preventing contrast medium-induced nephrotoxicity. A report from Italy has suggested that intravenous saline 0.4 before and after administration of the contrast medium, an infusion of dopamine 3 μg/kg/min for 24 hours after the contrast medium, intravenous furosemide 80 mg 30 minutes before the contrast medium, or intravenous mannitol (20%) 250 ml 1 hour before and 1 hour after the contrast medium each prevented the reduction in renal function caused by the non-ionic agents iobitridol, ioversol, or iodixanol (16[c]). However, the protocol of the study was not described, and previous studies have shown that dopamine, furosemide, and mannitol do not offer good protection against contrast media-induced nephrotoxicity. On the other hand, volume expansion with intravenous saline has been found to offer some protection (17[C]).

More recently a study from Germany has shown that the antioxidant acetylcysteine plus intravenous saline 0.45% prevented the reduction in renal function induced by contrast media (17[C]). The authors prospectively studied 83 patients with chronic renal impairment (creatinine clearance under 50 ml/min). The patients took oral acetylcysteine 600 mg bd for 1 day before and 1 day after the contrast medium. Saline 0.45% was given intravenously at a rate of 1 ml/kg/hour for 12 hours before and 12 hours after intravenous iopromide 300 mg I/ml, 75 ml. All the patients were encouraged to drink if they were thirsty. A matched control group received placebo and saline. The mean serum creatinine in the control group (42 patients mean age 65 years) rose from a mean of 212 to 226 μmol/l 48 hours after contrast injection. In those given acetylcysteine (41 patients, mean age 66 years) the serum creatinine was 220 μmol/l before contrast injection and 186 μmol/l 48 hours after. One patient given acetylcysteine and nine controls developed contrast-induced nephrotoxicity. This suggests that the prophylactic oral administration of the antioxidant acetylcysteine in patients who are adequately hydrated with saline prevents contrast-induced nephrotoxicity in patients with chronic renal insufficiency. The main limitation of this study was the relatively small dose of intravenous contrast medium used (75 ml). It is important to determine whether acetylcysteine plus saline would still offer the same protection if higher doses of contrast media were used or if the agent was given intra-arterially.

Although endothelin is considered to be an important mediator of the renal effects of contrast media, a recent report from the USA has shown that prophylactic administration of a non-selective endothelin receptor antagonist not only did not protect against contrast nephrotoxicity but exacerbated it (18[C]). In this study 158 patients with chronic renal insufficiency (mean serum creatinine 242 μmol/l) undergoing cardiac angiography were randomized to receive either the non-selective endothelin antagonist SB290670 (mean age 65 years, 51 men, 26 women) or placebo (mean age 67 years, 59 men, 22 women). The mean doses of contrast medium were 104 ml in the SB290670 group and 122 ml in the placebo group. Only low-osmolar radiographic contrast media were used. The dose of SB290670 was 100 μg/kg over 10 minutes followed by an infusion of 1 μg/kg/min starting 30–150 minutes before administration of contrast medium and continuing for 12 hours after. All the patients received intravenous hydration with saline 0.45% (1 ml/kg/hour) beginning 2–12 hours before contrast medium and continuing for at least 12 hours after. The mean increase in serum creatinine 48 hours after angiography was higher with SB290670 than placebo (64 vs 34 μmol/l). The incidence of radiocontrast nephrotoxicity was significantly higher with SB290670 than placebo (56% vs 29%). The authors concluded that a non-selective endothelin receptor antagonist may increase the incidence of contrast media nephrotoxicity and they questioned the role of endothelin in mediating the renal effects of contrast media. However, there were flaws in the design of this study. First, the endothelin receptor antagonist was administered only for a maximum of 12 hours after contrast examination – a longer period (2–3 days) should have been considered, since the reduction in renal function after contrast examination peaks at 48–78 hours, and in previous studies a single dose of nitrendipine 20 mg did not prevent contrast nephrotoxicity whereas 20 mg/day for 3 days offered good protection. Second, a non-selective endothelin receptor antagonist is probably not suitable for the prevention of contrast nephrotoxicity. Blocking endothelin B receptors does not offer an advantage, since these receptors mediate renal vasodilatation and they also act as clearance receptors for endothelin. B receptor blockade could have caused the raised plasma endothelin concentrations that were observed in the treated group and may explain why the non-selective endothelin antagonist exacerbated contrast medium nephropathy. A selective endothelin A receptor antagonist should be studied before a role for this class of drugs in preventing contrast nephrotoxicity is excluded.

Skin Delayed skin reactions after contrast media have the features of true delayed hypersensitivity reactions, including positive skin tests (SEDA-24, 523). A *generalized macular rash* 24 hours after injection of ioversol with positive skin tests has been reported (19[A]).

A 61-year-old man received ioversol during a CT examination and 1 day later developed a generalized macular rash, which lasted for 2 weeks. Prick, intradermal, and patch tests with different types of non-ionic contrast media showed a delayed hypersensitivity reaction to ioversol, which lasted for 7 days.

Drug formulations BR21 is a sterile pyrogen-free suspension containing iomeprol, both free in solution and entrapped in liposomal vesicles. The ideal strength of the suspension is 320 mg I/ml and the osmolality is 560 mosmol/kg. The liposomes are 0.4 μm unilamellar vesicles in which the membrane is made of phospholipid. The total lipid concentration of the suspension is about 20 mg/ml. About 40 mg I/ml are trapped within the liposomal vesicles and there is 280 mg I/ml in the external phase. BR21 is taken up by the reticuloendothelial system and can enhance normal liver tissue, whereas neoplastic lesions, which lack reticuloendothelial cells, are not enhanced.

The safety and pharmacokinetics of intravenous BR21 have been evaluated in 30 healthy adult men in a phase I, single-blind, placebo-controlled, ascending-dose study (20[C]). Four volunteers each received a single intravenous dose of BR21 (0.5, 1.0, 1.5, 2.0, or 2.5 ml/kg), and for each dose of BR21 two volunteers received saline 0.9%. All adverse events (headache, metallic taste, nausea, back pain, dizziness, tremors, sweating) were minor or mild and resolved rapidly without treatment. There was no difference in the incidence of adverse events from dose to dose of BR21 or between

BR21 and saline. There were no significant changes in vital signs, electrocardiography, or laboratory findings.

Interference with diagnostic tests Water-soluble contrast media are used to examine the pancreas and bile ducts during endoscopic retrograde cholangiopancreatography (ERCP). A recent report has suggested that contrast media can affect the examination of bile for microlithiasis (21[C]). Bile contaminated with contrast media during ERCP had pseudo-microlithiasis, mimicking calcium bilirubinate granules. This effect was observed with both the high-osmolar contrast medium sodium amidotrizoate and the low-osmolar medium iohexol. The authors concluded that bile collected during ERCP to be examined for microlithiasis should be collected without contamination by contrast agents. If this is not possible, pathologists should be aware that contrast media can cause pseudo-microlithiasis. Awareness of this effect of may prevent unnecessary cholecystectomy.

ALTERNATIVES TO WATER-SOLUBLE IODINATE CONTRAST AGENTS

Carbon dioxide *(SEDA-24, 526)*

Carbon dioxide (CO_2), which is a highly soluble gas, can be used as a negative contrast agent for angiographic examinations when the use of iodinated contrast media is contraindicated (22[C]). The safety of CO_2 in vena cavography has been investigated in 119 patients (aged 17–89 years, 65 men). Patients with intracardiac shunts, severe pulmonary compromise, or non-dialysis dependent renal insufficiency were excluded. Two patients developed mild adverse effects: one had *nausea* that resolved spontaneously and the other *vomited* several minutes after the administration of CO_2 but needed no treatment. The diagnostic quality of the venography was comparable to that with iodinated contrast media. The authors concluded that CO_2 cavography is well tolerated and is specially valuable in patients with a history of a reaction to iodinated contrast material or renal insufficiency.

Iofendylate

Iofendylate (Myodil), an oily iodine formulation, was the standard contrast agent for myelography before the introduction of the low-osmolar non-ionic water-soluble contrast media. *Arachnoiditis* is a well-recognized complication of intrathecal iofendylate. It is most commonly seen in the lumbar region but it can affect arachnoid tissue at other sites. Arachnoiditis is often related to retention of iofendylate in the subarachnoid space and can develop several years after the procedure. Other factors can contribute, such as spinal trauma, surgery, intervertebral disc collapse, and the presence of subarachnoid blood. A case of iofendylate cyst causing a thoracic radiculopathy has been reported (23[A]).

A 45-year-old woman had severe root pain at T10, which had gradually become more intense over the preceding 4 years. She had undergone spinal myelography about 30 years before. Clinical examination was normal. A plain X-ray of the thoracic spine showed a radio-opaque abnormality at the level of T10, which axial CT showed was in the vertebral canal, compressing the left posterolateral margin of the theca. At thoracic laminectomy a well circumscribed subarachnoid extramedullary cyst was identified, from which a small volume of oily material was removed. The cyst collapsed and its posterior wall was excised. Histology confirmed a benign arachnoid cyst. Within 24 hours the thoracic root pain had gone.

MRI CONTRAST MEDIA

Gadolinium *(SEDA-20, 419; SEDA-22, 503; SEDA-24, 526)*

Gadolinium-based contrast media are to enhance magnetic resonance imaging (MRI) or as radiographic contrast agents. Gadolinium can sufficiently attenuate X-rays to be visualized with digital subtraction angiography, although the quality of the image is consistently poorer than with iodinated contrast agents (SEDA-22, 504; SEDA-23, 500).

The efficacy and the safety of gadolinium-DTPA-BMEA (Optimark) and gadolinium-DTPA (Magnavist) have been compared in a multicenter, randomized, double-blind, parallel-group study in patients with suspected central nervous system pathology who required MRI examination (24[C]). They were randomized to receive 0.1 mmol/kg of either gadolinium-DTPA-BMEA (*n* = 262, aged 12–80 years, mean volume of contrast medium injected 15 ml) or gadolinium-DTPA (*n* = 133, aged 20–73 years, mean volume of contrast medium injected 16 ml). There were no significant differences in adverse effects or diagnostic efficacy between the two groups. Of those given gadolinium-DTPA-BMEA, 71 patients (27%) had adverse events, severe in only five (1.9%). Of those given gadolinium-DTPA, 31 patients (23%) had adverse events, severe in only five (3.8%). The adverse effects included *headache*, *chest pain*, *taste disturbance*, and *leg cramps*.

Gadolinium has not yet been widely approved for intrathecal use. However, gadolinium-DTPA (1 ml mixed with 4 ml of 5% saline) has been used in myelocisternography in four patients (aged 28–62 years) to demonstrate the exact site of cerebrospinal fluid (CSF) leakage in patients with CSF rhinorrhea (25[c]). All tolerated the examination without adverse effects or complications.

Gadovist 1.0 is a new contrast medium for MRI. It is an extracellular neutral gadolinium chelate belonging to the class of macrocyclic neutral gadolinium complexes. It has the lowest osmolality of gadolinium-based contrast agents (1.60 osmol/kg). In preclinical evaluation there was good tolerance up to a dose of 0.5 mmol/kg, and this has been confirmed in phase I clinical studies. In a Phase II study 89 patients with suspected cerebrovascular insufficiency received Gadovist 1.0 in doses of 0.1 (*n* = 11), 0.2 (*n* = 21), 0.3 (*n* = 21), 0.4 (*n* = 21), or 0.5 (*n* = 15) mmol/kg (26[C]). There were no significant changes in vital signs or any serious adverse reactions. Two patients had *nausea* and *dry mouth*. A dose of 0.3 mmol/kg was diagnostically adequate.

Urinary tract The use of gadodiamide (Omniscan) in cerebral angiography has been reported in a 55-year-old woman with polycystic kidney disease and chronic renal impairment (serum creatinine concentration 181 μmol/l); there were no adverse effects and the serum creatinine was unchanged (27[A]). The authors concluded that gadodiamide is a safe alternative to iodinated contrast media in patients with renal impairment.

However, the use of large volumes of gadolinium-based contrast agents can cause *deterioration in renal function*, and the safety of these agents in relation to the kidney when a large volume is used is not known (27[A]).

The use of gadolinium-DTPA has been described in 28 patients (22 men, 6 women, mean age 51 years) for angiography (28[C]). The mean dose of gadolinium was 35 (range 20–60) ml. All the patients had renal impairment (serum creatinine over 133 μmol/l). Gadolinium was well tolerated, but 17 patients noted a mild heat sensation and one complained of transient pain during the injection. Only one patient, who received 40 ml, developed worse renal function, with an increase in serum creatinine from 360 to 450 μmol/l. Although the gadolinium was well tolerated in this group of patients, gadolinium-based contrast agents should be used with extreme care, particularly in patients with renal impairment, as they can be nephrotoxic in large doses.

A prospective, randomized, double-blind, placebo-controlled trial has also confirmed the safety of gadolinium infusion in 32 patients with renal impairment in dosages typically used during MRI examination (29[C]). Nine patients had moderate renal impairment (mean age 57 years, creatinine clearance 30–60 ml/min) and 11 had severe renal impairment (mean age 63 years, creatinine clearance 10–29 ml/min). They were given an intravenous bolus of gadolinium-BOPTA (dimeglumine) 0.2 mmol/kg. A comparable control group received an injection of isotonic saline. There was no significant deterioration in renal function in any group during the following 7 days.

Mangafodipir trisodium (MnDPDP)

Mangafodipir trisodium is a chelate complex containing manganese (II) ion bound to fodipir. After injection, mangafodipir trisodium undergoes net transmetalation with endogenous zinc (II) ion and removal of the two phosphate groups to give two metabolites, manganese dipyridoxal ethyldiamine diacetate and zinc dipyridoxal ethylenediamine diacetate. The transmetalation with zinc is associated with a transient reduction in serum zinc concentrations, which normalize within about 24 hours after injection. About 14–20% of the manganese is excreted in the urine and 52–61% is excreted in the feces over 4 days. About 92% of fodipir is eliminated within 24 hours. Liver and renal impairment might predispose patients to manganese retention and toxicity.

Mangafodipir trisodium is mainly indicated to enhance the MRI T1-weighted images that are used in the detection, localization, and characterization of hepatic lesions. Normal liver parenchyma takes up the manganese and becomes bright, resulting in clear demarcation of abnormal parenchymal lesions.

In a phase III study 546 patients with suspected or known focal liver lesions received intravenous mangafodipir trisodium 5 μmol/kg before MRI examination (30^C). There were 195 adverse effects in 123 (23%) patients; only 72 were considered to be related to the contrast medium. Most common were *nausea* (7%), *headache* (4%), *vomiting and abdominal pain* (2% each), *chest pain and palpitation* (1% each), and *hypertension*, *flushing*, *vasodilatation*, and *hypotension* (under 1% each). Injection-associated reactions included heat (49%) and flushing (39%). Most of the adverse events (65%) were moderate and 7% were severe. Changes in laboratory values (full blood count, electrolytes, serum creatinine, and liver function tests) and vital signs (pulse, blood pressure) were generally transient, not clinically significant, and did not require treatment. The authors concluded that exposure to mangafodipir trisodium is not associated with short term risks.

Superparamagnetic iron oxide (SPIO) MRI contrast agents

The SPIO contrast agent ferristene has been shown to be effective and safe in delineating the gastrointestinal tract after oral ingestion. Different rectal formulations of ferristene with different viscosities and iron concentrations have been evaluated in a phase II clinical study, in which ferristene enemas (200–500 ml) and intravenous gadodiamide (0.1 mmol/kg) were used in the evaluation and staging of rectal cancer in 113 patients (31^C). Five patients had 10 adverse events, including rectal pain, diarrhea, edema, a phobic reaction, nausea, and a skin rash; all recovered without further therapy. The high-viscosity formulation (70 g of granules/l) was better than the low-viscosity formulation in tumor staging, but the iron concentration (30 or 59 mg/l) of the contrast agent was less important.

ULTRASOUND CONTRAST MEDIA *(SED-14, 1625; SEDA-22, 498; SEDA-23, 501, SEDA-24, 529)*

The first generation of echo contrast agents comprises compounds made of air bubbles stabilized with human serum albumin or D-galactose, which pass through the lung capillaries and reach the left heart chambers. The second generation comprises agents made of stabilized microbubbles of gases of high molecular weight and low solubility in water, mainly fluorocarbons, which provide better resistance to pressure. The high molecular weight fluorocarbon gases have lower diffusivity and blood solubility and thus give better persistence of microbubbles in the circulation. These agents can actually be considered as blood pool agents. Other factors, such as the size and stability of the particles, play a major role in optimal examination. Microbubbles larger than 7 μm will not cross the pulmonary vasculature after intravenous administration and hence the mean size of the microbubbles should be 2–5 μm.

Non-thermal bioeffects can develop with ultrasound equipment with high acoustic input in the presence of ultrasound contrast agents with a high mechanical index. Mechanical index is defined as the maximal rarefactional acoustic pressure divided by the acoustic frequency. *Ventricular extra beats* have been reported in people subjected to strong ultrasound fields but not with diagnostic ultrasonography, which is generally considered safe and without adverse effects. However, new ultrasound machines can provide high acoustic pressures, and the maximum mechanical index currently allowed is 1.9 (32^c).

AIP10119

AIP10119 is a contrast agent that consists of heat-stabilized, air-filled, albumin microcapsules with a median diameter of 4 μm. It contains 1.5×10^8 microcapsules/ml after reconstitution with water for injection. It can be prepared in a formulation with a relatively high acoustic pressure (mechanical index 1.5).

Cardiovascular In a phase I study in healthy men (mean age 28 years) who received continuous infusions of 1 ml/min of AIP10119 (mechanical index 1.5) for 10 minutes ($n = 6$) or

20 minutes ($n = 4$) there was a significant dose-dependent increase in the number of *ventricular extra beats* during end-systolic imaging but not during end-diastolic imaging (32[C]). Nine volunteers received AIP10119 as a single infusion of 1 ml/min for 25 minutes (mechanical index 1.1) followed by three rapid bolus injections of 1 ml at least 5 minutes apart, the infusion and the series of bolus injections being separated by at least 2 hours; there was no increase in the number of ventricular extra beats. The authors concluded that precautionary measures would include using formulations with a low mechanical index or end-diastolic imaging.

Optison

Optison is a second-generation contrast agent based on sonicated human albumin. In 191 patients with chronic pulmonary disease and/or cardiomyopathy (aged 21–83 years) given intravenous Optison 0.2, 0.5, 3.0, and 5.0 ml, adverse effects were observed in 6.5% (33[C]). The most frequent adverse events were transient *alterations in taste* (2.5% of patients), *headache* (2.0%), and a *warm sensation/flushing* (2.0%). The adverse events were similar to those reported with first-generation ultrasound contrast agents.

Perflenapent

Perflenapent emulsion (EchoGen) is an ultrasound contrast agent for echocardiography. It is a liquid-in-liquid emulsion of dodecafluoropentane in water, which becomes a dispersion of microbubbles after hypobaric activation.

The safety of perflenapent has been evaluated in multicenter phase II studies in 146 patients with congestive heart failure (NYHA class III or IV, mean age 68 years), of whom 99 received perflenapent and 47 received isotonic saline, and in 134 patients with severe chronic obstructive pulmonary disease (FEV_1 no more than 60% of predicted, mean age 65 years), of whom 91 received perflenapent and 43 received isotonic saline (34[C]). Blood pressure, heart rate, respiratory rate, oxygen saturation, the electrocardiogram, FEV_1, complete serum biochemistry, hematology, and mental state were assessed. Adverse events were mild and required no treatment. There was no significant difference in the incidence of adverse reactions between those given perflenapent (15%) and those given placebo (11%). The most frequent adverse events with perflenapent were *vasodilatation* ($n = 8$), *taste disturbance* ($n = 6$), *nausea* ($n = 5$), and *headache* ($n = 3$).

Perflutren

Perflutren is an ultrasound agent that consists of perfluoropropane gas encapsulated in lipid microbubbles. It has been used in patients with suspected cardiac disease and suboptimal baseline echocardiography in doses of 5 μl/kg ($n = 85$) or 10 μl/kg ($n = 84$); 42 patients received isotonic saline (35[C]). The magnitude of clinically useful opacification was not dose-dependent, but its duration was 81 seconds with 5 μl/kg and 99 seconds with 10 μl/kg. There were no clinically significant changes in physical examination, vital signs, electrocardiography, biochemistry, or hematology. *Headache* was the most frequent averse event, in nine patients who received perflutren and in three controls.

Sono Vue (sulfur hexafluoride)

Sono Vue (BR1) is an ultrasound contrast medium that consists of microbubbles containing sulfur hexafluoride gas stabilized by phospholipids. The diameter of each microbubble is 2.5 μm and there are about 0.5×10^9 microbubbles/ml. It is isotonic with human plasma, has the same viscosity as blood, and has minimal antigenic potential, since it contains no protein material.

The pharmacokinetics of Sono Vue have been studied in 12 healthy volunteers (aged 20–36 years, seven men), who received two intravenous doses of 0.03 and 0.3 ml/kg in random order (36[C]). Sono Vue was rapidly cleared from the blood, with a half-life of 5–7 minutes. About 40–50% of the dose was eliminated in the expired air during the first minute after injection and 80–90% was eliminated by 11 minutes. Within 90 minutes sulfur hexafluoride could no longer be detected in the expired air in most cases. There were no adverse effects.

The diagnostic efficacy and the safety of Sono Vue has been assessed in 218 patients with suspected coronary artery disease who underwent echocardiography (37[C]). Each received intravenous Sono Vue 0.5, 1.0, 2.0, and 4.0 ml in random order at intervals of at least 5 minutes between injections. There were no clinically significant changes in physical examination, vital signs, or electrocardiography. There were no serious adverse effects, even in patients who had heart failure and a history of myocardial infarction. The non-serious adverse reactions were mild and transient and required no treatment. The most common adverse effects were *headache* (4%) and *nausea* (1.4%).

Assessment of vascularity can be useful in differentiating benign and malignant breast lesions using color Doppler examination. However, some neoplasms have low blood flow and Doppler may be suboptimal. In these cases ultrasound contrast may be beneficial. In a phase II/III, multicenter, randomized study 220 patients with breast lesions in different anatomical areas received intravenous Sono Vue 0.3, 0.6, 1.2, and 2.4 ml (38^C). Sono Vue improved the quality of Doppler blood flow information in both parenchymal and focal lesions. There were mild adverse events in two patients only; one complained of *nausea* and the other *discomfort*. It is not clear whether these events were related to the contrast agent or not.

REFERENCES

1. Dooley M, Jarvis B. Iomeprol: a review of its use as a contrast medium. Drugs 2000; 59: 1169–86.
2. Pelagatti V, Bagheri H, Fernandez P, Railhac N, Bregeon C, Railhac JJ, Montastruc JL. Effets indesirables des produits de contraste: bilan de 6 mois de suivi. Thérapie 2000; 55: 391–4.
3. Uppal R, Jhaj R, Malhotra S. Adverse drug reactions among inpatients in a north Indian referral hospital. Natl Med J India 2000; 13: 16–18.
4. Ono K, Haraguchi M, Kimura M, Fujii K, Matsuzaki M. A case of survival from severe non-cardiac pulmonary edema caused by non-ionic contrast media. Respir Circ 2000; 48: 193–7.
5. Jeng C-M, Wang Y-C, Wu C-Y, Kung C-H, Lee W-Y, Fan J. The necessity of preheating contrast media for IVP injection. Chin J Radiol 2000; 25: 153–7.
6. Bartolucci F, Cecarini M, Gabrielli G, Abbiati R, Barberio M. Delayed adverse drug reactions to iodinated contrast media (iopamidol prospective study). Radiol Med 2000; 100: 273–8.
7. Hoyosa T, Yamaguchi K, Akutsu T, Mitsuhashi Y, Kondo S, Sugai Y, Adachi M. Delayed adverse reactions to iodinated contrast media and their risk factors. Radiat Med Med Imaging Radiat Oncol 2000; 18: 39–45.
8. Bertrand ME, Esplugas E, Piessens J, Rasch W. Influence of a non ionic iso-osmolar contrast medium iodixanol versus ionic, low-osmolar contrast medium (ioxaglate) on major adverse cardiac events in patients undergoing percutaneous transluminal coronary angioplasty: a multicenter, randomized, double-blind study. Circulation 2000; 101: 131–6,
9. Flinck A, Selin K. Vectorcardiographic changes during cardioangiography with iodixanol and ioxaglate. Int J Cardiol 2000; 76: 173–80.
10. Cissoko H, Lemesle F, Jonville-Bera A-P, Autret-Leca E. Aseptic meningitis after iohexol myelography. Ann Pharmacother 2000; 34: 812–13.
11. Boyes LA, Tew K. Cortical blindness after subclavian arteriography. Australas Radiol 2000; 44: 315–17.
12. Dembinski J, Arpe V, Kroll M, Hieronimi G, Bartmann P. Thyroid function in very low birthweight infants after intravenous administration of the iodinated contrast medium iopromide. Arch Dis Child Fetal Neonatal Ed 2000; 82: F215–17.
13. De Meester A, Six C, Lismonde M, Lambot D, Vermonden J. Fatal disseminated intravascular coagulation during arteriography. Reanim Urgences 2000; 9: 141–4.
14. Goebel C, Hardt P, Doppl W, Temme H, Hackstein N, Klor HU. Frequency of pancreatitis after endoscopic retrograde cholangiopancreatography with iopromid or iotrolan: a randomized trial. Eur Radiol 2000; 10: 677–80.
15. Kohli HS, Bhaskaran MC, Muthukumar T, Thennarasu K, Sud K, Jha V, Gupta LK, Sakhuja V. Treatment related acute renal failure in the elderly: a hospital-based prospective study. Nephrol Dial Transplant 2000; 15: 212–17.
16. Spoto S, Galluzzo S, De Galasso L, Zobel B, Navajas MF. Prophylaxis for acute tubular necrosis after X-ray contrast i.v. administration. Clin Ter 2000; 151: 323–7.
17. Tepel M, Van der Giet M, Schwarzfeld C, Laufer U, Liermann D. Prevention of radiographic-contrast-agent-induced reductions in renal function by acetylcysteine. New Engl J Med 2000; 343: 180–4.
18. Wang A, Holcslaw T, Bashore TM, Freed MI, Miller D, Rudnick MR, Szerlip H, Thames MD, Davidson CJ, Shusterman N, Schwab SJ. Exacerbation of radiocontrast nephrotoxicity by endothelin receptor antagonism. Kidney Int 2000; 57: 1675–80.
19. Erdmann S, Roos T, Merk HF, Grussendorf-Conen E-II, Rubben A, Dahl T. Delayed hypersensitivity reaction to the non-ionic contrast medium ioversol. H G Z Hautkr 2000; 75: 169–71.
20. Spinazzi A, Ceriati S, Pianezzola P, Lorusso V,

Luzzani F. Safety and pharmacokinetics of a new liposomal liver-specific contrast agent for CT: results of clinical testing in non patient volunteers. Invest Radiol 2000; 35: 1–7.
21. Parasher VK, Romain K, Sukumar R, Jordan J. Can ERCP contrast agents cause pseudomicrolithiasis? Their effect on the final outcome of bile analysis in patients with suspected microlithiasis. Gastrointest Endosc 2000; 51: 401–4.
22. Dewald CL, Jensen CC, Park YH, Hanks SE, Harrell DS. Vena cavography with CO_2 versus with iodinated contrast material for inferior vena cava filter placement: a prospective evaluation. Radiology 2000; 216: 752–7.
23. Fitzpatrick MO, Goyal K, Johnston RA. Thoracic radiculopathy caused by a Myodil cyst. Br J Neurosurg 2000; 14: 351–3.
24. Grossman RI, Rubin DL, Hunter G, Haughton VM, Lee D, Sze G, Kuhn MJ, Maravilla K, Tu R, Heindel W, et al. Magnetic resonance imaging in patients with central venous system pathology: a comparision of Optimark (Gd-DTPA-BMEA) and Magnevist (Gd-DTPA). Invest Radiol 2000; 35: 412–19.
25. Wenzel R, Leppien A. Gadolinium–myelocisternography for cerebrospinal fluid rhinorrhoea. Neuroradiology 2000; 42: 874–80.
26. Benner T, Reimer P, Erb G, Schuierer G, Heiland S, Fischer C, Geens V, Sartor K, Forsting M. Cerebral MR perfusion imaging: first clinical application of a 1 M gadolinium chelate (Gadovist 1.0) in a double-blinded randomised dose-finding study. J Magn Reson Imaging 2000; 12: 371–80.
27. Slaba SG, El-Hajj LF, Abboud GA, Gebara VA. Selective angiography of cerebral aneurysm using gadodiamide in polycystic kidney disease with renal insufficiency. Am J Roentgenol 2000; 175: 1467–8.
28. Hammer FD, Malaise J, Goffette PP, Mathurin P. Gadolinium dimeglumine: an alternative contrast agent for digital subtraction angiography in patients with renal failure. Transplant Proc 2000; 32: 432–3.
29. Townsend RR, Cohen DL, Katholi R, Swan SK, Davies BE. Safety of intravenous gadolinium (Gd-BOPTA) infusion in patients with insufficiency. Am J Kidney Dis 2000; 36: 1207–12.
30. Federle MP, Chezmar JL, Rubin DL, Weinreb JC, Freeny PC, Semelka RC, Brown JJ, Borrello JA, Lee JKT, Mattrey R, et al. Safety and efficacy of mangafodipir trisodium (MnDPDP) injection for hepatic MRI in adults: results of the US Multicenter Phase III clinical trials (safety). J Magn Reson Imaging 2000; 12: 186–97.
31. Maier AG, Kersting-Sommerhoff B, Reeders JWAJ, Judamaier W. Staging of rectal cancer by double-contrast MR imaging using the rectally administered super paramagnetic iron oxide contrast agent ferristene and IV gadodiamide injection: results of a multicenter phase II trial. J Magn Reson Imaging 2000; 12: 651–60.
32. Van der Wouw PA, Brauns AC, Bailey SE, Powers JE, Wilde A. Premature ventricular contractions during triggered imaging with ultrasound contrast. J Am Soc Echocardiogr 2000; 13: 288–94.
33. Ellahham S, Hausnerova E, Gottdiener J. Intravenous Optison (FS069) enhances pulmonary vein flow velocity signals: a multicentre study. Clin Cardiol 2000; 23: 91–5.
34. Kitzman DW, Wesley DJ. Safety assessment of perflenapent emulsion for echocardiographic contrast enhancement in patients with congestive heart failure or chronic obstructive pulmonary disease. Am Heart J 2000; 139: 1077–80.
35. Kitzman DW, Goldman ME, Gillam LD, Cohen JL, Aurigemma G. Efficacy and safety of the novel ultrasound contrast agent perflutren (Definity) in patients with suboptimal baseline left ventricular echocardiographic images. Am J Cardiol 2000; 86: 669–74.
36. Morel DR, Schwieger I, Hohn L, Terrettaz J, Llull JB. Human pharmacokinetics and safety evaluation of SonoVue™, a new contrast agent for ultrasound imaging. Invest Radiol 2000; 35: 80–5.
37. Senior R, Anderson O, Caidahl K, Carlens P, Herregods MC. Enhanced left ventricular endocardial border delineation with an intravenous injection of SonoVue, a new echocardiographic contrast agent. A European Multicenter Study. Echocardiography 2000; 17: 705–11.
38. Madjar H, Prompeler HJ, Del Favero C, Hackeloer BJ, Llull J. A new Doppler signal enhancing agent for flow assessment in breast lesions. Eur J Ultrasound 2000; 12: 123–30.

B.C.P. Polak

47 Drugs used in ocular treatment

ANTICHOLINERGIC DRUGS
(SED-14, 1640)

Cyclopentolate hydrochloride

Cyclopentolate hydrochloride is a widely used mydriatic, with few reported adverse effects. A case of *contact urticaria* has been reported (1^{A}).

A 72-year-old man, with a history of adverse reactions to sulfonamides, had erythema, edema, itching, burning of the eye, and an urticarial rash on his right cheek after the administration of several drugs to his right eye. Patch testing was performed and the cyclopentolate hydrochloride patch showed erythema after 15 minutes and an itching wheal after 30 minutes. No immediate or delayed reaction was observed with any of the other eye drops. Patch tests with cyclopentolate hydrochloride in eight healthy volunteers were negative.

ANTIHISTAMINES

Pheniramine maleate

A 30-year old woman using pheniramine maleate eye-drops for allergic oculorhinitis developed *eyelid dermatitis* (2^{A}). Patch testing showed positive reactions on days 2 and 3.

CORTICOSTEROIDS *(SED-14, 1640)*

Ophthalmic corticosteroids can cause local and systemic adverse effects in susceptible patients. These adverse reactions occur in children more often, more severely, and more rapidly than in adults, for unknown reasons. It could be that children have relatively immature chamber angles, giving rise to a rapidly increasing intraocular pressure (3^{Ar}).

Glaucoma has been reported after the use of a corticosteroid ointment in a young boy (3^{Ar}).

A 6-year-old boy underwent a resection of levator palpebrae superioris for congenital blepharoptosis. Postoperatively an ointment containing 0.1% dexamethasone and neomycin (Maxitrol) was applied to the operated eyelid three times a day to reduce lid edema. Four days later the surgical correction was satisfactory and there were no symptoms, but the intraocular pressure was raised to 44 mmHg in the operated eye, although normal in the other eye. The corticosteroid was withdrawn and topical ocular hypotensive agents were prescribed. The intraocular pressure returned to normal the next day, and the antiglaucoma treatments were maintained for 1 week and tapered over the next 2 weeks. Subsequent follow-up confirmed normal intraocular pressure and no glaucomatous damage.

The ocular hypertensive response in this case could have been due to systemic absorption of corticosteroid through the skin of the eyelid, especially when there was a surgical wound. Alternatively, a sufficient amount of ointment could have seeped over the eyelid margins to have caused the rise in intraocular pressure, similar to the application of eye-drops, as has been reported in another child, who also had *Cushing's syndrome*, a rare result of ophthalmic corticosteroids (4^{A}).

An 11-year-old boy with iridocyclitis developed Cushing's syndrome, a posterior subcapsular cataract, and increased intraocular pressure in both eyes after the topical administration of prednisolone acetate 1% eye-drops bilaterally for 6 months. The Cushing's syndrome was aggravated when periocular methylprednisolone acetate was started while bilateral posterior subtenon injections of 80 mg of sus-

---

Side Effects of Drugs, Annual 25
J.K. Aronson, ed.

pension were continued every 6 weeks for 6 months. He had not used systemic corticosteroids before.

NON-STEROIDAL ANTI-INFLAMMATORY DRUGS (NSAIDs)

NSAIDs are used locally in the eye to prevent and treat postoperative cystoid macular edema, to control postoperative ocular inflammation and pain, for example after radial keratotomy or photorefractive keratectomy, and for non-surgically induced inflammatory disorders, such as allergic conjunctivitis.

Diclofenac sodium

Diclofenac can cause *reduced corneal sensitivity*, starting from 15 minutes after instillation and measurable after 1 hour (5[c]). This corneal hypesthesia can be useful in reducing pain and discomfort in ocular inflammation and after surgery. In chronic treatment, however, the effect of diclofenac on corneal nerves can cause either an increased healing time of the corneal epithelium or a neurotrophic epitheliopathy in patients with conditions that predispose to epithelial damage, such as dry eyes. In contrast, flurbiprofen indomethacin, and ketorolac tromethamine did not cause corneal hypoesthesia.

CICLOSPORIN

Ciclosporin eye-drops are used after keratoplasty, in high-risk cases, to prevent graft rejection and to treat severe vernal conjunctivitis, keratoconjunctivitis sicca, and various immune-related corneal disorders. Despite its severe adverse effects after systemic use, topical ciclosporin can generally be used without serious adverse reactions (6[R], 7[C]).

Ciclosporin oil-in-water emulsion is a novel formulation for local treatment of moderate to severe dry eye disease. Chronic dry eye disease results from inflammation mediated by cytokines and receptors for autoimmune antibodies in the lacrimal glands. It affects the lacrimal gland acini and ducts, leading to abnormalities in the tear film, and ultimately disrupting the homeostasis of the ocular surface. Topical ciclosporin reduces the cell-mediated inflammatory response associated with inflammatory ocular surface diseases.

The efficacy, safety, tolerability, and optimal dose of ciclosporin eye-drops have been studied in a randomized, double-masked, vehicle-controlled multicenter trial in 162 patients with keratoconjunctivitis sicca with or without Sjögren's disease and refractory to conventional treatment (8[C]). Ciclosporin ophthalmic emulsion 0.05%, 0.1%, 0.2%, or 0.4%, or the vehicle alone was instilled twice daily into both eyes for 12 weeks, followed by a 4-week observation period. There was no clear dose-response relation; ciclosporin 0.1% emulsion produced the most consistent improvement in objective and subjective endpoints and ciclosporin 0.05% gave the most consistent improvement in symptoms. The vehicle also performed well, perhaps because of its long residence time on the ocular surface. There were no significant adverse effects, no microbial overgrowth, and no residence time of the vehicle emulsion on the ocular surface. All treatments were well tolerated and the highest ciclosporin blood concentration detected was 0.16 ng/ml.

To study the efficacy and safety of ciclosporin 0.05% and 0.1% ophthalmic emulsions and their vehicle in patients with moderate to severe dry eye disease two identical multicenter, randomized, double-masked, vehicle-controlled trials have been performed in 877 patients for 6 months (9[C]). More than 76% completed the course. Ciclosporin 0.05% or 0.1% eye-drops gave significantly greater improvement than the vehicle in two objective signs of dry eye disease (corneal staining and Schirmer values). Ciclosporin 0.05% also gave significantly greater improvement in three subjective measures (blurred vision, need for concomitant artificial tears, and the physician's evaluation of global response to treatment). There was no dose-response effect and there were no topical or systemic adverse findings.

Corneal deposition of ciclosporin can occur (10[A]).

A 45-year-old woman with dry eye syndrome caused by graft-vs-host disease after bone-marrow transplantation for acute leukemia was given systemic ciclosporin and topical 0.1% sodium hyaluronate, 0.3% ofloxacin, 0.1% fluorometholone, and isotonic saline. She was also given 0.4% oxybuprocaine for the relief of severe ocular pain. The bilateral corneal epithelial defects persisted even after the application of punctal plugs, and

2% ciclosporin in olive oil was added as eye-drops three times a day bilaterally. Five days later she complained of severe visual loss in association with bilateral corneal opacities, which covered the pupil and the punctal plugs bilaterally. As she did not agree to keratectomy, infrared spectroscopy and X-ray analysis were conducted on the deposits on the plugs. The spectroscopic pattern and X-ray analysis showed that the deposits had the properties of ciclosporin. As the corneal deposits did not decrease after withdrawal of the ciclosporin eye-drops, the systemic ciclosporin as well as its topical use may have contributed to the deposits. One should be aware that precipitation of ciclosporin on a compromised cornea can lead to severe visual impairment.

REFERENCES

1. Muñoz-Bellido FJ, Beltrán A, Bellido J. Contact urticaria due to cyclopentolate hydrochloride. Allergy Eur J Allergy Clin Immunol 2000; 55: 198–9.
2. Parente G, Pazzaglia M, Vincenzi C, Tosti A. Contact dermatitis from pheniramine maleate in eyedrops. Contact Dermatitis 1999; 40: 338.
3. Chua JKH, Fan DSP, Leung ATS, Lam DSC. Accelerated ocular hypertensive response after application of corticosteroid ointment to a child's eyelid. Mayo Clin Proc 2000; 75: 539.
4. Ozerdem U, Levi L, Cheng L, Song MK, Scher C, Freeman WR. Systemic toxicity of topical and periocular corticosteroid therapy in an 11-year-old male with posterior uveitis. Am J Ophthalmol 2000; 130: 240–1.
5. Aragona P, Tripodi G, Spinella R, Lagana E, Ferreri G. The effects of the topical administration of non-steroidal anti-inflammatory drugs on corneal epithelium and corneal sensitivity in normal subjects. Eye 2000; 14: 206–10.
6. Ben Ezra D, Pe'er J, Brodsky M. Cyclosporine eyedrops for the treatment of severe vernal keratoconjunctivitis. Am J Ophthalmol 1986; 101: 278–82.
7. Zierhut M, Thiel HJ, Weidle EG, Waetjen R, Pleyer U. Topical treatment of severe corneal ulcers with cyclosporin A. Graefe's Arch Clin Exp Ophthalmol 1989; 227: 30–5.
8. Stevenson D, Tauber J, Reis BL, and the Cyclosporin A Phase 2 Study Group. Efficacy and safety of cyclosporin A ophthalmic emulsion in the treatment of moderate-to-severe dry eye disease. Ophthalmology 2000; 107: 967–74.
9. Sall K, Stevenson OD, Mundorf TK, Reis BL, and the Cyclosporin A Phase 3 Study Group. Two multicenter, randomized studies of the efficacy and safety of cyclosporin ophthalmic emulsion in moderate-to-severe dry eye disease. Ophthalmology 2000; 107: 631–9.
10. Kachi S, Hirano K, Takesue Y, Miura M. Unusual corneal deposit after the topical use of cyclosporine as eyedrops. Am J Ophthalmol 2000; 130: 667–9.

E. Ernst

48 Treatments used in complementary and alternative medicine

A flurry of survey data have shown that complementary medicine is rapidly rising in popularity (1[C]). Research into related safety issues has therefore greatly increased. This has also led to a substantial rise in reports of adverse effects. The steadily growing size of this chapter over recent years is an expression of this phenomenon.

HERBAL MEDICAMENTS

(SED-14, 1651; SEDA-22, 511; SEDA-23, 506; SEDA-24, 537)

Several general reviews have been published, including reviews on the adverse effects of herbal antidepressants (2[R]), adverse effects of herbal medicaments on the skin (3[R]) or the liver (4[R]), of Chinese herbal medicaments (5[R]), and on herbal medicaments in general (6[R]). Herb–drug interactions have also been discussed (7[R]–15[R]).

A particularly important report from the Uppsala Monitoring Centre of the WHO has summarized all suspected adverse reactions to herbal medicaments reported from 55 countries worldwide over the past 20 years (16[M]). A total of 8985 case reports were on record. Most originated from Germany (20%), followed by France (17%), the USA (17%), and the UK (12%). *Allergic reactions* were the most frequent serious adverse events and there were 21 deaths. The authors pointed out that adverse reactions to herbal medicaments constitute only about 0.5% of all adverse reactions on record.

Side Effects of Drugs, Annual 25
J.K. Aronson, ed.

Drug formulations Quality control for herbal medicaments that are sold as dietary supplements in most countries is poor (17[r], 18[r]). Thus, considerable variations in the contents of active ingredients have been reported, with lot to lot variations of up to 1000% (19[r]).

Chinese herbal medicines

When 1100 Australian practitioners of traditional Chinese medicine were asked to complete questionnaires about the adverse effects of Chinese herbal mixtures, they reported 860 adverse events, including 19 deaths (20[C]). It was calculated that each practitioner had encountered an average of 1.4 adverse events during each year of full-time practice.

Liver A physician prospectively monitored all 1265 patients taking traditional Chinese medicines at his clinic during 33 months (21[C]). Liver enzymes were measured before the start of therapy and 3 and 10 weeks later. *Alanine aminotransferase activity was raised* in 107 patients (8.5%) who initially had normal values. Of these patients, about 25% reported symptoms such as *abdominal discomfort*, *looseness of bowels*, *loss of appetite*, or *fatigue*.

Drug contamination Some herbal medicaments are contaminated with pesticides (22[r]) and some, particularly Chinese herbal medicines, with *conventional synthetic drugs* (23[c]).

Cases of contamination with the heavy metals *mercury* (24[A]) and *lead* (25[A]) have been reported.

A 5-year-old Chinese boy developed motor and vocal tics. His parents had given him a Chinese herbal spray to treat mouth ulcers. The spray contained mercury 878 ppm. Mercury poisoning was confirmed by the blood mercury concentration (183 nmol/l, normal value for adults under 50 nmol/l).

A 5-year-old boy of Indian origin with encephalopathy, seizures, and developmental delay developed persistent anemia. The more obvious causes were ruled out and his blood lead concentration was high (860 μg/l). He was treated with chelation therapy and his blood lead concentration fell. For the previous 4 years his parents had given him "Tibetan Herbal Vitamins", produced in India, which contained large amounts of lead. The investigators calculated that over that time he had ingested around 63 g of lead.

The California Department of Health Services Food and Drug Branch has issued a warning to consumers that they should immediately stop using five herbal products because they contain two prescription drugs that are not listed as ingredients and that are unsafe without monitoring by a physician (26[S]). The products are Diabetes Hypoglucose Capsules, Pearl Hypoglycemic Capsules, Tongyi Tang Diabetes Angel Pearl Hypoglycemic Capsules, Tongyi Tang Diabetes Angel Hypoglycemic Capsules, and Zhen Qi Capsules. The products are available by mail order and can be purchased by telephone or via the Internet. Their manufacturers claim that they contain only natural Chinese herbal ingredients. However, after a diabetic patient in Northern California had had several episodes of hypoglycemia after taking Diabetes Hypoglucose Capsules, an investigation by the Department showed that they contain the antidiabetic drugs glibenclamide (glyburide) and phenformin. Consumers should stop using these products and seek medical advice, especially if they are currently taking other hypoglycemic drugs or if they have symptoms of fatigue, excessive hunger, profuse sweating, or numbness of the limbs. They should return the products to the seller or dispose of them safely, to prevent exposure of children.

Japanese (Kampo) herbal mixtures

Japanese (Kampo) herbal mixtures historically developed from traditional Chinese medicine and have grown into a popular form of treatment in Japan.

Sensory systems *Corneal opacities* causing photophobia have been attributed to a Kampo medicine (27[A]).

A 30-year-old Japanese woman developed bilateral photophobia. There were dust-like opacities in both corneae. She had a superficial keratectomy, and electron microscopy identified the opacities as lipid-like particles. She had intermittently taken a Kampo medicine composed of 18 different herbal ingredients. Her photophobia coincided with episodes of taking this medicine. The remedy was withdrawn and her symptoms subsequently subsided. She then abstained from the Kampo medicine without recurrence.

Liver Severe liver damage has been attributed to a Kampo medicine (28[A]).

A 50-year-old Japanese woman with a 20-year history of asthma was taking steroids and bronchodilators when she started self-medicating with a Kampo mixture called "Saiko–Keishi–Kankyo–To". Two months later, she developed acute severe liver damage. The Kampo mixture was withdrawn and she promptly recovered.

The authors attributed the liver damage to one ingredient of the mixture Trichosanthis radix, a Chinese medicament that is prepared from the root of *Trichosanthis kirilowii maxim* (Tian-hua-fen).

Aristolochia species

Urinary tract Since rapidly progressive *renal insufficiency* or "Chinese herb nephropathy" has been repeatedly reported in patients taking herbal medicaments containing *Aristolochia*, the UK Medicines Control Agency has banned its medicinal use in the UK. Several review articles have covered the toxicology of *Aristolochia* (29[r]–32[r]).

In Japan two cases of Chinese herb nephropathy were associated with chronic use of *Aristolochia manchuriensis* (Kan-mokutsu) (33[A]). The diagnosis was confirmed by renal biopsy and the toxic constituents were identified as aristolochic acids I, II, and D.

Taiwanese authors have reported 12 cases of suspected Chinese herb nephropathy, confirmed by renal biopsy (34[A]). Renal function deteriorated rapidly in most patients, despite withdrawal of the *Aristolochia*. Seven patients underwent dialysis and the rest had slowly progressive renal insufficiency. One patient was subsequently found to have a bladder carcinoma.

Because of fear of malignancies the Belgian researchers who first described the condition have advocated prophylactic removal of the kidneys and ureters in patients with Chinese herb nephropathy. Of 39 patients who agreed to this, 18 (46%) had *urothelial carcinoma*, 19 of the others had mild to moderate urothelial dysplasia, and only two had normal urothelium (35[C]). All tissue samples contained aristolochic acid-related DNA in adducts. The original dose of *Aristolochia* correlated positively with the risk of urothelial carcinoma.

Another case of renal fibrosis has been reported (96[C]).

Cascara sagrada

Liver *Cascara sagrada* has been reported to cause liver damage (36[A]).

A 48-year old man developed cholestatic hepatitis and hypertension shortly after he started to use the herbal laxative *Cascara sagrada*, which contains an anthracene glycoside. He took 1 capsule (425 mg of aged *Cascara sagrada* bark) tds for 3 days and subsequently developed right upper quadrant pain, nausea, abdominal bloating, anorexia, and jaundice. The *Cascara* was withdrawn, but his symptoms persisted and his liver function tests were abnormal. One week later, he developed ascites and jaundice and underwent liver biopsy, which showed moderately severe portal inflammation, intracanalicular bile stasis, portal bridging fibrosis, and mild steatosis. He gradually improved without specific treatment and 3 months later his ascites and jaundice had resolved.

Datura suaveolens (angel's trumpet)

Angel's trumpet is a popular ornamental plant, sometimes used for its alleged hallucinogenic effects. *Anticholinergic effects* can result from the hyoscine, hyoscyamine, and atropine that angel's trumpet contains (37[A]).

A 53-year-old woman was admitted to hospital with vertigo, blurred vision, palpitation, mydriasis of the right eye, and tachycardia (120/min). She reported that she had been cutting leaves from an angel's trumpet when a drop of sap had entered her right eye.

Ecbalium elaterium (squirting cucumber)

A report from a poisons unit in Israel included 13 patients who had used the juice of the squirting cucumber, either orally or topically, for unreported reasons (38[c]). They subsequently had *edema of the pharynx*, *dyspnea*, *drooling*, *dysphagia*, *vomiting*, and *conjunctivitis*. With symptomatic treatment they recovered within a few days.

Echinacea (coneflower)

Teratogenicity Of 412 pregnant Canadian women who contacted a specialized information service between 1996 and 1998 with concerns about the use of *Echinacea* during pregnancy, 206 had already taken the remedy and the other 206 eventually decided not to use it (39[C]). In the *Echinacea* group, 54% had taken it during the first trimester of pregnancy; 12 babies had malformations, six major and six minor. The figures in the control group were seven and seven respectively. Thus, there was no difference in the incidence of birth defects. However, the study lacked sufficient power to generate reliable data.

Ephedra sinica (Ma huang)

Ephedra is used to treat asthma, nasal congestion, fever, obesity, and anhidrosis. It is also abused as a recreational drug. Of 140 reports of adverse events related to *Ephedra* supplements submitted to the FDA between June 1997 and March 1999, 31% were definitely or probably causally related to *Ephedra* (40[c]). In 47% of the cases, there were *cardiovascular symptoms* and in 18% *central nervous system effects*; 10 patients died.

Glycyrrhiza glabra (licorice)

The active ingredients of licorice inhibit the breakdown of mineralocorticoids by inhibition of 11β-hydroxysteroid dehydrogenase type 2, and its adverse effects relate mainly to *mineralocorticoid excess*, with sodium retention, potassium loss, and inhibition of the renin–angiotensin–aldosterone system (41[R]).

In two cases prolonged intake of relatively small amounts of licorice resulted in *hypertension*, *encephalopathy*, and *pseudohyperaldosteronism* (42[A]). Both patients were highly susceptible to the adverse effects of glycyrrhizic acid because of 11β-hydroxysteroid dehydrogenase deficiency.

Sensory systems Five patients who had consumed large amounts (0.25–2 lbs) of licorice subsequently had *transient visual* *loss/aberrations* (43[A]). Glycyrrhetinic acid in licorice causes vasoconstriction in vascular smooth muscle and the authors therefore speculated that vasospasm of the retinal or occipital artery had caused the problems.

Hypericum perforatum (St John's wort)

Nervous system The mechanism of action of St John's wort in depression is not yet understood, but serotonin re-uptake inhibition is one possibility, for which evidence is increasing. In one case this may have led to the *serotonin syndrome* in a 33-year-old woman who developed extreme acute anxiety after taking only three doses of extracts of St John's wort and recovered after withdrawal (44[A]).

Skin Of 43 users of St John's wort surveyed by telephone, 47% reported adverse effects that they related to the remedy (45[c]). The only potentially serious complaint was *photosensitivity*, which was noted by four individuals.

An Australian dermatologist has reported three cases of phototoxic reactions to St John's wort (46[A]). The patients were fair-skinned and had had significant exposure to ultraviolet light. In two cases St John's wort was applied topically. In all cases complete recovery occurred after withdrawal of St John's wort and cessation of exposure to ultraviolet light.

Drug interactions Following reports about the potential for herb–drug interactions, many national regulatory agencies have issued warnings about the use of St John's wort, and its safety has been reviewed (47[R], 48[R]).

The mechanism of hepatic enzyme induction by St John's wort has been intensively researched (49[E], 50[E]). Treatment of human hepatocytes with extracts of St John's wort or with hyperforin (one of its active constituents) resulted in induction of CYP3A4 expression (51[E]). Because CYP3A4 is involved in the oxidative metabolism of more than 50% of all drugs, this suggests the possibility of a wide range of herb–drug interactions. Several reports have shown that such interactions are more than a theoretical possibility.

Ciclosporin In 30 patients a fall in ciclosporin concentrations by 33–62% after self-medication with St John's wort necessitated a gradual increase in the dose of ciclosporin of 187% (range 84–292%) (52[c]). No patient suffered any permanent consequences as a result.

There have also been further anecdotal reports of interactions of ciclosporin with St John's wort.

A 29-year-old woman, who had received a cadaveric kidney and pancreas transplant, had stable organ function with ciclosporin when she decided to take St John's wort (53[A]). Subsequently her ciclosporin concentrations became subtherapeutic and she developed signs of organ rejection. St John's wort was withdrawn and her ciclosporin concentrations returned to the target range. However, she developed chronic kidney rejection and had to return to dialysis.

A 63-year-old patient with a liver allograft developed severe acute rejection 14 months after transplantation (54[A]). Two weeks before he had taken St John's wort, which significantly reduced his ciclosporin concentration. The dose of ciclosporin was doubled, at the expense of adverse effects. The patient recovered fully after St John's wort was withdrawn.

A 55-year-old woman, who had received a kidney transplant and had stable organ function with ciclosporin, took St John's wort and 4 weeks later her ciclosporin concentration fell sharply (55[A]). The concentration rose again on withdrawal of St John's wort and fell on rechallenge. As the problem was identified early enough, the patient incurred no serious consequences.

Digoxin In a randomized, placebo-controlled, double-blind study volunteers with steady-state digoxin concentrations took either placebo, a standardized extract of St John's wort, encapsulated St John's wort powder, St John's wort tea, or an encapsulated fatty oil formulation of St John's wort (56[C]). The extract and the powder caused marked reductions in digoxin concentrations but the tea and the fatty oil formulation did not. The mechanism was not discussed, and it is not clear why the different formulations had different effects.

SSRIs Inhibition of serotonin re-uptake by St John's wort may lead to interactions with SSRIs (57[A]).

A 28-year-old man without a previous psychiatric history was given sertraline 50 mg/day for depression after bilateral orchidectomy. Against medical advice, he also took St John's wort and subsequently became manic. The authors suggested that inhibition of serotonin re-uptake by sertraline had been potentiated by the use of St John's wort.

Morinda citrifoli (noni)

Electrolyte balance Noni juice has been reported to cause *hyperkalemia*; the mechanism was not discussed (58[A]).

A man with chronic renal insufficiency who followed dietary restriction of potassium developed a raised serum potassium concentration (5.8 mmol/l). He insisted that he had followed his dietary regimen as usual, except for taking noni juice, purchased from a health food store. He was treated with sodium polystyrene sulfonate and told to stop taking noni juice. At the next check-up his potassium was still raised; he said that he would never stop taking noni juice and that his physicians did not understand its healing power.

Passiflora incarnata (passion flower)

Cardiovascular Passion flower is widely touted as a herbal sedative. It has reportedly caused *prolongation of the QT interval* (59[A]).

A 34-year-old woman developed nausea, vomiting, drowsiness, a prolonged QT interval, and episodes of non-sustained ventricular tachycardia following self-medication of passion flower for 1 day. She made a full recovery after withdrawal of the passion flower.

The authors suggested that the adverse event had been caused by harman alkaloids from *Passiflora incarnata*, but did not discuss the mechanism.

Piper methysticum (kava)

Liver Kava, which is used as an anxiolytic, has recently been associated with toxic *liver damage* in six cases reported from Switzerland (60[cr]). The authors pointed out that a total of nine such cases are now on record. In one patient, the liver damage was so extensive that liver transplantation became necessary. Histological data from four patients were consistent with an allergic mechanism. In several cases, other medications with hepatotoxic potential had been taken concurrently. Symptoms generally occurred at between 3 weeks and 4 months and involved daily doses that contained kavapyrones 60–210 mg. Most instances involved acetone extracts. The leading kava extract, Laitan, has subsequently been withdrawn from the Swiss market.

Skin Kava has reportedly caused a *skin rash* (61[A]).

A 36-year-old woman presented with a generalized rash, severe itching with erythema, and papules 4 days after discontinuing a kava formulation (Antares®), which she had taken in a dosage of 120 mg/day for 3 weeks. The condition improved with corticosteroids and antihistamines, but the itching lasted several weeks. Patch tests with the kava extract were positive.

Musculoskeletal *Rhabdomyolysis* has been attributed to kava (62[A]).

A 29-year-old man developed severe diffuse muscle pain and passed dark urine a few hours after taking a herbal combination product containing guarana 500 mg, *Ginkgo biloba* 200 mg, and kava 100 mg. His blood creatine kinase activity and myoglobin concentration were raised and there were no signs of an underlying metabolic myopathy. His condition improved within 6 weeks.

The authors suggested that the methylxanthine-like effects of guarana and the antidopaminergic and neuromuscular blocking properties of kava had caused the rhabdomyolysis in this patient.

Drug overdose A 34-year-old Tongan man complained of *sore eyes*, *headache*, *generalized muscle weakness*, and *abdominal pain* (63[A]). He was disoriented and hallucinating. His family reported that he had been drinking large quantities of kava daily for about 14 years. Chronic kava intoxication was treated with intravenous Plasmalyte (a crystalloid solution) and he recovered within a day.

Pyrrolizidine alkaloids

Pyrrolizidine alkaloids are present in several plants, for instance *Senecio* and *Crotalaria* species commonly used for medicinal purposes in Africa and elsewhere.

Liver In a South African study 20 children were identified as suffering from *hepatic veno-occlusive disease* thought to be caused by the administration of traditional remedies (64[C]). The predominant clinical presentation was ascites and hepatomegaly. Nine children died. The surviving patients progressed to cirrhosis and portal hypertension. In four cases early urine specimens were available, and in all of these the presence of pyrrolizidine alkaloids was confirmed.

Ranunculus damascenus (buttercup)

Skin Buttercup is used topically for abscess drainage, hemorrhoids, and burns. It has been reported to cause *skin damage* (65[A]).

A 45-year-old Turkish woman developed open wounds on the abdomen, right knee, and neck. She had used buttercup topically and orally for pain relief. She was treated with antibiotics and adequate wound care. Complete healing was achieved within 10 days.

The authors argued that protoanemonin, a constituent of *Ranunculus damascenus*, which inhibits mitosis in plants, had caused this severe reaction.

Rhus (lacquer)

Rhus is used as a traditional remedy for gastrointestinal complaints in Korea, where 31 patients with *Rhus* allergy have been seen over a 10-year period (66[c]). The clinical manifestations included *maculopapular eruptions* (65%), *erythema multiforme* (32%), *erythroderma* (19%) *pustules*, *purpura*, *wheals*, and *blisters*. All patients had generalized or localized *pruritus*, and other symptoms included *gastrointestinal problems* (32%), *fever* (26%), *chills*, and *headache*. Many developed a leukocytosis (70%) with neutrophilia (88%), and some had *toxic effects on the liver or kidneys*. All responded to corticosteroids or antihistamines.

PROPRIETARY HERBAL MIXTURES

Numerous herbal mixtures are being promoted worldwide, e.g. through the Internet. In many cases their herbal ingredients are not disclosed.

Essiac

Body temperature Essiac is a Canadian herbal mixture promoted as a cancer cure. It has been reported to have caused *fever* (67[A]).

A 46-year-old woman with a squamous cell carcinoma of the cervix developed neutropenic fever during radiation therapy, 10 days after taking Essiac. The fever resolved after antibiotic therapy, but it delayed her radiation therapy for 9 days and required 4 days of hospitalization.

The authors felt that Essiac had caused this problem, but causality was uncertain, not least because she also took four other herbal medicaments.

Herbalife

Herbalife is a complex herbal formula that is promoted for weight loss. *Acute mania* has been attributed to it (68[A]).

A 39-year-old man developed classic symptoms of mania within 4–72 hours of taking Herbalife. He continued to take it and after several days became psychotic, paranoid, and out of control, culminating in a high-speed car chase with the police. Bipolar disorder was diagnosed and treated, including withdrawal of the Herbalife, and he remained free of symptoms 3 months later.

The author thought it likely that the herbal mixture had caused the psychotic illness in a man who had no previous history of mental disturbance.

Isabgol

Liver Isabgol is an Italian herbal mixture that is promoted for constipation. *Syncytial giant cell hepatitis* occurred in a 26-year-old woman who used Isabgol (69[A]). Autoimmune disease and viral infections were excluded. The authors felt that the causative role of the Isabgol was supported by the spontaneous and dramatic clinical, biochemical, and histological improvement that followed the withdrawal of Isabgol without any further therapy.

Rio Hair Naturalizer System

Rio Hair Naturalizer System is a complex mixture of metallic salts and botanical extracts promoted to straighten curled hair. The product has been popular with African Americans in the USA. A survey of 464 individuals who had complained to the FDA about this remedy showed that 95% had experienced *hair breakage and hair loss* (70[C]). Three-quarters of those who had hair loss had lost 40% or more; regrowth took 8 months on average.

HOMEOPATHY *(SED-14, 1668)*

Homeopathic remedies are often highly dilute and are therefore usually viewed as being devoid of adverse effects. A systematic review of all data on the safety of such medicines have challenged this view (71[M]). It showed that in placebo-controlled trials the mean incidence of adverse effects of homeopathic remedies was 9.4%, higher than that of placebo (6.1%). All the adverse effects were minor and transient. Anecdotal reports of more serious adverse effects mainly related to aggravation of presenting symptoms, which, from the homeopathic point of view, can be looked on as confirmation that the optimal remedy has been found, and thus interpreted as a positive event.

Harm can also be done when an ineffective homeopathic intervention replaces an effective conventional one (72[A]).

A 40-year-old woman traveling to a malaria-infested region took her homeopath's advice and was "immunized" with homeopathic remedies (*Ledum palustre* 5CH and *Malaria officinalis* 4CH) instead of taking conventional protection. She contracted malaria and had to be treated for 2 months in intensive care for multiple organ system failure due to *P. falciparum*.

Seven Israeli children were seriously harmed when their parents used homeopaths and other providers of complementary medicine instead of conventional doctors; four died (73[c]). Similarly, it has been reported that seeing a traditional healer in Kenya increased the risk of dying from an acute pneumonia by 5.3 times (74[R]).

AROMATHERAPY *(SED-14, 1668; SEDA-22, 516)*

Aromatherapy is a highly popular form of complementary medicine usually entailing the application of essential plant oils to the skin by gentle massage. It has been shown to have relaxing effects but other claims have not been substantiated by reliable trials evidence (75[R]).

Immunologic A survey of UK aromatherapists (no details provided) yielded 11 reports of adverse effects (76[c]). Most of these cases seemed to relate to *allergic reactions* to the essential oils. A therapist also reportedly developed an allergy to ylang–ylang oil used in aromatherapy (77[A]).

Japanese dermatologists have reported an increase in positive patch tests to lavender oil from 1.1% in 1990 to 14% in 1998 (78[C]). The authors argued that this rise coincided with a similar increase in the use of lavender aromatherapy in Japan and that the latter caused the former.

ACUPUNCTURE *(SED-14, 1673; SEDA-22, 516; SEDA-23, 511; SEDA-24, 540)*

Acupuncture keeps being associated with serious adverse events (79[R]), and several attempts to define the size of this problem more closely have been published.

A Japanese survey of 391 patients who received acupuncture in 1441 treatment sessions involving a total of 30 338 needle insertions showed the following systemic adverse effects: *tiredness* (8.2%), *drowsiness* (2.8%), *aggravation of the presenting condition* (2.8%), *itching in the punctured region* (1.0%), *dizziness or vertigo* (0.8%), *faintness or nausea* during treatment (0.8%), *headache* (0.5%), and *chest pain* (0.3%) (80[C]). The incidences of local reactions were: *minor bleeding after withdrawal of the needle* (2.6%), *pain on insertion of the needle* (0.7%), *petechiae or ecchymoses* (0.3%), *local pain after treatment* (0.1%), *subcutaneous hematomas* (0.1%).

Norwegian researchers sent questionnaires about acupuncture to a random sample of the Norwegian general population (81[C]). Of the 653 respondents, 7% claimed to have had adverse effects. The most common were *dizziness*, *fatigue*, and *pain from the needles*. No serious adverse effects were reported.

In a prospective UK survey of members of the medical and physiotherapy acupuncture organizations in Britain the preliminary data included 25 500 treatments given by 77 acupuncturists (82[C]). There were 29 major events, including four episodes of *loss of consciousness* and one *tonic–clonic seizure*. The most common minor events were *bleeding or hematoma*

(3%), *aggravation of symptoms* (1%), and *pain during needling* (0.9%).

In the above-mentioned survey of 1100 Australian providers of traditional Chinese medicine the adverse events of acupuncture were also monitored (20[C]). There were 3222 events, including 64 cases of *pneumothorax* and 80 *convulsions*. No deaths were recorded.

A systematic review of case reports from the Japanese literature yielded 105 cases of suspected acupuncture adverse effects not previously reported in Western publications (83[M]). These included 21 *spinal lesions*, 21 cases of *pneumothorax*, 19 *infections*, 15 cases of *foreign bodies in organs*, 10 instances of *argyria*, 10 *neural injuries*, and 11 other adverse events, including two cases of *cardiac tamponade*.

Cardiovascular Acupuncture has been associated with *hemopericardium* due to ventricular puncture (84[A]).

An 83-year-old Austrian woman developed syncope and cardiogenic shock shortly after acupuncture over the sternum. Echocardiography showed cardiac tamponade, and pericardiocentesis revealed hemopericardium. At operation a small bleeding perforation of the right ventricle was found and closed. The acupuncture at the point "Ren 17" was above a sternal foramen, which allowed the needle to penetrate the heart.

Nervous system Acupuncture has been associated with *subarachnoid hemorrhage* due to arterial puncture (85[A]).

A 44-year-old Chinese man had severe occipital headache, nausea, and vomiting during acupuncture in the posterior neck. A CT scan showed hemorrhage in the third, fourth, and lateral ventricles, and blood was found in the lumbar fluid. The problem was due to puncture of a branch of the vertebral artery at the "feng fu" point, which coincides with the site for performing cisternal puncture. The patient made a spontaneous full recovery within 28 days.

Skin *Local reactions* can occur to acupuncture needles (86[A]).

A 55-year-old Japanese woman developed papules at sites where she had had acupuncture 4 years and 3 weeks before. Histological examination showed that the papules were silicone granulomas. The authors postulated that the papules were reactions to the silicone from the coating of the acupuncture needles.

Infection risk Acupuncture needles can transmit infection (87[A]).

A 67-year-old Japanese man was treated with "depot acupuncture", an unusual technique involving the implantation of a sheep gut thread through a spinal anesthesia needle into the abdomen. He subsequently developed intractable pain, high fever, and other signs of infection. A CT scan showed a low density mass in the left psoas muscle and the ventral portion of the distal aorta, corresponding to an abscess and a false infected aneurysm. The affected part of the aorta was replaced with a Gore-Tex graft and the patient was treated with antibiotics. He eventually made a full recovery.

After a patient of a London doctor (who practiced an unusual acupuncture technique involving re-injection of native blood) acquired *hepatitis B*, 352 of his patients treated by this method were investigated; 33 were positive for hepatitis B antigen and 30 showed complete nucleotide identity in the DNA segments derived from the surface and core genes (88[C]). Contaminated saline used in the treatment was identified as the probable vehicle of transmission.

Korean epidemiologists have studied the prevalence of *hepatitis C* virus infection in a rural population ($n = 1033$) with a high incidence of liver cancer (89[C]). They noted that the strongest associations in a multivariate analysis were with anti-HCV positivity and the use of acupuncture (OR = 2.2, 95%CI = 1.0, 4.7).

Similarly, French investigators have evaluated the presence of serum markers of *hepatitis A, B,* and *C* viruses in a rural population of 303 volunteers (90[C]). The main risk factors for positivity were past hospitalizations (72%), acupuncture (18%), conjugal unfaithfulness (11%), blood transfusion (9.4%), tattoos (5.8%), homosexuality (1.1%), and intravenous drug addiction (0.73%).

Miscellaneous A 52-year-old man received acupuncture in the backs of both hands for chronic back pain and subsequently developed *bilateral swelling of both hands and fingers* (91[A]). No reason for this adverse effect could be found, and the authors considered infection or allergy as the most likely cause, but without finding strong evidence of either.

SPINAL MANIPULATION

(SED-14, 1674; SEDA-22, 516; SEDA-23, 512; SEDA-24, 540)

Spinal manipulation is carried out by chiropractors, osteopaths, physiotherapists, and other healthcare professionals to treat back and neck pain as well as other (predominantly musculoskeletal) disorders. Serious adverse effects of spinal manipulation have been repeatedly reported, but prospective studies to define the incidence of such events are scarce.

In the UK 108 consecutive patients of chiropractors were asked to complete a questionnaire, which 80% of them returned (92^C). Of the questionnaires 68% were suitable for analysis. Adverse effects at 1 hour after treatment were reported by 28 patients and eight had adverse effects the morning after treatment. The most common adverse effects were extra *local pain* or *radiating pain*. No serious adverse effects were reported.

When all 26 cases of *vertebral artery dissection* during the period 1989–99 were retrospectively analyzed in a tertiary Canadian academic center, possible precipitating factors were identified in 14 patients (93^C). Chiropractic spinal manipulation and sporting activity were the most common factors (11% and 15% respectively).

There are also indirect risks associated with the use of chiropractic. For instance, some chiropractors tend to advise clients against any type of immunization. The basis of this attitude seems to lie in early chiropractic philosophy. Eschewing the germ theory of infectious disease, this philosophy considered any disease to be the result of spinal nerve dysfunction caused by misalignment of vertebrae (94^R). When 150 US chiropractors were questioned about their attitude towards immunization, only 30% reported recommending childhood immunizations (95^c).

REFERENCES

1. Ernst E, White AR. The BBC survey of complementary medicine use in the UK. Complement Ther Med 2000; 8: 32–6.
2. Pies R. Adverse neuropsychiatric reactions to herbal and over-the-counter "antidepressants". J Clin Psychiatry 2000; 61: 815–20.
3. Ernst E. Adverse effects of herbal drugs in dermatology. Br J Dermatol 2000; 143: 923–9.
4. Chitturi S, Farrell GC. Herbal hepatotoxicity: an expanding but poorly defined problem. J Gastroenterol Hepatol 2000; 15: 1093–9.
5. Tomlinson B, Chan TYK, Chan JCN, Critchley JAJH, But PPH. Toxicity of complementary therapies: an Eastern perspective. J Clin Pharmacol 2000; 40: 451–6.
6. Calixto JB. Efficacy, safety, quality control, marketing and regulatory guidelines for herbal medicines (phytotherapeutic agents). Braz J Med Biol Res 2000; 33: 179–89.
7. Boullata JI, Nace AM. Safety issues with herbal medicine. Pharmacotherapy 2000; 20: 257–69.
8. Shapiro R. Safety assessment of botanicals. Nutraceuticals World 2000; July/August: 52–63.
9. Saller R, Iten F, Reichling J. Unerwünschte Wirkungen und Wechselwirkungen von Phytotherapeutika. Erfahrungsheilkunde 2000; 6: 369–76.
10. Pennachio DL. Drug–herb interactions: how vigilant should you be? Patient Care 2000; 19: 41–68.
11. Ernst E. Possible interactions between synthetic and herbal medicinal products. Part 1: a systematic review of the indirect evidence. Perfusion 2000; 13: 4–6, 8.
12. Ernst E. Interactions between synthetic and herbal medicinal products. Part 2: a systematic review of the direct evidence. Perfusion 2000; 13: 60–70.
13. Blumenthal M. Interactions between herbs and conventional drugs: introductory considerations. Herbal Gram 2000; 49: 52–63.
14. Ernst E. Herb–drug interactions: potentially important but woefully under-researched. Eur J Clin Pharmacol 2000; 56: 523–4.
15. De Smet PAGM, Touw DJ. Sint–janskruid op de balans van werking en interacties. Pharm Weekbl 2000; 135: 455–62.
16. Farah MH, Edwards R, Lindquist M, Leon C, Shaw D. International monitoring of adverse health effects associated with herbal medicines. Pharmacoepidemiol Drug Saf 2000; 9: 105–12.
17. Murch SJ, KrishnaRaj S, Saxena PK. Phytopharmaceuticals: problems, limitations, and solutions. Sci Rev Altern Med 2000; 4: 33–7.
18. Tyler VE. Product definition deficiencies in clinical studies of herbal medicines. Sci Rev Altern Med 2000; 4: 17–21.
19. Gurley BJ, Gardner SF, Hubbard MA. Content versus label claims in *Ephedra*-containing dietary supplements. Am J Health-Syst Pharm 2000; 57: 963–9.
20. Bensoussan A, Myers SP, Carlton AL. Risks associated with the practice of traditional Chinese medicine: an Australian study. Arch Fam Med 2000; 9: 1071–8.
21. Al-Khafaji M. Monitoring of liver enzymes in patients on Chinese medicine. J Chin Med 2000; 62: 6–10.

22. Zuin VG, Vilegas JHY. Pesticide residues in medicinal plants and phytomedicines. Phytother Res 2000; 14: 73–8.
23. Lau KK, Lai CK, Chan AYW. Phenytoin poisoning after using Chinese proprietary medicines. Hum Exp Toxicol 2000; 19: 385–6.
24. Li AM, Chan MHM, Leung TF, Cheung RCK, Lam CWK, Fok TF. Mercury intoxication presenting with tics. Arch Dis Child 2000; 83: 174–5.
25. Moore C, Adler R. Herbal vitamins: lead toxicity and developmental delay. Pediatrics 2000; 106: 600–2.
26. Anonymous. Herbal medicines. Warning: found to contain antidiabetics. WHO Newslett 2000; 2: 4–5.
27. Akatsu T, Santo RM, Nakayasu K, Kanai A. Oriental herbal medicine induced epithelial keratopathy. Br J Ophthalmol 2000; 84: 934.
28. Hanawa T. A case of bronchial asthma with liver dysfunction caused by Kampo medicine, saiko–keisi–kankyo–to, and recovered smoothly in general through natural course. Phytomedicine 2000; SII: 123.
29. Chen JK. Nephropathy associated with the use of *Aristolochia*. Herbal Gram 2000; 48: 44–5.
30. Pokhrel PK, Ergil KV. Aristolochic acid: a toxicological review. Clin Acupunct Orient Med 2000; 1: 161–6.
31. Hammes MG. Anmerkungen zu *Aristolochia* – eine Recherche in chinesischen Originaltexten. Dtsch Z Akupunkt 2000; 3: 198–200.
32. Wiebrecht A. Über die *Aristolochia* – Nephropathie. Dtsch Z Akupunkt 2000; 3: 187–97.
33. Tanaka A, Nishida R, Maeda K, Sugawara A, Kuwahara T. Chinese herb nephropathy in Japan presents adult-onset Fanconi syndrome: could different components of aristolochic acids cause a different type of Chinese herb nephropathy? Clin Nephrol 2000; 53: 301–6.
34. Yang C-S, Lin C-H, Chang S-H, Hsu H-C. Rapidly progressing fibrosing interstitial nephritis associated with Chinese herbal drugs. Am J Kidney Dis 2000; 35: 313–18.
35. Nortier JL, Martinez MCM, Schmeiser HH, Arlt VM, Bieler CA, Petein M, Depierreux MF, De-Fauw L, Abramowicz D, Vereerstraeten P, Vanherweghem J-L. Urolethial carcinoma associated with the use of a Chinese herb (*Arictolochia fangchi*). New Engl J Med 2000; 342: 1686–92.
36. Nadir A, Reddy D, Van Thiel DH. *Cascara sagrada*-induced intrahepatic cholestasis causing portal hypertension: case report and review of herbal hepatotoxicity. Am J Gastroenterol 2000; 95: 3634–7.
37. Roemer HC, Both HV, Foellmann W, Golka K. Angel's trumpet and the eye. J R Soc Med 2000; 93: 319.
38. Raikhlin-Eisenkraft B, Bentur Y. *Ecbalium elaterium* (squirting cucumber) – remedy or poison? Clin Toxicol 2000; 38: 305–8.
39. Gallo M, Sarkar M, Au W, Pietrzak K, Comas B, Smith M, Jaeger TV, Einarson A, Koren G. Pregnancy outcome following gestational exposure to echinacea: a prospective controlled study. Arch Intern Med 2000; 160: 3141–3.
40. Haller CA, Benowitz NL. Adverse cardiovascular and central nervous system events associated with dietary supplements containing *Ephedra* alkaloids. New Engl J Med 2000; 343: 1833–8.
41. Olukoga A, Donaldson D. Liquorice and its health implications. J R Soc Promot Health 2000; 120: 83–9.
42. Russo S, Mastropasqua M, Mosetti MA, Persegani C, Paggi A. Low doses of liquorice can induce hypertension encephalopathy. Am J Nephrol 2000; 20: 145–8.
43. Dobbins KRB, Saul RF. Transient visual loss after licorice ingestion. J Neuro-Ophthalmol 2000; 20: 38–41.
44. Brown TM. Acute St John's wort toxicity. Am J Emerg Med 2000; 18: 532–3.
45. Beckman SE, Sommi RW, Switzer J. Consumer use of St John's wort: a survey on effectiveness, safety, and tolerability. Pharmacotherapy 2000; 20: 568–74.
46. Lane-Brown MM. Photosensitivity associated with herbal preparations of St John's wort (*Hypericum perforatum*). Med J Aust 2000; 172: 302.
47. Biffignandi PM, Bilia AR. The growing knowledge of St John's wort (*Hypericum perforatum* L.) drug interactions and their clinical significance. Curr Ther Res Clin Exp 2000; 61: 389–94.
48. Schulz V. Häufigkeit und klinische Relevanz der Interaktionen und Nebenwirkungen von *Hypericum* – Präparaten. Schweiz Rundsch Med Prax 2000; 89: 2131–40.
49. Budzinski JW, Foster BC, Vandenhoek S, Arnason JT. An in vitro evaluation of human cytochrome P450 3A4 inhibition by selected commercial herbal extracts and tinctures. Phytomedicine 2000; 7: 273–82.
50. Obach RS. Inhibition of human cytochrome P450 enzymes by constituents of St John's wort, an herbal preparation used in the treatment of depression. J Pharmacol Exp Ther 2000; 294: 88–95.
51. Moore LB, Goodwin B, Jones SA, Wisely GB, Serabjit-Singh CJ, Willson TM, Collins JL, Kliewer SA. St John's wort induces hepatic drug metabolism through activation of the pregnane X receptor. Proc Natl Acad Sci USA 2000; 97: 7500–2.
52. Breidenbach Th, Kliem V, Burg M, Radermacher J, Hoffmann MW, Klempnauer J. Profound drop of cyclosporin A whole blood trough levels caused by St John's wort (*Hypericum perforatum*). Transplantation 2000; 69: 2229–32.
53. Barone GW, Gurley BJ, Ketel BL, Lightfoot ML, Abul-Ezz SR. Drug interaction between St John's wort and cyclosporine. Ann Pharmacother 2000; 34: 1013–16.
54. Karliova M, Treichel U, Malagò M, Frilling A, Gerken G, Broelsch CE. Interaction of *Hypericum perforatum* (St John's wort) with cyclosporin A metabolism in a patient after liver transplantation. J Hepatol 2000; 33: 853–5.

55. Mai I, Krüger H, Budde K, Johne A, Brockmöller J, Neumayer H-H, Roots I. Hazardous pharmacokinetic interaction of Saint John's wort (*Hypericum perforatum*) with the immunosuppressant cyclosporin. Int J Clin Pharmacol Ther 2000; 38: 500–2.
56. Uehleke B, Mueller SC, Woehling H, Petzsch M, Riethling A-K, Drewelow B. Interaction of St John's wort with digoxin in relation to dosage and formulation. Phytomedicine 2000; SII: 20.
57. Barbenel DM, Yusufi B, O'Shea D, Bench CJ. Mania in a patient receiving testosterone replacement post-orchidectomy taking St John's wort and sertraline. J Psychopharmacol 2000; 14: 84–6.
58. Mueller BA, Scott MK, Sowinski KM, Prag KA. Noni juice (*Morinda citrifolia*): hidden potential for hyperkalemia? Am J Kidney Dis 2000; 35: 310–12.
59. Fisher AA, Purcell P, Le Couteur DG. Toxicity of *Passiflora incarnata* L. Clin Toxicol 2000; 38: 63–6.
60. Stoller A. Leberschädigungen unter Kava-Extrakten. Schweiz Ärztez 2000; 24: 1335–6.
61. Schmidt P, Boehncke WH. Delayed-type hypersensitivity reaction to kava–kava extract. Contact Dermatitis 2000; 42: 363–4.
62. Donadio V, Bonsi P, Zele I, Monari L, Liguori R, Vetrugno R, Albani F, Montagna P. Myoglobinuria after ingestion of extracts of guarana, *Ginkgo biloba* and kava. Neurol Sci 2000; 21: 124.
63. Chanwai LG. Kava toxicity. Emerg Med 2000; 12: 142–5.
64. Steenkamp V, Stewart MJ, Zuckerman M. Clinical and analytical aspects of pyrrolizidine poisoning caused by South African traditional medicines. Ther Drug Monit 2000; 22: 302–6.
65. Metin A, Alka Ö, Behçet L, Yildrim E. Phytodermis from *Ranunculus damascenus*. Contact Dermatitis 2001; 44: 183.
66. Park SD, Lee S-W, Chun J-H, Cha S-H. Clinical features of 31 patients with systemic contact dermatitis due to the ingestion of *Rhus* (lacquer). Br J Dermatol 2000; 142: 937–42.
67. Von Gruenigen VE, Hopkins MP. Alternative medicine in gynecologic oncology: a case report. Gynecol Oncol 2000; 77: 190–2.
68. Katz JL. A psychotic manic state induced by an herbal preparation. Psychosomatics 2000; 41: 73–4.
69. Fraquelli M, Colli A, Cocciolo MCD. Adult syncytial giant cell, chronic hepatitis due to herbal remedy. J Hepatol 2000; 33: 505–8.
70. Swee W, Klontz KC, Lambert M. A nationwide outbreak of alopecia associated with the use of a hair-relaxing formulation. Arch Dermatol 2000; 136: 1104–8.
71. Dantas F, Rampes H. Do homeopathic medicines provoke adverse effects? A systematic review. Br Homeopath J 2000; 89: S35–8.
72. Delaunay P. Homoeopathy may not be effective in preventing malaria. Br Med J 2000; 321: 1288.
73. Luder AS, Friedman G. The mortality and morbidity of non-medical (alternative) treatment for minors. Int J Adolesc Med Health 2000; 12: 295–305.
74. Scott JAG, Hall AJ, Muyodi C, Lowe B, Ross M, Chohan B, Mandaliya K, Getambu E, Gleeson F, Drobniewski F. Aetiology, outcome, and risk factors for mortality among adults with acute pneumonia in Kenya. Lancet 2000; 355: 1225–30.
75. Cooke B, Ernst E. Aromatherapy: a systematic review. Br J Gen Pract 2000; 50: 493–6.
76. Smith I. Suspected adverse reaction to essential oils. Aromatherapy World 2000; September: 7.
77. Romaguera C, Vilaplana J. Occupational contact dermatitis from ylang–ylang oil. Contact Dermatitis 2000; 43: 251.
78. Sugiura M, Hayakawa R, Kato Y, Sugiura K, Hashimoto R. Results of patch testing with lavender oil in Japan. Contact Dermatitis 2000; 43: 157–60.
79. Ernst E, White AR. Acupuncture may be associated with serious adverse events. Br Med J 2000; 320: 513–14.
80. Yamashita H, Tsukayama H, Hori N, Kimura T, Tanno Y. Incidence of adverse reactions associated with acupuncture. J Altern Complement Med 2000; 6: 345–50.
81. Norheim AJ, Fonnebo V. A survey of acupuncture patients: results from a questionnaire among a random sample in the general population in Norway. Complement Ther Med 2000; 8: 187–92.
82. White AR, Ernst E. Survey of adverse events following acupuncture (SAFA). Forsch Komplementarmed 2000; 7: 29–58.
83. Yamashita H, Tsukayama H, White AR, Ernst E, Tanno Y, Sugishita C. Systematic review of case reports on acupuncture adverse events in the Japanese literature. Forsch Komplementarmed 2000; 7: 57.
84. Kirchgatterer A, Schwarz CD, Höller E, Punzengruber C, Hartl P, Eber B. Cardiac tamponade following acupuncture. Chest 2000; 117: 1510–11.
85. Choo DCA, Yue G. Acute intracranial hemorrhage caused by acupuncture. Headache 2000; 40: 397–8.
86. Yanagihara M, Fujii T, Wakamatu N, Ishizaki H, Takehara T, Nawate K. Silicone granuloma on the entry points of acupuncture, venepuncture and surgical needles. J Cutan Pathol 2000; 27: 301–5.
87. Origuchi N, Komiyama T, Ohyama K, Wakabayashi T, Shigematsu H. Infectious aneurysm formation after depot acupuncture. Eur J Vasc Endovasc Surg 2000; 20: 211–13.
88. Webster GJM, Hallett R, Whalley SA, Mletzer M, Balogun K, Brown D, Farrington CP, Sharma S, Hamilton G, Farrow SC, Ramsay ME, Teo C-G, Dusheiko GM. Molecular epidemiology of a large outbreak of hepatitis B linked to autohaemotherapy. Lancet 2000; 356: 379–84.
89. Shin HR, Kim JY, Ohno T, Cao K, Mizokami M, Risch H, Kim SR. Prevalence and risk factors of hepatitis C virus infection among Koreans in rural area of Korea. Hepatol Res 2000; 17: 185–96.
90. Nalpas B, Zylberberg H, Dubois F, Presles

M-A, Gillant J-C, Lienard M, Delemotte B, Bréchot C. Prévalence des infections par les virus hépatotropes en milieu rural. Gastroenterol Clin Biol 2000; 24: 536–40.
91. McCartney CJL, Herriot R, Chambers WA. Bilateral hand oedema related to acupuncture. Pain 2000; 84: 429–30.
92. Barrett AJ, Breen AC. Adverse effects of spinal manipulation. J R Soc Med 2000; 93: 258–9.
93. Bin Saeed A, Shuaib A, Al-Sulatti G, Emery D. Vertebral artery dissection: warning symptoms, clinical features and prognosis in 20 patients. Can J Neurol Sci 2000; 27: 292–6.
94. Campbell JB, Busse JW, Injevan S. Chiropractors and vaccination. A historical perspective. Pediatrics 2000; 105: 43–51.
95. Lee ACC, Li DH, Kemper KJ. Chiropractic care for children. Arch Pediatr Adolesc Med 2000; 154: 401–7.
96. Anonymous. Aristolochic acid. Warning concerning interstitial renal fibrosis. WHO Newslett 2000; 2: 1.

N.H. Choulis

49 Miscellaneous drugs, materials, and medical devices

Aspartame

Two patients reported *Raynaud's phenomenon* (1[A]) and one man had *fibromyalgia*. All three described regular keyboarding to the extent of 30 hours per week but had used wrist rests, "stretch breaks", and other steps to optimize their work practices. Each had used aspartame 6–15 g/day (0.12–0.16 mg/kg/day) as well as a dietary drink containing aspartame, and no other risk factors were identified. Complete resolution of symptoms occurred over 2 weeks after they had eliminated aspartame from the diet, despite no changes in the intensity of keyboarding or other work practices. Nerve conduction velocities had been within normal limits before the withdrawal of aspartame and were not repeated.

Nervous system In three non-obese individuals (two women and one man) it was suspected that heavy use of the artificial sweetener aspartame (Nutra Sweet®) was causally related to symptoms of *carpal tunnel syndrome* (2[A]). All three reported moderate pain and tingling in the hands, especially at night, using a self-administered questionnaire for the assessment of severity of symptoms and functional status (3[c]). Given the ubiquity of aspartame–one manufacturer has stated that it is used in 5000 products–physicians may want to inquire about its use in patients who report symptoms of carpal tunnel syndrome.

Aspartame is completely hydrolysed in the gastrointestinal tract to methanol, aspartic acid, and phenylalanine (4[E]). It has been associated with other neuropsychological conditions, including *brain tumors*, *mood disturbances*, and *seizures*, but only anecdotally (5[A]). Evidence of a causal connection with *headache* in susceptible individuals is more suggestive.

Bisphosphonates

In a long term follow-up of two randomized placebo-controlled trials of pamidronate in women with breast carcinoma and osteolytic bone metastases adverse events caused premature withdrawal of therapy in 22% of 367 patients taking pamidronate 90 mg/day and 20% of 38 patients taking placebo (6[C]). A 75-year-old woman was withdrawn after developing an *allergic reaction* in her left eye possibly related to pamidronate. Another patient discontinued pamidronate after an episode of symptomatic *hypocalcemia*. Two other serious and unexpected adverse events occurred in patients taking pamidronate. A 45-year-old woman who had been taking placebo developed an *interstitial pulmonary infiltrate and dyspnea* 4 days after taking pamidronate on a compassionate basis after completing the study. An 83-year-old woman developed increased *weakness*, *fatigue*, and *dyspnea* 3 weeks after her last dose of pamidronate. These adverse events were both assessed by the treating physician as being possibly related to pamidronate. *Fatigue* related to the study drug was reported slightly more often by patients taking pamidronate (40%) than those taking placebo (29%). Fever related to the study drug was reported in 14% of pamidronate patients and in 5% of placebo patients.

Sensory systems *Uveitis* is an underrecognized albeit uncommon adverse effect of pamidronate. The first case was reported in 1993 (7[A]). A review of reports published as of 1994 (8[R]) found 23 cases, including seven cases of anterior uveitis, three of episcleritis or scleritis, and 13 of non-specific

Side Effects of Drugs, Annual 25
J.K. Aronson, ed.

transient conjunctivitis. Since then, 11 new cases of anterior uveitis have been reported (9[c], 10[c]).

Of 16 cases of pamidronate-induced anterior uveitis (9[c], 10[c]), 11 were bilateral and five unilateral. In most cases, the onset was within 24–48 hours of initiation of the pamidronate infusion, although in one patient the interval was 17 days. The severity, when specified, ranged from mild to severe. Treatment was by watchful waiting in two patients, oral glucocorticoid therapy or hospital admission in four, and topical glucocorticoids with or without cycloplegic agents in nine. The time to recovery, when specified, ranged from a few days to a month. The cumulative pamidronate dose was 30–240 mg.

Gastrointestinal Pamidronate is an aminobisphosphonate that contains a nitrate derivative. It is used intravenously because it is not well absorbed from the gut. However, the effect of oral pamidronate on bone mineral density and its adverse effect profile has been investigated in a double-blind placebo-controlled study in 122 patients aged 55–75 years with established vertebral osteoporosis (11[C]). The patients took disodium pamidronate 300 mg/day for 4 weeks every 16 weeks (group A), 150 mg/day for 4 weeks every 8 weeks (group B), or placebo (group C). All also took calcium 500 mg/day and vitamin D 400 IU/day. In groups A and B there were significant reductions in serum osteocalcin and urinary deoxypuridinoline and an excess of *gastrointestinal adverse effects*, particularly in group A. The authors concluded that intermittent pamidronate therapy can prevent bone loss in both the lumbar spine and femoral neck in patients with established vertebral osteoporosis, although the 300 mg dose did not appear suitable for clinical use because of gastrointestinal adverse effects.

Severe *esophagitis* or *esophageal ulceration* have been reported in seven patients taking bisphosphonates (six alendronate and one etidronate); the lesions healed on withdrawal (12[c]).

Disulfiram

Liver Disulfiram can cause severe *liver damage*. The Swedish adverse drug reactions register, SWEDIS, has received 149 case reports of 157 adverse reactions associated with disulfiram since 1971, of which 63 cited disorders of the liver and biliary tract (13[A]). Of these 63 reports, seven were classified as serious. In three cases of severe liver damage with a fatal outcome disulfiram was suspected to have caused the reaction. If signs of liver damage appear, it is recommended that disulfiram be withdrawn and liver function tests performed.

Skin A 49-year-old woman developed *pruritic erythema* 2 weeks after the implantation of Esperal® (Kela NV, Belgium) in her left buttock (14[A]). Three months later she started drinking alcohol and developed generalized erythema with numerous papules on her face and limbs; the dermatitis at the site of the implant became more severe. The serum ethanol concentration was 270 mg/dl. Methanol was not detected.

Hydrazine sulfate

Hydrazine sulfate is sometimes promoted as an alternative cancer cure. It has been reported to cause *liver damage* (15[A]).

A 55-year-old man with maxillary sinus cancer declined conventional therapy and opted to treat his condition with hydrazine sulfate obtained via the Internet. He had followed the recommended regimen for 4 months when he developed fulminant hepatorenal failure, hepatic encephalopathy, and profound coagulopathy. He died of severe gastrointestinal hemorrhage.

Nicotine

Smoking is negatively associated with ulcerative colitis and positively associated with *Crohn's disease*; it is the most striking and firmly established epidemiological factor associated with the two conditions. The first association of non-smoking with ulcerative colitis was made 17 years ago (16[r]), and was followed within 2 years by the observation that patients with Crohn's disease were more often smokers (17[R]). Smoking also has opposite effects on the clinical course of the two conditions, with possible benefit in ulcerative colitis (18[C]) and a detrimental effect in Crohn's disease (19[R]). Nicotine is probably the principal active ingredient in smoking responsible for these associations.

Nervous system In another study in 53

subjects two- and three-dimensional analyses of nicotine-induced eye movements were performed to evaluate whether they were primarily of vestibular or oculomotor origin (20[C]). Nicotine-induced *nystagmus* was detected in 27 subjects (51%). These findings suggest that nicotine causes an imbalance in the vestibulo-ocular reflex.

Phosphates

A 39-year-old woman with oncogenic osteomalacia caused by an osteosarcoma of the right scapula developed *tertiary hyperparathyroidism* after taking oral phosphate and vitamin D (21[A]). The uniqueness of this case was the coexistence of hyperparathyroidism and oncogenic osteomalacia. All patients previously reported as having developed tertiary hyperparathyroidism with phosphate supplements had taken them for 10–14 years before diagnosis, but this patient had taken it for only 2 years. The proposed mechanism is that exogenous phosphate stimulates parathyroid activity through sequestration of calcium.

Phosphate enemas are used in preparing children's bowels for colonoscopy and have been described as being safe and ideal for this purpose (22[R]). However, phosphate toxicity associated with enteral sodium phosphate has previously been reported in more than 20 children (23[C], 24[C]). Two died, and one had severe neurological sequelae; these three children had either gastrointestinal or renal abnormalities, and one was very premature. Fatal phosphate toxicity has been reported in a 17-month-old child who had no apparent renal or gastrointestinal abnormality after a relatively small dose of hypertonic phosphate enema (25[A]).

Polyethylene glycol

Polyethylene glycol is a high molecular weight inert molecule that is commonly combined with electrolytes (potassium chloride, sodium bicarbonate, sodium chloride, and sodium sulfate) in colonic lavage systems. Owing to the osmotic properties of these solutions, there is little absorption or secretion of electrolytes or water, although small amounts of polyethylene glycol and sulfates have been detected in the urine of healthy patients and higher concentrations in the urine of patients with inflammatory bowel disease (26[R]). Common adverse effects of solutions containing polyethylene glycol and electrolytes include *nausea*, *abdominal fullness*, and *bloating* in up to 50% of patients. These solutions are contraindicated in patients with gastric outlet obstruction or gastroparesis, gastrointestinal obstruction or perforation, ileus, or toxic colitis (27[R]).

Pancreas Severe acute *pancreatitis* has been reported in a 75-year-old woman who had been given polyethylene glycol 4 l rectally (28[A]).

Sodium citrate

The FDA has issued an urgent warning to all hospital pharmacies and hemodialysis units that triCitrasol, an unapproved formulation of sodium citrate that has been used as an anticoagulant to keep intravascular lines open, can cause *death* after intravenous infusion. TriCitrasol is marketed in individual sterile 30 ml glass vials, distributed both individually and in hemodialysis kits (29[R]). A patient died of cardiac arrest shortly after the injection of triCitrasol 46.7% into a permanent hemodialysis blood access catheter that had just been implanted. Rapid or excessive infusion of citrate solutions can cause fatal cardiac dysrhythmias, seizures, or bleeding due to sequestration of blood calcium.

TriCitrasol is manufactured by Cytosol Laboratories, and is distributed by Medcomp (previously by Citra Anticoagulants, Inc). Both Cytosol Labs and Medcomp have voluntarily recalled triCitrasol for use with blood access catheters. On 9 April 2000, Medcomp announced in a letter to its customers that it was recalling its kits (or trays) containing triCitrasol and the Medcomp Ash Split Catheter II for hemodialysis or apheresis, a blood separation and retransfusion process. About 3000 Medcomp catheter kits with triCitrasol were distributed nationwide. They were also distributed in Puerto Rico and Canada.

The FDA has urged hospital pharmacies and hemodialysis units across the USA to stop using the product. Alternative 4% solutions of citrate are available for use in these and most other medical settings.

Because there is a need for this product in some procedures to prepare white cells for transfusion, the FDA is working with the company to ensure that the product currently remains available for this use, which involves dilution.

Vinegar

Vinegar was used topically in a Turkish neonate with suspected sepsis (30[A]). The child was treated with antibiotics and his grandmother decided in addition to rub his upper thorax, back, and arms with vinegar. As a result the child developed *chemical burns* on the treated areas. Fortunately he made a full recovery after the grandmother stopped the treatment.

EXCIPIENTS AND PRESERVATIVES

Dimethylsulfoxide

In preparation for bone-marrow transplantation, autologous hemopietic stem cells are normally frozen in liquid nitrogen after harvesting. However, a cryoprotective agent is required, normally dimethylsulfoxide. During and immediately after stem cell infusion, many adverse effects, which may be severe or life-threatening, have been reported. These include *hypotension* and *hypertension*, *anaphylactic reactions*, and *cardiac and respiratory failure*, all possibly due to dimethylsulfoxide, *hemolysis* induced by cryopreservation and thawing, and *fluid overload*.

In a retrospective study 30 children were reviewed after bone-marrow or peripheral autologous hemopoietic transplantation (31[C]). At the time of infusion, hydrocortisone, chlorpheniramine, and hyperhydration were administered to all patients, and furosemide and tropiseptron to most. Vital signs and symptoms were monitored for 6 hours after infusion. Thawing was performed rapidly at the bedside in a 42° C water-bath, and the cells were infused through a central venous catheter at 10 ml/min. All 32 procedures were well tolerated; there were infusion-related adverse effects in 15 of 32 infusions, but none required specific therapy. There was mild *bradycardia* in nine patients, one reported *abdominal pain*, two reported *headache*, and three had *hemoglobinuria*.

The authors concluded that a single-step cryopreservation technique aimed at limiting the total amount of dimethylsulfoxide is effective in avoiding most toxicity while not compromising post-thawing viability.

Oak moss resin

Conventional soluble oils or coolants are oil/water emulsions used during metal-working to reduce the amount of frictional heat generated by these processes. Oak moss resin is an extract of *Evernia prunasti* found in many aftershave lotions and some perfumes (32[R]). It is usually reported as a contact allergen in those who use perfumed products, but is also reported in rural and forestry workers (33[R]). Perfumes are recognized as being potential sensitizers in soluble oils (34[R]), but oak moss as a specific sensitizer within a coolant has not previously been reported.

A 47-year-old atopic man gave a 3-year history of dermatitis of his hands, forearms, and face (35[A]). He had worked for 24 years as an engineer, grinding components for printing presses. During an enforced absence from work, he noticed that his rash had resolved, but it relapsed within 2 days of his return. Further remissions were noted during his annual holidays, but the rash would always recur within 2 days of returning to work. His skin eruption continued to deteriorate until the coolant used during the grinding process was withdrawn. His rash subsequently resolved and did not recur. Patch testing with standard series, oils and coolants, the constituents of fragrance mix, and his own coolant gave strong positive reactions to fragrance mix, balsam of Peru (*Myroxylon pereirae*), sodium metabisulfite, diethanolamine, and oak moss, and a smaller reaction to his own coolant. The manufacturer of the coolant was contacted for information on the individual constituents of the oil. Further patch tests were then carried out with these components plus the individual components of the fragrance used within it. There were strong positive reactions to oak moss resin and monoethanolamine.

This case highlights the importance of patch testing with individual components of a suspected product in *occupational dermatitis*. This reduces the chance of false positive reactions and of missing a relevant allergen.

Polyvinylpyrrolidone

Polyvinylpyrrolidone (Povidone, Kollidon, poly-*N*-vinyl-lactam) is widely used as a suspending and coating agent in tablets, for its film-forming properties in eye drops, and as a carrier molecule for iodine in disinfectants. About 20% of all tablets on the market contain polyvinylpyrrolidone. It is also used in the cosmetics industry as a dispersing agent and as a lubricant in ointments. It has been reported to cause anaphylaxis (36[A]).

A 32-year-old man took paracetamol (in Doregrippin®) for flu-like symptoms, and about 10 minutes later developed generalized urticaria, angioedema, hypotonia, and tachycardia, and became semiconscious. His symptoms were rapidly relieved by intravenous antihistamines and steroids. This was the first time he had taken Doregrippin®, but he had previously taken paracetamol-containing formulations, which had been well tolerated. He was not taking any regular medication. Subsequent testing of the various constituents of the analgesic tablets identified polyvinylpyrrolidone as the cause of the anaphylactic reaction.

This report demonstrates a rare case of a type I allergic reaction towards a commonly used ingredient of tablets and widely used disinfectants.

MATERIALS

Silicone

Many severe complications have been reported from direct injection of liquid silicone, and the practice of injecting liquid silicone has largely been abandoned by plastic surgeons (37[R]). Unfortunately, there are still people who perform these injections injudiciously (38[C]).

A 26-year-old male-to-female transsexual received an injection of 100 ml of liquid silicone of unknown grade into her upper lateral thighs to gain female contours (39[A]). Four years later she developed pain and a massively swollen right ankle with signs of inflammation. An MRI scan showed massive diffuse and localized silicone infiltration throughout the soft tissues of the legs.

This case provides further evidence that severe morbidity can be associated with the subcutaneous injection of large volumes of liquid silicone.

Talc

Respiratory Talc is one of the agents most commonly used for producing a pleurodesis in patients with either a spontaneous pneumothorax or a recurrent pleural effusion. However, questions have been raised concerning its safety. In particular, there have been reports of the *acute respiratory distress syndrome* after intrapleural talc either as a slurry (40[R]) or insufflated (41[R], 42[R]). The literature on acute respiratory failure after intrapleural talc has been reviewed, with recommendations on whether talc should continue to be used to produce pleurodesis (43[R]).

There have been at least 32 reported cases of acute respiratory distress syndrome after intrapleural talc. The mechanism is not known, but it may be related to systemic absorption of talc. Since there are effective alternatives for producing pleurodesis (mechanical abrasion if thoracoscopy is performed; tetracycline derivatives or bleomycin if chest tubes are used), intrapleural talc should not be used to produce a pleurodesis.

Thiuram

Three Chinese national servicemen developed an itchy postauricular *rash* (44[A]). None had a history of atopy and all three reported prior use of rubberized spectacle retainers as a curved pliable extension to the posterior ends of the earpieces of their spectacles, to stabilize them while undergoing rigorous military physical training. They were all patch-tested with the National Skin Center standard series and were positive to thiuram mix and the rubberized spectacle retainers. They were treated with topical corticosteroids and were advised to stop wearing their rubberized spectacle retainers.

MEDICAL DEVICES

Catheters

Totally implantable venous devices are being increasingly used in patients who require long-term continuous parenteral drug therapy, especially in cancer chemotherapy. Inevitably there have been complications, the most recent of which was *catheter fracture*, as a consequence of "pinchoff" syndrome (45[A]).

A 67-year-old woman was provided with a totally implantable venous device in the right subclavian vein by the Seldinger technique with a peel-away sheath. The device was used for a course of chemotherapy. After about 1 month there was subcutaneous extravasation of the drug. A chest X-ray showed that the silicone catheter had fractured below the clavicle and the distal portion of the catheter had embolized into the right atrium. The fragments were removed.

This "pinchoff" effect has been reported before. It appears to be due to narrowing of the catheter as it passes over the first rib and beneath the clavicle, when using the Seldinger technique, but it is usually only observed after long-term use. The authors recommend that the cephalic cut-down (Seldinger) technique is best avoided.

Continuous venous access for extended periods is commonly required in patients with cancer for chemotherapy delivery. Transcutaneously tunnelled central venous lines provide one means for the administration of such therapy, although they account for significant costs and morbidity (46[c]). In a prospective study, 923 central venous tunnelled catheters in 791 patients were evaluated for device-specific events. The most important adverse events included 11 insertion complications. Subsequent to placement, a proven or suspected devise-specific complication occurred in 540 lines. For every 10 000 catheter days there were 17.6 *episodes of infection*, 8.1 *thrombotic complications*, 6.9 instances of *catheter breakage*, 3.5 accidental or inadvertent cases of *catheter displacement*, and 0.6 *device leaks*. The devices were in position for a median of 365 days, but the median duration of device-specific complications was 167 days, reflecting a highly significant device salvage rate after complications. The authors concluded that central lines can be placed safely for use in long-term administration of cancer chemotherapy. Factors determining outcome are related to where the device is placed as well as the patient's disease.

Migration of a catheter caused failure of parenteral nutrition in a baby (47[A]).

A premature small 4-day-old girl (34 weeks gestation, birthweight 1000 g) received parenteral nutrition for necrotizing enterocolitis. On day 7, among several septic spots that developed on the skin, an abscess developed on the left shoulder and ruptured spontaneously, leaving a superficial ulcer with purulent discharge. This was cleaned daily with isotonic saline and covered with gauze. On day 11, the blood glucose fell to 1.3 mmol/l and 10% glucose was given. Four further episodes of hypoglycemia during the next 12 hours were similarly treated. Over the next 12 hours the baby became lethargic, hypothermic, and apneic. Her blood glucose remained low (0.9–1.6 mmol/l). Several hours later she became bradycardic and hypotensive. It was then noticed that her bed linen was wet, and some fluid was seen trickling from the ulcer on her shoulder. A chest X-ray showed that the catheter tip had migrated to the left cephalic vein adjacent to the site of the ulcer. Despite rigorous resuscitation she died.

The authors speculated that the catheter tip had spontaneously migrated because the ulcer on the left shoulder had eroded deeply to form a venocutaneous fistula with the left cephalic vein. Continuous leakage of parenteral nutrition fluid through the fistula was soaked up by the gauze pads used to cover the ulcer, preventing early recognition of the problem.

Umbilical venous catheters are commonly used in neonatal care for drug administration and parenteral nutrition. However, many risks are associated with their use. *Ascites* associated with parenteral nutrition has been reported (48[A]).

A girl weighing 1488 g was born by emergency Ceserean section at 28 weeks gestation. An umbilical venous catheter was inserted as sole venous access. An abdominal X-ray showed that the catheter was at the level of T11/T12 in the midline. Owing to complications with oral feeding, parenteral nutrition was begun on day 2. The baby developed necrotizing enterocolitis and had to be ventilated. An abdominal X-ray suggested abdominal ascites. A diagnostic paracentesis produced 90 ml of blood-stained opalescent fluid, which settled to show a white layer on the surface (presumed to be fat emulsion). Following this procedure, respiratory status improved. Ultrasound and aerated saline tests on the umbilical venous catheter suggested that it had not migrated to the peritoneal cavity. However, it was removed and the abdominal distention resolved. The baby was extubated 3 days later and subsequently thrived with no further abdominal problems.

Infection risk Catheter infections in recipients of parenteral nutrition continue cause of concern, especially in children. Such infections can result in line removal, deep vein thrombosis, or an increased risk of liver disease. The incidence of catheter-related infections in 47 children receiving long-term parenteral nutrition has been studied retrospectively, one goal being to identify potential risk factors (49[C]). The children had 125 catheters and 207 catheter-years. The average infection rate was 2.1/1000 parenteral nutrition days. The only factor identified was that early onset of infection after starting parenteral nutrition appeared to predict a poor prognosis.

One of the most prevalent complications of central venous catheters is line-related infection, and HIV-positive subjects are expected to be at even greater risk. A recent prospective study of 212 subjects with HIV infection with 327 central venous catheters has provided evidence of this enhanced risk (50[C]). Over the period 1994-7, 33% were suspected as being infected, although only 61 episodes were diagnosed as catheter-related sepsis. Three variables affected the rate of sepsis: parenteral nutrition, low numbers of circulating CD^+ cells, and a high Apache score.

In a prospective double-blind study, the use of either vancomycin + heparin + ciprofloxacin or vancomycin + heparin flush solution, compared with heparin alone, significantly reduced the infective complications associated with tunneled central venous lines in immunocompromised children. Neither antibiotic could be detected after flushing, and there were no adverse events (51[C]).

Hemodiafiltration

Intensive high-flux hemodiafiltration can be used in the management of drug toxicity. However, this therapy may be associated with *hypophosphatemia*, as demonstrated in two reports of patients with vancomycin toxicity. One patient was treated with an intravenous phosphorus infusion, and in the other hypophosphatemia was corrected by use of a phosphorus-enriched dialysate; this was more efficient than intravenous phosphate (52[A]).

Intrauterine contraceptive devices

Intrauterine contraceptive devices can migrate in the body. Another report of this has appeared (53[A]).

A 29-year-old woman who had had a Copper 7 intrauterine contraceptive device inserted 3 years before developed amenorrhea. The intrauterine contraceptive was not in the uterine cavity and X-ray showed that it was positioned over the sacrum just to the right of the midline and outside the uterus. It later moved to the cecum and became completely embedded in the muscular layer after penetrating the serosal surface.

Vacuum devices

Vacuum tumescence constriction therapy is the use of an external device that creates a vacuum to cause an erection, which is then maintained by a constriction band. It produces rigidity sufficient for intercourse in 91% of men, with satisfaction in 80%.

Adverse effects of this procedure have been reported (54[R]): *ecchymosis* (37%), *discomfort* (28%), *hematoma* (10%), *numbness* (6.9%), *penile skin irritation*, and *edema*. Subcutaneous penile hematoma occurred in two patients using anticoagulants and penile gangrene occurred in one patient; all had worn the constriction band overnight (55[A]). The current recommendation is to apply the constriction band for not more than 30 min.

A 55-year-old African–American, tetraplegic after a motor vehicle accident in 1969, had been using an erection aid device for 4–5 years (56[A]). He used the device, but forgot the constricting ring, which remained on overnight. The next morning his penis was markedly swollen and 2 days later he developed a septicemia. He had a gangrenous penis and necrotizing fasciitis with a foul smelling discharge.

Internet drug sites

The Food and Drug Administration has issued cyber letters (letters sent electronically via the Internet) to a dozen operators of foreign-based Internet sites that offer to sell online drugs that may be illegal (57[S]). The letters warn these website operators that they may be engaged in illegal activities, and inform them of the laws that govern drug sales in the USA. This is the first time that the FDA has used the Internet as a means for reaching those who are potentially violating the Federal Food, Drug, and Cosmetic Act, and it represents a new stage in the Agency's efforts to protect the public against illegal and potentially dangerous products sold through web sites.

The cyber letters are electronic versions similar to traditional warning or untitled letters that the Agency has for a long time sent to organizations or individuals it believes are engaged in illegal activities. These letters usually outline the nature of the alleged violation and request a formal response.

Consumers who want information about online pharmacies, or who want to report web

Table 1. *Miscellaneous reports*

Drug	Adverse effect(s)	Reference
Amaranth	Allergic reactions (asthma etc)	(58[R])
Collagen	Foreign body reactions	(59[c])
Dimethylacetamide	Hallucinations, delusions, pulmonary edema	(60[c])
Ethylenediamine	Allergy, occupational asthma	(61[c])
Fluoride	Dental and skeletal fluorosis; impaired development of intelligence	(62[R])
Glycerol	Rotatory vertigo with vertical nystagmus	(63[c])
Indigo carmine	Anaphylactoid reaction; cardiac arrest	(64[c])
Methylene blue	Severe hemolytic reactions	(65[r])
Parathion	Acute intoxication	(66[R])
Polyoxyethylene lauryl ether	Follicular contact dermatitis	(67[c])
Potassium chloride	Drug-induced esophagitis	(68[c])
Sodium prasterone sulfate	Anaphylactic reactions	(69[C])
Sorbic acid	Systemic contact dermatitis	(70[c])
Titanium alloy prosthesis	Cytogenic damage	(71[R])

sites that they believe may be acting illegally, can contact the FDA through its web site at www.fda.gov/oc/buyonline/.

MISCELLANEOUS

Miscellaneous reports are listed in Table 1.

REFERENCES

1. Pal B, Keenan J, Misra HN, Moussa K, Morris J. Raynaud's phenomenon in idiopathic carpal tunnel syndrome. Scand J Rheumatol 1996; 25: 143–5.
2. Robbins PI, Raymond L. Aspartame and symptoms of carpal tunnel syndrome. J Occup Environ Med 1994; 41: 418.
3. Levine DW, Simmons BP, Koris MJ. A self-administered questionnaire for the assessment of severity of symptoms and functional status in carpal tunnel syndrome. J Bone Joint Surg Am 1993; 75: 1585–92.
4. Trefz F, De Sonneville L, Matthis P, Benninger C, Lanz-Englert B, Bickl H. Neuropsychological and biochemical investigations in heterozygotes for phenylketonuria during ingestion of high dose aspartame (a sweetener containing phenylalanine). Hum Genet 1994; 93: 369–74.
5. Koehler SM, Glaros A. The effect of aspartame on migraine headache. Headache 1988; 28: 10–13.
6. Lipton A, Theriault RL, Hortobagyi GM, Simeone J, Knight RD, Mellars K, Reitsma DJ, Heffernan M, Seaman JJ. Pamidronate prevents skeletal complications and is effective palliative treatment in women with breast carcinoma and osteolytic bone metstases. Cancer 2000; 88: 1082–90.
7. Siris ES. Biphosphonates and iritis. Lancet 1993; 341: 436–7.
8. Macarol V, Fraunfelder FT. Pamidronate disodium and possible ocular adverse drug reactions. Am J Ophthalmol 1994; 118: 220–4.
9. Ghose K, Waterworth R, Trolove P, Highton J. Uveitis associated with pamidronate. Aust NZ J Med 1994; 24: 320.
10. O'Donnell NP, Rao GP, Aguis-Fernandez A. Paget's disease: ocular complications of disodium pamidronate treatment. Br J Clin Pract 1995; 49: 272–3.
11. Ryan PJ, Blake GM, Davie M, Haddaway M, Gibson T, Fogelman I. Intermittent oral disodium pamidronate in established osteoporosis: a 2-year double-masked placebo-controlled study of efficacy and safety. Osteoporosis Int 2000; 11: 171–6.
12. Larsen K-O, Stray N, Engh V, Sandnes D. Oesophagus lesions associated with biphosphonates. Tidsskr Nor Laegeforen 2000; 120: 2397–9.
13. Anonymous. Disulfiram. Liver reactions. WHO Newslett 2000; 4: 11.
14. Kiec Swierczynska M, Krecisz B, Fabicka B. Systemic contact dermatitis from implanted disulfiram. Contact Dermatitis 2000; 43: 246–7.

15. Hainer MI, Naoky T, Komura ST, Chiu C. Fatal hepatorenal failure associated with hydrazine sulfate. Ann Intern Med 2000; 133: 877–80.
16. Harries AD, Baird A, Rhodes J. Non-smoking: a feature of ulcerative colitis. Br Med J 1982; 284: 706.
17. Sommerville KW, Logan RFA, Edmond M. Smoking and Crohn's disease. Br Med J 1984; 289: 954–6.
18. Green JT, Rhodes J, Thomas GAO. Clinical status of current smokers with ulcerative colitis. Am J Gastroenterol 1998; 93: 1463–7.
19. Cottone M, Rosselli M, Orlando A. Smoking habits and recurrence in Crohn's disease. Gastroenterology 1994; 106: 643–8.
20. Pereira CB, Strupp M, Eggert T. Straube A, Brandt T. Nicotine induced nystagmus: three-dimensional analysis and dependence on head position. Neurology 2000; 55: 1563–5.
21. Huang QL, Feig DS, Blackstein ME. Development of tertiary hyperparathyroidism after phosphate supplementation in oncogenic osteomalacia. J Endocrinol Invest 2000; 23: 263–7.
22. Abubakar K, Goggin N, Gormallly S, Durnin M, Drumm B. Preparing the bowel for colonoscopy. Arch Dis Child 1995; 73: 459–61.
23. Craig JC, Hodson EM, Martin HCO. Phosphate enema poisoning in children. Med J Aust 1994; 160: 347–51.
24. Helikson MA, Parham WS, Tobias JD. Hypocalcemia and hyperphosphatemia after phosphate enema use in a child. J Pediatr Surg 1997; 32: 1244–6.
25. Ismail EAR, Al-Mutairi G, Al-Anzy H. A fatal small dose of phosphate enema in a young child with no renal or gastrointestinal abnormality. J Pediatr Gastroenterol Nutr 2000; 30: 220–1.
26. Brady CE III, DiPalma JA, Morawski SG, Santa Ana CS, Fordtran JS. Urinary excretion of polyethylene glycol 3350 and sulfate after gut lavage solution. Gastroenterology 1986; 90: 1914–18.
27. Anonymous. PEG electrolyte lavage solutions: drug evaluation monograph. Englewood (CO): Micromedex Inc, 1999: 1–21.
28. Franga DL, Harris JA. Polyethylene glycol-induced pancreatitis. Gastrointest Endosc 2000; 52: 789–91.
29. Anonymous. Sodium citrate (triCitrasol). Warning: cardiac arrest. WHO Newslett 2000; 2: 6.
30. Korkmaz A, Sahiner Ü, Yurdakök M. Chemical burn caused by topical vinegar application in a newborn infant. Pediatr Dermatol 2000; 17: 34–6.
31. Perseghin P, Balduzzi A, Bonanomi S, Dasi M, Buscemi F. Infusion-related side-effects in children undergoing autologous hematopoietic stem cell transplantation for acute leukemia. Bone Marrow Transplant 2000; 26: 116–18.
32. Held JL, Ruszkowski AM, Deleo VA. Consort contact dermatitis due to oak moss. Arch Dermatol 1988; 124: 261–2.
33. Gonçalo S, Cabral F, Gonçalo M. Contact sensitivity to oak moss. Contact Dermatitis 1988: 19: 355–7.
34. Hodgson G. Eczemas associated with lubricants and metal-working fluids. Dermatol Dig 1976: Oct: 11–15.
35. Owen CM, August PJ, Beck MH. Contact allergy to oak moss resin in a soluble oil. Contact Dermatitis 2000; 43: 112.
36. Ronnau AC, Wulferink M, Gleichmann E, Unver E, Ruzicka T, Krutmann J, Grewe M. Anaphylaxis to polyvinylpyrrolidone in an analgesic preparation. Br J Dermatol 2000; 143: 1055–8.
37. Behar TA, Anderson EE, Barwick WJ, Mohler JL. Sclerosing lipogranulomatosis: a case report of scrotal injection of automobile transmission fluid and literature review of subcutaneous injection of oils. Plast Reconstr Surg 1993; 91: 352–61.
38. Chen TH. Silicone injection granulomas of the breast: treatment by subcutaneous mastectomy and immediate subpectoral breast implant. Br J Plast Surg 1995; 48: 71–6.
39. Hofer SOP, Damen A, Nicolai CPA. Large volume liquid silicone injection in the upper thighs: a never ending story. Eur J Plast Surg 2000; 23: 241–4.
40. Rinaldo JE, Owens GR, Rogers RM. Adult respiratory distress syndrome following intrapleural instillation of talc. J Thorac Cardiovasc Surg 1983; 85: 523–6.
41. Rehse DH, Aye RW, Florence MG. Respiratory failure following talc pleurodesis. Am J Surg 1999; 177: 437–40.
42. Nandy P. Recurrent spontaneous pneumothorax: an effective method of talc poudrage. Chest 1980; 77: 493–5.
43. Light RW. Diseases of the pleura: the use of talc for pleurodesis. Curr Opin Pulm Med 2000; 6: 255–8.
44. Leow Y-H, Ng S-K, Goh C-L. An unusual cause of post-auricular dermatitis. Contact Dermatitis 2000; 42: 308.
45. Carlo I, Fisichella P, Russello D, Puleo S, Latteri F. Catheter fracture and cardiac migration: a rare complication of totally implantable venous devices. J Surg Oncol 2000; 73: 172–3.
46. Schwartz RE, Coit DG, Groeger JS. Transcutaneously tunneled central venous lines in cancer patients: an analysis of device-related morbidity factors based on prospective data collection. Ann Surg Oncol 2000; 7: 441–9.
47. Cheah F-C, Boo N-Y. An unusual case of refractory hypoglycaemia in a neonate receiving total parenteral nutrition. Acta Paediatr 2000; 89: 497–8.
48. Panetta J, Morley C, Betheras R. Ascites in a premature baby due to parenteral nutrition from an umbilical venous catheter. J Paediatr Child Health 2000; 36: 197–8.
49. Colomb V, Fabeiro M, Dabbas M, Goulet O, Merckx J, Ricour C. Central venous catheter-related infections in children on long-term home parenteral nutrition: incidence and risk factors. Clin Nutr 2000. 19: 355–9.
50. Tacconelli E, Tumbarello M, de Gaetano-Donati K, Bertagnolio S, Pittiruti M, Leone F, Morace G, Cauda R. Morbidity associated with

central venous catheter-use in a cohort of 212 hospitalized subjects with HIV infection. J Hosp Infect 2000; 44: 186–92.

51. Henrickson KJ, Axtell RA, Hoover SM, Kuhn SM, Pritchett J, Kehl SC, Klein JP. Prevention of central venous catheter-related infections and thrombotic events in immunocompromised children by the use of vancomycin/ciprofloxacin/heparin flush solution: a randomized, multicenter, double-blind trial. J Clin Oncol 2000; 18: 1269–78.
52. Gatchalian RA, Popli A, Ejaz AA, Leehey DJ, Kjellstrand CM, Ing TS. Management of hypophosphatemia induced by high-flux hemodiafiltration for the treatment of vancomycin toxicity: intravenous phosphorus therapy versus use of a phosphorus-enriched dialysate. Am J Kidney Dis 2000; 36: 1262–6.
53. Sarkar P. Translocation of a Copper 7 intrauterine contraceptive device with subsequent penetration of the caecum: case report and review. Br J Fam Plann 2000: 26; 161.
54. Witherington R. Vacuum constriction device for management of erectile impotence. J Urol 1989; 141: 320–2.
55. Rivas DA, Chancellor MD. Complications associated with the use of vacuum constriction devices for erectile dysfunction in spinal cord injured patients. J Am Paraplegia Soc 1994; 17: 136–9.
56. Eltorai I, Mentory R, Laurente. F. Gangrene of the penis in a tetraplegic due to the use of vacuum constriction device for erection. Sex Disabil 2000; 18: 105-14.
57. Anonymous. Illegal internet drug sites. Cautionary "cyber" letters sent. WHO Newslett 2000; 2: 5.
58. Bossert J, Wahl R. Amaranth: a new allergen in bakeries. Allergologie 2000; 23: 448–57.
59. Moody BR, Sengelmann RD, Klein AW. Self-limited adverse reaction to human-derived collagen injectable product. Dermatol Surg 2000; 26: 936–8.
60. Su TC, Lin PH, Chin MJ, Chu TS, Chang MJW, Wang JD, Cheng TJ. Dimethylacetamide, ethylenediamine, and diphenylmethane diisocyanate poisoning manifest as acute psychosis and pulmonary edema: treatment with hemoperfusion. J Toxicol Clin Toxicol 2000; 38: 429–33.
61. Asakawa H, Araki T, Yamamoto N, Imai I, Yamane M, Tsutsumi Y, Kawakami F. Allergy to ethylenediamine and steroid. J Invest Allergol Clin Immunol 2000; 10: 372–4.
62. Lu Y, Sun ZR, Wu LN, Wang X, Lu W, Liu SS. Effect of high-fluoride water on intelligence in children. Fluoride 2000; 33: 74–8.
63. Mizuta K, Furuta M, Ito Y, Sawai S, Fujigaki M, Horibe M, Miyata H. A case of Menière's disease with vertical nystagmus after administration of glycerol. Auris Nasus Larynx 2000; 27: 271–4.
64. Gousse AE, Safir MH, Madjar S, Ziadlourad F, Raz S. Life-threatening anaphylactoid reaction associated with indigo carmine intravenous injection. Urology 2000; 56: 508iii–508iv.
65. Gauthier TW. Methylene blue-induced hyperbilirubinemia in neonatal glucose-6-phosphate dehydrogenase (G6PD) deficiency. J Matern-Fetal Med 2000; 9: 252–4.
66. Marques EGP, Oliveira MM, Monsanto PV, Proenca P, Castanheira F, Vieira DN. Parathion and acute intoxication. The importance of toxicological analytic tests. Z Zagodnien Nauk Sadowych 2000; 43: 157–63.
67. Kimura M, Kawada A. Follicular contact dermatitis due to polyoxyethylene laurylether. J Am Acad Dermatol 2000; 42: 879–80.
68. O'Donnell J. Drug-induced esophagitis. J Pharm Pract 2000; 13: 290–6.
69. Anonymous. Sodium prasterone sulfate: anaphylactoid reactions. WHO Newslett 2000; 2: 6.
70. Raison Peron N, Maynadier JM, Maynadier J. Sorbic acid: an unusual cause of systemic contact dermatitis in an infant. Contact Dermatitis 2000; 43: 247–8.
71. Stea S, Visentin M, Granchi D, Savarino L, Dallari D, Gualtieri G, Rollo G, Toni A, Pizzoferrato A, Montanaro L. Sister chrometic exchange in patients with joint prostheses. J Arthroplasty 2000; 15: 772–7.

I. Ralph Edwards and Sten Olsson

50 The WHO International Drug Monitoring Programme

History

The WHO International Drug Monitoring Programme was established in 1968 as a pilot project, with the participation of ten countries that had organized national pharmacovigilance systems at that time. The intention was to develop international collaboration to make it easier to detect rare adverse drug reactions not revealed during clinical trials. The International Drug Monitoring Centre was moved from WHO headquarters in Geneva, Switzerland, to a WHO Collaborating Centre for International Drug Monitoring in Uppsala, Sweden, in 1978. This was the result of an agreement between the WHO and the Swedish Government, by which Sweden assumed the operational responsibility for the Programme. WHO headquarters, Geneva, retained the responsibility for policy matters. The Collaborating Centre is often referred to as the Uppsala Monitoring Centre (UMC). Information about the WHO and the UMC can be obtained from their websites: www.who.int and www.who-umc.org.

A new negotiation between the WHO and Swedish Government is complete, and the Uppsala Monitoring Centre is now a non-profit-making foundation, with a Board appointed partly by the WHO and partly by the Swedish Government, as well as having a jointly agreed Director.

Vision and goals of the Uppsala Monitoring Centre

It is the aim of the Uppsala Monitoring Centre to support WHO's leadership in the field of world health by providing excellence:

- in the science and concepts of all aspects of pharmacovigilance;
- to prevent harm to humans from the effects of medicines;
- to gather and share objective intelligence and opinion in the field of drug safety through open and transparent means of communication;
- to support the promotion of the rational use of drugs, and the achievement of improved patient therapy and public health;
- in global education and communications in benefit, harm, effectiveness, and risk in medical therapy.

This will be achieved by the following activities:

- developing leading-edge systems and science for the identification and communication of safety hazards from drugs and other substances used in medicine;
- carrying out research that pushes forward the ethical, intellectual, and scientific boundaries of theory and practice in pharmacovigilance;
- pursuing active collaboration and communication with all stakeholders;
- pursuing the goal of a single global database for drug safety data.

The Uppsala Monitoring Centre will particularly:

- ensure that effective, timely, international collective effort will never miss a signal of a potential hazard;
- ensure that all stakeholders evaluate and learn from decisions and actions through positive impact-assessment, follow-up, and debate;
- encourage the growth of pharmacovigilance

Side Effects of Drugs, Annual 25
J.K. Aronson, ed.

activities around the world, in particular the establishment of new National Centres;
- promote existing National Centres and other stakeholders in the field;
- contribute actively to the global vision of the WHO Programme;
- use and share available information openly and transparently;
- sponsor and support others in their pharmacovigilance activities;
- exploit fully the resources of the Uppsala Monitoring Centre ;
- stimulate the development of coherent, harmonized systems worldwide for pharmacovigilance, through education, training, promoting and participating in international forums, promoting best practice, and the publication of guidelines;
- maintain and develop useful products, services, and tools in pursuit of the vision and goals of the WHO Programme and the Uppsala Monitoring Centre.

Current programme structure

At present 67 countries are active members of the WHO Programme. Several countries each year have formally applied for membership, and they are considered associated members while the issue of the technical compatibility of their reports with the WHO requirements is established. Member countries and associated member countries are listed in Table 1.

In each country a national centre or system, designated by the competent health authority, is responsible for collection, processing, and evaluation of adverse reaction case reports submitted by health professionals. Information obtained from these reports is passed back to the professionals on a national basis, but is also submitted to the WHO Centre for inclusion in the international database. Collectively the centres annually provide over 200 000 individual reports to WHO of reactions suspected of being drug-induced. The cumulative data base of the WHO Programme now comprises nearly 3 million case reports.

Case reports submitted to the WHO centre according to an agreed format are checked for technical correctness and then incorporated into the international database in a weekly routine. The material is screened at least four times a year for new and serious reactions, as well as the reporting frequencies of associations of particular interest. Many additional examinations of the data are made on an ad hoc basis. A new database has been constructed that will allow the storage of much more information, as proposed by the Council of Organizations of Medical Sciences (CIOMS) monograph 1(a) (1^S) and adapted by the International Conference on Harmonization (ICH), project E2B.

Signal finding

Each national centre reasonably focuses on its own country's issues and data, turning to international information for secondary support. The WHO Programme has the only international repository of adverse drug reactions reports in which one can look at the pooled information for signals on all reported medicinal products from around the world. The need for automated tools to help deal with all this information is great, but the tools must be such that they do not obscure the tentative nature of the information and conclusions. The tools must aid human review and not replace it. It is a truism that people do not cope with large amounts of information, let alone multiple variables, missing data, and data of variable quality. A combination of automatic signaling devices and scanning by experienced medical personnel is now considered by the Uppsala Monitoring Centre most advantageous in successfully fulfilling the original aim of the programme, i.e. the early identification of new adverse drug reactions. In 1998 new methods developed at the Uppsala Monitoring Centre, using a Bayesian Confidence Propagation Neural Network (BCPNN) (2, 3) in analysing the database, were put into routine use. These methods provide a quantitative measure of the strength of association of a drug/reaction combination in the database (4). The BCPNN method has been tested as a routine tool for finding new adverse drug reactions in the WHO database; its positive predictive value is a little less than 50%, but its negative predictive value is about 85% (5).

When the new data have been processed and entered into the database, a BCPNN scan is run to generate statistical measurements for each combination of drug and adverse reaction. The resulting Combinations database is made available to national centres and pharmaceutical companies, in the latter case including only information on the company's own patented products. The database is presented in a

Table 1. *Members of the WHO International Drug Monitoring Programme and their year of entry*

Country	Year of entry	Country	Year of entry	Country	Year of entry
Argentina	1994	Greece	1990	Portugal	1993
Armenia	2001	Hungary	1990	Romania	1976
Australia	1968	Iceland	1990	Russia	1998
Austria	1991	India	1998	Singapore	1993
Belgium	1977	Indonesia	1990	Slovak Republic	1993
Brazil	2001	Iran	1998	South Africa	1992
Bulgaria	1975	Ireland	1968	Spain	1984
Canada	1968	Israel	1973	Sri Lanka	2000
Chile	1996	Italy	1975	Sweden	1968
China, PR	1998	Japan	1972	Switzerland	1991
Costa Rica	1991	Korea, Republic of	1992	Tanzania	1993
Croatia	1992	Latvia	2002	Thailand	1984
Cuba	1994	Macedonia	2000	Tunisia	1993
Cyprus	2000	Malaysia	1990	Turkey	1987
Czech Republic	1992	Mexico	1998	Ukraine	2002
Denmark	1968	Morocco	1992	United Kingdom	1968
Egypt	2001	Netherlands	1968	Uruguay	2002
Estonia	1998	New Zealand	1968	USA	1968
Fiji Islands	1999	Norway	1971	Venezuela	1995
Finland	1974	Oman	1995	Vietnam	1999
France	1986	Peru	2002	Yugoslavia FR	2000
Germany	1968	Philippines	1995	Zimbabwe	1998
Ghana	2001	Poland	1972		
Associated member countries					
Bahrain		Moldova		Pakistan	
Kyrgyz Republic		Netherlands Antilles			

computerized form, which facilitates searching and sorting of the information.

An associations database is generated by selecting those combinations that pass a preset threshold. Based on the results of the test runs of the BCPNN, the threshold level for associations is that of the lower 95% confidence limit of the Information Component crossing zero when a new batch of reports is added. The Information Component in information theory is a measure of disproportionality, indicating how strongly a data field or complex of data fields stands out from the background of information value.

All associations are followed automatically for 2 years, the data being checked at 6-monthly intervals. After the final listing, an association may be reintroduced for another 2-year follow-up. The associations are also copied to a cumulative log file (history file), which serves as a filter to exclude combinations that have in previous quarters passed the threshold level. This will prevent drug–reaction combinations with a confidence limit that fluctuates around zero from being repeatedly fed into the review process.

The associations database is sent to the expert review panel for evaluation. Before distributing the database, associations are checked against standard reference sources (e.g. the Physician's Desk Reference, Martindale's Extra Pharmacopoeia), and the published literature (using, for example, Medline and Reactions Weekly). This facilitates the review and identifies those associations that have at least been identified previously, even if they are not generally known.

Up to the Associations stage the process is purely quantitative, but clinical knowledge and judgement is necessary for the evaluation of associations, and is provided by the national centres and expert reviewers. The Uppsala Monitoring Centre triages case reports sent out for review into different categories of interest, such as "new drugs associated with serious reactions and rapidly changing Information Component values" and "drugs associated with agranulocytosis/rhabdomyolysis/etc". This allows reviewers to focus on their interest areas and thereby to reduce their workload.

Short summaries of reviewers' findings are circulated to participating national centres in a memorandum called "Signal". An investigation has shown that the WHO Programme is successful in finding new drug–reaction associations at an early stage and in providing useful information about them to national centres. Individualized sections of the Signal document can be provided to companies on a subscription basis (only on their patented products).

As with the associations, all signals will be automatically reassessed on a 6-monthly basis, for 2 years, with a possibility of re-introduction for follow-up, and also copied to a history file for easy tracking. The follow-up system also allows renewed consideration of associations for which there was initially not enough information to merit signaling. Signals that are later supported by new evidence can also be highlighted. The nature of the signal will determine what measures need be taken in terms of follow-up.

A larger numbers of variables than the routine drug–reaction combinations can also be considered using the Bayesian approach described above. Searching and sorting of the associations data can be done, not only on drug, adverse reaction, and the various statistical measurements, but also on System Organ Class and on therapeutic drug groups using the Anatomical–Therapeutic–Chemical (ATC) classification (6).

The system can be used in other ways. For example, a specific pair of adverse reactions can be highly associated with a specific drug, or the effects can be determined of any other report variable or combination of variables on the "information component" values. In addition, the effects of including drugs reported as "concomitant medications" can be studied using the BCPNN. One of the outcomes of these analyses might be to identify patient subgroups at particularly high risk of a specific adverse reaction to a specific drug. Another possibility is to establish that a drug safety problem is related to a particular country, or region, or a certain time period. However, it should be pointed out that, in order for these data to be useful, a substantial number of case reports is required.

The BCPNN has also been used for the first time for "unsupervised pattern recognition" of multiple variables in the database. This is being developed into a routine tool.

Reference source and database

The database of the WHO Programme is a unique reference source that is used in many different circumstances. When a national centre receives the first report of an unfamiliar drug–reaction association the WHO database is often consulted to find out whether a similar observation has been made elsewhere in the world. If so, the initial signal may be strengthened. National centres are provided with an annual reference document that provides summary figures of suspected drug–reaction associations reported to the WHO. On-line search facilities are also at the disposal of national centres for up-to-date checking of what has been reported.

A new database will allow better access for external searching, coming into operation during the second half of 2002. New search tools will also be introduced.

In order to speed up the accrual of useful case data, a primary consideration is the structure of databases. In the past, database structure has been limited in the number of fields provided, partly because of limited computer storage capacity, but also because single-sheet reporting forms have been thought to be user friendly and that reporters would be put off reporting by what appeared to be a lengthy questionnaire.

This has meant that the information sent to national centres has been limited by the design of the forms used, and that sent to the WHO database has been further limited because of storage capacity. In the modern world all that has changed. It is possible to capture information for reporting from the doctor's notes and prescribing information in an automated way, thus making the reporting of more data much easier. We have collaborated with ICH on international agreement on information technology standards for the transmission of data in a secure way. With first CIOMS (1) and then with

ICH we have developed a comprehensive set of data fields; these have been included in our new database, which is now complete (7, 8). The new database has great complexity, and it seems unlikely that many of the available fields will be completed until a "paperless" system comes into operation in several countries. The new database is fully compatible with the old one. To provide flexibility for users with varying requirements and sophistication is a great challenge, but we are hopeful that the new database will pave the way for the international availability of much more useful case data, without recourse to the original provider for more details.

Quantification

There is a general need to quantify adverse drug reactions information. Under-reporting of adverse reactions in routine monitoring is the norm. However, the degree of under-reporting differ from time to time, from place to place, and from drug to drug. The WHO centre is working jointly with IMS International, to analyse adverse reaction reports together with drug use data from different countries. This allows national differences in reporting rates to be further analysed for reasons that may be due to differences in indications for use, medical practice, demographics, etc. Several new signals have been evaluated in this way, often making it clearer what biases might be present both geographically and over time. Bearing such problems in mind, cautious comparisons of reporting rates between medicinal products are often revealing (9–12). This type of analysis of international data serves as a guide to the need for more precise pharmacoepidemiological investigations.

A clearing house for information

The Uppsala Monitoring Centre has an important role to play as a communication centre – a clearing house for information on drug safety at the service of drug regulatory agencies, the pharmaceutical industry, researchers, and other groups in need of drug safety information (13, 14). Requests for special database searches and investigations are received from the these parties at a rate of around 275 per year. In addition, flexible on-line retrieval programmes are made available, by which the database users may perform a variety of standardized searches by themselves. Access for non-member parties is subjected to confidentiality restrictions agreed by Programme members. Countries have the right to refuse the release of their own information if they so wish, and some do. Use of the information released is subject to a caveat document as to its proper use. Detailed manuals for the on-line service and the customized retrievals on request are available from the Uppsala centre.

National centres are provided with the WHO Pharmaceuticals Newsletter, distributed by the Health Technology & Pharmaceuticals department of WHO headquarters. The Uppsala Monitoring Centre is responsible for the information that is included in the drug safety section of this newsletter, leading to wide distribution of the information to all member countries of the WHO. An agreement with ADIS Press has allowed information from newsletters produced by members of the WHO Programme to be printed in "Reactions Weekly". This journal is made available to national centres and greatly enhances their access to up-to-the-minute information on adverse drug reactions.

"Uppsala Reports" is the name of a bulletin that is made freely available to all interested parties by the Uppsala Monitoring Centre. It provides an easy-to-read account of news about pharmacovigilance, the WHO Programme, and its members and services.

Communications within the WHO Programme have improved with the increasing use of electronic communications media. The Uppsala Monitoring Centre maintains an e-mail discussion group called "Vigimed", which allows rapid exchange of information around the world on drug safety matters. Membership is restricted to persons connected with national pharmacovigilance centres.

The Internet home page of the WHO Programme (http://www.who-umc.org) was introduced in 1996. It is intended to be developed into a dynamic tool for communications with all clients of the Uppsala Monitoring Centre. Recently Internet-based seminars and training courses were introduced on the Uppsala Monitoring Centre web site.

The Uppsala Monitoring Centre publishes a book, "National Pharmacovigilance Systems – Country Profiles and Overview" (15), in which the operating procedures of the national centres that participate in the WHO Programme are described.

Terminologies and standards

The WHO Programme has assumed responsibility for developing a standardized adverse reactions terminology (WHO–ART) and a comprehensive index of reported drugs (WHO–DD), both of which have a utility beyond their importance to the monitoring system. These tools are used in the premarketing safety area, as well as for postmarketing studies by many pharmaceutical companies. WHO–ART has also been adopted by the International Programme on Chemical Safety as the medical terminology to describe poisoning incidents.

The WHO Drug Dictionary (WHO–DD) is unique in its coverage of drugs marketed throughout the world. It is available in hard copy or as computer files. The Uppsala Centre is developing it further, to incorporate more detailed information and make it compatible with the prestandard proposed by the European Committee for Standardization (CEN). In response to the challenge to safety monitoring offered by traditional herbal remedies, the WHO centre has taken initiatives to improve the classification systems for such medicines. In a joint project (16–19) with institutions such as the Royal Botanical Gardens, Kew, in the UK, others in South Africa and in the Netherlands, and including the phytotherapy industry, a system compatible with the ATC system used for modern synthetic medicines has been developed. This will soon be added to the WHO–DD. Input from experts from all parts of the world, representing different therapeutic traditions, will be indispensable for the further development of this project.

The way in which adverse drug reactions terminology is used is an important factor in data mining. The development of definitions and guidelines for the use of terms is paramount. We have worked with CIOMS in this area, resulting in the publication of definitions that are useful in pharmacovigilance (20). It is hoped that this work can be extended. In data mining, the hierarchical linkage between terms is less important. On the other hand we are aware of the need by many people for some harmony in this area. The advent of MedDRA as a commercial terminology has caused some difficulties, since it is not yet clear that it represents a clear improvement over all. The WHO and Uppsala Monitoring Centre are actively looking at ways in which the different terminologies can be used in a parallel fashion, while we find a way forward that will offer clear benefits. One obvious proposal is to link WHO–ART with the world standard, the International Classification of Disease (ICD 9 and 10). This we are pursuing, since ICD has the advantage of having a core structure onto which variants can be grafted in a transparent way. There are already domain versions of ICD, for example in neurology and psychiatry, which follow the common ICD logic. Definitions for terms are already available in ICD. The advantage to WHO in maintaining such a unbiased, normative terminology, which can be used for any aspect of public health epidemiology in any country in the world, and at minimal cost, must be clear.

Within the WHO Programme a number of definitions of commonly used terms, like adverse reaction, side effect, adverse event, signal, have been worked out. These definitions contribute to a harmonized way of communicating both inside and outside the Programme (21). However, approaches to, and the extent of, pharmacovigilance are being considered all the time. New definitions therefore need to be considered (22^{R}).

Education

In order to foster education and communication in pharmacovigilance, every second year the WHO Centre offers a 2-week training course in "Pharmacovigilance – the Study of Adverse Drug Reactions" in Uppsala, to which 25 health-care professionals are accepted. The course is divided into two modules. The first is about spontaneous monitoring and the practicalities of managing a drug monitoring centre. This section also offers hands-on experience in using the database of the WHO Programme. The second module is an introduction to wider issues in pharmacoepidemiology.

There is an increasing trend towards local and regional meetings and courses in pharmacovigilance. The WHO Programme often takes part in such meetings, particularly those organized in developing countries, to provide support and technical advice.

Support to national centres

Along with the provision of the new database (which is also offered as a single-stop repository for industry reports, rather than their sending them to each national centre), we are planning to give more active support to national centres for the development of information technology (IT). Many delays in transmission of reports to the WHO are secondary to a variety of technical difficulties, which must be minimized.

Through a consortium of IT providers directed by the Uppsala Monitoring Centre, it is possible to provide a relatively inexpensive IT solution for national centres and others, which is compatible with the WHO database and conforms to ICH standards.

Harm and risk

The consideration of benefit/effectiveness versus harm/risk has so far been almost entirely at a descriptive level. Most of the work so far in this area is confined to describing the benefits and the risks separately for each medicinal product. The more difficult task of deriving a useful analysis and then a synthesis of the information is accorded much less attention.

The situation is changing and there is an increasing effort to give semi-quantitative tabular summaries of information for all medicines that might be used for a specific indication. On the other hand, there is a need for an improved conceptual approach to what is benefit and harm, effectiveness and risk, as well as more technical thinking over how to improve comparisons between medicinal products (23–25).

We are also working on publications and guidelines that will aid the everyday diagnosis of adverse drug reactions and their management.

Communication

Through its consultants, the Uppsala Monitoring Centre continues to offer advice and training on all aspects of the communication of the complex messages of benefit and harm, effectiveness and risk to all stakeholders in drug safety (26). The WHO and Uppsala Monitoring Centre are working on new guidelines and publications, which will be ready early in 2002 to try to improve knowledge of pharmacovigilance, and to expand the horizons beyond searching for new signals to new medicinal products. This includes issues that vary from new professional concerns (such as poisoning by drugs, fraudulent drugs, and adverse reactions to herbal remedies) to promoting the view that consumer reports have unique importance in telling us what patients feel about the adverse events they experience. They may not be telling us about new adverse reactions, but they are giving us their concerns, which must be considered and acted upon (27, 28). A new CIOMS monograph on key issues of communication in the medicines safety area will be available in 2002.

Annual meetings

Every year representatives of national centres are invited to a meeting arranged jointly by the WHO and one of the participating countries. At these meetings technical issues are discussed, in relation to how to improve global drug monitoring in general and concerning individual drug safety problems. Since the meetings have very high attendance rates, they are important for establishment and maintenance of personal relationships and subsequently contribute to good communications.

Collaboration with other organizations

Cooperation with organizations that are interested in developing early signals of significance is of importance in achieving safer drug therapy. The International Society for Pharmacoepidemiology (ISPE) is specifically interested in the science of pharmacovigilance, and the Council for International Organizations of Medical Sciences (CIOMS) is pivotal in bringing interested parties together to mount various collaborative projects. Much support has been given to the International Society of Pharmacovigilance (ISOP).

WHO is also involved in the ICH processes, as observers at all meetings, and the Uppsala Monitoring Centre provides additional technical advice to WHO when required.

Developments needed in the immediate future

Given the considerations above, the biggest challenge we face is how to manage efficiently the large amount of risk information that accumulates while a medicinal product is being aggressively marketed (29). Our failure to cope with this challenge can have two opposite consequences: failure to recognize a signal early and the unnecessary exposure of patients to harm, and deletion of a medicinal product due to hasty action on poorly considered information.

Many will argue that pharmacoepidemiology and the use of, mainly, case-control studies will provide a surer answer to safety questions. The extent to which this is true is very limited, for the following reasons. Most medicines safety signals, including those that arise from how the particular product was used, come from experience contained in accumulated single case reports. It is not possible to perform an epidemiological analysis of each signal: the cost is prohibitive. Case–control studies suffer from biases, just as case reports do. Case–control studies, while very suitable for rare events, often have problems of power from a practical standpoint. Rare but clinically serious events are not easily investigated without long multicentre studies, and sometimes cannot be reasonably investigated at all by this method.

The use of continuous, comprehensive, and rigorously collected data on medicinal products and their use to provide information on benefit and harm, has long been seen as attractive. Post-marketing surveillance of a restricted number of medicines (used as a continuous method in New Zealand and the UK) has provided useful new information on a limited range of medical products, with limited comparative opportunities. Health-care databases mainly in the USA and UK have also been useful. Their limitations are size and their structure, which does not necessarily allow all the relevant information to be collected, nor for the finding of new signals relating to properties of medicines or their use: their role has been restricted to hypothesis testing using nested studies.

Almost the whole effort of this vast collection machinery for clinical case report information is directed towards finding new adverse reactions signals. Little use is made of the data for other signal work, such as finding at-risk groups (do some adverse reactions occur disproportionately with age?), interactions (do known reactions occur more frequently with certain drug combinations?), or use-related adverse reactions (do certain reactions occur more often in certain countries? at higher doses?). This is not surprising, since the quantity of data is so great and most national centres have few resources.

Several needs are apparent if we are to meet the challenges of the future. Amongst the most important are:

I. To encourage clinicians to report clinical experience. The concentration only on new and rare adverse reactions to new drugs is not going to help us get information that will allow us to tackle avoidable reactions adequately (30).
II. To give advice about the diagnosis and management of adverse reactions.
III. To improve the rapid transmission of quality information to national centres and industry, and thence to the WHO database.
IV. To bridge the gap between a tentative signal from raw adverse reactions data to observational studies that use specific protocols and to clinical outcomes (31).
V. To link genetic information with adverse reactions.

The USA is already reacting to the need to find ways to reduce the avoidable burden of adverse drug reactions, and in an African meeting the need to consider monitoring all adverse reactions, and not only the new and rare, was regarded as a priority. Whether or not this kind of work should be linked to the current work of national regulatory agencies and the WHO Programme for International Drug Monitoring is a consideration. Perhaps, the overlap in the work will be regarded as large enough to warrant using the existing adverse reactions monitoring machinery, but much depends on how far there will be monitoring of other medical misadventures and the attitude of national monitoring agencies.

It is clear to any clinical pharmacologist that causation of disease by medicines is often missed in the differential diagnosis. Failure to take an adequate medication history is one reason, but the complexities of polypharmacy in elderly patients with multiple diseases make diagnosis difficult. Education of undergraduates and postgraduates in the logical approach to a diagnosis of medicine-related injury has been neglected.

The reasons for failure to report adverse drug reactions is an old topic. Redoubled efforts with new initiatives are required. Modern communications theory throws some light on reasons for under-reporting. Failure to understand the motivation of doctors and the need for health professionals to understand the adverse drug reactions reporting schemes and to see why they are important to them in their clinical practice, are critical issues.

It is likely that modern information technology can contribute to better reporting in some countries. This need not be only in the most developed countries. Argentina had one of the first e-mail adverse drug reactions reporting systems to function on a routine basis, linking regional centres, based in hospitals, to the national regulatory authority.

The gap between the analysis of raw data to find a signal and the need to perform more formal studies is of great importance. The decision to perform the latter must be based on the seriousness of the event, the strength of the causal relation, and an idea of the medicine-related fraction of that event. The latter piece of information is much helped by having information on the where, how, and how widely a medicine is used. Unfortunately, there still seem to be problems in obtaining full information on the use of medicines.

The advent of genotyping technology throws open the possibility of not only genotyping for pharmacokinetic phenotypic variation, but also of examining pharmacodynamic phenotypes. This should allow the identification of people at risk and the possibility of preventing some adverse reactions.

REFERENCES

1. CIOMS. Harmonization of data fields for electronic transmission of case-report information internationally. Public report. Geneva: CIOMS 1995.
2. Orre R, Lansner A, Bate A, Lindquist M. Bayesian neural networks with confidence estimations applied to data mining. Comput Stat Data Analysis 2000; 34: 473–93.
3. Bate A, Lindquist M, Edwards IR, Olsson S, Orre R, Lansner A, De Freitas RM. A Bayesian neural network method for adverse drug reaction signal generation. Eur J Clin Pharmacol 1998; 54: 315–21.
4. Lindquist M, Edwards IR, Bate A, Fucik H, Nunes AM, Ståhl M. From Association to Alert – a revised approach to International Signal Analysis. Pharmacoepidemiol Drug Saf 1999; 8: S15–25.
5. Lindquist M, Ståhl M, Bate A, Edwards IR, Meyboom RHB. A retrospective evaluation of a data mining approach to aid finding new adverse drug reaction signals in the WHO international database. Drug Saf 2000; 23: 533–42.
6. Lindquist M. ATC – a useful tool in ADR monitoring. Pharm Weekbl (Sci) 1987; 9: 331.
7. Lindquist M, Edwards IR. The WHO Programme for International Drug Monitoring, its database, and the technical support of the Uppsala Monitoring Center. J Rheumatol 2001; 28: 1180–7.
8. Lindquist M. The WHO Programme for International Drug Monitoring: the Present and Future. In: Mitchard M, editor. Electronic Communication Technologies. Buffalo Grove: Interpharm Press Inc, 1998: 527–49.
9. Lindquist M, Edwards IR. Risks of non-sedating antihistamines. Lancet 1997; 349: 1322.
10. Lindquist M, Pettersson M, Edwards IR, Sanderson J, Taylor N, Fletcher P, Schou J, Fraunfelder FT. Omeprazole and visual disorders: seeing alternatives. Pharmacoepidemiol Drug Saf 1996; 5: 27–32.
11. Lindquist M, Pettersson M, Edwards IR, Sanderson J, Taylor N, Fletcher P, Schou JS, Savage R. How does cystitis affect a comparative risk profile of tiaprofenic acid with other non-steroidal antiinflammatory drugs? An international study based on spontaneous reports and drug usage data. Pharmacol Toxicol 1997; 80: 211–17.
12. Lindquist M, Sanderson J, Claesson C, Imbs JL, Rohan A, Edwards IR. New pharmacovigilance information on an old drug – an international study of spontaneous reports on digoxin. Drug Invest 1994; 8: 73–80.
13. Olsson S. Support to developing countries from the WHO Drug Monitoring Centre. In: Abstracts from the DIA 30th Annual Meeting, Washington DC, 5–9 June 1994: 103.
14. Olsson, S. The role of the WHO Programme on International Drug Monitoring in coordinating worldwide drug safety efforts. Drug Saf 1998; 19: 1–10.
15. Olsson S, editor. National Pharmacovigilance Systems: Uppsala Monitoring Centre. 2nd edition. Uppsala: The Uppsala Monitoring Centre, 1999.
16. Edwards IR. Monitoring the safety of herbal remedies: WHO project is under way. Br Med J 1995; 311: 1569–70.
17. Farah MH. Consumer protection and herbal remedies. WHO Drug Inf 1998; 12: 141.
18. Farah MH, Edwards IR, Lindquist M, Leon

C, Shaw D. International monitoring of adverse health effects associated with herbal medicines. Pharmacoepidemiol Drug Saf 2000; 9: 105–12.
19. Fucik H, Farah MH, Meyboom RHB, Lindquist M, Edwards IR, Olsson S. Vigilance of herbal medicines at the Uppsala Monitoring Centre. Minerva Med 2001; 92: 24–6.
20. CIOMS. Reporting of adverse drug reactions: definitions of terms and criteria for their use. Report No. 9290360712. Geneva: CIOMS 1999.
21. Edwards IR, Biriell C. Harmonisation in pharmacovigilance. Drug Saf 1994; 10: 93–102.
22. Edwards IR, Aronson JK. Adverse drug reactions: definitions, diagnosis, and management. Lancet 2000; 356: 1255–9.
23. Edwards IR, Lindquist, M. Understanding and communication of key concepts in therapeutics. In: Velo G, editor. Moments of truth – communicating drug safety. Verona: Elsevier Science, 2000: 9-14.
24. Edwards IR, Wiholm B-E, Martinez C. Concepts in risk–benefit assessment. Drug Saf 1996; 15: 1–7.
25. CIOMS, editor. Benefit-risk balance for marketed drugs: evaluating safety signals, 1st edition. Geneva: World Health Organization 1998.
26. Edwards IR, Hugman B. The challenge of effectively communicating risk–benefit information. Drug Saf 1997; 17: 216–27.
27. Edwards IR. Who cares about pharmacovigilance? Eur J Clin Pharmacol 1997; 53: 83–8.
28. Edwards IR. Spontaneous reporting – of what? Clinical concerns about drugs. Br J Clin Pharmacol 1999; 48: 138–41.
29. Edwards IR. The accelerating need for pharmacovigilance. J R Coll Phys London 2000; 34: 48–51.
30. Biriell C, Edwards IR. Reasons for reporting adverse drug reactions – some thoughts based on an international review. Pharmacoepidemiol Drug Saf 1997; 6: 21–6.
31. Edwards IR, Fucik H. Impact and credibility of the WHO adverse reaction signals. Drug Inf J 1996; 30: 461–4.

Address list of national centres that participate in the WHO drug monitoring programme

Argentina (ARG)
Dr Mabel Teresa Foppiano
Head
Tel: +54-1-340 0866
Fax: +54-1-340 0866
E-mail: snfvg@anmat.gov.ar
Website: anmat.gov.ar

Administración Nacional de Medicamento, Alimentos y Tecnologia Medica (ANMAT)
Sistema Nacional de Farmacovigilancia
Avenida de Mayo 869, piso 11o
(1084) Buenos Aires, Argentina

Armenia (ARM)
Dr Samvel Azatyan
Head
Tel: +374-1-584 020, 584 120
Fax: +374-1-151 697
E-mail: azatyan@pharm.am
Website: pharm.am

Department of Pharmacovigilance and Rational Use of Drugs
Armenian Drug and Medical Technology Agency
15, Moskowian Street
Yerevan 375001, Armenia

Australia (AUS)
Dr John McEwen
Director
Tel: +61-2-6232 8113
Fax: +61-2-6232 8392
E-mail: john.Mcewen@health.gov.au
Website: www.health.gov.au/

Therapeutic Goods Administration
Adverse Drug Reactions Unit
PO Box 100
Woden, ACT 2606, Australia

Austria (AUT)
Ms Renate Jentzsch
Head
Tel: +43-1-711 00, ext 4638
Fax: +43-1-712 0823
E-mail: viiia3@bmsg.gv.at
Website: bmsg.gv.at

Federal Ministry for Social Security and Generations
Pharmacovigilance Unit VIII/A/3
Radetzkystrasse 2
A-1031 Vienna, Austria

Belgium (BEL)
Mr André Pauwels
Head
Tel: +32-2-227 5567
Fax: +32-2-227 5528
E-mail: andre.pauwels@afigp.fgov.be

Ministry of Health, Pharmacy General Inspectorate
Centre National de Pharmacovigilance
Vesale Building
20 rue Montagne de l'Oratoire, 3rd Floor
B-1010 Brussels, Belgium

Brazil (BRA)
Mr Murilo Freitas Dias
Tel: +55-61-448 1219
Fax: +55-61-448 1275
E-mail: murilo.freitas@anvisa.gov.br

Unidade de Farmacovigilancia (UFARM)
Agência Nacional de Vigilância
Sanitárita
SEPN 515 Bl.B Ed. Omega 2 Andar
CEP 70770-502 Brasilia DF, Brazil

Bulgaria (BUL)
Ms Daniela Encheva
Head
Tel: +359-2-4347 356
Fax: +359-2-9434 487
E-mail: pharmacovig@bda.bg
Website: bda.bg

Bulgarian Drug Agency
Department of Pharmacovigilance
Eurointegration and Pharmacopoeia
26, Yanko Sakazov Boulevard
BG-1504 Sofia, Bulgaria

Canada (VAR)
Dr Wikke Walop
Head, Vaccine Safety Epidemiologist
Tel: +1-613-954 5590
Fax: +1-613-957 1340 or 998 6413
E-mail: Wikke.Walop@hc-sc.gc.ca
Website: hc-sc.gc.ca

VAAE Surveillance Section, Division of Immunization
Centre for Infectious Diseases, Prevention & Control
Population and Public Health Branch
Tunney's Pasture 0603EI
Ottawa, Ontario K1A OL2, Canada

Canada (CAN)
Dr Christopher Turner
Acting Director General
Tel: +1-613-954 6522
Fax: +1-613-952 7738
E-mail: cadrmp@hc-sc.gc.ca
Website: www.hc-sc.gc.ca

Marketed Health Product Directorate
Health Products and Food Branch
Health Canada
Room D-162, Finance Building
Tunney's Pasture AL 0201C1
Ottawa, Ontario K1A 1B9, Canada

Chile (CHL)
Dr Q F Cecilia Morgado-Cadiz
Head
Tel: +56-2-239 8769
Fax: +56-2-239 8760
E-mail: cmorgado@ispch.cl

CENIMEF Instituto de Salud Publica de Chile
Avenida Marathon 1000
3 piso, Nuñoa-Casilla 48, Santiago, Chile

China, People's Republic of (CHN)
Prof Li Shaoli
Director-General
Tel: +86-10-6716 4982
Fax: +86-10-6716 4984
E-mail: l_shaoli@263.net
Website: cdr.gov.cn

Center for Drug Re-evaluation (CDR)
National Center for ADR Monitoring
Building 11, Fa-Hua-Na-Li Chongwen District
Beijing 100061, People's Republic of China

Costa Rica (COR)
Jetty Murillo Ocampo
Tel: +506-222 1878
Fax: +506-257 7004
E-mail: jettymurillo@hotmail.com

Caja Costarricense de Seguro Social
Centro Nacional de Farmacovigilancia
Avda. Segunda
San José 1000, Costa Rica

Croatia (CRO)
Prof Bozidar Vrhovac
Head
Tel: +385-1-2421 875 or 2388 284
Fax: +385-1-2421 875
E-mail: bozidar.vrhovac@zg.hinet.hr

National Adverse Drug Reactions Monitoring Centre
Section of Clinical Pharmacology
Department of Medicine
University Hospital Centre
12 Kispaticeva, 41000 Zagreb, Croatia

Cuba (CUB)
Francisco Debesa
Head
Tel: +53-7-24 09 24
Fax: +53-7-24 72 27
E-mail: frank@mcdf.sld.cu

Pharmacoepidemiology Development Center
44 No 502 esq 5a Ave
Miramar, Playa
Havana CP 11300, Cuba

Cyprus (CYP)
Dr Athos Tsinontides
Clinical Pharmacist
Tel: +357-240 7101
Fax: +357-233 9623
E-mail: dipcc@cytanet.com.cy

Pharmaceutical Services
Ministry of Health
1475 Lefkosia, Cyprus

Czech Republic (CZE)
Dr Ivana Koblikova
Head
Tel: +42-02-7218 5848, 7218 5111
Fax: +42-02-7143 2377, 7218 5816
E-mail: klinhodn@sukl.cz

Branch of Clinical Trials and Pharmacovigilance
State Institute for Drug Control
Srobarova 48
10041 Prague 10, Czech Republic

Denmark (DEN)
Ms Margit Handlos
Tel: +45-44-88 91 11
Fax: +45-44-91 73 73
E-mail: mh@dkma.dk
Website: www.dkma.dk

Danish Medicines Agency
Medicines Control Division
378, Frederikssundsvej
DK-2700 Brønshøj, Denmark

Egypt (EGY)
Prof Abdulla Molokhia
Chairman, NODCAR
Tel: +20-2-7484 989
Fax: +20-2-3379 445
E-mail: molokhia@pharmaco.sti.sci.eg

Ministry of Health
National Organization for Drug Control and Research
PO Box 29
Cairo, Egypt

Estonia (EST)
Dr Maia Uusküla
Head
Tel: +372-7-374 140
Fax: +372-7-374 142
E-mail: maia.uuskula@sam.ee
Website: sam.ee

Ravimiamet
State Agency of Medicines
19 Ravila Street
50411 Tartu, Estonia

Fiji (FJI)
Mr Peter Zinck
Chief Pharmacist
Tel: +679-315 022
Fax: +679-304 199
E-mail: pzinck@healthfiji.gov.fj

Government Pharmacy
GP Box 106, Suva, Fiji

Finland (FIN)
Prof Erkki Palva
Research Director
Tel: +358-9-4733 4288
Fax: +358-9-4733 4297
E-mail: erkki.palva@nam.fi
Website: nam.fi

National Agency for Medicines—Lääkelaitos
Drug Information Centre
P.O. Box 55, Mannerheimintie 166
SF-00301 Helsinki, Finland

France (FRA)
Dr Carmen Kreft Jaïs
Head
Tel: +33-1-5587 3533
Fax: +33-1-5587 3532
E-mail:
fr-h.pharmacovigilance@fr-h.eudra.org
Website:
agmed.sante.gouv.fr/fr/htm/2/2000.htm

Agence de Médicament
Unité de Pharmacovigilance
143–145, Boulevard Anatole France
F-93285 Saint–Denis, Cedex, France

Germany (GFR)
Dr Jürgen Beckmann
Head
Tel: +49-30-4548 3311
Fax: +49-30-4548 3515
E-mail: j.beckmann@bfarm.de
Website: bfarm.de

Federal Institute for Drugs and Medical Devices
Bundesinstitut für Arzneimittel und
Medizinprodukte
Seestraße 10, D-13353 Berlin, Germany

Ghana (GHA)
Dr Alex Dodoo
Tel: +233-21-675 885
Fax: +233-21-666 8219
E-mail: alexooo@yahoo.com

Centre for Tropical Clinical Pharmacology
& Therapeutics
University of Ghana Medical School
Korle-Bu Teaching Hospital, Accra, Ghana

Greece (GRC)
Dr Georgia Athanassiou
Head of Pharmacovigilance Unit
Tel: +30-1-6507 337
Fax: +30-1-654 9585
E-mail: adr@eof.gr
Website: eof.gr

National Organization for Medicines
Adverse Drug Reactions Section
284 Messogion Avenue
GR-155 62 Athens–Holargos, Greece

Hungary (HUN)
Dr Sándor Elek
Head
Tel: +36-1-215 4462
Fax: +36-1-215 8977
E-mail: sandor.elek@nip.hu

National Institute of Pharmacy
Adverse Drug Reactions Monitoring Centre
Zrínyi u 3-1051, PO Box 450
H-1372 Budapest, Hungary

Iceland (ICE)
Prof. Magnús Jóhannsson
Tel: +354-5-20 2114
Fax: +354-5-61 2170
E-mail:
magnus.johannsson@lyfjastofnun.is
Website: lyfjastofnun.is

The Icelandic Medicines Control Agency
Eidistorg 13–15,
172 Seltjarnarnes, Iceland

India (IND)

Prof Suresh K Gupta
Chief
Tel: +91-11-659 3633
Fax: +91-11-686 2663 or 652 10 41
E-mails: skgup@hotmail.com;
skgupta@medinst.ernet.in

National Pharmacovigilance Centre
Department of Pharmacology
All India Institute of Medical Sciences
Ansari Nagar
New Delhi 110029, India

Indonesia (INO)

Dr Engko Sosialine M
Head
Tel: +62-21-4245 459
Fax: +62-21-4243 605
E-mail: engkosm@yahoo.com

Section of Adverse Drug Reaction Surveillance
Directorate of Drug and Biological Product Evaluation
National Agency of Drug and Food Control
Jalan Percetakan Negara 23
Jakarta 10560, Indonesia

Iran, Islamic Republic of (IRN)

Dr Gloria Shalviri
Tel: +98-21-640 5569
Fax: +98-21-641 7252
E-mail: shalviri_g@yahoo.com

Ministry of Health and Medical Education
Iranian ADR Centre
Under-Secretary for Food and Drug Affairs
Building no. 3, Fakhre Razi Enghlab Ave
Tehran 13145, Islamic Republic of Iran

Ireland (IRE)

Ms Niamh Arthur
Pharmacovigilance Co-ordinator
Tel: +353-1-676 4971
Fax: +353-1-676 7836
E-mail: niamh.arthur@imb.ie
Website: imb.ie

Pharmacovigilance Unit
Irish Medicines Board
Earlsfort Centre, Earlsfort Terrace
Dublin 2, Ireland

Israel (ISR)

Dr Dina Hemo
Head
Tel: +972-2-568 1219
Fax: +972-2-672 5820
E-mail: dina.hemo@moh.health.gov.il

Ministry of Health
Department of Clinical Pharmacology
Drug Monitoring Center
29 Rivka Street, PO Box 1176
Jerusalem 91010, Israel

Italy (ITA)

Dr Roberto Raschetti
Tel: +39-6-5994 3212
Fax: +39-6-5994 3554
E-mail: roras@iss.it

Ministry of Health Medicines Evaluation and Pharmacovigilance General Direction
Pharmacovigilance Centre
Via della Civiltá Romana 7
I-00144 Roma, Italy

Japan (JPN)

Dr Tatsuo Kurokawa
Director, Safety Division
Tel: +81-3-3595 2435
Fax: +81-3-3508 4364

Ministry of Health and Welfare
Pharmaceutical and Medical Safety Bureau
Safety Division 1-2-2
Kasumigaseki, Chiyoda-Ku
Tokyo 100-8045, Japan

Korea, Republic of (KOR)
Dr Soo-Young Choi
Head
Tel: +82-2-382 0185
Fax: +82-2-383 2870
E-mail: syc1047@kfda.go.kr
Website: kfda.go.kr

Korea Food and Drug Administration
Pharmaceutical Safety Bureau
5 Nokbun–dong, Eunpyong–ku
Seoul 122-704, Republic of Korea

Latvia (LVA)
Dr Inese Studere
Tel: +371-2-781 2611
Fax: +371-2-711 2848
E-mail: inese.studere@vza.gov.lv

Pharmacological Department
State Agency of Medicine of Latvia
Jersikas St. 15, LV-1003 Riga, Latvia

Macedonia, Republic of (MKD)
Ms Biljana Celevska
Tel: +389-2-11 93 75, 23 76 69
Fax: +389-2-23 08 57, 11 30 14

Ministry of Health
ul. 50 Divizija b.b.
1000 Skopje, Republic of Macedonia

Malaysia (MAL)
Mr Mohd Zin Che Awang
Director of Pharmaceutical Services
Tel: +60-3-4045 7389
E-mail: zin@bpfk.gov.my
Website: madrac.gov.my/madrac

Pharmaceutical Services Division
Ministry of Health
11th floor
Bangunan Perkim Jalan IPOM
51200 Kuala Lumpar, Malaysia

Mexico (MEX)
Dr Carmen Becerril Martinez
Head
Tel: +52-5-203 4378
Fax: +52-5-203 4378
E-mail: mcbecerril@mail.ssa.gob.mx

Ministry of Health
Gauss No 4, 7 piso
Col. Casa Blanca
Mexico City, DF CP 11590, Mexico

Morocco (MOR)
Dr Rachida Soulaymani-Bencheikh
Head
Tel: +212-7-68 64 64
Fax: +212-7-772 067
E-mail: ismailia@iam.net.ma

Institut National d'Hygiène
Centre Anti Poisons et de Pharmacovigilance
Avenue Ibn Batouta 27
BP 769, Agdal, M-11400 Rabat, Morocco

Netherlands (NET)
Dr A C van Grootheest
Director
Tel: +31-73-646 9700
Fax: +31-73-642 6136
E-mail: ac.vangrootheest@lareb.nl
Website: lareb.nl

Netherlands Pharmacovigilance Foundation LAREB
Goudsbloemvallei 7
NL-5237 MH s'Hertogenbosch, The Netherlands

Netherlands (NET1)
Dr Hans van Bronswijk
Head of Pharmacovigilance
Tel: +31-70-356 7400
Fax: +31-70-356 7515
E-mail: h.v.bronswijk@cbg-meb.nl
Website: cbg-meb.nl
Medicines Evaluation Board
PO Box 16229
Kalvermarkt 53
NL-2500 BE, The Hague, The Netherlands

New Zealand (NEZ)
Dr David Coulter
Head
Tel: +64-3-479 7249
Fax: +64-3-477 0509
E-mail: david.coulter@stonebow.otago.ac.nz
Centre for Adverse Reactions Monitoring
Dunedin School of Medicine
PO Box 913 9001
Dunedin 9000, New Zealand

Norway (NOR)
Ms Ingebjorg Buajordet
Head
Tel: +47-22-897 700
Fax: +47-22-897 799
E-mail:
Ingebjorg.Buajordet@legemiddelverket.no
Website: slk.no
Norwegian Medicines Control Authority
Statens Legemiddelskontroll (SLK)
Adverse Drug Reaction Section
Sven Oftedals vei 6
N-0950 Oslo 9, Norway

Oman (OMN)
Dr Sawsan Ahmad Jaffar
Head
Tel: +968-600 016
Fax: +968-602 287
E-mail: mohphar@omantel.net.om
Ministry of Health
Directorate General of Pharmaceutical Affairs and Drug Control
PO Box 393, Muscat, Sultanate of Oman 113

Peru (PER)
Ms Susana Vasquez
Jefe de CENAFIM
Tel: +51-14-71 62 46
Fax: +51-14-71 63 53
E-mail: SVASQUEZ@digemid.gob.pe
Website: minsa.gob.pe
Presidenta del Comite Tecnico Nacional de Farmacovigilancia CENAFIM
DIGEMID
Ministerio de Salud
Avenue Arenales #1302—Of. 318-319
Lima 11, Peru

Philippines (PHL)
Ms Marissa Macaraeg
Information Officer
Tel: +63-2-807 8517
Fax: +63-2-8078 285
E-mail: mariz_phl@hotmail.com
Adverse Drug Reaction Monitoring Bureau of Food and Drugs
Department of Health
Filinvest Corporate City, Alabang
Muntinlupa City 1770, Philippines

Poland (POL)
Dr Agata Maciejczyk
Head
Tel: +48-22-8416 742
Fax: +48-22-8514 366
E-mail: magat@il.waw.pl
Website: il.waw.pl
Drug Institute
Pharmacoepidemiology Centre
Centre for Adverse Drug Reactions Monitoring
30/34 Chelmska Street
PL-00725 Warsaw, Poland

Portugal (POR)
Dr António M N Faria Vaz
Head
Tel: +351-21-798 7140
Fax: +351-21-798 7155, 795 9069
E-mail: faria.vaz@infarmed.pt
Website: infarmed.pt

Centro Nacional de Farmacovigilancia
Instituto Nacional da Farmácia e do Medicamento (INFARMED)
Parque de Saúde de Lisboa
Avenida do Brasil, no. 53
1749-048 Lisboa, Portugal

Romania (ROM)
Dr Juliana Daniela Stanciu
Head
Tel: +40-1-224 1102, 224 1710
Fax: +40-1-230 5083
E-mail: daniela.stanciu@anm.kappa.ro

National Medicines Agency
Str Aviator Sanatescu no 48, Sector 1
R-71 324 Bucuresti, Romania

Russia (RUS)
Prof Victor Cheltsov
Head
Tel: +7-95-434 52 44
Fax: +7-95-434 02 92
E-mail: rfcadr@med.pfu.edu.ru

Department of Clinical Pharmacology
Miklukho–Maklay Street, 8
117198 Moscow, Russia

Singapore (SIN)
Ms Chan Cheng Leng
Head of Pharmacovigilance
Tel: +65-325 5604, 325 5610
Fax: +65-325 5448
E-mail: chan_cheng_leng@hsa.gov.sg

Health Sciences Authority
Pharmacovigilance Unit Centre for Pharmaceutical Administration
No. 2 Jalan Bukit Merah
Singapore 169547

Slovakia (SVK)
Dr Pavol Gibala
Head
Tel: +421-2-5293 1735, 5293 1732
Fax: +421-2-5293 1734
E-mail: sukl@cnit.sk
Website: sukl.sk

National Centre for Monitoring Adverse Reactions to Drugs
State Institute for Drug Control
Kvetná 11, 825 08 Bratislava 26, Slovakia

South Africa (SOA)
Ms Ushma Mehta
Head
Tel: +27-21-447 1618
Fax: +27-21-448 6181
E-mail: umehta@uctgsh1.uct.ac.za

National Adverse Drug Event Monitoring Centre
c/o Department of Pharmacology
Faculty of Medicine
University of Cape Town
K45 Old Main Building
Observatory 7925, South Africa

Spain (SPA)
Dr Fransisco José de Abajo
Head
Tel: +34-91-596 7711
Fax: +34-91-596 7891
E-mail: fabajo@agemed.es
Website: msc.es/agemed

Agencia Española del Medicamento
División de Farmacoepidemiología y Farmacovigilancia
Carretera a Pozuelo, Km 2
E-28220 Majadahonda (Madrid), Spain

Sri Lanka (LKA)
Dr Bernadette Mignonne Rohini Fernandopulle
Senior Lecturer
Tel: +94-1-695 300 ext. 41 03 17
Fax: +94-1-695 300
E-mail: phrm_cmb@slt.lk
Faculty of Medicine
University of Colombo
Kynsey Road
PO Box 271
Colombo 8, Sri Lanka

Sweden (SWE)
Ingemar Persson
Head
Tel: +46-18-17 46 44
Fax: +46-18-54 85 66
E-mail: Ingemar.Persson@mpa.se
Website: mpa.se
Adverse Drug Reaction Section
Medical Product Agency
PO Box 26
S-751 03 Uppsala, Sweden

Switzerland (SCH)
Ruedi Stoller
Head
Tel: +41-31-322 0348
Fax: +41-31-322 0418
E-mail: vigilance@iks.admin.ch
Website: iks.ch
Interkantonale Kontrollstelle für Heilmittel
Pharmacovigilance Centre
Erlachstrasse 8
CH-3000 Bern 9, Switzerland

Tanzania (TAN)
Mr Henry Irunde
Tel: +255-22-2450 512, 2450 929
Fax: +255-22-2450 793
E-mail: tadatis@twiga.com
Tanzania Drug and Toxicology Information Service (TADATIS)
PO Box 77150
Dar Es Salaam, Tanzania

Thailand (THA)
Ms Pornpit Silkavute
Director
Tel: +66-2-590 7281
Fax: +66-2-591 8497
E-mail: pornpit@health.moph.go.th
Drug Information Center and ADRMC
Technical Division
National Adverse Drug Reaction Monitoring Centre
Ministry of Public Health
Food and Drug Administration
Ti–wa–nondh Rd
Nonthaburi, Thailand

Tunisia (TUN)
Prof Chalbi Belkahia
Head
Tel: +216-1-562 098
Fax: +216-1-571 390 or 57 81 96
E-mail: chalbi.belkahia@rns.tn
Centre National de Pharmacovigilance
Sis Hôpital Ch Nicolle
Bd du 9 Avril
Tunis 1006, Tunisia

Turkey (TUR)
Prof Dr Orban Canbolat
Head
Tel: +90-312-230 1674, 230 2769
Fax: +90-312-230 1610
E-mail: orban@celik.net.tr
Ministry of Health
General Directorate of Drugs and Pharmacy
Ilkiz Sokak No 4
Sihhiye, Ankara 06430, Turkey

Ukraine (UKR)
Dr Marina Sharayeva
E-mail: vigilance@pharma-center.kiev.ua
State Pharmacological Center
Ministry of Health of Ukraine
8 Hrushevsky Str., Kiev, Ukraine

United Kingdom (UNK)
Dr June Raine
Head
Tel: +44-207-273 0400
Fax: +44-207-273 0282, 273 0675
E-mail: june.raine@mca.gov.uk
Website: open.gov.uk/mca/
Medicines Control Agency
Pharmacovigilance
Department of Health
Market Towers, 1 Nine Elms Lane
Vauxhall, London SW8 5NQ, UK

United States of America (USAV)
Dr M Miles Braun
Director
Tel: +1-301-827 3974
Fax: +1-301-827 3529
E-mail: braunm@cber.fda.gov
Food and Drug Administration
Center for Biologics Evaluation and Research
Division of Epidemiology
1401 Rockville Pike, HFM-220
Rockville, MD 20852-1448, USA

United States of America (USA)
Dr Paul Seligman
E-mail: Seligmanp@cder.fda.gov
Center for Drug Evaluation and Research
Food and Drug Administration
5600 Fishers Lane, Room 17-65
Rockville, MD 20857, USA

Uruguay (URY)
Dr Carolina Seade Fournie
Tel: +598-487 27 02
E-mail: cseade@montevideo.com.uy
Depto de Farmacologia
Hospital de Clinicas Avda Italia s/n
piso 1, 11600 Montevideo, Uruguay

Uruguay (URY)
Dr Mabel Burger
Tel: +598-2-480 4000
Fax: +598-2-487 0300
E-mail: hcciat@hc.edu.uy
Website: ciat.hc.edu.uy
Deptartamento de Toxicologia
Hospital de Clínicas Avda Italia s/n
piso 7, 11600 Montevideo, Uruguay

Venezuela (VEN)
Dr Jesús Querales Castillo
Head
Tel: +58-2-6624 797
Fax: +58-2-6624 797, 693 1455
Instituto Nactional de Higiene "Rafael Rangel" Presidente
Apartado Postal 60.412-Ofic. del Este
Ciudad Universitaria, Caracas, Venezuela

Vietnam (VNM)
Prof Hoang Tich Huyên
Head
Tel: +84-4-245 292
Fax: +84-4-823 1253
E-mail: adpcl@hn.vnn.vn
Adverse Drug Reaction Centre
Institute for Drug Quality Control
Ministry of Health
48 Hai Ba Trung Street, Hanoi, Vietnam

Yugoslavia, Federal Republic of (YUG)
Prof Vaso Antunovic
Head
Tel: +381-11-361 5531
Fax: +381-11-361 5630
Clinical Centre of Serbia
National Centre for Adverse Drug Reactions
Visegradska 26
YU-11000 Belgrade, Fed Rep of Yugoslavia

Zimbabwe (ZWE)
Dr Obet Mguni
Regulatory Officer
Tel: +263-4-736 981/5
Fax: +263-4-736 980
E-mail: mcaz@africaonline.co.zw

Medicines Control Authority of Zimbabwe
106 Baines Ave
Harare, Zimbabwe

Associate Member Countries

Bahrain (BHR)
Ms Layla Abdur-Rahman
Director
Tel: +973-25 86 68
Fax: +973-27 93 57
E-mail: lmohammed1@health.gov.bh

Ministry of Health
Pharmacy and Drug Control
P.O. Box 12, Manama, Bahrain

Kyrgyz, Republic of (KGZ)
Ms Nazgul Chokmorova
Fax: +996-312 542910
E-mail: DIC@elcat.kg

Ministry of Health
Drug Information Centre
Logvinenko str 8
Bishkek, Kyrgyz Republic

Moldova (MDA)
Dr V. I. Ghicavii

National Institute of Pharmacy
Ministerul Sanatatii al Republicii Moldova
str Vasile Alecsandri 1
2009 Chisinau, Moldova

Netherlands Antilles (ANT)
Msc Zjumira G M Wout
Tel: +599-9-737 4877
Fax: +599-9-737 4844
E-mail: zwout@hotmail.com

Bureau of Pharmaceutical Affairs
Groot Davelaar K-139-140
Fokkerweg #26
PO Box 3824
Curacao, Netherlands Antilles

Pakistan (PAK)
Prof Akhlaque Un-Nabi Khan
Tel: +92-21-588 2997, 589 2801
Fax: +92-21-588 1444, 589 3062
E-mail: cpsp@super.net.pk

College of Physicians & Surgeons
Pakistan (CPSP)
Department of Clinical Pharmacology
7th Central Street
Phase II, Defence Housing Authority
Karachi 75500, Pakistan

Institutions

EMEA
Ms Priya Bahri
Tel: +44-207-418 8454
Fax: +44-207-418 8551
E-mail: priya.bahri@emea.eudra.org

EMEA-The European Agency for the Evaluation
of Medicinal Products
Pharmacovigilance Section
7 Westferry Circus, Canary Wharf
London E14 4HB, UK

EC

Emer Cooke
Tel: +32-2-296 7072
Fax: +32-2-296 1520
E-mail: Emer.Cooke@cec.eu.int

European Commission
Directorate General III-Industry
Rue de la Loi 200
B-1049 Brussels, Belgium

WHO

Dr Mary Couper
Tel: +41-22-791 3643
Fax: +41-22-791 4730
E-mail: couperm@who.ch

World Health Organization
Policy, Access and Rational Use, EDM-HTP
CH-1211 Geneva 27, Switzerland

Index of drugs

Page numbers in **bold** indicate where the given drug is discussed in detail.

Index of adverse effects

Complementary to this volume:

SIDE EFFECTS OF DRUGS ANNUALS 1–24 (1977–2001)
Edited by M.N.G. Dukes (Annuals 1–16) and J.K. Aronson (Annuals 15–24)

MEYLER'S SIDE EFFECTS OF DRUGS, 14th EDITION (2000)
Edited by M.N.G. Dukes and J.K. Aronson

UNWANTED EFFECTS OF COSMETICS AND DRUGS USED IN DERMATOLOGY, 3rd EDITION (1994)
A.C. de Groot, J.W. Weyland and J.P. Nater

DRUGS AND HUMAN LACTATION, 2nd Edition (1996)
P.N. Bennett

PHARMACOLOGICAL AND CHEMICAL SYNONYMS, 10th Edition (1994)
E.E.J. Marler

A MANUAL OF ADVERSE DRUG INTERACTIONS, 5th Edition (1997)
J.P. Griffin and P.F. D'Arcy

A DICTIONARY OF PHARMACOLOGY AND ALLIED TOPICS (1998)
D.R. Laurence and J. Carpenter

DRUGS DURING PREGNANCY AND LACTATION (2001)
C. Schaefer

The Website of the Side Effects of Drugs Annual 25, edited by Jeffrey K. Aronson, can be viewed at http://www.elsevier.com/locate/isbn/0444506748